Acute Heart Failure

Alexandre Mebazaa, Mihai Gheorghiade,
Faiez M. Zannad, and Joseph E. Parrillo (Eds.)

Acute Heart Failure

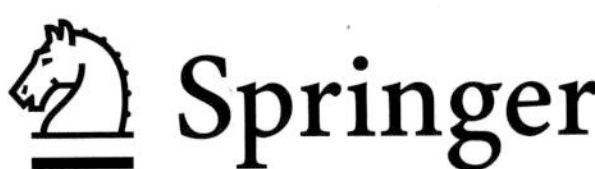

Alexandre Mebazaa, MD, PhD
Professor of Medicine
Université Paris Diderot
Department of Anesthesiology and Critical Care Medicine
Lariboisière University Hospital
Assistance Publique-Hôpitaux de Paris
Paris, France

Mihai Gheorghiade, MD, FACC
Professor of Medicine and Surgery
Associate Chief, Division of Cardiology
Chief, Cardiology Clinical Service
Northwestern University
Feinberg School of Medicine
Chicago, IL, USA

Faiez M. Zannad, MD, PhD, FESC
Professor of Medicine
University Henri Poincaré
Department of Cardiology
Centre d'Investigation Clinique (CIC)
INSERM U-684
Centre Hospitalier Universitaire
Nancy, France

Joseph E. Parrillo, MD
Professor of Medicine
Robert Wood Johnson Medical School
University of Medicine and Dentistry of New Jersey
Chief, Department of Medicine
Edward D. Viner MD Chair, Department of Medicine
Director, Cooper Heart Institute
Cooper University Hospital
Camden, NJ, USA

Project Coordinator
Wendy A. Gattis Stough, PharmD
Department of Clinical Research
Campbell University School of Pharmacy
Cary, NC, USA

British Library Cataloguing in Publication Data
Acute heart failure
1. Heart failure – Treatment 2. Heart failure
I. Mebazaa, Alexandre
616.1´2906
ISBN-13: 9781846287817

Library of Congress Control Number: 2007929111

ISBN: 978-1-84628-781-7 e-ISBN: 978-1-84628-782-4

9 8 7 6 5 4 3 2 1

Springer Science+Business Media
springer.com

Foreword

Acute heart failure is a leading cause of morbidity and mortality worldwide, and its incidence is increasing as the population ages. This represents a huge clinical and economic burden for all health care systems. With its high prevalence and associated morbidity and mortality, acute heart failure requires better therapies. Greater awareness of the disease process, better understanding of the underlying mechanisms, and improved management of patients with heart failure are urgently needed to ensure that the outcomes of patients with acute heart failure are optimized.

In recent years, the concept of acute heart failure as a single disease entity has changed, and the definition and classification of acute heart failure have gradually been modified with the increased realization that the term *acute heart failure* incorporates several acute heart failure syndromes, which differ in presentation, etiology, pathophysiology, and outcome. Clinicians and investigators around the world are now collaborating to establish more uniform definitions, collect relevant epidemiologic data, and develop more standardized guidelines and recommendations for the management of patients with acute heart failure. Recent epidemiologic studies have helped delineate key characteristics of patients with acute heart failure, highlight important risk factors, and identify national and international approaches to management.

This new book on acute heart failure is thus very timely, drawing together the most recent data and concepts in this field, and providing a fresh look at the complexities of acute heart failure. The editors, who are indeed authorities in the field, have succeeded in producing a truly complete review of this vast and important subject. The book is divided into two main parts, the first concentrating largely on epidemiology and pathophysiology, and the second focusing on diagnosis and management. In addition to the chapters covering the more traditional features of heart failure, other chapters address the nutritional, psychological, and ethical aspects. The text is supported throughout by ample and appropriate imaging and relevant references.

The 85 chapters are written by a broad cross-section of recognized experts from the different clinical arenas involved in the investigation and treatment of patients with acute heart failure, including cardiologists, cardiac and thoracic surgeons, intensivists, anesthesiologists, pharmacologists, nephrologists, and pulmonologists. The wide range of specialties represented by the authors highlights the multidisciplinary nature of this disease process, which can affect almost all organ systems, creating a heterogeneous and complex entity. In addition, the international nature of the authors, including contributors from some 15 countries, helps make this text relevant for clinicians worldwide.

This highly comprehensive book is an important contribution to the literature in this field and will serve as a valuable text for all those involved in the care of patients with acute heart failure.

Jean-Louis Vincent
Head
Department of Intensive Care
Erasme Hospital
Free University of Brussels Belgium
Belgium

Preface

One challenge in editing a textbook is that by the time the the book is published, it is outdated. We believe that the present textbook on AHFS stands up to this challenge. AHFS is a new and rapidly evolving field. At present, we are just starting to learn about AHFS and to develop paradigms similar to those created in the early 1980s for chronic heart failure, one of the fastest changing areas in cardiovascular medicine during the last 20 years. Researchers have only started to measure how important a burden AHFS is on health care.

We are beginning to investigate some reasonable pathophysiological hypotheses. Only recently, the ESC and ACC/AHA issued the first set of guidelines. None of these guidelines is truly evidence based, as only a few clinical trials have investigated new treatments for AHFS and even fewer have yielded positive results. Therefore, the editors felt the need to assemble in a single compendium a baseline document that establishes the current knowledge of this syndrome. In so doing, we have also tried to highlight unmet needs and to delineate areas for future research. Finally, the editors addressed the large heterogeneity of this syndrome by inviting a variety of contributors with different backgrounds and from different continents to participate.

Alexandre Mebazaa
Mihai Gheorghiade
Faiez M. Zannad
Joseph E. Parrillo

Contents

Section 1.3.4 Acute Heart Failure Syndromes in the Extreme Ages

Part 2 DIAGNOSTIC AND THERAPEUTIC MANAGEMENT OF SEVERE ACUTE HEART FAILURE SYNDROMES

Section 2.1 Procedures and Technology

Section 2.6 Anesthesia and Surgical Management of Acute Heart Failure Syndrome

Section 2.7 Management of Organ Dysfunction Associated with Acute Heart Failure Syndrome

Section 2.8 Rescue Management in Acute Heart Failure Syndrome

Contributors

Eric Abadie MD, MBA
French Health Products Safety Agency (Agence Française de Sécurité Sanitaire des Produits de Santé)
Saint-Denis, France

William T. Abraham, MD
Division of Cardiovascular Medicine
The Ohio State University
Columbus, OH, USA

Kirkwood F. Adams, Jr., MD
Heart Failure—Cardiology
University of North Carolina
Bolin Creek, NC, USA

Christophe Adrie, MD, PhD
General ICU
Delafontaine Hospital
Saint Denis, France

Nancy M. Albert, PhD
Nursing Research Innovation
Cleveland Clinic Foundation
Cleveland, OH, USA

François Alla, MD, PhD
Department of Epidemiology
University Hospital
Nancy, France

Roberto Aquilani, MD
Service of Metabolic-Nutritional Patho Physiology
Scientific Institute of Montescano (PV) "S.Maugeri"
Montescano, Pavia, Italy

Thomas R. Aversano, MD
Department of Medicine/Cardiology
Johns Hopkins Medical Institutions
Baltimore, MD, USA

Elie Azoulay, MD, PhD
Medical Intensive Care
Saint-Louis Hospital
Assistance Publique-Hôpitaux de Paris
Université Paris Diderot
Paris, France

Frédéric J. Baud, MD
Department of Medical and Toxicological Critical Care
Lariboisière University Hospital
Assistance Publique-Hôpitaux de Paris
Université Paris Diderot
Paris, France

Nadia Belmatoug
Service de Medecine Interne
Hopital Beaujon
Assistance Publique Hôpitaux de Paris
Clichy, France

Nadia Benyounes-Iglesias, MD
Department of Cardiology-Internal Medicine
Fondation Ophtalmologique de Rothschild
Paris, France

Guido Boerrigter, MD
Division of Cardiovascular Research
Mayo Clinic
Rochester, MN, USA

Robert C. Bourge, MD
Division of Cardiovascular Disease
University of Alabama at Birmingham
Birmingham
Jefferson, AL, USA

John H. Boyd, MD
Division of Critical Care
Department of Medicine
The University of British Columbia
St Paul's Hospital
Vancouver, BC, Canada

Filippo Brandimarte
Department of Cardiovascular, Respiratory and Morphological Sciences
University of Rome "La Sapienza"
Rome, Italy

Claire Broche, MD
Department of Anesthesiology and Critical Care
Lariboisière University Hospital
Assistance Publique-Hôpitaux de Paris
Université Paris Diderot
Paris, France

Dirk L. Brutsaert, MD, PhD
Cardiology Department
AZ Middelheim—University of Antwerp
Antwerp, Belgium

John C. Burnett, Jr., MD
Division of Cardiovascular Diseases
Mayo Clinic
Rochester, MN, USA

Vincent Caille, MD
Intensive Care Unit
Ambroise Pare Hospital
Boulogne, France

Cyril Charron, MD
Intensive Care Unit
Ambroise Pare Hospital
Boulogne, France

Juhsien Chen
Department of Cardiovascular Medicine
Duke University Medical Center
Durham, NC, USA

Alexandru B. Chicos, MD
Department of Cardiology
Northwestern University
Chicago, IL, USA

Bernard P. Cholley, MD, PhD
Anesthesiology and Critical Care Medicine
Lariboisière University Hospital
Assistance Publique-Hôpitaux de Paris
Université Paris Diderot
Paris, France

John G.F. Cleland, MD
Department of Cardiology
University of Hull
Kingston upon Hull
East Yorkshire, UK

Dagmar Cobaugh, MD
Department of Thoracic and Cardiovascular Surgery
Heart and Diabetes Centre North-Rhine Westphalia
Bad Oeymhausen, Germany

Ariel A. Cohen, MD, PhD, FESC, FACC
Cardiology Department
Assistance-Publique-Hôpitaux de Paris
Saint-Antoine University and Medical School
Assistance Publique-Hôpitaux de Paris
and
Université Pierre et Marie Curie
St-Antoine, Paris, France

Iris Cohen, MD
The Non Invasive Echocardiography Laboratory
The European Hospital Georges Pompidou
Paris, France

Alain Cohen Solal, MD, PhD
Department of Cardiology
Lariboisière University Hospital
Assistance Publique-Hôpitaux de Paris
Université Paris Diderot
Paris, France

Martin J. Cook, MBChB, MRCP, FRCA
St George's Hospital
London, UK

Maria Rosa Costanzo, MD
Centre for Advanced Heart Failure
Edward Hospital—Midwest Heart Specialists
Naperville, IL, USA

Stefan G. De Hert, MD, PhD
Department of Anaesthesiology
University of Antwerp
Antwerp University Hospital
Edegem, Belgium

Nathalie Dervaux, MD
Centre de Médecine Préventive Cardiovasculaire
Centre Hospitalier Hôpital Européen Georges Pompidou-Broussais
Assistance Publique-Hôpitaux de Paris
Paris, France

Nicolas Deye, MD
Department of Medical and Toxicological Critical Care
Lariboisière University Hospital
Assistance Publique-Hôpitaux de Paris
Université Paris Diderot
Paris, France

Ioanna Dimopoulou, MD
Department of Critical Care Medicine
Attikon University Hospital
Athens University, Medical School
Chaidari, Athens, Greece

Stavros G. Drakos, MD
Clinical Therapeutics
University of Athens
Athens, Attica, Greece

Laurent Ducros, MD
Department of Anaesthesiology and Intensive Care
Lariboisière University Hospital
Assistance Publique-Hôpitaux de Paris
Université Paris Diderot
Paris, France

François Durand, MD
Hepatology Unit
Hospital Beaujon
Assistance Publique-Hôpitaux de Paris
Université Paris Diderot
Clichy, France

Aly El-Banayosy, MD
Department of Thoracic and Cardiovascular Surgery
Heart and Diabetes Centre North-Rhine Westphalia
Bad Oeymhausen, Germany

Fabrice Extramiana, MD, PhD
Department of Cardiology
Lariboisière University Hospital
Assistance Publique-Hôpitaux de Paris
Université Paris Diderot
Paris, France

Thomas Fassier, MD
Medical and Respiratory Intensive Care Unit
Croix Rousse Hospital
Lyon, France

Brian Feingold, MD
School of Medicine
Department of Paediatrics
Division of Cardiology
University of Pittsburgh
Children's Hospital Pittsburgh
Pittsburgh, PA, USA

Gerasimos S. Filippatos, MD
2nd University Department of Cardiology
University of Athens Hospital, Attikon
Athens, Greece

Lee A. Fleisher, MD, FACC
Department of Anaesthesiology and Critical Care
University of Pennsylvania
Philadelphia, PA, USA

Gregg C. Fonarow, MD
UCLA Division of Cardiology
David Geffen School of Medicine at UCLA
Los Angeles, CA, USA

Etienne Gayat, MD
Department of Anesthesiology and Critical Care
Lariboisière University Hospital
Assistance Publique-Hôpitaux de Paris
Université Paris Diderot
Paris, France

Mihai Gheorghiade, MD, FACC
Division of Cardiology
Northwestern University
Feinberg School of Medicine
Chicago, IL, USA

Fredric Ginsberg, MD
Department of Cardiovascular Disease and Critical Care Medicine
Cooper University Hospital
Camden, NJ, USA

Abdeddayem Haggui, MD
Department of Cardiology
Lariboisière University Hospital
Assistance Publique-Hôpitaux de Paris
Université Paris Diderot
Paris, France

Jesse B. Hall, MD, FCCP
Department of Medicine
University of Chicago
Chicago, IL, USA

Patrick Henry, MD, PhD
Department of Cardiology
Lariboisière University Hospital
Assistance Publique-Hôpitaux de Paris
Université Paris Diderot
Paris, France

Steven M. Hollenberg, MD
Coronary Care Unit
Cooper University Hospital
Camden, NJ, USA

Paolo Iadarola, PhD
Department of Biochemistry
University of Pavia
Pavia, Italy

Adrian Iaina, MD
Department of Nephrology
A.P.C Health Specialists Clinic Ltd.
Qiriat Ono, Israel

Carole Ichai, MD, PhD
Department of Anesthesiology and Intensive Care Unit
Hôpital Saint-Roch
Nice, France

Ioannis Ilias, MD, PhD
Department of Pharmacology
Medical School
University of Patras
Rion, Achaia, Greece

François Jardin, MD
Intensive Care Unit
Ambroise Pare Hospital
Boulogne, France

Wei Jiang, MD
Psychiatric and Behavioural Sciences/Medicine
Duke University Medical Center
Durham, NC, USA

Hani Jneid, MD
Division of Cardiology
Massachusetts General Hospital
and
Harvard Medical School
Boston, MA, USA

Karen E. Joynt, MD
Internal Medicine
Duke University Medical Centre
Durham, NC, USA

Alan H. Kadish, MD
Department of Cardiology
Northwestern University
Chicago, IL, USA

Vijay Karajala, MD
Department of Critical Care Medicine
University of Pittsburgh School of Medicine
Pittsburgh, PA, USA

John A. Kellum, MD, FACP, FCCM, FCCP
Department of Critical Care Medicine
University of Pittsburgh School of Medicine
Pittsburgh, PA, USA

Gilles W. De Keulenaer, MD, PhD
Department of Cardiology
AZ Middelheim
Antwerp, Belgium

Rami N. Khayat, MD
Department of Internal Medicine
Ohio State University
Columbus, OH, USA

Reiner Koerfer, MD
Department of Thoracic and Cardiovascular Surgery
Heart and Diabetes Centre North-Rhine Westphalia
Bad Oeymhausen, Germany

Tal H. Kopel, MD
Department of Internal Medicine
Jewish General Hospital, McGill University
Montreal, QC, Canada

Dimitrios Th. Kremastinos, MD, PhD
2nd Cardiology Department
University of Athens Medical School
University General Hospital "Attikon"
Athens, Greece

Anand Kumar, MD
Section of Critical Care Medicine
Health Sciences Centre
University of Manitoba
Winnipeg, MB, Canada

Aseem Kumar, BSc, MSc, PhD
Biomolecular Sciences Programme
Laurentian University
Sudbury, ON, Canada

Ivan Laurent, MD
Intensive Care Medicine
Institut Jacques Cartier
Massy, France

Antoine Leenhardt, MD
Department of Cardiology
Lariboisière University Hospital
Assistance Publique-Hôpitaux de Paris
Université Paris Diderot
Paris, France

Carl V. Leier, MD
Cardiovascular Division, Internal Medicine
Ohio State University
Columbus, OH, USA

Diane Lena, MD
Department of Anesthesiology and Intensive Care Unit
Hôpital Saint-Roch
Nice, France

Xavier Leverve, MD, PhD
Department of Anesthesiology and Intensive Care Unit
Hôpital Saint-Roch
Nice, France

Damien Logeart, MD, PhD
Department of Cardiology
Lariboisière Hospital
Paris, France

Dan Longrois, MD, PhD
Department of Anesthesiology and Critical Care
Centre Hospitalier Universitaire de Nancy
Vandoeuvre-les-Nancy, France

Esteban López de Sá
Coronary Care Unit
Hospital Universitario La Paz
Madrid, Spain

Jose López-Sendón, MD, PhD
Department of Cariology
Hospital Universitario La Paz
Madrid, Spain

Marie-Reine Losser, MD, PhD
Anaesthesia and Critical Medicine
Lariboisière University Hospital
Assistance Publique-Hôpitaux de Paris
Université Paris Diderot
Paris, France

Donata Lucci, MS
ANMCO Research Centre
ANMCO (Italian Association of Hospital Cardiologist)
Florence, Italy

Keith G. Lurie, MD
University of Minnesota
Department of Emergency Medicine
Hennepin County Medical Center
Eden Prairie, MN, USA

Hartmut Lüss, MD
Cardiopep Pharma GmbH
Hannover, Germany

Aldo Pietro Maggioni, MD
ANMCO Research Centre
ANMCO (Italian Association of Hospital Cardiologist)
Florence, Italy

Andrew O. Maree, MSc, MB BCh
Division of Cardiology
Department of Medicine
Massachusetts General Hospital
and
Harvard Medical School
Boston, MA, USA

Fernando L. Martin, MD
Division of Cardiovascular Research
Mayo Clinic
Rochester, MN, USA

Anthony S. McLean, MB, ChB, BSc (Hons), FRACP
Department of Intensive Care Medicine
Nepean Hospital
Penrith, Sydney, Australia

Alexandre Mebazaa, MD, PhD
Department of Anesthesiology and Critical Care Medicine
Lariboisière University Hospital
Assistance Publique-Hôpitaux de Paris
Université Paris Diderot
Paris, France
and
School of Medicine of Tunis
Tunis, Tunisia

Bruno Mégarbane, MD, PhD
Department of Medical and Toxicological Critical Care
Lariboisière University Hospital
Assistance Publique-Hôpitaux de Paris
Université Paris Diderot
Paris, France

Rohit Mehta, MD
Cardiovascular Division, Internal Medicine
The Ohio State University
Columbus, OH, USA

Jean-Jaques Mercadier, MD, PhD
Department of Physiology
Groupe Hospitalier Bichat-Claude Bernard
Assistance Publique-Hôpitaux de Paris
Université Paris Diderot
Paris, France

Paul Michel Mertes, PU-PH
Service d'Anesthésie Réanimation Chirurgicale
Chu de Nancy—Hôpital Central
Nancy Cedex, France

Anja K. Metzger, PhD
University of Minnesota
Department of Emergency Medicine
Hennepin County Medical Center
Eden Prairie, MN, USA

Markus Meyer, MD, PhD
Cardiopep Pharma GmbH
Hannover, Germany

Nuala J. Meyer, MD
Section of Pulmonary and Critical Care
Department of Medicine
University of Chicago
Chicago, IL, USA

Karima Mezaïb, MD
Department of Emergency Medicine
Lariboisière University Hospital
Assistance-Publique Hôpitaux de Paris
Paris, France

Paul Milliez, MD, PhD
Department of Cardiology
Lariboisière University Hospital
Assistance Publique-Hôpitaux de Paris
Université Paris Diderot
Paris, France

Veselin Mitrovic, MD
Department of Cardiology
Kerckhoff-Klinik GmbH
Bad Nauheim, Germany

Mehran Monchi, MD
Intensive Care Medicine
Intitut Jacques Cartier
Massy, France

Xavier Monnet, MD, PhD
Medical ICU
Bicêtre University Hospital
Assistance Publique-Hôpitaux de Paris
Le Kremlin-Bicêtre, France

Laurence Monnier-Cholley, MD
Department of Radiology
Hôpital Saint-Antoine
Assistance Publique-Hôpitaux de Paris
Paris, France

Gilles Montalescot, MD, PhD
Institut de Cardiologie
Groupe Hospitalier Pitié-Salpétrière
Assistance Publique-Hôpitaux de Paris
Paris, France

John N. Nanas, MD, PhD
Department of Clinical Therapeutics
University of Athens School of Medicine
Athens, Greece

Tien M.H. Ng, BSPharm, PharmD
Pharmacy
University of Southern California
Los Angeles, USA

Markku S. Nieminen, MD, PhD
Department of Medicine
University Central Hospital
Helsinki, Finland

Christopher M. O'Connor
Duke University Medical Center
Durham, NC, USA

Cristina Opasich, MD
Cardiology Division
Sc. Institute of Pavia
S. Maugeri Foundation
Pavia, Italy

Jean-Christophe Orban, MD
Department of Anaesthesiology and Intensive Care Unit
Hôpital Saint-Roch
Nice, France

Cesare Orlandi, MD
Otsuka Maryland Research Institute
Rockville, MD, USA

Igor F. Palacios, MD
Division of Cardiology
Department of Medicine
Massachusetts General Hospital
and
Harvard Medical School
Boston, MA, USA

Salpy V. Pamboukian, MD, MSPH
Division of Cardiovascular Disease
University of Alabama at Birmingham
Birmingham
Jefferson, AL, USA

Ioannis A. Paraskevaidis, MD
Department of Cardiology
Athens University Hospital Attikon
Athens, Greece

John T. Parissis, MD
Second Department of Cardiology and Heart Failure Unit
University of Athens
Athens, Greece

Joseph E. Parrillo, MD
Robert Wood Johnson Medical School
University of Medicine and Dentistry of New Jersey
Chief, Department of Medicine
Edward D. Viner MD Chair, Department of Medicine
Director, Cooper Heart Institute
Cooper University Hospital
Camden, NJ, USA

Evasio Pasini, MD
Cardiology Division
Sc. Institute of Gussago
S. Maugeri Foundation
Gussago (BS), Italy

J. Herbert Patterson, PharmD
School of Pharmacy
University of North Carolina
Chapel Hill, NC, USA

Didier Payen de La Garanderie, MD, PhD
Department of Anesthesiology and Critical Care Medicine
Lariboisière University Hospital
Assistance Publique-Hôpitaux de Paris
Université Paris Diderot
Paris, France

Louis Peeters, MD, PhD
Ob-Gyn Department
University Hospital Maastricht
Maastricht, The Netherlands

Paul E. Pepe, MD, MPH
Department of Surgery
UT Southwestern Medical Center at Dallas
Dallas, TX, USA

Clément R. Picard, MD
Department of Respiratory Disease
Saint-Louise Teaching Hospital
Paris, France

Ileana L. Piña, MD
Department of Medicine
Case Western Reserve University
Cleveland, OH, USA

Michael R. Pinsky, MD, CM, Dr, hc
Department of Critical Care Medicine
University of Pittsburgh
Pittsburgh, PA, USA

Patrick I. Plaisance, MD, PhD
Department of Emergency Medicine
Lariboisière University Hospital
Assistance Publique-Hôpitaux de Paris
Université Paris Diderot
Paris, France

Piero Pollesello, PhD
Department of Cardiology and Critical Care
Orion Pharma
Espoo, Finland

Christophe Rabuel, MD
Department of Anaesthesiology and Critical Care Medicine
Lariboisière University Hospital
Assistance Publique-Hôpitaux de Paris
Université Paris Diderot
Paris, France

Murugan Raghavan, MD, MRCP
Department of Critical Care Medicine
University of Pittsburgh School of Medicine
Pittsburgh, PA, USA

Andrew Rhodes, MRCP, FRCA
St George's Hospital
London, UK

Jean-Damien Ricard, MD, PhD
Service de Réanimation Médicale
Hôpital Louis Mourier
Assistance Publique-Hôpitaux de Paris
Université Paris Diderot
Colombes, France

Michael W. Rich, MD
Cardiovascular Division
Department of Medicine
Washington University, School of Medicine
St. Louis, MO, USA

Howard A. Rockman, MD
Department of Cardiovascular Medicine
Duke University Center
Durham, NC, USA

Jo E. Rodgers, PharmD
School of Pharmacy
University of North Carolina
Chapel Hill, NC, USA

Edmond Roland, MD, FAHA
French Health Products Safety Agency (Agence Française de Sécurité Sanitaire des Produits de Santé)
Saint-Denis Cedex, France

Damien Roux, MD, MSc
INSERM U722
Université Paris Diderot
Paris, France

Doron Schwartz, MD
Department of Nephrology
Tel Aviv Sourasky Medical Centre
Tel Aviv, Israel

Ajay M. Shah, MD, FRCP, FMedSci
Department of Cardiology, Cardiovascular Division
King's College London School of Medicine
London, UK

Donald S. Silverberg, MD, FRCPCC
Department of Nephrology
Tel Aviv Medical Centre
Tel Aviv, Israel

Marc A. Simon, MD
Department of Medicine
University of Pittsburgh
Pittsburgh, PA, USA

Wendy A. Gattis Stough, PharmD
Department of Clinical Research
Campbell University School of Pharmacy
Cary, NC, USA

José A. Tallaj, MD
Division of Cardiovascular Disease
University of Alabama at Birmingham
Birmingham
Jefferson, AL, USA

Shari L. Targum, MD
Division of Cardio-Renal Products
Center for Drug Evaluation and Research, Food and Drug Administration
Silver Springer London Ltd.
Silver Spring, MD, USA

Jean-Michel Tartière, MD
Lariboisière Hospital
Assistance Publique-Hôpitaux de Paris
Université Paris Diderot
Paris, France

Luigi Tavazzi, MD
Department of Cardiology
Istituti di Ricovero e Cura a Carattere Scientifico
Policlinico S Matteo
University Hospital
Pavia, Italy

Abdellatif Tazi, MD, PhD
Department of Respiratory Disease
Saint-Louis Teaching Hospital
Assistance Publique-Hôpitaux de Paris
Université Paris Diderot
Paris, France

Jean-Louise Teboul, MD, PhD
Medical ICU
Bicetre University Hospital
Assistance Publique-Hôpitaux de Paris
Le Kremlin-Bicêtre, France

John R. Teerlink, MD, FACC, FAHA, FESC
Section of Cardiology
San Francisco Veterans Affairs Medical Center
University of California
San Francisco, CA, USA

Olivier Thomas, MD
Cardiology Department
Ambroise Pare Clinic
Neuilly Sur Seine, France

Andrew Tillyard, B.Apple.Sc, FRCA
St George's Hospital
London, UK

Eleftheria P. Tsagalou, MD
Department of Clinical Therapeutics
University of Athens
Athens, Attica, Greece

Stylianos Tsagarakis, MD, PhD
Department of Endocrinology
Athens Polyclinic
Athens, Greece

Elias Tsolakis, MD
Department of Clinical Therapeutics
University of Athens
Athens, Attica, Greece

Martin A. Valdivia-Arenas, MD
Internal Medicine, Division of Pulmonary, Critical Care, Allergy and Sleep Medicine
The Ohio State University
Columbus
Franklin, OH, USA

Greet Van den Berghe, MD, PhD
Intensive Care Unit
Catholic University of Leuven
Leuven, Belguim

Walther N.K.A. van Mook, MD
Intensive Care
University Hospital Maastricht
Maastricht, The Netherlands

Ramesh Venkataraman, MD
Department of Critical Care Medicine
University of Pittsburgh School of Medicine
Pittsburgh, PA, USA

Antoine Vieillard-Baron, MD, Phd
Medical Intensive Care Unit
Hopital Ambroise Pare
Assistance Publique-Hôpitaux de Paris
Boulogne, France

Simona Viglio, PhD
Department of Biochemistry
University of Pavia
Pavia, Italy

Philippe Vignon, MD, PhD
Medical Surgical Intensive Care Unit
Dupuytren Teaching Hospital
Limoges, France

Fábio Vilas-Boas, MD, PhD
Department of Cardiology
Hospital Espanhol
Salvador, Bahia, Brazil

Dirk Vlasselaers, MD
Intensive Care Unit
Catholic University of Leuven
Leuven, Belguim

Gorazd Voga, MD, PhD
Department for Intensive Internal Medicine
General and Teaching Hospital
Celje, Slovenia

Keith R. Walley, MD
Division of Critical Care
Department of Medicine
The University of British Columbia
St Paul's Hospital
Vancouver, BC, Canada

Todd A. Watson, MD
Department of Anesthesiology
and Critical Care
University of Pennsylvania
Philadelphia, PA, USA

Steven A. Webber, MBChB, MRCP
School of Medicine
Department of Paediatrics
Division of Cardiology
University of Pittsburgh
Children's Hospital Pittsburgh
Pittsburgh, PA, USA

Dov Wexler, MD
Department of Cardiology
Tel Aviv Sourasky Medical Centre
Tel Aviv, Israel

Jane G. Wiggington, MD
Department of Surgery
UT Southwestern Medical Center at Dallas
Dallas, TX, USA

Clyde W. Yancy, MD, FACC, FAHA, FACP
Baylor Heart and Vascular Institute
Baylor University Medical Center
Dallas, TX, USA

Demetris Yannopoulos, MD
Department of Cardiology
University of Minnesota
Minneapolis, MN, USA

Faiez M. Zannad, MD, PhD, FESC
Heart Failure and Hypertension Unit
Department of Cardiology
Centre d'Investigation Clinique (CIC)
INSERM U-684
Centre Hospitalier Universitaire
University Henri Poincaré
Nancy, France
and
School of Medicine of Tunis
Tunis, Tunisia

Min Zhang, MD, PhD
Department of Cardiology
Cardiovascular Division
London, UK

1
Acute Heart Failure Syndromes: From Epidemiology to Clinical Practice

1.1
Epidemiology and Definitions

1
Definitions of Acute Heart Failure Syndromes

Alexandre Mebazaa, Mihai Gheorghiade, Faiez M. Zannad, and Joseph E. Parrillo

Old Concepts

Acute heart failure is likely one of the oldest described diseases. However, although clinical signs, such as paroxysmal nocturnal dyspnea and crackles, are known by any physician, the epidemiology of acute heart failure was only recently assessed (1). In most textbooks of cardiology or intensive care in the last 40 years, acute heart failure is considered a mixture including acute pulmonary edema following an increased arterial blood pressure and a cardiogenic shock related to acute myocardial infarction.

The word *heart* in *acute heart failure* is indeed confusing. Many young physicians still believe that during an acute heart failure episode, the heart, and likely its systolic function, is not working properly; we know today that this is not true.

In addition, as pulmonary edema was described in the 1950s in patients with a long history of heart failure, and called "congestive heart failure" for years, physicians left with the impression that pulmonary edema is always associated with increased blood volume and that pulmonary edema should be always treated with diuretics. However, we know today that most acute pulmonary edema appears in patients with a long history of hypertension and who are rather normovolaemic.

New Concept: Acute Heart Failure Syndromes

Acute heart failure syndromes (AHFS) may be defined as heart failure with a relatively rapid onset of signs and symptoms, resulting in hospitalization or unplanned office or emergency department visits (1). As the term *acute heart failure syndromes* indicates, acute heart failure can result from a variety of different pathophysiologic conditions.

The Heart Failure Society of America (2) recently distinguished patients in three categories: (1) The majority of patients hospitalized with acute heart failure have evidence of systemic hypertension on admission and commonly have preserved left ventricular ejection fraction (LVEF). (2) Most hospitalized patients have volume overload and congestive symptoms predominates. (3) A distinct minority have severely impaired systolic function, reduced blood pressure, and symptoms from poor end-organ perfusion.

We recently proposed, based on pathophysiologic targets, distinguishing between "vascular" and "cardiac" acute heart failure, each with a different initial clinical presentation (Table 1.1) (3).

The European Society of Cardiology and the European Society of Intensive Care Medicine further classified acute heart failure patients in six categories (Table 1.2) (4). This is the basis of the new concept of acute heart failure syndromes. These categories have been shown to also represent a different outcome: hypertensive acute pulmonary edema has a lower mortality rate compared to decompensated heart failure or cardiogenic shock (5). In addition, outcome is likely different when AHFS appears de novo or in a context of decompensated heart failure (6).

Table 1.1. Initial clinical presentation of acute heart failure syndrome

Vascular failure	Cardiac failure
High blood pressure	Normal blood pressure
Rapid worsening	Gradual worsening (days)
Pulmonary congestion	Systemic rather than pulmonary
PCWP acutely increased	PCWP chronically high
Rales: present	Rales: may be absent
Severe radiographic congestion	Radiographic congestion may be absent
Weight gain minimal	Weight gain significant (edema)
LVEF relatively preserved	LVEF usually low
Response to therapy: relatively rapid	Response to therapy: continue to have systemic congestion in spite of the initial symptomatic response

LVEF, left ventricular ejection fraction; PCWP: pulmonary artery wedged pressure.
Source: Gheorghiade et al. (3), with permission.

Table 1.2. Classification of acute heart failure syndrome based on clinical presentation from the most frequent to the less frequent

Hypertensive acute HF: signs and symptoms of HF are accompanied by high blood pressure and relatively preserved left ventricular function, with a chest radiograph compatible with acute pulmonary edema.
Pulmonary edema (verified by chest x-ray) accompanied by severe respiratory distress, with crackles over lung orthopnea, with O_2 saturation usually <90% on room air before treatment.
Acute decomposed HF (de novo or as decomposition of chronic HF): signs and symptoms of acute HF that are mild do not fulfill the criteria for cardiogenic shock, pulmonary edema, or hypertensive crisis.
Cardiogenic shock: cardiogenic shock is defined as evidence of tissue hypoperfusion induced by HF after correction of preload. There is no clear definition for hemodynamic parameters, but cardiogenic shock is usually characterized by reduced blood pressure (systolic blood pressure <90 mm Hg or a drop of mean arterial pressure >30 mm Hg) and/or low urine output (<0.5 mL/kg per hour), with a pulse rate >60 beats per minute with or without evidence of organ congestion. There is a continuum from low cardiac output syndrome to cardiogenic shock.
High output failure is characterized by high cardiac output usually with high heart rate (caused by arrhythmias, thyrotoxicosis, anemia, Paget disease, or iatrogenic or other mechanisms), with warm peripheries, pulmonary congestion, and sometimes low blood pressure, as in septic shock.
Right HF is characterized by low output syndrome with increased jugular venous pressure, increased live size, and hypotension.

HF, heart failure.
Note: These scenarios can be seen in acute de novo or chronic decomposed heart failure (HF) (4).

References

1. Gheorghiade M, Mebazaa A. Introduction to acute heart failure syndromes. Am J Cardiol 2005; 96(suppl):1G–4G.
2. HFSA. Evaluation and management of patients with acute decompensated heart failure. J Cardiac Failure 2006;12:e86–e103.
3. Gheorghiade M, De Luca L, Fonarow GC, Filippatos, Metra M, Francis G. Pathophysiologic targets in the early phase of acute heart failure syndromes. Am J Cardiol 2005;96(suppl):11G–17G.
4. Nieminen MS, Bohm M, Cowie MR, et al.; ESC Committee for Practice Guideline (CPG). Executive summary of the guidelines on the diagnosis and treatment of acute heart failure: the Task Force on Acute Heart Failure of the European Society of Cardiology. Eur Heart J 2005;26:384–416.
5. Zannad F, Adamopoulos C, Mebazaa A, Gheorghiade M. The challenge of acute decompensated heart failure. Heart Fail Rev 2006;11:135–139.
6. Nieminen MS, Brutsaert D, Dickstein K, et al. EuroHeart Failure Survey II (EHFS II): a survey on hospitalized acute heart failure patients: description of population. Eur Heart J 2006:27:2725–2736.

2
Risk Stratification Models and Predictors of Mortality in Acute Heart Failure Syndromes, Based on United States Registries

Gregg C. Fonarow

Heart failure causes considerable morbidity and mortality and produces a tremendous burden on health care systems worldwide. In the United States, heart failure resulted in 1.1 million hospitalizations and entailed an annual estimated cost of $29 to $56 billion.(1) The in-hospital mortality rates reported for acute heart failure has varied greatly, ranging from 2% to 20%. Prognosis is also reported to be very poor postdischarge; the mortality risk after acute heart failure hospitalization has been reported to be as high as 11.3% at 30 days and 33.1% at 1 year.(2) In addition, patients also face a high risk of rehospitalization. In a study of almost 18,000 Medicare recipients, approximately 44% were rehospitalized at least once in the 6 months following their index hospitalization.(3) These statistics emphasize the need for clinically practical methods of risk stratification for patients hospitalized with acute heart failure syndromes as well as the need to develop and implement more effective strategies to manage heart failure.

Risk Stratification Models

Clinical risk prediction tools may be helpful in guiding medical decision making. In patients hospitalized with acute heart failure, those estimated to be at lower risk may be managed with less intensive monitoring and therapies available on a telemetry unit or hospital ward, whereas patients estimated to be at higher risk may require more intensive management in an intensive or coronary care unit. Despite the large number of patients impacted and the mortality risk, integrated models for the risk stratification of patients hospitalized with heart failure were not available until recently. A number of individual variables that are associated with increased mortality among patients hospitalized with heart failure have been identified. These include, among many others, patient age, gender, and race; ischemic etiology; comorbid conditions, such as cerebrovascular disease, dementia, chronic obstructive pulmonary disease, hepatic cirrhosis, and cancer; and measurement of systolic blood pressure (SBP), heart rate, respiratory rate, left ventricular ejection fraction (LVEF), serum sodium concentration, serum creatinine concentration, blood urea nitrogen (BUN), hemoglobin, and B-type natriuretic peptide (BNP) concentration.(4) Because multiple risk factors can exist in the same patient, to be meaningful, the risk factor analysis must consider factors in combination rather than isolation. Because most evaluations tended to treat these factors as isolated entities, they had not produced a clinically practical way of integrating various factors to stratify risk in heart failure patients. A number of recent studies have developed and validated models to enable clinicians to reliably identify patients at low, medium, and high risk for mortality based on patient characteristics, vital signs, and laboratories at the time of admission.

EFFECT Risk Tool

A retrospective study of 4031 community-based patients presenting with heart failure at multiple hospitals in Ontario, Canada, from 1997 to 2001 identified as part of the Enhanced Feedback for Effective Cardiac Treatment (EFFECT) study was used to identify predictors of mortality and to develop and to validate a model using information available at hospital presentation.(2) In hospital, 30-day and 1-year all-cause mortality rates for the cohort were 8.9% in hospital, 10.7% at 30 days, and 32.9% at 1 year. Multivariable predictors of mortality at both 30 days and 1 year included older age, lower SBP, higher respiratory rate, higher urea nitrogen level (all $p < .001$), and hyponatremia ($p < .01$) (Table 2.1).(2) Comorbid conditions associated with mortality included cerebrovascular disease (30-day mortality odds ratio [OR], 1.43; 95% confidence interval [CI], 1.03–1.98; $p = .03$), chronic obstructive pulmonary disease (OR, 1.66; 95% CI, 1.22–2.27; $p = .002$), hepatic cirrhosis (OR, 3.22; 95% CI, 1.08–9.65; $p = .04$), dementia (OR, 2.54; 95% CI, 1.77–3.65; $p < .001$), and cancer (OR, 1.86; 95% CI, 1.28–2.70; $p = .001$). A risk index was developed to stratify the risk of death and identify low- and high-risk individuals. Patients with very low-risk scores (≤60) had a mortality rate of 0.4% at 30 days and 7.8% at 1 year. Patients with very high risk scores (>150) had a mortality rate of 59.0% at 30 days and 78.8% at 1 year.(2) Patients with higher 1-year risk scores had reduced survival at all times up to 1 year (log-rank, $p < .001$). For the derivation cohort, the area under the receiver operating characteristic curve for the model was 0.80 for 30-day mortality and 0.77 for 1-year mortality. Thus, among community-based heart failure patients, factors identifiable within hours of hospital presentation predicted mortality risk at 30 days and 1 year. The externally validated

TABLE 2.1. Heart failure risk scoring system[a]

Variable	No. of points	
	30-day score[b]	1-year score[c]
Age. years	+Age (in years)	+Age (in years)
Respiratory rate, minutes (minimal 20; maximum 45)[d]	+Rate (in breaths/min)	+Rate (in breaths/min)
Systolic blood pressure, mm Hg[e]		
≥180	−60	−50
160–179	−55	−45
140–159	−50	−40
120–139	−45	−35
100–119	−40	−30
90–99	−35	−25
<90	−30	−20
Urea nitrogen (maximum, 60 mg/dL)[d,f]	+Level (in mg/dL)	+Level (in mg/dL)
Sodium concentration <136 mEq/L	+10	+10
Cerebrovascular disease	+10	+10
Dementia	+20	+15
Chronic obstructive pulmonary disease	+10	+10
Hepatic cirrhosis	+25	+35
Cancer	+15	+15
Hemoglobin < 10.0 g/dL (<100 g/L)	NA	+10

NA, not applicable to 30 day model.

[a]An electronic version of the risk scoring system is available at http://www. ccort.ca/CHFriskmodel.asp.

[b]Calculated as age + respiratory rate + systolic blood pressure + urea nitrogen + sodium points + cerebrovascular disease points + dementia points + chronic obstructive pulmonary disease points + hepatic cirrhosis points + cancer points.

[c]Calculated as age + respiratory rate + systolic blood pressure + urea nitrogen + sodium points + cerebrovascular disease points + dementia points + chronic obstructive pulmonary disease points + hepatic cirrhosis points + cancer points + hemoglobin points.

[d]Values higher than maximum or lower than minimum are assigned the listed maximum or minimum values.

[e]Increases were protective in both mortality models. Points are subtracted for higher blood pressure measurements.

[f]Maximum value is equivalent to 21 mmol/L. Score calculated using value in mg/dL.

Source: Lee et al. (2), with permission. Copyright © 2003, American Medical Association.

predictive index may assist clinicians in estimating heart failure mortality risk and in providing quantitative guidance for decision making in heart failure care.

ADHERE Risk Tool

The Acute Decompensated Heart Failure National Registry (ADHERE) patient records were used to develop and validate a practical and user-friendly method of risk stratification for in-hospital mortality admitted with heart failure that could be applicable to the bedside.(5) Overall, in-hospital mortality was 4.1%. In ADHERE, of 39 variables, BUN level of 43 mg/dL or higher, serum creatinine level of 2.75 mg/dL or higher, and SBP of less than 115 mmHg were independent predictors of high risk for in-hospital mortality in a Classification and Regression Tree (CART) analysis.(5) The mortality risk varied more than 10-fold (from 2.1% to 21.9%) based on the patient's initial SBP and BUN and creatinine (Cr) levels (Fig. 2.1). With this validated risk tool, low-, intermediate-, and high-risk patients could be readily identified.

In a multivariate analysis of the same data set, blood pressure (BP), heart rate, serum creatinine, serum sodium, and liver disease were highly predictive of in-hospital mortality.(5) Multivariate logistic regression identified BUN, SBP, heart rate, and age as the most significant mortality risk predictors, and adding as many as 24 additional predictors did not meaningfully increase the accuracy of this model. Based on the area under the receiver operator curves, the accuracy of the CART model (0.67) was only modestly less than that of the more complicated logistic regression model (0.76). Acutely decompensated heart failure patients at low, intermediate, and high risk for in-hospital mortality can be easily identified using vital sign and laboratory data obtained on

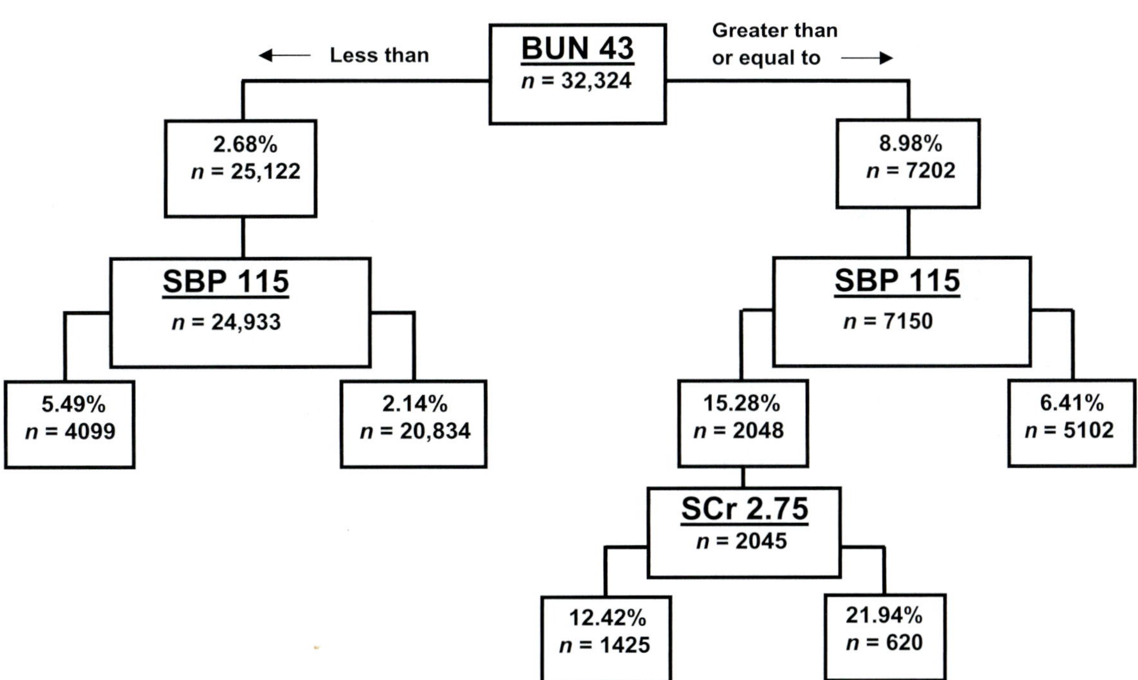

FIGURE 2.1. Predictors of in-hospital mortality and risk stratification identified by the Acute Decompensated Heart Failure National Registry (ADHERE) using Classification and Regression Tree (CART) analysis. Each node is based on available data from registry patient hospitalizations for each predictive variable presented. Percentages indicate crude mortality for each terminal node. BUN, blood urea nitrogen; SBP, systolic blood pressure; SCr, serum creatinine.

hospital admission with the model. The ADHERE risk tree provides clinicians with a validated, practical bedside tool for mortality risk stratification.

In a subsequent analysis of >100,000 hospitalizations from ADHERE, CART analysis identified elevated BUN, lower SBP, low sodium, older age, elevated creatinine, the presence of dyspnea at rest, and the absence of chronic beta-blocker use as mortality risk factors.(6) Among these variables, the two main contributors to higher mortality (the top splits in the tree) were BUN >37 mg/dL and SBP ≤125 mm Hg. When the CART analysis was carried out in heart failure patients with preserved systolic function (LVEF ≥0.40) and separately in those with systolic dysfunction, elevated BUN and lower systolic BP were confirmed as the most important mortality predictors within each group. In addition, increased heart rate was identified as a mortality predictor in patient episodes of heart failure with preserved systolic function, but not in patient episodes of heart failure with systolic dysfunction.(6) Thus mortality risk can be reliably predicted for both preserved systolic function and systolic dysfunction heart failure patients equally well.

Other Risk Models

The Outcomes of a Prospective Trial of Intravenous Milrinone for Exacerbations of Chronic Heart Failure (OPTIME-CHF) study found that in 949 patients with decompensated heart failure (HF), the variables at presentation that predicted death at 60 days were older age, lower SBP, New York Heart Association (NYHA) class IV symptoms, elevated BUN, and decreased sodium.(7) Hospitalization data have been used to develop a risk score for HF readmission. This risk score, which is based on 16 parameters, was moderately predictive in the derivative cohort, but it has not been independently validated in a second cohort. Medicare claims data from 1998 to 2001 were used to develop and validate a hierarchical regression model to predict hospital risk-standardized 30-day mortality rates using medical chart review data.(8) This model was then compared to an administrative claims model. The final model included 24 variables. The model had an area under the receiver operating characteristic curve of 0.70. This administrative claims-based model produced estimates of risk-standardized state mortality that appeared to be a reasonable surrogate for estimates derived from a medical record model. This model may be useful in facilitating quality assessment and improvement efforts.

Although the variables retained in specific acute heart failure risk models vary, multiple evaluations have demonstrated the prognostic value of SBP and indices of renal function. In EFFECT, higher BUN and lower SBP were significant and independent predictors of both 30-day and 1-year mortality. In ADHERE, the SBP, BUN, and creatinine were the three variables most predictive of in-hospital mortality. In OPTIME, the SBP and BUN were significant and independent predictors of death or rehospitalization. Similarly, in a retrospective review of 1004 patients hospitalized for heart failure at 11 hospitals, worsening renal function was associated with a 7.5-fold increase in the adjusted risk of in-hospital mortality. Thus the assessment of blood pressure and determining renal function are essential in the risk-stratifying patients presenting with acute decompensated heart failure.

The use of biomarkers as prognostic indicators for patients hospitalized with heart failure has been of interest. Several studies have suggested that markers of myocardial damage such as cardiac troponin I and T are elevated in patients hospitalized with heart failure in the absence of an acute coronary syndrome and provide prognostic information. Admission BNP and N-terminal pro-BNP has been show to predict in-hospital and postdischarge mortality, independent of other prognostic variables. These biomarkers can be used in conjunction with the clinical risk tools or as more data become available integrated into the risk models.

Clinical Applicability of Different Models

A significant disadvantage of multivariate-generated risk scores is their complexity. The number of parameters and mathematical functions involved frequently require access to a computer or electronic calculator to generate the score and determine the risk, making them potentially impractical for bedside assessment. Even when converted to point scores, the tools derived from a multivariate model still require a nomogram reference to convert the point score to risk. The CART methodology can detect interactions between variables and yields a decision tree that is relatively easy to apply at the bedside. In the ADHERE CART analysis, three variables were found to be the most significant predictors of in-hospital mortality risk.(5) In a simple two- to three-step process, these variables permit identification of patients with low, intermediate, or high risk for in-hospital mortality. The CART-based analysis of the ADHERE registry has created a simple robust tool to predict in-hospital mortality that is easy to use, can be readily applied at the bedside, and has good discriminative ability. For clinicians with bedside access to computers or personal digital assistants, using logistic regression model calculation or point score determination for prediction of heart failure patient risk may be preferred.

There have also been risk tools developed for outpatients with heart failure. A heart failure survival score has been developed and independently validated for ambulatory outpatients with HF.(9) This score, based on seven parameters—heart failure etiology, heart rate, blood pressure, serum sodium concentration, intraventricular conduction time, LVEF, and peak oxygen consumption—stratifies patients into low (16%), medium (39%), and high (50%) mortality risk categories. The Seattle Heart Failure Model was derived in a cohort of 1125 heart failure patients with the use of a multivariate Cox model.(10) This model predicted 1-, 2-, and 3-year survival in heart failure patients using characteristics relating to clinical status, therapy (pharmacologic as well as devices), and laboratory parameters. For the lowest score, the 2-year survival was 92.8% compared with 88.7%, 77.8%, 58.1%, 29.5%, and 10.8% for scores of 0, 1, 2, 3, and 4, respectively.(1) The overall receiver operating characteristic area under the curve was 0.73. This model also allowed estimation of the benefit of adding medications or devices to an individual patient's therapeutic regimen. The utility of these models to assess risks in patients hospitalized with acute decompensated heart failure has not been assessed.

Role in Clinical Management

These validated hospital models should aid medical decision making in patients hospitalized with acute decompensated heart failure.(5) Patients judged to be at higher risk may receive higher-level monitoring and earlier, more intensive treatment for acute decompensated heart failure, while patients estimated to be at lower risk may be reassured and managed less intensively. Furthermore, high-risk patients can be identified for whom very resource-intensive interventions designed to improve outcomes as described in other chapters in this book may be justified. If is important to recognize that these model should be used to enhance, not replace, physician assessment. These models have also been useful in demonstrating that there is a risk-treatment mismatch in heart failure. The EFFECT model medication administration rates at hospital discharge and 90 days after discharge were assessed in patients in the low-, intermediate-, and high-risk groups.(11) It was shown that the highest-risk heart failure patients were much less likely to receive lifesaving therapies. Low-risk patients were more likely to receive angiotensin-converting enzyme (ACE) inhibitors or angiotensin receptor blockers (adjusted hazard ratio [HR], 1.61; 95% CI, 1.49–1.74) and beta-receptor antagonists (HR, 1.80; 95% CI, 1.60–2.01) compared with high-risk patients (both $p < .001$). In addition, these models should prove to be valuable in designing clinical trials to evaluate heart failure therapies, allowing for development of trial inclusion criteria to enroll only patients at high risk for in-hospital mortality.

Conclusion

In patients hospitalized with acute heart failure syndromes, the risk of in-hospital, 30-day, and 1-year mortality can be quickly and effectively determined using admission clinical and laboratory parameters. On the basis of these parameters, acute heart failure syndrome patients can be readily stratified into groups at low-, intermediate-, and high-risk for mortality. The finding that indices of renal status and systolic blood pressure are among the best mortality risk discrimination underscores the importance of renal function and systolic blood pressure in acute heart failure syndrome patients. The continued high mortality for patients hospitalized with acute heart failure syndrome provides a compelling indication to apply risk prediction tools to improve the evaluation, management, and outcomes of these patients.

References

1. Hunt SA, Abraham WT, Chin MH, et al. ACC/AHA 2005 Guideline Update for the Diagnosis and Management of Chronic Heart Failure in the Adult: a report of the American College of Cardiology/American Heart Association Task Force on Practice Guidelines (Writing Committee to Update the 2001 Guidelines for the Evaluation and Management of Heart Failure). Circulation 2005;112:e154–235.
2. Lee DS, Austin PC, Rouleau JL, Liu PP, Naimark D, Tu JV. Predicting mortality among patients hospitalized for heart failure: derivation and validation of a clinical model. JAMA 2003;290:2581–2587.
3. Krumholz HM, Wang Y, Parent EM, et al. Quality of care for elderly patients hospitalized with heart failure. Arch Intern Med 1997;157:2242–2247.
4. Gheorghiade M, Zannad F, Sopko G, et al. Acute heart failure syndromes: current state and framework for future research. Circulation 2005;112: 3958–3968.
5. Fonarow GC, Adams KF Jr, Abraham WT, Yancy CW, Boscardin WJ. Risk stratification for in-hospital mortality in acutely decompensated heart failure: classification and regression tree analysis. JAMA 2005;293:572–580.
6. Yancy CW, Lopatin M, Stevenson LW, De Marco T, Fonarow GC. Clinical presentation, management, and in-hospital outcomes of patients admitted with acute decompensated heart failure with preserved systolic function: a report from the Acute Decompensated Heart Failure National Registry (ADHERE) Database. J Am Coll Cardiol 2006;47:76–84.
7. Klein L, O'Connor CM, Leimberger JD, et al. Lower serum sodium is associated with increased short-term mortality in hospitalized patients with worsening heart failure: results from the Outcomes of a Prospective Trial of Intravenous Milrinone for Exacerbations of Chronic Heart Failure (OPTIME-CHF) study. Circulation 2005;111:2454–2460.
8. Krumholz HM, Wang Y, Mattera JA, et al. An administrative claims model suitable for profiling hospital performance based on 30-day mortality rates among patients with heart failure. Circulation 2006;113:1693–1701.
9. Aaronson KD, Schwartz JS, Chen TM, Wong KL, Goin JE, Mancini DM. Development and prospective validation of a clinical index to predict survival in ambulatory patients referred for cardiac transplant evaluation. Circulation 1997;95:2660–2667.
10. Levy WC, Mozaffarian D, Linker DT, et al. The Seattle Heart Failure Model: prediction of survival in heart failure. Circulation 2006;113:1424–1433.
11. Lee DS, Tu JV, Juurlink DN, et al. Risk-treatment mismatch in the pharmacotherapy of heart failure. JAMA 2005;294:1240–1247.

3
Epidemiology and Management of Acute Heart Failure Syndromes in Europe

François Alla and Faiez M. Zannad

Guidelines on the diagnosis and treatment of acute heart failure (AHF) were recently published by the European Society of Cardiology (ESC)[1]. These guidelines were published after a major European epidemiologic study was done, the Euro Heart Failure Survey Programme (EuroHF), which provided a description of clinical characteristics and management of patients hospitalized for AHF syndromes across Europe. This program was conducted in 115 hospitals in 24 countries, which have included 11,327 patients with suspected or confirmed AHF[2–4]. Another major European study was EFICA, *Etude Française de l'Insuffisance Cardiaque Aigue* (French Study of Acute Heart Failure), which have included 581 patients admitted to 60 intensive care units (ICUs) or coronary care units (CCU) randomly selected among French centers[5]. Finally, a nationwide survey on AHF syndromes in Italy was recently published. During the 3-month inclusion period, 206 cardiology centers with intensive CCUs have recruited 2807 patients[6].

Beyond differences in disease definitions, methods used, and recruiting conditions, these studies present a coherent epidemiologic picture of patients hospitalized with AHF syndrome.

We will not describe AHF syndromes within the setting of acute myocardial infarction. Indeed, this other distinct entity has been already well studied.

Clinical Characteristic of Patients Hospitalized with Acute Heart Failure Syndrome

The results of these studies allow us to show an accurate picture of patients admitted with AHF syndrome (Table 3.1). These were old patients (mean age from 71 to 73 years), with a balanced sex ratio (from 41% to 47% female patients).

These studies reveal similarly the significant proportion of morbidity and cardiovascular risk factors such as ischemic heart disease (from 46% to 68%); arterial hypertension (from 53% to 66%); diabetes (from 27% to 38%); arrhythmia, especially atrial fibrillation (from 21% to 42%); and renal insufficiency (from 17% to 53%). Besides these cardiovascular diseases, these patients also suffered from other serious morbidities, such as cancer (8% of patients included in EFICA), cirrhosis or hepatic insufficiency (3% in EFICA), or chronic obstructive pulmonary disease (19% in EFICA).

Type, Etiology, and Clinical Presentation

There are many types of classification for AHF syndromes[5,7,8]. Indeed, the AHF syndromes may be classified according to mechanism

Table 3.1. Clinical characteristic of patients hospitalized with acute heart failure syndrome

	Euro Heart Failure Survey Programme(3)	EFICA(4)	AHF in Italy(5)
Geographic zone	24 countries	France	Italy
Inclusion period	2000–01	2001	2004
Number of included patients	11,327	581	2807
Mean age (years)	71	73 ± 13	73 ± 11
Men	53%	59%	59%
Admitted in ICU/CCU	7%	100%	69%
Cardiogenic shock	<1%	32%	8%
Known CHF	65%	66%	56%
Previous AHF hospitalization	44%	35%	–
History and cardiovascular risk factors (%)			
Ischemic heart disease (myocardial infarction history)	68% (39%)	46% (22%)	46%* (37%)
Arterial hypertension	53%	60%	66%
Diabetes mellitus	27%	27%	38%
Renal insufficiency (creatine serum levels >2 mg/dL)	17%	53%	25%
Evolution			
Mean length of hospitalization (days)	11	15	9
In-hospital mortality	7%	28%	7%

*Heart failure etiology.

AHF, acute heart failure CCU, coronary care unit; CHF, congestive heart failure; EFICA, *Etude Fran çaise de l'Insuffisance Cardiaque Aigue* (French Study of Acute Heart Failure); HF, heart failure; ICU, intensive care unit.

(decompensated chronic heart failure or de novo heart failure), according to the underlying etiology, or according to the clinical presentation. Classification according to presentation is pragmatic and appears to be the most adequate from a clinical point of view[5], while the other two, which reveal the underlying mechanisms, also have definite epidemiological importance.

Mechanism and Etiology: Acute Decompensated Chronic Heart Failure

Decompensated chronic heart failure represents two thirds of AHF syndromes (65% of patients in EuroHF, 66% in EFICA, and 56% in Italian study had known HF). These HF cases were generally associated with depressed systolic function (54% of patients in EuroHF, 27% in EFICA, and 29% in Italian study have a left ventricular ejection fraction [LVEF] >40). As it has been already extensively illustrated, heart failure with preserved systolic function concerned mainly women (37% vs. 16% of men in EFICA) and elderly patients (29% of those 80 or older vs. 21% before the age of 80 in EFICA).

As demonstrated by many descriptive studies, generally carried out on inpatients, the etiology of known heart failure was ischemic in half of the cases. In the EFICA study, the proportion of ischemic etiology in patients with preexisting HF failure was 58%. The main triggering factors for these patients were ischemia (49% of ischemic etiology HF, 9% of others), arrhythmias and conduction disorders (22% of ischemic etiology HF, 35% of others), and infections (19% of ischemic etiology HF, 25% of other).

Mechanism and Etiology: De Novo Acute Heart Failure

About a third of the episodes were de novo AHF (35% in EuroHF, 34% in EFICA, and 44% in Italian study). They appeared in the great majority during an acute coronary syndrome. In the EFICA study, 66% of de novo HF were thus recognized as being of ischemic etiology.

Clinical Presentation

The presence or absence of cardiogenic shock, which greatly influences short-term prognosis and determines therapeutic management, is the predominant clinical characteristic. The proportion of AHFS with shock differed according to the studies depending on recruiting sites. In the EFICA study, conducted in ICU/CCU, 29% of patients were admitted with a cardiogenic shock. In the EuroHF study, only 7% of patients were admitted in ICU/CCU, and less than 1% of patients were in cardiogenic shock.

In the French study, de novo HF patients presented more often a shock, compared to the decompensated chronic HF (36% vs. 25%), especially ischemic AHF syndromes (38%).

Initial In-Hospital Outcome

Length of Hospitalization

In the EuroHF study, the mean duration of the index hospitalization was 11 days. In the Italian study, this duration was 9 days. These data were similar to those provided by hospital administrative databases. For example, in France in 2004, the mean duration for HF hospitalizations was also 11 days[9]. The hospitalization duration is twice as long in Europe when compared to the United States. This disparity probably reflects the continental differences as far as organization, health system functioning, and care management.

In the EFICA study, which has included more severe patients, hospitalization length was 15 days, of which 6 were spent in ICU/CCU.

In-Hospital Mortality

In-hospital mortality was 6.9% in the EuroHF study. As well, the in-hospital mortality was 7.3% in the Italian study, and 8% in the Rudiger study, which was conducted in two hospitals from Switzerland and Finland[10].

Globally, the etiology and the precipitating factors had little impact on in-hospital outcome. The clinical presentation remains the most important determinant of early lethality. Acute heart failure syndrome with shock was the most serious presentation, as shown by EFICA results: initial hospitalization lethality was 58% for patients with shock, as opposed to 16% for patients without shock (Fig. 3.1). Rudiger et al.[10] observed comparable results: the mortality after 30 days was 46% for patients with shock and 9% for patients without shock.

In the absence of shock, the association of high blood pressure and pulmonary edema represented the most favorable prognosis, with a 4-week mortality rate of 7% in the EFICA study. In the same way, the Rudiger study showed a 4-week mortality rate of 6.5% in patients with high blood pressure history.

Preadmission Mortality

We know that in-hospital mortality is only the tip of the iceberg. Indeed, some patients die before admission to wards, be it at home, during transportation, or in the emergency department. However, there are only a few data available regarding the prehospitalization mortality. Thus, the need for an ancillary study from EFICA that has provided the total mortality rate of AHF

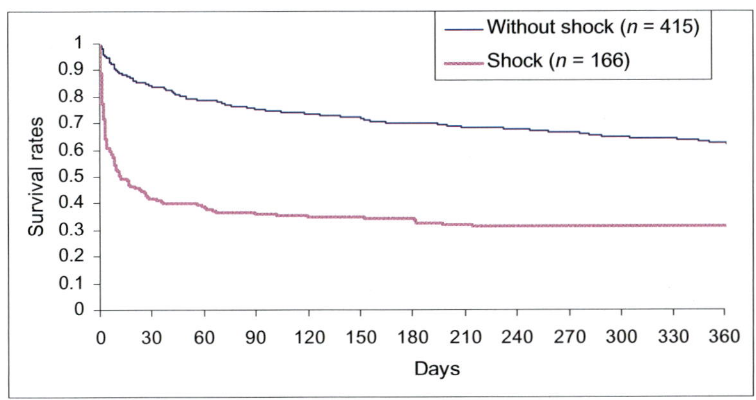

Figure 3.1. One-year survival rate, comparison between patients with or without shock during index hospitalization ($n = 581$, EFICA study data, not published).

syndromes by analyzing registries of patients who have been referred or admitted to the emergency services of establishments participating in the study (excluding deaths occurring at home prior to specialized transport care). When including these deaths, the estimated total 4-week mortality rate rose from 27.4% to 43.2%.

Management of Patients with Acute Heart Failure Syndromes

Investigations

In the EuroHF program, 95% of patients were reported to have had an electrocardiogram (ECG). A chest x-ray report was available for 92% of patients. Other investigations, which guidelines on heart failure suggest should be routine, including hemoglobin, electrolytes, and renal function, were measured in >90% of patients. Sixty-three percents of patients had an LVEF reported by at least one imaging test, most often echocardiography. There was substantial international variation across Europe in the use of echocardiography, with patients in northern Europe being generally less likely to be investigated. Other investigations that may be considered in patients with heart failure but are not recommended as a routine in the guidelines were conducted less frequently. Coronary arteriography (16% during the index hospitalization, 32% total), exercise testing, and pulmonary function tests were conducted on a substantial minority of patients. Stress-imaging tests for myocardial ischemia and viability and exercise testing with metabolic gas exchange were rarely performed. There was evidence of considerable international variation in the use of coronary arteriography (e.g., 60% in Germany vs. 4% in the United Kingdom during the index hospitalization).

Heart Failure Drug Therapies

The EuroHF program has confirmed previous reports that suggested that guidelines for the pharmacologic treatment of HF are not closely adhered to. Indeed, this study reported the drug therapy prescribed during the index hospitalization across European countries[4]. Diuretics (mainly loop diuretics) were the most commonly prescribed class of agent (86.9%). Overall, angiotensin-converting enzyme (ACE) inhibitors were used in 61.8% of patients and almost 80% of those with reduced LVEF. The respective figures for beta-blockers were less widely used overall (36.9%) and in patients with reduced LVEF (49%). Other prescribed drugs were cardiac glycosides (35.7%), nitrates (32.1%), calcium channel blockers (21.2%), and spironolactone (20.5%). Nearly half (44.6%) of the population used four or more different drugs. Only 17.2% were under the combination of diuretic, ACE inhibitors, and beta-blockers. Moreover, daily dosages of ACE inhibitors reached 50% to 60% of the target recommended dose except for captopril, which was prescribed at much lower doses, whereas the daily dosage of beta-blockers were far below the target dose used in randomized trials. Finally, important variations between countries, and according to the type of hospital wards, were found in the rate of prescription of ACE inhibitors and particularly beta-blockers.

Intensive Care Unit/Coronary Care Unit Management

In the EFICA study, depending on the patient's condition, ventilatory support was provided in 59% of cases (invasive ventilation, 35%; noninvasive positive pressure ventilation, 24%). Central venous catheterization was performed in 33% of cases and catecholamines administered in 53% of cases.

Medium-Term Outcome

Hospitalization

One particular feature of AHF syndromes is the high frequency of rehospitalizations. In the EuroHS survey, 24% of patients were rehospitalized at least once during the 3 months following discharge from index hospitalization.

Mortality and Prognosis Factors

The 1-year mortality rate in EFICA study was 43.2%. The Rudiger study observed a 1-year

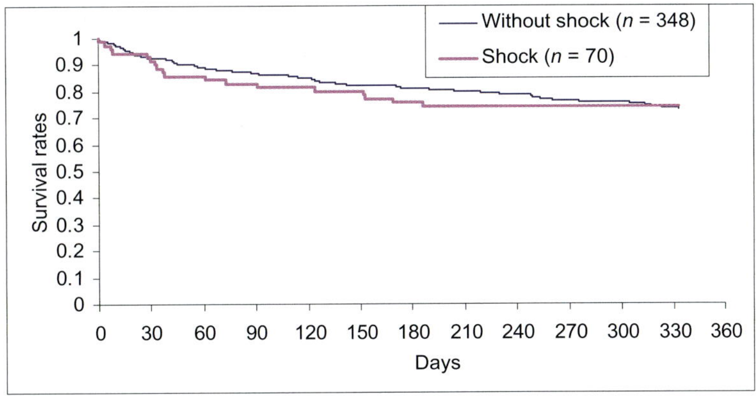

FIGURE 3.2. One-year survival rate for survivors at 28 days, comparison between patients with or without shock during index hospitalization ($n = 418$, EFICA study data, not published).

mortality rate of 29%. Prognostic factors of middle-term mortality differ from those of short-term. Notably, the presence or absence of shock, which is the major prognostic factor during the hospitalization, did not have influence after the acute phase (Fig. 3.2). Mortality after 1 year among survivors at 28 days in the EFICA study was of 24.6% for patients with shock at the index hospitalization compared to 26.7% for the other patients.

However, the existence of known HF seems to be a major prognostic factor for medium-term outcome. Mortality at 1 year for survivors at 28 days in the EFICA study was 19.3% in patients without preexistent HF, 23.3% in patients with a presence of New York Heart Association (NYHA) class I or II symptoms, and 38.6% in patients with NYHA class III or IV symptoms (Fig. 3.3). These results are compatible with those observed in HF cohorts. For example, the EPidémiologie de L'Insuffisance Cardiaque Avancée en Lorraine (EPICAL) study, which has recruited patients in France with NYHA class III/IV symptoms, found a 1-year mortality rate of 35.4%, a value comparable to that of patients in the EFICA study at the same classes[11].

Even so, if one takes into account early mortality, the 1 year prognosis is substantially impaired for patients with shock: in the EFICA study 68.2% of patients with shock had died the year following inclusion, compared to 37.9% of other patients. In the same way, in the Rudiger study, the 1-year mortality rate was 62% in patients with shock

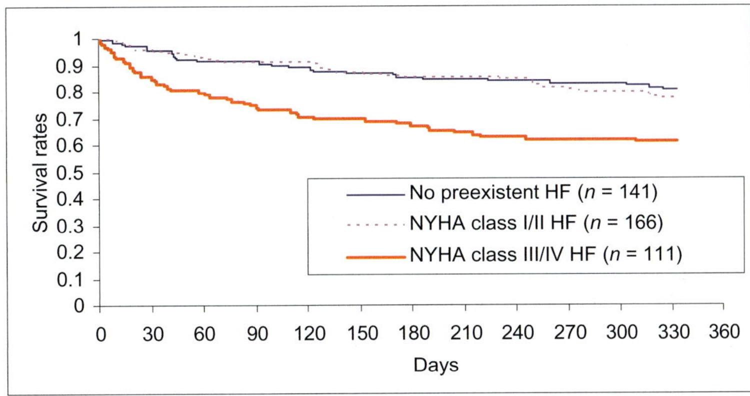

FIGURE 3.3. One-year survival rate for survivors at 28 days, comparison between patients with or without preexistent heart failure (n = 418, EFICA study data, not published). NYHA, New York Heart Association.

versus about 28% in patients without shock during the index hospitalization.

Incidence of Acute Heart Failure Syndrome

The incidence of AHF syndromes is defined by nonscheduled hospitalizations or admissions to the emergency departments for AHF syndromes. The principal sources used are hospital administrative databases. Some methodology problems are related to the use of these data for an epidemiologic objective. Indeed, this information was not collected with an epidemiologic objective in mind but served mainly accounting purposes. These databases are event based, not person based; it is therefore usually not possible to estimate directly the number of patients that presented at least one episode during a given period (one patient could be hospitalized several times during a given period). What's more, the AHF syndromes may not be identified as such but coded according to the underlying diagnosis or the triggering factor (for example, myocardial infarct or atrial fibrillation).

However, we still can find consistent results across various European countries. For example, the number of HF hospitalizations was 4.7/1000 in women and 5.1/1000 in men in Scotland[12], 5.1/1000 in Spain[13], 3.6/1000 adults in France (approximation)[9], and 4.2/1000 in Sweden (approximation)[14].

In Europe, heart failure represents 1% to 2% of all hospitalization, which makes it the leading cause of hospitalization for people 65 and over. This hospitalization percentage is rising[8,12]. The increase may be tied to the aging of the general population and to the increase in patient life expectancy, especially after myocardial infarction.

Economic Consequences

The social burden of HF is very significant in Europe. The direct cost of care management is estimated to be 26 million Euros per one million inhabitants in the U.K., 37 in Germany, and 39 in France. These figures represent between 1% and 2% of total health care costs[15,16]. This makes HF the leading pathology in terms of health care expenditures, ahead of cancer and myocardial infarct for example.

Due to their frequency and seriousness, hospitalizations represent the bulk of the cost (between 60% and 74% depending on country)[16]. For example, the average cost for one hospitalization surpasses €4000 in France[9].

Conclusion

Acute heart failure syndrome is a condition that most severely affects patient prognosis in the short and medium terms. It involves a great number of people. It is probable that the number of people suffering from HF will be increasing with the aging of the population, the increase in the prevalence of risk factors, and the better management of myocardial infarction.

In addition to the human cost, AHF syndrome represents a very high social burden: it is the first cause of hospitalization for old people, and is the leading health care cost in Europe.

However, and this is a true paradox, this affliction is relatively little known. The results of the Study on Heart failure Awareness and Perception in Europe (SHAPE) study, from a random sample of 7958 inhabitants in nine European countries are a good case in point[17]. These people were surveyed about their knowledge of HF (symptoms, prevalence, severity, treatment, cost), by comparing it to their knowledge of other cardiovascular pathologies. The SHAPE study has shown, for example, that 31% of subjects could identify coronary disease, and 51% could identify cerebralvascular pathology from their symptoms, but only 3% could identify HF. Moreover, the public underestimated the seriousness of this syndrome.

Parallel to this low level of awareness and poor perception of the disease by the public, epidemiologic and clinical research in this field is lacking substantially compared to other cardiology research (HF is 30 times less cited on Medline, and is 50 times less likely to be the object of clinical trials when compared to myocardial infarction[18]).

The recent recognition of the syndrome by the medical and scientific community, as is evidenced by the very recent publications of European recommendations[6], should foster more clinical and epidemiologic research in the field. This research is most needed for a better understanding of the mechanisms as well as for an improvement in prevention and treatment of this syndrome.

References

1. The Task Force on Acute Heart Failure of the ESC. Executive summary of the guideline on the diagnosis and treatment of acute heart failure. European Heart Journal 2005;26:384–416.
2. Cleland JGF, Swedberg K, Cohen-Solal A, et al. A survey on the quality of care among patients with heart failure in Europe. European Heart Journal 2000;24:123–32.
3. Cleland JGF, Swedberg K, Follath F, et al. The Euro-Heart Failure survey programme—a survey on the quality of care among patients with heart failure in Europe. Part 1: patient characteristics and diagnosis. European Heart Journal 2003;24:442–63.
4. Komajda M, Follath F, Swedberg K, et al. The Euro-Heart Failure survey programme—a survey on the quality of care among patients with heart failure in Europe. Part 2: treatment. European Heart Journal 2003;24:464–74.
5. Zannad F, Mebazaa A, Juillière Y, et al., for the EFICA Investigators. Clinical profile, contemporary management and one-year mortality in patients with severe acute heart failure syndromes: The EFICA study. Eur J Heart Fail 2006;8(7):697–705.
6. Tavazzi L, Maggioni AP, Lucci D, et al. Nationwide survey on acute heart failure in cardiology ward services in Italy. European Heart Journal 2006; 27(10):1207–15.
7. Felker GM, Adams KF, Konstam MA, O'Connor CM, Gheorghiade M. The problem of decompensated heart failure: nomenclature, classification, and risk stratification. American Heart Journal 2003;145:S18–25.
8. Nieminen MS, Veli-Pekka H. Definition and epidemiology of acute heart failure syndromes. American Journal of Cardiology 2005;96(suppl): 5G–10G.
9. Agence technique de l'information sur l'hospitalisation. http://www.atih.sante.fr.
10. Rudiger A, Harjola VP, Müller A, et al. Acute heart failure: clinical presentation, one-year mortality and prognostic factors. European Journal of Heart Failure 2005;7:662–70.
11. Zannad F, Briançon S, Juillière Y, et al., and the EPICAL Investigators. Incidence, clinical and etiologic features, and outcomes of advanced chronic heart failure: the EPICAL study. J Am Coll Cardiol 1999;33:734–42.
12. Stewart S, MacIntyre K, MacLeod MMC, et al. Trends in hospitalization for heart failure in Scotland, 1990–1996. European Heart Journal 2001; 22:209–17.
13. Rodriguez-Artalejo F, Guallar-Castillon P, Banegas Banegas JR, del Rey Calero J. Trends in hospitalization and mortality for heart failure in Spain, 1980–1993. European Heart Journal 1997;18(11): 1771–9.
14. Ryden-Bergsten T, Andersson F. The health care costs of heart failure in Sweden. Journal of Internal Medicine 1999;246(3):275–84.
15. Bundkirchen A, Schwinger RHG. Epidemiology and economic burden of chronic heart failure. European Heart Journal Supplements 2004;6(suppl D):D57–60.
16. Berry C, Murdoch DR, McMurray JVJ. Economics of chronic heart failure. European Journal of Heart Failure 2001;3:283–91.
17. Remme WJ, McMurray JJ, Rauch B, et al. Public awareness of heart failure in Europe: first results from SHAPE. European Heart Journal 2005; 26(22):2413–21.
18. Zannad F. Acute heart failure syndromes: the "Cinderella" of heart failure research. European Heart Journal Supplements 2005;7(supplement B): B8–12.

4

Epidemiology and Management of Acute Decompensating Heart Failure in the Asia–Pacific Region

Anthony S. McLean

Heart failure is a huge challenge worldwide, with acute decompensating heart failure syndromes being at the frontline of the problem. Health patterns are changing, with cardiovascular disease becoming the leading cause of mortality in developing countries, resulting globally in more heart failure, specifically in the Asia–Pacific region.

Epidemiology

General Epidemiology

The Asia–Pacific region is an extraordinary region with a huge diversity in living standards, ethnicity, and populations. Country populations range from the small pacific island nations with total populations of less than 20,000 to the largest in the world with a population in China of 1.2 billion people. India has in excess of 1 billion. Over 2 billion people live north of Australia alone. Some countries such as Australia and New Zealand have experienced large migration flows resulting in ethnically diverse populations, while others like Japan are remarkably homogeneous. Economic diversity also abounds with Japan boasting the second biggest economy in the world, yet others are some of the poorest countries in the world. Per capita income ranges from high income countries like Japan ($30,400 in U.S. dollars) and Australia ($32,000 U.S.) down to poorest in the world, that of East Timor ($400 U.S.). Numerous countries such as India, Nepal, Myanmar, Vietnam, Indonesia, and Laos have per capita incomes less than $5000 U.S. per annum[1]. The overall quality and availability of medical care generally mirrors the economic status of an individual country.

Epidemiology of Cardiovascular Disease

Published information on the prevalence and clinical course of chronic heart failure patients in the Asia–Pacific region is scarce, with available data about acute decompensating heart failure syndromes (AHFSs) being nonexistent. Epidemiologic data on published studies with relevance to cardiovascular disease and chronic heart failure in the region do provide a glimpse of what is relevant for AHFS. In a comprehensive study on the global significance of cardiovascular disease, Leeder et al.[2] examined the premature loss of life in people 35 to 64 years of age. As can be seen in Table 4.1 the numbers in Asia are enormous now and are set to rise to dramatic levels by the years 2030.

The proportion of deaths from cardiovascular disease (CVD) ranges from less than 20% in Thailand, Philippines, and Indonesia, to 20% to 30% in urban China, Hong Kong, Japan, Korea, and Malaysia. New Zealand, Australia, and Singapore have relatively high rates that exceed 35%[3]. However, mortality from CVD is dropping in the latter countries while increasing in the former. By 2020 it is anticipated that noncommunicable diseases will account for 7 of 10 deaths in the developing countries, compared with half that amount today.

The risk factors for coronary artery disease are similar to those found in Western countries[4,5]. The INTERHEART was a global study examining

TABLE 4.1. Total years of life lost due to cardiovascular disease (CVD) among populations aged 35 to 64 for five study and two comparator countries 2000 and 2030, and the years-lost rates per 100,000 (assuming current CVD rates)

	2000		2030	
	Years lost	Rate/100,000	Years lost	Rate/100,000
Brazil	1,060,840	2,121	1,741,620	1,957
S. Africa	302,265	2,753	391,980	2,667
Russia	3,314,014	5,684	3,208,265	5,887
China	6,666,990	1,595	10,460,030	1,863
India	9,221,165	3,572	17,937,070	3,707
Subtotal	20,565,274		33,738,965	
U.S.	1,631,825	1,267	1,972,215	1,661
Portugal	40,880	1,103	53,125	1,317
Subtotal	1,672,705		2,025,340	

Source: Leeder et al.[2]

potentially modifiable risk factors associated with myocardial infarction, which found that the same nine risk factors were responsible in all countries, with cigarette smoking and elevated lipids being the most important two. Public health practices aimed at controlling these factors are more advanced in Australia and New Zealand[6]. A comparison of mortality from coronary heart disease (CHD) in middle-aged men from Japan, South Korea, Taiwan, and the United States found that Japan had the lowest mortality especially when compared with the U.S. However, the proportion of deaths from heart failure to overall cardiovascular disease in Japan was over 70% compared with less than 5% in the U.S. (Fig. 4.1)[7]. Death from coronary artery disease is also increasing in Korea and Taiwan, but decreasing in the U.S. and Japan. The Thai population have lower prevalence of CHD and adjustable risk factors than in other developing countries[8].

It can be assumed that genetic factors play some role, in that certain ethnic groups like the Okinawans are noted for their longevity and low rate of heart disease. Even here, however, the known risk factors in Western countries still are important[9]. Interestingly for some countries there appears to be more information on heart disease in expatriates settled in Western countries than in the home country[10,11]. Information in the literature on heart disease among Indians has multiple publications on expatriate populations, usually by comparing different ethnic populations in the country studied. Indians have a higher hospital admission rate for congestive heart failure compared with the Chinese population in Singapore[12]. In Britain, Galasko and colleagues[13] showed that South Asians had a higher prevalence of coronary artery disease (CAD) as the underlying cause of left ventricular systolic dysfunction than do white patients[13]. Included in the limited published data on the management of heart failure in India is the very important consideration of patient compliance following the prescription of appropriate treatment[14].

Epidemiology of Heart Failure

In contrast to the more visible cardiac pathology of ischemic heart disease including incidence and management of CAD, there are limited published data available on heart failure and essentially none on acute heart failure. The data available indicates that the overall burden of cardiac disease is growing and also that cardiac failure is treated with the same therapies used in the more developed countries[15]. The underlying etiologies of heart failure in this Indonesian study showed less CAD (47%) compared with Australia, and more valvular disease (15%), with hypertensive heart disease responsible for 27% and cardiomyopathy 8%. Some unique types of heart failure such as beriberi appear in less developed countries. Although data are scarce, it appears that these conditions make up only a very small proportion of heart failure patients. A study from Singapore highlights the role of infectious endocarditis as a cause of heart failure[16]. It is likely that heart failure resulting from rheumatic valvular disease represents a sizable cohort, albeit with little or no data on the prevalence, in various countries.

New Zealand, with a relatively small population of 4 million people, has no comprehensive data on AHFS but does have a reputation for being a pioneer in the use of natriuretic peptides in the diagnosis of chronic heart failure, in addition to research on ethnic and social influences on the risk of developing heart failure[17]. Davis et al.[18] showed that the most common comorbidities in CHF was chronic pulmonary disease and this was more common in Maori than non-Maori populations. The disparity between the prevalence in CHF rates between the Maori and non-Maori

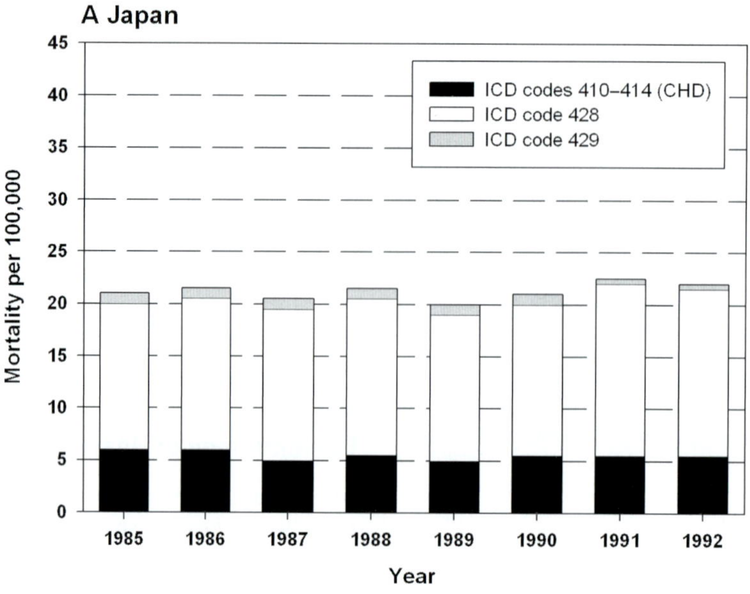

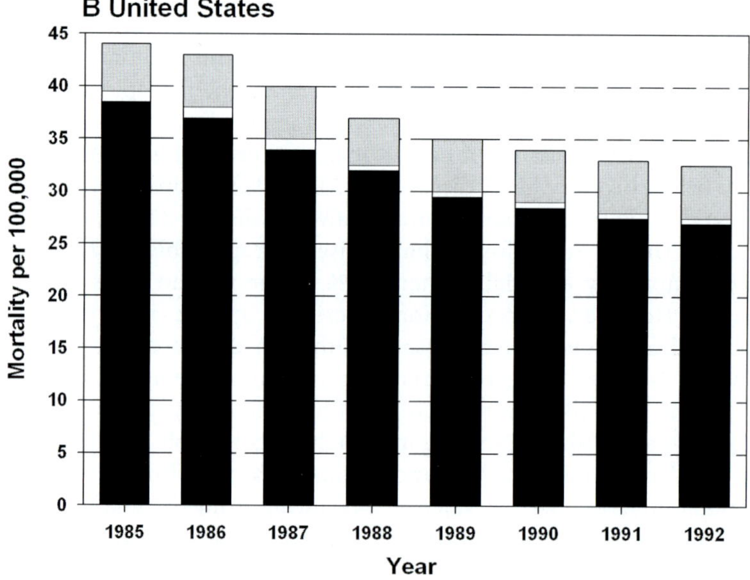

FIGURE 4.1. Trends in the mortality from coronary heart disease (International Classification of Diseases [ICD] codes 410–414), heart failure (ICD code 428), and defined description and complications of heart disease (ICD code 429) in men aged 35 to 55 in Japan (A) and the United States (B), 1985–1992. (From Sekikawa et al.[7])

population is accentuated in other studies[19,20]. A study in Australia examined the important link between CHF and AHFS, reviewing the multiple hospital admissions in patients with known CHF. Eighty-eight patients admitted with a diagnosis of CHF were followed over a 4-month period. There were subsequently 26 CHF-related readmissions. The mean length of stay was 13.8 days, accounting for 4.2% of bed days for all inpatients over the age of 65 years[21]. The expectation of increasing heart failure morbidity and mortality in Western countries is shared in Australia[22]. The difference between incidence and prevalence is important because death certificate information in Australia shows that death from heart failure is remaining constant[23]. However, the increasing longevity resulting from improved therapies, including pharmacologic and heart failure teams, increases the prevalence of both CHF and AHFS.

Diagnosis of Acute Decompensating Heart Failure Syndrome

Acute decompensating heart failure syndrome refers to a disease state where there are new or worsening signs or symptoms of failure requiring treatment. This definition includes patients who have an exacerbation of chronic stable heart failure with significant worsening of symptoms, those who develop acute ventricular failure of sudden onset with no prior history, and those who are severely symptomatic and refractory to state-of-the-art therapy. Precipitating factors for decompensated heart failure are numerous and include myocardial ischemia, postoperative myocardial damage, cardiac arrhythmias, hypo- or hypertension, hypo- or hyperthyroidism, pulmonary embolism, drug or alcohol abuse, diet or medication noncompliance, anemia, and infections.

Making the diagnosis of AHFS can be very difficult. Many patients with the symptoms and signs of AHFS present to an emergency department, in many cases with preceding prehospital care by ambulance services with varying degrees of sophistication. Many countries, however, have no or minimal prehospital services. At the more sophisticated end of the prehospital care system, intravenous cannulation, diuretic and morphine administration, and intubation with assisted ventilation are available.

The diagnosis of AHFS rests upon history and clinical signs with selected investigations such as chest radiography, electrocardiography, serum electrolytes, and arterial blood gases playing an important role. Two major advances in assisting in the diagnosis of heart failure and differentiation from other conditions such as acute or chronic lung disease or noncardiogenic edema are serum biomarkers and Doppler echocardiography. Invasive procedures, such as insertion of a pulmonary artery catheter, can be helpful but are only necessary or available in a minority of cases. Here I concentrate on two areas where there is considerable history and development in the Asia–Pacific region: the development of biomarkers and the application of echocardiography in the critical care setting.

Biomarkers of Cardiac Failure

The search for a rapid and easy biomarker of heart failure, to diagnose, to prognosticate, and to guide management, has been underway for some years. The use of such biomarkers is still in its infancy, with a number of candidates being investigated (Table 4.2). A favorite candidate is type B natriuretic peptide (BNP), which has undergone intensive clinical evaluation in the attempt to clarify its role. Richards and colleagues[27] from New Zealand have explored for over a decade the role of BNP in the diagnosis and monitoring of CHF, demonstrating a useful place for it in clinical practice. Such research is not without cost, and output from the Asia–Pacific region is limited to few centers, primarily Japan, Australia, and New Zealand[24,25,26,27].

The benefit of BNP/N-terminal-proBNP is definite but still requires further exploration to

Table 4.2. Serum biomarkers of cardiac failure with diagnostic potential

Potential biomarker of cardiac failure		
Myocardial and matrix injury	Neuroendocrine	Inflammatory
H-FABP	ANP	CRP
Metalloproteinases	BNP	TNF-α
TIMP-1	NT-pro BNP	IL-6, -18
Myosin light chains	Norepinephrine	CA125
		CD40–CD154
Other		ST2
vWF		ICAM
Urocortin		P-selectin
		NF-κB

ANP, atrial natriuretic protein; BNP, B-type natriuretic peptide; CRP, C-reactive protein; ICAM, intercellular adhesion molecule; IL, interleukin; NK, natural killer; TIMP, tissue-inhibitor metalloproteinase; TNF-α, tumor necrosis factor-α; vWF, von Willebrand factor.

consolidate its role in the diagnosis and management of AHFS[28]. Other biomarkers of cardiac failure are being actively investigated. In particular, research on inflammatory markers is exciting, as they appear not only to have a potential role in diagnosis, but also to contribute greatly to our understanding of the underlying pathogenic mechanisms of heart failure. China and Japan have enthusiastic research programs in this field.

Echocardiography

Echocardiography is a vital tool in evaluating the patient with suspected or proven cardiac failure. It is of particular value in developing countries because of cost. The price of sophisticated machines is decreasing, and maintenance costs compare favorably with those of invasive alternatives. When compared with other potential bedside methods of directly assessing cardiac function such as thoracic electrical bioimpedance, nuclear-gated heart-pool scanning, pulmonary artery catheterization, esophageal Doppler, and contour cardiac output (PiCCO), the advantages of echocardiography are obvious. These include rapid application, widespread availability, and the fact that it is noninvasive.

A subjective assessment of overall cardiac output is usually obtainable in most patients and with good-quality images objective information, such as left ventricular ejection fraction (LVEF) and cardiac output, assists in formulating management. This can be achieved by the Simpson method using apical two- and four-chamber views[29]. Alternatively, combining Doppler with two-dimensional (2D) parameters across the left ventricular outflow tract (LVOT) is also accurate[30,31]. Although originally established with transthoracic echocardiography (TTE), these same methods have been validated with transesophageal echocardiography (TEE)[32].

The presence of a normal LVEF on echocardiography does not rule out heart failure, and indeed the prognosis may be worse in this group. A review of 2258 hospitalized patients with a diagnosis of heart failure identified one third with a normal LVEF. Their prognosis was worse despite fewer comorbidities[33].

Assessing right and left ventricular filling or preload is central to evaluating the patient with AHFS. A rapid subjective assessment is often possible with echocardiography. Review of chamber sizes is a crude but often helpful guide, especially where marked hypovolemia is suspected[34]. Decreased size of the cardiac chambers can be a quick guide to inadequate filling, especially when resuscitating the patient. In regard to elevated filling pressures, a simple guide is the fixed bowing of the interatrial septum, from left to right, during the cardiac cycle, indicating a pulmonary capillary wedge pressure (PCWP) greater than 18 mm Hg[35]. In the operating room, the use of left ventricular end-diastolic area (LVEDA) as a guide to volume status is well established, although in the critical care setting this parameter is not always so helpful, in that it is not influenced by fluid challenge or predictive of increasing stroke volume with a fluid challenge[36,37]. The principal tool used for the noninvasive estimation of left ventricular filling pressures is pulsed wave Doppler echocardiography, with a number of indices having been validated. A useful and succinct overview is that by Pozzoli and colleagues[38].

Analysis by Doppler of the mitral inflow and pulmonary vein waveforms, in addition to utilizing Doppler tissue imaging (DTI), has demonstrated good correlation to invasive measurements and that this technique is helpful in the clinical setting where experienced echocardiographers perform the procedure. A number of parameters used in identifying elevated left atrial pressure have been described[35,39,40,41,42,43,44]. For many years now, right atrial pressure (RAP) has been estimated using respiratory variation of inferior vena cava (IVC) and hepatic vein diameters[45]. The collapse of the IVC by >50% during inspiration indicates a RAP of <10 mm Hg.

A more relevant approach in the intubated patient with pump failure plus other organ dysfunction is to assess fluid responsiveness and optimize intravascular volume using variation of superior vena cava diameter with ventilation. Vieillard-Baron et al.[46] have done some elegant work in this area.

Echocardiography facilitates the evaluation of other cardiac causes of heart failure, in addition to left ventricular systolic and diastolic dysfunction. These include right ventricular dysfunction, pericardial tamponade, valvular dysfunction, mitral papillary muscle dysfunction, valvular endocarditis, intracardiac shunts, mural thrombi, and abnormalities of the thoracic aorta. Segmental wall defects indicating possible underlying ischemic heart disease may be seen.

Management of Acute Heart Failure Syndrome

Background

Emergency physicians, intensivists, and cardiologists are frequently the attending physicians. In countries where the speciality of emergency medicine is well established, the emergency department (ED) physician is usually the first contact for these patients. Intensivists increasingly offer life support to patients in whom severe heart failure appears reversible, either wholly or partially. Economic imperatives are relevant, particularly considering the daily cost of a patient in an intensive care unit (ICU), expensive medications that are not efficacious in all people, and the ever-increasing expectations of a population combined with more aggressive treatment like major surgery and chemotherapy for the elderly, in whom a comorbidity is often underlying heart failure. The tremendous success in treating CHF with angiotensin-converting enzyme inhibitors, beta-blockers, spironolactone, angiotensin receptor blockers, and cardiac resynchronization therapy, results in a higher prevalence of people who are at risk of decompensation when experiencing other illnesses. Indeed, such triggers may include physical as well as emotional stimuli. In a fascinating study, Wittstein and colleagues[47] demonstrated severe reversible left ventricular depression in the absence of underlying coronary disease with one exception, in 19 patients who had suffered marked emotional stress. A particular form of heart failure where the left ventricular apex develops reversible akinesis, known as Takotsubo cardiomyopathy, is thought to come from catecholamine excess or adrenoceptor hyperactivity[48]. The incidence of this increased immediately following a series of earthquakes in Niigata 2004[49].

Outline of Management

The management of AHFS in the Asia–Pacific region is no different from that practiced elsewhere in the world, or if there are countries where treatment is markedly different, then no published literature is readily available. It would appear that differences in management are dictated by available resources rather than cultural. Even the wealthier countries like Japan and Australia have considerable challenges in providing currently available therapies in the treatment of heart failure—the cost burden of cardiac resynchronization therapy and automatic implantable defibrillators in CHF being examples. Some of the new drugs used in AHFS cost in excess of $1000 (US) per treatment, well beyond the reach of many. A more educated population becomes aware of these more expensive options mentioned in the heart failure literature. Finding the balance between possible beneficial treatment and the cost of providing it will affect the prescribing habits of doctors.

The challenges in rapidly providing effective therapy to the distressed patient with AHFS comes not only in achieving rapid resolution of symptoms but also in reducing mortality and morbidity in the short and long term. Diagnosis and assessment of severity is usually performed concurrently with initiation of treatment, especially where life is endangered. There is an increasing scale of complexity in management, with the more heroic measures available to, and offered to, very few. Most patients are stabilized in the ED with basic measures. Where sophisticated resources are available, there is the same uncertainty surrounding treatment efficacy as experienced in Europe and the U.S. Once supplementary oxygen, diuretics, nitrates, and noninvasive ventilation in the form of continuous positive airway pressure (CPAP) have been given, the data on the use of other widely used therapies is somewhat contradictory or even condemnatory. Even with regularly used agents, dosage is important, as high-dose furosemide, for example, is associated with higher mortality[50]. In general the European guidelines on the management of acute decompensating heart failure are equally applicable in the Asia–Pacific region as in Europe[51].

Basic Management

Basic treatment consists of encouraging a sitting position; prescribing supplementary oxygen, morphine, diuretics, and nitrates; and controlling heart rhythm and rate where indicated. Bertini and colleagues,[52] in a retrospective study on the effect of nitrates on prehospital mortality in patients with acute pulmonary edema, found a reduction in mortality from 7.8% to 5.3%.

Noninvasive Ventilation in Acute Heart Failure Syndrome

Positive pressure ventilation has an established role in the treatment of AHFS. Few patients require intubation for ventilatory assistance, so the emphasis has centered on the application of non-invasive ventilation (NIV) in the ED, coronary care unit (CCU), and ICU, primarily in the form of CPAP. Bi-level positive airway pressure (BiPAP) has yet to prove superior to CPAP in acute decompensating heart failure and requires a higher level of nursing support[53]. From anecdotal evidence it appears that CPAP is more widely used for AHFS in Australia than in many other countries. It is standard equipment in most EDs, ICUs, CCUs, and cardiac wards. Kaye and colleagues[54,55] from Australia have examined the physiologic response to CPAP in heart failure patients. It reduces myocardial oxygen consumption and inhibits sympathetic tone.

Inotropes in Acute Heart Failure Syndrome

Only a small proportion of patients require more advanced therapy. There is a need to evaluate accurately the volume status of the patients, which may require invasive techniques. This is particularly the situation when significant comorbidities exist such as with the intensive care patient. Once preload is optimized and afterload minimized, inotropes need to be considered.

Although inotropes have been an integral part in the management of both CHF and AHFS, their use is under scrutiny, and some data indicate that they should not be used routinely. In a review, Felker and O'Conner[56] conclude that their only benefit is as a bridge to transplantation or revascularization. A meta-regression analysis between 1966 and 2000 of the effectiveness of intravenous inotropic drugs acting through the adrenergic pathways in patients with heart failure found little evidence of a beneficial effect; indeed, they may worsen the outcome[57]. There is a paucity of data, with a total of 632 patients enrolled in trials over this 34-year period. A larger study recently published was the Outcomes of a Prospective Trial of Intravenous Milrinone for Exacerbations of Chronic Heart Failure (OPTIME-CHF) trial in which 951 hospitalized patients with worsening heart failure were randomised to a single 48-hour infusion of milrinone or placebo. No benefit in morbidity or length of hospital stay was demonstrated, but there was an increase in adverse effects in the milrinone group[58]. Mortality in large placebo-controlled trials of oral inotropes indicates short-term hemodynamic benefit, but all have been associated with increased mortality. Also, trials of chronic inotropic therapy demonstrate conflicting results in regard to subsequent quality of life[56].

Levosimendan, available in Australia with restricted prescribing, is an inotrope described as a calcium sensitiser; it possesses theoretical advantages over the traditional inotropes[59]. It has been shown to be efficacious in a number of studies in acute heart failure[60,61,62]. However, two large recently presented studies, REVIVE and SURVIVE, while confirming clinical benefits, did not demonstrate a survival advantage over placebo or dobutamine[63]. One important advantage of levosimendan is the overcoming of therapeutic confusion that occurs when using catecholamines, where an intravenous beta-agonist is prescribed for a patient established on oral beta-blockers.

Other Therapies

Therapies using natriuretic analogues are currently not available for use in Australia, so the uncertainties surrounding the use of nesiritide are not an issue[64]. Some centers are involved in a multinational study trialing ularitide, a renal natriuretic peptide[65].

Extraordinary measures including left ventricular assist devices (LVADs) and cardiac transplantation are available in very few locations in the Asia–Pacific region and will not make a major impact on the management of AHFS in the region.

Conclusion

There are scant data on the incidence and management of AHFS in the Asia–Pacific region. Information regarding cardiovascular disease in the region strongly indicates that cardiovascular diseases generally and, by inference, more heart failure are going to become an enormous problem in the future. This is especially the case when examining the change of disease patterns in developing countries and the size of the populations in these countries. Management of AHFS is similar to that in other parts of the world, perhaps with greater emphasis on noninvasive ventilation than elsewhere. Fortunately, the majority of patients improve with basic measures, but there is a great need to identify therapies that not only improve symptoms but also the medium- and long-term outcome. Some centers in the Asia–Pacific region are actively engaged in research to achieve this end.

References

1. CIA-World Fact Book. www.cia.gov./publications.
2. Leeder S, Raymond S, Greenburg H. A Race Against Time: The Challenge of Cardiovascular Disease in Developing Economies. New York: The Earth Institute at Columbia University, 2004.
3. Khor GL. Cardiovascular epidemiology in the Asia-Pacific region. Asia Pacific J Clin Nutr 2001;10(20): 76–80.
4. Wang L, Yao D, Wu T. Prevalence of Overweight and smoking patients with coronary heart disease in rural China. Aust J Rural Health 2004;12:17.
5. Jiang H, Dongfeng G, Xigui W, et al. Major causes of death among men and women in China. N Engl J Med 2005;353:1124–1132.
6. Yusuf S, Hawkins S, Onupuu S, et al. Effect of potentially modifiable risk factors associated with myocardial infarction 52 countries (the INTERHEART study): case-control study. Lancet 2004;364: 937–952.
7. Sekikawa A, Kuller LH, Ueshima H, et al. Coronary heart disease mortality trends in men in the post World War II birth cohorts aged 35–44 in Japan, South Korea and Taiwan compared to the United States. Int J Epidemiology 1999;28:1044–1049.
8. Tatsanavivat P, Klungboonkrong V, Chirawatkul A, et al. Prevalence of coronary heart disease and major cardiovascular risk factors in Thailand. Int J Epidemiology 1998;27(3):405–409.
9. Tokuda Y. Risk factors for acute myocardial infarction among Okinawans. J Nutr Health Aging 2005; 9(40):272–276.
10. Ross MC, Duong D, Wiggins SD, et al. Descriptive study of hypercholesteremia in a Vietnamese population of the Gulf Coast. J Cultural Diversity 2000; 7(3):65–71.
11. Rissel C, Russel C. Heart disease risk factors in the Vietnamese community of southwest Sydney. Aust J Public Health 1993;17(1):71–73.
12. Ng TP, Niti M. Trends and ethnic differences in hospital admissions and mortality for congestive heart failure in the elderly in Singapore, 1992–1998. Heart 2003;89(8):865–870
13. Galasko GI, Senior R, Lahiri A. Ethnic differences in the prevalence and aetiology of left ventricular systolic dysfunction in the community: the Harrow heart failure watch. Heart 2005;91(15):595–600.
14. Joshi PP, Mohanan CJ, Sengupta SP, et al. Factors precipitating congestive heart failure—role of patient non-compliance. J Assoc Phys India 1999; 47(3):294–295.
15. Kalim H, Thosin A, Firman D, et al. Clinical profile and management of heart failure in a cardiac centre. Crit Care Shock 2002;5(4):229–234.
16. Lim MC, Tan TZ, Choo M, et al. Review of patients with infectious endocarditis of native valves over a five year period. Ann Acad Med 1993;22(3):296–299.
17. Yandle T, Fisher S, Livesey J, et al. Exponential increase in clinical use of plasma brain batriuretic peptide (BNP) assays. N Z Med J 2004;117(1197): U956.
18. Davis P, Lay-Yee R, Fitzjohn J, et al. Co-morbidity and Health outcomes in three Auckland hospitals. N Z Med J 2002;115(1153):211–125.
19. Carr J, Ronson B, Reid P, et al. Heart failure: ethnic differences in morbidity and mortality in NZ. N Z Med J 2002;115(1146):15–17.
20. Riddell T. Heart failure hospitalisations and deaths in New Zealand: pattern by deprivation and ethnicity. N Z Med J 2005;118(1208):U1254.
21. Blyth FM, Lazarus R, Ross D, et al. Burden and outcomes of hospitalisation for congestive heart failure. Med J Aust 1997:167(2):61–62.
22. Campbell DJ. Heart failure: how can we prevent the epidemic? Med J Aust 2003;179(8):422–425.
23. McLean AS, Eslick G, Coats AJ. The epidemiology of heart failure in Australia. Int J Cardiol 2007; 118:370–374.
24. Goto T, Takase H, Toriyama T, et al. Circulating concentrations of cardiac proteins indicate the severity of congestive heart failure. Heart 2003;89:1303–1307.
25. Yasue H, Yoshimura M, Sumida H, et al. Localisation and mechanism of secretion of B-type

natriuretic peptide in comparison with those of A-type natriuretic peptide in normal subjects and patients with heart failure. Circulation 1994;90:195–203.
26. McLean AS, Tang B, Nalos M, et al. Increased B-type natriuretic peptide (BNP) level is a strong predictor for cardiac dysfunction in the intensive care unit patients. Anaesth Intensive Care 2003;31: 21–27.
27. Richards AM, Crozier IG, Yandle TG, et al. Brain natriuretic factor: regional plasma concentrations and correlations with hemodynamic state in cardiac disease. Br Heart J 1993;69:414–417.
28. Mclean AS, Huang SJ. B-Type Natriuretic Peptide to Assess Cardiac Function in the Critically Ill. In: Vincent JL, ed. Yearbook of Intensive Care and Emergency Medicine. Berlin, Germany: Springer-Verlag, 2005:151–160.
29. Schiller NB, Shah PM, Crawford M, et al. Recommendations for quantification of the left ventricle by two-dimensional echocardiography. Am Soc Echo 1989;2(5):358–367.
30. Nishimura RA, Callahan MJ, Schaff HV, et al. Non-invasive measurement of cardiac output by continuous wave Doppler echocardiography: initial experience and review of the literature. Mayo Clin Proc 1984;59(7):484–489.
31. Hatle I, Angelsen BA. Doppler Ultrasound in Cardiology, 2nd ed. Philadelphia: Lea & Febiger, 1985.
32. Izzat MB, Regragui IA, Wilde P, et al. Transoesophageal echocardiography measurements of cardiac output in cardiac surgical patients. Ann Thorac Surg 1994;58:1486–1489.
33. Varadarajan P, Pai RG. Prognosis of congestive heart failure in patients with normal versus reduced ejection fractions: results from a cohort of 2,258 hospitalized patients. J Cardiac Failure 2003;9:107–112.
34. Leung JM, Levine EH. Left ventricular endsystolic cavity obliteration as an estimate of intraoperative hypovolaemia. Anesthesiology 1994;81:1102–1109.
35. Royse CF, Royse AG, Soeding PF, et al. Shape and movement of the interatrial septum predicts change in pulmonary capillary wedge pressure. Ann Thorac Cardiovasc Surg 2001;7:79–83.
36. Cheung AT, Savino JS, Weiss SJ, et al. Echocardiographic and hemodynamic indexes of left ventricular preload in patients with normal and abnormal ventricular function. Anesthesiology 1994;81:376 – 387.
37. Axler O, Tousignant C, Thompson CR, et al. Comparison of transesphageal echocardiographic, fick, and thermodilution cardiac output in critically ill patients. J Crit Care 1996;11:109–116.
38. Pozzoli M, Traversi E, Roelandt RTC. Noninvasive Estimation of left ventricular filling pressures by Doppler echocardiography. Eur J Echo 2002;3:75–79.
39. Giannuzzi P, Imparato A, Temporelli PL, et al. Doppler derived mitral deceleration time of early filling is a strong predictor of pulmonary capillary wedge pressure in postinfarction patients with left ventricular systolic dysfunction. J Am Coll Cardiol 1994;23:1630–1637
40. Pozzoli M, Capromolla S, Pinna G, et al. Doppler echocardiography reliably predicts pulmonary artery wedge pressure in patients with chronic heart failure with and without mitral regurgitation. J Am Coll Cardiol 1996;27:883–893
41. Ommen SR, Nishimura RA, Appleton CP, et al. Clinical utility of doppler echocardiography and tissue Doppler imaging in the estimation of left ventricular filling pressures. Circulation 2000;102:1788–1794
42. Rossvoll O, Hatle LK. Pulmonary flow velocities recorded by transthoracic Doppler ultrasound: relation to left ventricular diastolic. J Am Coll Cardiol 1993;21:1687–1696
43. Gonzalez-Vilchez F, Ayuela J, Miguel A, et al. Comparison of Doppler echocardiography, color M-mode Doppler and tissue imaging for the estimation of pulmonary capillary wedge pressure. J Am Soc Echo 2002;15:1245–1250.
44. Gorscan J, Snow FR, Paulson W, et al. Noninvasive estimation of left atrial pressure in patients with congestive heart failure and mitral regurgitation by Doppler echocardiography. Am Heart J 1991;121: 858–863.
45. Kircher BJ, Himelman RB, Schiller NB. Non-invasive estimation of right atrial pressure from the inspiratory collapse of the inferior vena cava. Am J Cardiol 1990;66:493.
46. Vieillard-Baron A, Chergui K, Rabilks A, et al. Superior venacava collapsibility as a gauge of volume status in ventilated septic patients. Intensive Care Med 2004;30:1734–1739.
47. Wittstein IS, Thiemann DR, Lima JA, et al. Neurohumoral features of myocardial stunning due to sudden emotional stress. N Engl J Med 2005;352:539–548.
48. Akashi YJ, Nakazawa K, Sakakibara M, et al. The Clinical features of Takotsubo cardiomyopathy. OJM 2003;96(8):563–573.
49. Watanabe H, Kodama M, Okura Y, et al. Impact of earthquake on Takotsuba cardiomyopathy. JAMA 2005;294(3):305–307.
50. Cotter G, Metzkor E, Kaluski E, et al. Randomised trial of high-dose isosorbide dinitrate plus low-dose furosemide versus high-dose furosemide plus low-dose isosorbide in severe pulmonary oedema. Lancet 1998;351:389–393.

51. Nieminen MS, Bohm M, Lowie MR, et al. Executive summary of the guidelines on the diagnosis and treatment of acute heart failure: the Taskforce on Acute Heart Failure of the ESC. Eur Heart J 2005;26:384–416.
52. Bertini G, Gilioli C, Biggeri A, et al. Intravenous nitrates in the prehospital management of acute pulmonary oedema. Ann Emerg Med 1998;31:493–499.
53. Panacek EA, Kirk JD. Role of non-invasive ventilation in the management of acutely decompensated heart failure. Rev Cardiovasc Med 2002;3(4):S35–S40.
54. Kaye DM, Mansfield D, Naughton MT. Continuous Positive airway pressure decreases myocardial oxygen consumption in heart failure. Clin Sci 2004;106(6):599–603.
55. Kaye DM, Mansfield D, Aggawal A, et al. Acute effects of continuous airway pressure on cardiac sympathetic tone in congestive heart failure. Circulation 2001;103(19):2336–2338.
56. Felker GM, O'Conner CM. Inotropic therapy for heart failure: an evidence-based approach. Am Heart J 2001;142:393–401.
57. Thackray S, Easthaugh J, Freemantle N, et al. The effectiveness and relative effectiveness of intravenous inotropic drugs acting through the adrenergic pathway in patients with heart failure—a meta-regression analysis. Eur J Heart Fail 2002;4:515–529.
58. Cuffe MS, Califf RM, Adams KF, et al. Short-term intravenous milrinone for acute exacerbation of chronic heart failure: a randomised controlled trial (OPTIME). JAMA 2002;287:1541–1547.
59. Ukkonen H, Saraste M, Akkila J, et al. Myocardial efficiency during calcium sensitisation with levosimendan; a non-invasive study with positron emission tomography and echocardiography in healthy volunteers. Clin Pharmacol Ther 1997;61:596–607.
60. Follath F, Cleland JGF, Just JGY, et al. Efficacy and safety of intravenous levosimendan compared to dobutamine in severe low-output heart failure: a randomised double-blind trial. Lancet 2002;360:196–202.
61. Moiseyev VS, Poder P, Andrejevs N, et al. Safety and efficacy of a novel calcium sensitiser, levosimendan, in patients with left ventricular failure due to an acute myocardial infarction. Eur Heart J 2002;23:1422–1432.
62. McLean AS, Huang SJ, Nalos M, et al. Duration of the beneficial effects of levosimendan in decompensated heart failure as measured by echocardiographic and B-type natriuretic peptide. J Cardiovasc Pharmacol 2005;46:830–835
63. Cleland JGF, Freemantle N, Coletta AP, et al. Clinical trials update from the American Heart Association. Eur J Heart Failure 2006;8:105–110.
64. Topol E. Nesiritide—not verified. N Engl J Med 2005;353:113–116.
65. Cleland JGF, Coletta AP, Lammiman M, et al. Clinical trials update from the European Society of Cardiology Meeting 2005. Eur J Heart Failure 2005;7:1070–1075.

5
Peculiarities of Acute Heart Failure Syndromes in Latin America and the Role of Chagas' Disease

Fábio Vilas-Boas

Heart failure (HF) is becoming a major health problem in developing and already-developed countries that requires more investment in human and physical resources. Taking Brazil, the largest country in Latin America, as representative of the continent, cardiovascular diseases are responsible for almost 30% of annual deaths. It is estimated that one third of these deaths are due to HF. These data are relevant, since they demonstrate that this syndrome is one of the main causes of death in this part of the world and consequently demand more attention from the medical community and public health authorities[1].

When we consider the total number of hospital admissions in 1 year, we perceive that from the total of 11,450,000 hospital admissions in Brazil, cardiovascular diseases represented almost 10%, or more than 1 million hospital admissions in the public health system alone. Heart failure is responsible for about one third of hospital admissions for cardiovascular causes, representing close to 380,000 admissions per year. If we consider that in Brazil, as in most of the countries in Latin America, the public health system is responsible for almost 80% of the hospital admissions, we can conclude that another 75,000 occur in the private health system, representing a total of almost half a million HF admissions in Brazil alone.

In Latin America this problem is aggravated by the presence of almost 11 million people with Chagas' heart disease[2]. Due to intense immigration from endemic areas, transfusion-related infection has been perceived as a potential threat in the United States[3].

Decompensated Heart Failure: Definition and Clinical Presentations

Decompensated heart failure (DHF) is a clinical syndrome that until recently has been poorly studied and not clearly defined. Heart failure specialists from 10 countries in Latin America published, on behalf of their national societies, the 1st Latin American Guidelines for the Assessment and Management of Decompensated Heart Failure[4]. In this document, DHF is generally defined as a clinical syndrome in which a structural or functional heart abnormality leads to the incapacity of the heart to eject or accommodate the blood within physiologic pressure values, thus causing functional limitation and requiring immediate therapeutic intervention. This broad definition encompasses three major points: a pathophysiologic explanation, a clinical presentation, and the need for urgent therapeutic intervention.

In these guidelines, acute decompensated heart failure (ADHF) was divided in three categories:

1. Acute HF (without a previous diagnosis): corresponds to the clinical situation in which a certain aggression triggers the development of the clinical syndrome of HF in patients with no previous signs and symptoms of HF
2. Chronic decompensated HF (acute exacerbation of a chronic condition): corresponds to the clinical situation in which there is acute or gradual exacerbation of signs and symptoms of HF in patients at rest with a previous diagnosis of HF that require additional and immediate therapy

3. Refractory chronic HF (chronic low output or various degrees of congestion): corresponds to the clinical situation in which patients with a previously known diagnosis of HF present low output, systemic congestion, or persistent functional limitation refractory to the best possible clinical treatment

Two other major clinical presentations were defined, due to ADHF's peculiarities:

1. Pulmonary edema: corresponds to the clinical situation in which there is a sudden increase in the pulmonary capillary pressure leading to an increase of fluid in the interstitial and alveolar pulmonary spaces, which causes sudden and intense dyspnea at rest
2. Cardiogenic shock: characterized by serious arterial hypotension (systolic pressure <90 mmHg or 30% below baseline levels) for a minimum period of 30 minutes, showing signs of tissue hypoperfusion and organic dysfunction (tachycardia, paleness, cold extremities, mental confusion, oliguria, and metabolic acidosis), from cardiac etiology (acute myocardial infarction, cardiomyopathy, valvular heart disease, arrhythmias)

In a Brazilian study of decompensated HF, the patient's clinical profile revealed congestion in 50% of cases. Another 34% had congestion and peripheral hypoperfusion and only 16% had isolated hypoperfusion[5].

Heart Failure Management in Latin America: Main Characteristics

The main differences between HF management in Latin America and that in other parts of the world are related to the quality of public health assistance and to the socioeconomic status of the population. Taking Brazil as an example, more than 80% of the population depends on the government health system, which is far from optimal. This means that whenever a decompensated HF patient requires hospital admission, it will not always be immediately possible. These patients do not have enough money to pay for their medications, and the government does not commonly provide them, at least to the extent that is needed.

Many international studies have identified the factors associated with hospital admissions for ADHF. However, in approximately 30% of the cases it is not possible to identify the reasons for clinical decompensation. Brazilian data indicate that there are important differences in etiology, in decompensation factors, and in the treatment and prognosis of patients with HF in different parts of the country.

Chagas' Heart Disease

One of the most important differences in HF in Latin America is the presence of Chagas' disease as an important etiology. Chronic Chagas' cardiomyopathy is one of the major causes of HF in Latin America. In this model of HF, characterized by persistent diffuse myocarditis, a cross-reactive autoimmunity component is responsible for the maintenance of cellular aggression (Fig. 5.1). In this form of disease the heart is affected globally, and patients may present signs and symptoms of both right and left HF. It is caused by a parasite,

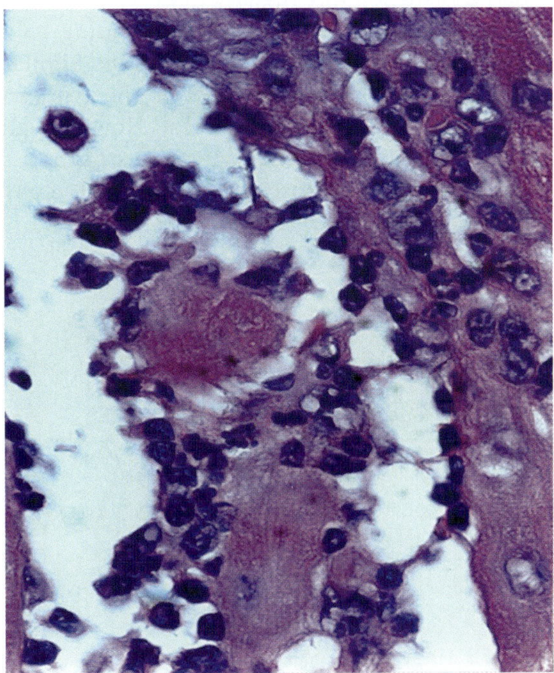

Figure 5.1. Intense inflammatory infiltrate in a heart infected by *Trypanosoma cruzi*.

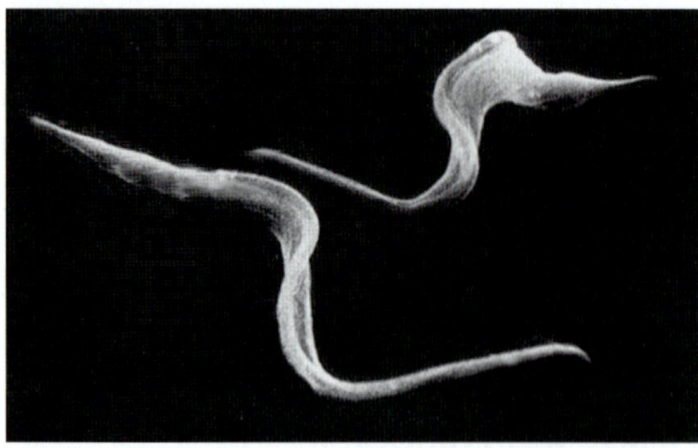

FIGURE 5.2. *Trypanosoma cruzi* showing developing trypomastigotes, which have a free flagellum.

Trypanosoma cruzi (Fig. 5.2), transmitted to humans by blood-sucking triatomine bugs (Fig. 5.3). *T. cruzi* also can be transmitted congenitally and through blood transfusion or organ transplantation. The infection lasts for the entire life but the majority of infected persons are asymptomatic, and their disease remains undiagnosed[6].

A coordinated multinational program in South America was responsible for controlling the transmission of Chagas' disease by vectors and by blood transfusion in Uruguay, Chile, and in eight of the 12 endemic states of Brazil leading to a decrease in the incidence of new infections. Similar initiatives have been launched in the Andean countries and in Central America[7]. However, all these efforts do not seem enough to stop transmission, since new cases still occurs in many countries[8].

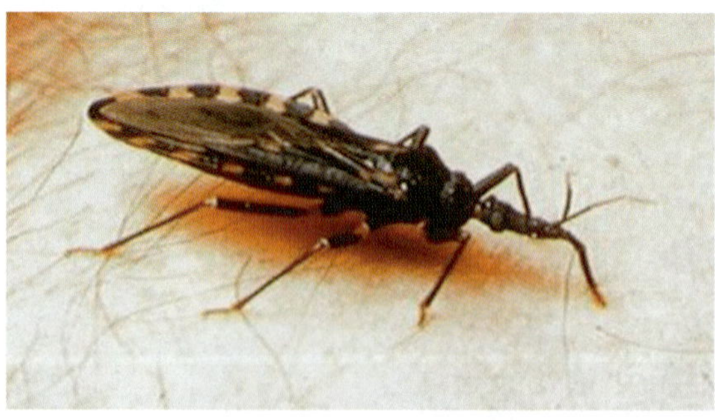

FIGURE 5.3. The vector of Chagas' disease: *Triatoma infestans*. The insect sucks blood through the skin and deposits feces with parasites, causing pruritus; after scrubbing the skin, the parasites take to the bloodstream.

Chagas' disease is becoming increasingly common outside Latin America. Seroprevalence studies using research tests have documented the presence of *T. cruzi* antibodies in U.S. blood and organ donor populations[9].

Acute Phase

After infection, the acute phase of Chagas' disease lasts 6 to 8 weeks, followed by a chronic phase (Table 5.1). Generally, Chagas' disease may resemble other types of myocarditis. Systemic manifestations may occur concomitantly with fever, tachycardia unrelated to the degree of hyperthermia, mild splenomegaly, lymphadenopathy, and edema. When the parasite penetrates the skin, local inflammation occurs. If the site of penetration is the eyes, conjunctivitis may occur, along with unilateral palpebral edema and preauricular satellite adenopathy (Romaña sign). Hematologic examination usually demonstrates lymphocytosis. The electrocardiogram can show sinus tachycardia, low QRS voltage, prolonged PR or QT intervals, and T-wave changes. Ventricular arrhythmias, atrial fibrillation, and right-branch block may occur in the acute phase, but they indicate a poor prognosis[10].

The acute phase usually occurs in children. Without treatment, about 5% to 10% of symptomatic patients die during this phase due to encephalomyelitis or severe cardiac failure, and rarely due to sudden death. After several years, around 30% of the infected individuals develop irreversible lesions of the heart, esophagus, or colon.

When the disease is congenitally transmitted, it may be associated with hepatosplenomegaly, jaundice, skin hemorrhages, and neurologic signs, especially in premature newborn infants.

TABLE 5.1. Clues to the diagnosis of acute Chagas' disease

Fever
Tachycardia not related to the degree of hyperthermia
Mild splenomegaly
Lymphadenopathy
Peripheral edema
Romaña sing (unilateral palpebral edema and preauricular satellite adenopathy)
ECG: low QRS voltage, prolonged PR or QT intervals, and T-wave changes; ventricular arrhythmias, atrial fibrillation, right-branch block
Antibodies against *Trypanosoma cruzi* antigens or serologic tests

Conditions that provoke immunosuppression may reactivate Chagas' disease, with parasite proliferation, necrotic or tumoral lesions in the brain, and intensification of myocarditis. This has frequently occurred with HIV co-infection and peripheral blood CD4 cells under 200/μL, and in organ transplantation. In AIDS, reactivation may occur in any form of the disease, with a marked increase in parasitemia, with no antibodies response. There is acute myocarditis and acute congestive HF. The clinical picture includes systemic manifestations, such as fever and symptoms related to meningoencephalitis. The main differential diagnosis is toxoplasmosis.

After a heart transplant, parasitemia occurs in chagasic patients as revealed by direct examination of peripheral blood in 30% to 80% of cases, and is difficult to differentiate from rejection and reactivation[11]. After renal transplantation, reactivation occurs in about 20% of patients, as revealed by fever and by the presence of *T. cruzi* by direct examination of peripheral blood or skin lesions containing the parasite.

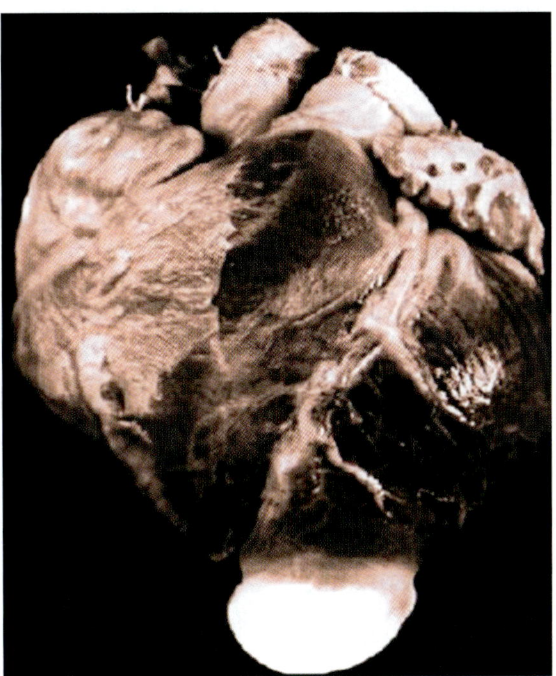

FIGURE 5.4. A large heart with a typical apical aneurysm.

Chronic Phase

In its chronic phase, Chagas' disease can present as an HF syndrome with arrhythmias and thromboembolism. Such presentations can occur isolated or in association; the concurrence of HF and arrhythmias is more frequent. Chronic HF usually appears 20 years or more after acute infection. Its most frequent presentation is a biventricular HF, with predominance of symptoms related to a larger compromise of the right ventricle (Fig. 5.4)[6]. Due to compromise of the right ventricle, it is often difficult to evaluate the volume status of patients with Chagas' disease HF, leading to potential overuse of diuretics.

Diagnosis

The diagnosis of Chagas' cardiomyopathy is based on epidemiologic data, direct demonstration of antibodies against *T. cruzi* antigens or serologic tests (indirect immunofluorescence test, indirect hemagglutination, complement fixation, and immunoenzymatic test)[12]. The diagnosis is suggested by the presence of total right bundle branch block and anterosuperior left bundle branch block in the electrocardiogram (ECG), the presence of an apical left ventricular aneurysm in echocardiogram, with or without a thrombus, and posterobasal akinesia. Patients with HF usually have a worse prognosis than other etiologies, a high prevalence of myocarditis, and conduction system disturbances or bradyarrhythmias. When HF occurs, chest x-ray usually already reveals severely enlarged hearts (Fig. 5.5).

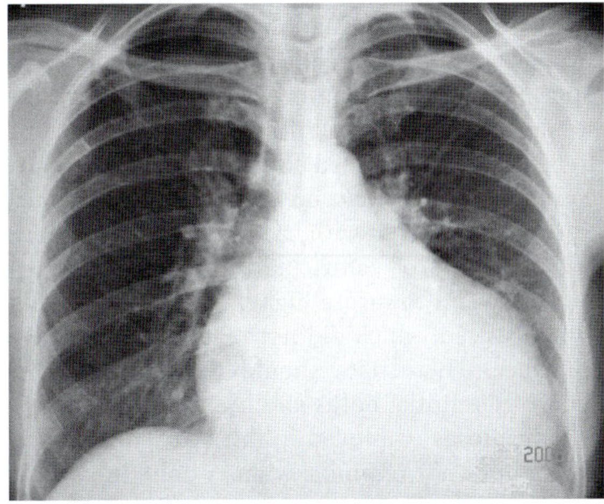

FIGURE 5.5. Chest x-ray of a patient with heart failure due to Chagas' disease showing severely enlarged heart.

Over the past few years B-type natriuretic peptide (BNP) has become an important tool in the diagnosis and risk stratification of patients with HF. The fact that BNP has been shown to be cost-effective in the diagnosis of HF is a relevant issue in developing countries. Only recently, BNP has been introduced as a clinical tool in South America, so there are few reports on BNP in Chagas' disease HF. The scarce available data indicate that patients with positive serology, but no heart compromise, have normal BNP levels[13]. Another report indicates that BNP levels are higher in Chagas' disease patients with apical aneurysm and complex ventricular arrhythmia than in those with apical aneurysm alone[14].

Decompensated Heart Failure General Treatment

Treatment options of DHF in Latin America are similar to those in other parts of the world, except for the unavailability of newer intravenous vasoactive drugs. Furthermore, the issue of pricing of newer drugs may be a major limitation in their application in the health system of developing countries[15].

The new calcium-sensitizing agent levosimendan is available in many countries in Latin America, as well as in Europe and Asia, and it has been reported to provide good clinical results in Latin America[16]. An observational study of its efficacy revealed that in Chagas' disease patients it has the same effects as in other etiologies[5]. The results of large international randomized trials showed that levosimendan was more effective than placebo in symptomatic improvement, but similar to dobutamine, despite a nonsignificant trend toward decreased short-term mortality. In comparison with placebo, hypotension episodes were more frequent with levosimendan, and there was an excess of ventricular and atrial arrhythmias. A trend toward a higher number of deaths was observed, which did not reach statistical significance. These data should be considered in light of the initial bolus and high uniform maintenance doses employed in this particular study, which does not resemble what is done in clinical practice in Latin America[5,16]. Also, levosimendan was used together with other vasodilators and phosphodiesterase inhibitors after intense diuresis, which may have led to unrecognized hypovolemia and massive vasodilatation.

The use of milrinone in Latin America is not as common as in the United States and other parts of the world. A possible reason for this is the cost as well as recent data indicating potential adverse effects in regard to mortality.

The synthetic natriuretic peptide nesiritide has promising initial results but is available only in selected countries in Latin America. Recently, questions regarding its safety have been raised. Retrospective data suggest potential adverse effects on renal function and mortality. A randomized controlled mortality clinical trial was recently announced to be started in 2007. Nesiritide remains a promising new agent, but its safety profile must be better demonstrated before widespread application.

Chagas' Disease Heart Failure

General Treatment

Treatment of DHF secondary to Chagas' disease normally follows the same treatment for other etiologies[4]. However, due to its peculiarities, it is possible that patients with DHF and Chagas' disease do not have the same therapeutic response[17].

These patients usually have lower blood pressures than other etiologies and it is common to present with right-sided heart failure (ascites and peripheral edema) in disproportion to the level of lung congestion. Diuretics are almost always needed in higher doses or in association of different mechanisms of action. Hypotension makes the up-titration of angiotensin-converting enzyme inhibitors (ACEIs) and beta-blockers very difficult. This disease occurs with a high prevalence of advanced atrioventricular blocks and bradyarrhythmias that can get worse with the use of beta-blockers. To date, there is no definite evidence regarding the efficacy and safety of the use of beta-blockers in Chagas' heart disease.

As mentioned before, an observational study of levosimendan revealed that in Chagas' disease patients it has the same efficacy as in other etiologies[5].

Because of the high incidence of thromboembolism in Chagas' heart disease, anticoagulants are recommended for patients with atrial fibrillation, previous embolic episodes, and apical aneurysm, although their efficacy has not been confirmed.

Severe bradyarrhythmias and atrioventricular (AV) block are common and pacemakers are frequently implanted. It is also very common to find atrial fibrillation and different kinds of atrial and ventricular arrhythmias. In sustained and non-sustained ventricular tachycardia, amiodarone is recommended, especially in the presence of ventricular dysfunction. For patients with recurrent sustained ventricular tachycardia and hemodynamic instability, or survivors of a cardiac arrest, the implant of an automatic cardioverter-defibrillator is proposed.

Heart transplant for the treatment of HF seems to have better results than other etiologies, despite reactivation and the possibility of neoplasia and rejection, suggesting that the presence of Chagas' disease either in the recipient or the donor should not represent a contraindication for organ transplantation[11].

Specific Treatment

Specific treatment for Chagas' disease is a matter of controversy. If left untreated, Chagas' disease is not cured spontaneously. Benznidazole, a nitroimidazole derivative, has been recommended for the treatment of acute and congenital Chagas' disease[18]. The use of benznidazole in the reactivation or in the acute phase should be mentioned. There is agreement about drug use in the following circumstances: first, in the prophylaxis of accidental contamination. Since the procedure of treating immediately those exposed to contagion and to continue treatment for at least 10 days was adopted, no new cases have been recorded in that group. Second, during the acute phase of the disease, there is improvement of symptoms, and the parasites disappear from peripheral blood after the 5th day of treatment. Later the serology becomes negative. Treatment applied some time after the acute phase may also produce good results, especially in children who also better tolerate the medication. In the reactivation of infection in immunosuppressed subjects, treatment may improve the clinical picture, turn parasitemia negative, cause regression of meningoencephalic lesions, and attenuate myocarditis.

In some cases side effects require suspension of the treatment. The most important are hypersensitivity (rash, fever, generalized edema, lymphadenopathy, and joint and muscle pain), bone marrow depression (neutropenia, thrombocytopenic purpura), and peripheral polyneuropathy. These side effects are highly dose-dependent. The daily dose for benznidazole is 5 to 7 mg/kg body weight for 30, or better yet, 60 days.

For secondary prophylaxis in AIDS co-infection, continuous treatment with 5 mg/kg of benznidazole three times a week is indicated. There is no agreement about primary prophylaxis. During the chronic phase, specific treatment is controversial. There is evidence indicating that it reduces parasitemia, as evaluated by xenodiagnosis, blood culture, and polymerase chain reaction (PCR), although parasites may be detected in the myocardium. The titers of *T. cruzi* antibodies may decrease, but this does not necessarily indicate a cure since in some patients long-term follow-up shows evolution of the disease[19].

Recently, stem cell therapy has been proposed as alternative treatment for severe heart failure syndromes. The initial results suggest that transplantation of bone marrow mononuclear cells to the myocardium of patients with heart failure due to Chagas' disease is feasible, potentially safe, and effective, bringing symptomatic relief and improving the quality of life of a significant portion of the population affected by Chagas' disease[20]. These results open new perspectives for the treatment of heart diseases through the regenerating capacity of stem cells. On the other hand, further studies focused on elucidating the mechanisms leading to improvement after therapy are clearly needed, as well as establishing more effective protocols and determining potential risks and limitations associated with the procedure.

Selecting an Intravenous Treatment Based on Clinical and Hemodynamic Parameters

The algorithm in Figure 5.6 provides a rationalization of the treatment of DHF from all etiologies, based on clinical and hemodynamic parameters[15].

Those patients who present with warm extremities and pulmonary or systemic congestion, without hypotension, are treated initially with

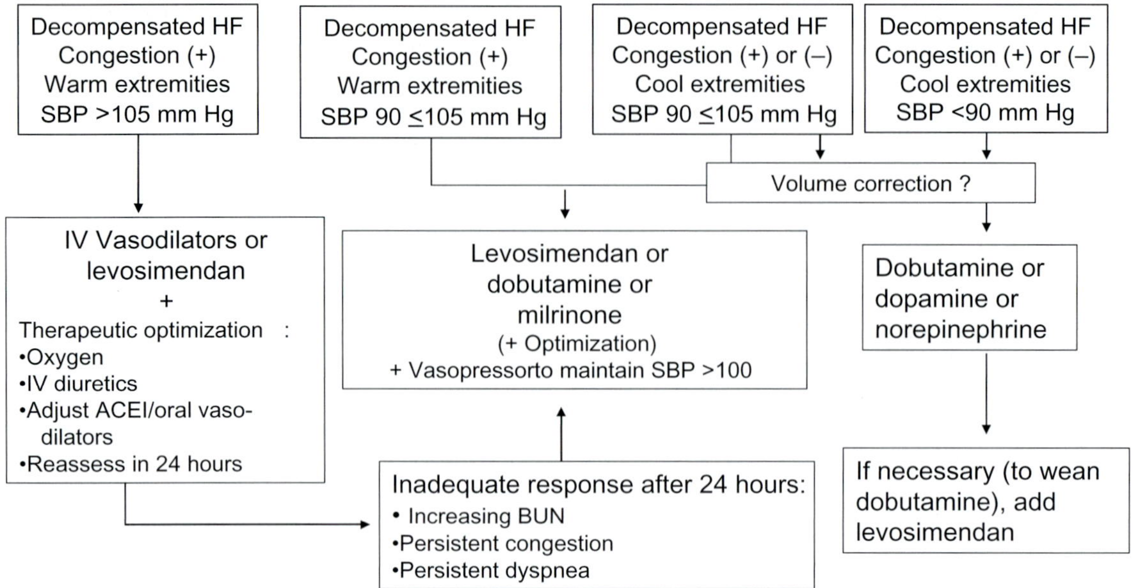

Figure 5.6. Algorithm for current intravenous (IV) therapies in decompensated heart failure (HF). BUN, blood urea nitrogen; SBP, systolic blood pressure.

intravenous diuretics and optimization of oral therapy. The use of intravenous vasodilators or levosimendan is optional. If the response to initial treatment is considered inadequate after 24 to 48 hours (worsening of renal function, persistent congestion, and dyspnea), levosimendan, if available and not used yet, should be the next option.

Patients with cool extremities, with or without hypotension, should have their volume status checked first. If the presence of congestion is not obvious, one should check for hypovolemia and the need for volume administration. For patients with systemic or pulmonary congestion, without hypotension, levosimendan or an intravenous vasodilator seems to be the best choice. However, if hypotension is present, the initial choice should rely on dobutamine associated with dopamine or norepinephrine. After initial stabilization, levosimendan can be added to wean the patient off of dobutamine. In patients already taking dobutamine, it is our practice to start levosimendan at 0.05 to 0.1 μg/kg/min and after 6 hours of simultaneous infusion, start the weaning process off of dobutamine so that, after 24 hours, it can be discontinued. If hypotension occurs, the infusion rate can be reduced; alternatively, we prefer to add, or increase the dose of, dopamine or norepinephrine.

For patients who are on chronic oral treatment with a beta-blocker, and there is a need for inotropic therapy, levosimendan or milrinone should be the preferred choice (since the mechanisms of action are postreceptor, and they are not attenuated by beta blockers).

Conclusion

Acute heart failure syndromes in Latin America are common and represent a major burden for the health systems of developing countries. Chagas' disease is one of the major causes of HF and, in the absence of definitive evidence, its treatment should be similar to that of other etiologies. Acute Chagas' disease is becoming progressively less common but still needs to be part of a differential diagnosis of acute heart failure in this part of the world. The role of new treatments must be better investigated in clinical trials designed specifically for this particular form of HF.

References

1. Mansur AP, Souza MFM, Timerman A, Ramires JAF. Tendência do risco de morte por doenças circulatórias, cerebrovasculares e isquêmicas do coração em 11 capitais do Brasil de 1980 a 1998. Arq Bras Cardiol 2002;79:269–276.
2. Dias JCP, Silveira AC, Schofield CJ. The impact of Chagas' disease control in Latin America: a review. Mem Inst Oswaldo Cruz 2002;97(5):603–612.
3. Shulman IA, Appleman MD, Saxena S, Hiti AL, Kirchhoff LV. Specific antibodies to Trypanosoma cruzi among blood donors in Los Angeles, California. Transfusion 1997;37:727–731.
4. Bocchi EA, Vilas-Boas F, Perrone S, et al. 1st Latin American Guidelines for the Assessment and Management of Decompensated Heart Failure. Arq Bras Cardiol 2005;85(suppl 3):1–94.
5. Pereira-Barretto AC, Rassi S, Vilas-Boas F, et al., for the Brazilian Evaluation of Levosimendan Infusion Efficacy (BELIEF) study investigators. Levosimendan treatment for acutely decompensated heart failure is as effective for Chagas disease patients as for patients with other etiologies. Crit Care 2003;7(suppl 3):P23.
6. Rassi Jr A, Rassi A, Little WC. Chagas' heart disease. Clin Cardiol 2000;23:883–889.
7. Moncayo A. Chagas disease: current epidemiological trends after the interruption of vectorial and transfusional transmission in the Southern Cone countries. Mem Inst Oswaldo Cruz 2003;98(5):577–591.
8. Coll-Cardenas R, Espinoza-Gomez F, Maldonado-Rodriguez A, Reyes-Lopez PA, Huerta-Viera M, Rojas-Larios F. Active transmission of human Chagas disease in Colima Mexico. Mem Inst Oswaldo Cruz 2004;99(4):363–368.
9. Nowicki MJ, Chinchilla C, Corado L, et al. Prevalence of antibodies to Trypanosoma cruzi among solid organ donors in Southern California: a population at risk. Transplantation 2006;81:477–479.
10. Prata A. Clinical and epidemiological apects of Chagas disease. Lancet Infect Dis 2000;1:92–100.
11. Bocchi EA, Bellotti G, Mocelin A, et al. Heart transplantation for chronic Chagas heart disease. Ann Thorac Surg 1996;61:1727–1733.
12. Alemida IC, Salles NA, Santos MLP, et al. Serum diagnosis of American trypanosomiasis in blood bank: a highly sensitive and specific carbohydrate rich trypomastigotes antigen and why there are so many inconclusive results. Mem Inst Oswaldo Cruz 1995;90(suppl):72–74.
13. Bezerra de Melo R, Parente GBO, Victor EG. Measurement of human brain natriuretic. Peptide in patients with Chagas' disease. Arq Bras Cardiol 2005;84(2):137–140.
14. Talvani A, Rocha MOC, Cogan J, et al. Brain natriuretic peptide and left ventricular dysfunction in chagasic cardiomyopathy. Mem Inst Oswaldo Cruz 2004;99(6):645–649.
15. Vilas-Boas F, Follath F. Current insights into the modern treatment of decompensated heart failure. Arq Bras Cardiol 2006;87:329–337.
16. Garrido M, Castano R, Antonio J, Estrada J, Gaxiola A. Levosimendan reduces length of hospital stay for patients with acutely decompensated heart failure. Eur J Heart Fail 2003;2(suppl 1):163(abstr).
17. Pinto Dias JC. The treatment of Chagas disease (South American trypanosomiasis). Ann Intern Med 2006;16;144(10):772–774.
18. Andrade ALS, Zicker F, Oliveira RM, et al. Randomised trial of efficacy of benznidazole in treatment of early Trypanosoma cruzi infection. Lancet 1996;348:1407–1413.
19. Viotti R, Vigliano C, Lococo B, et al. Long-term cardiac outcomes of treating chronic Chagas disease with benznidazole versus no treatment. A nonrandomized trial. Ann Intern Med 2006;144:724–734.
20. Vilas-Boas F, Feitosa GS, Soares MBP, et al. Early results of bone marrow cell transplantation to the myocardium of patients with heart failure due to Chagas disease. Arq Bras Cardiol 2006;87:545–552.

1.2
Transition from Normal Physiology to Pathophysiology

1.2.1
Cardiac Level

6
Normal Physiology and Pathophysiology of Left Ventricular Systole

Marc A. Simon and Michael R. Pinsky

Background

Left ventricular (LV) systole is defined as that part of the cardiac cycle wherein active contraction occurs. Contractile performance is a major determinant of overall cardiac function. The final end-systolic pressure and volume are a function of intrinsic cardiac contractility, myocardial energy state, and ventricular-arterial coupling, whereas the developed stroke volume and stroke work are a function of these factors plus end-diastolic volume. Since end-diastolic volume is a primary determinant of systolic function, through the Frank-Starling mechanism, diastolic dysfunction directly alters systolic performance. Diastolic dysfunction is discussed elsewhere in this volume. In this chapter we focus only on systolic events.

The beginning of systole can be defined in many ways. First, on a cellular level, systole starts with excitation-contraction coupling of the ventricular myocardium. However, one usually considers systole from a mechanical perspective because it is easier to identify. On a mechanical level, the start of systole can be defined as either that point during the initiation of contraction when the LV intraluminal pressure exceeds left atrial pressure, or when the mitral valve closes and isovolumic contraction occurs. In practice, these mechanical events occur within 20 ms of each other and so mitral valve closure is usually used to define the start of systole, as it is easier to identify clinically. Systole ends when active contraction ends. This usually occurs at the peak of ejection.

To understand the therapeutic approaches used to support LV ejection and aid acutely decompensated hearts, it is important to understand the mechanisms underpinning LV systole. For example, almost half of all patients presenting with acute decompensated heart failure have systolic dysfunction as their primary abnormality.[1] However, a small proportion of heart failure cases have preserved systolic function, such that their underlying pathology is diastolic dysfunction. Appropriate recognition of systolic dysfunction, including such physical findings as cool extremities and cyanosis, in addition to signs of volume overload such as edema and increased jugular venous pressure, guides the treatment. The main thrust of treatment is directed toward pharmacologically improving systolic function and reducing the impedance to ejection.

Definition and Diagnosis of Contractile Function

Systolic ventricular function is determined by preload, afterload, and contractility. Preload is the wall stress on the left ventricle prior to ejection. Operationally, we use LV end-diastolic volume to reflect this wall stress. Since measures of volumes can be difficult at the bedside, LV end-diastolic pressure, left atrial pressure, or pulmonary artery occlusion pressure is often used as a surrogate for LV end-diastolic volume. Afterload is the maximal LV wall stress during ejection. By Laplace's law, wall stress is proportional to the product of LV radius of curvature and transmural pressure. During isovolumic contraction, the radius of curvature remains constant and LV pressure rises.

However, during the ejection phase of systole, the LV radius of curvature progressively decreases while ejection pressure continues to rise. Importantly, under normal conditions the product LV radius of curvature and ejection pressure decreases markedly. Thus, under normal conditions maximal LV afterload occurs at the instant of aortic value opening. Furthermore, during ejection, the left ventricle actually unloads itself, hence the reason why systolic hypertension is usually well tolerated but diastolic hypertension rapidly leads to LV hypertrophy.

Furthermore, in subjects with dilated cardiomyopathies, and reduced ejection fractions, the LV radius of curvature does not decrease much during ejection while arterial pressure continues to rise. Accordingly, such ventricles do not unload during ejection and are more sensitive to small changes in arterial pressure in determining systolic function. Indeed, one can use a pressor test to identify such subjects. Contractility is a more difficult term to define and quantify. A reasonable definition is the amount of force capable of being produced by the contracting myocardium.[2] On a cellular level, contractility is related to the integrity of the actin-myocin coupling, intracellular calcium (Ca^{2+}) flux rate and quantity. Functionally, one measures contractility by varying preload and afterload. Numerous measures have been attempted to quantify contractility with varying degrees of success, depending on the degree of true independence they have from preload or afterload.

Force of Contraction Per Unit Time: *dP/dt*

The maximal rate of isovolumic pressure development, dP/dt_{max}, serves as an empirical index of ventricular contractility. All things being equal, a greater dP/dt_{max} for a constant preload, the higher the contractility and the greater the rate of work per unit time (power). However, increasing preload, coronary perfusion pressure, or energy substrate availability increases dP/dt_{max}. Furthermore, dP/dt_{max} has a wide range of normal values between individuals, and there is considerable overlap between normal subjects and patients with systolic dysfunction. Presumably, since myocardial fibers are not all oriented in the same direction within the ventricular wall and are not all activated at the same time, the mechanical event characterizing dP/dt_{max} becomes less sensitive to identifying systolic dysfunction.[3] Thus any measure of rate of contraction must take into consideration the preload, the variable direction of force vectors, and the time sequence of excitation when attempting to derive a sum measure of contractility.

The Frank-Starling Relationship

By the Frank-Starling relationship, also referred to as Starling's law of the heart, peak systolic activity, defined as maximal developed pressure, volume ejected, or the product of the two, is directly proportional to end-diastolic volume.[4] The cellular basis for this relation is that increased cell stretch is proportional to developed contractile force, which occurs due to increased inward Ca^{2+} flux. The Frank-Starling relationship described an intrinsic beat-to-beat variability in inotropy. Length-dependent activation of cardiomyocytes has fast and slow components. The fast component is due to increased myofilament Ca^{2+} sensitivity that is induced by stretch and the resultant change in interfilament spacing.[5] The slow component is due to increasing calcium transient following the action potential. Mechanical stretch produces autocrine release of angiotensin II, which induces endothelin release via stimulation of AT_1 receptors. Endothelin then increases intracellular Ca^{2+} via activation of the Na^+-H^+ exchanger that subsequently activates the Na^+-Ca^{2+} exchanger.[6] Still, for the same stroke work, myocardial O_2 consumption (MVO_2) varies depending on whether or not the stroke work comprises mainly flow work (lower MVO_2) or pressure work (greater MVO_2). This clinically relevant phenomenon cannot be explained by analysis of Frank-Starling relations alone.

Pressure-Volume Loops

The heart is a hydraulic pump, bringing in volume at low pressures and ejecting this volume under higher pressures. Thus, it is useful to describe this pumping behavior in the pressure-volume domain, wherein no time units exist. The LV pressure-volume loop (PV loop) displays the relationship of time-varying LV pressure (y-axis) and volume (x-axis) as a counterclockwise, rectangular loop. Four phases of the heart cycle can be distinguished in the loop, as illustrated in Figure 6.1. The lower limb of the loop is the diastolic filling phase, which terminates at the lower right corner, end-diastole. Diastolic filling starts when left atrial pressure exceeds LV intraluminal pressure during active LV diastolic relaxation. The left ventricle then passively fills aided at end-diastole by the atrial contraction, which allows LV end-diastolic volume to be greater than would have occurred passively and also allows this end-diastolic wall stress to occur only briefly prior to systole. This is followed by active myocardial contraction, which results first in isovolumic contraction (right ascending limb of the loop) and then in ejection (upper limb of the loop), which terminates at end-systole, the upper left corner. Finally, the isovolumic relaxation phase (left descending limb of the loop) completes the LV PV loop.

For a given ventricle, both preload and afterload alter ejection pressure, stroke volume, and end-systole. If one were to vary end-diastolic volumes, as may occur with sudden decreases in venous return, or suddenly increase ejection pressure, as may occur with arterial occlusion, then one would create a series of different LV PV loops, all having the same contractility. Importantly, the line derived by connecting the end-systolic points of all these separate LV PV loops would be straight (Fig. 6.1). This relationship is referred to as the LV end-systolic pressure-volume relation (ESPVR). Although the position on this line that a given end-systole resides will be a function of preload and afterload, the ESPVR domain will be a function of contractility. The slope of the ESPVR line describes the LV stiffness or elastance at end-systole and is referred to as end-systolic elastance (E_{es}). E_{es} changes in a directionally similar fashion to changes in contractility under most conditions that do not include remodeling or dyssynchrony. E_{es} is increased by treatment with positive inotropic agents and decreased by treatment with negative inotropic agents. Technically, it is often easier to define the point during end-ejection when the ratio of LV pressure to volume is maximal. This point is referred to as E_{max}. Usually E_{es} and E_{max} co-vary, and both are approximated by the end-systolic point on the PV loop (the upper left corner). However, if arterial impedance increases, then E_{max} may occur before E_{es}. Thus, E_{es} is a more accurate estimate of contractility and its change than is E_{max}, if arterial tone is varying. Operationally, the way the ESPVR is created is by rapidly varying LV filling. Inferior vena caval occlusion using a balloon catheter works in intact patients, and simple manual compression of the inferior vena cava work during open thoracotomy studies can be used in patients during cardiac surgery.

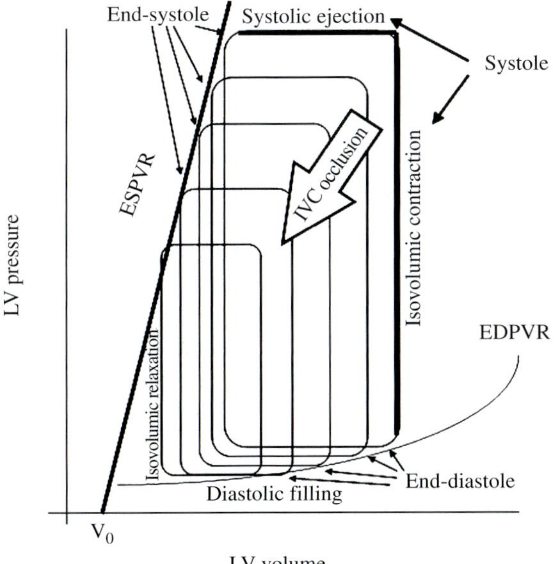

FIGURE 6.1. The pressure-volume loop and its component structures. LV, left ventricle; ESPVR, end-systolic pressure-volume relation; IVC, inferior vena cava; EDPVR, end-diastolic pressure-volume relation; V_0, ventricular volume extrapolated to correlate to a ventricular pressure of 0.

Interestingly, increasing afterload alters E_{es} independently of altering preload.[7] So, while increasing afterload would be expected to increase end-diastolic volume (preload) and thus result in the same alterations in PV loops as increasing preload, namely varying the position of end-systole linearly along the ESPVR, it instead results in a different ESPVR with a greater E_{es}. This may be explained by the Anrep effect, in which an abrupt increase in afterload results in a positive inotropic effect. Operationally, these findings translate into the reality that estimates of E_{es} need to be made using the same preload or afterload-altering maneuver over time, and not comparing E_{es} at one point using preload reduction with another measure of E_{es} using afterload reduction.

Another way to assess contractility using the E_{es} concept but not relying on exact measures of end-systole is to measure the entire external LV work done as a function of end-diastolic volume (preload) and then vary preload and note how stroke work varies. The slope of the stroke work to end-diastolic volume relation is referred to as preload-recruitable stroke work. The slope of this relation is also a measure of contractility.[8] Preload-recruitable stroke work has the added advantage over E_{es} as a measure of contractility in that it is a more robust measure, being less sensitive to minor measurement errors in defining accurately end-systole. Furthermore, if pulmonary artery occlusion pressure is substituted for preload, then one can use a pulmonary artery catheter to measure all the components needed to assess preload-recruitable stroke work at the bedside.

The energetics of the left ventricle can also be derived from the PV loop (Fig. 6.2). The area within a PV-loop is the stroke work (SW) and is the energy that the ventricle passes on to the arterial circuit to pump blood forward. However, even if no forward blood flow were to occur, as may be the case if arterial pressure were very high, the heart would still create a pressure and use oxygen. This non-external work aspect of systolic function is depicted in the triangular area defined by the isovolumic relaxation limb of the PV loop, and the ESPVR is the potential energy of the system. This potential energy is the minimal energy the ventricle consumes for contraction in absence of load. The sum of the potential energy and SW is known as the pressure-volume area (PVA), and represents all the energy that the ventricle needs to contract and pump blood under the given loading conditions. There is a very strong linear correlation between the PVA and MVO_2.[9]

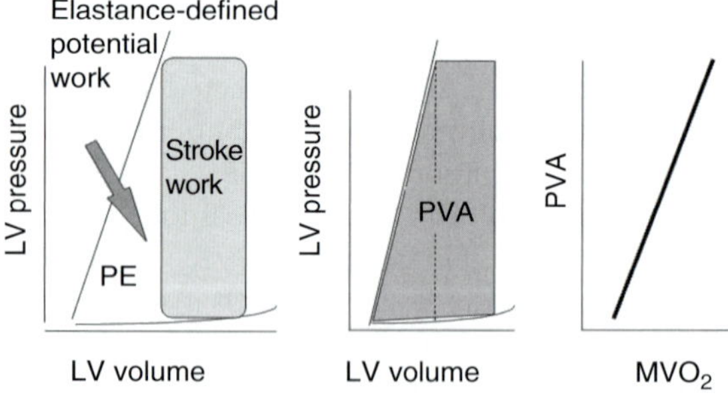

FIGURE 6.2. Energetics derived from the pressure-volume loop. LV, left ventricle; PE, potential energy; PVA, pressure-volume area; MVO_2, myocardial oxygen consumption.

Time-Varying Ventricular Elastance, $E(t)$, and E_{max}

Time-varying ventricular elastance, $E(t)$, is the ratio of the change in pressure to the change in volume ($\Delta P/\Delta V$) over time and represents changes in ventricular stiffness throughout the cardiac cycle. The actual equation is as follows:

$$E(t) = \frac{p(t)}{[V(t) - V_0]}$$

where $p(t)$ is time-varying LV pressure (mm Hg), $V(t)$ is time-varying LV volume (mL), and V_0 is the volume intercept of the ESPVR (mL). The numerator is simply $p(t)$ instead of $p(t) - p_0$ since $p_0 = 0$.

Mechanically speaking systole represents a progressive increase in ventricular wall stiffness as contraction proceeds from start to end of systole. $E(t)$ increases throughout ventricular systole as the ventricle stiffens (Fig. 6.3). End-systole can be defined as the time at which $E(t)$ reaches its maximum, E_{max}.[10] Suga et al.[11] defined $E(t)$ and demonstrated that it is independent of preload or afterload. They further showed that $E(t)$ is independent of ejection characteristics (isovolumic or ejecting) of the heart. Inotropic agents alter $E(t)$ such that E_{max} is increased and time to E_{max} (T_{max}) is shorter.[12] Work since then has shown that LV pressure cannot be completely accurately calculated by $E(t)$ and volume alone, leading to more complex calculations that take into consideration instantaneous ventricular flow, $Q(t)$, and ventricular resistance to flow.[13] Importantly, using echocardiographic estimates of LV volumes, one can measure $E(t)$ and preload-recruitable stroke work in patients and can demonstrate dynamic changes in contractility. Gorcsan et al.[14] used this approach to demonstrate that LV contractility was reduced following cardiopulmonary bypass, even though

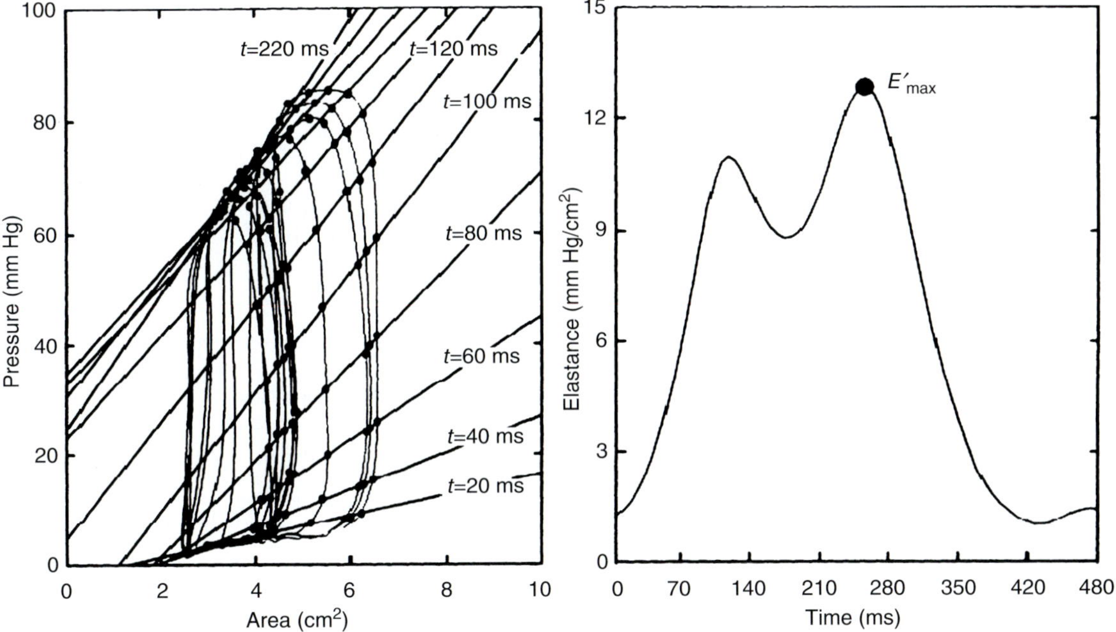

FIGURE 6.3. Time-varying elastance measured in a patient prior to cardiac surgery. (From Gorcsan et al.,[14] with permission.)

other measure of systolic function, like ejection fraction and dP/dt_{max} were not affected (Fig. 6.4).

Systolic Performance: Ventricular Emptying

Systolic performance is the ability of the LV to empty. This is a function of end-systolic volume; a commonly used calculation is the LV ejection fraction (effective ejection fraction in the case of valvular regurgitation). With increased inotropy, stroke volume (width of the PV loop) increases due predominantly to decreased end-systolic volume. Thus, at a given ejection pressure, end-systolic volume is inversely proportional to

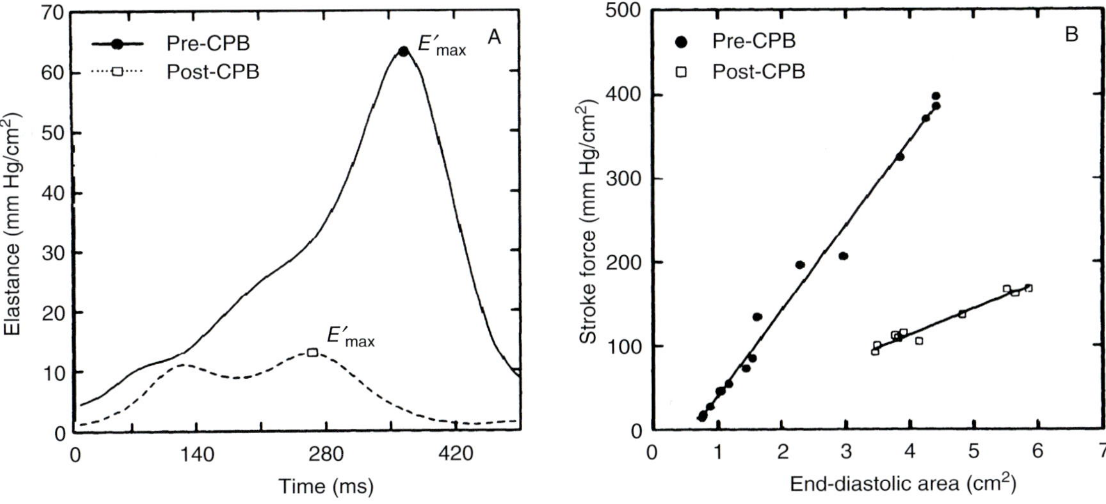

FIGURE 6.4. Time-varying elastance and preload-recruitable stroke work measured in one patient pre– and post–cardiopulmonary bypass (CPB). (From Gorcsan et al.,[14] with permission.)

contractility. Normal values depend on body size, so the range is large and overlaps considerably among disease states and normal values. Furthermore, end-systolic volume depends to a variable extent upon end-diastolic volume, particularly if LV ejection fraction is constant.

Force-Frequency Relation

A final determinant of systolic function is heart rate (HR). Faster stimulation of muscle fibers results in increased contraction. This has been shown in isolated cardiomyocytes from humans. The mechanism is thought to result from large intracellular Na^+ and Ca^{2+} shifts that overloads the Na^+-Ca^{2+} pump, leading to continued intracellular accumulation of Ca^{2+}.[15,16] Eventually, stimulation rate becomes too rapid and contractile force decreases.

Pathophysiology

Impaired myocardial contractility occurs due to a loss of functional myocytes or a decrease in function of viable myocytes. These processes may be due to primary myocardial dysfunction, in which permanent damage to the myocytes has generally occurred, or other conditions that adversely affect myocardial function and are generally reversible if the condition can be remedied. Loss of myocytes results from either necrosis (ischemia, toxic damage, or myocarditis) or the less understood process of apoptosis.

Conditions creating primary myocardial dysfunction are listed in Table 6.1. These are most likely due to myocardial ischemia and infarction or causes of nonischemic cardiomyopathies. Causes of secondary myocardial systolic dysfunction include valvular disease, hypertension, tachycardia, metabolic abnormalities (hypoglycemia, hypocalcemia), systemic infection or inflammation, and neuromuscular disorders, but are beyond the scope of this discussion. High-output heart failure syndromes represent failure of systole to meet the body's metabolic demands, usually due to a systemic illness, and is discussion elsewhere in this book.

Systolic dysfunction secondary to regional myocardial dyssynchrony warrants special attention. Contraction asynchrony is the most common clinical contractile abnormality seen, accounting for much of the observed clinically relevant increase in morbidity from heart disease. Regional myocardial asynchrony, characterized by regional wall motion abnormalities (RWMAs), is common in patients with both normal and abnormal cardiac physiology.[17,18,19,20,21,22,23] Initially, pacing was thought to have minimal effects of contraction synchrony, because when viewed from the perspective of the whole ventricle, little change could be ascertained when compared to normally conducted beats.[24] However, Badke et al.[25] observed marked regional differences in myocardial contraction when analyzed by multiple dimensions using ultrasonic crystals. Park et al.[26] showed that increasing contraction asynchrony, as exemplified by right ventricular (RV) and left ventricular (LV) pacing in their model, did not change E_{es} but did induce progressive LV dilation proportional to the degree of asynchrony. As described above, any process that results in an increased LV volume for a constant LV ejection pressure and stroke volume will also increase MVO_2. Subjects with heart failure have a close correlation between conduction delays and contraction asynchrony.[27] Thus, the finding that many patients with prolonged QRS heart failure treated with cardiac resynchronization therapy (CRT) demonstrate a decrease in LV end-diastolic volume without a change in ejection pressure or stroke volume,

Table 6.1. Common causes of primary myocardial dysfunction

- I. Ischemia
  - A. Acute
    - 1. Necrosis
    - 2. Stunned myocardium
  - B. Chronic
    - 1. Infarct/scar
    - 2. Hibernating myocardium
- II. Inflammation/infection (viral)
- III. Cardiac toxins
  - A. Alcohol
  - B. Cocaine
  - C. Chemotherapeutic agents: doxorubicin, cyclophosphamide
- IV. Genetic disorders
  - A. Hypertrophic cardiomyopathies
  - B. Familial dilated cardiomyopathies
  - C. Peripartum cardiomyopathy
  - D. Muscular dystrophies
- V. Idiopathic dilated cardiomyopathy

suggests that CRT improved ejection effectiveness by reducing contractile asynchrony.[28,29] Although redistribution of local work, reduced mitral regurgitation, and metabolism have all been suggested as possible mechanisms by which biventricular pacing improves LV performance in these subjects, the mechanism has not yet been defined.[30,31]

Left ventricular ejection reflects the summed contraction of a many cardiac muscle cells whose function is altered by LV volume, arterial impedance, coronary blood flow, and excitation-contraction coupling.[20,32,33] Left ventricular contraction is normally heterogeneous.[19,34] The apex and base differ in their onset of contraction and in their response to inotropes; the apex being slightly phase lagged in relation to the base region and somewhat more dynamic.[17,35] This degree of asynchrony is necessary for proper mechanical functioning of the mitral valve apparatus and causes minimal cardiac dilation. However, as LV contraction becomes more asynchronous among cardiac regions, LV ejection effectiveness (the ratio of global LV contraction to phase-specific regional LV contraction) decreases.

One need not have abnormally conducted beats to develop regional contraction asynchrony. Regional dyskinesis induced by sub-selective coronary artery infusion of esmolol in an acute canine model induced regional asynchrony, caused similar rightward shifts of the LV ESPVR but did not alter E_{es} (Fig. 6.5).[36]

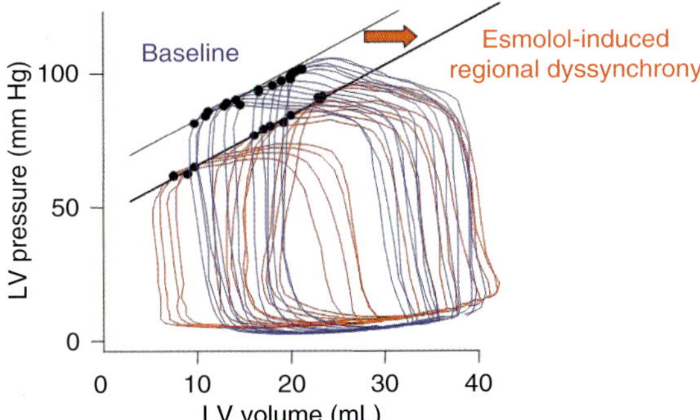

FIGURE 6.5. Effect of regional dyskinesis on global LV function. Esmolol was infused into the left anterior descending coronary artery affecting 25% of the total LV myocardium. (Data from Strum and Pinsky.[36])

The final common pathway of systolic dysfunction from any cause is positive ventricular remodeling if the damage occurs for a long enough time. Remodeling occurs as an adaptive process to prevent the heart from dying. One mechanism of ventricular remodeling is myocardial hypertrophy. Hypertrophy is an adaptive response to increased wall stress caused by increased volumes. By the law of Laplace, wall tension (T) can be calculated as: $T = (P \times R)2t$, where P is the intraventricular pressure, R is the ventricular radius, and t is the ventricular wall thickness.[37] By this relation, as the radius increases, so does wall tension, and this can be reduced by increasing wall thickness. Remodeling is further exacerbated by neurohormonal activation via adrenergic and renin-angiotensin pathways. Acutely, neurohormonal activation can improve hemodynamics but constitutive overactivation leads to a vicious cycle of remodeling, systolic dysfunction, ventricular dilation, and further stimulation.[38,39] Cytokine release also has been implicated in the progression of ventricular remodeling. In addition to cellular hypertrophy, changes in the interstitium characterize the remodeling process, including alterations in the complex balance of matrix metalloproteinases (MMPs) and their tissue inhibitors (tissue-inhibitor metalloproteinases, TIMPs), which are closely tied to fibroblast activity and are implicated in apoptosis.[40,41,42,43] Such changes have been observed after acute myocardial infarction associated with LV systolic dysfunction.[44] Changes in collagen type, amount, and cross-linking lead to fibrosis.[45,46]

Conclusion

Left ventricular systole is the determinant of cardiac function. It is defined by preload, afterload, and contractility. Contractility has been assessed by a number of different methods that highlight the complex interplay of physiological conditions, neurohormonal input, and cellular and subcellular mechanisms that together result in the contractile state. Measures of contractility include dP/dt, the Frank-Starling force-tension relation, the force-frequency relation, ESPVR and related variables, and $E(t)$. Many conditions can impair contractility, but the approach to management in the acute setting is based on an understanding of determinants of the contractile state and how they can be altered.

References

1. Fonarow GC, Adams KF Jr, Abraham WT, Yancy CW, Boscardin WJ. Risk stratification for in-hospital mortality in acutely decompensated heart failure: classification and regression tree analysis. JAMA 2005;293:572–580.
2. Noble MI. Problems concerning the application of concepts of muscle mechanics to the determination of the contractile state of the heart. Circulation 1972;45:252–255.
3. Sagawa K, Maughan WL, Sunagawa K, Suga H. Cardiac Contraction and the Pressure-Volume Relationship. New York: Oxford University Press, 1988:16–17.
4. Sagawa K, Maughan WL, Sunagawa K, Suga H. Cardiac Contraction and the Pressure-Volume Relationship. New York: Oxford University Press, 1988:8–13.
5. Fuchs F, Wang Y. Sarcomere length versus interfilament spacing as determinants of cardiac myofilament Ca^{2+} sensitivity and Ca^{2+} binding. J mol Cell Cardiol 1996;28:1375–1383.
6. Alverez BV, Perez NG, Ennis IL, Camilion de Hurtado MC, Cingolani HE. Mechanisms underlying the increase in force and Ca^{2+} transient that follow stretch of cardiac muscle: a possible explanation of the Anrep effect. Circ Res 1999;85:716–722.
7. Reyes M, Freeman GL, Escobedo D, Lee S, Steinhelper ME, Feldman MD. Enhancement of contractility with sustained afterload in the intact murine heart: blunting of length-dependent activation. Circulation 2003;107:2962–2968.
8. Glower DD, Spratt JA, Snow ND, et al. Linearity of the Frank-Starling relationship in the intact heart: the concept of preload recruitable stroke work. Circulation 1985;71(5):994–1009.
9. Suga H, Hayashi T, Shirahata M. Ventricular systolic pressure-volume area as predictor of cardiac oxygen consumption. Am J Physiol 1981;240:H39–H44.
10. Sagawa K, Maughan WL, Sunagawa K, Suga H. Cardiac Contraction and the Pressure-Volume Relationship. New York: Oxford University Press, 1988:38–39.
11. Suga H, Sagawa K, Shoukas AA. Load-independence of the instantaneous pressure-volume ratio of the canine left ventricle and effects of epinephrine and heart rate on the ratio. Circ Res 1973;32: 314–322.
12. Suga H, Sagawa K. Instantaneous pressure-volume relationships and their ratio in the excised supported canine left ventricle. Circ Res 1974;35:117–134.
13. Shroff SG, Janicki JS, Weber KT. Mechanical and energetic behavior of the intact left ventricle. In: Fozzard HA, et al., eds. The Heart and Cardiovascular System, 2nd ed. New York: Raven Press, 1992:129–150.
14. Gorcsan J 3rd, Gasior TA, Mandarino WA, Deneault LG, Hattler BG, Pinsky MR. Assessment of the immediate effects of cardiopulmonary bypass on left ventricular performance by on-line pressure-area relations. Circulation 1994;89:180–190.
15. Mulieri LA, Leavitt BJ, Martin BJ. Myocardial force-frequency defect in mitral regurgitation heart failure is reversed by forskolin. Circulation 1993; 88:2700–2704.
16. Hasenfuss G, Reinecke H, Studer R, et al. Relation between myocardial function and expression of sarcoplasmic reticulum Ca^{2+}-ATPase in failing and nonfailing human heart. Circ Res 1994;75:434–442.
17. Pandian NG, Skorton DJ, Collins SM, Falsetti HL, Burke ER, Kerber RE. Heterogeneity of left ventricular segmental wall thickening and excursion in 2-dimensional echocardiograms of normal human subjects. Am J Cardiol 1983;51:1667–1673.
18. Thys DM. The intraoperative assessment of regional myocardial performance: Is the cart before the horse? J Cardiothorac Anesth 1987;1:273–275.
19. LeWinter M, Kent R, Kroener J, Carew T, Covell J. Regional differences in myocardial performance in the left ventricle of the dog. Circ Res 1975;37:191–199.
20. Haendchen RV, Wyatt HL, Maurer G, Zwehl W, Bear M, Meerbaum S, Corday E. Quantification of regional cardiac function by two-dimensional echocardiography I. Patterns of contraction on the normal left ventricle. Circulation 1983;67:1234–1245.
21. Xiao HB, Roy C, Gibson DG. Nature of ventricular activation in patients with dilated cardiomyopathy: evidence for bilateral bundle branch block. Br Heart J 1994;72:167–174.
22. Bonow RO. Regional left ventricular nonuniformity: effects on left ventricular diastolic function in ischemic heart disease, hypertrophic cardiomyopathy, and the normal heart. Circulation 1990;81: III54–III65.
23. Little W, Reeves R, Arciniegas J, Katholi R, Rogers E. Mechanism of abnormal interventricular septal motion during delayed left ventricular activation. Circulation 1982;65:1486–1491.

24. Grover M, Glanz SA. Endocardial pacing affects left ventricular end-diastolic volume and performance in the intact anesthetized dog. Circ Res 1983;53: 72–83.
25. Badke FR, Boinay P, Covell JW. Effect of ventricular pacing on regional ventricular performance. Am J Physiol 1980;238:H858–H867.
26. Park RC, Little WC, O'Rourke RA. Effect of alteration of LV activation sequence on the LV end-systolic pressure-volume relation in closed-chest dogs. Circ Res 1985;57:706–717.
27. Toussaint JF, Lavergne T, Kerrou K, et al. Ventricular coupling of electrical and mechanical dyssynchronization in heart failure patients. Pacing Clin Electrophysiol 2002;25:178–182.
28. Kass DA, Chen C-H, Curry C, et al. Improved LV mechanics from acute VDD pacing in patients with dilated cardiomyopathy and ventricular conduction delay. Circulation 1999;99:1567–1573.
29. Mulukutta S, Stetten GD, Jacques DC, Gorcsan J. Quantification of left ventricular phase asynchrony in patients with left bundle branch block using tissue Doppler echocardiography. Circulation 2000;102:II-384.
30. Prinzen FW, Hunter WC, Wymann BT, McVeigh ER. Mapping of regional myocardial strain and work during ventricular pacing: Experimental study using magnetic imaging tagging. J Am Coll Cardiol 1999;33:1735–1742.
31. Delhass T, Arts T, Prinzen FW, Reneman RS. Relation between electrical activation time and subepicardial fiber strain in the canine left ventricle. Pflugers Arch 1993;423:78–87.
32. Miura T, Bhargava V, Guth BD, et al. Increased afterload intensifies asynchronous wall motion and impairs ventricular relaxation. J Appl Physiol 1993; 75:389–396.
33. Shroff SG, Naegelen D, Clark WA. Relation between left ventricular systolic resistance and ventricular rate processes. Am J Physiol 1990;258:H381–H394.
34. Diedericks J, Leone BJ, Foëx P. Regional differences in left ventricular wall motion in the anesthetized dog. Anesthesiology 1989;70:82–90.
35. Freedman RA, Alderman EL, Sheffield LT, Saporito M, Fisher LD. Bundle branch block in patients with chronic coronary artery disease: angiographic correlates and prognostic significance. J Am Coll Cardiol 1987;10:73–80.
36. Strum DP, Pinsky MR. Esmolol-induced regional wall motion abnormalities do not affect regional ventricular elastances. Anesth Analg 2000;90(2): 252–261.
37. Norton JM. Towards consistent definitions for preload and afterload. Adv Physiol Educ 2001;25: 53–61.
38. Francis GS, McDonald KM, Cohn JN. Neurohumoral activation in preclinical heart failure. Circulation 1993;87:IV-90–IV-96.
39. Remme WJ. Pharmacological modulation of cardiovascular remodeling: a guide to heart failure therapy. Cardiovasc Drugs Ther 2003;17(4):349–360.
40. Polyakova V, Hein S, Kostin S, Ziegelhoeffer T, Schaper J. Matrix metalloproteinases and their tissue inhibitors in pressure-overloaded human myocardium during heart failure progression. J Am Coll Cardiol 2004;44(8):1609–1618.
41. Fedak PW, Verma S, Weisel RD, Li RK. Cardiac remodeling and failure: from molecules to man (part II). Cardiovasc Pathol 2005;14(2):49–60.
42. Ovechkin AV, Tyagi N, Rodriguez WE, Hayden MR, Moshal KS, Tyagi SC. Role of matrix metalloproteinase-9 in endothelial apoptosis in chronic heart failure in mice. J Appl Physiol 2005;99:2390–2405.
43. Goldstein S, Ali AS, Sabbah H. Ventricular remodeling. Mechanisms and prevention. Cardiol Clin 1998;16(4):623–632, vii-viii.
44. Papadopoulos DP, Moyssakis I, Makris TK, et al. Clinical significance of matrix metalloproteinases activity in acute myocardial infarction. Eur Cytokine Netw 2005;16(2):152–160.
45. Katz AM. Cardiac interstitium in health and disease: the fibrillar collagen network. J Am Coll Cardiol 1989;13:1637–1652.
46. Woodiwiss AJ, Tsotetsi OJ, Sprott S, et al. Reduction in myocardial collagen cross-linking parallels left ventricular dilatation in rat models of systolic chamber dysfunction. Circulation 2001;103(1):155–160.

7
Normal Physiology and Pathophysiology of Left Ventricular Diastole

Gilles W. De Keulenaer and Dirk L. Brutsaert

The diastole of the heart has captured the imagination of scientists ever since antiquity. Not surprisingly, the meaning of the word *diastole* has often been changed, as most scientific words change when novel experimental observations lead to new theories and concepts. At some instants in history, some physiologists even insisted that the terms *systole* and *diastole* ought to be banished altogether due to the confusion about the meaning and exact delineation of both phases in the overall cardiac cycle (1). Wiggers's almost dogmatic subdivision of the cardiac cycle temporarily ended, however, an era of controversy, although he himself admitted that it was difficult to correlate end ejection with valve closure and to delineate where systole ceases and relaxation starts (Fig. 7.1).

Since the recognition of impaired relaxation and filling of the heart as an early and common feature in various cardiac diseases, however, there has been renewed interest in diastolic function of the heart. Meanwhile, our understanding of the function of the heart as a muscular pump—as opposed to the previous approach to the heart as a hemodynamic pump—has advanced substantially and has led us to revise the subdivision of the cardiac cycle (2–4). These considerations about the function of the heart as a muscular pump constitute the central concept behind this chapter on normal and abnormal diastolic function of the ventricle.

Diastole and Diastolic Dysfunction at the Level of the Ventricular Muscular Pump System

Any discussion about normal and abnormal diastolic function of the ventricle is inevitably linked to the fact that the heart is as much a muscle as it is a pump. When evaluating the function of this muscular pump, therefore, one should always take into account the mechanical properties of the cardiac muscle as well as those of the cardiac pump. As further illustrated in Figure 7.1, the most important physiologic consequence of these aspects of the cardiac muscular pump system, at least with respect to the analysis of cardiac diastole, is that the fall in pressure during ventricular isovolumic relaxation (that fully completes at end-systolic volumes) and the increase in ventricular volume during early rapid filling are inherent parts of the contraction-relaxation cycle of the cardiac muscular "systole" (2–4). Theoretically, "true" diastole of the "muscular" pump encompasses only diastasis and the atrial contraction phase and, hence, starts clearly after early rapid ventricular filling. In the in vivo ventricle, however, early rapid filling should be considered as a gray zone between systole and diastole, as its properties may slightly diverge from those of the rapid reextension of a relaxing isolated cardiac muscle due to the involvement of a number of

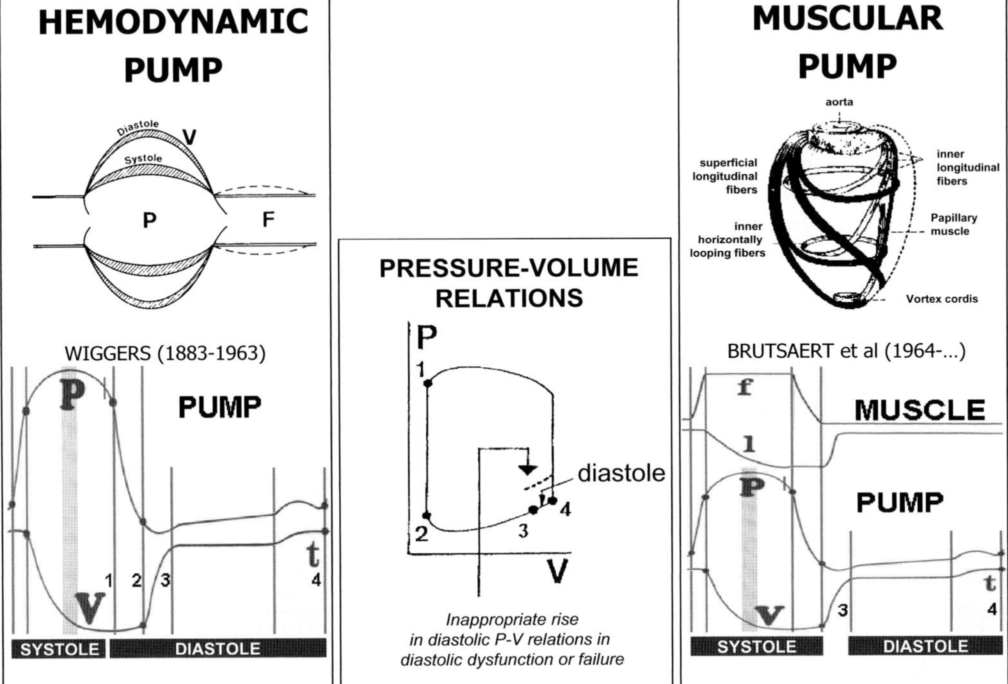

FIGURE 7.1. Subdivision of the cardiac cycle in a ventricular hemodynamic pump versus a ventricular muscular pump. (Left) Wiggers' traditional subdivision, with systole ending slightly prior to aortic valve closure. (Middle) Ventricular pressure-volume relations, illustrating upward shift at (end-) diastole in patients with diastolic dysfunction and/or diastolic failure. (Right) Novel insights, since the early 1960s, into the intracellular physiological and pathophysiological mechanisms of the heart as a muscular pump, which were obviously unknown in the Wiggers' era, have logically led to reconsidering the traditional Wiggers' subdivision of the cardiac cycle. The figure compares the time traces (*t*) of an afterloaded twitch in cardiac muscle (*f*, force; *l*, length) with the synchronized time traces of pressure (*P*) and volume (*V*) of a ventricular hemodynamic pump. The similarity between the corresponding time traces has led to the inclusion of isovolumic relaxation into systole of a ventricular muscular pump. Although the rapid filling phase should, on the same conceptual grounds, also be seen as part of systole, we prefer—because of a number of (non-muscular) hemodynamic, i.e. mostly flow-related variables—to consider this phase rather as a transition between systole and diastole. This subtle modification to our previous re-appraisal of the cardiac cycle emphasizes that during early rapid filling, the properties of a pump may indeed diverge somewhat from those of a muscle (2–4).

(nonmuscular) hemodynamic factors. By contrast, left ventricular (LV) isovolumic relaxation clearly belongs to systole of the ventricular muscular pump. At normal rest heart rates, diastole, that is, diastasis and atrial contraction, usually lasts for approximately 50% of the total time duration of the cardiac cycle. In a pressure-volume diagram, however, diastole represents only the last 5% to 15% of ventricular filling (points 3 to 4 in Fig. 7.1) (3, 4).

As a consequence, diastolic dysfunction should refer to a disease process that shifts the *end portion* of the pressure-volume diagram inappropriately upward so that LV filling pressures are increased disproportionally to the magnitude of LV dilatation. The causes of such a shift can be subdivided as follows:

1. Inappropriate tachycardia (e.g., transient atrial fibrillation, supraventricular tachyarrhythmias, resulting in inappropriate abbreviation of diastolic duration)
2. A decrease in ventricular diastolic compliance
3. Impairment in ventricular systolic relaxation, that is, impaired isovolumic pressure fall (and/or impaired early rapid filling)
4. A combination of 1, 2, and 3, as is usually the case

By extension of the above statements, it follows that impaired ventricular relaxation—as it is the last part of systole of the muscular pump—should not be called diastolic dysfunction, although it can itself be the cause of an inappropriate upward shift of the end portion of the pressure-volume diagram, and, therefore, of diastolic heart failure. *Instead, impaired ventricular relaxation should be retained as an early and isolated manifestation of systolic dysfunction.* Obviously, in daily clinical practice, it is not trivial to diagnose whether impaired ventricular relaxation (e.g., recorded on echo Doppler as a prolonged isovolumic relaxation time [IVRT] or reversed E-wave/A-wave relation) does or does not cause such an upward shift of the end portion of the pressure-volume diagram. Fortunately, there is emerging evidence that additional diagnostic efforts, for example by applying tissue Doppler or by assessing serum B-type natriuretic peptide (BNP) or N-terminal-pro-BNP, may help to scrutinize between these different clinical conditions.

Definition of Diastolic Heart Failure

Heart failure is a clinical syndrome characterized by symptoms and signs of decreased tissue perfusion and increased tissue water. Defining the cause of this syndrome requires measurements of both systolic and diastolic function. When abnormalities in diastolic function are predominant and abnormalities in hemodynamic pump function are absent or mild (e.g., preserved ejection fraction), this syndrome is called “diastolic heart failure” or “heart failure with preserved ejection fraction.”

Therefore, diastolic heart failure can be defined as a clinical syndrome characterized by the symptoms and signs of heart failure, a preserved ejection fraction, and diastolic dysfunction. Importantly, as we will see below, a preserved ejection fraction indicates that systolic hemodynamic pump performance (sometimes called “global pump” performance) is preserved, whereas contractile function of the myocardium may already be compromised. From a conceptual perspective, diastolic heart failure occurs when the ventricular chamber is unable to accept an adequate volume of blood during diastole, at normal diastolic pressures, and at volumes sufficient to maintain an appropriate stroke volume. These abnormalities are caused by impaired ventricular relaxation or by an increase in ventricular stiffness, both resulting in higher filling pressures at rest; more frequently, these impairments may produce elevated filling pressures during exercise or result in exercise dyspnea or so-called exercise intolerance.

Impaired Ventricular Relaxation and Decreased Compliance in Diastolic Heart Failure

Diastolic heart failure can be caused by impaired ventricular relaxation (in fact a process of systole but at the same time a possible cause of diastolic heart failure when disturbed, see above) and by decreased diastolic compliance (defined by the pressure-volume relationship). Causes of impaired relaxation or compliance (Table 7.1) can be divided into (1) factors intrinsic to the cardiomyocyte, (2) factors within the extracellular matrix that surrounds the cardiomyocytes, and (3) factors that activate the production of neurohormones and paracrine factors (5). To varying extents, these factors play a role in diastolic heart failure, but much remains to be learned about how these factors interplay, and to what extent therapeutic targeting would result in prognostic or symptomatic improvements.

Cardiomyocyte

Elements and processes intrinsic to the cardiomyocyte contributing to diastolic (dys)function have been summarized in Table 7.1. In general, these relate to processes responsible for calcium removal from the myocyte cytosol (calcium homeostasis), to processes involved in cross-bridge detachment, and to cytoskeletal functional elements. Changes in any of the processes and elements can lead to abnormalities in both active relaxation and passive stiffness. For a detailed discussion, the interested reader is

TABLE 7.1. Causes leading to diastolic dysfunction

Inappropriate tachycardia	Impaired systolic relaxation	Decreased compliance
Intermittent atrial fibrillation; atrial tachyarrhythmlas	➢ **Load-induced** ■ Pressure-volume overload ➢ **Impaired inactivation processes** ■ Calcium homeostasis ✓ calcium overload ✓ calcium transport (sarcolemma, SR) ✓ modifying proteins (phospholamban, calmodulin, . . .) ■ Myofilaments ✓ Tn-C calcium binding ✓ Tn-I phosphorylation ✓ myofilament calcium sensitivity ■ Energetics ✓ ADP/ATP ratio ✓ ADP and Pi concentration ➢ **Nonuniformity of load or inactivation processes in space or time** ■ E.g. "asynchrony" by conduction disturbances ➢ **Abnormal activity of RAAS, OS, ANP/BNP, cardiac endothelial system**	➢ **Extracellular matrix** ■ Fibrillar collagen ■ Basement membrane proteins ■ Proteoglycans ■ MMP/TIMP ➢ **Abnormal activity of cardiac endothelial system (especially NO)** ➢ **Cytoskeletal abnormalities** ■ Microtubules ■ Intermediates filaments (desmin) ■ Titin ■ Nebulin

ADP, adenosine diphosphate; ANP, atrial natriuretic protein; ATP, adenosine triphosphate; BNP, B-type natriuretic protein; MMP, matrix metaloproteinase; NO, nitric oxide; OS, orthosympathic nerve system; RAAS, renin-angiotensin-aldosterone system; Tn-C, troponin-C; Tn-I, troponin-I. Modified from Zile and Brutsaert (5).

referred to more extensive reviews on this topic (6).

Extracellular Matrix

Changes in the structures within the extracellular matrix (ECM) can also affect diastolic function. The myocardial ECM is composed of three important constituents: (1) fibrillar protein, such as collagen type I, type III, and elastin; (2) proteoglycans; and (3) basement membrane protein such as collagen type IV, laminin, and fibronectin. It has been hypothesized that the most important component within the ECM that contributes to the development of diastolic heart failure is fibrillar collagen (amount, geometry, distribution, degree of cross-linking, ratio of collagen type I to III) (7–9). Collagen synthesis is altered by load, both preload and afterload, by neurohormonal activation (e.g., the renin-angiotensin-aldosterone system [RAAS] and the sympathic nervous system), and by growth factors. Collagen degradation is under the control of proteolytic enzymes including matrix metalloproteinases. Any change in the regulatory processes affecting collagen degradation and synthesis can alter diastolic function.

Neurohormonal and Cardiac Endothelial Activation

Both acutely and chronically, neurohormonal and cardiac endothelial activation and inhibition have been shown to alter diastolic function. Chronic activation of the RAAS increases ECM fibrillar collagen, whereas inhibition of the RAAS prevents or reverses this increase. Generally but not consistently, these changes have been shown to affect myocardial stiffness. Acute activation of the cardiac endothelial system has been shown to alter relaxation and stiffness (10, 10a). These acute changes in endothelial function induce rapid responses too fast to involve the ECM; therefore, the cardiac endothelium seems to act on the cardiomyocyte directly (10a) and to affect one or more cellular determinants of diastolic function within a very short time frame. For example, in the heart there is cyclical release of nitric oxide (NO) that is most pronounced subendocardially and that peaks at the time of relaxation and filling. These brief bursts of NO release provide a beat-to-beat modulation of relaxation and stiffness (11).

Systolic Dysfunction in Diastolic Dysfunction and Failure

Recent observations with advanced imaging technology have revealed significant systolic abnormalities of the ventricular muscular pump in patients with diastolic dysfunction and failure. These abnormalities have been objectified by tissue Doppler imaging, radionuclide imaging, and magnetic resonance imaging (12–22) as ventricular segmental or longitudinal dysfunction (Fig. 7.2). Importantly, these systolic abnormalities occur at normal ventricular ejection fractions, reminding us that ejection fraction and parameters directly or indirectly related to it are indices of the ventricular hemodynamic pump, insensitive for measuring the performance of ventricular muscular pump (Table 7.2). A preserved ejection fraction merely indicates that the radial (or circumferential) fibers of the ventricle compensate for longitudinal LV dysfunction to preserve overall hemodynamic pump performance, but does not imply that the systolic function of the muscular pump is normal (23).

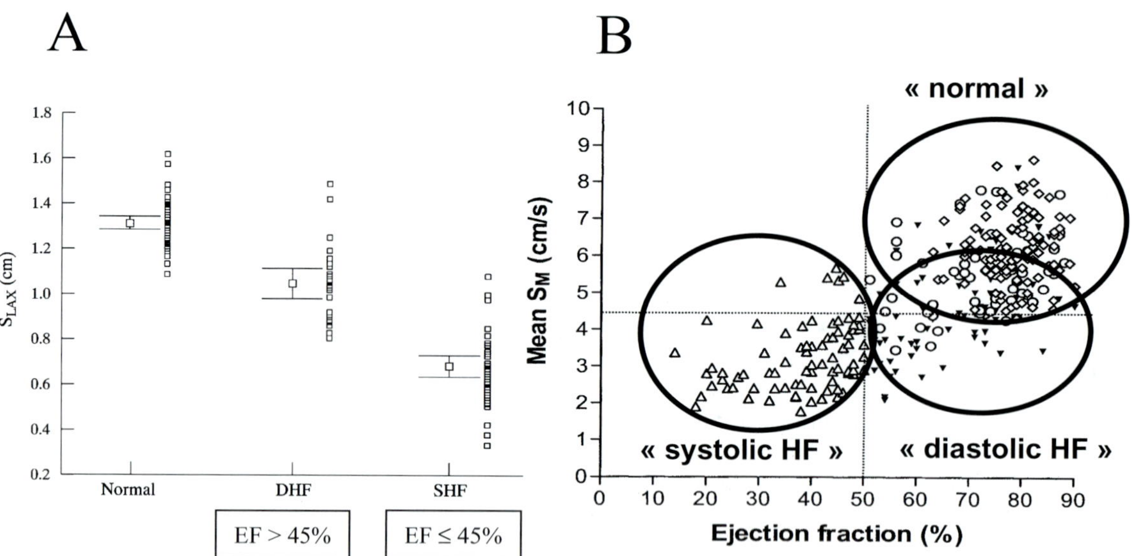

FIGURE 7.2. Heart failure with preserved ejection fraction (HFprEF) is commonly accompanied by various degrees of systolic dysfunction. In particular through excessive nonuniformities and impaired longitudinal myocardial function, the latter indicating radial compensation for longitudinal left ventricular (LV) dysfunction. (A) Systolic mitral annular amplitude by long axis M mode echo (S_{LAX}) reveals a significant decrease in patients with HFprEF despite a preserved left ventricular ejection fraction (LVEF) >45%. (Modified from Yip et al. [12].) (B) Scatter plot of mean regional myocardial sustained systolic velocity (mean SM) from a six–basal segmental model by tissue Doppler imaging (TDI) plotted as a function of LVEF; importantly, in the lower right quadrant, the mean SM has already significantly decreased in about 50% of patients with HFprEF ≥50%. DHF, diastolic heart failure; SHF, systolic heart failuce. (Modified from Yu et al. [17].)

TABLE 7.2. Assessment of left ventricular function

Cardiac input–output system	Ventricular hemodynamic pump	Ventricular muscular pump
SWANN-GANZ catheterization – cardiac output (CO) = stroke volume (SV) × HR – arterial pressure (Part) – peripheral resistance (R) – arterial elastance (Ea) – stroke work (SW) = Part × SV – Pven (rt atr P) – PCWP (*lt atr P; LVEDP*) – SW *vs* PCWP (LVEDP) **ventricular function curve**	➢ <u>– Time</u> – ventricular PRESSURE-VOLUME curves – ventricular wall stress-strain (Laplace Law) – **LVEDV; LVESV; LVmass** – LVMI/LVEDVI ratio – LVEDP/LVEDV ratio – **LV Ejection Fraction = (LVEDV – LVESV) / LVEDV** – preload recruitable stroke work (SW) = SW vs LVEDV (ventricular function curve) – elastance (Emax; Ees; Ed) – systolic blood pressure vs end-systolic LV diameter – Echo-Doppler E/A ratio; **Left atrial size** ➢ <u>+ Time</u> – peak(+)dP/dt; peak(–)dP/dt; tau – LV ejection rate; LV power (reserve) – time-varying elastance – **systolic time Intervals**; time interval ratio **PEP/ET** – arterial impedance – **Echo-Doppler** IVRT; early mitral inflow velocity E; deceleration time DT; A wave	NETWORK of MUSCLE FIBERS <u>**I. CONTRACTION**</u> myocardial (ventricular) contractility <u>**II. RELAXATION**</u> – **time to onset of relaxation** [t-end ejection; t-(–)dP/dt; Echo-Doppler or MRI time intervals] <u>**III. UNIFORMITY**</u> **TDI (MRI)** – ventricular twisting-untwisting – regional ventricular torsion – mitral annular shortening – mitral annular shortening velocity Em – E / Em ratio at rest and exercise (~LVEDP) – long axis vs radial shortening (& velocity) – myocardial segmental velocity – myocardial segmental strain (~local EF?) – myocardial strain rate – transmural myocardial strain rate profile – differences in regional or segmental time intervals of peak velocities and strains CELL COMMUNICATION – **Cardiac Cellular BIOMARKERS . . . BNP; NT-proBNP; Other?** – **Molecular Imaging Techniques**

LVEDP, left ventricular end-diastolic pressure: LVEDV, left ventricular end-diastolic volume; LVESV, left ventricular end-systolic volume; PEP/ET, pre-ejection period/ejection time. Modified from Brutsaert and DeKeulenaer (4, 23). Currently most frequently used indices are printed in bold.

Diastolic and Systolic Heart Failure Progress Along a Single Pathophysiological Time Trajectory

The observation with the newest cardiac imaging techniques of marked systolic abnormalities in patients with diastolic heart failure has led to reconsidering some traditional pathophysiologic paradigms of heart failure progression. Heart failure progression can now be presented, for example, in a time trajectory in which diastolic and systolic heart failure progress along a single pathophysiologic time line (Fig. 7.3). In this graph, progression of hemodynamic pump dysfunction (as calculated by ejection fraction) is plotted against time and as such can be subdivided into three somewhat arbitrary consecutive pathophysiologic phases: systolic activation, systolic dysfunction, and hemodynamic pump failure (Fig. 7.3 legend). The first two phases, systolic activation and systolic dysfunction, are phases of compensated hemodynamic pump function following cardiac stress, as indicated by the normal levels of ejection fraction, although ejection fraction may be slightly reduced already. A thorough understanding of the systolic-dysfunction phase in the presence of compensated (i.e., preserved) LV ejection fraction is an essential step in understanding diastolic dysfunction and failure.

The systolic activation phase is reversible and reflects activation of all adaptive mechanisms of cardiac performance, including homeometric (neurohormones) and heterometric (Starling's law) autoregulatory mechanisms or associated with early ventricular hypertrophy. A key feature of this phase consists of the capacity to modulate the time of onset of ventricular relaxation, and hence to adjust within the cardiac cycle the systolic time window during which the ventricle can deliver stroke work.

Gradually the above autoregulatory mechanisms become maladaptive, leading to the second stage of systolic dysfunction of the ventricular muscle pump (with impaired regional systolic function), occurring at still normal levels of LV

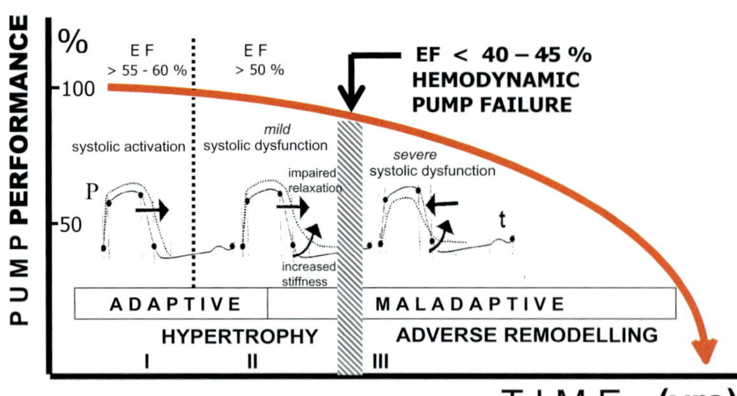

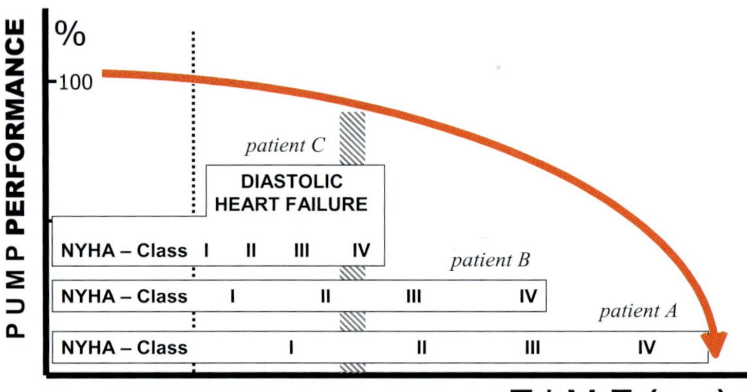

FIGURE 7.3. Time progression paradigm of chronic heart failure. Top: Pathophysiologic time progression. Deterioration of pump performance during the progression of chronic heart failure evolves in three successive, somewhat arbitrary, phases. Bottom: Clinical time progression. The clinical time progression, as evident from the superimposed clinical symptoms and signs of heart failure according to the New York Heart Association (NYHA) classification, paradoxically diverges from the pathophysiologic progression as depicted by a single time trajectory. (Modified from De Keulenaer and Brutsaert [34].)

ejection fraction. Though early in this stage the onset of ventricular relaxation is still delayed as part of the initial systolic activation process, this adaptive process gradually progresses into a maladaptive slowed rate of relaxation, with a progressive loss of the ventricle to modulate the timing of onset of relaxation. As explained above and reviewed in greater detail (2–4), slowed relaxation is caused by three major processes: (1) dysfunction of intracellular myocardial inactivation; (2) inappropriate volume or pressure loading, including those induced by arterial elastance abnormalities (24); and (3) and excessive nonuniformity (3, 4, 10a). Clearly at this stage, symptoms of heart failure may already be triggered or be continuously present (Fig. 7.3, lower part), leading to the diagnosis of so-called diastolic heart failure but in fact only presenting a premature clinical manifestation of systolic dysfunction of the muscular pump. These symptoms generally occur during exercise, during episodes of inappropriate tachycardia, during sudden increases in volume load, or at instants of increased diastolic LV stiffness (e.g., induced by ischemia) or further impairments of LV systolic relaxation (e.g., induced by hypertensive crises).

Finally, during a third stage, below a threshold LV ejection fraction of 45% to 50%, overt systolic-diastolic heart failure with severely compromised hemodynamic pump performance develops in about 50% to 60% of patients. Meanwhile, hypertrophy of the ventricle irreversibly evolves into so-called adverse remodeling. Adverse remodeling is still an ill-defined term indicating activation of a number of structural and functional abnormalities, which may result in myocardial fibrosis/necrosis and irreversible dilatation.

Divergent Symptom Time Trajectories Lead to a Spectrum of Chronic Heart Failure Phenotypes

Although in Figure 7.3 heart failure is presented as one disease with a single pathophysiologic time trajectory, the paradoxical divergence between the pathophysiologic progression of hemodynamic pump dysfunction and the time course of symptom progression is, as yet, unexplained. This paradox is manifested most clearly in patients with so-called diastolic heart failure, that is, heart failure at a preserved ejection fraction. In fact, heart failure symptoms may occur at any stage of hemodynamic pump dysfunction (i.e., any level of ejection fraction).

Therefore, in Figure 7.4, chronic heart failure is presented schematically as a disease with multiple, in the time spectrum diverging, clinical patient-specific trajectories. To the left of the spectrum, patients suffer from chronic heart failure, with end-stage nondilated ventricles and New York Heart Association (NYHA) class III to IV symptoms, but a normal ejection fraction. Although often considered as originating from pure diastolic dysfunction and failure, most if not all of these patients have regional myocardial systolic dysfunction, in particular of the longitudinal, mainly subendocardial myocardial fibers, unless they suffer from external pericardial constriction without cardiomyopathy, which clearly is a distinct disease.

To the right of the spectrum in Figure 7.4, patients suffer from chronic heart failure with dilated and highly remodeled ventricles, advanced muscular and hemodynamic pump dysfunction with low ejection fraction, and NYHA class III to IV symptoms. Again, these patients do not suffer from pure systolic dysfunction, as 80% of the patients studied in clinical trials (e.g., the SOLVD, Studies of Left ventricular Dysfunction study) have signs of diastolic dysfunction as well. In addition, Yotti et al. (25) recently reported that ventricular dilation itself impairs diastolic filling by enhancing convective deceleration. Along with slowed relaxation, reduced elastic recoil, and displacement onto the stiff portion of the left ventricular end-diastolic pressure (LVEDP)–left ventricular end-diastolic volume (LVEDV) relation, increased convective deceleration may thus also contribute to the substantial diastolic dysfunction observed in the patients (26).

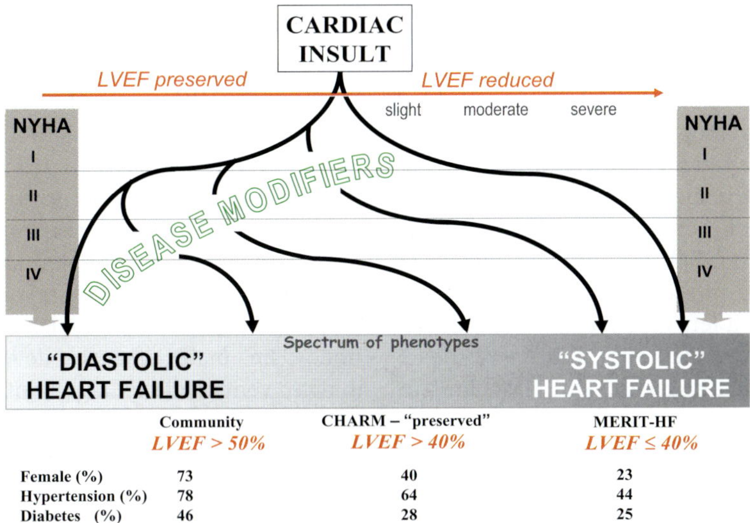

	Community	CHARM – "preserved"	MERIT-HF
	LVEF > 50%	*LVEF > 40%*	*LVEF ≤ 40%*
Female (%)	73	40	23
Hypertension (%)	78	64	44
Diabetes (%)	46	28	25

Figure 7.4. Phenotype paradigm of chronic heart failure. Chronic heart failure may from a phenotypical point of view progress along an infinite number of time trajectories, each one being unique for any individual patient; patients may thus develop signs and symptoms of heart failure over a wide range of pathophysiologic stages of the same disease, varying from stages with a preserved LVEF (left) to stages with a severely reduced LVEF (right) and leading to a spectrum of heart failure phenotypes. CHARM, Candesartan in Heart Failure Assessement of Reduction in Mortality and Morbidity. MERIT-HF, Metoprolol CR/XL Randomised Intervention Trial in Congestive Heart Failure. (Modified from De Keulenaer and Brutsaert [34].)

Accordingly, there is currently no basis to postulate that ejection fraction is an appropriate parameter to subdivide heart failure in two separate nonoverlapping disease identities. Instead, as evident from Figure 7.4, chronic heart failure is a disease characterized by a continuous spectrum of clinical phenotypes in which most if not all cases of heart failure are hybrids of so-called systolic and diastolic heart failure. Extreme forms of diastolic heart failure without systolic myocardial dysfunction or systolic heart failure without diastolic dysfunction are extremely rare or nonexistent and should not be presented as representative for the total heart failure population.

The Spectrum of Heart Failure Phenotypes Is Explained by Disease Modifiers

Current scientific evidence suggests that each patient's time trajectory within the heart failure spectrum depends on a number of disease modifiers that may be extrinsic or intrinsic to the heart. This hypothesis is derived from epidemiologic and clinical patient studies, as well as from experimental animal studies that have identified differences in genotypic or phenotypic characteristics of subpopulations with heart failure. First, epidemiologic studies and clinical trials have enabled comparing the demographic and the clinical characteristics of patients with heart failure at various degrees of hemodynamic pump dysfunction. In Figure 7.4, for example, gender, incidence of hypertension and diabetes, and age have been compared for three different groups of heart failure patients: those with left ventricular ejection fraction (LVEF) of more than 50%, those with LVEF more than 40%, and those with LVEF less than 40% (27–29). Strikingly, female gender, diabetes, and hypertension were more common in the first group, patients with heart failure at preserved ejection fraction, than in the third group, and at intermediate incidence in the second group. From this, it would appear as if these "modifying" conditions in patients with heart failure at preserved ejection fraction would somehow protect the heart from dilation, remodeling, and hemodynamic pump failure, but paradoxically not from developing symptoms of heart failure, thereby directing the patient's individual clinical trajectory toward the left in Figure 7.4.

A causative role for diabetes, female gender, and hypertension as modifiers of a patient's individual clinical trajectory is further endorsed by animal and clinical studies specifically addressing the impact of the above disease modifiers on ventricular remodeling and heart failure symptoms. For example, in a SAVE (Survivial and Ventricular Enlargement trial) substudy on 512 patients postinfarct, Solomon and coworkers (30) reported that, compared with nondiabetics, diabetics were at higher risk of developing heart failure (in 30% of the cases in diabetes patients vs. 17% in nondiabetes patients), but they were at the same time protected from ventricular systolic and diastolic dilatation (30). This observation is consistent with the hypothesis that diabetes has an important modifying impact on the clinical trajectory of heart failure after myocardial injury.

Similarly, in a prospective follow-up study of 953 patients successfully treated with primary percutaneous coronary intervention for acute myocardial infarction, Parodi et al. (31) found that hypertensive patients were at significantly higher risk of developing heart failure than normotensive patients, despite the fact that ventricular end-diastolic volume did not change in the hypertensives, whereas it did significantly increase in the normotensives. Hypertensive patients showed more hospitalizations for heart failure despite identical ventricular ejection fractions in hypertensive and normotensive patients.

Finally, in studies on the impact of gender in heart failure progression, female rats exposed to pressure overload (32) or myocardial infarction (33) were resistant to ventricular diastolic dilatation. The male animals developed, however, marked ventricular enlargement and concomitant reductions in ventricular ejection fraction and had a worse prognosis, consistent with a modifying role of gender on heart failure phenotype.

Thus it has been demonstrated that heart failure progression is critically dependent on a number of disease modifiers that profoundly influence the degree of ventricular remodeling and dilatation. At the same time, symptom progression after myocardial injury, often evolves, paradoxically, in an opposite direction (e.g., less remodeling but more symptoms of heart failure). The prevalence of these modifiers is distributed unevenly among patients at risk for heart failure. Intriguingly, the prevalence of numerous modifiers gradually increases when comparing groups of heart failure patients with increasing ejection fraction. This observation indicates that the effects of these modifiers are additive and as such lead to a spectrum of heart failure phenotypes, ranging from low to preserved ejection fraction.

Conclusion

We have focused on the physiology and pathophysiology of diastolic dysfunction and failure. Throughout the discussion, we have maintained a view of the heart as a muscular pump. From this conceptual approach, we have defined diastole as the very last part of the cardiac cycle (diastasis and atrial contraction) and of the pressure-volume relation, and introduced the conjecture that diastolic heart failure can result from abnormalities in both diastole and systole. The recent observations with novel cardiac imaging techniques of systolic dysfunction in patients with heart failure at preserved ejection fractions have further reinforced the conjecture that systolic and diastolic heart failure are more closely related than previously anticipated.

Hence, the binary view of chronic heart failure with two distinct phenotypes, systolic heart failure and diastolic heart failure, was replaced by a view that heart failure is a continuous spectrum of phenotypes in which the two extremes, i.e. (pure) diastolic and (pure) systolic heart failure, do probably not exist. The origin of this spectrum was explained by an uneven distribution of disease modifiers in patients at risk for heart failure, in which each of these modifiers affect ventricular remodeling and symptom progression during the progression of heart failure, paradoxically often in an opposite direction.

References

1. Edgren JG. Kardiographische und sphygmografische Studien. Skan Arch Physiol 1889;1:66–151.
2. Brutsaert DL, Sys SU. Diastolic dysfunction in heart failure. J Card Fail 1997;3:225–42.
3. Brutsaert DL, Sys SU. Relaxation and diastole of the heart. Physiol Rev 1989;69:1228–315.
4. Brutsaert DL. Cardiac dysfunction in heart failure: the cardiologist is love affair with time. Prog Cardiovasc Dis 2006;49:157–81.
5. Zile MR, Brutsaert DL. New concepts in diastolic dysfunction and diastolic heart failure: Part II: causal mechanisms and treatment. Circulation 2002;105:1503–8.
6. Kass DA, Bronzwaer JG, Paulus WJ. What mechanisms underlie diastolic dysfunction in heart failure? Circ Res 2004;94:1533–42.
7. Jalil JE, Doering CW, Janicki JS, Pick R, Shroff SG, Weber KT. Fibrillar collagen and myocardial stiffness in the intact hypertrophied rat left ventricle. Circ Res 1989;64:1041–50.
8. Weber KT, Janicki JS, Pick R, Capasso J, Anversa P. Myocardial fibrosis and pathologic hypertrophy in the rat with renovascular hypertension. Am J Cardiol 1990;65:1G–7G.
9. Kato S, Spinale FG, Tanaka R, Johnson W, Cooper G 4th, Zile MR. Inhibition of collagen cross-linking: effects on fibrillar collagen and ventricular diastolic function. Am J Physiol 1995;269: H863–8.
10. Paulus WJ, Vantrimpont PJ, Shah AM. Paracrine coronary endothelial control of left ventricular function in humans. Circulation 1995;92:2119–26.

10a. Brutsaert DL. Cardiac endothelial-myocardial signalling: its role in cardiac growth, contractile performance, and rhythmicity. Physiol Rev 2003; 83:59–115.

11. Pinsky DJ, Patton S, Mesaros S, et al. Mechanical transduction of nitric oxide synthesis in the beating heart. Circ Res 1997;81:372–9.
12. Yip G, Wang M, Zhang Y, Fung JW, Ho PY, Sanderson JE. Left ventricular long axis function in diastolic heart failure is reduced in both diastole and systole: time for a redefinition? Heart 2002;87:121–5.
13. Petrie MC, Caruana L, Berry C, McMurray JJ. "Diastolic heart failure" or heart failure caused by subtle left ventricular systolic dysfunction? Heart 2002;87:29–31.
14. Nikitin NP, Witte KK, Clark AL, Cleland JG. Color tissue Doppler-derived long-axis left ventricular function in heart failure with preserved global systolic function. Am J Cardiol 2002;90:1174–7.
15. Vinereanu D, Nicolaides E, Tweddel AC, Fraser AG. "Pure" diastolic dysfunction is associated with long-axis systolic dysfunction. Implications for the diagnosis and classification of heart failure. Eur J Heart Fail 2005;7:820–8.

16. Garcia EH, Perna ER, Farias EF, et al. Reduced systolic performance by tissue Doppler in patients with preserved and abnormal ejection fraction: New insights in chronic heart failure. Int J Cardiol 2006;108:181–8.
17. Yu CM, Lin H, Yang H, Kong SL, Zhang Q, Lee SW. Progression of systolic abnormalities in patients with "isolated" diastolic heart failure and diastolic dysfunction. Circulation 2002;105:1195–201.
18. Bruch C, Gradaus R, Gunia S, Breithardt G, Wichter T. Doppler tissue analysis of mitral annular velocities: evidence for systolic abnormalities in patients with diastolic heart failure. J Am Soc Echocardiogr 2003;16:1031–6.
19. Nagueh SF, McFalls J, Meyer D, et al. Tissue Doppler imaging predicts the development of hypertrophic cardiomyopathy in subjects with subclinical disease. Circulation 2003;108:395–8.
20. Rosen BD, Edvardsen T, Lai S, et al. Left ventricular concentric remodeling is associated with decreased global and regional systolic function: the Multi-Ethnic Study of Atherosclerosis. Circulation 2005;112:984–91.
21. Fonseca CG, Oxenham HC, Cowan BR, Occleshaw CJ, Young AA. Aging alters patterns of regional nonuniformity in LV strain relaxation: a 3-D MR tissue tagging study. Am J Physiol Heart Circ Physiol 2003;285:H621–30.
22. Rosen BD, Gerber BL, Edvardsen T, et al. Late systolic onset of regional LV relaxation demonstrated in three-dimensional space by MRI tissue tagging. Am J Physiol Heart Circ Physiol 2004;287: H1740–6.
23. Brutsaert DL, De Keulenaer GW. Diastolic heart failure: a myth. Curr Opin Cardiol 2006;21:240–248.
24. Kawaguchi M, Hay I, Fetics B, Kass DA. Combined ventricular systolic and arterial stiffening in patients with heart failure and preserved ejection fraction: implications for systolic and diastolic reserve limitations. Circulation 2003;107:714–20.
25. Yotti R, Bermejo J, Antoranz JC, et al. A noninvasive method for assessing impaired diastolic suction in patients with dilated cardiomyopathy. Circulation 2005;112:2921–9.
26. Little WC. Diastolic dysfunction beyond distensibility: adverse effects of ventricular dilatation. Circulation 2005;112:2888–90.
27. Klapholz M, Maurer M, Lowe AM, et al. Hospitalization for heart failure in the presence of a normal left ventricular ejection fraction: results of the New York Heart Failure Registry. J Am Coll Cardiol 2004;43:1432–8.
28. Yusuf S, Pfeffer MA, Swedberg K, et al. CHARM Investigators and Committees. Effects of candesartan in patients with chronic heart failure and preserved left-ventricular ejection fraction: the CHARM-Preserved Trial. Lancet 2003;362:777–81.
29. The Merit-HF study group. Effect of metoprolol CR/XL in chronic heart failure: Metoprolol CR/XL Randomised Intervention Trial in Congestive Heart Failure (MERIT-HF). Lancet 1999;353: 2001–7.
30. Solomon SD, St. John Sutton M, Lamas GA, et al. Ventricular remodeling does not accompany the development of heart failure in diabetic patients after myocardial infarction. Circulation 2002;106: 1251.
31. Parodi G, Carrabba N, Santoro GM, et al. Heart failure and left ventricular remodeling after reperfused acute myocardial infarction in patients with hypertension. Hypertension 2006;7:706–10.
32. Douglas PS, Katz SE, Weinberg EO, Chen MH, Bishop SP, Lorell BH. Hypertrophic remodeling: gender differences in the early response to left ventricular pressure overload. J Am Coll Cardiol 1998;32:1118–25.
33. Cavasin MA, Tao Z, Menon S, Yang XP. Gender differences in cardiac function during early remodeling after acute myocardial infarction in mice. Life Sci 2004;75:2181–92.
34. De Keulenaer GW, Brutsaert DL. Different Phenotypes of the Same Disease? Eur J Heart Failure 2007;9:136–43.

8
Normal Physiology and Pathophysiology of the Right Ventricle

Etienne Gayat and Alexandre Mebazaa

Until recently, the right ventricle (RV) was considered as a moderately passive conduit between the systemic and pulmonary circulations. This belief was supported by studies showing that complete destruction of the right ventricular free wall in dogs had no detectable impairment on overall cardiac performance (1). However, investigations in the 1970s demonstrated that right ventricular failure (RVF) has significant hemodynamic and cardiac performance effects (2).

Right ventricular failure has a similar incidence to that of left-sided heart failure, with each affecting about 1 in 20 of the population (3). In contrast with left-sided heart failure, which is often a chronic, progressive disease with a mortality four to eight times greater than that of age-matched general population (4), the outcome of RVF is broadly dependent on the underlying cause, resulting in either an acute or chronic condition. The importance of the right ventricular involvement in heart failure is illustrated by the fact that ischemia following a myocardial infarction involving both the right and the left ventricle results in a greater mortality than isolated left ventricular ischemia (5,6).

Normal Physiology of the Right Ventricle

The right ventricle provides low-pressure perfusion of the pulmonary vasculature, but is sensitive to changes in loading conditions and intrinsic contractility. Factors that affect right ventricular preload, right ventricular afterload, or left ventricular function can adversely influence the functioning of the RV and induce a worsen right ventricular failure (RVF).

Right Ventricular Preload

Preload can be defined as the initial stretching of the cardiac myocytes prior to contraction. In the normal heart, right ventricular preload is determined by the volume of blood that fills the RV at the end of passive filling and atrial contraction (i.e., the end-diastolic volume). Factors that can enhance ventricular preload include venous blood pressure (determined by venous blood volume and compliance), and the rate of venous return, which is influenced by blood volume, gravity, and mechanical activity of muscles and the respiratory system (Fig. 8.1).

Right Ventricular Afterload

The pressure-volume characteristics for the RV differ markedly from those of the left ventricle (7). The main difference is that the RV has only brief periods of isovolemic contraction and relaxation. There is sustained ejection during pressure development that, more importantly, continues during pressure decline. This prolonged low-pressure emptying implies that (1) blood is transferred from the venous bed to the pulmonary bed with a minimum of oxygen consumption, and (2) right ventricular emptying is very sensitive to changes in afterload. Thus, right ventricular function worsens parallel to elevation of the pulmonary

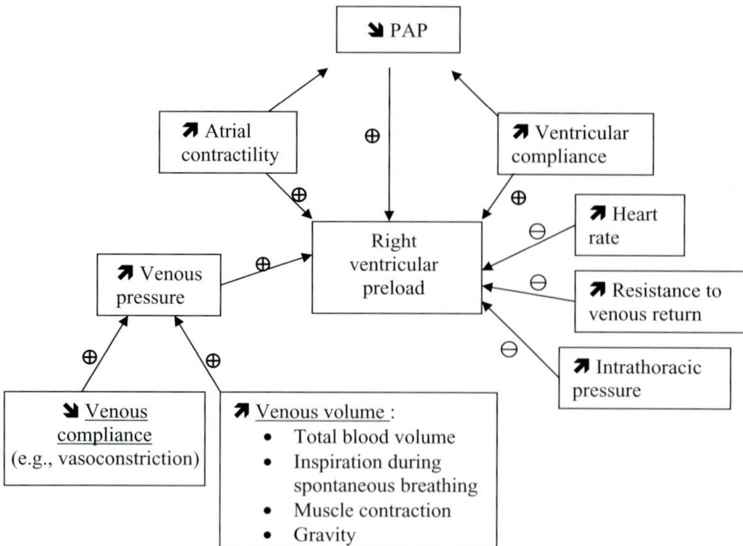

Figure 8.1. Factors determining right ventricular preload. The sign ⊕ means that the described factors lead to an increase in right ventricular preload. In contrast, the sign ⊕ means that the described factors lead to a fall of right ventricular preload. PAP, pulmonary arterial pressure.

arterial pressure (PAP), the main determinant of the right ventricular afterload.

The Right Heart Vascularization

Physiologically, right coronary artery perfusion occurs during both diastole and systole, in contrast to the left coronary artery, which supplies the left ventricular muscle mostly during diastole. However, if systolic PAP increases, right ventricular parietal pressure increases, occluding the right coronary artery during systole. Right coronary flow therefore predominantly occurs during diastole. In that condition, diastolic arterial pressure should be optimal in order to maintain sufficient right and left coronary blood flows (8).

Table 8.1. Normal right heart pressures

Variable	Value
Right atrial pressure*	
Mean	0–7 mm Hg
Right ventricular pressure	
Systolic	15–25 mm Hg
Diastolic	0–8 mm Hg
Pulmonary artery pressure	
Systolic	15–25 mm Hg
Diastolic	8–15 mm Hg
Mean	10–20 mm Hg
Wedge	6–12 mm Hg
Pulmonary vascular resistance	100–250 dyne/s per cm^5

*0–4 mm Hg in spontaneous breathing and 2–7 mm Hg in mechanical ventilation (normal lungs in zero end-expiratory pressure).

Normal Right Heart Pressure Values

The normal right heart pressure values are summarized in Table 8.1.

Pathophysiology of Right Heart Failure

Pathophysiologic changes in right heart failure vary according to the underlying cause, which are represented in Figure 8.2. Often, patients experience RVF secondary to a combination of decreased right ventricular contractility, increased right ventricular pressure, and increased right ventricular volume.

Right Ventricular Contractile Impairment

This condition occurs most often in cases of right ventricular ischemia and infarction. Usually, right ventricular infarction is due to proximal occlusion of the right coronary artery (RCA). In this condition, the RV is unable to contract against normal PAPs (Fig. 8.3). Accordingly, right ven-

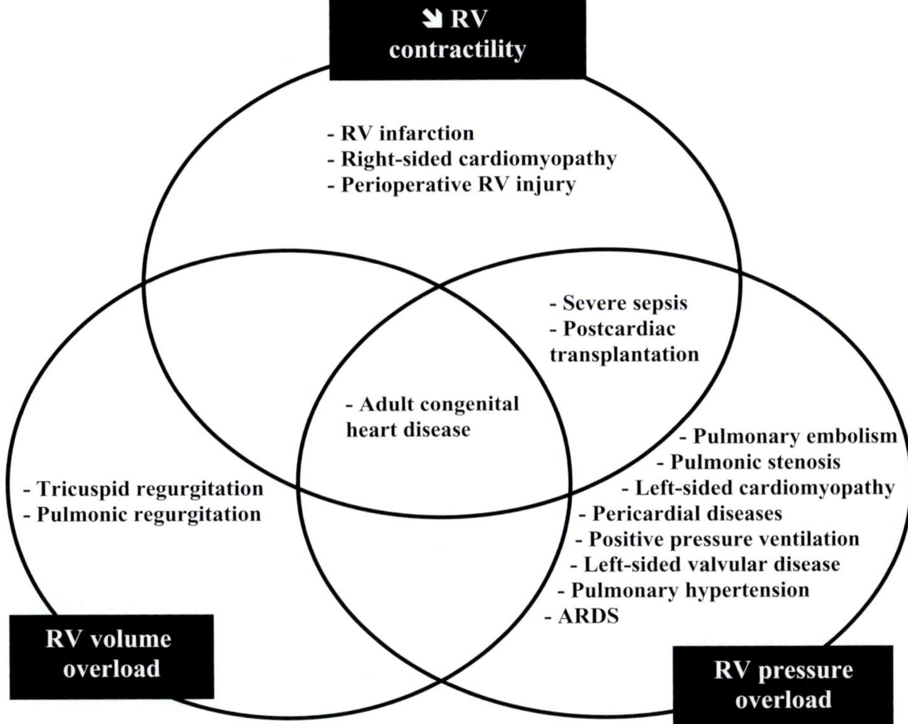

FIGURE 8.2. Conditions associated with right ventricular (RV) failure categorized by initial pathophysiology. ARDS, acute respiratory distress syndrome. (From Piazza and Goldhaber [20], with permission.)

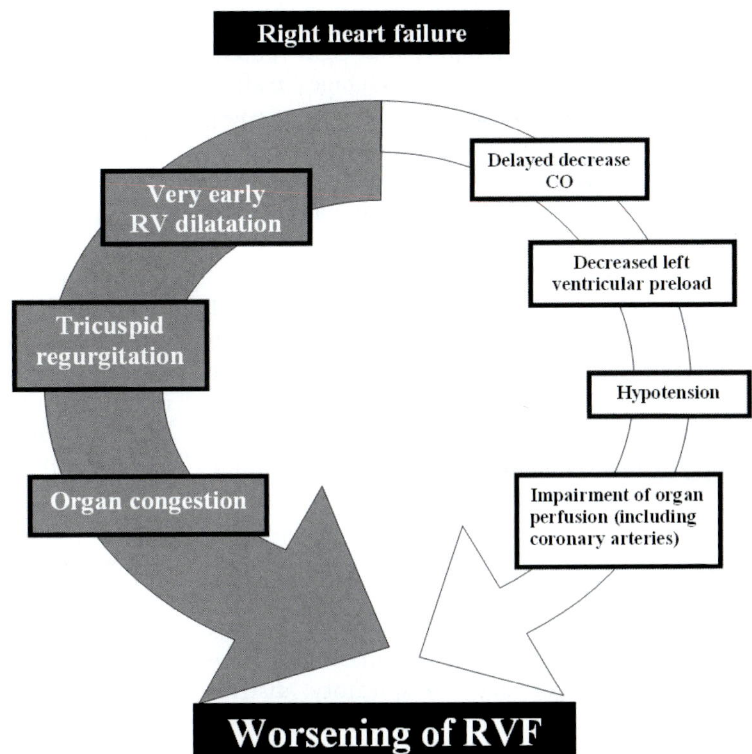

FIGURE 8.3. Vicious cycle of autoaggravation. This pathophysiologic pathway is specific to the right ventricle. This cascade of events must be prevented as soon as possible and implies that any sign of RVF should result in an immediate treatment in order to avoid this vicious cycle.

tricular ischemia rapidly leads to right ventricular dilatation with a concomitant rise in right ventricular diastolic pressure. Such elevation causes a shift of the interventricular septum toward an already underfilled left ventricle. Accordingly, right ventricular dilatation in the setting of limited pericardial compliance leads to increased intrapericardial pressures and an additional constraint on the RV but also on left ventricular filling (9). These changes in right ventricular mechanics lead to depressed right-sided output, decreased left ventricular preload, and subsequently a reduced overall cardiac output (10).

Effect of an Increase in Right Ventricular Afterload

Chronic Pulmonary Hypertension

As described above, increased PAP alters both coronary perfusion and ventricular function of the RV.

In normal condition, RCA perfusion occurs quasi-exclusively during diastole. A sudden increased in PAP reduces systolic perfusion, potentially reducing the oxygen supply to the RV during increased oxygen demand.

In addition, as already described, the prolonged low-pressure emptying implies that right ventricular emptying is very sensitive to changes in afterload. In a patient with pulmonary hypertension, the RV dilates to maintain the stroke volume, though the ejection fraction is reduced and the peristaltic contraction is lost, causing an accelerated worsening in RVF.

The increased afterload also prolongs the isovolemic contraction phase and ejection time and, therefore, the increased myocardial oxygen consumption. Accordingly, in a patient with decreased RCA perfusion, it is important to reduce right ventricular afterload to improve the oxygen supply/demand balance in the RV and maintain right ventricular function.

Acute Cor Pulmonale

Acute cor pulmonale relates to a sudden increase in afterload, most often due to a massive pulmonary embolism or acute respiratory distress syndrome (ARDS) in adults (11,12). In either setting, right ventricular outflow impedance is suddenly increased, right ventricular ejection is impaired, and the RV is enlarged. Thus, both systolic and diastolic right ventricular functions are impaired, which may cause or precipitate circulatory failure, particularly in critically ill patients.

In ARDS, circulating vasoconstrictors, increased sympathic tone, microvascular obstruction, and hypoxic vasoconstriction all increase the RV afterload (13).

Of note, acute cor pulmonale is reversible when the cause of increased afterload is removed.

Effect of an Increase in Right Ventricular Volume

Volume overload is common during RVF and volume loading may further dilate the RV, increase tricuspid regurgitation, and, consequently, worsen hepatic and renal congestion and RVF. Accordingly volume management is a difficult but important task in the treatment of RVF. Physiologically, volume loading may be useful in increasing preload, but in the large majority of RVF patients this compensatory mechanism is potentially limited beyond a mean pulmonary artery pressure of 30 mm Hg (14), and therefore caution is warranted when considering volume loading in any patient with suspected RVF (Fig. 8.4).

Ventricular Interdependence

There is a high degree of ventricular interdependence due to the role of the interventricular septum in the contraction of both ventricles, which is pronounced due the existence of pericardium (15). This close association between the cardiac cavities can be seen in echocardiography images of the four chambers (16).

Indeed, increases in the end-diastolic volume of the left ventricle are transmitted to the RV by movement of the interventricular septum toward the right cavity, increasing the end-diastolic pressure of the RV (17). Similarly, when right ventricular end-diastolic volume is increased, the interventricular septum shifts toward the left

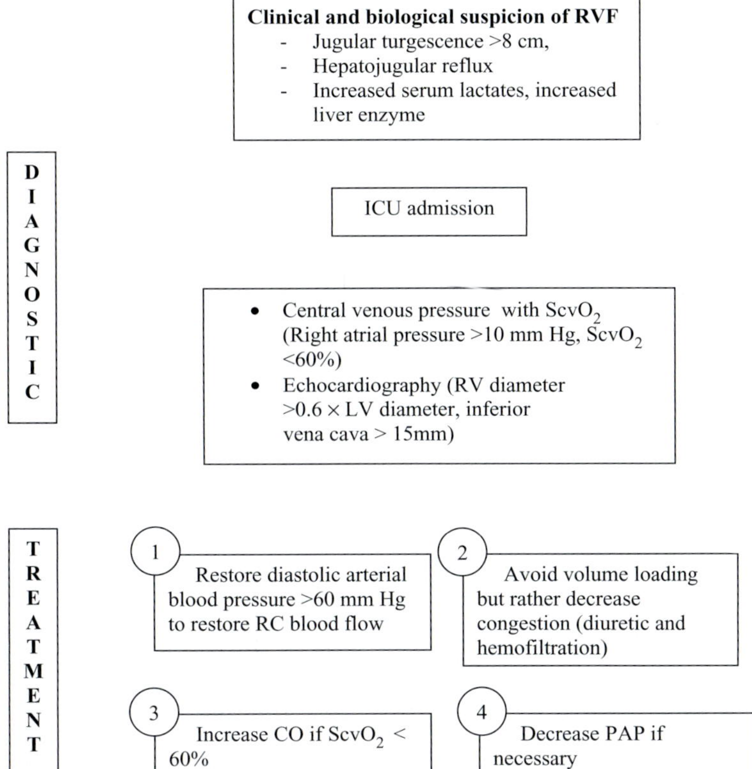

FIGURE 8.4. Example of management algorithm of right ventricular failure (RVF). ICU, intensive care unit; PAP, pulmonary arterial pressure; Scv, central venous oxygen saturation.

cavity during diastole due to restrictions imposed by the pericardium on the RV as the cavity volume increases. This leftward shift impairs the function of the left ventricle due to the reduction in left ventricle volume, decreasing both left ventricular filling and compliance, manifested as increased left ventricular muscle stiffness.

Ventricular interdependence can also cause RVF during left ventricular assist device support. As the left ventricular assist device unloads the left ventricle, the interventricular septum is shifted left. This alters the right ventricular compliance, decreasing force and the rate of contraction together with a decreased afterload and increased preload. In a healthy heart, cardiac output may be maintained, but with preexisting pathology, the decrease in contractility may result in RVF (18). It is therefore crucial to support right ventricular function during the first days following insertion of a left ventricular assist device.

The Vicious Cycle of Autoaggravation (Figs. 8.3 and 8.5)

Compared to the left ventricle, RVF progresses quickly from compensated to end-stage heart failure because of a vicious cycle of autoaggravation. This is unique to the RV and is rarely seen in isolated left ventricular failure.

As seen in Figure 8.3, a sudden increase, although modest, in right ventricular afterload (inhaled nitric oxide withdrawal) on an ischemic RV immediately dilates the RV, induces a tricuspid regurgitation, and decreases cardiac output.

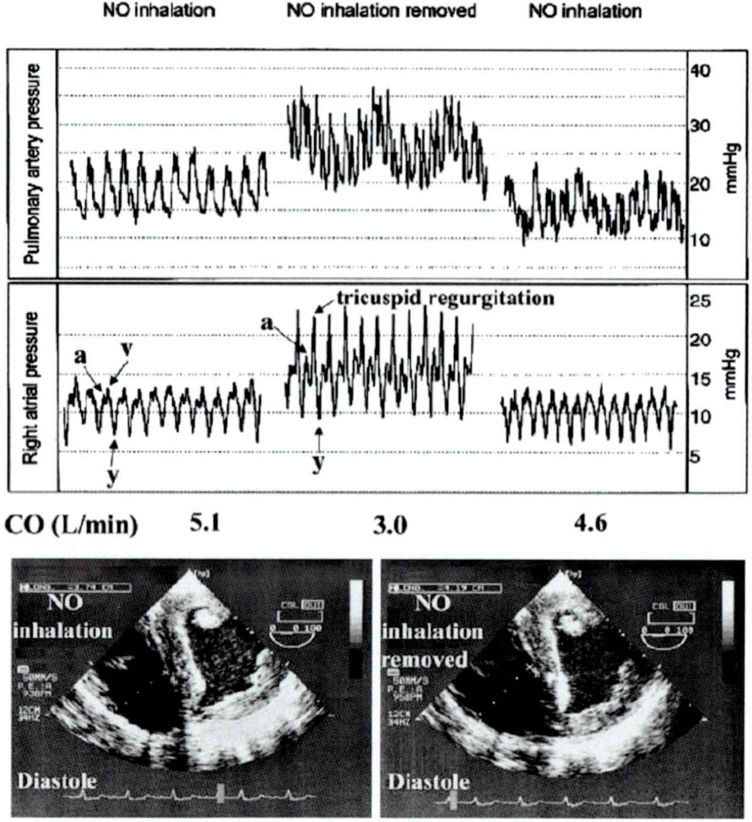

Figure 8.5. Patient hemodynamics with and without inhaled nitric oxide (NO). Inhaled NO withdrawal in this patient with ischemia-induced right ventricular failure increased mean pulmonary artery pressure from 18 to 25 mm Hg. During NO inhalation and preserved right ventricular function, right atrial pressure showed "a" waves (auricular contraction) followed by "v" waves (passive atrial filling due to venous return) and "y" waves (beginning of diastole: rapid ventricular filling and passive atrial emptying). When inhaled NO was removed, although pulmonary artery pressure remained in the normal range, the slight increase resulted in a deterioration of the right ventricular function and dilatation of the right ventricle. Right atrial pressure showed that tricuspid insufficiency emerged (positive waves) that worsened cardiac output despite the increase in auricular contraction (increase in "a" waves). Echocardiography shows the close association between the left and right ventricles separated by the interventricular septum. An enlargement of the right ventricle can be seen, with the end-diastolic diameter increasing from 37 to 42 mm when NO inhalation was removed. (From Mebazaa et al. [19], with permission.)

Conclusion

The RV plays a pivotal role in hemodynamic homeostasis, and changes in right ventricular function can have profound effects on the pulmonary and systemic circulation.

Understanding the normal physiology and physiopathology of the RV seems to be essential for the management of right ventricular failure. It should allow a quick and accurate diagnosis.

The principal therapeutic goals of the early management of RVF depend on its underlying etiology, but primarily involve breaking the vicious circle of reduced cardiac output. This will allow restoring adequate oxygen delivery to the myocardium and reducing right ventricular overload. Treatment of RVF, therefore, should focus on alleviating congestion (limit volume loading), increasing right coronary artery flow, improving right ventricular contractility, and reducing right ventricular afterload (avoiding mechanical ventilation and high airway pressure). An example of a management algorithm is shown in Figure 8.4.

References

1. Starr IJW, Meade RH. The absence of conspicuous increments of venous pressure after severe damage to the RV of the dog, with discussion of the relation between clinical congestive heart failure and heart disease. Am Heart J 1943;26:291–301.
2. Cohn JN, Guiha NH, Broder MI, Limas CJ. Right ventricular infarction. Clinical and hemodynamic features. Am J Cardiol 1974;33:209–14.
3. Encyclopaedia. Right-sided heart failure. http://www.healthcentral.com/mhc/top/000154.cfm, 2002.
4. Kannel WB, Belanger AJ. Epidemiology of heart failure. Am Heart J 1991;121:951–7.
5. Mehta SR, Eikelboom JW, Natarajan MK, et al. Impact of right ventricular involvement on mortality and morbidity in patients with inferior myocardial infarction. J Am Coll Cardiol 2001;37:37–43.
6. Lupi-Herrera E, Lasses LA, Cosio-Aranda J, et al. Acute right ventricular infarction: clinical spectrum, results of reperfusion therapy and short-term prognosis. Coron Artery Dis 2002;13:57–64.
7. Redington AN, Gray HH, Hodson ME, et al. Characterisation of the normal right ventricular pressure-volume relation by biplane angiography and simultaneous micromanometer pressure measurements. Br Heart J 1988;59:23–30.
8. Brooks H, Kirk ES, Vokonas PS, et al. Performance of the right ventricle under stress: relation to right coronary flow. J Clin Invest 1971;50:2176–83.
9. Goldstein JA. Pathophysiology and management of right heart ischemia. J Am Coll Cardiol 2002;40: 841–53.
10. Pfisterer M. Right ventricular involvement in myocardial infarction and cardiogenic shock. Lancet 2003;362:392–4.
11. Vieillard-Baron A, Schmitt JM, Augarde R, et al. Acute cor pulmonale in acute respiratory distress syndrome submitted to protective ventilation: incidence, clinical implications, and prognosis. Crit Care Med 2001;29:1551–5.
12. Vieillard-Baron A, Prin S, Chergui K, et al. Echo-Doppler demonstration of acute cor pulmonale at the bedside in the medical intensive care unit. Am J Respir Crit Care Med 2002;166:1310–9.
13. McNeil K, Dunning J, Morrell NW. The pulmonary physician in critical care. 13: the pulmonary circulation and right ventricular failure in the ITU. Thorax 2003;58:157–62.
14. Sibbald WJ, Driedger AA. Right ventricular function in acute disease states: pathophysiologic considerations. Crit Care Med 1983;11:339–45.
15. Visner MC, Arentzen CE, O'Connor MJ, et al. Alterations in left ventricular three-dimensional dynamic geometry and systolic function during acute right ventricular hypertension in the conscious dog. Circulation 1983;67:353–65.
16. Jardin F. Ventricular interdependence: how does it impact on hemodynamic evaluation in clinical practice? Intensive Care Med 2003;29: 361–3.
17. Taylor RR, Covell JW, Sonnenblick EH, Ross J Jr. Dependence of ventricular distensibility on filling of the opposite ventricle. Am J Physiol 1967;213: 711–8.
18. Santamore WP, Gray LA Jr. Left ventricular contributions to right ventricular systolic function during LVAD support. Ann Thorac Surg 1996;61: 350–6.
19. Mebazaa A, Karpati P, Renaud E, Algotsson L. Acute right ventricular failure—from pathophysiology to new treatments. Intensive Care Med 2004; 30:185–96.
20. Piazza G, Goldhaber SZ. The acutely decompensated right ventricle: pathways for diagnosis and management. Chest 2005;128:1836–52.

9 Myocardial Protection from Ischemia and Reperfusion Injury

Stefan G. De Hert

Prolonged and unresolved interruption of blood supply to the myocardium without reperfusion ultimately causes myocyte cell death. Early restoration of blood flow to the ischemic myocardium is therefore necessary to prevent myocardial cell death to occur. However, reperfusion itself may lead to additional tissue injury beyond that generated by the ischemic event. This phenomenon is called *reperfusion injury* and it may manifest as arrhythmias, reversible contractile dysfunction (myocardial stunning), endothelial dysfunction, and ultimately irreversible reperfusion injury with myocardial cell death. Irreversible reperfusion injury is defined as the injury caused by restoration of blood flow after an ischemic episode leading to the death of cells that were only reversibly injured during the preceding ischemic period (Fig. 9.1). This lethal reperfusion injury may result from two mechanisms: necrosis and apoptosis. Therefore, treatment of myocardial ischemia not only should be directed toward a prompt restoration of blood flow to the ischemic area but also should include measures to prevent or minimize the extent of reperfusion injury.

Mechanisms of Myocardial Reperfusion Injury

The cellular damage associated with reperfusion can be reversible or irreversible depending on the duration of ischemia (Fig. 9.2). If reperfusion is started within 20 minutes after the onset of ischemia, myocardial injury is reversible and characterized by a transient depression of myocardial function, which is termed myocardial stunning. Histologically and metabolically, the stunned myocardium exhibits no signs or irreversible injury and no evidence of myocardial necrosis. When ischemia lasts longer than 20 minutes, irreversible myocardial damage with cellular necrosis occurs. The extent of tissue necrosis that occurs during reperfusion is related to the duration of ischemia. Tissue necrosis starts in the subendocardial layer and extends to the subepicardial regions when duration of ischemia becomes longer [1].

The pathogenesis of reperfusion injury still is not fully elucidated but several mechanisms have been shown to be involved (Fig. 9.3). The major consistent metabolic abnormality that has been observed in the stunned myocardium is a reduction of the adenosine triphosphate (ATP) concentration in the cells [2]. Because this resolves with a time course that is roughly parallel to that of the functional recovery [3], emphasis was initially placed on a potential role of high-energy phosphate stores in the development of myocardial stunning. However, several lines of evidence have made it quite clear that ATP depletion has no major pathogenetic role in the development of reperfusion injury [4–6].

More recently the focus has turned to a potential role of reactive oxygen species (ROS) and the disruption of the normal intracellular calcium homeostasis as major mechanisms involved in the pathogenesis of reperfusion injury. The *oxygen paradox* hypothesis is based on the observation that oxygen, while essential for tissue survival, may also be harmful during reperfusion of

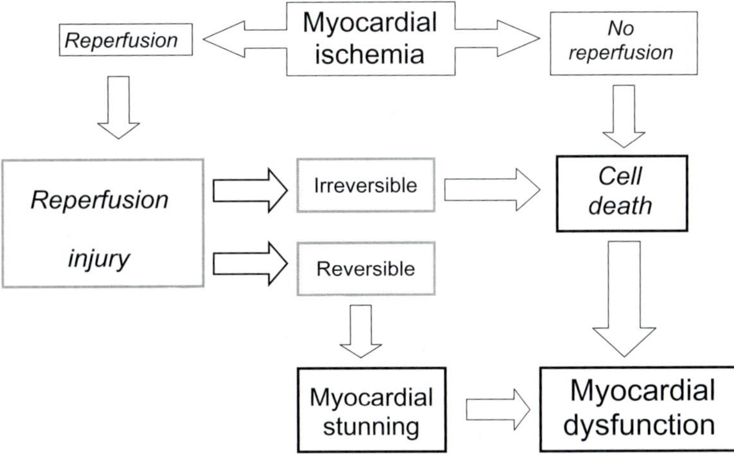

Figure 9.1. Schematic representation of the different possible pathways of myocardial dysfunction with myocardial ischemia.

the ischemic myocardium [1]. Indeed, upon reperfusion, molecular oxygen undergoes a sequential reduction with formation of ROS, which interact with cell membrane lipids and essential proteins. This results in myocardial cell damage, initially with depressed myocardial function but ultimately leading to irreversible tissue damage. Although the role of ROS in the pathogenesis of myocardial stunning has been established, the mechanisms by which oxygen-derived free radicals produce contractile dysfunction at the cellular level is still not fully established. Since calcium is the major ion involved in the force generation by the myocardium, it seems likely that a change in extracellular calcium influx, intracellular calcium release, or reuptake by the sarcoplasmatic reticulum or an alteration in myofilament sensitivity to calcium is also involved in the pathogenesis of depressed function with myocardial stunning [7].

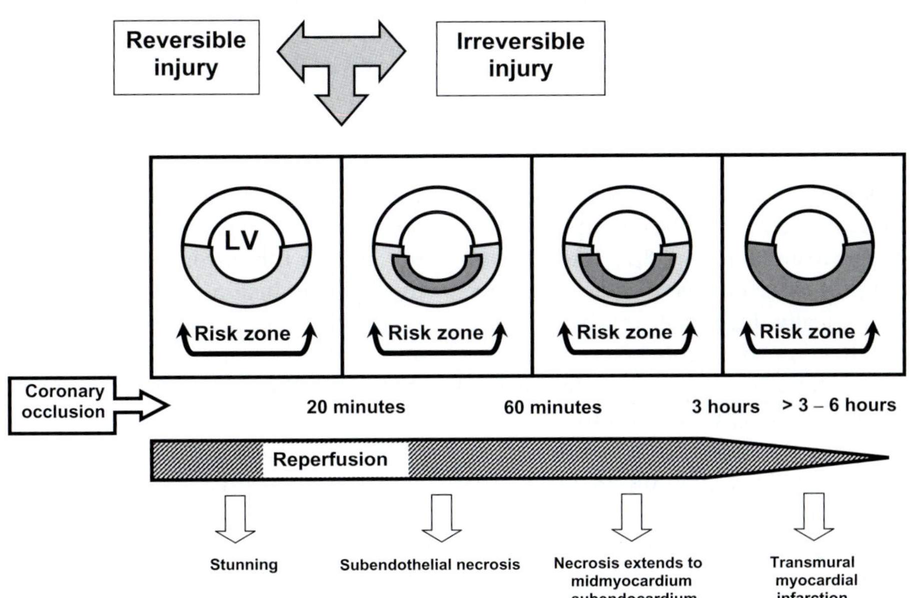

Figure 9.2. Schematic representation of the time course of myocardial damage associated with myocardial ischemia. LV, left ventricle. (Adapted from Kloner and Jennings [68].)

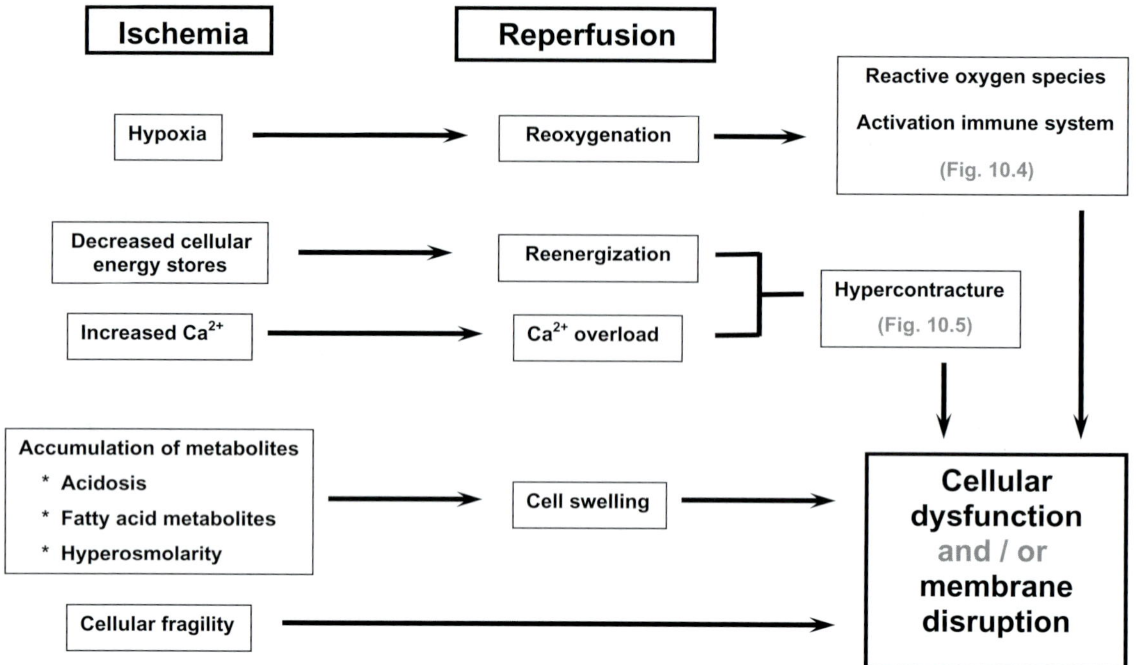

FIGURE 9.3. Schematic representation of the different factors contributing to myocardial dysfunction and damage with ischemia–reperfusion.

Role of Reactive Oxygen Species and the Immune System (Fig. 9.4)

Experimental studies have indicated that a burst of ROS occurs upon reintroduction of oxygen to an ischemic tissue. Most of the evidence is indirect, as it is derived from the observations that free radical scavengers are able to improve some aspects of reperfusion injury [4,8,9]. It is noteworthy that the protective effects of these scavengers seem to be critically dependent on the timing of their administration: the protective effects were seen only when the scavengers were administered 15 minutes prior to reperfusion and not when they were administered 15 minutes after reperfusion [10]. More direct measurements of free radical release have provided additional evidence for reactive oxygen species–induced reperfusion injury [11–14].

The sources responsible for the burst of ROS upon reperfusion are not clear at the moment. It has been shown that the site of ROS generation during ischemia was located along the electron transport chain in the mitochondria (more specifically at the ubisemiquinone site) [15]. Evidence indicates that the mitochondrial source of oxidants seen during ischemia is probably not the source of ROS during reperfusion, since, in contrast to ROS release during ischemia, inhibitors of the mitochondrial electron transport chain were not able to inhibit or decrease the burst of ROS during reperfusion [15]. The exact source of the reperfusion peak, therefore, remains uncertain and is the focus of ongoing research, but it seems that several sources contribute to the increased production of oxygen radicals with reperfusion injury [16]. These include blood-borne cells such as activated neutrophils, as well as constitutive cell of the myocardium such as cardiomyocytes and endothelial cells.

Neutrophils are an important component of the host defense system. They respond to myocardial ischemia-reperfusion injury in a manner similar to the bacterial invasion of a host. Although earlier studies have suggested that neutrophils are involved in causing postischemic myocardial stunning [17,18], subsequent studies demonstrated that neutrophil depletion did not prevent myocardial stunning from occurring, implying that neutrophils are not involved in the pathogenesis of stunning [19–21]. It is now widely accepted that neutrophils probably do not have an important role in the pathogenesis of reversible myocardial perfusion injury [22–24]. In contrast, in the pathogenesis of lethal reperfusion injury, neutrophils seem to be involved. There appears to be a specific recruitment of neutrophils to the ischemic-reperfused myocardium, resulting in a release of noxious products by the neutrophils that can directly injure the myocytes and the coronary vascular endothelial cells, with subsequent physiologic damage.

Neutrophils release numerous proteolytic enzymes. The primary target of these enzymes is the extracellular matrix and its collagen, elastin, proteoglycan, and glycoprotein constituents. Neutrophils are also the primary source of ROS. In the course of ischemia-reperfusion, ROS can interact with specific targets such as the complement component C5a, platelet-activating factor (PAF), tumor necrosis factor-α (TNF-α), and interleukins (ILs). Neutrophils are activated by a number of compounds derived from different cell types in the myocardium, such as endothelial cells, mast cells, and myocytes. These compounds include complement factors and cytokines [25,26], which act as activating and chemoattractant factors that stimulate neutrophil-related events in the reperfused myocardium.

Central to the pathogenesis of neutrophil-mediated injury is the interaction between neutrophils and the endothelial cells and myocytes [27–31]. The initial tethering of neutrophils to the vascular endothelium is selectin-dependent (Fig. 9.4, inset).

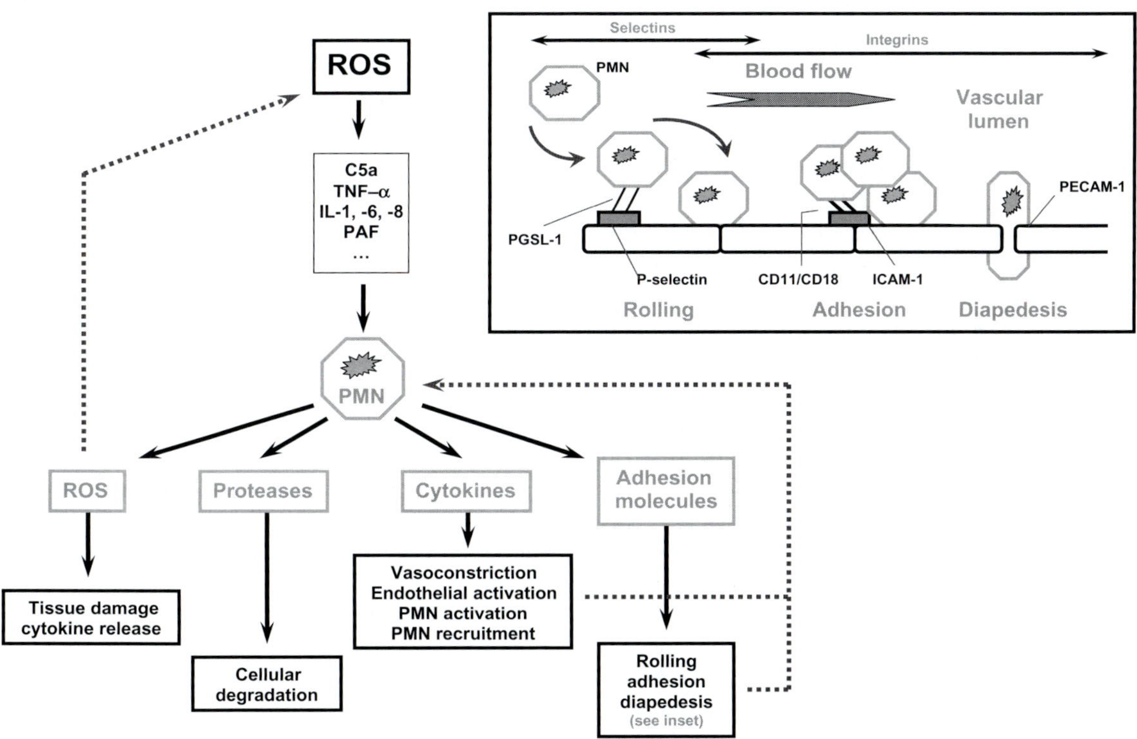

FIGURE 9.4. Schematic diagram of the pathways that participate in the release of reactive oxygen species (ROS) and the activation of neutrophils (polymorphonuclear, PMN) in the course of ischemia–reperfusion injury. The inset displays the different steps involved in the interaction between neutrophils and the endothelial layer. See text for abbreviations.

P-selectin is the predominant selectin involved in the recruitment of neutrophils during reperfusion, and it is expressed on the surface of the vascular endothelial cells within the first minutes of reperfusion [32]. The physiologic ligand for P-selectin on the endothelium is the P-selectin glycoprotein ligand-1 (PGSL-1) localized on neutrophils [33]. The interaction between P-selectin and PGSL-1 results in loose tethering and rolling of the neutrophils along the coronary endothelium, which is essential for the later stage of adherence and transendothelial migration [34]. Neutrophil rolling stimulates the upregulation of β_2-integrins—specifically the CD11/CD18 family of adhesion molecules—on their surface. The physiologic ligand of the CD11/CD18 complex on the neutrophils is the immunoglobulin intercellular adhesion molecule-1 (ICAM-1), which is located on the vascular endothelium. Adherence of the neutrophils to the endothelial cell is followed by extravasation of the neutrophils through the endocardial barrier into the underlying interstitial space and tissues. This migration requires the presence of platelet-endothelial cell adhesion molecule-1 (PECAM-1), which is located at the endothelial cell junctions [24].

Also at level of the myocytes, cytokines stimulate the upregulation of ICAM-1, resulting in the adherence of neutrophils to cardiomyocytes through a CD11/CD18–ICAM-1–dependent mechanism. Damage to the cardiomyocytes then may occur by release of cytotoxic oxidants and proteolytic enzymes by the neutrophils [35,36].

The neutrophil response during reperfusion seems to be distinct from the one during ischemia. Myocardial ischemia without reperfusion is associated with a slow infiltration of neutrophils in the area at risk starting with migration from the border of the infarction after 12 to 24 hours and peaking between 2 and 4 days after the start of the myocardial infarction [37]. In the absence of reperfusion, the neutrophil infiltration is limited to the outer border of the infarcted area with only a few neutrophils in the center of the necrotic zone. With reperfusion after reversible occlusion, however, neutrophil infiltration is accelerated, with a predominant accumulation in the subendocardium compared to the subepicardium [38]. Neutrophil adhesion to the coronary vascular endothelium occurs within minutes after the onset of reperfusion and is paralleled by a progressive decrease in endothelial function [39,40]. Accumulation is initially localized in the intravascular space of the myocardial area at risk for the first 6 hours after reperfusion, followed by a transendothelial migration over the following 24 hours, following a time course that parallels the progression of necrosis [41].

During ischemia and reperfusion injury, the *complement system* is activated. This results in the formation of the anaphylatoxins C3a, C4a, and C5a as well as the terminal complement system. The complement factors induce direct cell injury by increasing cell permeability and release of histamine and PAF. In addition, complement factors, especially C5a, are potent stimulators of neutrophil adherence and superoxide production [1].

Disruption in Calcium Homeostasis (Fig. 9.5)

With ischemia, myocardial cells become energy depleted and the cardiomyocytes start to accumulate Na^+ via various influx pathways including the Na^+ channel, the Na^+/H^+ exchanger, and the Na^+/HCO_3^- symporter. The normal Na^+ extrusion is inhibited since the activity of the Na^+/K^+–adenosine triphosphatase (ATPase) at the level of the sarcolemma is impaired because of the lack of ATP. In a depolarized Na^+ overloaded cell the Na^+/Ca^{2+} exchanger is turned in the reverse mode, leading to an intracellular accumulation of Ca^{2+}. If the ability of the mitochondria to resume ATP synthesis was not critically impaired during ischemia, reoxygenation with the start of reperfusion will lead to a rapid recovery of the oxidative energy production. The renewed synthesis of high-energy phosphates not only enables the myocytes to restore the normal intracellular ion gradients but also reactivates the contractile process. The restoration of contractile activity occurs faster than the restoration of the intracellular Ca^{2+} gradients, leading to oscillatory Ca^{2+} shifts with high peak Ca^{2+} concentrations and myocyte hypercontracture [42–45]. During this period, the transsarcolemmal Na^+ gradient is still reduced and the Na^+/Ca^{2+} exchanger still functions in reverse mode. In cells capable of reestablishing a normal intracellular ion homeostasis,

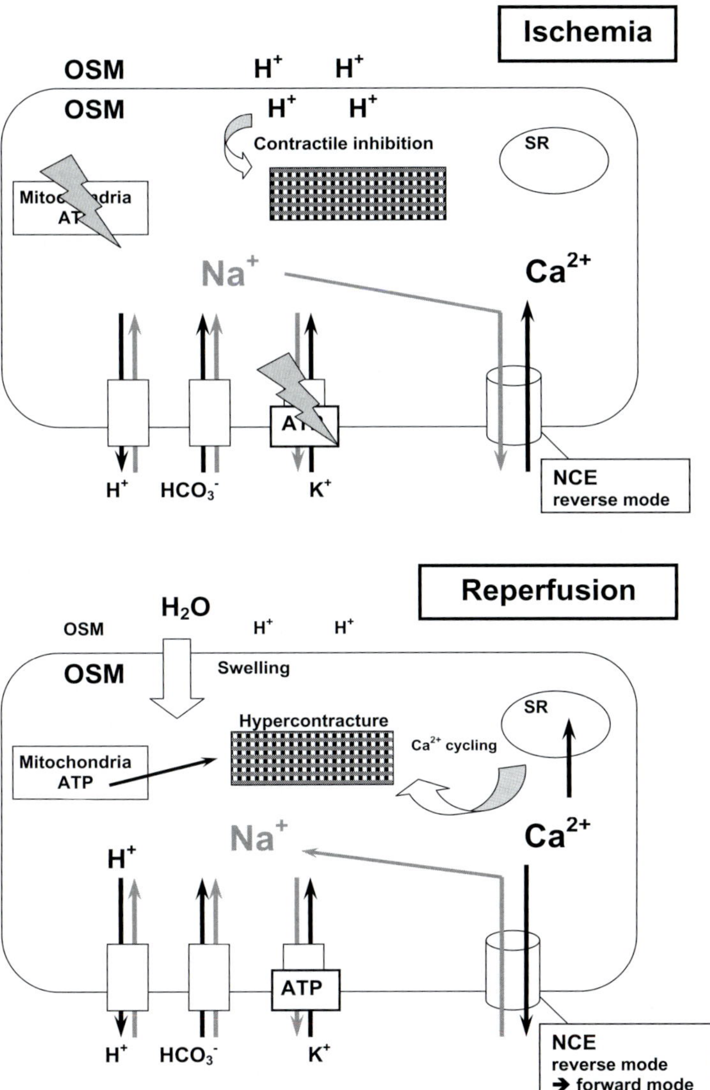

FIGURE 9.5. Schematic representation of the intracellular events occurring during myocardial ischemia (upper panel) and reperfusion (lower panel). Ischemia rapidly leads to a lack of oxygen and consequently to a dramatic fall in intracellular high-energy phosphates with accumulation of metabolites, with an increase in osmolality (OSM) and development of acidosis. With ischemia, cardiomyocytes accumulate Na^+ through various pathways such as the Na^+/H^+ exchanger and the Na^+/HCO_3^- symporter. Na^+ extrusion is inhibited because the Na^+/K^+ adenosine triphosphatase (ATPase) in the sarcolemma is impaired by the lack of adenosine triphosphate (ATP). The Na^+/Ca^{2+} exchanger (NCE) is turned in reverse mode leading to an extrusion of Na^+ and an influx of Ca^{2+}, resulting in Ca^{2+} overload. In the early phase of reperfusion, the NCE still is operating in the reverse mode. When the sarcoplasmatic reticulum (SR) is resupplied with ATP, it starts sequestering the excess cytosolic Ca^{2+}. Spontaneous release and reuptake leads to oscillations in intracellular Ca^{2+} concentrations. Once the Na^+/K^+-ATPase is resupplied with ATP, the transsarcolemmal Na^+ gradient switches again to the forward mode of the NCE, gradually removing the excess Ca^{2+} from the cell. Reactivation of oxidative phosphorylation in the mitochondria with reperfusion provides energy not only to the ion pumps but also to the contractile machinery. This energy supply in the presence of high cytosolic Ca^{2+} concentration causes uncontrolled contractile activation with hypercontracture and mechanical injury of cell structures. Upon reperfusion the accumulated extracellular H^+ concentration is rapidly reduced and thus a transsarcolemmal H^+ gradient is created. Excess H^+ is removed via the Na^+/H^+ exchanger and the Na^+/HCO_3^- symporter. As long as a high intracellular H^+ concentration is present, the contractile machinery is impaired and hypercontracture is prevented. With reperfusion, extracellular osmolality is also rapidly decreased, thereby creating a transsarcolemmal osmotic gradient. This results in water influx and cell swelling, which may augment fragility of the cellular structures and cause additional damage on reperfusion. Of note, lightning bolts (in the upper panel) mean markedly reduced activity.

recovery of the intracellular Ca^{2+} concentrations can be divided in two stages: an early stage during which the cytosolic Ca^{2+} level falls due to uptake of Ca^{2+} in the sarcoplasmatic reticulum, and a second stage during which Ca^{2+} is shifted in a oscillatory manner between sarcoplasmatic reticulum and cytosol until Ca^{2+} gradients across the sarcolemma can be restored by turning the Na^+/Ca^{2+} exchanger again in forward mode [46]. In fact, it is the resupply of energy to the myofibrillar elements in the presence of an increased concentration of cytosolic Ca^{2+} that may become harmful for the reoxygenated myocardium. Indeed, in the initial phase of reoxygenation, the cytosolic Ca^{2+} concentration is still elevated, and myofibrillar activation therefore results in excessive force generation with hypercontraction. This in turn results in severe damage to the cell by deformation of the cytoskeletal structures.

More recent evidence has indicated that the susceptibility of the reoxygenated cardiomyocytes to develop hypercontracture at a given Ca^{2+} concentration is increased after a prolonged period of hypoxic energy depletion [47]. This means that hypercontraction with reoxygenation may occur at cytosolic Ca^{2+} concentrations that would cause no harm in the normal cell. The reason for this phenomenon seems to be related to an increased fragility of the cytoskeleton that is no longer able to sustain the normal contraction forces.

A number of publications have indicated that the transient calcium overload in the stunned myocardium results in a deceased sensitivity or responsiveness of the cardiac myofilaments to intracellular calcium [48–50]. Although the mechanisms involved still are fully elucidated, there is evidence suggesting that proteolysis of the myofibrils due to activation of the calcium-dependent protease calpain I is involved [51,52] and a direct effect of oxygen free radicals on the myofilaments [53].

Other Intracellular Events (Fig. 9.5)

After ischemia, the cytosolic pH is decreased because anaerobic metabolism and the breakdown of ATP produce an excess of H^+ ions, which results in an acidification of both the intracellular and the interstitial space. Upon reperfusion, the pH in the interstitial space is rapidly normalized and a concentration gradient is generated between the cytosol, still containing a high H^+ concentration, and the interstitium, where the H^+ concentration is already normalized. This triggers the activation of the H^+ extruding mechanisms, which are the Na^+/H^+ exchanger and the Na^+/HCO_3^- symporter [54]. These mechanisms restore normal intracellular pH but may at the same time aggravate reperfusion injury. Indeed, intracellular acidosis inhibits the myofibrillar machinery, and this inhibition represents in fact a protective mechanism in the early vulnerable phase of reoxygenation [55]. Rapid extrusion of excess H^+ from the reoxygenated cell thus removes a potentially protective mechanism. Also, activation of the Na^+/H^+ exchanger causes a net influx of Na^+ into the cytosol, resulting potentially in an excess intracellular load of Na^+. This may activate the Na^+/Ca^{2+} exchange mechanism, transporting Na^+ out of the cell and Ca^{2+} in the cell, thereby even further increasing the already existing Ca^{2+} overload of the reperfused myocardial cell.

The cytosolic Na^+ overload is also one of the major causes of the edema of the ischemic-reperfused myocardial cell. With reperfusion, the accumulated osmotically active molecules are rapidly washed out, creating an osmotic gradient between the intracellular and the extracellular space [56,57]. Intracellular uptake of water in a myocardial cell in which the mechanical fragility is increased during the preceding energy depletion may further aggravate the mechanical stress on the intracellular structures and add up with the other sources of stress, resulting in further cell deterioration [58].

Mitochondria play an essential role in normal cellular function since their primary function is the provision of ATP through oxidative phosphorylation in order to meet the high-energy demands of the beating heart. However, latent within the mitochondria there exist mechanisms that, once activated, convert the mitochondria from organelles that support the life of the cells to those that actively induce both necrotic and apoptotic cell death. This switch is mediated by the opening of a nonspecific pore in the inner mitochondrial membrane, which is the mitochondrial permeability transition pore (MPTP). Normally this pore is closed, but in conditions of stress such as with reperfusion of the heart after a period of ischemia, the MPTP opens. This opening causes the mitochondria to become uncoupled, resulting in a loss of their ATP-generating capacity. Unrestrained, this leads to the loss of the ionic homeostasis and ultimately to necrotic cell death.

In addition to its role in the course of cell necrosis, transient opening and subsequent closure of the MPTP may occur and lead to the release of cytochrome c and other proapoptotic molecules that initiate the apoptotic cascade [59]. Apoptosis is a transcriptionally controlled cellular response to moderate cell injury. In contrast to necrotic cell death, which is the consequence of severe structural cell damage, cells that have entered the apoptotic process initially retain physical integrity of the sarcolemma. The point where the process becomes irreversible is the activation of endonucleases that target the genomic DNA. Several studies have indicated that apoptotic cell injury may also occur in the ischemic-reperfused myocardium [60–64].

Therapeutical Approaches for Protection Against Myocardial Reperfusion Injury

Based on the pathophysiologic mechanisms involved in ischemia-reperfusion injury, several potential therapeutic approaches can be proposed that may help to decrease the extent of myocardial reperfusion injury. Two factors are of importance to improve the outcome of patients with an acute myocardial ischemic event. First, infarct size needs to be limited since the prognosis of the patient depends on the amount of myocardium that is lost [65]. Therefore, timely reperfusion by thrombolysis, coronary angioplasty, or coronary surgery remains the cornerstone of the treatment of acute ischemic events. Second, therapy should be directed toward minimizing the extent of myocardial ischemia-reperfusion injury. The importance of limiting myocardial ischemia-reperfusion injury has been appreciated for more than three decades since the introduction of the idea that the extent and severity of tissue damage after coronary occlusion were not predetermined at the onset of ischemia but could be modified by therapeutic measures during ischemia [66]. Since then an ever-growing body of literature is available on potential therapeutic approaches to help treat the extent of myocardial ischemia-reperfusion injury in addition to the classic principles of treatment, which are based on the maintenance or restoration of myocardial oxygen supply and the control of determinants of myocardial oxygen demand.

Myocardial preconditioning (Fig. 9.6)

The heart possesses the remarkable ability to protect itself against the consequences of ischemia. In 1986, Murry et al. [67] reported that short episodes of ischemia and reperfusion before a sustained ischemic event—ischemic preconditioning—reduced infarct size. Preconditioning represents a potent and consistently reproducible method of protection against ischemia, which not only reduces infarct size but also alleviates postischemic cardiac dysfunction and arrhythmias. Ischemic preconditioning typically consists of two windows of cardioprotection: an early phase that occurs immediately and produces a strong protection but has a limited duration of about 2 hours, and a late phase or second window that occurs about 24 hours after the initial stimulus and induces less protection, but lasts for as long as 3 days. Several reviews have summarized the present knowledge on the underlying mechanisms involved in preconditioning [68–73]. Briefly, signaling substances bind to receptors and trigger the activation of several intracellular signaling pathways. These pathways mainly involve a posttranslational modification of proteins (translocation and phosphorylation). Protein kinase C plays a central role as intracellular mediator, but tyrosine kinase and mitogen-activated protein kinases are also involved.

During the early phase of preconditioning, the cellular memory is believed to be related to translocation of protein kinase C from cytosol to the different cellular membranes, which results in a more rapid activation of protein kinase C during the prolonged ischemic period. Several structures have been involved as end-effectors. However, the majority of experimental findings now indicate that preservation of mitochondrial function, which occurs as a consequence of mitochondrial K_{ATP} channel activation (opening), is of pivotal importance for the cardioprotective effect against

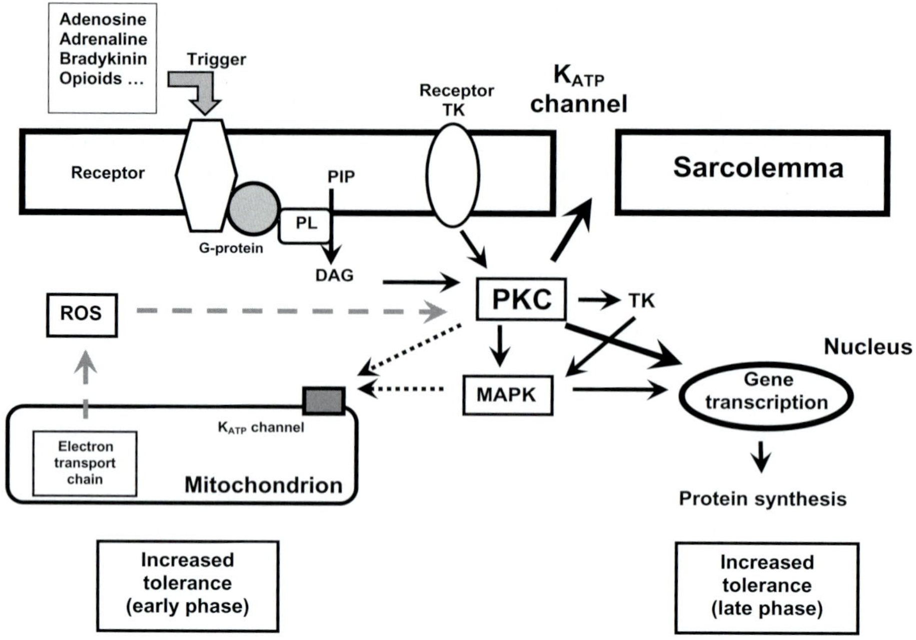

FIGURE 9.6. Schematic illustration of the proposed pathways involved in ischemic preconditioning. PL, phospholipase; PIP, phosphatidylinositol diphosphate; TK, tyrosine kinases; DAG, diacylglycerol; PKC, protein kinase C; MAPK, mitogen-activated kinases.

ischemia. This increased tolerance to myocardial ischemic damage has been attributed to a reduction of calcium overload, better preservation of energy stores, prevention of the activation of necrotic or apoptotic pathways, and an influence on the extent of oxidative stress.

During the late phase of preconditioning, cellular memory is thought to be related to the synthesis or activation of proteins that have a cytoprotective effect, such as the induction of several antioxidant enzymes, or the synthesis of heat-shock proteins that are involved in the stabilization of the cytoskeleton.

Several studies have indicated that ischemic preconditioning also occurs in humans [74–77] and a number of ischemic preconditioning protocols have been applied in the setting of cardiologic interventions and coronary artery bypass surgery, with varying results [78–86]. Although the clinical application of an ischemic preconditioning protocol might help to reduce the consequences of myocardial ischemia-reperfusion injury, it should be noted that rendering an already-diseased myocardium transiently ischemic implies the inherent risk to further jeopardize myocardial function and cell survival.

Different experimental studies have shown that ischemic preconditioning could be either abolished or mimicked by the use of pharmacologic agents that either block or stimulate certain steps in the intracellular cascade of events. This has led to the concept of pharmacologic preconditioning. However, the current use of pharmacologic compounds to induce preconditioning in the clinical setting is limited by their unwanted side effects, such as occurrence of hypotension (adenosine), arrhythmias (adenosine, K_{ATP} channel openers), or possible carcinogenic effects (protein kinase activators).

In recent years, both experimental and clinical evidence has increasingly demonstrated that volatile anesthetics are able to precondition the myocardium. The mechanisms involved in anesthetic preconditioning strongly resemble those involved in ischemic preconditioning, and have been subject of recent reviews [87–93]. The cardioprotective effects of a volatile anesthetic regimen have been demonstrated in cardiac surgery patients and were evident from a better-preserved postoperative myocardial function and a lower increase in biochemical markers of myocardial damage or dysfunction. Although no data are yet available on postoperative mortality or morbidity, there is some evidence that the perioperative use of a volatile anesthetic regimen decreases intensive care and hospital length of stay [94] and improves 1-year cardiovascular outcome [95].

Pharmacologic Modulation of Cardiac Energy Metabolism

In the heart, function and metabolism are intimately linked. To preserve its normal function, the heart consumes huge amounts of ATP, and an exact matching is present between rate of adenosine diphosphate phosphorylation and rate of ATP hydrolysis. With ischemia, this close matching becomes disrupted, and a depletion of high-energy phosphates occurs. Therefore, restoration or support of cardiac metabolism has become part of the possible therapeutic strategies in the treatment of ischemic heart disease. The primary goal of this therapeutic approach is to lessen the metabolic and functional consequences of ischemia and to redirect flux through the normal metabolic pathways by modulation of the regulatory enzymes and by replenishment of the depleted intermediates. It is beyond the scope of this chapter to discuss this therapeutic approach in detail, and the reader is referred to several reviews on this subject [96–101].

Among the different possible metabolic strategies, the use of the metabolic cocktail, *glucose-insulin-potassium*, appears to be associated with the most convincing clinical benefits. The current dogma is that the cardioprotective effect of this cocktail acts via the modulation of cardiac and circulating metabolites to provide the heart with an optimal metabolic milieu to resist ischemia and reperfusion injury. However, this may not be the only mechanism involved and it has been suggested that insulin may also exert direct cardiac cell survival effects in the context of ischemia and reperfusion injury [102]. For a number of years clinical data have supported a role of the glucose-insulin-potassium cocktail in reducing morbidity and mortality after myocardial infarction [103,104]. However, it seems that the extent of cardioprotective effects may depend on a number of variables, such as the extent of collateral circulation, the presence of heart failure, and the dosage scheme used [105–108]. Also in the course of cardiac surgery, the clinical benefits of glucose-insulin solutions seem to be related to patient characteristics [109,110].

Another compound that has been focus of intensive research is *adenosine*. It is a direct precursor of adenosine monophosphate and is therefore essential for raising a decreased myocardial adenine nucleotide pool. As such the supplementation of adenosine might be helpful to provide substrate for the necessary resynthesis of the depleted ATP pool with myocardial ischemia. In addition to this effect, adenosine has a number of other actions that are more directly related to a cardioprotective effect in the presence of ischemia-reperfusion injury. These actions include activation of the potassium-sensitive ATP channels, resulting in a preconditioning effect. Adenosine also strongly inhibits neutrophil function with a reduction in production of ROS, protease release, and coronary endothelial adherence, thereby attenuating neutrophil-mediated reperfusion injury. Several clinical studies have reported beneficial effects with adenosine treatment, but the effects were less obvious than those reported by experimental studies [111–115].

Modulation of Reactive Oxygen Species Release and of Immune System Activation

The generation of ROS is a key process in the development of reperfusion injury. If these free radicals can be captured or their release be prevented, this may attenuate the extent of reperfusion injury. Conflicting results with regard to the protective effects of these agents have been reported. Part of this controversy might be related to the duration of the myocardial ischemia and the interindividual variations of collateral flow, allowing the compound to reach the ischemic area [27,116–118].

Attempts to diminish neutrophil-mediated effects in the development of reperfusion injury have included depletion of neutrophils, direct inhibition of neutrophils, and inhibition of cell adhesion molecules on neutrophils and endothelial cells. Depletion by administration of specific antibodies against neutrophils or neutrophil-clearing filters have been shown—although not unequivocally—to have protective effects on the extent of ischemia-reperfusion injury. Also, in experimental studies, blocking of adhesion molecules with specific antibodies against ICAM-1, P-selectin, L-selectin, and PECAM-1 just before reperfusion appeared to be associated with a decrease in the extent of reperfusion injury. Neutrophils release serine proteases. The serine protease inhibitor aprotinin inhibits neutrophil migration and inhibits endothelial cell activation in response to proinflammatory stimuli. Protease inhibitors appear to reduce infarct size and apoptosis probably by attenuation or inhibition of neutrophil activation and recruitment either directly or by inhibition of cytokine generation [17–24, 27–29,32,118–121].

Another possible therapeutic target is the inhibition of the *complement cascade* by selective inhibition of the different complement proteins involved or by interference with complement receptors. Several experimental studies have indicated that inhibition of different steps in the complement cascade resulted in a reduction of infarction size following myocardial ischemia and reperfusion [1,118].

Modulation of Calcium Homeostasis

Since calcium overload plays a key role in the pathogenesis of myocardial ischemia-reperfusion injury, it can be hypothesized that modulation of the intracellular Ca^{2+} transients may have a protective effect in the course of ischemia-reperfusion injury. Calcium antagonists were shown to be cardioprotective when administered prior to the induction of ischemia. However, it was not possible from these studies to distinguish between protection against injury induced by ischemia or by reperfusion [122,123]. It was suggested that the beneficial effects of calcium antagonists were mainly related to the negative inotropic and chronotropic, and hence energy-sparing effects of these compounds. However, calcium antagonists may also act as antioxidants and nitric oxide synthase regulators. In addition, more recent studies indicated that calcium antagonists not only have antiischemic effects but also are protective against the myocardial injury induced by reperfusion itself [118,124,125].

In vitro data have shown that the reoxygenated myocardial cell may be protected from hypercontracture by damping the oscillatory intracellular movements of Ca^{2+}, thereby reducing the high peak concentrations of cytosolic Ca^{2+}. This can be achieved by specific blockade of the Ca^{2+} uptake (cyclopiazonic acid) or release (ryanodine) at the level of the sarcoplasmatic reticulum. Interestingly, the volatile anesthetic halothane also blocks these Ca^{2+} transients, thereby protecting the myocardial cells against hypercontracture and lethal reperfusion injury [42,126].

Other Therapeutic Possibilities

Of particular interest in the potential treatment modalities of ischemia-reperfusion injury is the therapeutic value of H^+ transport inhibition during the early phase of reperfusion. As described previously, activation of the Na^+/H^+ exchanger is associated with intracellular calcium accumulation. Inhibition of this exchanger, therefore, may attenuate the consequences of reperfusion injury. Although experimental and early clinical studies were suggestive of a protective effect, recently performed larger trials failed to demonstrate a clinical benefit [45,54,118,127].

In recent years, the potential use of nitric oxide (NO) as a therapeutic tool in the course of ischemia-reperfusion injury has gained wide interest. Nitric oxide is a powerful vasodilator and may improve blood flow during reperfusion. In addition, NO inhibits adherence of neutrophils to the vascular endothelium and may act as a scavenger of free oxygen radicals. During reperfusion after ischemia, bioavailability of NO is impaired due to enhanced inactivation of NO by ROS and to a reduced production of NO. Administration of NO or NO donors may attenuate the extent of ischemia-reperfusion injury. Also, pretreatment with drugs that enhance NO release, such as statins, certain calcium antagonists, angiotensin-converting enzyme inhibitors, endothelin-1 receptor antagonists, and dexamethasone, may protect the myocardium against ischemia-reperfusion injury [118,128,129].

Other therapeutic possibilities, related to the pathways known to be involved in the pathogenesis of ischemia-reperfusion injury, that have been explored include modulation of the reperfusion injury salvage kinase pathway [130], targeting the mitochondrial permeability transition pore [59], and also targeting the pathways involved in the apoptotic process [118].

Conclusion

Based on the different pathogenetic mechanisms involved in ischemia-reperfusion injury, it is possible to hypothesize a number of therapeutic approaches. Mainly experimental studies have demonstrated a beneficial role in containing the extent of reperfusion injury with a number of pharmacologic and nonpharmacologic approaches. Clinical data, however, are either not yet available or report conflicting results. Given the small size of most of these studies, larger clinical trials will be necessary to definitively demonstrate whether application of potential therapeutic approaches really translate into a better clinical outcome after ischemia-reperfusion injury. Significant resources have indeed been invested in studies that have often yielded inconclusive results. A new approach has been proposed that may help to obviate a number of the difficulties associated with translation of basic science findings. This implies a new focus on translational research that emphasizes efficacy and clinically relevant outcomes with the establishment of a system for rigorous preclinical testing of promising cardioprotective agents using clinical trial-like approaches (blinded, randomized, multicenter, sufficiently powered, standardized methodology). This can then be followed by a system that enables rational translation of important basic findings into clinical studies, ultimately leading to a well-founded application of new therapeutical strategies. [131]

References

(Note: key references are marked with *.)

*1. Park JL, Lucchesi BR. Mechanisms of myocardial reperfusion injury. Ann Thorac Surg 1999;68: 1905–12.
2. Kloner RA, Deboer LWV, Darsee JR, et al. Prolonged abnormalities of myocardium salvages by reperfusion. Am J Physiol 1981;241:H591–9.
3. Ellis SG, Henschke CI, Sandor T, et al. Time course of functional and biochemical recovery of myocardium salvaged by reperfusion. J Am Coll Cardiol 1983;1:1047–55.
4. Przyklenk K, Kloner RA. Superoxide dismutase plus catalase improve contractile function in the canine model of "stunned" myocardium. Circ Res 1986;58:148–56.
5. Ambrosio G, Jacobus WE, Mitchell MC, et al. Effects of ATP precursors on ATP and free ADP content and functional recovery of postischemic hearts. Am J Physiol 1989;256:H560–6.
6. Kusuoka H, Marban E. Cellular mechanisms of myocardial stunning. Annu Rev Physiol 1992;54: 243–56.
*7. Gross GJ, Kersten JR, Warltier DC. Mechanisms of postischemic contractile dysfunction. Ann Thorac Surg 1999:68:1898–904.
8. Myers ML, Bolli R, Lekich RF, et al. Enhancement of recovery of myocardial function by oxygen free-radical scavengers after reversible regional ischemia. Circulation 1985;72:915–21.
9. Gross GJ, Farber NE, Hardman HF, et al. Beneficial actions of superoxide dismutase and catalase in stunned myocardium of dogs. Am J Physiol 1986;250:H372–7.
10. Joly SR, Kane WJ, Bailie MB, et al. Canine myocardial reperfusion injury. Its reduction by the combined administration of superoxide dismutase and catalase. Circ Res 1984;54:277–85.
11. Zweier JL, Flaherty JT, Weisfeldt ML. Direct measurements of free radical generation following reperfusion of ischemic myocardium. Proc Natl Acad Sci USA 1987;84:1404–7.
12. Bolli R, Patel BS, Jeroudi MO, et al. Demonstration of free radical generation in "stunned" myocardium of intact dogs with the use of the spin trap α-phenyl-N-tertbutyl nitrone. J Clin Invest 1988;82:476–85.
13. Ambrosio G, Zweier JL, Flaherty JT. The relationship between oxygen radical generation and impairment of myocardial energy metabolism following post-ischemic reperfusion. J Mol Cell Cardiol 1991;23:1359–74.
14. Khalid MA, Ashraf M. Direct detection of endogenous hydroxyl radical production in adult cardiomyocytes during anoxia and reoxygenation: is the hydroxyl radical really the most important species? Circ Res 1993;72:725–36.
*15. Becker LB. New concepts in reactive oxygen species and cardiovascular reperfusion physiology. Cardiovasc Res 2004;61:461–70.
16. Piper HM, Garcia-Dorado D. Prime causes of rapid cardiomyocyte death during reperfusion. Ann Thorac Surg 1999;68:1913–9.
17. Eagler R, Covell JW. Granulocytes cause reperfusion ventricular dysfunction after 15-minute ischemia in the dog. Circ Res 1987;61: 20–8.

18. Westlin W, Mullane KM. Alleviation of myocardial stunning by leucocyte and platelet depletion. Circulation 1989;80:1828–36.
19. Jeremy RW, Becker LC. Neutrophil depletion does not prevent myocardial dysfunction after brief coronary occlusion. J Am Coll Cardiol 1989;13:1155–63.
20. O'Neill PG, Charlat ML, Michael LH, et al. Influence of neutrophil depletion on myocardial function and flow after reversible ischemia. Am J Physiol 1989;256:H341–51.
21. Juneau CF, Ito BR, del Balzo U, et al. Severe neutrophil depletion by leucocyte filters or cytotoxic drugs does not improve recovery of contractile function in stunned porcine myocardium. Cardiovasc Res 1993;27:720–7.
22. Becker LC. Do neutrophils contribute to myocardial stunning? Cardiovasc Drug Ther 1991;5:909–13.
23. Bolli R. Role of neutrophils in myocardial stunning after brief ischemia: the end of a six old controversy (1987–1993). Cardiovasc Res 1993;27:728–30.
24. Vinten-Johansen J. Involvement of neutrophils in the pathogenesis of lethal myocardial reperfusion injury. Cardiovasc Res 2004;61:481–97.
25. Vakeva AP, Agah A, Rollins SA, et al. Myocardial infarction and apoptosis after myocardial ischemia and reperfusion. Role of the terminal complement components and inhibition by anti-C5 therapy. Circulation 1998;97:2259–67.
26. Dörge H, Schulz R, Belosjorow S, et al. Coronary microembolization: the role of TNF-α in contractile dysfunction. J Mol Cell Cardiol 2002;34:51–62.
27. Forman MB, Puett DW, Virmani R. Endothelial and myocardial injury during ischemia and reperfusion: pathogenesis and therapeutic implications. J Am Coll Cardiol 1989;13:450–9.
28. Lefer AM, Weyrich AS, Buerke M. Role of selectins, a new family of adhesion molecules, in ischemia-reperfusion injury. Cardiovasc Res 1994;28:289–94.
29. Lefer AM. Role of selectins in myocardial ischemia-reperfusion injury. Ann Thorac Surg 1995;60:773–7.
30. Weyrich AC, Buerke M, Albertine KH, et al. Time course of coronary vascular endothelial adhesion molecule expression during reperfusion of the ischemic feline myocardium. J Leukoc Biol 1995;57:45–55.
31. Zhao Z-Q, Velez DA, Wang N-P, et al. Progressively developed myocardial apoptotic cell death during late phase of reperfusion. Apoptosis 2001;6:279–90.
*32. Collard CD, Gelman S. Pathophysiology, clinical manifestations, and prevention of ischemiareperfusion injury. Anesthesiology 2001;94:1133–8.
33. McEver RP, Cummings RD. Role of PSGL-1 binding to selectins in leucocyte recruitment. J Clin Invest 1997;100:485–92.
34. Bienvenu K, Granger DN. Molecular determinants of shear rate-dependent leucocyte adhesion in postcapillary venules. Am J Physiol 1993;264:H1504–8.
35. Entman ML, Youker K, Shappell SB, et al. Neutrophil adherence to isolated adult canine myocytes. Evidence for a CD18-dependent mechanism. J Clin Invest 1990;85:1497–506.
36. Entman ML, Youker K, Shoji T, et al. Neutrophil induced oxidative injury of cardiac myocytes. A compartmented system requiring CD11b/CD18—ICAM-1 adherence. J Clin Invest 1992;90:1335–45.
37. Reimer KA, Murry CE, Richard VJ. The role of neutrophils and free radicals in the ischemic-reperfused heart: why the confusion and controversy? J Mol Cell Cariol 1989;21:1225–39.
38. Chatelain P, Latour J-G, Tran D, et al. Neutrophil accumulation in experimental myocardial infarcts: relation with extent of injury and effect of reperfusion. Circulation 1987;75:1083–90.
39. Murohara T, Buerke M, Lefer AM. Polymorphonuclear leukocyte-induced vasoconstriction and endothelial dysfunction. Role of selectins. Arterioscler Thromb 1994;14:1509–19.
40. Sheridan FM, Cole PG, Ramage D. Leucocyte adhesion to the coronary microvasculature during ischemia and reperfusion in an vivo canine model. Circulation 1996;93:1784–7.
41. Zhao Z-Q, Nakamura M, Wang N-P, et al. Dynamic progression of contractile and endothelial dysfunction and infarct extension in the late phase of reperfusion. J Surg Res 2000;94:1–12.
42. Siegmund B, Schlack W, Ladilov YV, et al. Halothane protects cardiomyocytes against reoxygenation-induced hypercontracture. Circulation 1997;96:4372–9.
43. Piper HM, Garcia-Dorado D, Ovize M. A fresh look at reperfusion injury. Cardiovasc Res 1998;38:291–300.
44. Schäfer C, Ladilov YV, Inserte J, et al. Role of the reverse mode of the Na^+/Ca^{2+} exchanger in reoxygenation-induced cardiomyocyte injury. Cardiovasc Res 2001;51:241–50.
*45. Piper HM, Abdallah Y, Schäfer C. The first minutes of reperfusion: a window of opportunity for cardioprotection. Cardiovasc Res 2004;61:365–71.

46. Siegmund B, Zude R, Piper HM. Recovery of anoxic-reoxygenated cardiomyocytes from severe Ca^{2+} overload. Am J Physiol 1992;263:H1262–9.
47. Ladilov YV, Siegmund B, Piper HM. Simulated ischemia increases the susceptibility of rat cardiomyocytes to hypercontracture. Circ Res 1997; 80:69–75.
48. Carrozza JP, Bentivegna LA, Williams CP, et al. Decreased myofilament responsiveness in myocardial stunning follows transient calcium overload during ischemia and reperfusion. Circ Res 1992;71:1334–40.
49. Hofmann PA, Miller WP, Moss RL. Altered calcium sensitivity of isometric tension in myocyte-sized preparations of porcine postischemic stunned myocardium. Circ Res 1993;72:50–6.
50. Miller WP, McDonald KS, Moss RL. Onset of reduced Ca^{2+} sensitivity of tension during stunning in porcine myocardium. J Mol Cell Cardiol 1996;28:689–97.
51. Gao WD, Liu Y, Mellgren R, et al. Intrinsic myofilament alterations underlying the decreased contractility of stunned myocardium. A consequence of Ca^{2+}-dependent proteolysis? Circ Res 1996;78:455–65.
52. Gao WD, Atar D, Liu Y, et al. Role of troponin I proteolysis in the pathogenesis of stunned myocardium. Circ Res 1997;80:393–9.
53. Gao WD, Liu Y, Marban E. Selective effects of oxygen free radicals on excitation-contraction coupling in ventricular muscle. Implications for the mechanism of stunned myocardium. Circulation 1996;94:2597–604.
54. Piper HM, Balser C, Ladyloc YV, et al. The role of Na^+/H^+ exchange in ischemia-reperfusion. Basic Res Cardiol 1996;91:191–202.
55. Ladilov YV, Siegmund B, Piper HM. Protection of the reoxygenated cardiomyocyte against hypercontracture by inhibition of the Na^+/H^+ exchange. Am J Physiol 1995;268:H1531–9.
56. Garcia-Dorado D, Oliveras J. Myocardial edema: a preventable cause of reperfusion injury. Cardiovasc Res 1993;27:1555–63.
57. Inserte J, Garcia-Dorado D, Ruiz-Meana M, et al. The Na^+/H^+ exchange occurring during hypoxia in the genesis of reoxygenation-induced myocardial oedema. J Mol Cell Cardiol 1997;29: 1167–75.
58. Ruiz-Meana M, Garcia-Dorado, Gonzales MA, et al. Effect of osmotic stress on sarcolemmal integrity of isolated cardiomyocytes following transient metabolic inhibition. Cardiovasc Res 1995;30:64–9.
59. Halestrap AP, Clarke SJ, Javadov SA. Mitochondrial permeability transition pore opening during myocardial reperfusion—a target for cardioprotection. Cardiovasc Res 2004;61:372–85.
60. Gottlieb RA, Burleson KO, Kloner RA, et al. Reperfusion injury induces apoptosis in rabbit cardiomyocytes. J Clin Invest 1994;94:1621–8.
61. Veinot JP, Gattinger DA, Fliss H. Early apoptosis in human myocardial infarcts. Hum Pathol 1997;28:485–92.
62. Saraste A, Pulkki K, Kallajoki M, et al. Apoptosis in human acute myocardial infarction. Circulation 1997;95:320–3.
63. Zhao Z-Q, Vinten-Johansen J. Myocardial apoptosis and ischemic preconditioning. Cardiovasc Res 2002;55:438–55.
64. Valen G. The basic biology of apoptosis and its implications for cardiac function and viability. Ann Thorac Surg 2003;75:S656–60.
65. Miller TD, Christian TF, Hopfenspirger MR, et al. Infarct size after acute myocardial infarction measured by quantitative tomographic 99mTc sestamibi imaging predicts subsequent mortality. Circulation 1995;92:334–41.
66. Maroko PR, Kjekshus JK, Sobel BE, et al. Factors influencing infarct size following experimental coronary artery occlusions. Circulation 1971; 43:67–82.
67. Murry CE, Jennings RB, Reimer KA. Preconditioning with ischemia: a delay in lethal injury in ischemic myocardium. Circulation 1986;74:1124–36.
68. Kloner RA, Jennings RB. Consequences of brief ischemia: stunning, preconditioning, and their clinical implications. Part 1. Circulation 2001;104: 2981–9.
69. Kloner RA, Jennings RB. Consequences of brief ischemia: stunning, preconditioning, and their clinical implications. Part 2. Circulation 2001;104: 3158–67.
70. Laude K, Beauchamp P, Tuillez C, et al. Endothelial protective effects of preconditioning. Cardiovasc Res 2002;55:466–73.
71. Fryer RM, Auchampach JA, Gross GJ. Therapeutic receptor targets of ischemic preconditioning. Cardiovasc Res 2002;55:520–5.
72. Sommerschild HT, KirkebØen KA. Preconditioning—endogenous defence mechanisms of the heart. Acta Anaesthesiol Scand 2002;46:123–37.
*73. Yellon DM, Downey JM. Preconditioning the myocardium: from cellular physiology to clinical cardiology. Physiol Rev 2003;83:1113–51.
74. Deutsch E, Berger M, Kussmaul WG, et al. Adaptation to ischemia during percutaneous

transluminal angioplasty. Clinical, hemodynamic, and metabolic features. Circulation 1990;82:2044–51.
75. Kloner RA, Shook T, Przyklenk K, et al. Previous angina alters in-hospital outcome in TIMI 4. A clinical correlate to preconditioning? Circulation 1995;91:37–45.
76. Laskey WK. Beneficial impact of preconditioning during PTCA on creatine kinase release. Circulation 1999;99:2085–9.
77. Ottani F, Galvani M, Ferrini D, et al. Prodromal angina limits infarct size. A role for ischemic preconditioning. Circulation 1995;91:291–7.
78. Perrault LP, Menasché P, Bel A, et al. Ischemic preconditioning in cardiac surgery: a word of caution. J Thorac Cardiovasc Surg 1996;112:1378–86.
79. Jenkins DP, Pugsley WB, Alkhulaifi AM, et al. Ischaemic preconditioning reduces troponin T release in patients undergoing coronary artery bypass surgery. Heart 1997;77:314–8.
80. Jacobson E, Young CJ, Aronson S, et al. The role of ischemic preconditioning during minimally invasive coronary artery bypass surgery. J Cardiothorac Vasc Anesth 1997;11:787–92.
81. Illes RW, Swoyer KD. Prospective, randomized clinical study of ischemic preconditioning as an adjunct to intermittent cold blood cardioplegia. Ann Thorac Surg 1998;65:748–52.
82. Lu EX, Chen SX, Hu TH, et al. Preconditioning enhances myocardial protection in patients undergoing open heart surgery. Thorac Cardiovasc Surg 1998;46:28–32.
83. Lucchetti V, Caputo M, Suleiman MS, et al. Beating heart coronary revascularization without metabolic myocardial damage. Eur J Cardiothorac Surg 1998;14:443–4.
84. Malkowski MJ, Kramer CM, Parvizi ST, et al. Transient ischemia does not limit subsequent ischemic regional dysfunction in humans: a transesophageal echocardiographic study during minimally invasive coronary artery bypass surgery. J Am Coll Cardiol 1998;31:1035–9.
85. Laurikka J, WU Z-K, Lisalo P, et al. Regional ischemic preconditioning enhances myocardial performance in off-pump coronary artery bypass grafting. Chest 2002;121:1183–9.
86. Vaage J, Valen G. Preconditioning and cardiac surgery. Ann Thorac Surg 2003;75:S709–14.
87. Ross S, Foëx P. Protective effects of anaesthetics in reversible and irreversible ischaemia-reperfusion injury. Br J Anaesth 1999;82:622–32.
88. Zaugg M, Lucchinetti E, Uecker M, et al. Anaesthetics and cardiac preconditioning. Part 1. Signalling and cytoprotective mechanisms. Br J Anaesth 2003;91:552–65.
89. Zaugg M, Lucchinetti E, Garcia C, et al. Anaesthetics and cardiac preconditioning. Part 2. Clinical implications. Br J Anaesth 2003;91:566–76.
90. De Hert SG. Cardioprotection with volatile anaesthetics: clinical relevance. Curr Opin Anaesthesiol 2004;17:57–62.
91. Tanaka K, Ludwig LM, Kersten JR, et al. Mechanisms of cardioprotection by volatile anesthetics. Anesthesiology 2004;100:707–21.
*92. De Hert SG, Turani F, Mathur S, et al. Cardioprotection with volatile anesthetics: mechanisms and clinical implications. Anesth Analg 2005;100:1584–93.
93. De Hert SG. The concept of anaesthetic-induced cardioprotection: clinical relevance. Best Pract Res Clin Anaesthesiol 2005;19:445–59.
94. De Hert SG, Van der Linden PJ, Cromheecke S, et al. Choice of primary anesthetic regimen can influence intensive care unit length of stay after coronary surgery with cardiopulmonary bypass. Anesthesiology 2004;101:9–20.
95. Garcia C, Julier K, Bestmann L, et al. Preconditioning with sevoflurane decreases PECAM-1 expression and improves one-year cardiovascular outcome in coronary artery bypass graft surgery. Br J Anaesth 2005;94:159–65.
96. Taegtmeyer H. Energy metabolism of the heart: from basic concepts to clinical implications. Curr Probl Cardiol 1994;19:59–113.
97. Stanley WC, Lopaschuk GD, Hall JL, et al. Regulation of myocardial carbohydrate metabolism under normal and ischaemic conditions. Potential for pharmacological interventions. Cardiovasc Res 1997;33:243–57.
98. Ferrari R, Pepi P, Ferrari F, et al. Metabolic derangement in ischemic heart disease and its therapeutic control. Am J Cardiol 1998;82:K2–13.
99. Lopaschuk GD. Treating ischemic heart disease by pharmacologically improving cardiac energy metabolism. Am J Cardiol 1998;82:K14–17.
100. Taegtmeyer H, King LM, Jones BE. Energy substrate metabolism, myocardial ischemia, and targets for pharmacotherapy. Am J Cardiol 1998;82:K54–60.
*101. Lee L, Horowitz J, Frenneaux M. Metabolic manipulation in ischaemic heart disease, a novel approach to treatment. Eur Heart J 2004;25:634–41.
102. Sack MN, Yellon DM. Insulin therapy as an adjunct to reperfusion after acute coronary

ischemia. A proposed direct myocardial cell survival effect independent of metabolic modulation. J Am Coll Cardiol 2003;41:1404–7.
103. Fath-Ordoubadi F, Beatt KJ. Glucose-insulin-potassium therapy for treatment of acute myocardial infarction: an overview of randomized placebo-controlled trials. Circulation 1997;96: 1152–6.
104. Diaz R, Paolasso EA, Piegas LS, et al. Metabolic modulation of acute myocardial infarction. The ECLA Collaborative Group. Circulation 1998;98: 2227–34.
105. Apstein CS, Opie LH. Glucose-insulin-potassium (GIK) for acute myocardial infarction: a negative study with a positive value. Cardiovasc Drug Ther 1999;13:185–90.
106. Ceremuzynski L, Budaj A, Czepiel A, et al. Low-dose glucose-insulin-potassium is ineffective in acute myocardial infarction: results of a randomized multicenter Pol-GIK trial. Cardiovasc Drugs Ther 1999;13:191–200.
107. van der Horst ICC, Zijstra F, van't Hof AWJ, et al. Glucose-insulin-potassium infusion in patients treated with primary angioplasty for acute myocardial infarction. J Am Coll Cardiol 2003;42:784–91.
108. Apstein CS. The benefits of glucose-insulin-potassium for acute myocardial infarction (and some concerns). J Am Coll Cardiol 2003;42: 792–5.
109. Nicolini F, Beghi C, Muscari C, et al. Myocardial protection in adult cardiac surgery: current options and future challenges. Eur J Cardiothorac Surg 2003;24:986–93.
110. Doenst T, Bothe W, Beyersdorf F. Therapy with insulin in cardiac surgery: controversies and possible solutions. Ann Thorac Surg 2003;75: S721–8.
111. Forman MB, Velasco CE. Role of adenosine in the treatment of myocardial stunning. Cardiovasc Drugs Ther 1991;5:901–8.
112. Mubagwa K, Flameng W. Adenosine, adenosine receptors and myocardial protection: an updated review. Cardiovasc Res 2001;52: 25–39.
113. Obata T. Adenosine production and its interaction with protection of ischemic and reperfusion injury of the myocardium. Life Sciences 2002;71: 2083–103.
114. Donato M, Gelpi RJ. Adenosine and cardioprotection during reperfusion—an overview. Mol Cell Biochem 2003;251:153–9.
115. Vinten-Johansen J, Zhao Z-Q, Corvera JS, et al. Adenosine in myocardial protection in on-pump and off-pump cardiac surgery. Ann Thorac Surg 2003;75:S691–9.
116. Bolli R. Oxygen-derived free radicals and postischemic myocardial dysfunction ("stunned myocardium"). J Am Coll Cardiol 1988;12:239–49.
117. Kukreja RC, Janin Y. Reperfusion injury: basic concepts and protection strategies. J Thromb Thrombolysis 1997;4:7–24.
*118. Wang Q-D, Pernow J, Sjöquist P-O, et al. Pharmacological possibilities for protection against myocardial reperfusion injury. Cardiovasc Res 2002;55:25–37.
119. Hansen PR. Role of neutrophils in myocardial ischemia and reperfusion. Circulation 1995;91: 1872–85.
120. Jordan JE, Zhao Z-Q, Vinten-Johansen J. The role of neutrophils in myocardial ischemia-reperfusion injury. Cardiovasc Res 1999;43:860–78.
121. Bull DA, Maurer J. Aprotinin and preservation of myocardial function after ischemia-reperfusion injury. Ann Thorac Surg 2003;75:S735–9.
122. Garcia-Dorado D, Theroux D, Fernandez-Aviles F, et al. Diltiazem and progression of myocardial ischemic damage during coronary artery occlusion and reperfusion in porcine hearts. J Am Coll Cardiol 1987;10:906–11.
123. Vatner SF, Patrick TA, Knight DR, et al. Effects of calcium channel blocker on responses of blood flow, function, arrhythmias, and extent of infarction following reperfusion in conscious baboons. Circ Res 1988;62:105–15.
124. Herzog WR, Vogel RA, Schlossberg ML, et al. Short-term low dose intracoronary diltiazem administered at the onset of reperfusion reduces myocardial infarct size. Int J Cardiol 1997;59: 21–7.
125. Smart SC, Sagar KB, Warltier DC. Differential roles of myocardial Ca^{2+} channels and Na^+/Ca^{2+} exchange in myocardial reperfusion injury in open chest dogs: relative roles during ischemia and reperfusion. Cardiovasc Res 1997;36:337–46.
126. Schlack W, Hollmann M, Stunneck J, et al. Effect of halothane on myocardial reoxygenation injury in the isolated rat heart. Br J Anaesth 1996;76: 860–7.
127. Mentzer RM, Lasley RD, Jessel A, et al. Intracellular sodium hydrogen exchange inhibition and clinical myocardial protection. Ann Thorac Surg 2003;75:S700–8.
128. Bolli R. Cardioprotective function of inducible nitric oxide synthase and role of nitric oxide in myocardial ischemia and preconditioning: an

overview of a decade of research. J Mol Cell Cardiol 2001;33:1897–918.

129. Schulz R, Kelm M, Heusch G. Nitric oxide in myocardial ischemia/reperfusion injury. Cardiovasc Res 2004;61:402–13.

130. Hausenloy DJ, Yellon DM. New directions for protecting the heart against ischaemia-reperfusion injury: targeting the Reperfusion Injury Salvage Kinase (RISK)-pathway. Cardiovasc Res 2004;61:448–60.

131. Bolli R, Becker L, Gross G, et al. Myocardial protection at a crossroads: the need for translation into clinical therapy. Circ Res 2004;95: 125–34.

1.2.2
Cellular and Organ System Level

10
Receptor Signaling Pathways in Heart Failure: Transgenic Mouse Models

Juhsien Chen and Howard A. Rockman

With increasing prevalence and high mortality, heart failure (HF) emerges as a major health problem. The heart often undergoes myocardial hypertrophy in response to increased load demand, and acute or chronic HF occurs when the heart acutely or gradually decompensates in the setting of new pathologic stresses. In addition to hypertrophy, the heart also undergoes other maladaptive modifications in response to pathogenic stresses that include altered contractility, cardiomyocyte survival, and transcriptional gene expressions. These changes are mediated, in part, by plasma membrane receptors that transduce extracellular signals to multiple complex intracellular signaling pathways that regulate cardiac gene expression. These various signaling pathways implicated in the pathophysiology of HF have been extensively studied, and genetically modified mouse models have been crucial in elucidating these pathways. This chapter discusses the signaling mechanisms underlying cardiac hypertrophy and failure and the transgenic mouse models that have been used to study these signaling pathways, with emphasis on G-protein–coupled receptors, growth factor receptors, and the convergence of extracellular signaling pathways in intracellular and transcriptional regulation of hypertrophy and HF.

G-Protein–Coupled Receptor Signaling

G-protein–coupled receptors (GPCRs) are a conserved class of seven-transmembrane receptors that play an important role in cardiovascular homeostasis. The GPCRs that are particularly crucial for cardiovascular function include the adrenergic, angiotensin II, endothelin, and muscarinic cholinergic receptors.[1] Upon extracellular ligand binding, GPCRs undergo conformational change and coupling of their intracellular domain with a heterotrimeric guanine-nucleotide-binding regulatory protein (G protein). The coupling allows for the exchange of guanosine diphosphate (GDP) to guanosine triphosphate (GTP) on the G-protein α subunit and results in G-protein dissociation into Gα and G$\beta\gamma$ subunits. Classic GPCR signaling is activated by the coupling of the Gα subunit to an effector molecule such as adenylyl cyclase, phospholipase C β (PLCβ), or ion channels.[1,2]

G proteins are classified into four major families based on the α subunits: Gs, Gi, Gq/11, and Gα12/13. Specifically, the Gs class activates the enzyme adenylyl cyclase to generate second-messenger cyclic adenosine monophosphate (cAMP),[3] leading to the sequential activation of protein kinase A (PKA) and L-type Ca^{2+} channels and increased contractility of the heart.[4–6] The Gi class comprises inhibitory G proteins that diminish agonist-stimulated cAMP production. Coupled to α_1-adrenergic, angiotensin II, and endothelin-1 receptors, Gq activates PLCβ, resulting in the production of inositol-1,4,5-triphosphate (IP_3) and diacylglycerol; IP_3 leads to the release of Ca^{2+} from sarcoplasmic reticulum and activation of Ca^{2+}/calmodulin kinase, which then mediates hypertrophic gene expression.[7] Diacylglycerol activates serine/threonine protein kinase C (PKC) that participates in various downstream pathways.

Gα12/13 signals via small G-protein Rho and regulates cellular responses such as cytoskeletal changes and cellular growth.[8]

Desensitization, a process in which the receptor response is attenuated in the presence of persistent agonist stimulation, plays a crucial role in GPCR downregulation. Three families of regulatory molecules are involved in GPCR desensitization: second messenger-regulated kinases (PKA, PKC), G-protein–coupled receptor kinases (GRKs), and arrestins. Protein kinases A and C, when activated, participate in feedback regulation by phosphorylating the third intracellular loop of the receptor, thus uncoupling the receptor from G protein.[1,2] In contrast, GRKs participate in desensitization by phosphorylating the receptor in an agonist-dependent manner. Subsequently, the arrestin proteins are recruited to displace the receptor from G protein and sterically interdict further G-protein coupling. Desensitization also results from receptor downregulation via receptor internalization, receptor degradation, decreased receptor synthesis, or destabilization of receptor messenger RNA (mRNA).[9] Arrestin molecules participate in receptor internalization via clathrin-coated vesicles by serving as an adaptor protein that links the receptors to clathrin and other internalization apparatus.[10,11] In addition, arrestin serves as scaffold protein for GPCR-mediated cellular signaling.[12,13] Finally, receptor downregulation also serves to resensitize the receptor by dephosphorylating the receptor before it is recycled back to the plasma membrane.[14,15]

β-Adrenergic Receptors

The adrenergic receptors are an important class of GPCRs that regulates chronotropy, inotropy, and cardiac growth in response to catecholamine stimulation. Of the three subtypes of β-adrenergic receptors (ARs) (β_1, β_2, and β_3), β_1-ARs are the predominant subtype found in mammalian heart, and regulates heart rate, contractility, and conduction velocity.[1,16] β_2-ARs are located primarily in the smooth muscles of the vasculature, bronchial, gastrointestinal, and urinary systems, as well as the skeletal muscles, and mediate smooth muscle relaxation and glycogenesis. β_3-ARs play a role in lipolysis and thermogenesis and may have negative inotropic effects on the heart.[17,18]

The heart responds to injury by activating the sympathetic nervous system. In the failing heart, chronic catecholamine stimulation results in β-AR desensitization and downregulation.[19–21] More specifically, β_1-AR is selectively downregulated, leading to a β_1-AR/β_2-AR ratio of 60:40 in the failing heart instead of the normal 80:20 ratio.[22,23] Both β_1-AR and β_2-AR are uncoupled from G proteins.[19] The abnormal β-AR signaling results in abnormal contractile function and allows the receptors to couple to other signaling pathways involved in ventricular hypertrophy such as mitogen-activated protein kinases (MAPK) and phosphoinositide-3-kinase (PI3K) cascades.[24,25]

Several transgenic murine models have been generated to help elucidate the mechanistic role of β-ARs in HF. Mice with 5- to 15-fold cardiac-specific overexpression of β_1-AR have increased sensitivity to catecholamine stimulation and initially exhibit improved cardiac contractility, but later develop progressive hypertrophy and early HF, with pathologic changes similar to that seen in human HF.[26] β_1-AR knockout (KO) mice have high embryonic lethality, and those that do survive exhibit no inotropic or chronotropic response to exercise or β-agonist stimulation despite normal basal heart rate and blood pressure and the presence of β_2-AR in the heart.[27] In contrast, cardiac-specific β_2-AR overexpression up to 200-fold results in enhanced contractile function even beyond 1 year of age with few signs of HF,[28,29] but a high level of β_2-AR overexpression (>200-fold) leads to rapid development of hypertrophy and HF.[28] The enhanced basal cardiac function in β_2-AR–overexpressing mice is likely attributed to an increased fraction of spontaneously isomerized receptors that are maximally activated in a ligand-independent manner when highly expressed, as these mice showed no response to β-agonist stimulation.[29] β_2-AR has also been shown to couple to Gi proteins since treating β_2-AR–overexpressing myocytes with the Gi-inhibitory pertussis toxin restores β-AR responsiveness.[30] β_2-AR KO mice display normal development and resting cardiovascular function but develop hypertension in response to exercise and epinephrine stimulation.[31]

Taken together, these mouse models demonstrate that β_1-ARs, which couple to Gαs, are the main mediator of positive chronotropic and inotropic response to catecholamine stimulation. On the other hand, β_2-ARs, which signal via both Gαs and Gαi, mainly regulate peripheral vascular relaxation, energy metabolism, cell differentiation, and survival, as β_2-AR KO mice display longer exercise endurance.[24,30,31] Overexpression of β_1-ARs, though initially augments cardiac function, eventually leads to deleterious effects on the heart similar to HF. Only high levels of β_2-AR overexpression are deleterious for the heart, while moderate overexpression confers beneficial cardiac effects.[32] The different phenotypes of the transgenic mice highlight the different functions of the β-ARs and the different downstream signaling each receptor is coupled to.

α_1-Adrenergic Receptors

All three α_1-adrenergic receptors (α_{1A}, α_{1B}, and α_{1D}) are found in the heart but in smaller 1:10 ratio compared to β-AR. α_1-ARs couple to Gq in response to norepinephrine and phenylephrine and signal via the PLC/PKC pathway to mobilize Ca^{2+} entry into intracellular compartment, resulting in cardiac inotropic and growth responses.[33] Mice with cardiac-targeted α_{1A}-AR overexpression display increased cardiac contractility without evidence of hypertrophy, implicating α_{1A}-AR in cardiac inotropy.[34] Cardiac-specific overexpression of wild-type α_{1B}-AR in mice results in left ventricular dysfunction and dilated cardiomyopathy without hypertrophy.[35] Interestingly, these mice have a blunted in vivo response to β-AR agonist isoproterenol; this is likely attributed to the ability of overexpressed α_{1B}-ARs to couple to pertussis toxin–sensitive Gi protein and to depress β-AR signaling by upregulating GRKs.[35] In contrast to wild-type receptors, cardiac-specific overexpression of constitutively active mutant α_{1B}-AR in mice results in activation of PLC and a hypertrophic phenotype,[36] while α_{1B}-AR KO mice show blunted hypertrophy in response to chronic norepinephrine stimulation.[37] α_{1B}-AR KO mice also fail to increase their blood pressure in response to α_1-AR agonist phenylephrine.[38] Together these studies demonstrate that α_1-ARs actively regulate inotropic and cardiac hypertrophic response as well as blood pressure in vivo.

G Proteins

Transgenic mice have also been used to study the role of G proteins in the pathogenesis of HF. Gαs transduces the inotropic and chronotropic response of the β-AR stimulation via cAMP and adenylyl cyclase.[1] Transgenic mice with cardiac-specific Gαs overexpression display increased heart rate and contractility in response to catecholamine stimulation initially, but eventually develop histologic evidence of myocardial damage such as cellular hypertrophy, fibrosis, and necrosis at older age.[39,40] This is consistent with the results obtained from studies of enhanced β-AR signaling.

Gαq mediates cardiac hypertrophy in response to adrenergic, angiotensin, and endothelin receptors stimulation.[1] While modest overexpression of wild-type Gαq[41] or constitutively active mutant of Gαq[42] both result in cardiac hypertrophy and modest cardiac dysfunction, high overexpression of Gαq lead to overt HF.[41] In addition, Gαq-overexpressing mice subjected to pressure overload by transverse aortic constriction develop rapidly decompensating eccentric ventricular hypertrophy.[43] The failing hearts of these mice show significant apoptosis, which could be the cellular mechanism for the transition from hypertrophy to failure.[44] Furthermore, cardiac-specific overexpression of a Gαq inhibitory peptide that interferes with Gq coupling to multiple receptors prevents the development of cardiac hypertrophy and ventricular dysfunction in pressure-overloaded mice (Fig. 10.1).[45,46] Collectively, these data demonstrate that Gαq is an important common mediator of cardiac hypertrophy in response to different GPCRs.

Gi couples with A1 adenosine and M2 muscarinic receptors in the heart and decreases cAMP levels, contractility, and heart rate. A transgenic mouse model with cardiac-specific and conditionally expressed Gi-coupled receptor Ro1 that is modified from human κ-opioid receptor illustrates that increased Gi signaling results in abnormal cardiac contractility, ventricular conduction delay, as well as dilated cardiomyopathy with high mortality at 16 weeks.[47,48] Suppression of Ro1 expression partially reverses the cardiac dysfunction. Although increased Gi activity was previously thought to be a compensatory response to

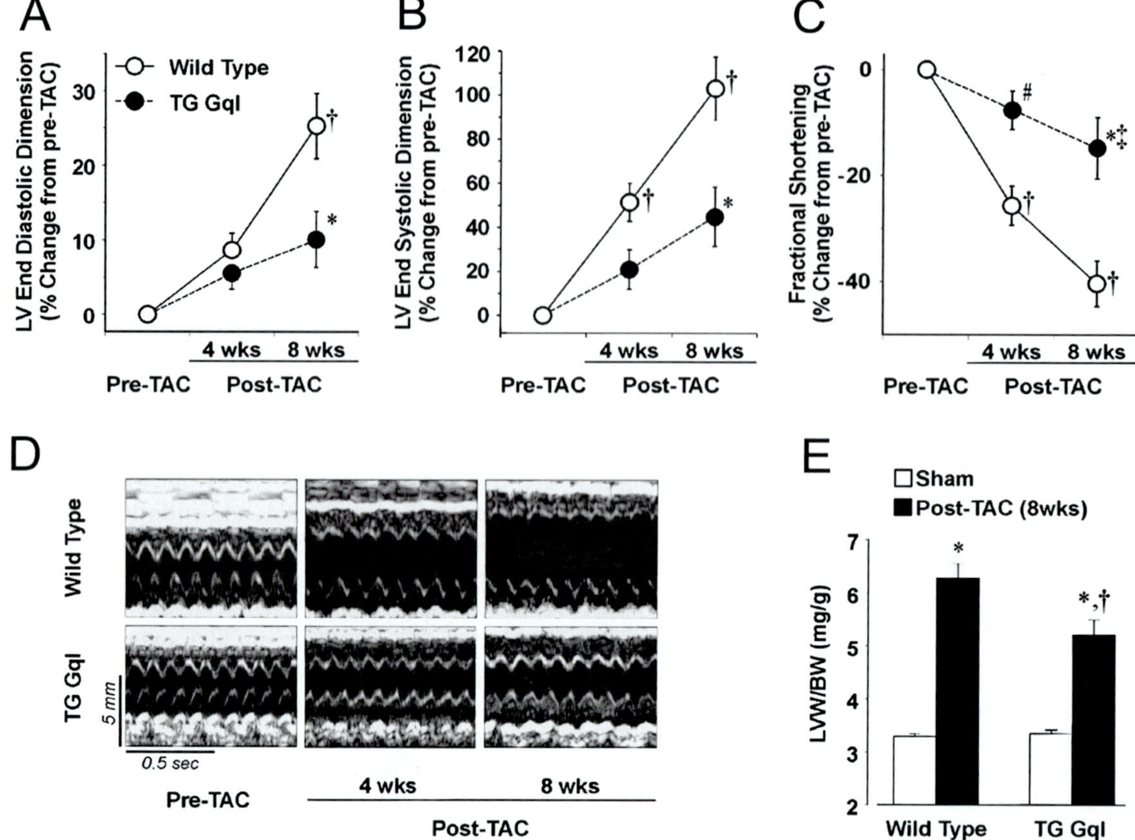

FIGURE 10.1. Serial echocardiography in conscious wild-type and transgenic mice overexpressing a Gαq inhibitory peptide (TgGql) prior to and after chronic pressure overload via transverse aortic constriction (TAC). TgGql mice have attenuated ventricular hypertrophy and did not develop cardiac dysfunction after chronic pressure overload. LVW/BW, left ventricle to body weight ratio. (From Esposito et al.,[46] with permission.)

the increased catecholamine stimulation in failing hearts, the Ro1 transgenic mouse implies a possible causative role for Gi in dilated cardiomyopathy.[47]

G-Protein–Coupled Receptor Kinases (GRKs)

The GRKs desensitize GPCRs by agonist-dependent phosphorylation of the receptor, which leads to subsequent recruitment of arrestins, which interfere with the binding of receptors to G proteins. GRK-mediated desensitization may be an important mechanism for catecholamine unresponsiveness in failing hearts. Of seven GRKs types, GRK2 (commonly known as β-AR kinase 1 or β-ARK1) and GRK5 are the predominant forms expressed in the heart.[49] Elevated levels of β-ARK1 have been observed in human HF and hypertrophy.[23,50] Mice overexpressing β-ARK1 in the heart have attenuated response to isoproterenol stimulation.[51] In contrast, mice overexpressing a peptide inhibitor of β-ARK1, β-ARKct, which inhibits β-ARK1 activity by competitively interfering with β-ARK1 binding to Gβγ, display increased left ventricular contractility and enhanced β-AR response to isoproterenol.[51,52] Homozygous β-ARK1 KO mice exhibit early embryonic death and cardiac malformation, while heterozygous β-ARK1 KO mice, though normal at baseline, display increased contractile response to isoproterenol stimulation.[53,54] Thus, β-ARK1 not only is important for embryonic cardiac development but also is a critical regulator of the heart's contractile function and sympathetic response.[51,53]

Many studies have examined the effects of cross-breeding β-ARKct transgenic mice with various mouse models of HF, including mice with KO of muscle LIM protein,[55,56] cardiac overexpression of calsequestrin (CSQ),[57] and overexpression of mutant cardiac α-myosin heavy chain.[58] Interestingly, in each hybrid transgenic model, overexpressing β-ARKct is able to rescue hypertrophic phenotype and the progression to HF, augment exercise tolerance, and reverse βAR signaling dysfunction (Fig. 10.2).[1] In addition, these beneficial effects are found to be synergistic with the effects of beta-blockers, and even partial inhibition of β-ARK1 may potentially improve cardiac function in response to sympathetic stimulation.[59–62] These studies demonstrate potential therapeutic use of β-ARK1ct in treatment of HF.

The functions of GRK5 and GRK3, which are expressed at low levels in the heart, have also been studied. Overexpression of GRK5 in mice results in similar phenotype as β-ARK1-overexpressing mice, exhibiting β-AR desensitization and depressed contractile function.[63] GRK3 overexpression, however, appears to attenuate cardiac signaling via the thrombin receptor.[64]

Angiotensin II Receptors

Angiotensin II (Ang II) is a neuroactive peptide known to stimulate vascular smooth muscle contraction and aldosterone release as well as an autocrine/paracrine mediator of myocardial growth and hypertrophy.[65] Ang II signals primarily via the Gq-coupled Ang II type 1 receptor

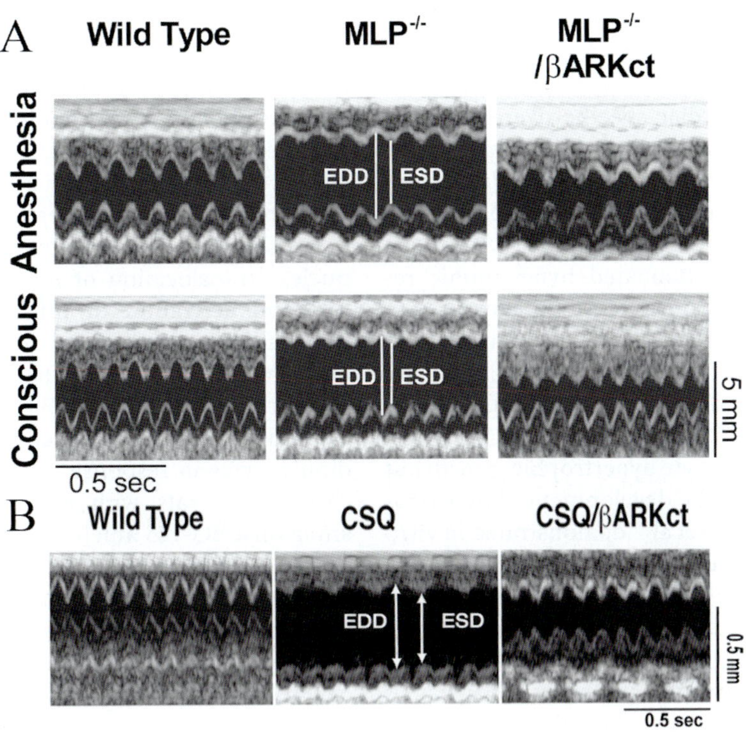

FIGURE 10.2. β-ARKct rescues hypertrophic phenotype and progression to heart failure (HF). (A) Representative M-mode echocardiographic images of conscious and anesthetized wild-type mice, muscle LIM protein knockout mice (MLP–/–), and MLP–/–/β-ARKct mice. The white lines represent left ventricular end-diastolic dimension (EDD) and end-systolic dimension (ESD). While MLP–/– mice show evidence of dilated cardiomyopathy, chamber dimension and cardiac performance in MLP–/–/β-ARKct mice remain normal. (B) Similarly, representative echocardiography of wild-type, CSQ, and CSQ/β-ARKct mice are shown. CSQ/β-ARKct mice have moderate chamber dilation and slightly reduced cardiac function compared to wild-type, while CSQ mice have marked chamber dilation and impaired cardiac function. (From Esposito et al.,[55] and Harding et al.,[57] with permission.)

(AT1R) and less of the Ang II type 2 receptor (AT2R), and downstream signaling is mediated via the MAPK pathways.[66] In rodents, of the two AT1R subtypes ($AT1_AR$ and $AT1_BR$), $AT1_AR$ is more abundant.[67,68]

Ang II and angiotensin-converting enzyme (ACE) levels are found to be elevated in cardiac hypertrophy and HF in both rodents and humans.[69–71] In vivo infusion of Ang II in rats results in ventricular hypertrophy accompanied by extracellular matrix deposition, which are blocked by AT1R antagonism.[72,73] In addition, ACE inhibitors and angiotensin receptor blockers can prevent the development of pressure overload hypertrophy in mice and ameliorate cardiac hypertrophy and HF in both mice and humans.[74–77] Interestingly, in an in vitro model of load-induced cardiac hypertrophy, Ang II is secreted from cardiomyocytes in response to mechanical stretch.[78] Overall, Ang II appears to mediate cardiac hypertrophy via autocrine/paracrine pathway in response to passive mechanical stretch.

Several studies have examined the role of $AT1_AR$ in hypertrophy. Cardiac-specific overexpression of $AT1_ARs$ in mice results in cardiac hypertrophy and fibrosis at baseline and premature death from HF, as well as enhanced hypertrophic response to pressure overload.[79] $AT1_AR$ KO mice with intact $AT1_BR$ levels have attenuated hypertrophic response to subpressor doses of Ang II compared to wild-type mice.[80,81] However, these mice still develop hypertrophy in response to pressure overload, that is indistinguishable from that seen in wild-type mice,[80] suggesting that $AT1_AR$ can stimulate cardiomyocyte hypertrophic growth but is not necessary for the development of hypertrophy. In addition, Zou et al.[82] demonstrated in vitro that mechanical stretch activates AT1R independent of angiotensin II. These data suggest a possible role for $AT1_BRs$ in the hypertrophic response and the possible existence for other AT1R-independent hypertrophic pathways.[65,83]

In contrast to $AT1_ARs$, the role of AT2Rs in cardiac hypertrophy is controversial. Various in vivo studies of AT2R KO or overexpressing transgenic mice produce conflicting results.[84–89] Because AT2Rs are known to be important in fetal mouse development, Metcalfe et al.[89] attempted to bypass the potential deleterious effects of AT2R deficiency on development by using viral gene therapy in rats to study the effects of AT2Rs on the heart. They showed that viral-mediated AT2R overexpression is able to prevent hypertrophy in spontaneously hypertensive rats. In addition, it has been observed that in failing or ischemic hearts, downregulation of AT1Rs leads to increased AT2: AT1 receptor ratio.[90] Though more studies are needed, the present evidence suggests that AT2Rs may oppose AT1R-mediated growth responses in cardiomyocytes.

Endothelin Receptors

Endothelin is a powerful vasoconstrictor and hypertrophic promoting growth factor, in addition to mediating its several other physiologic effects.[91,92] While endothelin levels are found to be elevated in HF, it is not clear what function it plays in the disease.[93–95] Of the three isoforms, endothelin-1 (ET-1) is expressed in the cardiovascular system and signals via the Gq-coupled ET-1 receptor.[94] Nontargeted overexpression of ET-1 in mice results in either embryonic death or no obvious cardiac phenotype.[92] Conditional and cardiac-specific overexpression of ET-1, however, in adult mice results in myocardial inflammation and hypertrophy and early death from HF.[92] Overexpression of ET-1 also results in concurrent nuclear translocation of nuclear factor-κB (NF-κB) and activation of inflammatory cytokine, implicating a potential role of ET-1 in initiating an inflammatory cascade that ultimately leads to myocardial damage and HF.[92] Interestingly, it has been shown that ET-1 is secreted by cultured cardiomyocytes in response to stretch, and treating chronic HF rats with an endothelin receptor antagonist BQ-123 ameliorates heart function.[94,96] This suggests that ET-1 is involved in the autocrine/paracrine stimulation of cardiac hypertrophy in response to mechanical stress, much like the effects of angiotensin II.

Growth Factors and Their Receptors

Growth factors regulate cell growth and proliferation, differentiation, survival, and apoptosis, and participate in cardiac hypertrophic responses in vivo. In particular, the receptor tyrosine kinases and cytokines are discussed here.

Receptor Tyrosine Kinases and Their Growth Factors

Receptor tyrosine kinases (RTKs) are a major type of cell-surface receptors that mediate a wide variety of functions including cell proliferation, differentiation, survival, and metabolism.[97] They comprise an extracellular domain for ligand binding, a single hydrophobic transmembrane domain, and a cytosolic domain with protein-tyrosine kinase activity. When stimulated by growth factors, RTKs dimerize and the intracellular domains autophosphorylate.[98]

Several growth factors that signal via RTKs are implicated in the pathogenesis of cardiac hypertrophy and HF. Targeted deletion of fibroblast growth factor (FGF) in mice prevents the development of hypertrophy in response to pressure overload.[99] Fibroblast growth factor is thought to mediate hypertrophy via the MAPK pathways as its downstream signals.[100] Insulin-like growth factor-I (IGF-I) levels are increased in hypertrophic hearts in humans and animal models.[100–102] Likewise, transforming growth factor-β (TGF-β) mRNA levels are elevated in hypertrophy in rodents and humans, particularly during the transition from stable cardiac hypertrophy to HF.[103–105] Transforming growth factor-β overexpression in mice leads to cardiac hypertrophy with extracellular matrix deposition and interstitial fibrosis, enhanced β-adrenergic signaling, and induction of fetal contractile protein expression.[106,107]

Cardiac-specific overexpression of platelet-derived growth factor (PDGF) in mice, interestingly, results in a different cardiac phenotype between males and females.[108] Although both sexes exhibit myocardial interstitial fibrosis, altered vasculature, and decreased capillary density by 3 months of age, males develop fibrosis and hypertrophy while females develop more severe, dilated cardiomyopathy, implicating a role of PDGF in fibrosis and vascularization of the heart.[108]

Further illustrating the importance of cardiac angiogenesis in HF, vascular endothelial growth factor (VEGF), a potent paracrine angiogenic factor, and its receptor levels are reduced in both human and animal models of dilated cardiomyopathy.[109,110] Decreased VEGF levels in a mouse (Akt-induced) model of pathologic cardiac hypertrophy have been found to contribute not only to decreased capillary density but also to contractile dysfunction.[111] Furthermore, cardiomyocyte-targeted VEGF KO mice develop reduced capillary density in the heart, impaired contractility, and dilated cardiomyopathy.[112] Vascular endothelial growth factor–mediated angiogenesis in the heart appears to involve the signal transducer and activator of transcription 3 (STAT3) and mammalian target of rapamycin (mTOR) signaling pathways.[113] Interestingly, restoration of VEGF expression using plasmid gene therapy in rat models of diabetic cardiomyopathy results in improved cardiac function.[110] These studies illustrate the importance of myocardial angiogenic response in the pathology of HF.

Cytokines

In addition to its role in mounting immune responses, cytokines are also important players in the heart. In particular, gp130, a common signal transducing subunit of cytokine receptor complex, has been implicated in HF.[114] In response to various cytokines such as the leukemia inhibitory factor/ciliary neurotrophic factor/interleukin-6 (IL-6) family of cytokines,[115] gp130 dimerizes and activates Janus kinase (JAK), which in turn phosphorylates gp130 and activates many downstream pathways that include STAT, c-Src tyrosine family kinases, MAPK, and PI3K.[116] Ventricular-targeted gp130 KO mice show normal cardiac structure and function at baseline but rapidly develop dilated cardiomyopathy and significant cardiomyocyte apoptosis, particularly when exposed to increased biomechanical stress.[117] Constitutive expression of gp130 results in ventricular hypertrophy,[118] while cardiac-specific dominant-negative mutant gp130 results in blunted hypertrophy in response to pressure overload.[119] Cardiotrophin-1 is a cytokine of the IL-6 family that has been shown to induce cardiomyocyte hypertrophy in vitro by activating antiapoptotic signaling pathways.[120,121] In hypertensive transgenic mice, both cardiotrophin-1 and gp130 are elevated during the distinct transition from ventricular hypertrophy to HF.[122] These studies highlight gp130's critical role in cardiomyocyte apoptosis and the transition from compensated hypertrophy to HF.

Circulating levels of tumor necrosis factor-α (TNF-α) and other proinflammatory cytokines have been found to be elevated in patients with chronic HF,[123–125] with higher levels found in those with more advanced disease, suggesting that cytokines are secreted at a relatively late stage of CHF.[124,126] In vitro, TNF-α induces cardiomyocyte hypertrophy with accompanying fetal gene reexpression and extracellular matrix remodeling in response to mechanical load.[127] Transgenic mice overexpressing TNF-α in the heart develop early progressive dilated cardiomyopathy and myocarditis, with an associated increase in matrix metalloproteinase activity and decreased myocardial fibrillar collagen content.[128–131] Tumor necrosis factor-α is also found to have negative inotropic effects on the heart via nitric oxide (NO)-dependent pathways.[127] Thus, TNF-α appears to contribute to HF in several ways by altering hypertrophic response, extracellular matrix remodeling, as well as contractility.

Intracellular Signaling Pathways in Hypertrophy and Heart Failure

The various receptors described above transmit extracellular signals into intricately integrated intracellular signaling pathways to mediate cellular processes involved in cardiac hypertrophy and HF. Four of these pathways are discussed here: (1) MAPK; (2) JAK-STAT; (3) Ca^{2+}-sensitive signaling pathways; and (4) phosphoinositide-3-kinase pathways.

Mitogen-Activated Protein Kinases

Mitogen-activated protein kinases are a superfamily of serine/threonine kinases that regulate diverse cellular processes such as cell differentiation, proliferation, and apoptosis.[132,133] When activated by tyrosine and threonine phosphorylation, MAPKs translocate into the nucleus to phosphorylate various transcription factors. The MAPK cascades are composed of three sequentially activated kinases. MKK kinases (MKKKs) phosphorylate and activate MAPK kinases (MKKs), which in turn activates MAPK (Fig. 10.3).[134] Three main pathways of MAPKs exist: extracellular regulated kinases (ERKs) and the two stress-activated protein kinases (SAPKs), c-Jun N-terminal kinases (JNKs) and p38 MAPKs. All three pathways have been shown to participate in the development of cardiac hypertrophy.[135] The specific roles of each MAPK pathway are briefly discussed below.

Extracellular Regulated Kinases

Of the six subtypes of ERKs, ERK1 and ERK2 are the predominant isoforms found in the heart.[136] The upstream activator of ERK is the small G protein Ras, which activates Raf (MKKK), leading to sequential phosphorylation of MEK1/2 and ERK1/2. ERK then activates transcription factors to regulate cell growth, proliferation, and differentiation.[135] In the heart ERK is activated by Gq/11-protein–coupled receptors (in response to phenylephrine, angiotensin II, and endothelin-1) and receptor tyrosine kinases (in response to peptide growth factors).[135] In addition to several in vitro studies supporting MEK-ERK signaling in agonist-induced cardiomyocyte hypertrophy, data from transgenic mice further strengthen this observation.[137] Gq-mediated ERK activation is observed in pressure overload hypertrophy in mice.[138,139] Nine separate transgenic mouse lines with cardiac-specific, constitutively active MEK1 expression, which results in preferential ERK activation, demonstrate enhanced cardiac function, concentric hypertrophy with no signs of deterioration over time, as well as resistance to apoptosis in ischemia/reperfusion injury.[140,141] Although downstream targets of ERKs in the heart are numerous and unclearly defined, ERK has been shown to activate the transcription factor GATA4, a critical regulator of cardiac structural and hypertrophic genes.[142,143] Overall, these studies suggest that ERK exert cardioprotective effects by regulating compensatory hypertrophy and apoptosis.

Stress-Activated Protein Kinases: c-Jun N-Terminal Kinases and p38

The stress-activated MAPKs (SAPKs), c-Jun N-terminal kinases (JNK) and p38, are both activated by cellular stresses, such as pH/oxidative changes or heat, and by GPCR in response to phenylephrine, endothelin-1, and angiotensin II in cardiomyocytes.[135,144] When activated, these kinases modulate gene expression by interacting with a variety of transcription factors.[145,146] Of the

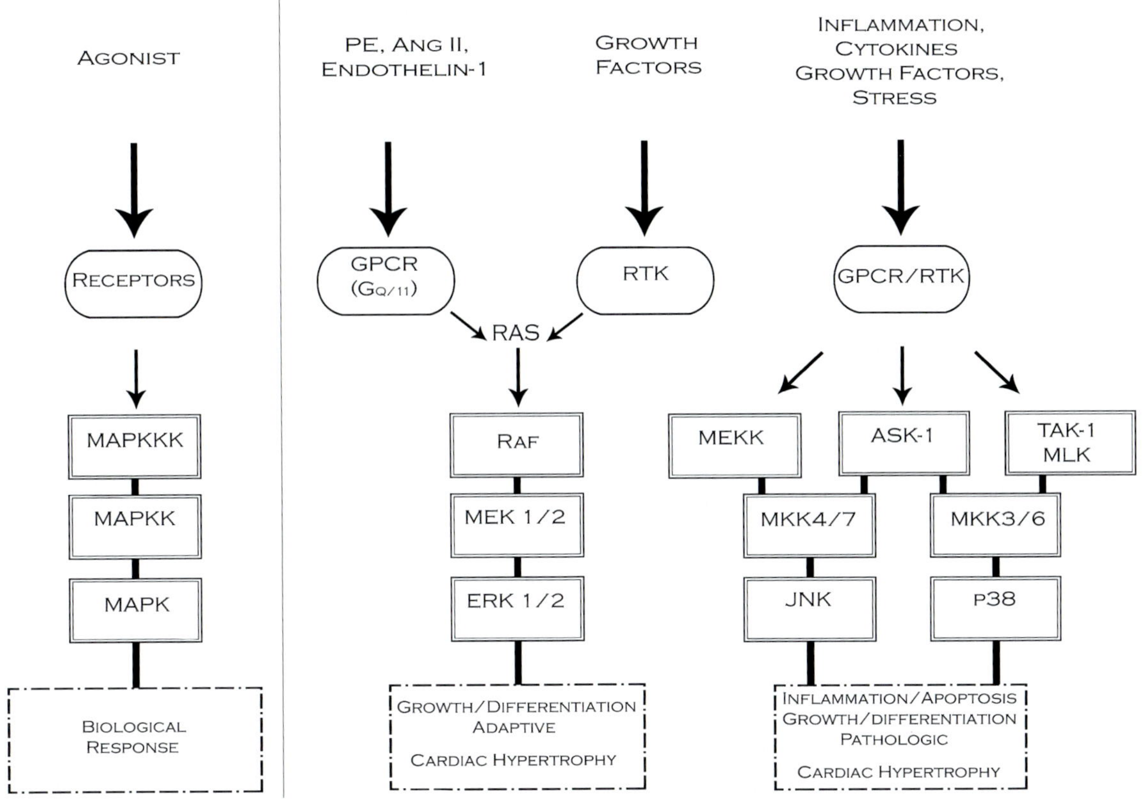

Figure 10.3. A summary of mitogen-activated protein kinase (MAPK) signaling pathways. Each of the three cascades, ERK, JNK, and p38 are organized into three sequentially activated kinases. MAPKKK phosphorylates and activates MAPKK, which then phosphorylates and activates MAPK. (Adapted from Suvarna et al. Receptor-signaling pathways in heart failure. In: Runge MS, Patterson C, eds. Contemporary Cardiology: Principles of Molecular Cardiology. Totowa, NJ: Humana Press, 2004:123–143.)

three JNK isoforms (JNK1, 2, 3) and four p38α isoforms (p38α, β, γ, δ), JNK1/2, p38α/β are the predominant forms found in the heart.[144,147] The upstream regulator of JNK and p38 kinase cascades are not well defined but appear to involve the Rho family of small G proteins such as Rac and cdc42.[148] In the kinase cascade, MKKK includes MEKK1, TAK-1, and ASK-1, while MKK includes MKK4, MKK7, MKK3, and MKK6. The MEKK1-MKK4/7 specifically activates JNK while TAK-1-MKK3/6 activates p38.[149] ASK-1 is able to activate both JNK and p38 pathways.[148]

The role of SAPKs in cardiac hypertrophy and HF has been extensively studied, but the results are often contradictory. In vitro studies using activated or dominant-negative (dn) mutants of MKKs overall demonstrate that p38 and JNK modulate hypertrophy in cultured cardiomyocytes.[144,149] These in vitro studies show that it is p38β that promotes hypertrophy while p38α participates in apoptosis.[150] In contrast, the overall in vivo evidence suggests that both SAPKs have little or antagonistic effects on cardiac hypertrophy.[144,149] In p38 signaling, mice with overexpression of constitutively activated MKK3/6 die prematurely from HF with characteristics of marked interstitial cardiac fibrosis, restrictive diastolic abnormalities, and contractile depression.[151,152] Interestingly, although these mice show fetal gene expression characteristic of cardiac hypertrophy, no hypertrophy is observed.[152] Moreover, mice expressing dn mutants of p38α/β and MKK3/6 show increased hypertrophic response to pressure overload.[153] As for JNK, cardiac-targeted MKK7 overexpression in mice leads to premature death from lethal cardiomyopathy with loss of a gap junction protein connexin 43 but no signs of hypertrophy.[154] Pressure-overloaded mice with MEKK1 deletion still develop hypertrophy and show increased mortality compared to wild-type mice.[155] Similar to p38, JNK gene deletion and JNK dn mutant expression result in enhanced hypertrophic response following pressure overload.[156] Together, these in vivo studies suggest that p38 and JNK have little role in promoting cardiac hypertrophy, but in fact may have antihypertrophic effects. Although the antihypertrophic effects of p38 and JNK could be protective during initial cardiac stress, prolonged kinase activation may later lead to pathologic changes in the heart, such as dilated cardiomyopathy.[149,151] Numerous studies suggest an additional role for p38 and JNK in the pathophysiology of HF such as cardiac fibrosis/matrix remodeling, contractility, and apoptosis.[144,149,151,152,157,158]

Interestingly, the antihypertrophic effect of SAPKs have been attributed to their ability to inhibit nuclear factor of activated T cells (NFAT) nuclear translocation and hence NFAT's prohypertrophic effects in cardiac myocytes.[144] This hypothesis is supported by the observation that dn-p38 transgenic mice show increased NFAT transcriptional activity in the heart.[153] Hypertrophy induced by cardiac-specific expression of calcineurin, an upstream activator of NFAT, is reversed by overexpression of a MKK7-JNK1 fusion protein in the heart.[156] Moreover, calcineurin Aβ gene disruption attenuates the hypertrophic phenotype of dn-p38 and JNK-inhibited mice individually (Fig. 10.4).[153,156] Taken together, p38 and JNK appear to indirectly influence hypertrophy via crosstalk with the calcineurin-NFAT pathway.

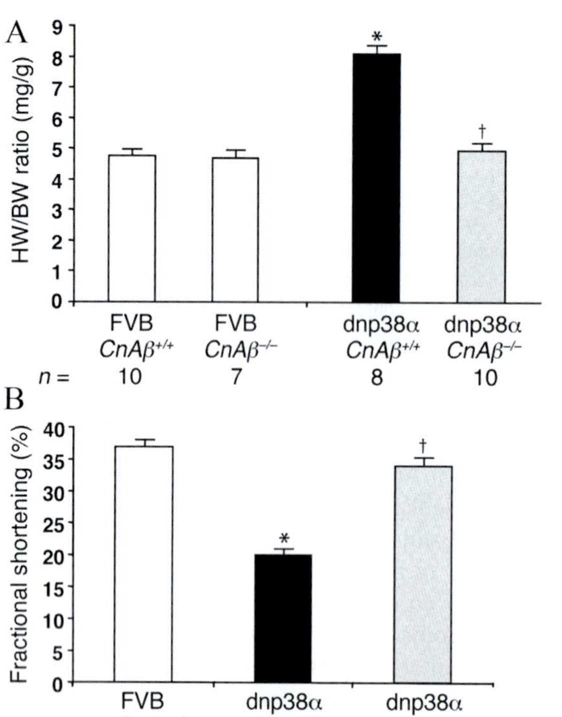

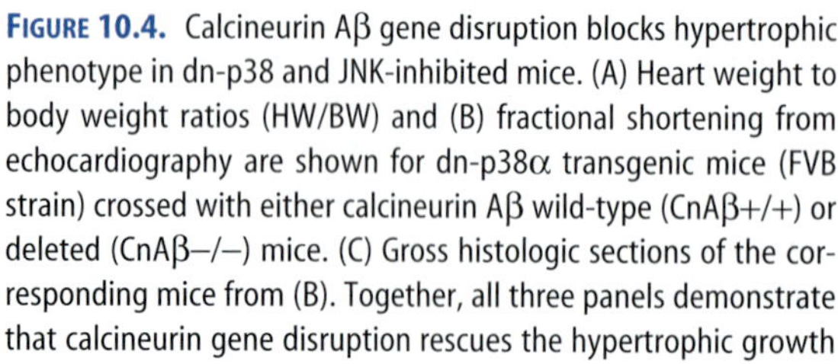

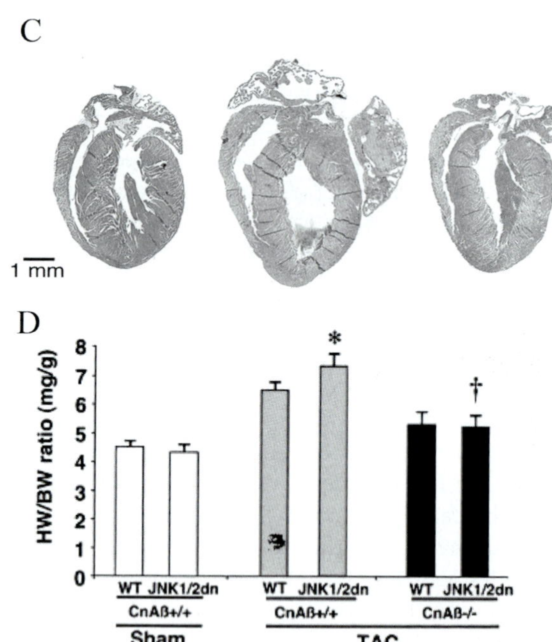

FIGURE 10.4. Calcineurin Aβ gene disruption blocks hypertrophic phenotype in dn-p38 and JNK-inhibited mice. (A) Heart weight to body weight ratios (HW/BW) and (B) fractional shortening from echocardiography are shown for dn-p38α transgenic mice (FVB strain) crossed with either calcineurin Aβ wild-type (CnAβ+/+) or deleted (CnAβ−/−) mice. (C) Gross histologic sections of the corresponding mice from (B). Together, all three panels demonstrate that calcineurin gene disruption rescues the hypertrophic growth associated with p38 inhibition. (D) HW/BW are shown for wild-type and JNK1/2 deleted mice (JNK1/2dn) crossed with either CnAβ+/+ or CnAβ−/− under sham and pressure overload conditions by transverse aortic constriction (TAC). Similarly, JNK1/2dn mice show attenuated hypertrophic response to pressure overload when crossed with CnAβ deleted mice. (From Braz et al.,[153] and Liang et al.,[156] with permission.)

As briefly delineated above, the role of MAPKs in regulating hypertrophy and HF is complex. While Haq et al.[159] report that all three MAPKs are elevated in the human HF but not during compensated hypertrophy, Esposito et al.[138] found that all three kinases are activated in pressure overload-induced hypertrophy in mice in sequential phases, with JNK activated acutely followed by p38 at day 3 and ERK at day 7 of aortic constriction. In human HF secondary to ischemic disease, JNK and p38 activity is found to be preferentially activated but not ERK.[160] Thus, MAPKs appear to be differentially activated during hypertrophy and HF, but their precise role and sequence of activation is unclear. However, the overall evidence suggests that ERK participates in adaptive hypertrophy and confers cardioprotective effects while the SAPKs JNK and p38 contribute to pathologic cardiac remodeling.[161]

JAK/STAT

The JAK/STAT signaling pathway mediates multiple immune and nonimmune biologic processes in response to cytokines, interferons, and growth factors.[115,162] Cytokine receptors appear to be the most important transducer activator of JAK/STAT, including the gp130 receptor described above.[114] JAKs become phosphorylated upon receptor activation. JAKs in turn phosphorylates STAT proteins, which are transcription factors that translocate into the nucleus to modify gene expression.[162,163] JAK is also known to activate the MAPK and PI3K pathways.

In a rat model of acute pressure overload, JAK/STAT is activated, which is partially dependent on the autocrine/paracrine effects of secreted angiotensin II.[164] Mice with STAT3 overexpression in the heart manifest cardiac hypertrophy at 12 weeks of age with fetal gene expression.[165] When these animals are treated with doxorubicin intraperitoneally, they have better survival than control mice treated with doxorubicin.[165] STAT3 also appears to exert antiapoptotic effects in myocardial infarction as well as induce proangiogenic factor expression in the heart.[113,166] Mice with cardiac-specific overexpression of STAT3 show increased capillary density and VEGF levels in the heart,[167] while cardiac-specific deletion of STAT3 results in decreased capillary density, increased susceptibility to ischemia/reperfusion injury, and premature death from dilated cardiomyopathy.[168] Taken together, these findings indicate that STAT3 not only induces a hypertrophic signal but also exerts a cardioprotective effect by stimulating angiogenesis.

Calcium-Sensitive Signaling Pathways

Calcium-dependent signaling is critical for cardiac muscle contraction and involves various components such as L-type Ca^{2+} channel, calsequestrin, phospholamban, sarcoplasmic reticulum (SR) Ca^{2+} ATPase pump, and PKC. Altered intracellular Ca^{2+} handling has been implicated in cardiac hypertrophy and HF.[169] Calcineurin is a serine-threonine phosphatase that is activated by sustained elevations in intracellular Ca^{2+} in response to the stimulation of various receptors including the antigen and Fc receptors on lymphocytes and GPCRs.[170,171] Calcineurin is composed of a catalytic subunit calcineurin A and two Ca^{2+} binding protein calcineurin B and calmodulin.[172] Activated calcineurin dephosphorylates the NFAT transcription factor family, leading to NFAT nuclear translocation and subsequent gene regulation.[171]

Cardiac-specific activation of calcineurin or NFAT in mice results in substantial cardiac hypertrophy and rapidly progressive HF within 2 to 3 months.[173] Overexpressing various inhibitors of the calcineurin-NFAT pathways (Cain, AKAP79, MCIP1, and GSK-3β mutants) attenuate cardiac hypertrophy in various transgenic mouse models.[174] Furthermore, deletion of calcineurin Aβ gene or one of the NFAT genes in transgenic mice results in impaired hypertrophic response to various pathologic hypertrophic stimuli.[174] In addition, pharmacologic inhibition of calcineurin and NFAT nuclear translocation by cyclosporin A and tacrolimus (FK-506) have been shown to reverse the hypertrophic and dilated cardiomyopathic phenotypes seen in various mouse model of hypertrophy and HF.[174,175] As mentioned above, the calcineurin-NFAT pathway interacts with other signaling pathways such as MAPK to regulate cardiac hypertrophy. Recent studies also imply a potential role of calcineurin in cardiomyocyte apoptosis.[7] Interestingly, evidence suggests that the calcineurin-NFAT pathway may be preferentially activated in pathologic hypertrophy. Transgenic mice with NFAT expressed under a luciferase reporter gene show increased NFAT activity in pressure-overloaded hypertrophy or postmyocardial infarction HF, but no increased activity in three other models of physiologic hypertrophy (i.e., exercise induced).[176]

Another important regulator of myocardial Ca^{2+} handling, the ryanodine receptor (RyR2) is a major Ca^{2+} release channel on the SR required for excitation-contraction coupling in cardiomyocytes.[177] Cyclic adenosine monophosphate (cAMP)-dependent PKA associates with RyR2 in a macromolecular signaling complex.[5,177] Phosphorylation of RyR2 by PKA dissociates a stabilizing FK-506 binding protein from the complex, resulting in increased channel activity (i.e., Ca^{2+} release).[5] Phosphodiesterase 4D (PDE4D), a molecule that regulates cAMP access to PKA in cardiomyocytes, is also found to be part of the RyR2 signaling complex and, interestingly, is found in reduced levels in failing human heart.[178] A recent study showed that PDE4D-deficient mice develop dilated cardiomyopathy and accelerated progression to HF after myocardial infarction as a result of RyR2 hyperphosphorylation by PKA and increased diastolic SR Ca^{2+} leak.[178] Thus defective Ca^{2+} regulation by dysfunctional RyR2 contributes to the pathogenesis of HF.

Phosphoinositide-3-Kinase

Phosphoinositide-3-kinase (PI3K) is a family of ubiquitous enzymes containing both lipid and protein kinase activities that mediate a variety of processes, such as cell proliferation, cytoskeletal trafficking, and endocytosis via its many downstream effectors PKB/Akt, GSK3β, and $p70^{S6K}$.[179,180] Class I PI3K is the best studied and comprises class I_A (PI3Kα) and I_B (PI3Kγ).[181] PI3Kα, which is activated by RTKs, is primarily involved in regulating cardiomyocyte size, while PI3Kγ, activated by Gβγ subunits of G proteins, mediates cardiac hypertrophy and contractility.[46,182,183] Mice with cardiac-specific expression of constitutively active PI3Kα demonstrate increased heart size and PKB/Akt levels, while those with expression of dn-PI3Kα have smaller heart size.[184] Similarly, cardiac-targeted overexpression of PKB/Akt also results in larger heart in mice.[185,186]

Phosphoinositide-3-kinase-γ and PKB/Akt are activated in both short- and long-term pressure overload via transverse aortic constriction in mice.[46,183] Cardiac expression of β-ARKct, which interferes with PI3Kγ binding to Gβγ, and a Gαq inhibitor peptide both block PI3Kγ activation,[183] while long-term pressure overload in two transgenic mouse models with attenuated hypertrophic responses to pressure overload results in no increased PI3Kγ activity.[46] These studies demonstrate that PI3Kγ is activated in pressure overload hypertrophy in a Gβγ-dependent manner. In addition, PI3Kγ has also been shown to regulate contractility by negatively regulating adenylyl cyclase activity and phospholamban.[187] Targeted deletion of PI3Kγ in mouse heart results in enhanced contractility with increased cAMP levels.[182] Conditional KO of PTEN (phosphatase and tensin homologue), a negative regulator of PKB/Akt and PI3K, results in spontaneous cardiac hypertrophy and impaired contractility. The cardiac contractility but not hypertrophy was rescued by breeding conditional PTEN-deficient mice with PI3Kγ-KO mice.[182]

The elevated PI3Kγ activity in hypertrophic hearts possibly contributes to β-AR dysfunction seen in HF by promoting β-AR internalization and impaired receptor coupling (Fig. 10.5A). More specifically, β-ARK1 interacts with PI3K via the phosphoinositide kinase (PIK) domain.[188,189] Upon agonist stimulation via Gq-coupled receptors, β-ARK1 translocates PI3K to β-ARs to generate phosphatidylinositol-3,4,5-triphosphate (PtdIns-3,4,5-P_3), which then mediates receptor internalization via clathrin-coated pits by recruiting phosphoinositide-binding endocytic proteins such as β-arrestin and activator protein 2 (AP-2).[189,190] Recent studies show that the lipid kinase activity of PI3K is required for AP-2 recruitment, while the protein kinase phosphorylation of nonmuscle tropomyosin is essential for receptor endocytosis by regulating actin filament rearrangement.[191] Mice with cardiac-specific overexpression of a catalytically inactive mutant of PI3Kγ, in which PI3K recruitment to β-AR is disrupted, show preserved cardiac function in chronic pressure overload and no β-AR downregulation in response to chronic catecholamine stimulation (Fig. 10.5B).[190] Mice overexpressing the PIK domain, which interferes with β-ARK1

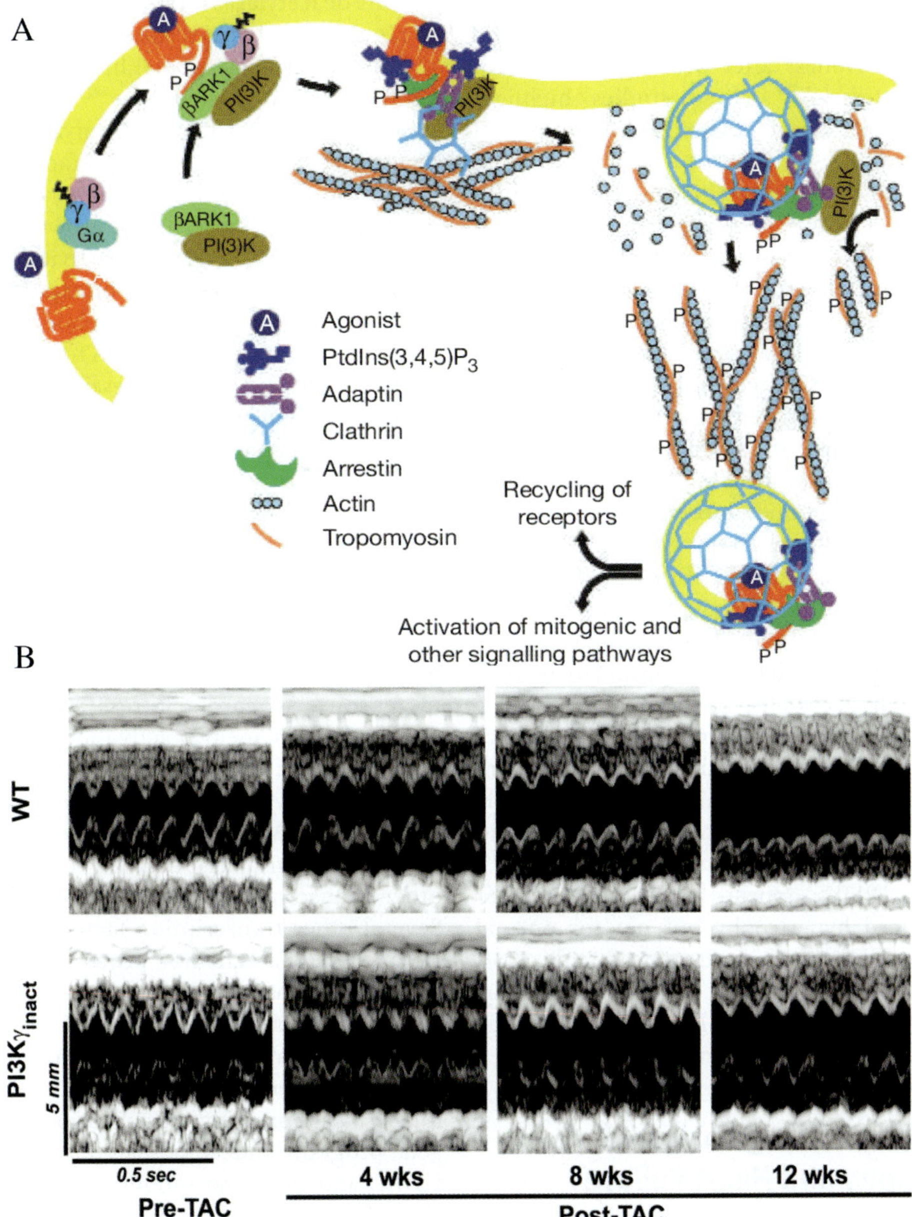

FIGURE 10.5. (A) Schematic diagram depicting phosphoinositide-3-kinase (PI3K)-mediated β-AR endocytosis. Agonist stimulation of β-ARs leads to the release of Gβγ subunit from the G protein. Gβγ in turn activates β-ARK1 and facilitates its translocation to the agonist-occupied receptor. β-ARK1 also interacts with PI3K and facilitates PI3K translocation to the receptor. Phosphorylation of the receptor by β-ARK1 leads to β-arrestin recruitment. PI3K generates PtdIns(3,4,5)P3 via its lipid kinase, leading to recruitment of AP-2 adaptor protein and targeting the receptor complex to clathrin-coated pits. The protein kinase activity of PI3K, on the other hand, phosphorylates nonmuscle tropomyosin, leading to changes in actin filament arrangement critical for endocytosis. (B) Representative serial echocardiography in conscious wild-type mice and mice with cardiac-specific overexpression of a catalytically inactive mutant of PI3Kγ (PI3Kγinact) before and after chronic pressure overload induced by TAC. PI3Kγinact mice show delayed development of HF following chronic pressure overload. (From Naga Prasad et al.,[191] and Nienaber et al.,[190] with permission.)

binding to PI3K, also show decreased β-AR downregulation and internalization and preserved β-AR responsiveness after prolonged treatment with isoproterenol.[192] These studies highlight PI3Kγ's critical role in β-AR signaling and heart function.

Further downstream of PKB/Akt are GSK-3β and mTOR. GSK-3β is a negative regulator of hypertrophy that acts by inhibiting the activity of many transcription factors important in cardiac growth.[161] The NFAT family of transcription factors is an example, as overexpression of GSK-3β in calcineurin-transgenic mice results in attenuated hypertrophic response.[161,193] mTOR, a mammalian target of rapamycin, is a protein kinase involved in translation regulation. Rapamycin treatment in mice reverses cardiac hypertrophy induced by pressure overload.[161,194]

Interestingly, as with the differential involvement of MAPK in physiologic versus pathologic hypertrophy, PI3Kα appears to mediate physiologic hypertrophy, while PI3Kγ appears to mediate pathologic hypertrophy.[161] McMullen et al.[195] demonstrate that dominant-negative PI3Kα mice display hypertrophy only in response to pressure overload, not to exercise training. Constitutively active PI3Kα mice develop hypertrophy that did not transition into maladaptive hypertrophy.[184] Conversely, PI3Kγ appears to be required for stress-induced hypertrophy but not for normal cardiac growth.[182,196] Thus, it appears that PI3K contributes to the regulation of pathologic versus adaptive hypertrophic responses of the heart via the two different PI3K isoforms.

Transcriptional Regulation of Hypertrophy and Heart Failure

The various extracellular and intracellular signaling pathways discussed above ultimately converge in the nucleus to mediate cardiac gene expression in response to stress signals. It is well known that the expressions of a number of genes are altered in the failing heart. β-myosin heavy chain (β-MHC), natriuretic peptide atrial natriuretic factor (ANF), and B-type natriuretic peptide (BNP) are upregulated while α-MHC and the sarcoplasmic reticulum Ca^{2+} ATPase (SERCA) are downregulated.[197] Histone acetyltransferases (HATs) and histone deacetylases (HDACs) are proteins known to regulate DNA transcription by modulating the acetylation of nucleosomal histones and thus the conformation of nucleosome.[197–200] Class II HDAC is known to associate with myocyte enhancer factor-2 (MEF2) transcription factor and other transcription factors to repress expression of genes associated with cardiac growth and remodeling.[201] Histone deacetylase activity is regulated via its nuclear translocation or export by various protein kinases.[198,199,202] Phosphorylated HDAC leaves the nucleus, allowing HAT to associate with MEF2 to activate gene expression.[203,204] Calcium/calmodulin-dependent protein kinase has been found to phosphorylate HDAC and activate its nuclear export.[205] Similarly, PKC activation by hypertrophic agonists leads to activation of PKD, which directly phosphorylates HDAC and induces its nuclear export.[199] Overexpression of class II HDACs in cardiomyocytes prevents agonist-induced hypertrophy, while HDAC gene deletion predisposes mice to develop hypertrophy and HF in response to cardiac stress such as pressure overload or calcineurin activation.[198–200,206]

In addition, the NFAT transcription factors described above have been shown to recruit HAT to NFAT and MEF-2 binding sites in the nucleus and activate transcription in cooperation with other transcription factors such as GATA4.[207] Several other transcription factors implicated in HF include the activator protein 1 (AP-1) transcription factor, which is activated by JNK, and STAT downstream of cytokine-JAK pathway.[114] Transcriptional control of cardiac hypertrophy and HF may provide potential therapeutic target for HF by suppressing the activation of pathologic gene program. Indeed, a search for inhibitors for HDAC and PKD and modulators of calcineurin/NFAT axis is already underway.[197]

Conclusion

The intracellular signaling pathways involved in regulation of the hypertrophic response and pathogenesis of HF are complex. Our understanding of these intricate mechanisms has made great strides with the aid of transgenic mouse technologies. Although too numerous to detail, the transgenic mouse models examined above illustrate that they are valuable tools in dissecting the distinct function of individual genes and proteins in the signaling pathway in vivo. It is important to keep in mind that HF is a result of dysfunction of multiple signaling pathways, and that these signaling pathways "communicate" through a complex network of interactions. Thus, novel therapies for HF will likely involve modulation of more than one of these signaling pathways.

References

1. Rockman HA, Koch WJ, Lefkowitz RJ. Seven-transmembrane-spanning receptors and heart function. Nature 2002;415(6868):206–12.
2. Lefkowitz RJ. G protein-coupled receptors. III. New roles for receptor kinases and beta-arrestins in receptor signaling and desensitization. J Biol Chem 1998;273(30):18677–80.
3. Barki-Harrington L, Perrino C, Rockman HA. Network integration of the adrenergic system in cardiac hypertrophy. Cardiovasc Res 2004;63(3): 391–402.
4. Kamp TJ, Hell JW. Regulation of cardiac L-type calcium channels by protein kinase A and protein kinase C. Circ Res 2000;87(12):1095–102.
5. Marx SO, Reiken S, Hisamatsu Y, et al. PKA phosphorylation dissociates FKBP12.6 from the calcium release channel (ryanodine receptor): defective regulation in failing hearts. Cell 2000;101(4): 365–76.
6. Tada M, Toyofuku T. SR Ca(2+)-ATPase/phospholamban in cardiomyocyte function. J Card Fail 1996;2(4 suppl):S77–85.
7. Molkentin JD. Calcineurin-NFAT signaling regulates the cardiac hypertrophic response in coordination with the MAPKs. Cardiovasc Res 2004;63(3): 467–75.
8. Kurose H. Galpha12 and Galpha13 as key regulatory mediator in signal transduction. Life Sci 2003;74(2–3):155–61.
9. Pitcher JA, Freedman NJ, Lefkowitz RJ. G protein-coupled receptor kinases. Annu Rev Biochem 1998;67:653–92.
10. Claing A, Laporte SA, Caron MG, Lefkowitz RJ. Endocytosis of G protein-coupled receptors: roles of G protein-coupled receptor kinases and beta-arrestin proteins. Prog Neurobiol 2002;66(2): 61–79.
11. Luttrell LM, Lefkowitz RJ. The role of beta-arrestins in the termination and transduction of G-protein-coupled receptor signals. J Cell Sci 2002; 115(pt 3):455–65.
12. McDonald PH, Chow CW, Miller WE, et al. Beta-arrestin 2: a receptor-regulated MAPK scaffold for the activation of JNK3. Science 2000;290(5496): 1574–7.
13. Luttrell LM, Roudabush FL, Choy EW, et al. Activation and targeting of extracellular signal-regulated kinases by beta-arrestin scaffolds. Proc Natl Acad Sci USA 2001;98(5):2449–54.
14. Sibley DR, Strasser RH, Benovic JL, Daniel K, Lefkowitz RJ. Phosphorylation/dephosphorylation of the beta-adrenergic receptor regulates its functional coupling to adenylate cyclase and subcellular distribution. Proc Natl Acad Sci USA 1986;83(24):9408–12.
15. Yu SS, Lefkowitz RJ, Hausdorff WP. Beta-adrenergic receptor sequestration. A potential mechanism of receptor resensitization. J Biol Chem 1993; 268(1):337–41.
16. Brodde OE, Michel MC. Adrenergic and muscarinic receptors in the human heart. Pharmacol Rev 1999;51(4):651–90.
17. Gauthier C, Leblais V, Kobzik L, et al. The negative inotropic effect of beta3-adrenoceptor stimulation is mediated by activation of a nitric oxide synthase pathway in human ventricle. J Clin Invest 1998;102(7):1377–84.
18. Gauthier C, Tavernier G, Charpentier F, Langin D, Le Marec H. Functional beta3-adrenoceptor in the human heart. J Clin Invest 1996;98(2):556–62.
19. Bristow MR. Why does the myocardium fail? Insights from basic science. Lancet 1998;352(suppl 1):SI8–14.
20. Bristow MR, Ginsburg R, Minobe W, et al. Decreased catecholamine sensitivity and beta-adrenergic-receptor density in failing human hearts. N Engl J Med 1982;307(4):205–11.
21. Bristow MR, Hershberger RE, Port JD, Minobe W, Rasmussen R. Beta 1- and beta 2-adrenergic receptor-mediated adenylate cyclase stimulation in nonfailing and failing human ventricular myocardium. Mol Pharmacol 1989;35(3):295–303.
22. Bristow MR, Minobe WA, Raynolds MV, et al. Reduced beta 1 receptor messenger RNA abundance in the failing human heart. J Clin Invest 1993;92(6):2737–45.
23. Ungerer M, Bohm M, Elce JS, Erdmann E, Lohse MJ. Altered expression of beta-adrenergic receptor kinase and beta 1-adrenergic receptors in the failing human heart. Circulation 1993;87(2): 454–63.
24. Zhu WZ, Zheng M, Koch WJ, Lefkowitz RJ, Kobilka BK, Xiao RP. Dual modulation of cell survival and cell death by beta(2)-adrenergic signaling in adult

mouse cardiac myocytes. Proc Natl Acad Sci USA 2001;98(4):1607–12.
25. Daaka Y, Luttrell LM, Lefkowitz RJ. Switching of the coupling of the beta2-adrenergic receptor to different G proteins by protein kinase A. Nature 1997;390(6655):88–91.
26. Engelhardt S, Hein L, Wiesmann F, Lohse MJ. Progressive hypertrophy and heart failure in beta1-adrenergic receptor transgenic mice. Proc Natl Acad Sci USA 1999;96(12):7059–64.
27. Rohrer DK, Desai KH, Jasper JR, et al. Targeted disruption of the mouse beta1-adrenergic receptor gene: developmental and cardiovascular effects. Proc Natl Acad Sci USA 1996;93(14): 7375–80.
28. Liggett SB, Tepe NM, Lorenz JN, et al. Early and delayed consequences of beta(2)-adrenergic receptor overexpression in mouse hearts: critical role for expression level. Circulation 2000;101(14): 1707–14.
29. Milano CA, Allen LF, Rockman HA, et al. Enhanced myocardial function in transgenic mice overexpressing the beta 2-adrenergic receptor. Science 1994;264(5158):582–6.
30. Xiao RP, Avdonin P, Zhou YY, et al. Coupling of beta2-adrenoceptor to Gi proteins and its physiological relevance in murine cardiac myocytes. Circ Res 1999;84(1):43–52.
31. Chruscinski AJ, Rohrer DK, Schauble E, Desai KH, Bernstein D, Kobilka BK. Targeted disruption of the beta2 adrenergic receptor gene. J Biol Chem 1999;274(24):16694–700.
32. Dorn GW, 2nd, Tepe NM, Lorenz JN, Koch WJ, Liggett SB. Low- and high-level transgenic expression of beta2-adrenergic receptors differentially affect cardiac hypertrophy and function in Galphaq-overexpressing mice. Proc Natl Acad Sci USA 1999;96(11):6400–5.
33. Exton JH. Mechanisms involved in alpha-adrenergic phenomena. Am J Physiol 1985;248(6 pt 1): E633–47.
34. Lin F, Owens WA, Chen S, et al. Targeted alpha(1A)-adrenergic receptor overexpression induces enhanced cardiac contractility but not hypertrophy. Circ Res 2001;89(4):343–50.
35. Akhter SA, Milano CA, Shotwell KF, et al. Transgenic mice with cardiac overexpression of alpha1B-adrenergic receptors. In vivo alpha1-adrenergic receptor-mediated regulation of beta-adrenergic signaling. J Biol Chem 1997;272(34):21253–9.
36. Milano CA, Dolber PC, Rockman HA, et al. Myocardial expression of a constitutively active alpha 1B-adrenergic receptor in transgenic mice induces cardiac hypertrophy. Proc Natl Acad Sci USA 1994;91(21):10109–13.
37. Vecchione C, Fratta L, Rizzoni D, et al. Cardiovascular influences of alpha1b-adrenergic receptor defect in mice. Circulation 2002;105(14):1700–7.
38. Cavalli A, Lattion AL, Hummler E, et al. Decreased blood pressure response in mice deficient of the alpha1b-adrenergic receptor. Proc Natl Acad Sci USA 1997;94(21):11589–94.
39. Gaudin C, Ishikawa Y, Wight DC, et al. Overexpression of Gs alpha protein in the hearts of transgenic mice. J Clin Invest 1995;95(4):1676–83.
40. Iwase M, Bishop SP, Uechi M, et al. Adverse effects of chronic endogenous sympathetic drive induced by cardiac GS alpha overexpression. Circ Res 1996;78(4):517–24.
41. D'Angelo DD, Sakata Y, Lorenz JN, et al. Transgenic Galphaq overexpression induces cardiac contractile failure in mice. Proc Natl Acad Sci USA 1997;94(15):8121–6.
42. Mende U, Kagen A, Cohen A, Aramburu J, Schoen FJ, Neer EJ. Transient cardiac expression of constitutively active Galphaq leads to hypertrophy and dilated cardiomyopathy by calcineurin-dependent and independent pathways. Proc Natl Acad Sci USA 1998;95(23):13893–8.
43. Sakata Y, Hoit BD, Liggett SB, Walsh RA, Dorn GW, 2nd. Decompensation of pressure-overload hypertrophy in G alpha q-overexpressing mice. Circulation 1998;97(15):1488–95.
44. Adams JW, Sakata Y, Davis MG, et al. Enhanced Galphaq signaling: a common pathway mediates cardiac hypertrophy and apoptotic heart failure. Proc Natl Acad Sci USA 1998;95(17):10140–5.
45. Akhter SA, Luttrell LM, Rockman HA, Iaccarino G, Lefkowitz RJ, Koch WJ. Targeting the receptor-Gq interface to inhibit in vivo pressure overload myocardial hypertrophy. Science 1998;280(5363): 574–7.
46. Esposito G, Rapacciuolo A, Naga Prasad SV, et al. Genetic alterations that inhibit in vivo pressure-overload hypertrophy prevent cardiac dysfunction despite increased wall stress. Circulation 2002;105(1):85–92.
47. Redfern CH, Degtyarev MY, Kwa AT, et al. Conditional expression of a Gi-coupled receptor causes ventricular conduction delay and a lethal cardiomyopathy. Proc Natl Acad Sci USA 2000;97(9): 4826–31.
48. Baker AJ, Redfern CH, Harwood MD, Simpson PC, Conklin BR. Abnormal contraction caused by expression of G(i)-coupled receptor in transgenic model of dilated cardiomyopathy. Am J Physiol Heart Circ Physiol 2001;280(4):H1653–9.
49. Inglese J, Freedman NJ, Koch WJ, Lefkowitz RJ. Structure and mechanism of the G protein-coupled receptor kinases. J Biol Chem 1993;268(32):23735–8.

50. Choi DJ, Koch WJ, Hunter JJ, Rockman HA. Mechanism of beta-adrenergic receptor desensitization in cardiac hypertrophy is increased beta-adrenergic receptor kinase. J Biol Chem 1997;272(27): 17223–9.
51. Koch WJ, Rockman HA, Samama P, et al. Cardiac function in mice overexpressing the beta-adrenergic receptor kinase or a beta ARK inhibitor. Science 1995;268(5215):1350–3.
52. Korzick DH, Xiao RP, Ziman BD, Koch WJ, Lefkowitz RJ, Lakatta EG. Transgenic manipulation of beta-adrenergic receptor kinase modifies cardiac myocyte contraction to norepinephrine. Am J Physiol 1997;272(1 pt 2): H590–6.
53. Jaber M, Koch WJ, Rockman H, et al. Essential role of beta-adrenergic receptor kinase 1 in cardiac development and function. Proc Natl Acad Sci USA 1996;93(23):12974–9.
54. Rockman HA, Choi DJ, Akhter SA, et al. Control of myocardial contractile function by the level of beta-adrenergic receptor kinase 1 in gene-targeted mice. J Biol Chem 1998;273(29):18180–4.
55. Esposito G, Santana LF, Dilly K, et al. Cellular and functional defects in a mouse model of heart failure. Am J Physiol Heart Circ Physiol 2000;279(6): H3101–12.
56. Rockman HA, Chien KR, Choi DJ, et al. Expression of a beta-adrenergic receptor kinase 1 inhibitor prevents the development of myocardial failure in gene-targeted mice. Proc Natl Acad Sci USA 1998;95(12):7000–5.
57. Harding VB, Jones LR, Lefkowitz RJ, Koch WJ, Rockman HA. Cardiac beta ARK1 inhibition prolongs survival and augments beta blocker therapy in a mouse model of severe heart failure. Proc Natl Acad Sci USA 2001;98(10): 5809–14.
58. Freeman K, Colon-Rivera C, Olsson MC, et al. Progression from hypertrophic to dilated cardiomyopathy in mice that express a mutant myosin transgene. Am J Physiol Heart Circ Physiol 2001;280(1):H151–9.
59. The Cardiac Insufficiency Bisoprolol Study II (CIBIS-II): a randomised trial. Lancet 1999; 353(9146):9–13.
60. Effect of metoprolol CR/XL in chronic heart failure: Metoprolol CR/XL Randomised Intervention Trial in Congestive Heart Failure (MERIT-HF). Lancet 1999;353(9169):2001–7.
61. Packer M, Bristow MR, Cohn JN, et al. The effect of carvedilol on morbidity and mortality in patients with chronic heart failure. U.S. Carvedilol Heart Failure Study Group. N Engl J Med 1996;334(21): 1349–55.
62. Packer M, Coats AJ, Fowler MB, et al. Effect of carvedilol on survival in severe chronic heart failure. N Engl J Med 2001;344(22):1651–8.
63. Rockman HA, Choi DJ, Rahman NU, Akhter SA, Lefkowitz RJ, Koch WJ. Receptor-specific in vivo desensitization by the G protein-coupled receptor kinase-5 in transgenic mice. Proc Natl Acad Sci USA 1996;93(18):9954–9.
64. Iaccarino G, Rockman HA, Shotwell KF, Tomhave ED, Koch WJ. Myocardial overexpression of GRK3 in transgenic mice: evidence for in vivo selectivity of GRKs. Am J Physiol 1998;275(4 Pt 2):H1298–306.
65. Wollert KC, Drexler H. The renin-angiotensin system and experimental heart failure. Cardiovasc Res 1999;43(4):838–49.
66. Touyz RM, Schiffrin EL. Signal transduction mechanisms mediating the physiological and pathophysiological actions of angiotensin II in vascular smooth muscle cells. Pharmacol Rev 2000;52(4):639–72.
67. Burson JM, Aguilera G, Gross KW, Sigmund CD. Differential expression of angiotensin receptor 1A and 1B in mouse. Am J Physiol 1994;267(2 Pt 1): E260–7.
68. Nio Y, Matsubara H, Murasawa S, Kanasaki M, Inada M. Regulation of gene transcription of angiotensin II receptor subtypes in myocardial infarction. J Clin Invest 1995;95(1):46–54.
69. Schunkert H, Dzau VJ, Tang SS, Hirsch AT, Apstein CS, Lorell BH. Increased rat cardiac angiotensin converting enzyme activity and mRNA expression in pressure overload left ventricular hypertrophy. Effects on coronary resistance, contractility, and relaxation. J Clin Invest 1990;86(6):1913–20.
70. Schunkert H, Jackson B, Tang SS, et al. Distribution and functional significance of cardiac angiotensin converting enzyme in hypertrophied rat hearts. Circulation 1993;87(4):1328–39.
71. Studer R, Reinecke H, Muller B, Holtz J, Just H, Drexler H. Increased angiotensin-I converting enzyme gene expression in the failing human heart. Quantification by competitive RNA polymerase chain reaction. J Clin Invest 1994;94(1): 301–10.
72. Kim S, Ohta K, Hamaguchi A, Yukimura T, Miura K, Iwao H. Angiotensin II induces cardiac phenotypic modulation and remodeling in vivo in rats. Hypertension 1995;25(6):1252–9.
73. Lijnen P, Petrov V. Antagonism of the renin-angiotensin-aldosterone system and collagen metabolism in cardiac fibroblasts. Methods Find Exp Clin Pharmacol 1999;21(3):215–27.

74. Cohn JN, Tognoni G. A randomized trial of the angiotensin-receptor blocker valsartan in chronic heart failure. N Engl J Med 2001;345(23):1667–75.
75. Lindholm LH, Ibsen H, Dahlof B, et al. Cardiovascular morbidity and mortality in patients with diabetes in the Losartan Intervention For Endpoint reduction in hypertension study (LIFE): a randomised trial against atenolol. Lancet 2002; 359(9311):1004–10.
76. Pitt B, Poole-Wilson PA, Segal R, et al. Effect of losartan compared with captopril on mortality in patients with symptomatic heart failure: randomised trial—the Losartan Heart Failure Survival Study ELITE II. Lancet 2000;355(9215): 1582–7.
77. Rockman HA, Wachhorst SP, Mao L, Ross J, Jr. ANG II receptor blockade prevents ventricular hypertrophy and ANF gene expression with pressure overload in mice. Am J Physiol 1994;266(6 pt 2):H2468–75.
78. Sadoshima J, Izumo S. Mechanical stretch rapidly activates multiple signal transduction pathways in cardiac myocytes: potential involvement of an autocrine/paracrine mechanism. Embo J 1993; 12(4):1681–92.
79. Paradis P, Dali-Youcef N, Paradis FW, Thibault G, Nemer M. Overexpression of angiotensin II type I receptor in cardiomyocytes induces cardiac hypertrophy and remodeling. Proc Natl Acad Sci USA 2000;97(2):931–6.
80. Harada K, Komuro I, Shiojima I, et al. Pressure overload induces cardiac hypertrophy in angiotensin II type 1A receptor knockout mice. Circulation 1998;97(19):1952–9.
81. Harada K, Komuro I, Zou Y, et al. Acute pressure overload could induce hypertrophic responses in the heart of angiotensin II type 1a knockout mice. Circ Res 1998;82(7):779–85.
82. Zou Y, Akazawa H, Qin Y, et al. Mechanical stress activates angiotensin II type 1 receptor without the involvement of angiotensin II. Nat Cell Biol 2004;6(6):499–506.
83. Lorell BH. Role of angiotensin AT1, and AT2 receptors in cardiac hypertrophy and disease. Am J Cardiol 1999;83(12A):48H–52H.
84. Ichihara S, Senbonmatsu T, Price E Jr, Ichiki T, Gaffney FA, Inagami T. Angiotensin II type 2 receptor is essential for left ventricular hypertrophy and cardiac fibrosis in chronic angiotensin II-induced hypertension. Circulation 2001;104(3): 346–51.
85. Masaki H, Kurihara T, Yamaki A, et al. Cardiac-specific overexpression of angiotensin II AT2 receptor causes attenuated response to AT1 receptor-mediated pressor and chronotropic effects. J Clin Invest 1998;101(3):527–35.
86. Senbonmatsu T, Ichihara S, Price E Jr, Gaffney FA, Inagami T. Evidence for angiotensin II type 2 receptor-mediated cardiac myocyte enlargement during in vivo pressure overload. J Clin Invest 2000;106(3):R25–9.
87. Akishita M, Iwai M, Wu L, et al. Inhibitory effect of angiotensin II type 2 receptor on coronary arterial remodeling after aortic banding in mice. Circulation 2000;102(14):1684–9.
88. Kurisu S, Ozono R, Oshima T, et al. Cardiac angiotensin II type 2 receptor activates the kinin/NO system and inhibits fibrosis. Hypertension 2003; 41(1):99–107.
89. Metcalfe BL, Huentelman MJ, Parilak LD, et al. Prevention of cardiac hypertrophy by angiotensin II type-2 receptor gene transfer. Hypertension 2004;43(6):1233–8.
90. Matsubara H. Pathophysiological role of angiotensin II type 2 receptor in cardiovascular and renal diseases. Circ Res 1998;83(12):1182–91.
91. Yanagisawa M, Kurihara H, Kimura S, et al. A novel potent vasoconstrictor peptide produced by vascular endothelial cells. Nature 1988;332(6163): 411–5.
92. Yang LL, Gros R, Kabir MG, et al. Conditional cardiac overexpression of endothelin-1 induces inflammation and dilated cardiomyopathy in mice. Circulation 2004;109(2):255–61.
93. Sakai S, Miyauchi T, Sakurai T, et al. Endogenous endothelin-1 participates in the maintenance of cardiac function in rats with congestive heart failure. Marked increase in endothelin-1 production in the failing heart. Circulation 1996;93(6): 1214–22.
94. Yamazaki T, Komuro I, Kudoh S, et al. Endothelin-1 is involved in mechanical stress-induced cardiomyocyte hypertrophy. J Biol Chem 1996;271(6): 3221–8.
95. Stewart DJ, Cernacek P, Costello KB, Rouleau JL. Elevated endothelin-1 in heart failure and loss of normal response to postural change. Circulation 1992;85(2):510–7.
96. Sakai S, Miyauchi T, Kobayashi M, Yamaguchi I, Goto K, Sugishita Y. Inhibition of myocardial endothelin pathway improves long-term survival in heart failure. Nature 1996;384(6607):353–5.
97. Waltenberger J. Modulation of growth factor action: implications for the treatment of cardiovascular diseases. Circulation 1997;96(11):4083–94.

98. Schlessinger J, Ullrich A. Growth factor signaling by receptor tyrosine kinases. Neuron 1992;9(3):383–91.
99. Schultz JE, Witt SA, Nieman ML, et al. Fibroblast growth factor-2 mediates pressure-induced hypertrophic response. J Clin Invest 1999;104(6):709–19.
100. Bogoyevitch MA, Glennon PE, Andersson MB, et al. Endothelin-1 and fibroblast growth factors stimulate the mitogen-activated protein kinase signaling cascade in cardiac myocytes. The potential role of the cascade in the integration of two signaling pathways leading to myocyte hypertrophy. J Biol Chem 1994;269(2):1110–9.
101. Li RK, Li G, Mickle DA, et al. Overexpression of transforming growth factor-beta1 and insulin-like growth factor-I in patients with idiopathic hypertrophic cardiomyopathy. Circulation 1997;96(3):874–81.
102. Serneri GG, Modesti PA, Boddi M, et al. Cardiac growth factors in human hypertrophy. Relations with myocardial contractility and wall stress. Circ Res 1999;85(1):57–67.
103. Song H FA, Conte JV, and Chi-Ming W. Presentation and localization of transforming growth factor beta isoforms and its receptor subtypes in human myocardium in the absence and presence of heart failure. Circulation 1997;197(Suppl I):I-362.
104. Takahashi N, Calderone A, Izzo NJ Jr, Maki TM, Marsh JD, Colucci WS. Hypertrophic stimuli induce transforming growth factor-beta 1 expression in rat ventricular myocytes. J Clin Invest 1994;94(4):1470–6.
105. Villarreal FJ, Dillmann WH. Cardiac hypertrophy-induced changes in mRNA levels for TGF-beta 1, fibronectin, and collagen. Am J Physiol 1992;262(6 Pt 2):H1861–6.
106. Parker TG, Packer SE, Schneider MD. Peptide growth factors can provoke "fetal" contractile protein gene expression in rat cardiac myocytes. J Clin Invest 1990;85(2):507–14.
107. Rosenkranz S, Flesch M, Amann K, et al. Alterations of beta-adrenergic signaling and cardiac hypertrophy in transgenic mice overexpressing TGF-beta(1). Am J Physiol Heart Circ Physiol 2002;283(3):H1253–62.
108. Ponten A, Li X, Thoren P, et al. Transgenic overexpression of platelet-derived growth factor-C in the mouse heart induces cardiac fibrosis, hypertrophy, and dilated cardiomyopathy. Am J Pathol 2003;163(2):673–82.
109. Abraham D, Hofbauer R, Schafer R, et al. Selective downregulation of VEGF-A(165), VEGF-R(1), and decreased capillary density in patients with dilative but not ischemic cardiomyopathy. Circ Res 2000;87(8):644–7.
110. Yoon YS, Uchida S, Masuo O, et al. Progressive attenuation of myocardial vascular endothelial growth factor expression is a seminal event in diabetic cardiomyopathy: restoration of microvascular homeostasis and recovery of cardiac function in diabetic cardiomyopathy after replenishment of local vascular endothelial growth factor. Circulation 2005;111(16):2073–85.
111. Shiojima I, Sato K, Izumiya Y, et al. Disruption of coordinated cardiac hypertrophy and angiogenesis contributes to the transition to heart failure. J Clin Invest 2005;115(8):2108–18.
112. Giordano FJ, Gerber HP, Williams SP, et al. A cardiac myocyte vascular endothelial growth factor paracrine pathway is required to maintain cardiac function. Proc Natl Acad Sci USA 2001;98(10):5780–5.
113. Hilfiker-Kleiner D, Limbourg A, Drexler H. STAT3-mediated activation of myocardial capillary growth. Trends Cardiovasc Med 2005;15(4):152–7.
114. Yamauchi-Takihara K, Kishimoto T. A novel role for STAT3 in cardiac remodeling. Trends Cardiovasc Med 2000;10(7):298–303.
115. Kishimoto T, Taga T, Akira S. Cytokine signal transduction. Cell 1994;76(2):253–62.
116. Hirano T, Nakajima, Koichi, Hibi, Masahiko. Signaling mechanisms through gp130: a model of the cytokine system. Cytokine & Growth Factor Reviews 1997;8(4):241–52.
117. Hirota H, Chen J, Betz UA, et al. Loss of a gp130 cardiac muscle cell survival pathway is a critical event in the onset of heart failure during biomechanical stress. Cell 1999;97(2):189–98.
118. Hirota H, Yoshida K, Kishimoto T, Taga T. Continuous activation of gp130, a signal-transducing receptor component for interleukin 6-related cytokines, causes myocardial hypertrophy in mice. Proc Natl Acad Sci USA 1995;92(11):4862–6.
119. Uozumi H, Hiroi Y, Zou Y, et al. gp130 plays a critical role in pressure overload-induced cardiac hypertrophy. J Biol Chem 2001;276(25):23115–9.
120. Pennica D, King KL, Shaw KJ, et al. Expression cloning of cardiotrophin 1, a cytokine that induces cardiac myocyte hypertrophy. Proc Natl Acad Sci USA 1995;92(4):1142–6.
121. Sheng Z, Knowlton K, Chen J, Hoshijima M, Brown JH, Chien KR. Cardiotrophin 1 (CT-1) inhibition of cardiac myocyte apoptosis via a mitogen-activated protein kinase-dependent pathway. Divergence from downstream CT-1 signals for

myocardial cell hypertrophy. J Biol Chem 1997; 272(9):5783–91.
122. Takimoto Y, Aoyama T, Iwanaga Y, et al. Increased expression of cardiotrophin-1 during ventricular remodeling in hypertensive rats. Am J Physiol Heart Circ Physiol 2002;282(3):H896–901.
123. Habib FM, Springall DR, Davies GJ, Oakley CM, Yacoub MH, Polak JM. Tumour necrosis factor and inducible nitric oxide synthase in dilated cardiomyopathy. Lancet 1996;347(9009): 1151–5.
124. Levine B, Kalman J, Mayer L, Fillit HM, Packer M. Elevated circulating levels of tumor necrosis factor in severe chronic heart failure. N Engl J Med 1990;323(4):236–41.
125. Torre-Amione G, Kapadia S, Benedict C, Oral H, Young JB, Mann DL. Proinflammatory cytokine levels in patients with depressed left ventricular ejection fraction: a report from the Studies of Left Ventricular Dysfunction (SOLVD). J Am Coll Cardiol 1996;27(5):1201–6.
126. Kubota T, Miyagishima M, Alvarez RJ, et al. Expression of proinflammatory cytokines in the failing human heart: comparison of recent-onset and end-stage congestive heart failure. J Heart Lung Transplant 2000;19(9):819–24.
127. Sack MN, Smith RM, Opie LH. Tumor necrosis factor in myocardial hypertrophy and ischaemia–an anti-apoptotic perspective. Cardiovasc Res 2000;45(3):688–95.
128. Kubota T, McTiernan CF, Frye CS, Demetris AJ, Feldman AM. Cardiac-specific overexpression of tumor necrosis factor-alpha causes lethal myocarditis in transgenic mice. J Card Fail 1997;3(2): 117–24.
129. Kubota T, McTiernan CF, Frye CS, et al. Dilated cardiomyopathy in transgenic mice with cardiac-specific overexpression of tumor necrosis factor-alpha. Circ Res 1997;81(4):627–35.
130. Li X, Moody MR, Engel D, et al. Cardiac-specific overexpression of tumor necrosis factor-alpha causes oxidative stress and contractile dysfunction in mouse diaphragm. Circulation 2000;102(14): 1690–6.
131. Sivasubramanian N, Coker ML, Kurrelmeyer KM, et al. Left ventricular remodeling in transgenic mice with cardiac restricted overexpression of tumor necrosis factor. Circulation 2001;104(7): 826–31.
132. Seger R, Krebs EG. The MAPK signaling cascade. Faseb J 1995;9(9):726–35.
133. Davis RJ. The mitogen-activated protein kinase signal transduction pathway. J Biol Chem 1993; 268(20):14553–6.
134. Garrington TP, Johnson GL. Organization and regulation of mitogen-activated protein kinase signaling pathways. Curr Opin Cell Biol 1999;11(2) :211–8.
135. Sugden PH, Clerk A. Cellular mechanisms of cardiac hypertrophy. J Mol Med 1998;76(11): 725–46.
136. Boulton TG, Nye SH, Robbins DJ, et al. ERKs: a family of protein-serine/threonine kinases that are activated and tyrosine phosphorylated in response to insulin and NGF. Cell 1991;65(4): 663–75.
137. Bueno OF, Molkentin JD. Involvement of extracellular signal-regulated kinases 1/2 in cardiac hypertrophy and cell death. Circ Res 2002;91(9):776–81.
138. Esposito G, Prasad SV, Rapacciuolo A, Mao L, Koch WJ, Rockman HA. Cardiac overexpression of a G(q) inhibitor blocks induction of extracellular signal-regulated kinase and c-Jun NH(2)-terminal kinase activity in in vivo pressure overload. Circulation 2001;103(10):1453–8.
139. Rapacciuolo A, Esposito G, Caron K, Mao L, Thomas SA, Rockman HA. Important role of endogenous norepinephrine and epinephrine in the development of in vivo pressure-overload cardiac hypertrophy. J Am Coll Cardiol 2001;38(3): 876–82.
140. Bueno OF, De Windt LJ, Tymitz KM, et al. The MEK1–ERK1/2 signaling pathway promotes compensated cardiac hypertrophy in transgenic mice. Embo J 2000;19(23):6341–50.
141. Wang LX, Ideishi M, Yahiro E, Urata H, Arakawa K, Saku K. Mechanism of the cardioprotective effect of inhibition of the renin-angiotensin system on ischemia/reperfusion-induced myocardial injury. Hypertens Res 2001;24(2):179–87.
142. Liang Q, Wiese RJ, Bueno OF, Dai YS, Markham BE, Molkentin JD. The transcription factor GATA4 is activated by extracellular signal-regulated kinase 1- and 2-mediated phosphorylation of serine 105 in cardiomyocytes. Mol Cell Biol 2001; 21(21):7460–9.
143. Molkentin JD. The zinc finger-containing transcription factors GATA-4, -5, and -6. Ubiquitously expressed regulators of tissue-specific gene expression. J Biol Chem 2000;275(50):38949–52.
144. Liang Q, Molkentin JD. Redefining the roles of p38 and JNK signaling in cardiac hypertrophy: dichotomy between cultured myocytes and animal models. J Mol Cell Cardiol 2003;35(12):1385–94.
145. Barr RK, Bogoyevitch MA. The c-Jun N-terminal protein kinase family of mitogen-activated protein kinases (JNK MAPKs). Int J Biochem Cell Biol 2001;33(11):1047–63.

146. Ono K, Han J. The p38 signal transduction pathway: activation and function. Cell Signal 2000;12(1):1–13.
147. Jiang Y, Gram H, Zhao M, et al. Characterization of the structure and function of the fourth member of p38 group mitogen-activated protein kinases, p38delta. J Biol Chem 1997;272(48):30122–8.
148. Davis RJ. Signal transduction by the JNK group of MAP kinases. Cell 2000;103(2):239–52.
149. Petrich BG, Wang Y. Stress-activated MAP kinases in cardiac remodeling and heart failure; new insights from transgenic studies. Trends Cardiovasc Med 2004;14(2):50–5.
150. Wang Y, Huang S, Sah VP, et al. Cardiac muscle cell hypertrophy and apoptosis induced by distinct members of the p38 mitogen-activated protein kinase family. J Biol Chem 1998;273(4):2161–8.
151. Liao P, Georgakopoulos D, Kovacs A, et al. The in vivo role of p38 MAP kinases in cardiac remodeling and restrictive cardiomyopathy. Proc Natl Acad Sci USA 2001;98(21):12283–8.
152. Liao P, Wang SQ, Wang S, et al. p38 Mitogen-activated protein kinase mediates a negative inotropic effect in cardiac myocytes. Circ Res 2002;90(2):190–6.
153. Braz JC, Bueno OF, Liang Q, et al. Targeted inhibition of p38 MAPK promotes hypertrophic cardiomyopathy through upregulation of calcineurin-NFAT signaling. J Clin Invest 2003;111(10):1475–86.
154. Petrich BG, Molkentin JD, Wang Y. Temporal activation of c-Jun N-terminal kinase in adult transgenic heart via cre-loxP-mediated DNA recombination. Faseb J 2003;17(6):749–51.
155. Sadoshima J, Montagne O, Wang Q, et al. The MEKK1-JNK pathway plays a protective role in pressure overload but does not mediate cardiac hypertrophy. J Clin Invest 2002;110(2):271–9.
156. Liang Q, Bueno OF, Wilkins BJ, Kuan CY, Xia Y, Molkentin JD. c-Jun N-terminal kinases (JNK) antagonize cardiac growth through cross-talk with calcineurin-NFAT signaling. Embo J 2003;22(19):5079–89.
157. Zhang S, Weinheimer C, Courtois M, et al. The role of the Grb2–p38 MAPK signaling pathway in cardiac hypertrophy and fibrosis. J Clin Invest 2003;111(6):833–41.
158. Petrich BG, Eloff BC, Lerner DL, et al. Targeted activation of c-Jun N-terminal kinase in vivo induces restrictive cardiomyopathy and conduction defects. J Biol Chem 2004;279(15):15330–8.
159. Haq S, Choukroun G, Lim H, et al. Differential activation of signal transduction pathways in human hearts with hypertrophy versus advanced heart failure. Circulation 2001;103(5):670–7.
160. Cook SA, Sugden PH, Clerk A. Activation of c-Jun N-terminal kinases and p38-mitogen-activated protein kinases in human heart failure secondary to ischaemic heart disease. J Mol Cell Cardiol 1999;31(8):1429–34.
161. Dorn GW, 2nd, Force T. Protein kinase cascades in the regulation of cardiac hypertrophy. J Clin Invest 2005;115(3):527–37.
162. Igaz P, Toth S, Falus A. Biological and clinical significance of the JAK-STAT pathway; lessons from knockout mice. Inflamm Res 2001;50(9):435–41.
163. Imada K, Leonard WJ. The Jak-STAT pathway. Mol Immunol 2000;37(1–2):1–11.
164. Pan J, Fukuda K, Kodama H, et al. Role of angiotensin II in activation of the JAK/STAT pathway induced by acute pressure overload in the rat heart. Circ Res 1997;81(4):611–7.
165. Kunisada K, Negoro S, Tone E, et al. Signal transducer and activator of transcription 3 in the heart transduces not only a hypertrophic signal but a protective signal against doxorubicin-induced cardiomyopathy. Proc Natl Acad Sci USA 2000;97(1):315–9.
166. Negoro S, Kunisada K, Tone E, et al. Activation of JAK/STAT pathway transduces cytoprotective signal in rat acute myocardial infarction. Cardiovasc Res 2000;47(4):797–805.
167. Osugi T, Oshima Y, Fujio Y, et al. Cardiac-specific activation of signal transducer and activator of transcription 3 promotes vascular formation in the heart. J Biol Chem 2002;277(8):6676–81.
168. Hilfiker-Kleiner D, Hilfiker A, Fuchs M, et al. Signal transducer and activator of transcription 3 is required for myocardial capillary growth, control of interstitial matrix deposition, and heart protection from ischemic injury. Circ Res 2004;95(2):187–95.
169. Balke CW, Shorofsky SR. Alterations in calcium handling in cardiac hypertrophy and heart failure. Cardiovasc Res 1998;37(2):290–9.
170. Rao A, Luo C, Hogan PG. Transcription factors of the NFAT family: regulation and function. Annu Rev Immunol 1997;15:707–47.
171. Molkentin JD, Dorn IG 2nd. Cytoplasmic signaling pathways that regulate cardiac hypertrophy. Annu Rev Physiol 2001;63:391–426.
172. Klee CB, Ren H, Wang X. Regulation of the calmodulin-stimulated protein phosphatase, calcineurin. J Biol Chem 1998;273(22):13367–70.
173. Molkentin JD, Lu JR, Antos CL, et al. A calcineurin-dependent transcriptional pathway for cardiac hypertrophy. Cell 1998;93(2):215–28.

174. Wilkins BJ, Molkentin JD. Calcium-calcineurin signaling in the regulation of cardiac hypertrophy. Biochem Biophys Res Commun 2004;322(4):1178–91.
175. Sussman MA, Lim HW, Gude N, et al. Prevention of cardiac hypertrophy in mice by calcineurin inhibition. Science 1998;281(5383):1690–3.
176. Wilkins BJ, Dai YS, Bueno OF, et al. Calcineurin/NFAT coupling participates in pathological, but not physiological, cardiac hypertrophy. Circ Res 2004;94(1):110–8.
177. Wehrens XH, Lehnart SE, Huang F, et al. FKBP12.6 deficiency and defective calcium release channel (ryanodine receptor) function linked to exercise-induced sudden cardiac death. Cell 2003;113(7):829–40.
178. Lehnart SE, Wehrens XH, Reiken S, et al. Phosphodiesterase 4D deficiency in the ryanodine-receptor complex promotes heart failure and arrhythmias. Cell 2005;123(1):25–35.
179. Prasad SV, Perrino C, Rockman HA. Role of phosphoinositide 3-kinase in cardiac function and heart failure. Trends Cardiovasc Med 2003;13(5):206–12.
180. Lawlor MA, Alessi DR. PKB/Akt: a key mediator of cell proliferation, survival and insulin responses? J Cell Sci 2001;114(Pt 16):2903–10.
181. Martin TF. Phosphoinositide lipids as signaling molecules: common themes for signal transduction, cytoskeletal regulation, and membrane trafficking. Annu Rev Cell Dev Biol 1998;14:231–64.
182. Crackower MA, Oudit GY, Kozieradzki I, et al. Regulation of myocardial contractility and cell size by distinct PI3K-PTEN signaling pathways. Cell 2002;110(6):737–49.
183. Naga Prasad SV, Esposito G, Mao L, Koch WJ, Rockman HA. Gbetagamma-dependent phosphoinositide 3-kinase activation in hearts with in vivo pressure overload hypertrophy. J Biol Chem 2000;275(7):4693–8.
184. Shioi T, Kang PM, Douglas PS, et al. The conserved phosphoinositide 3-kinase pathway determines heart size in mice. Embo J 2000;19(11):2537–48.
185. Condorelli G, Drusco A, Stassi G, et al. Akt induces enhanced myocardial contractility and cell size in vivo in transgenic mice. Proc Natl Acad Sci USA 2002;99(19):12333–8.
186. Shioi T, McMullen JR, Kang PM, et al. Akt/protein kinase B promotes organ growth in transgenic mice. Mol Cell Biol 2002;22(8):2799–809.
187. Jo SH, Leblais V, Wang PH, Crow MT, Xiao RP. Phosphatidylinositol 3-kinase functionally compartmentalizes the concurrent G(s) signaling during beta2-adrenergic stimulation. Circ Res 2002;91(1):46–53.
188. Naga Prasad SV, Barak LS, Rapacciuolo A, Caron MG, Rockman HA. Agonist-dependent recruitment of phosphoinositide 3-kinase to the membrane by beta-adrenergic receptor kinase 1. A role in receptor sequestration. J Biol Chem 2001;276(22):18953–9.
189. Naga Prasad SV, Laporte SA, Chamberlain D, Caron MG, Barak L, Rockman HA. Phosphoinositide 3-kinase regulates beta2-adrenergic receptor endocytosis by AP-2 recruitment to the receptor/beta-arrestin complex. J Cell Biol 2002;158(3):563–75.
190. Nienaber JJ, Tachibana H, Naga Prasad SV, et al. Inhibition of receptor-localized PI3K preserves cardiac beta-adrenergic receptor function and ameliorates pressure overload heart failure. J Clin Invest 2003;112(7):1067–79.
191. Naga Prasad SV, Jayatilleke A, Madamanchi A, Rockman HA. Protein kinase activity of phosphoinositide 3-kinase regulates beta-adrenergic receptor endocytosis. Nat Cell Biol 2005;7(8):785–96.
192. Perrino C, Naga Prasad SV, Schroder JN, Hata JA, Milano C, Rockman HA. Restoration of beta-adrenergic receptor signaling and contractile function in heart failure by disruption of the betaARK1/phosphoinositide 3-kinase complex. Circulation 2005;111(20):2579–87.
193. Antos CL, McKinsey TA, Frey N, et al. Activated glycogen synthase-3 beta suppresses cardiac hypertrophy in vivo. Proc Natl Acad Sci USA 2002;99(2):907–12.
194. McMullen JR, Sherwood MC, Tarnavski O, et al. Inhibition of mTOR signaling with rapamycin regresses established cardiac hypertrophy induced by pressure overload. Circulation 2004;109(24):3050–5.
195. McMullen JR, Shioi T, Zhang L, et al. Phosphoinositide 3-kinase(p110alpha) plays a critical role for the induction of physiological, but not pathological, cardiac hypertrophy. Proc Natl Acad Sci USA 2003;100(21):12355–60.
196. Patrucco E, Notte A, Barberis L, et al. PI3Kgamma modulates the cardiac response to chronic pressure overload by distinct kinase-dependent and -independent effects. Cell 2004;118(3):375–87.
197. McKinsey TA, Olson EN. Toward transcriptional therapies for the failing heart: chemical screens to modulate genes. J Clin Invest 2005;115(3):538–46.

198. Bush E, Fielitz J, Melvin L, et al. A small molecular activator of cardiac hypertrophy uncovered in a chemical screen for modifiers of the calcineurin signaling pathway. Proc Natl Acad Sci USA 2004;101(9):2870–5.
199. Vega RB, Harrison BC, Meadows E, et al. Protein kinases C and D mediate agonist-dependent cardiac hypertrophy through nuclear export of histone deacetylase 5. Mol Cell Biol 2004;24(19): 8374–85.
200. Zhang CL, McKinsey TA, Chang S, Antos CL, Hill JA, Olson EN. Class II histone deacetylases act as signal-responsive repressors of cardiac hypertrophy. Cell 2002;110(4):479–88.
201. McKinsey TA, Zhang CL, Olson EN. MEF2: a calcium-dependent regulator of cell division, differentiation and death. Trends Biochem Sci 2002;27(1):40–7.
202. Harrison BC, Roberts CR, Hood DB, et al. The CRM1 nuclear export receptor controls pathological cardiac gene expression. Mol Cell Biol 2004; 24(24):10636–49.
203. Han A, Pan F, Stroud JC, Youn HD, Liu JO, Chen L. Sequence-specific recruitment of transcriptional co-repressor Cabin1 by myocyte enhancer factor-2. Nature 2003;422(6933):730–4.
204. Youn HD, Grozinger CM, Liu JO. Calcium regulates transcriptional repression of myocyte enhancer factor 2 by histone deacetylase 4. J Biol Chem 2000;275(29):22563–7.
205. McKinsey TA, Zhang CL, Lu J, Olson EN. Signal-dependent nuclear export of a histone deacetylase regulates muscle differentiation. Nature 2000; 408(6808):106–11.
206. Chang S, McKinsey TA, Zhang CL, Richardson JA, Hill JA, Olson EN. Histone deacetylases 5 and 9 govern responsiveness of the heart to a subset of stress signals and play redundant roles in heart development. Mol Cell Biol 2004;24(19): 8467–76.
207. Youn HD, Chatila TA, Liu JO. Integration of calcineurin and MEF2 signals by the coactivator p300 during T-cell apoptosis. Embo J 2000;19(16):4323–31.

11
Acute Heart Failure and Cardiac Remodeling

Jean-Jacques Mercadier

Acute heart failure, as with chronic heart failure, is a clinical syndrome that has many different etiologies and as such, it is the result of very diverse pathophysiologic processes. From a theoretical point of view, the heart, ventricles, myocardium, cardiac myocytes, and constituting proteins can be strictly normal when the episode of acute heart failure occurs. In this case, heart failure is the result of the failure of the cardiac pump while myocardial structure and function are normal. Alternatively, each and often several of the above-described structures may have been subjected previously to a more or less severe and long-standing remodeling process due to very diverse chronic pathophysiologic mechanisms.

The most illustrative example of the first situation is acute heart failure resulting from a large anterior myocardial infarct occurring in a previously healthy heart. A few seconds before the coronary artery occlusion, the heart structure and function is normal; a few seconds or minutes after coronary occlusion, a large portion of the anterior wall has become functionally inactive and the rest of the ventricular myocardium (the noninfarcted myocardium, also called the remote area) is suddenly exposed to an increase in its hemodynamic load (it has to perform the work of the whole ventricle, including the ischemic/infracted area) under very unfavorable biologic conditions called "biomechanical stress" (see below). In this case, acute heart failure is simply resulting from an acute dysfunction of the cardiac pump as a whole, with an associated hyperfunction of the remote area that tries to compensate for the loss of function of the ischemic/infracted myocardial area. Another example of this situation of acute heart failure with no previous cardiac remodeling is acute mitral regurgitation due to chordae rupture.

The most typical example of the second situation, which is also the most common, is an episode of acute heart failure occurring as a more or less sudden decompensation of a thus far well-compensated chronically failing heart. In this case, the heart, ventricles, myocardium, and myocytes have been more or less severely remodeled by weeks, months, years, and sometimes decades of a more or less severe biomechanical stress resulting from the originating disease. It is clear that in such a situation, the dysfunction of the cardiac pump is the result of myocardial dysfunction, itself resulting, at least in part, from myocyte dysfunction due to the so-called maladaptive remodeling (see below). In such a situation, the heart is placed in a unfavorable situation when, being previously weakened by a long process of detrimental remodeling, it is unable to compensate for the often mild insult at the origin of the acute decompensation such as, for instance, an episode of atrial fibrillation.

Schematically in this second category, two types of anatomic remodeling of the left ventricle (LV) can be opposed: first, the concentric LV remodeling seen in hypertrophic cardiomyopathies of any etiology, most often resulting from untreated chronic hypertension. In this case, the remodeling process concerns more the ventricle itself (its shape and the thickness and stiffness of its wall) than the myocardium and myocytes, whose contractile function is generally mildly altered if at all.

This type of remodeling is essentially at the origin of acute diastolic heart failure due to alterations in the so-called passive properties of the LV, with little remodeling of cardiac myocytes.

The second types of anatomic remodeling is the eccentric remodeling of dilated cardiomyopathies of any etiology (genetic, toxic, etc.) in which LV dilation is associated with an insufficiently thickened and hypocontractile myocardium. This is also the case with large myocardial infarcts when they have reached the stage of chronic heart failure. In this case, chronic biomechanical stress has led to a profound remodeling of the structure and function of cardiac myocytes, a process responsible for the contractile dysfunction and also the ventricular arrhythmias often seen in this setting (see below).

This chapter briefly summarizes the triggers and signaling mechanisms of cardiac remodeling in general and then focuses on the pathophysiology of this second type of remodeling, the identification and understanding of which is especially important behind the often stereotyped presentation of an acute heart failure episode, since it will largely guide the therapeutic intervention and condition the short and long-term prognosis.

Biomechanical Stress and the Resulting Detrimental (Maladaptive) Cardiac Remodeling

Cardiac remodeling results from two types of triggers: mechanical and neurohumoral. Each cardiac disease associates various degrees of these two factor types. Again, myocardial infarction well illustrates this situation: immediately after the constitution of the infarct and even the ischemia, the decrease in LV performance leads to a rise in LV diastolic pressures and wall stress, resulting in myocardial and myocyte stretch. Left ventricular dilation also increases LV systolic wall stress and the decrease, even small, of mean arterial pressure that results from LV dysfunction, activates systemic neurohumoral systems, first the sympathetic system and then the renin-angiotensin-aldosterone system.

Myocyte stretch, catecholamines, angiotensin II, endothelin I, aldosterone, and diverse growth factors and cytokines (fibroblast growth factor [FGF], nerve growth factor [NGF], platelet-derived growth factor [PDGF], transforming growth factor-β [TGF-β], insulin-like growth factor-I [IGF-I], calcitonin [CT], leukemia inhibitory factor (LIF), interleukin-6 [IL-6], and others), produced either systemically or locally, are like many signals—depending on each disease and pathophysiologic process, they act on various types of receptors located on the plasma membrane or inside myocytes that trigger the reprogramming of myocyte gene expression. This leads to remodeling of myocytes of the noninfarcted area, a process that starts during the first seconds or minutes following coronary artery occlusion. These signals activate a host of complex intracellular signal transduction pathways (also called cascades), often interconnected as a web, which finally activate (or block) a number of transcription factors, thus modulating gene expression, while other factors modulate messenger RNA (mRNA) translation into proteins (see Mercadier[1] for a review). These processes, which also take place in nonmuscle cells, are responsible for myocyte/myocardial hypertrophy and remodeling of the extracellular matrix. In cardiac myocytes, they lead a specific alteration in protein phenotype known as "reexpression of the fetal program" (also called the hypertrophic phenotype). One typical example of this process is the production of natriuretic peptides (atrial natriuretic peptide [ANP] and B-type natriuretic peptide [BNP]) by ventricular myocytes, a production that occurred in the fetal ventricle and ceased shortly after birth. Although it has long been controversial, it is now well accepted that this remodeling process, although possibly beneficial in the short term, is detrimental in the long term, being responsible for the progression to heart failure[1].

The Remodeled Heart

The Remodeled Myocyte

The molecular remodeling that concerns potentially all myocyte proteins is not discussed here. Gene reprogramming may simply result in quantitative changes, such as the overall increase in protein synthesis and the increased expression in natriuretic peptides described above. Alternatively, the pattern of expression of multigenic protein families may be changed by up- and downregulation of specific isoforms as is the case for the α- to β-myosin heavy chain (MHC) or creatine phosphokinase (CPK)-M to CPK-B transitions.

However, the most important aspect of cardiac myocyte remodeling is that of calcium cycling. Briefly, myocyte contraction is due to an activation of myofibrillar proteins by Ca^{2+} originating from sarcoplasmic reticulum (SR)[2]. Ca^{2+} release out of the SR is triggered by the Ca^{2+} current (ICa^{2+}) that enters into the cell through L-type Ca^{2+} channels during the action potential plateau (Fig. 11.1). The process, called Ca^{2+}-induced Ca^{2+} release, implies that the small amount of Ca^{2+} entering the cell via ICa^{2+} is "sensed" by the SR Ca^{2+} channels (also called ryanodine receptors [RyRs]) that thereby open and release large amounts of Ca^{2+} into the cytosol, which activates the myofibrils. Myocyte relaxation is due to pumping of Ca^{2+} back into the SR due to a Ca^{2+}–adenosine triphosphatase (ATPase) called SERCA (for sarcoendoplasmic reticulum Ca^{2+}-ATPase). This SERCA is activated by high cytoplasmic free Ca^{2+} concentrations ($[Ca^{2+}]_i$, around 1 mM) and inhibited by a protein called phospholamban (PLB) when bound to the pump[3]. Phospholamban phosphorylation resulting from catecholamine stimulation unbinds PLB from SERCA, thereby activating its pumping function and accelerating relaxation[3].

Remodeling of myocyte Ca^{2+} cycling schematically consists in two major pathophysiological processes: (1) a decrease in Ca^{2+} pumping capacity into the SR due to a decreased expression of SERCA,[4] and its increased inhibition by a largely dephosphorylated PLB[3,5]; (2) a Ca^{2+} leak out of the SR during diastole through RyRs due to a complex, still controversial, pathophysiologic mechanism possibly implying RyR hyperphosphorylation and decreased binding of calstabin 2 (also known as FKBP12.6)[6,7]. The association of these two patho-

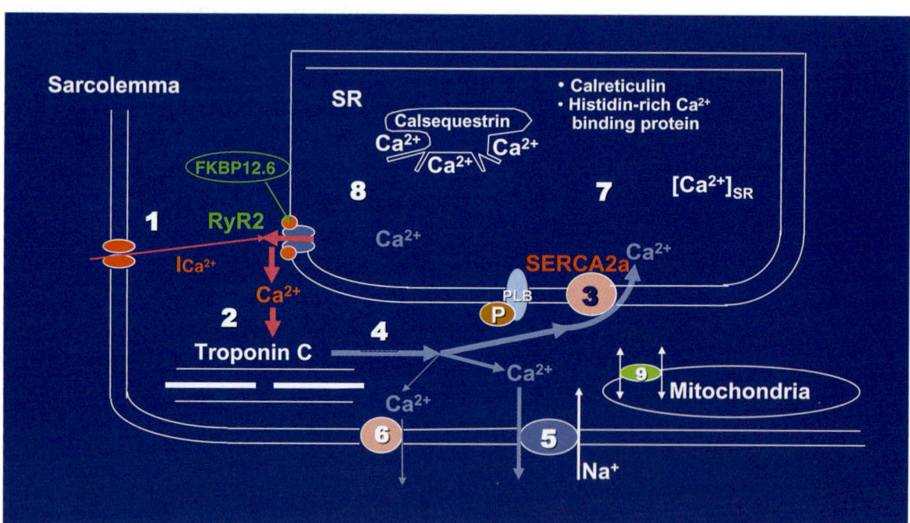

FIGURE 11.1. Excitation-contraction-relaxation of normal cardiac myocytes. Steps 1 and 2: Excitation-contraction coupling mechanism. Steps 3 and 4: Myocyte relaxation due to sarcoendoplasmic reticulum (SR) Ca^{2+}-ATPase (SERCA2a) that pumps Ca^{2+} back into the SR; this action is completed by that of the Na^+-Ca^{2+} exchanger (NCX) (step 5), that of the plasma membrane Ca2+-ATPase (PMCA, step 6) and mitochondria (step 9). Phospholamban (PLB), when phosphorylated by a cyclic adenosine monophosphate (cAMP)-dependent protein kinase (PKA), unbinds from SERCA, which activates Ca^{2+} uptake into the SR and myocyte relaxation. Once in the SR, Ca^{2+} binds to calsequestrin (step 8) and other Ca^{2+}-binding protein, waiting for its extrusion through the ryanodine receptor (RyR2) at the next beat. See details in the text.

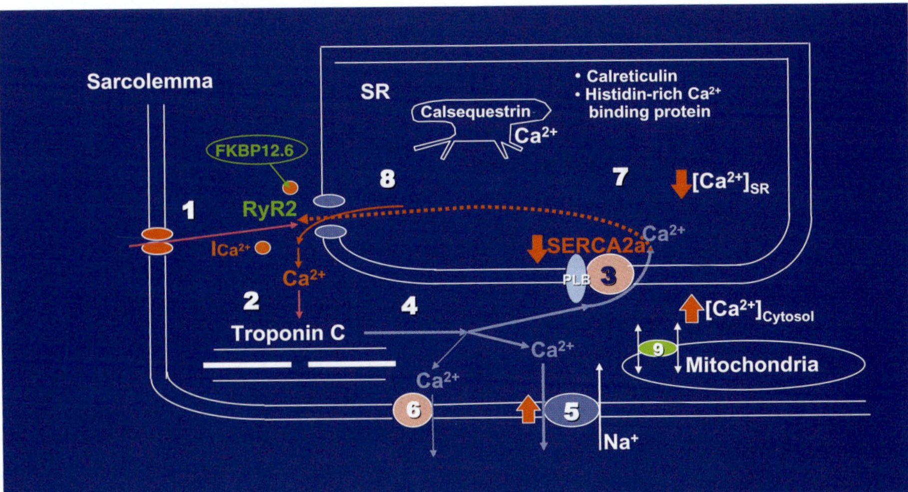

FIGURE 11.2. Excitation-contraction-relaxation of remodeled/failing cardiac myocytes. Two major mechanisms participate in the alteration of myocyte contraction and relaxation during chronic heart failure: defective Ca^{2+} pumping capacity into the SR due to downregulation of SERCA2a expression and its inhibition by a dephosphorylated PLB; and a leaky RyR due to its hyperphosphorylation by a protein kinase A (PKA)- or Ca^{2+}-calmodulin-dependent kinase (CaMK) resulting in FKBP12.6 dissociation. Addition of the two pathophysiologic mechanisms leads to a Ca^{2+}-depleted SR and increased cytosolic-free Ca^{2+} levels during diastole. See the text for details.

physiologic mechanisms transforms the SR into a sort of Danaides's barrel in which the small amount of Ca^{2+} pumped by SERCA is immediately lost through leaky RyRs (Fig. 11.2). This is associated with an increased activity/expression of the Na^{+}-Ca^{2+} exchanger (NCX) that extrudes Ca^{2+} out of the cell during diastole in exchange for an entry of Na^{+}. Together with the SR Ca^{2+} leak, this process worsens SR Ca^{2+} depletion, leading to a decreased SR Ca^{2+} store and therefore to decreased activating Ca^{2+} during systole responsible for the systolic dysfunction. Together with the deficient pumping function of SERCA, the RyR leak is also responsible for an increased $[Ca^{2+}]_i$ during diastole (above the normal value of 100 nM) responsible for an incomplete diastolic relaxation that contributes to increase myocardial stiffness, further deteriorating LV diastolic filling. Moreover, since NCX extrudes 1 Ca^{2+} out of the cell in exchange of the entrance of 3 Na^{+}, the exchanger is electrogenic, thus leading to a depolarizing current during diastole, a process largely contributing to the occurrence of ventricular arrhythmias.

Another important aspect of cardiac myocyte remodeling relates to alterations in energy production and utilization that worsen Ca^{2+} cycling dysfunction. During the early stages of cardiac remodeling, there is a transition from a predominantly fatty acid to a glucose consumption associated with the CPK isoform redistribution described above. Unfortunately, progression toward chronic heart failure (HF) is not accompanied by a sufficient expression of glycolytic enzymes, and other alterations also occur: altered mitochondrial adenosine triphosphate (ATP) production, decreased phosphocreatine (PCr)/ATP ratio, increased adenosine diphosphate (ADP) concentration, and decreased ATP supply to the SR and especially SERCA. Myocyte energy shortage and altered Ca^{2+} cycling results in a very deleterious vicious circle that is worsened during effort[8].

Whether the above-described alterations are the cause or consequence of the transition to overt chronic HF has long been a matter of controversy. As pointed out above, it is now clear that they belong to the remodeling process that starts very early (for instance at the onset of myocardial infarction) and worsens at each acute heart failure attack.

The Remodeled Myocardium

Schematically, the remodeled myocardium is composed of bigger myocytes that are either thickened in the case of chronic pressure overload, or lengthened in the case of chronic volume overload, or both. During the phase of compensated hypertrophy, that is, before the stage of chronic heart failure, their proliferation index is very low and is not greater than that observed in normal myocardium, whereas an increased proliferation would occur during chronic HF[9]. During hypertrophy, an insufficient angiogenesis may result in a certain degree of hypoxia for those myocytes situated far from capillaries, a process more severe for the subendocardial half than for the subepicardial half of the myocardium, further worsened during decompensated HF when increased left ventricular filling pressures hinder blood circulation in the subendocardium during diastole. Cardiac myocyte apoptosis, the importance of which has long been controversial[10,11], most probably plays a significant role in decreasing the myocyte numbers during progression of the disease, and especially at the occasion of HF attacks. This coexists with various degrees of proliferation of the nonmuscle cells and extracellular matrix remodeling, characterized by interstitial and perivascular fibrosis favored by an imbalance between the activity of the matrix metalloproteinases (MMPs) and their inhibitors (tissue-inhibitor metalloproteinases, TIMPs)[12]. Moreover, myocardial fibrosis increases myocardial stiffness (and decreases myocardial compliance).

The Remodeled Ventricle

The consequences of myocyte and myocardial remodeling for left ventricular function differ according to the type of remodeling considered. Concentric LV hypertrophy resulting from hypertrophic cardiomyopathies or chronic hypertension is responsible for an increased LV stiffness (and decreased LV compliance) due to LV wall thickening, often—but not necessarily—associated with an increased myocardial stiffness. This results in an up- and leftward deviation of the LV pressure/volume relationship. Together with the absence of significant LV systolic dysfunction, which is often the case in this pathophysiologic setting, this characterizes diastolic HF.

Functional consequences of dilative LV remodeling depend very much on the causal disease. Leaking valvular diseases are responsible for a chronic volume overload that can be compared to the LV dilative remodeling seen during sustained physical training during which no detrimental myocardial/myocyte remodeling is seen for a long period of time. This is why such remodeling is well tolerated for a long time, in all events as long as LV dilation remains moderate. An example of the opposite situation is the dilated cardiomyopathy due to a mutation in the gene of the muscle LIM protein (MLP)[13]. This mutation in the gene coding for a major mechanical sensor of cardiac myocytes makes them totally unable to hypertrophy, especially to compensate for LV dilation. This leads rapidly to very high diastolic and systolic wall stress, which accelerate molecular and cellular remodeling, and the occurrence of major systolic dysfunction. In this respect, it is important to note that dilated cardiomyopathies due to gene mutation(s) are associated with increased LV pre- and afterload due to LV dilation, a mechanism responsible for a "secondary" remodeling process similar to that seen in cardiopathies of extrinsic origin. This adds its own pathophysiologic process to that due to the originating mutation(s) responsible for a "primary" remodeling. Finally, the dilated and LV, with an insufficiently thickened wall as compared to its increased radius, is the converging point of all cardiopathies, a stage at which the biomechanical stress is maximal with its severely deleterious, rapidly evolving pathophysiologic consequences in the absence of therapeutic intervention. Therefore, all efforts should be made to prevent LV dilation and, when it is established, to reduce it.

Synthesis

The complexity of acute heart failure is that it occurs on a heart and myocardium, the intrinsic quality of which is often unknown. After the first therapeutic interventions usually performed in emergency, it becomes rapidly important to have an idea of the quality of the underlying myocardium, that is, of the age and severity of the remodeling process. Very schematically, acute heart failure occurring on small hearts is generally a problem of loading of a stiff LV whose myocyte functional characteristics (contraction and relaxation) are normal or little altered. By contrast, acute heart failure occurring on enlarged hearts, which may also result, at least in part, from a problem of LV loading, result from myocyte/myocardial dysfunction due to a more or less severe and long-standing remodeling process. Even if a sympathetic support may be beneficial for a short period of time in this setting, large clinical trials have clearly shown that such a support is deleterious in the long term because it worsens remodeling. In the long term, all efforts must be made to suppress triggers and block pathways of detrimental remodeling, starting with heart size reduction.

References

1. Mercadier JJ. Determinants of cardiac hypertrophy and progression to heart failure. In: Hosenpud JD, Greenberg BH, eds. Congestive Heart Failure. Philadelphia: Lippincott Williams & Wilkins, in press.
2. Bers DM. Cardiac excitation-contraction coupling. Nature 2002;415:198–205.
3. MacLennan DH, Kranias EG. Phospholamban: a crucial regulator of cardiac contractility. Nat Rev Mol Cell Biol 2003;4:566–77.
4. Mercadier JJ, Lompre AM, Duc P, et al. Altered sarcoplasmic reticulum Ca2(+)-ATPase gene expression in the human ventricle during end-stage heart failure. J Clin Invest 1990;85:305–9.
5. Pathak A, del Monte F, Zhao W, et al. Enhancement of cardiac function and suppression of heart failure progression by inhibition of protein phosphatase 1. Circ Res 2005;96:756–66.
6. Marx SO, Reiken S, Hisamatsu Y, et al. PKA phosphorylation dissociates FKBP12.6 from the calcium release channel (ryanodine receptor): defective regulation in failing hearts. Cell 2000;101: 365–76.
7. Wehrens XH, Lehnart SE, Reiken S, Vest JA, Wronska A, Marks AR. Ryanodine receptor/calcium release channel PKA phosphorylation: a critical mediator of heart failure progression. Proc Natl Acad Sci U S A 2006;103:511–18.
8. Ventura-Clapier R, Garnier A, Veksler V. Energy metabolism in heart failure. J Physiol 2004;555: 1–13.
9. Nadal-Ginard B, Kajstura J, Leri A, Anversa P. Myocyte death, growth, and regeneration in cardiac hypertrophy and failure. Circ Res 2003;92: 139–50.
10. Schaper J, Elsasser A, Kostin S. The role of cell death in heart failure. Circ Res 1999;85:867–9.
11. Kostin S, Pool L, Elsasser A, et al. Myocytes die by multiple mechanisms in failing human hearts. Circ Res 2003;92:715–24.
12. Polyakova V, Hein S, Kostin S, Ziegelhoeffer T, Schaper J. Matrix metalloproteinases and their tissue inhibitors in pressure-overloaded human myocardium during heart failure progression. J Am Coll Cardiol 2004;44:1609–18.
13. Knoll R, Hoshijima M, Hoffman HM, et al. The cardiac mechanical stretch sensor machinery involves a Z disc complex that is defective in a subset of human dilated cardiomyopathy. Cell 2002;111:943–55.

12
Reactive Oxygen Species in Heart Failure

Min Zhang and Ajay M. Shah

A constant supply of oxygen is indispensable for cardiac viability and function. However, oxygen is also central to the generation of reactive oxygen species (ROS). Indeed, it is estimated that up to 5% of the oxygen normally consumed by tissues can be transformed into ROS. Recent studies point to crucial roles of increased ROS in the pathophysiology of heart failure.[1]

Generation and Counterbalancing of Reactive Oxygen Species

Reactive oxygen species, such as superoxide ($O_2^-\cdot$), hydrogen peroxide (H_2O_2), peroxynitrite ($ONOO\cdot^-$), and hydroxyl radicals ($\cdot OH$), are highly reactive molecules with unpaired electrons in their outer orbit. $O_2^-\cdot$ is produced by the one-electron reduction of molecular O_2; it has a half-life of only a few seconds and is rapidly dismutated to H_2O_2. The diffusion capacity of $O_2^-\cdot$ is limited due to its poor membrane permeability, and therefore its actions are generally restricted to the intracellular compartment of production. In contrast, H_2O_2 is more stable and more cell membrane-permeable than $O_2^-\cdot$ and may therefore have the potential to act at more distant sites. The most reactive oxygen free radical is $\cdot OH$, which is formed from H_2O_2 via the Fenton or Haber-Weiss reactions. Normally, $\cdot OH$ is formed in negligible amounts, but in pathologic conditions (e.g., ischemia-reperfusion) it is generated in high amounts and contributes to oxidative stress-associated cellular damage. In settings where the level of the signaling molecule nitric oxide (NO) is in the high nanomolar range, $O_2^-\cdot$ may react with NO to generate the potent oxidant $ONOO\cdot^-$, this reaction also resulting in inactivation of NO.

In health, these basally generated ROS are efficiently counterbalanced by several enzymatic and nonenzymatic pathways. Among the best-characterized endogenous antioxidant pathways are the superoxide dismutases (SODs), catalase, and glutathione peroxidase enzymes. The SOD isoenzymes efficiently convert $O_2^-\cdot$ to H_2O_2 in vivo, with manganese SOD (Mn SOD) present in high concentration in mitochondria, copper/zinc (Cu/Zn) SOD in the cytosol, and extracellular (SOD) at the plasma membrane or in the extracellular compartment. H_2O_2 levels are tightly regulated by cellular catalase and glutathione peroxidase, which scavenge H_2O_2 to water. In addition, thioredoxin and thioredoxin reductase can catalyze the regeneration of many antioxidant molecules, including ubiquinone (Q10), lipoic acid, and ascorbic acid, and as such constitute an important antioxidant defense against ROS. Nonenzymatic mechanisms include intracellular antioxidants such as the vitamins E, C, and β-carotene (a precursor to vitamin A), ubiquinone, lipoic acid, urate, and glutathione; the latter acts as a reducing substrate for the enzymatic activity of glutathione peroxidase.

The Biologic Significance of Reactive Oxygen Species

Reactive oxygen species can exert either potentially beneficial or detrimental effects that contribute to cardiac dysfunction and death. On the one hand, when levels of ROS are elevated dramatically to overwhelm the cellular antioxidant defenses, they react directly with membrane lipids, proteins, and nucleic acid, causing cellular dysfunction and death (both through apoptosis and necrosis). The cellular production of one ROS may lead to the production of several others via radical chain reactions. For example, reactions between radicals and polyunsaturated fatty acids within cell membranes may result in a fatty acid peroxyl radical that can attack adjacent fatty acid side chains and initiate production of other lipid radicals. Lipid radicals produced in this chain reaction accumulate in the cell membrane and may have a myriad of effects on cellular function, including leakiness of the plasmalemma and dysfunction of membrane-bound receptors. Reactive oxygen species can contribute to mutagenesis of DNA by inducing strand breaks, purine oxidation, and protein-DNA cross-linking, which may significantly affect gene expression. Reactive oxygen species may also induce denaturation that renders proteins nonfunctional.

On the other hand, ROS can function as second messengers or regulatory mediators downstream of specific ligands, such as angiotensin II (AngII), endothelin, growth factors (fibroblast growth factor-2 [FGF-2], platelet-derived growth factor [PDGF]), cytokines (transforming growth factor-β1 [TGF-β1], tumor necrosis factor-α [TNF-α]), and many others (so-called redox signaling). Reactive oxygen species involved in signaling can activate various redox-sensitive protein kinases, inactivate protein tyrosine phosphatases, and modulate the activities of transcription factors such as activator protein 1 (AP-1), nuclear factor (NF)-κB and hypoxia-inducible factor-1 (HIF-1), thereby inducing specific changes in gene expression and cell phenotype. Such redox-regulated effects underlie the essential roles of ROS in biologic processes such as normal cell proliferation and growth. They may also contribute to pathophysiologic processes, for example, the induction of cardiomyocyte hypertrophy through the activation of NF-κB.

In cardiomyocytes, ROS may also exert specific direct effects on ion channels and membrane ion pumps, including L-type calcium channels, sodium channels, potassium channels, and the Na/Ca exchanger, which are critical for normal cardiac excitation-contraction coupling and function. Reactive oxygen species may alter the activity of the sarcoplasmic reticulum Ca^{2+}–adenosine triphosphatase (ATPase) (SERCA2) as well as reduce myofilament calcium sensitivity, both of which are important determinants of myocardial contractility. Another major mode of ROS action is by affecting the function of proteins involved in energy metabolism, thereby inducing energetic deficit. It is also worth mentioning that ROS may promote autocrine/paracrine interactions by altering the secretion of bioactive agents. For example, fibroblasts stimulated by ROS increase their secretion of TGF-β, which may have significant effects on adjacent cardiomyocytes. Therefore, ROS has a host of potential actions within the myocardium.

Sources of Reactive Oxygen Species in Cardiac Cells

Potential sources of ROS include the mitochondrial respiratory chain, xanthine oxidase (XO), reduced nicotinamide adenine dinucleotide phosphate (NADPH) oxidases, lipoxygenase, cytochrome P-450s, NO synthases, peroxidases, and other hemoproteins. All these enzymes system are present in the three major cardiac cell types: cardiac myocytes, fibroblasts, and endothelial cells. Although their exact relative contributions to the generation of ROS is not known, it has become clear that mitochondria, XO, and NADPH oxidases are the predominant sources of ROS that may be involved in the pathophysiology of heart failure.

Mitochondrial Reactive Oxygen Species

Reactive oxygen species can be formed during oxidative phosphorylation in the mitochondria as a by-product of normal cellular aerobic metabolism.[2] Thus, the major process by which the heart derives energy can also result in the production of ROS. During the Krebs cycle, electrons derived from reduced nicotinamide adenine dinucleotide ($NADH_2$) and flavin adenine dinucleotide (reduced form; $FADH_2$) flow along the respiratory transport chain through a series of cytochrome-based enzymes (complexes I, III, IV), which transport electrons finally to molecular O_2. Normally, the high free energy of the electrons is gradually extracted and converted into adenosine triphosphate (ATP), and only 1% or less of electrons "leak" to form $O_2^{-}\cdot$. Most of this $O_2^{-}\cdot$ is rapidly scavenged by mitochondrial MnSOD. However, during hypoxia-reoxygenation or ischemia-reperfusion, the electron chain transfer is blocked at the level of complex I or III and electrons are inappropriately diverted directly to O_2, resulting in a large amount of $O_2^{-}\cdot$ formation. The importance of the mitochondrial ROS in heart failure is emphasized by the finding that complete genetic deficiency of mitochondrial SOD in mice results in severe dilated cardiomyopathy and postnatal death.

Xanthine Oxidase

Xanthine oxidoreductase (XOR) is a molybdoenzyme capable of catalyzing the oxidation of hypoxanthine and xanthine in the process of purine metabolism. Xanthine oxidoreductase exists as one of two interconvertible yet functionally distinct forms, namely xanthine dehydrogenase (XD) or xanthine oxidase (XO). The former reduces the oxidized form of nicotinamide adenine dinucleotide (NAD^+), whereas the latter prefers molecular oxygen, leading to the production of both $O_2^{-}\cdot$ and H_2O_2. The conversion of XD to XO occurs either through reversible thiol oxidation of sulfhydryl residues on XD or via rapid and irreversible proteolytic cleavage of a segment of XD during hypoxia, ischemia, or in the presence of various proinflammatory mediators. Although XO-mediated $O_2^{-}\cdot$ production (usually assessed by inhibition by allopurinol or oxypurinol) can be documented in several cardiac pathophysiologic settings, constitutive XOR activity is apparently very low. It has been suggested that endogenous XO synthesis in the heart may be low but that it may be released from XO-rich organs such as liver and intestine under pathophysiologic conditions and may subsequently bind to endothelial cells in situ in the heart.[3]

Many experimental studies support an important role for XO-derived ROS generation in myocardial ischemia-reperfusion injury, although there may be a relatively narrow window in which this can be therapeutically targeted. During ischemia, irreversible proteolytic cleavage converts XD to XO, thereby priming the system for the triggering of microvascular inflammation by the generation of ROS upon the subsequent delivery of oxygen at reperfusion. The ROS thereby generated from XO could trigger the local accumulation and activation of neutrophils, leading to further bursts of ROS production and ultimately cardiac dysfunction. Increases in expression or activity of XO have been documented both in experimental canine heart failure and in end-stage failing human heart tissue, and treatment with the XO inhibitor allopurinol is reported to improve contractile function of failing hearts.

Nicotinamide Adenine Dinucleotide Phosphate Oxidases

Recently, a large body of evidence has indicated that an especially important source of ROS in cardiovascular system is a family of complex enzymes termed NADPH oxidases.[4] The prototypic NADPH oxidase was first characterized in neutrophils, where it plays an essential role in nonspecific host defense against invading microbes during the process of phagocytosis. NADPH oxidase is a multimeric complex with a core membrane-bound cytochrome b_{558} that catalyzes electron transfer from NADPH to molecular oxygen, thereby generating $O_2^{-}\cdot$. The cytochrome is a heterodimer made up of a catalytic Nox (for NADPH oxidase) subunit and a $p22^{phox}$ subunit. Several Nox isoforms (Nox1-5) have recently been identified; endothelial cells, cardiomyocytes, and fibroblasts express Nox2 and Nox4, whereas vascular smooth muscle cells express mainly Nox4 and Nox1. Interestingly, Nox1 and Nox2 require cytosolic subunits (termed $p47^{phox}$, $p67^{phox}$, and $p40^{phox}$) and the small G-protein Rac1 for their activation, whereas current evidence suggests that Nox4 does not depend on these subunits. Reduced nicotinamide adenine dinucleotide phosphate oxidases in cardiovascular (and other nonphagocytic) cells continuously generate a low level of $O_2^{-}\cdot$; however, the level of $O_2^{-}\cdot$ production is significantly increased by several pathophysiologic stimuli, such as AngII, α-adrenergic agonists, endothelin-1, tumor necrosis factor-α, and mechanical stress. A substantial proportion of the $O_2^{-}\cdot$ generated by NADPH oxidases in cardiovascular cells is produced intracellularly (in contrast to neutrophils) and is thought to be involved in redox signaling.[4]

Accumulating evidence suggests that NADPH oxidase-derived ROS play an important role in many cardiovascular diseases, including myocardial infarction and heart failure. Myocardial NADPH oxidase expression and activity are reported to be increased after acute myocardial infarction and in heart failure, both experimentally and in human disease.[5] Interestingly, the upregulation of NADPH oxidase-mediated ROS production in the failing myocardium of patients with dilated cardiomyopathy and ischemic cardiomyopathy was associated with increased rac1 activity, which potentially can be inhibited by treatment with statins.

The Role of Reactive Oxygen Species in Heart Failure

Acute Myocardial Infarction

The production of large amounts of ROS during reperfusion has traditionally been suggested to contribute to reperfusion injury and cell death in the context of myocardial infarction (MI). For example, in ischemia-reperfused rat hearts, maximum oxidant production was detected with electron paramagnetic resonance (EPR) at 10 to 30 seconds after reperfusion. Similarly, in humans, EPR spin trapping has been used in conjunction with coronary artery bypass graft (CABG) surgery to show that ROSs are increased in the first 5 minutes after reperfusion. It is suggested that up to 60% of cardiac myocyte death in the early stages of reperfusion may be attributable to oxidative injury. These patients may have elevated serum markers of oxidative stress such as thiobarbituric acid reactive substances (TBARS), and a significant proportion may go on to develop heart failure.[6]

In experimental animals, pretreatment with antioxidants/enzymes (such as SOD) or the genetic overexpression of these enzymes affords protection against reperfusion injury. A frequently studied antioxidant agent is *N*-2-mercaptopropionyl glycine (MPG), which is thought to work by directly reacting with free-radical species, promoting the resynthesis of glutathione, or acting as an alternative substrate for glutathione peroxidase, thereby limiting the cytotoxic effects of H_2O_2 and lipid peroxides. *N*-2-mercaptopropionyl glycine has been shown to significantly reduce MI size for as long as 48 hours after reperfusion. Other antioxidant agents shown to exert some cardioprotective action in animal models of MI include N-acetylcysteine (NAC), dimethylthiourea, and desferrioxamine. In canines, a combination of SOD and catalase significantly reduced MI size after 90 minutes of coronary artery ischemia and 24 hours of reflow. Interestingly, administration of the XO inhibitor allopurinol in the setting of rat acute MI attenuated stunning and ameliorated excitation-contraction uncoupling. However, such therapies have not achieved clinical usage as yet.

The genetic overexpression of glutathione peroxidase (GSHPx) also protected against myocardial ischemia-reperfusion, whereas GSHPx knockout mice were more susceptible to myocardial reperfusion injury compared with their wild-type counterparts.

Postmyocardial Infarction Remodeling

Increased oxidative stress is recognized to promote adverse LV remodeling post-MI (i.e., chronic ventricular dilatation and contractile dysfunction), a major precursor to heart failure. Experimentally, treatment with the antioxidants probucol or dimethylthiourea can ameliorate adverse LV remodeling and improve contractile function. Consistent with these data, post-MI remodeling was prevented in mice overexpressing glutathione peroxidase. Recent data from our laboratory suggest that Nox2 contributes significantly to the adverse remodeling observed after MI, whereas another study implicates XO.

Reactive Oxygen Species in the Diabetic Heart

Diabetes is an established risk factor for cardiovascular events, and the mortality from ischemic heart disease of diabetic patients is three times higher than that of nondiabetics. There is an increasing recognition that diabetic patients may have additional specific myocardial problems independent of coronary artery disease, age, hypertension, obesity, or hyperlipidemia, termed "diabetic cardiomyopathy." Prominent functional consequences include diastolic and systolic dysfunction and heart failure, with an annual mortality of 15% to 20%. While the mechanisms underlying diabetic heart muscle disease are not fully understood, a considerable body of evidence implicates oxidative stress as an important pathogenic factor.[7]

In animal models of streptozotocin-induced type I diabetes, the production of ROS in the heart has been shown to be increased in association with a reduction in number of left ventricular cardiomyocytes. Of importance, the antioxidant NAC could prevent this reduction in myocyte number. In experimental type 2 diabetes, the impairment of cardiomyocyte contractility can be ameliorated by overexpression of the antioxidant protein metallothionein or the antioxidant enzyme catalase. Human patients with type 2 diabetes also have elevated levels of oxidative stress markers in the plasma, although the effects of antioxidants on cardiac function have not been defined.

The sources of ROS generation in diabetes are of interest. Hyperglycemia can stimulate ROS generation directly through effects on various cellular enzymes. In endothelial cells, the increased ROS production appears to be mitochondrial in origin, whereas in adult rat cardiomyocytes the ROS seem to be generated by NADPH oxidases, and this is inhibited by the oxidase inhibitor apocynin both in vitro and in vivo. Hyperglycemia also promotes the formation of glucose-modified proteins such as early glycated Amadori products and advanced glycation end-products (AGEs). The two main types of Amadori products in blood are hemoglobin A_{1c} (HbA_{1c}) and fructosamine, both of which are used to assess the degree of glucose control. There is a positive relationship between the levels of glycated products and diabetic heart disease, with each 1% increase in HbA_{1c} being associated with an 8% increase in the risk of heart failure or death. Interestingly, both early and late glycation end-products can stimulate ROS generation in several cell types. In endothelial cells and cardiomyocytes, a large proportion of this ROS production emanates from activated NADPH oxidase. In the latter cell type, Nox2 NADPH oxidase-derived ROS led to NF-κB activation and the upregulation of atrial natriuretic factor (ANF) mRNA.

Alcoholic Cardiomyopathy

Long-term misuse of alcohol or binge drinking is recognized to lead to cardiac dysfunction and failure, characterized as a unique type of dilated cardiomyopathy termed alcoholic cardiomyopathy. A cardinal feature of this cardiomyopathy is its precipitation by alcohol abuse and the significant rates of recovery following abstinence. Although several hypotheses have been postulated to mechanistically explain the occurrence of this condition, enhanced oxidative stress seems to be central in explaining the toxicity of ethanol and its metabolite acetaldehyde.[8] Three main metabolic pathways for ethanol have so far been described in the human body, which involve alcohol dehydrogenase (ADH), microsomal ethanol oxidation system, and catalase. Each of these pathways is able to generate free radicals, including $O_2^{-}\cdot$, hydroxyl, acetyl, and methyl radicals. Acetaldehyde is formed by the oxidation of ethanol by ADH and is subsequently oxidized to acetic acid mainly through ADH, a process accompanied by ROS generation. Most evidence supporting an etiologic role for oxidant stress in alcoholic cardiomyopathy comes from animal experiments. For example, a recent study showed that transgenic mice with cardiac overexpression of catalase displayed preserved cardiac function and improved intracellular Ca^{2+} handling against ethanol-induced damage. However, convincing data from human studies remain lacking.

Reactive Oxygen Species in Cardiac Hypertrophy

Prolonged cardiac hypertrophy is a common precursor to heart failure, while cardiomyocyte hypertrophy is also a prominent feature of adverse LV remodeling following MI. Cardiac hypertrophy occurs in response to diverse stimuli, including mechanical stretch and neurohormones, which subsequently trigger various downstream signaling pathways such as the protein kinases C (PKCs), mitogen activated protein kinases (MAPKs), protein kinase B or Akt, calcineurin, and the transcription factors AP-1 and NF-κB.

Extensive experimental studies support a role of oxidant signaling in the development of cardiac hypertrophy. Interestingly, recent studies suggest that NADPH oxidase-derived ROS are important in this regard. For example, the induction of cardiomyocyte hypertrophy by short-term infusion of angiotensin II in vivo has been shown to involve the activation of Nox2 NADPH oxidase, with mice deficient in Nox2 demonstrating substantially reduced angiotensin II–induced cardiac hypertrophy and interstitial fibrosis compared with wild-type animals.[9]

Clinical Utility of Antioxidants?

Despite the wealth of experimental data and the theoretical arguments regarding the involvement of increased oxidative stress in the pathogenesis of heart failure, the therapeutic potential of free radical–directed drugs has not yet been realized. Clinical trials of antioxidant therapy have been less than compelling. For example, recombinant human SOD failed to improve recovery of ventricular function in patients undergoing thrombolysis for anterior wall acute myocardial infarction. The heart outcomes prevention evaluation (HOPE) investigators found no protective effect of vitamin E in reducing death or cardiovascular events in at-risk patients over a 4.5-year period. However, several issues are worth noting with regard to the clinical potential of antioxidant therapies: (1) Many antioxidants that have been studied to date (e.g., vitamin E) are essentially scavengers of already-formed intracellular oxidants and therefore may be considered to be "symptomatic" rather than causal treatments. (2) The levels of relevant tissue oxidative stress in most patients included in clinical trials have been unquantified while the dosages of antioxidants have been arbitrary. (3) The relationship between ROS and heart failure is probably too complex to be addressed by a single nonspecific intervention. Interestingly, however, many current therapies that are effective in heart failure (such as angiotensin-converting enzyme inhibitors, angiotensin receptor antagonists, beta-blockers, and statins) have in common the property that they are all "antioxidant" in some way. These findings provide an opportunity to reconsider the therapeutic potential of antioxidant agents in patients with heart failure, perhaps by targeting specific sources of ROS generation rather than relatively blunt nonspecific approaches.[10]

Acknowledgment. The authors' work is supported by the British Heart Foundation (BHF). A.M.S holds the BHF Chair of Cardiology.

References

1. Giordano FJ. Oxygen, oxidative stress, hypoxia, and heart failure. J Clin Invest 2005;115:500–8.
2. Lenaz G. Role of mitochondria in oxidative stress and ageing. Biochim Biophys Acta 1998;1366: 53–67.
3. Meneshian A, Bulkley GB. The physiology of endothelial xanthine oxidase: from urate catabolism to reperfusion injury to inflammatory signal transduction. Microcirculation 2002;9:161–75.
4. Lambeth JD. Nox Enzymes and the biology of reactive oxygen. Nat Rev Immunol 2004;4:181–89.
5. Heymes C, Bendall JK, Ratajczak P, et al. Increased myocardial NADPH oxidase activity in human heart failure. J Am Coll Cardiol 2003;41:2164–71.
6. Lefer DJ, Granger DN. Oxidative stress and cardiac disease. Am J Med 2000;109:315–23.
7. Hayden MR, Tyagi SC. Myocardial redox stress and remodeling in metabolic syndrome, type 2 diabetes mellitus, and congestive heart failure. Med Sci Monit 2003;9:SR35–SR52.
8. Zhang X, Li SY, Brown RA, Ren J. Ethanol and acetaldehyde in alcoholic cardiomyopathy: from bad to ugly en route to oxidative stress. Alcohol 2004;32:175–86.
9. Bendall JK, Cave AC, Heymes C, Gall N, Shah AM. Pivotal role of a gp91(phox)-containing NADPH oxidase in angiotensin II-induced cardiac hypertrophy in mice. Circulation 2002;105:293–96.
10. Ceriello A, Motz E. Is oxidative stress the pathogenic mechanism underlying insulin resistance, diabetes, and cardiovascular disease? The common soil hypothesis revisited. Arterioscler Thromb Vasc Biol 2004;24:816–23.

13 Mitochondrion: Key Factors in Acute Heart Failure

Christophe Rabuel

Mitochondria are largely abundant in the myocardium, not only because they provide the large part of energy in an organ that consumes a lot of adenosine triphosphate (ATP) for its mechanical activity and its cellular processes, but also because mitochondria play a potent role in cardiac homeostasis. Acute heart failure (AHF), defined as a reversible incapacity of the myocardium to provide a sufficient output for cellular metabolism of all the organs, is very common. Mechanisms leading to AHF have been largely investigated. Because the mitochondrial functional state is able to modulate force development and then pump function [1], impairment in cardiac contractile functions, as seen in AHF, may be the consequence of alterations in mitochondria function and metabolism. The role of mitochondria in AHF has been largely studied after ischemia-reperfusion injury and in septic shock. Besides these two situations, evidence of the role of mitochondria in AHF comes also from carbon monoxide (CO) poisoning where swollen mitochondria with rupture of mitochondrial cristae were described [2]. This chapter provides evidence of the involvement of mitochondria in AHF and describes abnormalities that can be used as targets for the development of new therapeutics for AHF.

Physiologic Roles of Mitochondria (Fig. 13.1)

Heart muscle is a highly oxidative tissue that produces more than 90% of its energy from mitochondrial respiration. Mitochondria occupy over 30% of cardiomyocyte space and are well organized under the sarcolemma space and in rows between myofilaments such that a constant diffusion distance exists between mitochondria and the core of myofilaments. Energy production is a major role for mitochondria. Mitochondria energy production depends on genetic factors that modulate normal mitochondria function, including enzyme activity and cofactor availability, and environmental factors, including the availability of fuels (e.g., sugars, fats, and proteins) and oxygen. Fatty acids are the primary energy substrate for heart muscle ATP generation by the mitochondrial respiratory chain. The supply of ATP from other sources, for example glycolytic metabolism, is limited in normal cardiac tissue. Fatty acid β-oxidation and the oxidation of carbohydrates through the Krebs cycle generate the majority of intramitochondrial reduced nicotinamide adenine dinucleotide (NADH) and reduced flavin adenine dinucleotide (FADH), which are the direct source of electrons for the electron transport chain. Electrons derived from intermediary metabolism are channeled to oxygen through the respiratory chain (complex I to IV) in a process coupled to H^+ ejection on the redox H^+ pumps. H^+ ejection results in the establishment of an electrochemical gradient ($\Delta\mu H$). $\Delta\mu H$ is utilized for ATP synthesis via the F0F1 adenosine triphosphatase (ATPase or complex V).

Under particular circumstances such as ischemia-reperfusion, energized mitochondria may undergo a sudden permeability increase of the inner membrane to solutes of molecular mass up to 1500 Da. This loss of $\Delta\varphi_m$, also called mitochon-

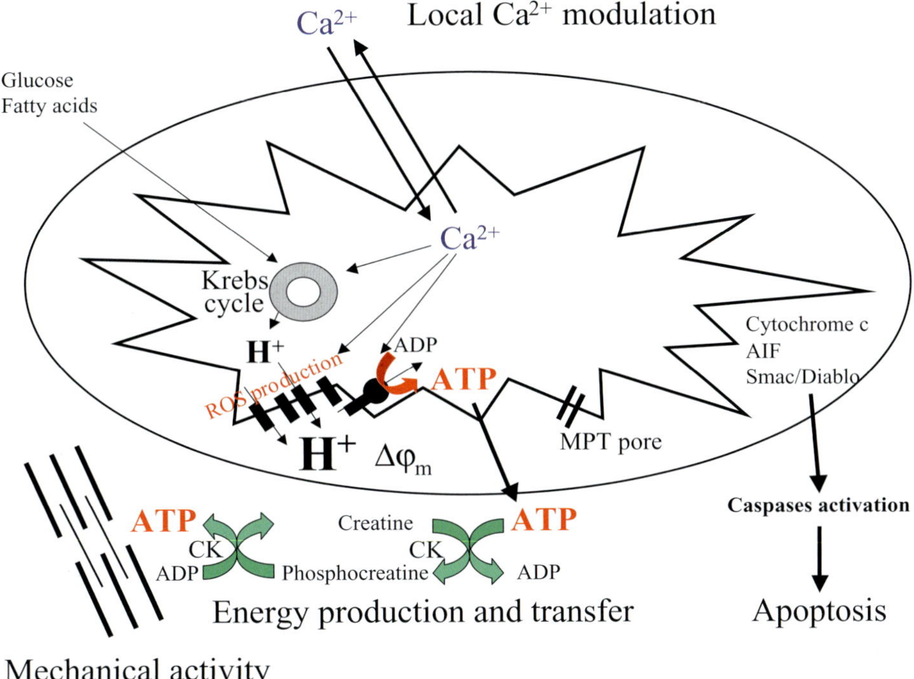

FIGURE 13.1. Roles of mitochondria in the cardiomyocyte. Mitochondria are largely involved in adenosine triphosphate (ATP) production by oxidative phosphorylation, providing energy for contractile and metabolic activities, reactive oxygen species (ROS) production linked to electron transfer throughout the respiratory chain, local calcium modulation by buffering locally, and temporally cytosolic calcium and apoptosis by releasing proapoptotic factors such as cytochrome c, AIF, Smac/Diablo. ADP, adenosine diphosphate; CK, creatine kinase; MPT, mitochondrial permeability transition.

drial permeability transition (MPT), is mediated by opening of a specific, nonselective high-conductance megachannel, the MTP pore. The only primary consequence of MTP pore opening is mitochondrial depolarization, followed by equilibration of the electrochemical gradients of ions and of solutes. Swelling results from solute and water flux to the matrix and can lead to outer membrane rupture.

Calcium metabolism is also largely influenced by mitochondria. Mitochondria are able to buffer cytosolic calcium, modulating locally and temporally the calcium level. Mitochondria calcium increases with an increase in cytosolic calcium. This close relationship between cytosolic and mitochondrial calcium concentration suggests that calcium may be responsible for the close coupling between aerobic metabolism and cardiac work. An increase in mitochondria calcium level activates the major mitochondrial dehydrogenases (pyruvate dehydrogenase, isocitrate dehydrogenase and α-ketoglutarate dehydrogenase [3]), F0-F1 ATP synthase [4], and electron transport, stimulating ATP production. Moreover, calcium is believed to be one of the major inductor of MPT [5]. However, these results were obtained mostly in isolated mitochondria and were not confirmed in isolated cardiomyocytes [6].

Reactive oxygen species (ROS) are mainly produced by mitochondria during the process of ATP generation. Reactive oxygen species have either unpaired electrons (i.e., $O_2\cdot$, $OH\cdot$) or the ability to attract electrons from other molecules (i.e., H_2O_2). Antioxidant systems, such as superoxide dismutase (SOD), catalase, and glutathione peroxidase, and endogenous antioxidants, such as vitamin E, ascorbic acid, and cysteine, have been developed to scavenge and detoxify these unwanted and toxic oxygen species.

The intrinsic pathway of apoptosis involves mitochondria and is characterized by the permeabilization of the outer mitochondrial membrane and the release of several proapoptotic factors from the intermembrane space into the cytosol. These include mainly cytochrome c, Smac/Diablo, and apoptosis inducing factor (AIF). Once released, these factors activate the caspases cascade and then initiate cell death.

Proofs of Mitochondria Involvement in Acute Heart Failure

Energetics Failure

In acute heart failure (AHF), as in chronic heart failure [7], the myocardial contents of high-energy phosphates (HEPs)—mainly of a creatine phosphate (CP) and to a much lesser extent of ATP—are reduced [8] and responsible for myocardial failure [9, 10]. Similarly, in the "stunned" myocardium, a form of reversible acute heart failure after ischemia-reperfusion, the ATP levels are depressed and recover slowly [11]. It has been suggested that this postischemic dysfunction might result from an inability of the myocardium to resynthesize enough HEPs to sustain contractile function [12]. However, this hypothesis has been challenged by the lack of correlation between myocardial ATP levels and the recovery of contractility, the normal or supranormal (CP overshoot) content in CP in the myocardium, the failure of increase in ATP levels in the stunned myocardium to restore myocardial function, and the response of stunned myocardium to inotropic stimuli without an abnormal decrease in ATP and CP stores [13].

Similarly, in sepsis-induced cardiac failure, ATP, creatinine phosphate (CrP), and glycogen levels are reduced.

A decrease in energy level is due to a decrease in energy production induced by alteration in mitochondria function. Indeed, immediate postmortem ultrastructural analysis of patients heart revealed mitochondrial swelling and degeneration of mitochondrial membranes [14]. This mitochondria depression has a prognostic value. It has been reported that sepsis nonsurvivors can be distinguished from control and sepsis survivors by lower concentrations of ATP [15]. Moreover, mitochondrial injury is positively correlated with indices of heart failure severity such as plasma norepinephrine, left ventricular (LV) end-diastolic pressure, and ejection fraction [16].

Several mechanisms of mitochondrial injury explaining this decrease in HEP levels have been described. A decrease in ATP production may be explained by a decrease in the activity of complexes of the respiratory chain or Krebs cycle enzymes. Activity of complex I + III, complex II + III, complex I, and complex IV is reduced in septic heart [15]. Limited exposure to nitric oxide (NO) produced by inducible NO synthase is capable of reversibly inhibiting complex IV (in competition with O_2), whereas prolonged exposures to NO can irreversibly inhibit complex I activity, presumably due to nitrosylation of thiols [17]. Peroxynitrite, produced by the combination of NO with superoxide anion, causes nitration of tyrosine residues, which can impair proteins activity. Peroxynitrite and the increased ROS can therefore decrease activities of pyruvate dehydrogenase [18], complex I + III, complex II + III, and glycolytic enzymes [19]. Peroxynitrite can also modify cellular energy production by activating poly–adenosine diphosphate (ADP) ribosyl polymerase (PARP) pathway. The PARP pathway further reduces the utilization of oxygen by diverting energy substrate (NADH) to repair DNA damage.

Besides these abnormalities in ATP production, an impairment in energy transfer and utilization may also be involved. A decrease in creatine kinase (CK) activity, an alteration in the isoenzyme pattern, and decreased CK fluxes have been described. This energy signaling impairment is responsible for altered energy fluxes and lower phosphocreatine (PCr)/ATP ratio, and for the incapacity of the failing heart to adapt its energy production to energy utilization and to mobilize its contractile reserve [20, 21].

Myocardial energetic failure is also involved in diastolic dysfunction. Indeed, diastolic distensibility is influenced by myocardial energetics. Hypoxia increases isovolumic resting tension in isolated guinea pig hearts [22] and raises the diastolic pressure-volume (PV) curve in humans during balloon coronary angioplasty [23]. An increase in the cytosolic ADP content or inhibition of creatine kinase activity results in an increase in ventricular end-diastolic pressure (EDP) and delayed relaxation [24–26].

However, energetic failure as a cause of impaired contractility in acute heart failure has been challenged, especially in sepsis-induced cardiomyopathy. Tavernier et al. [27] reported that 36 hours after endotoxin intravenous injection (at a time when cardiac contractility was consistently decreased in papillary muscles), the intrinsic functional properties of myocardial mitochondria and CK isoform activities were normal. These findings suggest that depression of cardiac contractility may occur without any impairment in cellular energy generation or transport during sepsis. Similarly, CK remodeling in the failing heart may be an adaptive mechanism. By decreasing the CK shuttle, excitation-contraction coupling becomes uncoupled from mitochondrial energy production and by this means preserves ATP production for other metabolic processes necessary for the survival of critically damaged cardiomyocytes but at the expense of contractile activity [28].

Oxidant-Mediated Mitochondrial Injury and Dysfunction [29]

Altered mitochondrial function and morphology have been attributed to generation of ROS. Indeed, exposure of isolated mitochondria to free radical-generating solutions disrupted matrix- and membrane-bound enzymes, altered MPT pore and mitochondrial membrane permeability, and produced mitochondrial swelling and the oxidized form of nicotinamide adenine dinucleotide (NAD^+)/NADH leakage.

Oxidative stress occurs in mitochondria during AHF and there is an inverse correlation between the degree of oxidative stress and the recovery of hemodynamic function after cardiac surgery [30]. Oxidative stress occurs in AHF because ROS production is increased (impaired respiratory chain function) and because the scavenger systems fail. As a consequence, electrons that would normally flow through the electron transport chain generate supranormal amounts of ROS with toxic consequences on lipid membranes, including mitochondrial components, promoting further mitochondrial damage and presumably more ROS formation.

Oxidative stress has major consequences on mitochondria and cell functions, particularly on mitochondrial enzyme complexes containing iron-sulfur clusters, which become subject to oxidative deactivation and thereby reducing enzyme activity [31, 32], and on lipids, which can induce apoptosis [33, 34]. Apoptosis may be also induced by the induction of MPT by the ROS (ROS-induced ROS release) [35].

Calcium Pathway

As mitochondria provide a Ca-buffering compartment, a persistent increase in cytosolic Ca^{2+} and persistent mitochondrial Ca^{2+} accumulation lead to excessive Ca^{2+} cycling by the mitochondria and alterations in membrane potential. A high concentration of cytosolic Ca^{2+} leads to mitochondrial Ca^{2+} overload, which in turn may activate the MPT pore in certain conditions. As calcium drives enzymes activity, altered mitochondrial Ca^{2+} homeostasis may affect cellular function, including oxidative phosphorylation.

Improving the Mitochondrial Function in Acute Heart Failure: Toward a Mitochondrial Medication

Substrates

It was the merit of Taegtmeyer and Gradinak in Houston in the late 1980s to recognize the therapeutic impact of metabolic support/energetic stimulation of the heart by objective measurement of hemodynamic and clinical parameters in patients with low output failure following coronary artery bypass surgery. They assigned patients with refractory left ventricular failure after cardiopulmonary bypass for coronary artery bypass graft (CABG) surgery to a regimen consisting of intraaortic balloon counterpulsation plus either intravenous inotropic drugs (control) or inotropic drugs with glucose–insulin–potassium (GIK) infusion for the first 48 hours after surgery [36, 37]. The study showed a favorable outcome of patients with GIK-therapy with shorter duration on intraaortic balloon counterpulsation and reduced mortality.

The therapeutic benefit of the glucose–insulin infusion in myocardial infarction may be attributed to an inhibition of fatty acid metabolism with a reduction of circulating free fatty acids and metabolites which are deleterious in ischemic myocardium, by increasing myocardial oxygen requirement, by impairing calcium homeostasis, and by increasing the production of free radicals, ultimately leading to electrical instability and depression of contractility [38]. The beneficial effects of GIK infusion may also result from an improvement of impaired substrate supply in low-flow ischemia or infarction, which hinges on the fact that glucose can be metabolized anaerobically and can thereby provide glycolytic ATP in the cytosolic compartment.

Under normal aerobic conditions with a normal substrate supply, amino acid oxidation accounts for less than 5% of myocardial energy production. L-glutamate is the only amino acid that is substantially metabolized by normal myocardium. During ischemia and reperfusion, glutamate and aspartate may become preferred fuels. In ischemic and stunned animal myocardium, several studies have shown beneficial effects of a high-dose glutamate infusion [39, 40]. Glutamate-enriched or α-ketoglutarate–enriched cardioplegic solutions resulted in moderately improved hemodynamics in patients undergoing coronary bypass surgery, and a combination of glutamate and GIK was successful in treatment of postoperative low-output failure or cardiogenic shock after CABG [41–43]. It has been postulated that amino acid supplementation was successful by activating the malate–aspartate shuttle, which induces the translocation of reducing equivalents (NADH) from the cytoplasm into the mitochondrial matrix where they enter the respiratory chain generating ATP. Furthermore, glutamate may be transaminated to form α-ketoglutarate, which can directly enter the citric acid cycle [44].

Exogenous pyruvate may prevent postischemic or reperfusion contractile failure by providing a significant positive inotropic effect [45]. Namely, pyruvate increases stroke volume index, decreases pulmonary capillary wedge pressure, and modulates intracellular pH and cytosolic redox state [45–47] as well as antioxidative effects [48–50]. Moreover, pyruvate increases flux through the Krebs cycle, supplementing oxidative phosphorylation by entering the Krebs cycle as a substrate following decarboxylation by pyruvate dehydrogenase. Lactic acid also should be considered an important substrate for oxidative metabolism in the setting of shock [51]. Stimulation of lactate and glucose oxidation in the experimental settings of ischemia and reperfusion [52], hemorrhagic shock [53], and septic shock [54] improves cardiac metabolic efficiency and contractile function. It could become a new approach to improve cardiac function.

Drugs Able to Preserve the Mitochondrial Energy Production

Carvedilol is a beta-blocker that has been used in patients with left ventricular dysfunction after an acute myocardial infarction (Carvedilol Port Infarct Survival Control in Left Ventricular Dysfunction–CAPRICORN-study). In this study, patients treated with carvedilol showed a significant decrease in total mortality, cardiovascular mortality, and nonfatal reinfarction [55]. These beneficial effects of carvedilol may be explained by its ability to improve energy production during acute myocardial ischemia. Indeed, carvedilol generates greater energy reserve by enhancing mitochondrial phosphorylation (greater and faster generation of ATP) as soon as oxygen became available after ischemia. Mechanisms by which carvedilol preserves mitochondrial functions are not clearly understood, but some hypotheses have been reported. Carvedilol may act as an antioxidant, suppressing the oxidative damage to mitochondria and inhibiting lipid peroxidation. It may also inhibit the cardiac exogenous NADH dehydrogenase and behave as an uncoupler of mitochondrial respiration, decreasing the ROS production.

In chronic heart failure, inhibitors of fatty acid oxidation, such as trimetazidine (TMZ) [56], increase glucose oxidation and production of ATP and then enhance cardiac mechanical function [57]. Trimetazidine may also decrease the fatty acid–induced uncoupling of respiration, which could be in part implicated in contractile impairment.

Calcium and Potassium Metabolism

Mitochondrial calcium overload is well established as a cause of mitochondrial damage. Despite a plethora of bench studies showing that calcium channel blockers reduce cellular and mitochondrial calcium overload, the clinical application of these agents to reduce reperfusion injury and myocardial infarction has been disappointing.

Nicorandil is able to decrease the size of infarction. It attenuates the ouabain-induced Ca^{2+} overload and this protective effect is abolished by both 5 hydroxy decanoate acid and glibenclamide, suggesting that nicorandil activates the mitochondrial ATP-sensitive K^+ channel that plays an essential role in ischemic cardioprotection [58].

Cardioprotective strategies such as preconditioning are able to decrease the infarct size and to attenuate the postischemic contractile failure. Ischemic preconditioning or pharmacologic preconditioning inhibit MPT pore opening and then cardiomyocyte apoptosis. Two different pathways are involved in cardioprotection signaling: the memory-associated signaling or "preconditioning," and the memory-lacking signaling. The memory-associated pathway involves mitochondria. Drugs that enhance mitochondria potassium influx directly, such as diazoxide, or indirectly, are protective because they increase the mitochondrial potassium influx, which induces mitochondria swelling and then activation of respiration, ROS production, protein kinase C activation, glycogen synthetase kinase 3β inhibition, and finally inhibition of the MPT pore opening, which provides protection [6]. Preconditioning preserves mitochondrial function by diminishing the oxidation of both mitochondrial and cytosolic proteins, leading to diminished damage [59].

Reactive Oxygen Species

Because MPT is promoted by the presence of oxygen radicals formed during oxidative stress, it is clear that antioxidants might be useful to prevent the progression of mitochondrial injury. However, it remains to be determined if this targeted approach of providing antioxidants to mitochondria would provide significant protection in clinical settings.

Poly(ADP-Ribose) Synthetase Inhibition

Inhibitors of poly(ADP-ribose) synthetase (PARS) prevent the depletion of NADH and preserve cellular energy metabolism [60, 61] and reduce apoptotic cell death [62]. Inhibitors of PARS activity have been shown to be efficacious in models of ischemia and reperfusion of heart [63].

Apoptosis Regulators

As apoptosis may be considered a mechanism involved in acute heart failure, inhibition of apoptosis could provide an interesting therapeutic target. It has been shown that inhibition of caspase-3 reduces cardiac dysfunction in animal models of sepsis [64, 65]. Cyclosporine, which prevents MPT and release of cytochrome c, prevents the mitochondrial pathway for apoptosis, reduces cardiac injury from ischemia and reperfusion, and dramatically extends the window of organ preservation with full recovery of cardiac function for heart transplantation [66].

Protection Afforded by Heat Shock Proteins

Heat shock treatment reduces the degree of the downregulation of the mitochondrial respiratory chain enzyme activities observed during sepsis. As a result, the ATP content is preserved and the severity of mitochondrial deformity is alleviated. Moreover, ultrastructure deformity of mitochondria induced by sepsis is attenuated by heat shock response. Grp75, one of the heat shock proteins (HSPs) in mitochondria, may contribute to the maintenance of mitochondrial function during sepsis [67]. Attenuation of oxidative stress may explain the protective effects induced by HSPs. They may play the vital role of a free radical scavenger [68] and increase the expression or the activity of endogenous scavengers of ROS such as catalase or superoxide dismutase, thus protecting mitochondrial respiratory ability [69, 70].

The HSPs also modulate the apoptosis cascade. By inhibiting the proteolytic maturation or activity of caspases and the cleavage of their target substrates [71, 72], they are able to suppress the engagement of apoptosis. They can also regulate the release of proapoptotic factors from mitochondria [72]. Hsp27 is known to suppress Bid translocation to the mitochondria and inhibit cytochrome c release [73], and Hsp70 can inhibit the formation of a functionally competent apoptosome [74].

Conclusion

Mitochondria are largely involved in the pathogenesis of acute heart failure, and these small intracytosolic structures not only provide fuel for the entire cell, permitting cardiac contraction and relaxation or enzymatic reactions, but also control cell survival or calcium metabolism, which are critical for cardiomyocytes. Carvedilol provides strong evidence that drugs targeting mitochondria may improve their function, opening a new field, the mitochondrial medicine. Mechanisms described in this chapter are the most widely recognized, but some others exist. Particularly, it has been reported that an autoantibody against adenosine nucleotide transferase (a key enzyme controlling ATP transfer) leads to AHF in viral myocarditis [75]. Better understanding of the physiologic role of mitochondria and their defects in pathologic states is necessary to develop new therapeutics. For example, in most of the cases, β-adrenergic agonists such as dobutamine are used as a treatment in AHF. These agents increase mitochondria metabolism at a moment where mitochondria energetic fails and therefore use of these agents may not be adequate. Therefore, new alternative therapeutics that do not impair mitochondria function that is already compromised have been developed or are still under investigation. New approaches based on apoptosis regulation, ROS scavenging, or modulation of HSPs may constitute alternative treatment of AHF in the near future.

References

1. Kaasik A, Joubert F, Ventura-Clapier R, et al. A novel mechanism of regulation of cardiac contractility by mitochondrial functional state. FASEB J 2004;18:1219–27.
2. Tritapepe L, Macchiarelli G, Rocco M, et al. Functional and ultrastructural evidence of myocardial stunning after acute carbon monoxide poisoning. Crit Care Med 1998;26:797–801.
3. McCormack JG, Halestrap AP, Denton RM. Role of calcium ions in regulation of mammalian intramitochondrial metabolism. Physiol Rev 1990;70:391–425.
4. Territo PR, French SA, Dunleavy MC, et al. Calcium activation of heart mitochondrial oxidative phosphorylation: rapid kinetics of mVO2, NADH, AND light scattering. J Biol Chem 2001;276:2586–99.
5. Bernardi P. Mitochondrial transport of cations: channels, exchangers, and permeability transition. Physiol Rev 1999;79:1127–55.
6. Juhaszova M, Zorov DB, Kim SH, et al. Glycogen synthase kinase-3beta mediates convergence of protection signaling to inhibit the mitochondrial permeability transition pore. J Clin Invest 2004; 113:1535–49.
7. Starling RC, Hammer DF, Altschuld RA. Human myocardial ATP content and in vivo contractile function. Mol Cell Biochem 1998;180:171–7.
8. Kübler W, Mäurer W, Dietz R, et al. Metabolic aspects of compensatory mechanisms in cardiac failure. In: Gross F, ed. Modulation of Sympathetic Tone in the Treatment of Cardiovascular Disease. Hans Huber Publishers, Bern, Vienna, Stuttgart, 1979:197–77.
9. Beer M, Seyfarth T, Sandstede J, et al. Absolute concentrations of high-energy phosphate metabolites in normal, hypertrophied, and failing human myocardium measured noninvasively with (31)P-SLOOP magnetic resonance spectroscopy. J Am Coll Cardiol 2002;40:1267–1274.
10. Kapelo V, Kuproyanov V, Novikova N, et al. The cardiac contractile failure induced by chronic creatine and phosphocreatine deficiency. J Mol Cell Cardiol 1988;20:465–79.
11. Ellis S, Henschke C, Sandor T, et al. Time course of functional and biochemical recovery of myocardium salvaged by reperfusion. J Am Coll Cardiol 1983;1:1047–55.
12. Reimer K, Hill M, Jennings R. Prolonged depletion of ATP and of the adenine nucleotide pool due to delayed resynthesis of adenine nucleotide following reversible myocardial ischemic injury in dogs. J Mol Cell Cardiol 1981;13:229–39.
13. Vogt AM, Kubler W. Heart failure: is there an energy deficit contributing to contractile dysfunction? Basic Res Cardiol 1998;93:1–10.
14. Cowley RA, Mergner WJ, Fisher RS, et al. The subcellular pathology of shock in trauma patients: studies using the immediate autopsy. Am Surg 1979;45:255–69.
15. Brealey D, Brand M, Hargreaves I, et al. Association between mitochondrial dysfunction and severity and outcome of septic shock. Lancet 2002;360: 219–23.
16. Sabbah HN, Sharov V, Riddle JM, et al. Mitochondrial abnormalities in myocardium of dogs with chronic heart failure. J Mol Cell Cardiol 1992;24: 1333–47.

17. Richter C, Gogvadze V, Laffranchi R, et al. Oxidants in mitochondria: from physiology to disease. Biochim Biophys Acta 1995;1271:67–74.
18. Zell R, Geck P, Werdan K, et al. TNF-alpha and IL-1 alpha inhibit both pyruvate dehydrogenase activity and mitochondrial function in cardiomyocytes: evidence for primary impairment of mitochondrial function. Mol Cell Biochem 1997;177:61–7.
19. Gellerich FN, Trumbeckaite S, Hertel K, et al. Impaired energy metabolism in hearts of septic baboons: diminished activities of complex I and complex II of the mitochondrial respiratory chain. Shock 1999;11:336–41.
20. Ingwall JS. Is cardiac failure a consequence of decreased energy reserved? Circulation 1993;67: VII58–VII62.
21. Liao RL, Nascinben L, Friedrich J, et al. Decreased energy reserve in animal model of dilated cardiomyopathy-relationship to contractile performance. Circ Res 1996;78:893–902.
22. Nayler WG, Yepez CE, Poole-Wilson PA. The effect of beta-adrenoceptor and Ca2+ antagonist drugs on the hypoxia-induced increased in resting tension. Cardiovasc Res 1978;12:666–74.
23. De Bruyne B, Bronzwaer JG, Heyndrickx GR, et al. Comparative effects of ischemia and hypoxemia on left ventricular systolic and diastolic function in humans. Circulation 1993;88:461–71.
24. Tian R, Christe ME, Spindler M, et al. Role of MgADP in the development of diastolic dysfunction in the intact beating rat heart. J Clin Invest 1997;99:745–51.
25. Tian R, Nascimben L, Ingwall JS, et al. Failure to maintain a low ADP concentration impairs diastolic function in hypertrophied rat hearts. Circulation 1997;96:1313–19.
26. Tian R, Christie ME, Spindler M, et al. Role of MgADP in the development of diastolic dysfunction in the intact beating heart. J Clin Invest 1997;99:745–51.
27. Tavernier B, Mebazaa A, Mateo P, et al. Phosphorylation-dependent alteration in myofilament Ca2+ sensitivity but normal mitochondrial function in septic heart. Am J Respir Crit Care Med 2001;163: 362–7.
28. Ventura-Clapier R, Kuznetsov A, Veksler V, et al. Functional coupling of creatine kinases in muscles: species and tissue specificity. Mol Cell Biochem 1998;184:231–47.
29. Giordano FJ. Oxygen, oxidative stress, hypoxia, and heart failure. J Clin Invest 2005;115:500–8.
30. Ferrari R, Alfieri O, Curello S, et al. Occurrence of oxidative stress during reperfusion of the human heart. Circulation 1990;81:201–11.
31. Melov S, Coskun P, Patel M, et al. Mitochondrial disease in superoxide dismutase 2 mutant mice. Proc Natl Acad Sci USA 1999;96:846–51.
32. Szabo C, O'Connor M, Salzman AL: Endogenously produced peroxynitrite induces the oxidation of mitochondrial and nuclear proteins in immunostimulated macrophages. FEBS Lett 1997 409:147–50.
33. Kroener G, Petit P, Zamzami N, et al. The biochemistry of programmed cell death. FASEB J 1995;9: 1277–87.
34. Buttke TM, Sandstrom PA. Oxidative stress as a mediator of apoptosis. Immunology Today 1994;15: 7–10.
35. Zorov DB, Filburn CR, Klotz LO, et al. Reactive oxygen species (ROS)-induced ROS release: a new phenomenon accompanying induction of the mitochondrial permeability transition in cardiac myocytes. J Exp Med 2000;192:1001–14.
36. Gradinak S, Coleman GM, Taegtmeyer H, et al. Improved cardiac function with glucose-insulin-potassium after coronary bypass surgery. Ann Thorac Surg 1989;48:484–9.
37. Taegtmeyer H. Metabolic support for the postischemic heart. Lancet 1995;345:1552–5.
38. Oliver MF, Opie LH. Effects of glucose and fatty acids on myocardial ischemia and arrhythmias. Lancet 1994;343:155–8.
39. Rau EE, Shine KI, Gervais A, et al. Enhanced mechanical recovery of anoxic and ischemic myocardium by amino acid perfusion. Am J Physiol 1979;236: H873–9.
40. Pisarenko OI, Solomatina ES, Studneva JM, et al. Protective effect of glutamic acid on cardiac function and metabolism during cardioplegia and reperfusion. Basic Res Cardiol 1983;78:534–43.
41. Kjellman U, Bjork K, Ekroth R. Alpha-ketoglutarate for myocardial protection in heart surgery. Lancet 1995;345:552–3.
42. Svedjeholm R, Huljebrant I, Hakanson E, et al. Glutamate and high-dose glucose–insulin–potassium in the treatment of severe cardiac failure after cardiac operations. Ann Thorac Surg 1995;59: 523–30.
43. Beyersdorf F, Kirsh M, Buckberg GD, et al. Warm glutamate/aspartate-enriched blood cardioplegic solution for perioperative sudden death. J Thorac Cardiovasc Surg 1992;104:1141–7.
44. Pisarenko OI, Solomatina ES, Ivanov VE, et al. On the mechanism of enhanced ATP formation in hypoxic myocardium caused by glutamic acid. Basic Res Cardiol 1985;80:126–34.
45. Bünger R, Mallet RT, Hartman DA. Pyruvate-enhanced phosphorylation potential and

inotropism in normoxic and postischemic isolated working heart. Eur J Biochem 1988;180:221–33.

46. Scholz TD, Laughlin MR, Balaban RS, et al. Effect of substrate on mitochondrial NADH, cytosolic redox state, and phosphorylated compounds in isolated hearts. Am J Physiol 1995;268:H82–91.
47. Laughlin MR, Heineman FW. The relationship between phosphorylation potential and redox state in the isolated working rat heart. J Mol Cell Cardiol 1994;26:1525–31.
48. Deboer LWV, Bekx PA, Han L, et al. Pyruvate enhances recovery of rat hearts after ischemia and reperfusion by preventing free radical generation. Am J Physiol (Heart Circ Physiol) 1993;265: H1571–6.
49. Bassenge E, Sommer O, Schwemmer M, et al. Antioxidant pyruvate inhibits cardiac formation of reactive oxygen species through changes in redox state. Am J Physiol (Heart Circ Physiol) 2000;279: H2431–8.
50. Tejero-Taldo MI, Caffrey JL, Sun J, Mallet RT. Antioxidant properties of pyruvate mediate its potentiation of β-adrenergic inotropism in stunned myocardium. J Mol Cell Cardiol 1999;31: 1863–72.
51. Rivers E, Nguyen B, Havstad S, et al. Early goal-directed therapy in the treatment of severe sepsis and septic shock. N Engl J Med 2001; 345:1368–77.
52. Taniguchi M, Wilson C, Hunter CA, et al. Dichloroacetate improves cardiac efficiency after ischemia independent of changes in mitochondrial proton leak. Am J Phys Heart Circ Phys 2001;280: H1762–9.
53. Kline JA, Maiorano PC, Schroeder JD, et al. Activation of pyruvate dehydrogenase improves heart function and metabolism after hemorrhagic shock. J Mol Cell Cardiol 1997;29:2465–74.
54. Burns AH, Summer WR, Burns LA, et al. Inotropic interactions of dichloroacetate with amrinone and ouabain in isolated hearts from endotoxin-shocked rats. J Cardiovasc Pharmacol 1988;11:379–86.
55. Dargie HJ. Effect of carvedilol on outcome after myocardial infarction in patients with left-ventricular dysfunction: the CAPRICORN randomized trial. Lancet 2001;357:1385–90.
56. Lopaschuk GD, Barr R, Thomas PD, et al. Beneficial effects of trimetazidine in ex vivo working ischemic hearts are due to a stimulation of glucose oxidation secondary to inhibition of long-chain 3-ketoacyl coenzyme a thiolase. Circ Res 2003;93:e33–7.
57. Chandler MP, Stanley WC, Morita H, et al. Short-term treatment with ranolazine improves mechanical efficiency in dogs with chronic heart failure. Circ Res 2002;91:278–80.
58. Garlid KD, Dos Santos P, Xie ZJ, et al. Mitochondrial potassium transport: the role of the mitochondrial ATP-sensitive K(+) channel in cardiac function and cardioprotection. Biochim Biophys Acta 2003;1606:1–21.
59. Khaliulin I, Schwalb H, Wang P, et al. Preconditioning improves postischemic mitochondrial function and diminishes oxidation of mitochondrial proteins. Free Radic Biol Med 2004;37:1–9.
60. Szabo C, Dawson VL. Role of poly(ADP-ribose) synthetase in inflammation and ischaemia-reperfusion. Trends Pharmacol Sci 1998;19:287–98.
61. Virag L, Szabo C. The therapeutic potential of poly(ADPribose) polymerase inhibitors. Pharmacol Rev 2002;54:375–429.
62. Virag L, Marmer DJ, Szabo C. Crucial role of apopain in the peroxynitrite-induced apoptotic DNA fragmentation. Free Radic Biol Med 1998; 25:1075–82.
63. Zingarelli B, Cuzzocrea S, Zsengeller Z, et al. Protection against myocardial ischemia and reperfusion injury by 3-aminobenzamide, an inhibitor of poly (ADP-ribose) synthetase. Cardiovasc Res 1997;36:205–15.
64. Nevière R, Fauvel H, Chopin C, et al. Caspase inhibition prevents cardiac dysfunction and heart apoptosis in a rat model of sepsis. Am J Respir Crit Care Med 2001;163:218–25.
65. Fauvel H, Marchetti P, Chopin C, et al. Differential effects of caspase inhibitors on endotoxin-induced myocardial dysfunction and heart apoptosis. Am J Physiol Heart Circ Physiol 2001;280:H1608–14.
66. Masters TN, Fokin AA, Schaper J, et al. Extending myocardial preservation with cyclosporin A treatment. J Heart Lung Transplant 2001;20:182.
67. Hsiang-Wen Chen, Chin Hsu, Tzong-Shi Lu, et al. Heat shock pretreatment prevents cardiac mitochondrial dysfunction during sepsis. Shock 2003; 20:274–9.
68. Jacquier-Sarlin MR, Fuller K, Dinh-Xuan A, et al. Protective effects of Hsp70 in inflammation. Experientia 1994;50:1031–8.
69. Bornman L, Steinmann CM, Gericke GS, et al. In vivo heat shock protects rat myocardial mitochondria. Biochem Biophys Res Commun 1998;246: 836–40.
70. Polla BS, Stubbe H, Kantengwa S, et al. Differential induction of stress proteins and functional effects of heat shock in human phagocytes. Inflammation 1995;19:363–78.
71. Garrido C, Bruey JM, Fromentin, A, et al. HSP27 inhibits cytochrome c-dependent activation of procaspase-9. FASEB J 1999;13:2061–70.

72. Mosser DD, Caron AW, Bourget L, et al. The chaperone function of Hsp70 is required for protection against stress-induced apoptosis. Mol Cell Biol 2000;20:7146–59.
73. Gabai VL, Mabuchi K, Mosser DD et al. Hsp72 and stress kinase c-jun N-terminal kinase regulate the bid-dependent pathway in tumor necrosis factor-induced apoptosis. Mol Cell Biol 2002;22:3415–24.
74. Beere HM, Wolf BB, Cain K, et al. Heat-shock protein 70 inhibits apoptosis by preventing recruitment of procaspase-9 to the apaf-1 apoptosome. Nat Cell Biol 2000;2:469–75.
75. Schulze K, Witzenbichler B, Christmann C, et al. Disturbance of myocardial energy metabolism in experimental virus myocarditis by antibodies against the adenine nucleotide translocator. Cardiovasc Res 1999;44:91–100.

14
Immune System Alterations in Acute Heart Failure

Kirkwood F. Adams, Jr., and Tien M.H. Ng

Acute heart failure has emerged as a major public health problem, with over 1 million hospitalizations annually, but debate continues concerning the pathophysiology of this syndrome. Whether there are unique and important mechanisms that mediate decompensation distinct from those operative in chronic heart failure or whether mechanisms in common to both play a more prominent role in acute heart failure remains to be determined. Maladaptive regulatory responses have been recognized as critical in the development and progression of acute and chronic heart failure, especially upregulation of a number of key neurohormonal systems. Relevant to this review, not only has activation of many mediators of the inflammatory response cascade now been demonstrated in patients with chronic heart failure, but also recent studies indicate abnormal activation in acute heart failure. The possibility that inflammatory activation could play a unique role in the pathophysiology of acute heart failure continues to be investigated.

Experimental studies have clearly documented the deleterious effects of inflammatory activation on damaged myocardium, and association studies suggest that adverse outcomes in patients are significantly more common when inflammatory processes are upregulated. Although to date pharmacologic inhibition of immune activation in heart failure has not been documented to be of clear clinical benefit, a number of strategies for immune modulation are still in development and may yet prove effective. This chapter considers a number of aspects of the inflammatory and immune response in heart failure, with particular emphasis on recent findings in patients hospitalized for worsening heart failure.

Inflammatory and Immune System Pathophysiology

Basic Mechanisms

A general consideration of the process of wound healing and the nature of the inflammatory response is important as background to understanding the potential pathogenic role of these body defenses in heart failure (1). Although these adaptive processes are familiar from everyday experience, at first thought they seem unlikely to be related to the pathophysiology of heart failure. Certainly, the ability to recover from wounds and to ward off tissue invasion by unwanted pathogens are two key aspects of maintaining health. These two processes are key elements of the inflammatory response, a highly complex array of molecular and cellular reactions that provide for host defense and aid in the recover from physical trauma. But, despite these common benefits from the inflammatory response system, the adverse consequences resulting from activation of this cascade of normally adaptive processes are now well recognized in the form of autoimmune disease (2). The further identification of an inflammatory response in patients with heart failure, acute coronary syndromes, and myocardial infarction has raised the possibility that activation of the immune system in these settings could make a significant contribution to the pathophysiology of cardiovascular disease as well (1–3).

Inflammatory Response in Cardiovascular Disease

Physically detectable hallmarks of the inflammatory process, like fever, have long been recognized as components of acute myocardial infarction and recently heart failure. But the molecular and cellular processes underlying such signs have remained obscure until relatively recently. The discovery that heart failure, particularly, but not only when severe, is often characterized elevation of the cytokine tumor necrosis factor-α (TNF-α), initiated a period of intense investigation that has demonstrated a wide array of immune abnormalities are present in this syndrome (4). Presently, alterations in a number of components of the inflammatory system have been described in detail. In the humoral domain these include upregulation of the protein families of chemokines and cytokines, and in the cellular domain activation of monocytes, lymphocytes, and macrophages (5). This chapter focuses mainly on the role of inflammatory molecules and the emerging data on the relationship of cellular immune response to the pathophysiology of heart failure.

Contrasts and Similarities in Cardiovascular Regulatory Systems

The important contrasts among the origin, interrelationships, nature of the activation of the humoral inflammatory response, and key neuroendocrine system have been elucidated well by Mann (6). Evidence has accumulated that many if not all nucleated cell types have the capacity to synthesize the protein constituents of the humoral response, creating a generalized relationship of many cells to one inflammatory mediator. This generality contrasts with the typical pattern of specific cell for specific hormone in neuroendocrine systems (7). The pathways to neurohormonal production tend to be linear and typically do not have significant redundancy, aspects common to the inflammatory process. In at least one critical aspect, the dysregulation is similar between the activation of inflammatory and neuroendocrine systems in heart failure. In both cases, activity of these systems is sustained, in marked contrast to the short-term increases in activity seen in healthy individuals faced with stress. Clearly, long-term upregulation of these systems may be associated with a pathologic effect on target cells whether short-term activation is beneficial or not.

Myocardial Infarction and Inflammation

As elegantly reviewed by Frangogiannis (1), acute myocardial infarction, featuring essentially all the aspects of wound healing process, represents a readily comprehensible example of the role of the inflammatory response in cardiovascular disease. The temporally and physically discrete injury created by the ischemic insult is readily identifiable as an initiator of the inflammatory and wound healing response. Indeed, all aspects of these processes appear to play a role in this form of physical injury, clearly a lot different from the traumatic damage frequently encountered by our ancestors in periods like the Ice Age.

Inflammatory Mechanisms in Heart Failure

In contrast to acute myocardial infarction, understanding the role of inflammation in chronic heart failure has proven more difficult to conceptualize. Except in the relatively rare instances where acute or chronic infection is evident (i.e., viral myocarditis) and despite a number of plausible hypotheses, the stimulus for the immune response in heart failure remains unknown (8). Clearly, recent studies have demonstrated that the presence of a classic immune stimulus, defined as an abnormally expressed protein that is immunogenic or endotoxin from gastrointestinal flora, is not essential to cause the elaboration of inflammatory molecules by cells of the immune system. Ample evidence demonstrates that all cellular elements of the myocardium may elaborate inflammatory molecules under conditions of cellular stress. What is interesting is the recognition that stress created by stimuli very different from those normally responsible for immune activation may in fact initiate the inflammatory response (9).

Classic Immune Activation

Immune activation can be due to direct antigenic stimulation in cases of acute myocarditis, which remains an uncommon cause of acute and chronic heart failure. The following sequence is proposed to explain the occurrence of abnormal inflammatory activation in patients with heart failure due to other causes. Antigenic stimulation is provoked by the changes that accompany myocardial damage due to a variety of insults. In this scheme, cardiac antigens not normally in contact with the immune system become exposed during myocardial damage from ischemia or other factors. This process is best understood in the setting of myocardial infarction, where antibodies to a variety of cardiac proteins develop including myosin, complement is activated, and a typical inflammatory response evolves. Speculation continues that pathologic hypertrophy or damage from fibrosis may trigger a similar response.

Pathogenic Mechanisms

Given that inflammatory and wound healing processes are activated in heart failure, what reasonable adverse effects could be attributed to their upregulation? The essential deleterious adaptations by the myocardium to stress and injury are few in number. The principal one, ventricular remodeling, is an example of one of these essential disease causing or aggravating processes. Potential mechanisms by which the inflammatory response might adversely alter the structure and function of the heart through maladaptive ventricular remodeling include inappropriate fibrosis, cardiomyocyte apoptosis, and pathologic cardiomyocyte hypertrophy. A number of experimental studies have demonstrated that activation of cytokines and other inflammatory molecules may be associated with pathologic ventricular remodeling involving essentially all of these potential pathways of adverse structural change (3).

Caution is necessary, however, as the pleomorphic cellular effects of cytokines and other humoral mediator of the immune response make it more difficult to predict or determine experimentally the consequences of their activation in states like heart failure and myocardial infarction. The cytokine TNF-α represents a well-documented example of a single cytokine that can have either beneficial or deleterious effects. It has two distinct receptors whose intracellular signaling effects are harmful or salutary respectively when stimulated in the setting of acute myocardial infarction. The majority of the deleterious myocardial effects of TNF-α appear to be mediated by tumor necrosis factor receptor type 1 (TNFR1) while activation of tumor necrosis factor receptor type 2 (TNFR2) may have beneficial effects on the myocardium during periods of ischemic injury (10, 11).

Neurohormones and Immune System Regulation

Renin-Angiotensin-Aldosterone System

Not surprisingly, there is significant communication between the adrenergic system and renin-angiotensin-aldosterone system (RAAS) and the immune system. Although the interaction between the sympathetic nervous system and immune system has been recognized for some time, less is known about how the RAAS and immune system interact. Accumulating evidence suggests that these two systems significantly influence the activity of each other. It has been demonstrated that angiotensin II activates nuclear factor (NF)-κB, the transcription factor responsible for upregulating numerous inflammatory mediators (12). In the isolated perfused heart and isolated cardiomyocyte myocyte studies, angiotensin II stimulation results in increased TNF-α messenger RNA (mRNA) (13, 14). This effect appears mediated through the AT-1 receptor as evidenced by lack of a similar effect under blockade by the angiotensin II receptor blocker losartan (14). In a separate study, pretreatment with quinapril attenuated the increase in mRNA of multiple proinflammatory cytokines (15). A reduction in adhesion molecule expression has also been demonstrated with either angiotensin-converting enzyme inhibition or AT-1 receptor blockade (16, 17). There is also evidence that cytokines influence activity of the renin-angiotensin system. Tumor necrosis factor-α has been shown to increase AT-1 receptor expression as well as cardiac angiotensin II concentrations in cardiac fibroblasts and in a murine model (18–20). It has been proposed that both systems potentiate each other through the common signal transduction pathways of mitogen activated protein kinases (MAPKs) and a similar response to reactive oxygen species (21).

Sympathetic Nervous System

Inflammatory cytokine expression is known to be regulated by the adrenergic nervous system. In models of sepsis, brain injury, and hemorrhage, adrenergic activation has been associated with attenuation of the inflammatory response, including decreased TNF-α and increased interleukin-10 (IL-10) expression (22–27). Binding of norepinephrine and epinephrine to adrenergic receptors is purported to decrease lipopolysaccharide (LPS)-induced TNF-α expression at the transcriptional level possibly via a cyclic adenosine monophosphate (cAMP)-dependent mechanism (22, 23, 28, 29). Several investigations have been performed to characterize these actions using pharmacologic agents. Isoproterenol, a pure β-agonist, reduced LPS-induced TNF-α gene expression in renal resident macrophages (22). Its effects were blocked by propranolol, a nonselective β-antagonist, but not by atenolol, a β_1-selective antagonist. In a murine hemorrhage model, pulmonary mononuclear cell production of TNF-α mRNA was blocked by phentolamine, an $\alpha_{1,2}$-antagonist, whereas propranolol enhanced its production (27). In lung neutrophils, LPS-induced TNF-α expression was enhanced by phenylephrine, an α_1-agonist, and reduced by phentolamine (26). These results were confirmed in other studies with cultured THP-1 monocytes, whole blood, and murine models (23, 24, 28–31). Overall, these experiments suggest that β_2-agonism produces anti–TNF-α effects, whereas α-agonism enhances TNF-α expression. Although less well characterized, catecholamines appear to increase IL-10 expression via a β_2-receptor mediated pathway (25). The antiinflammatory activity of IL-10 would be consistent with the previously described effects of adrenergic action on the immune system.

In a preliminary clinical study, a reduction in norepinephrine's ability to counterregulate inflammatory cytokine production in symptomatic heart failure was observed (32). In monocytes isolated from heart failure patients, attenuation of TNF-α production by norepinephrine was diminished compared to that seen in monocytes from healthy individuals. Augmentation of IL-10 production by norepinephrine was also reduced in heart failure patients. Diminution of the normal physiologic actions of the adrenergic nervous system in heart failure may be secondary to the general downregulation of the activity of this system in heart failure. These results require confirmation, but provide some evidence that communication between the adrenergic and immune systems may indeed be altered in heart failure, thus contributing to the overall proinflammatory state.

Humoral Inflammatory Mediators

Cytokine Activation in Acute Heart Failure

Previous work has amply demonstrated that chronic heart failure is associated with activation of a number of cytokines (33, 34). In contrast, activation of humoral elements of the inflammatory cascade in acute heart failure has only recently been described. Peschel et al. (35) demonstrated elevation of multiple cytokines including TNF-α and IL-6 in patients admitted to an intensive care unit with acute heart failure due to left ventricular dysfunction. The work of Milo et al. (36) demonstrated that cytokine activation can occur in the setting of acute heart associated with hypertension and pulmonary edema where systolic dysfunction may be present or not. These authors found that cytokine activation persisted in patients with these clinical forms of acute heart failure even 60 days after follow-up, well after most patients had been released from hospital.

C-Reactive Protein in Acute Heart Failure

There is growing evidence that multiple aspects of the inflammatory response are upregulated in acute heart failure. C-reactive protein (CRP) is an inflammatory protein synthesized in the liver that activates the complement cascade and contributes to opsonization by immune cells. Serum CRP levels have also been shown to help predict the development of heart failure in patients at risk. Increased circulating levels of CRP have been demonstrated in both acute and chronic heart failure (37–41). Despite the involvement of CRP with ischemic heart disease, there are conflicting data on whether levels differ based on heart failure etiology.

The exact role of CRP in heart failure remains to be fully defined. However, studies consistently demonstrate that elevated serum levels of CRP are independently predictive of poor clinical outcome (38, 40, 41). In the largest study to date, post-hoc analysis of the Valsartan Heart Failure Trial demonstrated approximately a 50% increase in mortality among study patients with serum CRP levels in the highest quartile (≥7.32 mg/L) versus the lowest quartile (≤1.42 mg/L) with a hazard ratio of 1.51 (95% confidence interval, 1.2–1.9) (41). A single admission CRP level was found to be predictive of progression to heart failure in acute myocardial infarction patients (42). Higher serial levels were also predictive of hypertrophy and heart failure development in patients on hemodialysis or those with cerebrovascular disease (43, 44). A potential causative role for CRP is also supported by the observation that CRP levels show a strong inversion correlation with left ventricular ejection fraction and correlated directly with left ventricular end-diastolic pressure (42, 45).

One study confirmed that levels increase in acute decompensation and decrease with symptomatic improvement (37). More recently, Mueller et al. (38) detected increased levels of CRP in patients hospitalized with acute heart failure. These investigators found that increases in CRP were associated with a significant increase in the risk of death and rehospitalization over approximately a 2-year period after discharge. This adverse association was seen after adjustment for a number of characteristics predictive of poor outcome in the study population.

The mechanism for the increased serum CRP levels in heart failure is not clear. However, IL-6, a known stimulant of CRP synthesis, is also elevated in heart failure and provides a plausible explanation. In support of this mechanism, a correlation between CRP levels and IL-6 was demonstrated in one study (37). Treatment with angiotensin-converting enzyme inhibitors, angiotensin receptor blockers, or beta-blockers has been shown to attenuate serum CRP levels in various settings (41, 46, 47). Whether a reduction in CRP from these therapies results in improved outcomes is unknown.

Potential Pathogenic Role Inflammatory Response in Acute Heart Failure

Recent findings of inflammatory activation in acute heart failure have led Felker and Cotter (48) to speculate that this systemic response may contribute to the pathophysiology of decompensation leading to hospitalization in this syndrome. Experimental studies have documented that acute administration of cytokines can induce a pathophysiologic picture typical of acute heart failure with ventricular dysfunction, increased diastolic stiffness, and pulmonary edema (49, 50). The recent demonstration in humans that vaccination with *Salmonella typhi* may be associated with acute increases in IL-6 and the induction of abnormal arterial stiffness further supports the potential role of the inflammatory response in acute heart failure (51).

Other Humoral Mediators Related to Inflammatory Response

Nitric Oxide

Nitric oxide (NO) is formed from the conversion of L-arginine via the Ca^{2+}-dependent enzyme system nitric oxide synthetase (NOS). This enzyme system consists of three isoforms: constitutively expressed endothelial-derived (eNOS), neuronal (nNOS), and inducible (iNOS) (52). Current evidence suggests that NO plays a dual role in the failing heart, with the potential to act as both a pathologic and protective factor. Excessive or reduced production of NO influences the function of many components critical to the circulation. These effects include myocardial actions (apoptosis, changes in chronotropic and inotropic response, matrix metalloproteinases, myocyte damage), vascular systems (endothelial function, platelet function), and neurohormonal systems (including the sympathetic nervous system and renin-angiotensin system). Ongoing research continues to elucidate mechanisms and consequences of NO up- and downregulation in the failing heart. The regulation of NO in heart failure is complex, and the net balance of NO up- and downregulation in a given individual depends on several factors. For example, heart failure is associated with greater expression of iNOS and this could lead to upregulation of NO production (53–57). Known sources of NO include myocytes, coronary and endocardial endothelial cells, and cardiac neuronal cells (58). As part of its metabolism, NO reacts with superoxide anion to form the free radicals peroxynitrite (ONOO–) and superoxide (O_2–). Formation of these free radicals results in increased oxidative stress and a negative feedback system that may further decrease availability of NO.

Increased NO, and subsequently peroxynitrite production, has the potential to contribute to heart failure pathophysiology via numerous mechanisms. Increased lipid peroxidation contributes to the atherosclerotic process and ischemic heart disease risk. Nitric oxide is also cardiodepressant, possibly due to inhibition of ion pumps and oxidation of contractile proteins. Evidence also demonstrates NO activates nuclear factor (NF)-κB, contributing to increased inflammatory responses such as increased expression of adhesion molecules. Nitric oxide is also a modulator of cardiac remodeling. Potential mechanisms include caspase activation and induction of apoptosis, activation of matrix metalloproteinases, activation of poly(ADP-ribose) polymerase, and direct oxidative damage to myocytes. In addition, NO is a known inhibitor of platelet adhesion and aggregation, and depletion may contribute to the procoagulant state in heart failure (59, 60). Other potential mechanisms for detrimental effects include disturbances in signal transduction pathways, interference with mitochondrial function, and antioxidant depletion. In support of these pathophysiologic mechanisms, animal studies have demonstrated significant correlations between iNOS gene expression and left ventricular ejection fraction, ventricular dilatation, and conduction defects (61).

In contrast, there are indications that heart failure may be characterized by reduced NO production, and this could have a variety of deleterious effects. Reduced bioavailability of NO impairs endothelial function through cyclic guanosine monophosphate–mediated smooth muscle relaxation. It has also been proposed that NO has an important regulatory role in reducing sympathetic outflow, along with inhibition of the central nervous system effects of angiotensin II (62). Human studies also show that pharmacologic manipulation of NO pathways via supplementation of L-arginine, boosting concentrations with NO donors such as isosorbide dinitrate and hydralazine, or by increasing synthesis through eNOS with spironolactone, is associated with improved endothelial function and cardiac contractility (63, 64). Most importantly, recent studies in self-described African Americans with heart failure support a major beneficial effect of the hydralazine-nitrate combination in reducing mortality and morbidity in this subgroup of patients with heart failure due to left ventricular systolic dysfunction (65).

Adhesion Molecules

Adhesion molecules comprise several distinct groups: intercellular adhesion molecule (ICAM), vascular adhesion molecule (VCAM), platelet endothelial cell adhesion molecule (PECAM), integrins, and selectins. These molecules bind with cell surface receptors integral in the interaction between immune cells such as leukocytes, and other cell types such as endothelial cells and the extracellular matrix. Their role in heart failure has been studied to a limited extent.

Several studies have demonstrated an increased expression of various adhesion molecules in chronic heart failure. Early work found elevated expression of ICAM-1, VCAM-1, PECAM-1, P-selectin, and E-selectin in myocardial tissue from cardiac transplant recipients. Increased serum levels of these soluble forms were also found in patients with myocarditis, idiopathic dilated cardiomyopathy, and ischemic cardiomyopathy (66–68). No differences were detected based on etiology. Subsequent studies have correlated elevated expression of cellular adhesion molecules to the severity of heart failure as assessed by functional ability and ejection fraction (69, 70). One study reported an increase in the combined endpoint of death, heart transplantation, and hospitalization for worsening heart failure over a median follow-up of 240 days in patients with higher soluble adhesion molecule concentrations (69).

Immune system activation is one proposed reason for the increased adhesion molecule expression in heart failure, although the exact mechanism is unknown. Angiotensin II is another known stimulus for the expression of adhesion molecules in cardiac fibroblasts (71). Finally, it has also been proposed that increased soluble levels occur due to shedding of protein from cytokine activated endothelial cells (72).

Nuclear Factor-κB

Nuclear factor κB (NF-κB) is a transcription factor implicated in the regulation of inflammation through gene expression of various cytokines, adhesion molecules, and chemokines. It is found in the cytoplasm of resting cells bound to inhibitory proteins, known as inhibitory κB (I-κB), which exist in various forms (73). Activation of NF-κB occurs when these inhibitory proteins are phosphorylated by a multimeric complex known as I-κB kinase (IKK), resulting in free NF-κB, which translocates into the nucleus and binds with promoter or enhancer regions of a specific gene (74). Apart from regulation of inflammatory mediators, NF-κB also appears to modulate apoptosis and cardiac remodeling (75–82).

Nuclear factor κB has been implicated in the pathophysiology of numerous disease states, such as autoimmune arthritis, septic shock, inflammatory bowel disease, asthma, atherosclerosis, and myocardial ischemia (73). There is mounting evidence that NF-κB is also activated in the failing heart. Immunohistologic studies have demonstrated increased activation of NF-κB in the myocardium and peripheral blood leukocytes from heart failure patients compared to healthy individuals (83–86). Elevated NF-κB activity appears to correlate with the severity of heart failure, but not with etiology (83, 84). In addition, proportionate elevations in I-κBs and IKK have recently been demonstrated (83).

The pathophysiologic and clinical implications of increased NF-κB activation remain uncertain. The rationale for a detrimental pathophysiologic effect stems from experimental evidence demonstrating induction of proinflammatory cytokines, promotion of cardiac fibrosis and remodeling, and an association between NF-κB and infarct size during reperfusion. Consistent with these findings, blockade of NF-κB in transgenic mouse models resulted in regression of hypertrophy, improved ventricular function, and survival (87–89). In contrast, there is evidence that NF-κB may be protective due to induction of antiapoptotic factors, and may promote ischemic preconditioning (90, 91). As a further example of the complexity of the actions of NF-κB, a recent study evaluated potential gene targets for this signaling molecule in the failing heart (83). Using a gene array, the investigators were able to identify over 50 genes up regulated in failing hearts, many of which were related to cytokines, growth factors, interferons, adhesion molecules, and other regulatory proteins. Whether changes in gene regulation due to upregulation by NF-κB are related to the pathophysiology of heart failure remains to be determined.

Humoral and Cellular Immune Response in Heart Failure

Innate Immunity Autoantibodies

There is growing evidence for a role of autoantibodies in the pathogenesis of at least some forms of cardiomyopathy. Cardiac autoantibodies have been found in circulation in idiopathic dilated cardiomyopathy and myocarditis (92). It has also long been recognized that autoantibodies to the β-adrenergic receptor are present in Chagas disease and idiopathic and ischemic cardiomyopathy, but not in valvular or hypertensive heart disease (93–95). These autoantibodies exert agonist activity on β_1-adrenergic receptors and it has been hypothesized that they contribute to chronic activation of these receptors, with subsequent receptor desensitization.

The pathologic role of β_1-adrenergic receptor autoantibodies is supported by experimental studies demonstrating the development of cardiomyopathy induced by injection of anti–β_1-adrenergic receptor antiserum, and improvement in cardiac hemodynamic parameters such as cardiac index and ejection fraction with removal of immunoglobulin G (IgG) by immunoadsorption (96,97). There has also been evidence that antibodies to cardiac troponin I can lead to development of experimental cardiomyopathy and that antimyosin antibodies may be associated with myocarditis in humans (98, 99).

Immune Cells

Overall, there is limited literature on the expression of immune cell types and alterations in heart failure. However, research continues to identify altered function of various immune cells and their possible roles in the development and progression of declining cardiac function.

Leukocytes

Much of the available literature on lymphocyte subsets in heart failure is derived from experimental autoimmune myocarditis. Infiltration of CD4 and CD8 cells has been demonstrated in myocardial biopsies in myocarditis and idiopathic dilated cardiomyopathy (100). Evidence suggests CD4 levels are proportionately higher than CD8, and that CD8 depletion may contribute to the disease (100). Increases in CD4 cell number has been shown to correlate with left ventricular systolic function in a murine model of myocarditis (101). Some preliminary studies also suggest a role of lymphocytes in modulating diastolic function (102, 103).

There is evidence to suggest phenotypic alterations occur in T lymphocytes in heart failure. Enhanced gene expression of inflammatory proteins (chemokines, interferon-γ, IL-18, and TNF superfamily ligands) has been demonstrated in these cells taken from patients in moderate to severe heart failure regardless of etiology (104). These cells also exhibited increased CD69 and CD25 expression. The peripheral CD4 subset has also been shown to be proportionately increased, compared to CD3 and CD8 subsets, in symptomatic heart failure patients (105). The increases in CD4 correlated with plasma TNF-α levels and the subpopulation of TNF-α producing monocytes.

In two preliminary clinical studies, percentage of plasma lymphocytes and lymphocyte G-protein receptor kinase-2 (GRK2) expression were found to correlate with incidence of cardiac events and increasing New York Heart Association functional class, respectively (106, 107). Importantly, lymphocyte GRK2 activity correlated with myocardial GRK2 activity.

Monocytes

There are several lines of evidence suggesting mononuclear cells may be important to the pathophysiology of heart failure, although overall the data are limited. Monocytes may contribute to the development of cardiomyopathy and heart failure. Peripheral monocytosis has been linked in left ventricular remodeling in reperfused patients post–Q-wave myocardial infarction (108). Peak increases in monocyte count were higher in patients experiencing complications such as left ventricular aneurysm or pump failure. Peak monocyte count was also positively associated with left ventricular end-diastolic volume and inversely with ejection fraction. In a separate study, monocytes from post–myocardial infarction patients who develop heart failure expressed increased levels of basal and stimulated Toll-like receptor-4 and inflammatory cytokines, compared to patients who did not develop heart failure or healthy subjects (109).

Monocyte-mediated cardiac damage is thought to be secondary to proinflammatory cytokine expression. Monocyte production and expression of inflammatory cytokines such as interferon-β, IL-6, and TNF-α, and CD14 has been demonstrated to be elevated in heart failure patients, although not universally (110, 111, 104). Basal and stimulated elevations appear proportional to the severity of heart failure as assessed by traditional functional classification (111). Additional experimental data suggest that monocyte chemoattractant protein-1 is essential for the development of autoimmune myocarditis and subsequent development of heart failure through inflammatory mediated apoptotic pathways (112, 113).

Mast Cells

Mast cell granules are known to contain various proteases and TNF-α. Limited evidence is available to suggest that these cells could contribute to the development and progression of heart failure through several mechanisms. In experimental models, mast cells are capable of inducing cardiomyocyte apoptosis and activating matrix metalloproteinases, thus potentially contributing to cardiac remodeling (114, 115). They may also be a significant source of growth factors such as transforming growth factor-β_1 and basic fibroblast growth factor, which may contribute to myocardial fibrosis (116). Despite these interesting preliminary data, the extent to which mast cells contribute to the pathophysiology of heart failure remains to be determined.

Therapeutic Implications

Despite the elegant data supporting the pathophysiologic importance of the inflammatory response in experimental heart failure and preliminary data from pilot studies in patients with chronic heart failure, the therapeutic benefits of antiinflammatory therapy have yet to be established in chronic heart failure and there is no available evidence to support this approach in acute heart failure (117–121). Review of the trials conducted to date suggests some potential explanations for the failure of tested approaches. One strategy, which focused on the use of etanercept to specifically inhibition of TNF-α, may have been rendered ineffective through redundancy in the immune response system, which would allow other upregulation of other cytokines (6). Work with another compound, infliximab, illustrates the complexity of drug action, which may prevent clinical success in heart failure. This compound is directly cytotoxic to cells producing TNF-α, which may be beneficial in inflammatory bowel disease but harmful in heart failure (6). Recently, a trial of a nonpharmacologic approach to immune modulation has been completed, and full analysis of the trial results may yet demonstrate evidence of benefit (120). It is hoped that these and other ongoing research efforts provide support for the therapeutic role of inflammatory modulation in the management of patients with acute and chronic heart failure.

References

1. Frangogiannis NG. Targeting the inflammatory response in healing myocardial infarcts. Current Medicinal Chemistry, 2006;13:1877–93.
2. Aukrust P, Gullestad L, Ueland T, Damås JK, Yndestad A. Inflammatory and anti-inflammatory cytokines in chronic heart failure: potential therapeutic implications. Ann Med 2005;37:74–85.
3. Mann DL. Activation of inflammatory mediators in heart failure. Heart Failure 2004;11:159–80.
4. Levine B, Kalman J, Mayer L, et al. Elevated circulating levels of tumor necrosis factor in severe chronic heart failure. N Engl J Med 1990;223:236–41.
5. Knuefermann P, Vallejo J, Mann DL. The role of innate immune responses in the heart in health and disease. Trends Cardiovasc Med 2004;14:1–7.
6. Mann DL. Targeted anticytokine therapy and the failing heart. Am J Cardiol 2005;95(S):9C–16C.
7. Rafiee P, Shi Y, Pritchard Jr KA, et al. Cellular redistribution of the inducible Hsp70 protein in the human and rabbit heart in response to the stress of chronic hypoxia: role of protein kinases. J Biol Chem 2003;278:43636–44.
8. Torre-Amione G. Immune activation in chronic heart failure. Am J Cardiol 2005;95(S):3C–8C.
9. Pomerantz BJ, Reznikov LL, Harken AH, et al. Inhibition of caspase 1 reduces human myocardial ischemic dysfunction via inhibition of IL-18 and IL-1β. Proc Natl Acad Sci 2001;98:2871–6.
10. Torre-Amione G, Kapadia S, Lee J, et al. Expression and functional significance of tumor necrosis factor receptors in human myocardium. Circulation 1995;92:1487–93.
11. Nakano M, Knowlton AA, Dibbs Z, et al. Tumor necrosis factor-α confers resistance to injury induced by hypoxic injury in the adult mammalian cardiac myocyte. Circulation 1998;97:1392–1400.
12. Brasier AR, Jamaluddin M, Han Y, Patterson C, Runge MS. Angiotensin II induces gene transcription through cell-type-dependent effects on the nuclear factor-kappaB (NF-kappaB) transcription factor. Mol Cell Biochem 2000;212(1–2):155–69.
13. Frolkis I, Gurevitch J, Yuhas Y, et al. Interaction between paracrine tumor necrosis factor-alpha and paracrine angiotensin II during myocardial ischemia. J Am Coll Cardiol 2001;37(1):316–22.
14. Kalra D, Baumgarten G, Dibbs Z, Seta Y, Sivasubramanian N, Mann DL. Nitric oxide provokes tumor necrosis factor-alpha expression in adult feline myocardium through a cGMP-dependent pathway. Circulation 2000;102(11):1302–7.
15. Wei GC, Sirois MG, Qu R, Liu P, Rouleau JL. Subacute and chronic effects of quinapril on cardiac cytokine expression, remodeling, and function after myocardial infarction in the rat. J Cardiovasc Pharmacol 2002;39(6):842–50.
16. Gullestad L, Aukrust P, Ueland T, et al. Effect of high- versus low-dose angiotensin converting enzyme inhibition on cytokine levels in chronic heart failure. J Am Coll Cardiol 1999;34(7):2061–7.

17. Gurlek A, Kilickap M, Dincer I, Dandachi R, Tutkak H, Oral D. Effect of losartan on circulating TNFalpha levels and left ventricular systolic performance in patients with heart failure. J Cardiovasc Risk 2001;8(5):279–82.
18. Gurantz D, Cowling RT, Villarreal FJ, Greenberg BH. Tumor necrosis factor-alpha upregulates angiotensin II type 1 receptors on cardiac fibroblasts. Circ Res 1999;85(3):272–9.
19. Peng J, Gurantz D, Tran V, Cowling RT, Greenberg BH. Tumor necrosis factor-alpha-induced AT1 receptor upregulation enhances angiotensin II-mediated cardiac fibroblast responses that favor fibrosis. Circ Res 2002;91(12):1119–26.
20. Flesch M, Hoper A, Dell'Italia L, et al. Activation and functional significance of the renin-angiotensin system in mice with cardiac restricted overexpression of tumor necrosis factor. Circulation 2003;108(5):598–604.
21. Sekiguchi K, Li X, Coker M, et al. Cross-regulation between the renin-angiotensin system and inflammatory mediators in cardiac hypertrophy and failure. Cardiovasc Res 2004;63(3):433–42.
22. Nakamura A, Johns EJ, Imaizumi A, Yanagawa Y, Kohsaka T. Effect of beta(2)-adrenoceptor activation and angiotensin II on tumour necrosis factor and interleukin 6 gene transcription in the rat renal resident macrophage cells. Cytokine 1999; 11(10):759–65.
23. Yoshimura T, Kurita C, Nagao T, et al. Inhibition of tumor necrosis factor-alpha and interleukin-1-beta production by beta-adrenoceptor agonists from lipopolysaccharide-stimulated human peripheral blood mononuclear cells. Pharmacology 1997;54(3):144–52.
24. Hasko G, Elenkov IJ, Kvetan V, Vizi ES. Differential effect of selective block of alpha 2-adrenoreceptors on plasma levels of tumour necrosis factor-alpha, interleukin-6 and corticosterone induced by bacterial lipopolysaccharide in mice. J Endocrinol 1995;144(3):457–62.
25. Szabo C, Hasko G, Zingarelli B, et al. Isoproterenol regulates tumour necrosis factor, interleukin-10, interleukin-6 and nitric oxide production and protects against the development of vascular hyporeactivity in endotoxaemia. Immunology 1997;90(1):95–100.
26. Abraham E, Kaneko DJ, Shenkar R. Effects of endogenous and exogenous catecholamines on LPS-induced neutrophil trafficking and activation. Am J Physiol 1999;276(1 pt 1):L1–8.
27. Le Tulzo Y, Shenkar R, Kaneko D, et al. Hemorrhage increases cytokine expression in lung mononuclear cells in mice: involvement of catecholamines in nuclear factor-kappaB regulation and cytokine expression. J Clin Invest 1997;99(7): 1516–24.
28. Guirao X, Kumar A, Katz J, et al. Catecholamines increase monocyte TNF receptors and inhibit TNF through beta 2-adrenoreceptor activation. Am J Physiol 1997;273(6 pt 1):E1203–8.
29. Severn A, Rapson NT, Hunter CA, Liew FY. Regulation of tumor necrosis factor production by adrenaline and beta-adrenergic agonists. J Immunol 1992;148(11):3441–5.
30. Spengler RN, Allen RM, Remick DG, Strieter RM, Kunkel SL. Stimulation of alpha-adrenergic receptor augments the production of macrophage-derived tumor necrosis factor. J Immunol 1990; 145(5):1430–4.
31. Bloksma N, Hofhuis F, Benaissa-Trouw B, Willers J. Endotoxin-induced release of tumour necrosis factor and interferon in vivo is inhibited by prior adrenoceptor blockade. Cancer Immunol Immunother 1982;14(1):41–5.
32. Ng T, Vrana A, Sears T. Sympathetic regulation of monocyte TNF-alpha/IL-10 balance is impaired in severe heart failure. J Card Fail 2002;8(4 suppl): s3.
33. Petretta M, Condorelli GL, Spinelli L, et al. Circulating levels of cytokines and their site of production in patients with mild to severe chronic heart failure. Am Heart J 2000;140:E28.
34. Maeda K, Tsutamoto T, Wada A, et al. High levels of plasma brain natriuretic peptide and interleukin-6 after optimized treatment for heart failure are independent risk factors for morbidity and mortality in patients with congestive heart failure. J Am Coll Cardiol 2000;36:1587–93.
35. Peschel T, Schönauer M, Thiele H, Anker S, Schuler G, Niebauer J. Invasive assessment of bacterial endotoxin and inflammatory cytokines in patients with acute heart failure. Eur J Heart Failure 2003;5:609–14.
36. Milo O, Cotter G, Kaluski E, et al. Comparison of inflammatory and neurohormonal activation in cardiogenic pulmonary edema secondary to ischemic versus nonischemic causes. Am J Cardiol 2003;92:222–6.
37. Sato Y, Takatsu Y, Kataoka K, et al. Serial circulating concentrations of C-reactive protein, interleukin (IL)-4, and IL-6 in patients with acute left heart decompensation. Clin Cardiol 1999;22(12): 811–3.
38. Mueller C, Laule-Kilian K, Christ A, Brunner-La Rocca HP, Perruchoud AP. Inflammation and long-term mortality in acute congestive heart failure. Am Heart J 2006;151(4):845–50.

39. Alonso-Martinez JL, Llorente-Diez B, Echegaray-Agara M, Olaz-Preciado F, Urbieta-Echezarreta M, Gonzalez-Arencibia C. C-reactive protein as a predictor of improvement and readmission in heart failure. Eur J Heart Fail 2002;4(3):331–6.
40. Yin WH, Chen JW, Jen HL, et al. Independent prognostic value of elevated high-sensitivity C-reactive protein in chronic heart failure. Am Heart J 2004;147(5):931–8.
41. Anand IS, Latini R, Florea VG, et al. C-reactive protein in heart failure: prognostic value and the effect of valsartan. Circulation 2005;112(10):1428–34.
42. Berton G, Cordiano R, Palmieri R, Pianca S, Pagliara V, Palatini P. C-reactive protein in acute myocardial infarction: association with heart failure. Am Heart J 2003;145(6):1094–101.
43. Kim BS, Jeon DS, Shin MJ, et al. Persistent elevation of C-reactive protein may predict cardiac hypertrophy and dysfunction in patients maintained on hemodialysis. Am J Nephrol 2005;25(3):189–95.
44. Campbell DJ, Woodward M, Chalmers JP, et al. Prediction of heart failure by amino terminal-pro-B-type natriuretic peptide and C-reactive protein in subjects with cerebrovascular disease. Hypertension 2005;45(1):69–74.
45. Shah SJ, Marcus GM, Gerber IL, et al. High-sensitivity C-reactive protein and parameters of left ventricular dysfunction. J Card Fail 2006;12(1):61–5.
46. Anzai T, Yoshikawa T, Takahashi T, et al. Early use of beta-blockers is associated with attenuation of serum C-reactive protein elevation and favorable short-term prognosis after acute myocardial infarction. Cardiology 2003;99(1):47–53.
47. Joynt KE, Gattis WA, Hasselblad V, et al. Effect of angiotensin-converting enzyme inhibitors, beta blockers, statins, and aspirin on C-reactive protein levels in outpatients with heart failure. Am J Cardiol 2004;93(6):783–5.
48. Felker GM, Cotter G. Unraveling the pathophysiology of acute heart failure: An inflammatory proposal. Am Heart J 2006;151:765–7.
49. Pagni FD, Baker LS, His C, et al. Left ventricular systolic and diastolic dysfunction after infusion of tumor necrosis factor-alpha in conscious dogs. J Clin Invest 1992;90:389–98.
50. Janssen SPM, Gayan-Ramirez G, Van Den Bergh A, et al. Interleukin-6 causes myocardial failure and skeletal muscle atrophy in rats. Circulation 2005;111:996–1005.
51. Vlachopoulos C, Dima I, Aznaouridis K, et al. Acute systemic inflammation increases arterial stiffness and decreases wave reflections in healthy individuals. Circulation 2005;112:2193–200.
52. Malinski T. Understanding nitric oxide physiology in the heart: a nanomedical approach. Am J Cardiol 2005;96(7B):13i-24i.
53. Ferrari R, Guardigli G, Mele D, Percoco GF, Ceconi C, Curello S. Oxidative stress during myocardial ischaemia and heart failure. Curr Pharm Des 2004;10(14):1699–711.
54. Mihm MJ, Coyle CM, Schanbacher BL, Weinstein DM, Bauer JA. Peroxynitrite induced nitration and inactivation of myofibrillar creatine kinase in experimental heart failure. Cardiovasc Res 2001;49(4):798–807.
55. Turko IV, Murad F. Protein nitration in cardiovascular diseases. Pharmacol Rev 2002;54(4):619–34.
56. Heymes C, Bendall JK, Ratajczak P, et al. Increased myocardial NADPH oxidase activity in human heart failure. J Am Coll Cardiol 2003;41(12):2164–71.
57. Hare JM, Stamler JS. NO/redox disequilibrium in the failing heart and cardiovascular system. J Clin Invest 2005;115(3):509–17.
58. Damy T, Ratajczak P, Shah AM, et al. Increased neuronal nitric oxide synthase-derived NO production in the failing human heart. Lancet 2004;363(9418):1365–7.
59. Radomski MW, Moncada S. Regulation of vascular homeostasis by nitric oxide. Thromb Haemost 1993;70(1):36–41.
60. Chung AW, Radomski A, Alonso-Escolano D, et al. Platelet-leukocyte aggregation induced by PAR agonists: regulation by nitric oxide and matrix metalloproteinases. Br J Pharmacol 2004;143(7):845–55.
61. Mungrue IN, Gros R, You X, et al. Cardiomyocyte overexpression of iNOS in mice results in peroxynitrite generation, heart block, and sudden death. J Clin Invest 2002;109(6):735–43.
62. Zucker IH, Liu JL. Angiotensin II–nitric oxide interactions in the control of sympathetic outflow in heart failure. Heart Fail Rev 2000;5(1):27–43.
63. Thai HM, Do BQ, Tran TD, Gaballa MA, Goldman S. Aldosterone antagonism improves endothelial-dependent vasorelaxation in heart failure via upregulation of endothelial nitric oxide synthase production. J Card Fail 2006;12(3):240–5.
64. Steppan J, Ryoo S, Schuleri KH, et al. Arginase modulates myocardial contractility by a nitric oxide synthase 1–dependent mechanism. Proc Natl Acad Sci U S A 2006;103(12):4759–64.
65. Taylor AL, Ziesche S, Yancy C, et al. Combination of isosorbide dinitrate and hydralazine in blacks

with heart failure. N Engl J Med 2004;351: 2049–57.

66. Devaux B, Scholz D, Hirche A, Klovekorn WP, Schaper J. Upregulation of cell adhesion molecules and the presence of low grade inflammation in human chronic heart failure. Eur Heart J 1997; 18(3):470–9.
67. Andreassen AK, Nordoy I, Simonsen S, et al. Levels of circulating adhesion molecules in congestive heart failure and after heart transplantation. Am J Cardiol 1998;81(5):604–8.
68. Serebruany VL, Murugesan SR, Pothula A, et al. Increased soluble platelet/endothelial cellular adhesion molecule-1 and osteonectin levels in patients with severe congestive heart failure. Independence of disease etiology, and antecedent aspirin therapy. Eur J Heart Fail 1999;1(3): 243–9.
69. Yin WH, Chen JW, Jen HL, et al. The prognostic value of circulating soluble cell adhesion molecules in patients with chronic congestive heart failure. Eur J Heart Fail 2003;5(4):507–16.
70. Tousoulis D, Homaei H, Ahmed N, et al. Increased plasma adhesion molecule levels in patients with heart failure who have ischemic heart disease and dilated cardiomyopathy. Am Heart J 2001;141(2): 277–80.
71. Schnee JM, Hsueh WA. Angiotensin II, adhesion, and cardiac fibrosis. Cardiovasc Res 2000;46(2): 264–8.
72. Pigott R, Dillon LP, Hemingway IH, Gearing AJ. Soluble forms of E-selectin, ICAM-1 and VCAM-1 are present in the supernatants of cytokine activated cultured endothelial cells. Biochem Biophys Res Commun 1992;187(2):584–9.
73. Valen G, Yan ZQ, Hansson GK. Nuclear factor kappa-B and the heart. J Am Coll Cardiol 2001;38(2):307–14.
74. Thurberg BL, Collins T. The nuclear factor-kappa B/inhibitor of kappa B autoregulatory system and atherosclerosis. Curr Opin Lipidol 1998;9(5): 387–96.
75. Van Antwerp DJ, Martin SJ, Kafri T, Green DR, Verma IM. Suppression of TNF-alpha-induced apoptosis by NF-kappaB. Science 1996;274(5288): 787–9.
76. Erl W, Hansson GK, de Martin R, Draude G, Weber KS, Weber C. Nuclear factor-kappa B regulates induction of apoptosis and inhibitor of apoptosis protein-1 expression in vascular smooth muscle cells. Circ Res 1999;84(6):668–77.
77. Beg AA, Baltimore D. An essential role for NF-kappaB in preventing TNF-alpha-induced cell death. Science 1996;274(5288):782–4.
78. Stehlik C, de Martin R, Kumabashiri I, Schmid JA, Binder BR, Lipp J. Nuclear factor (NF)-kappaB-regulated X-chromosome-linked iap gene expression protects endothelial cells from tumor necrosis factor alpha-induced apoptosis. J Exp Med 1998; 188(1):211–6.
79. Maulik N, Goswami S, Galang N, Das DK. Differential regulation of Bcl-2, AP-1 and NF-kappaB on cardiomyocyte apoptosis during myocardial ischemic stress adaptation. FEBS Letter 1999;443(3): 331–6.
80. Martinon F, Holler N, Richard C, Tschopp J. Activation of a pro-apoptotic amplification loop through inhibition of NF-kappaB-dependent survival signals by caspase-mediated inactivation of RIP. FEBS Lett 2000;468(2–3):134–6.
81. Schneider A, Martin-Villalba A, Weih F, Vogel J, Wirth T, Schwaninger M. NF-kappaB is activated and promotes cell death in focal cerebral ischemia. Nat Med 1999;5(5):554–9.
82. Frantz S, Kelly RA, Bourcier T. Role of TLR-2 in the activation of nuclear factor kappaB by oxidative stress in cardiac myocytes. J Biol Chem 2001;276(7):5197–203.
83. Gupta S, Sen S. Role of the NF-kappaB signaling cascade and NF-kappaB-targeted genes in failing human hearts. J Mol Med 2005;83(12):993–1004.
84. Jankowska EA, von Haehling S, Czarny A, et al. Activation of the NF-kappaB system in peripheral blood leukocytes from patients with chronic heart failure. Eur J Heart Fail 2005;7(6):984–90.
85. Wong SC, Fukuchi M, Melnyk P, Rodger I, Giaid A. Induction of cyclooxygenase-2 and activation of nuclear factor-kappaB in myocardium of patients with congestive heart failure. Circulation 1998;98(2):100–3.
86. Fukuchi M, Hussain SN, Giaid A. Heterogeneous expression and activity of endothelial and inducible nitric oxide synthases in end-stage human heart failure: their relation to lesion site and beta-adrenergic receptor therapy. Circulation 1998; 98(2):132–9.
87. Gupta S, Young D, Sen S. Inhibition of NF-kappaB induces regression of cardiac hypertrophy, independent of blood pressure control, in spontaneously hypertensive rats. Am J Physiol Heart Circ Physiol 2005;289(1):H20–9.
88. Kawamura N, Kubota T, Kawano S, et al. Blockade of NF-kappaB improves cardiac function and survival without affecting inflammation in TNF-alpha-induced cardiomyopathy. Cardiovasc Res 2005;66(3):520–9.
89. Kawano S, Kubota T, Monden Y, et al. Blockade of NF-κB improves cardiac function and survival

after myocardial infarction. Am J Physiol Heart Circ Physiol 2006.
90. Xuan YT, Tang XL, Banerjee S, et al. Nuclear factor-kappaB plays an essential role in the late phase of ischemic preconditioning in conscious rabbits. Circ Res 1999;84(9):1095–109.
91. Morgan EN, Boyle EM Jr, Yun W, et al. An essential role for NF-kappaB in the cardioadaptive response to ischemia. Ann Thorac Surg 1999;68(2):377–82.
92. Caforio AL, Mahon NJ, Tona F, McKenna WJ. Circulating cardiac autoantibodies in dilated cardiomyopathy and myocarditis: pathogenetic and clinical significance. Eur J Heart Fail 2002;4(4): 411–7.
93. Limas CJ, Goldenberg IF, Limas C. Autoantibodies against beta-adrenoceptors in human idiopathic dilated cardiomyopathy. Circ Res 1989;64(1): 97–103.
94. Jahns R, Boivin V, Siegmund C, Inselmann G, Lohse MJ, Boege F. Autoantibodies activating human beta1-adrenergic receptors are associated with reduced cardiac function in chronic heart failure. Circulation 1999;99(5):649–54.
95. Jahns R, Boivin V, Siegmund C, Boege F, Lohse MJ, Inselmann G. Activating beta-1-adrenoceptor antibodies are not associated with cardiomyopathies secondary to valvular or hypertensive heart disease. J Am Coll Cardiol 1999;34(5):1545–51.
96. Jahns R, Boivin V, Hein L, et al. Direct evidence for a beta 1-adrenergic receptor-directed autoimmune attack as a cause of idiopathic dilated cardiomyopathy. J Clin Invest 2004;113(10):1419–29.
97. Mobini R, Staudt A, Felix SB, et al. Hemodynamic improvement and removal of autoantibodies against beta1-adrenergic receptor by immunoadsorption therapy in dilated cardiomyopathy. J Autoimmun 2003;20(4):345–50.
98. Okazaki T, Tanaka Y, Nishio R, et al. Autoantibodies against cardiac troponin I are responsible for dilated cardiomyopathy in PD-1-deficient mice. Nat Med 2003;9(12):1477–83.
99. Lauer B, Schannwell M, Kuhl U, Strauer BE, Schultheiss HP. Antimyosin autoantibodies are associated with deterioration of systolic and diastolic left ventricular function in patients with chronic myocarditis. J Am Coll Cardiol 2000;35(1):11–8.
100. Afanasyeva M, Georgakopoulos D, Rose NR. Autoimmune myocarditis: cellular mediators of cardiac dysfunction. Autoimmun Rev 2004;3(7–8): 476–86.
101. Afanasyeva M, Georgakopoulos D, Belardi DF, et al. Quantitative analysis of myocardial inflammation by flow cytometry in murine autoimmune myocarditis: correlation with cardiac function. Am J Pathol 2004;164(3):807–15.
102. Yu Q, Watson RR, Marchalonis JJ, Larson DF. A role for T lymphocytes in mediating cardiac diastolic function. Am J Physiol Heart Circ Physiol 2005;289(2):H643–51.
103. Afanasyeva M, Georgakopoulos D, Belardi DF, et al. Impaired up-regulation of CD25 on CD4+ T cells in IFN-gamma knockout mice is associated with progression of myocarditis to heart failure. Proc Natl Acad Sci USA 2005;102(1): 180–5.
104. Yndestad A, Holm AM, Muller F, et al. Enhanced expression of inflammatory cytokines and activation markers in T-cells from patients with chronic heart failure. Cardiovasc Res 2003;60(1):141–6.
105. Satoh S, Oyama JI, Suematsu N, et al. Increased productivity of tumor necrosis factor-alpha in helper T cells in patients with systolic heart failure. Int J Cardiol 2006;111:405–12.
106. Sakatani T, Hadase M, Kawasaki T, Kamitani T, Kawasaki S, Sugihara H. Usefulness of the percentage of plasma lymphocytes as a prognostic marker in patients with congestive heart failure. Jpn Heart J 2004;45(2):275–84.
107. Iaccarino G, Barbato E, Cipolletta E, et al. Elevated myocardial and lymphocyte GRK2 expression and activity in human heart failure. Eur Heart J 2005;26(17):1752–8.
108. Maekawa Y, Anzai T, Yoshikawa T, et al. Prognostic significance of peripheral monocytosis after reperfused acute myocardial infarction: a possible role for left ventricular remodeling. J Am Coll Cardiol 2002;39(2):241–6.
109. Satoh M, Shimoda Y, Maesawa C, et al. Activated toll-like receptor 4 in monocytes is associated with heart failure after acute myocardial infarction. Int J Cardiol 2006;109(2):226–34.
110. Zhao SP, Xu TD. Elevated tumor necrosis factor alpha of blood mononuclear cells in patients with congestive heart failure. Int J Cardiol 1999; 71(3):257–61.
111. Conraads VM, Bosmans JM, Schuerwegh AJ, et al. Intracellular monocyte cytokine production and CD 14 expression are up-regulated in severe vs mild chronic heart failure. J Heart Lung Transplant 2005;24(7):854–9.
112. Goser S, Ottl R, Brodner A, et al. Critical role for monocyte chemoattractant protein-1 and macrophage inflammatory protein-1alpha in induction of experimental autoimmune myocarditis and effective anti-monocyte chemoattractant protein-1 gene therapy. Circulation 2005;112(22): 3400–7.

113. Niu J, Azfer A, Kolattukudy PE. Monocyte-specific Bcl-2 expression attenuates inflammation and heart failure in monocyte chemoattractant protein-1 (MCP-1)-induced cardiomyopathy. Cardiovasc Res 2006.
114. Hara M, Matsumori A, Ono K, et al. Mast cells cause apoptosis of cardiomyocytes and proliferation of other intramyocardial cells in vitro. Circulation 1999;100(13):1443–9.
115. Chancey AL, Brower GL, Janicki JS. Cardiac mast cell-mediated activation of gelatinase and alteration of ventricular diastolic function. Am J Physiol Heart Circ Physiol 2002;282(6): H2152–8.
116. Shiota N, Rysa J, Kovanen PT, Ruskoaho H, Kokkonen JO, Lindstedt KA. A role for cardiac mast cells in the pathogenesis of hypertensive heart disease. J Hypertens 2003;21(10):1935–44.
117. Engel D, Peshock R, Armstrong RC, Sivasubramanian N, Mann DL. Cardiac myocyte apoptosis provokes adverse cardiac remodeling in transgenic mice with targeted TNF over expression. Am J Physiol 2004;287:H1303–11.
118. Singh U, Devaraj S, Dasu MR, Ciobanu D, Reusch J, Jialal I. C-reactive protein decreases interleukin-10 secretion in activated human monocyte-derived macrophages via inhibition of cyclic AMP production. Arterioscler Thromb Vasc Biol 2006;26: 2469–75.
119. Verma S, Szmitko PE, Ridker PM. C-reactive protein comes of age. Cardiovascular Medicine 2005;2:29–36.
120. Torre-Amione G, Sestier F, Radovancevic B, Young J. Broad modulation of tissue responses (immune activation) by celacade may favorably influence pathologic processes associated with heart failure progression. Am J Cardiol 2005; 95(S):30C–37C.
121. Yndestad A, Kristian DJ, Oie E, Ueland T, Gullstad L, Aukrust P. Systemic inflammation in heart failure—the whys and wherefores. Heart Fail Rev 2006;11:83–92.

15
Organ Perfusion in Acute Heart Failure Syndromes

Tal H. Kopel and Marie-Reine Losser

Acute heart failure syndromes (AHFSs) are associated with some degree of perfusion abnormality that is not necessarily evident. Cardiogenic shock is among the most important manifestations of the AHFS and is defined by clinically obvious or measured inadequate end-organ perfusion and tissue hypoxia with mortality in the range of 50%[1]. Causes of death are not only cardiogenic shock but also various organ failures despite normalized cardiac index[2]. Renal dysfunction, for example, is the most frequent and apparent organ dysfunction and is a powerful adverse prognostic factor (reviewed in Gheorghiade et al.[3]). Low organ perfusion during AHFS (Fig. 15.1) may result from a "forward" failure (acute coronary syndrome, myocardial failure with cardiogenic shock of various etiologies), from a "backward" failure with congestion due to global or right heart failure, or from a maladapted peripheral vasoconstriction (hypertensive acute heart failure). Regional redistribution of blood flow toward various vascular beds in the setting of AHFS has been seldom addressed over the last three decades compared to other acute states such as sepsis or hemorrhage, and consequently this chapter focuses on low-output AHFS.

Systemic Perfusion/ Neurohormonal Pathways

Heart failure is characterized by an aberrant neurohormonal response within the vasculature. Decreased forward output by the failing left ventricle leads to diminished activation of mechanoreceptors in the myocardium, carotid sinus, aortic arch, and kidneys. This stimulates sympathetic outflow, activation of the renin-angiotensin-aldosterone system, nonosmotic release of vasopressin, and the counterregulatory natriuretic peptides (atrial natriuretic peptide, brain natriuretic peptide, C-type natriuretic peptide)[4]. Indeed, when comparing septic shock patients with cardiogenic shock patients with similar hypotension but very different cardiac output (CO), there is an increased plasma vasopressin level in cardiogenic but not in septic shock[5]. The result of this activation tips the balance toward a vasoconstrictor and salt-retaining state. In acute heart failure, patients are dependent on this system for maintaining viability, especially regarding the perfusion of the coronary and cerebral circulations. In experimental cardiogenic shock in monkeys, blood flow, however, is significantly reduced in the cerebral and coronary circulation even as the percentage of the CO is increased to the cerebral vasculature[6]. In a dog model of tamponade (acute congestion), the 70% decrease in cardiac output associated with profound hypotension (systolic arterial pressure of 55 mm Hg) induced a decrease in brain, liver, and nonrespiratory muscle blood flow during the first hour only in spontaneously breathing animals[7]. In established congestive heart failure (CHF), blood flow in patients has been shown to be decreased in the splanchnic, renal, and cutaneous vascular beds in the effort to preserve central blood flow[8].

Macrovascular alterations during experimental induction of heart failure include a general reduction of flow with preponderance toward the

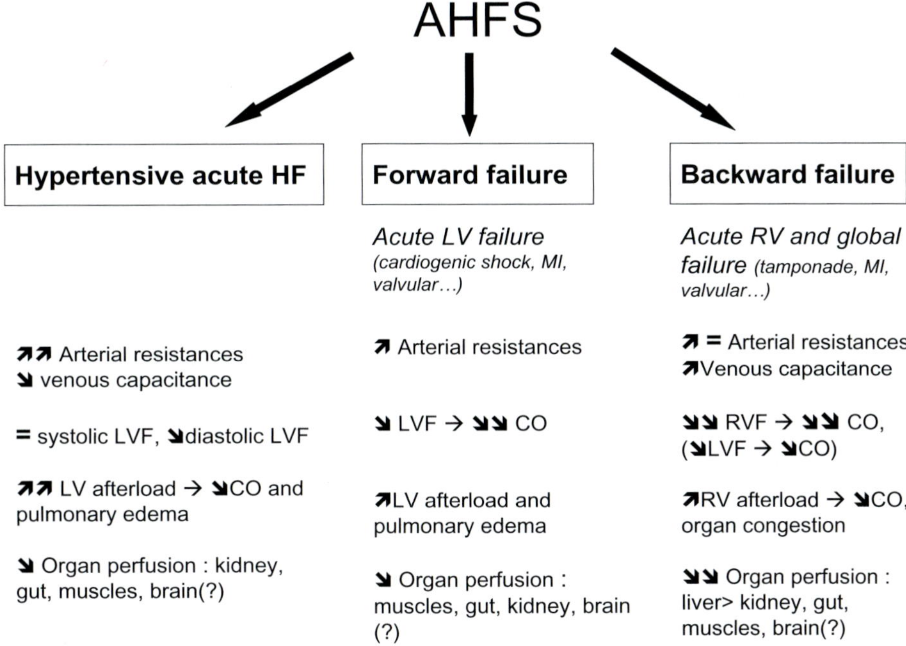

FIGURE 15.1. Different hemodynamic pattern responsible for acute heart failure syndrome (AHFS). CO, cardiac output; HF, heart failure; LVF, left ventricular function; MI, myocardial infarction; RVF, right ventricular function. ↗, increase; ↗↗, strong increase; ↘, decrease; ↘↘,strong decrease; =, stable.

carotid and femoral circulations[9]. Venous congestion in isolation may significantly reduce limb venous volume as well as resting blood flow[10]. Moreover, there is a markedly attenuated ability for peripheral vasodilatation that was first demonstrated experimentally in chronic heart failure and more recently in the setting of cardiogenic shock[11]. In experimental pacing-induced chronic heart failure in conscious dogs, it was shown that peripheral vascular responsiveness to β-agonist stimulation was decreased. It was associated with significantly decreased β-adrenergic receptor density in the vasculature, independent of an altered endothelium-mediated peripheral vasodilation[12]. However, macrovascular alterations may be poor predictors of downstream flow.

Within the microvascular circulation, the proportion of perfused vessels is decreased in severe heart failure and cardiogenic shock as compared with otherwise healthy adults[13]. Several mechanisms have been proposed to explain the incapacity of the peripheral microvasculature to maximally dilate in response to potent stimuli such as tissue hypoxia, including decreased red blood cell deformability, increased stiffness related to a higher local sodium concentration, and the mechanical influence of increased tissue edema. Recent data in chronic heart failure suggest that there is an inflammatory component as well, induced by cytokine release[14], which would be expected to occur in the acute setting.

Curiously, the response of regional vascular beds also shows disturbances in the ability to respond to hypotension induced by "pump failure." There was no expected vasoconstrictor response in renal, mesenteric, and carotid circulations after experimental induction of cardiogenic shock in anesthetized dogs, whereas the opposite response was documented in vagally induced hypotension[15]. This may help explain the hypotensive state in severe acute heart failure. The absence of appropriate vasoconstriction or even a vasodilator response termed "endogenous impedance reduction" may simply reflect timing and severity of the insult. It has been documented that systemic vasomotor responses become vasoconstrictor only later in the disease process, as typically seen in patients with chronic congestive heart failure or acutely when there is extensive myocardial damage from infarction[16].

Regional Circulations

It is important to recognize that analyzing regional organ perfusion in isolation is somewhat artificial, as many systemic and local mechanisms do interfere in an integrated system (Table 15.1).

Kidney

The determinants of renal blood flow (RBF) in acute heart failure have been investigated. It has been found that although low output induces marked increases in plasma renin and norepinephrine both systemically and intrarenally, there is no concomitant increase in renal vascular tone. However, levels of prostaglandin E_2 increased significantly in the renal venous system in acute heart failure induced by preventing venous return (heart unloading) in anesthetized ventilated dogs, and inhibition of prostaglandin synthesis led to markedly reduced renal blood flow[17]. These results suggest that renal blood flow is maintained by enhanced renal prostaglandin synthesis in acute failure to oppose systemic vasoconstrictor mechanisms. The implication of the nitric oxide (NO) pathway in these mechanisms remains to be fully clarified. Further, in low-output acute cardiac failure, renal perfusion pressure rather than the intrarenal renin-angiotensin system appears to be the predominant determinant of renal hemodynamics and the natriuretic response to atrial natriuretic peptide[18]. In a chronic model of heart failure in the rat, physiologic levels of atrial natriuretic peptide do not seem to result in increased diuresis, and in fact there may be an attenuated renal response secondary to eventual renal perfusion alterations[19,20].

Table 15.1. Summary of regional circulation modifications during acute heart failure syndrome

Target organ system	Flow	Mechanism
Kidney	↘ =	Prostaglandins, NO?
Respiratory muscles	↗	Sympathetic system
Hepatosplanchnic	↘↘	Sympathetic system, endothelin-1, renin-angiotensin system, congestion (liver)
Brain	↘ =	?
Musculocutaneous	=	Anaerobic metabolism secondary to impaired O_2 utilization, NO

NO, nitric oxide; ↗, increase; ↘↘, strong decrease; ↘, decrease; =, stable.

Although RBF decreases with acute heart failure, it is within proportion (i.e., not greater than expected) to the fall in cardiac output in experimental acute ischemic left ventricular failure in ventilated anesthetized dogs[21,22] or considerably less in unanesthetized dogs[23].

In nonventilated patients with severe congestive heart failure, there is a reduced RBF greater than expected as renal fraction of cardiac output was decreased[24]. Renal blood flow becomes the chief determinant of renal function, as measured by glomerular filtration rate (GFR), indicating dependence of GFR on afferent, rather than efferent vasoconstriction, under conditions of low renal perfusion. The greatest impairment of GFR was observed in elderly CHF patients, as RBF and function demonstrated an age-dependent decline, in addition to the adverse effects of CHF[24]. In conscious nonventilated patients with acute cardiogenic pulmonary edema, while cardiac index was low with preserved blood pressure, renal as well as brachial and hepatosplanchnic blood flow were decreased[25].

Thoracic

In the hemodynamic model of CHF, there is a venous reservoir that is under sympathetic nervous control. Cardiac preload is elevated with high filling pressure in the right heart and congested large pulmonary veins (reviewed in Freis[26]). Early studies with ganglionic blockers[27] showed the impact of peripheral dilatation: by decreasing the left ventricle afterload, the increased left ventricular output contributed to unloading the right heart and central veins, while the venodilatation permitted redistribution of blood volume from the congested thoracic area to the abdominal venous reservoir.

Respiratory muscle activity that sustains rhythmic contractions is dependent on muscle blood flow. In a model of severe acute tamponade in dogs, Viires et al.[7] showed the importance of spontaneous breathing in flow redistribution during this low flow state. Respiratory muscles consumed 21% of CO during heart failure conditions (and induced hyperventilation, which showed a threefold increase from baseline), while it represented 3% of CO in paralyzed animals under mechanical ventilation, with no decrease in other organ blood flows. It is concluded that the ventilatory failure of cardiogenic shock is due to an impairment of the contractile process of the respiratory muscles[28] leading to eventual muscle fatigue. The increased blood flow to respiratory muscles, especially the diaphragm, is unable to meet the increased metabolic demands and contributes to the lactic acidosis that appears in severe cardiogenic shock. Artificial ventilation, therefore, avoids respiratory failure and flow redistribution, while muscle paralysis limits the lactate production by ischemic muscles[29].

Hepatosplanchnic

The reduction in intestinal flow that occurs in a rabbit model of acute heart failure is proportionally larger than the fall in cardiac output, a response that is not seen in other vascular beds[22]. In lambs, the hepatic vasculature does receive a constant proportion of the cardiac output in the failing heart model; however, hepatic oxygen delivery falls more rapidly than systemic oxygen delivery, which is explained by the increased oxygen extraction by the intestinal tract that leads to oxygen poorer blood in the portal vein[30].

Mesenteric vasoconstriction is an active compensation for the hemodynamic changes induced in experimental cardiogenic shock. The response diverts blood flow to more critical and ischemic prone regional beds. The nature of the mediators of mesenteric vasoconstriction has been studied. Using a potent α-antagonist in a dog model of cardiac shock caused significantly higher mesenteric flows than in control animals, suggesting that sympathetic stimulation plays an important role[31]. One study demonstrated the specific regional influence of endothelin-1 induced vasoconstriction of the mesenteric bed in low cardiac output states[32]. Endothelin-1 is a potent vasoconstrictor produced in endothelial cells. Other mediators may be relatively more important in specific regional beds. The renin-angiotensin system has been shown to be the primary vasoconstrictor in the pancreatic and hepatic resistance vasculature with very little influence from either the α-adrenergic system or vasopressin in experimental cardiac tamponade[33,34]. The same appears to be true for the celiac vascular bed as a whole and the stomach vessels in particular. In this experimental model of tamponade- mediated cardiogenic shock in anesthetized pigs, it was clearly demonstrated that the dramatically decreased blood flows were secondary to profound vasospasm of the splanchnic circulation mediated primarily by the renin-angiotensin axis, rather than simply to a passive response to a reduced CO[35].

Despite the compensatory mesenteric vasoconstriction in response to decreased cardiac output, there is also interest in the role of the gut vasculature as a capacitance vessel. Splanchnic blood flow is not evenly distributed. In a model of anesthetized and denervated pigs (vagotomy and carotid denervation), hepatic blood volume increased after rapid atrial pacing. This was passively induced by the increased right atrial pressure and downstream caval pressure[36]. Using enalaprilat, an angiotensin-converting enzyme inhibitor, it is possible to further increase hepatic volume. The mechanism, however, is active, as demonstrated in the decreased hepatic and portal venous pressures associated with increased hepatic volume, which in turns serves to decrease left ventricular end-diastolic pressure in the failing heart of anesthetized dogs[37].

The hepatic circulation is especially sensitive to backward congestion rather than to forward hypoperfusion. This is due to the vascular architecture of the organ: two-thirds of its supply is dependent on the low pressure portal inflow. In a very illustrative case of global CHF, it was shown that adequate liver oxygenation could only be restored by unloading the right heart (using hemofiltration and nitric oxide inhalation). This case also stressed the adverse effect of mechanical ventilation. By generating positive pressure in the thorax, there was an increase in the right-sided afterload, worsening backward hepatic congestion[38].

Brain

Chronic heart failure patients (New York Heart Association functional classes II to IV) demonstrate decreased global cerebral blood flow[39], and more recently it was shown that there are specific regional blood flow abnormalities in the posterior cortical areas of the brain at rest[40]. In acute heart failure syndromes these changes are expected to be amplified. In normotensive patients in acute heart failure, there is evidence of decreased cerebral oxygen saturation as measured by nearinfrared spectrophotometry[41]. However, this technique has major limitations in adults because of scalp and skull interference in the signal.

Common carotid diameter and flow were markedly decreased in cardiogenic pulmonary edema patients as compared with healthy volunteers, probably more related to the musculocutaneous external carotid territory than to the internal carotid flow[25]. The impact on intracerebral hemodynamics can only be speculative, and is probably well preserved due to the strong autoregulation in this vascular bed. In a model of tamponade described above[7], muscle paralysis and mechanical ventilation avoided the large CO redistribution at the expense of the brain when compared to spontaneous breathing animals.

Musculocutaneous

Much interest has been generated surrounding decreased exercise tolerance in chronic heart failure[42]. In particular, impaired vasodilatation in the muscular vasculature has been the subject of several studies. There is considerably much less literature on acute heart failure syndromes and muscle perfusion. We can extrapolate results from chronic heart failure investigations. For example, stimulated release but not basal release of nitric oxide is impaired in established heart failure, leading to significant downstream peripheral vasculature resistance[43]. In chronic heart failure, small-muscle exercise is surprisingly not limited by tissue hypoperfusion and hypoxia but rather from impaired mitochondrial utilization of oxygen[44,45]. It is more likely that in acute heart failure, a smaller percentage of the cardiac output is redistributed to exercising skeletal muscles so that increased anaerobic metabolism is a combination of relative hypoxia and impaired oxygen utilization. In low cardiac output states, nonrespiratory muscle blood flow was drastically decreased in this model during spontaneous breathing, but to a lesser extent when the animals were paralyzed and mechanically ventilated[7], thus probably helping to minimize the participation of muscles in the occurrence of lactic acidosis. There is one human study of severe left ventricular failure and cardiogenic shock that demonstrated marked anaerobic muscle metabolism with a magnitude that was directly correlated with the clinical severity of the disease[46].

Blood flow to the adipose tissue decreases to a greater extent than the decrease in cardiac output with probable trapping of free fatty acids in the poorly perfused tissue[21].

Impact of Acute Heart Failure Syndrome Treatment

Treatment targets in acute heart failure have been the subject of recent reviews[3,47].

Ventilation, especially positive end expiratory pressure (PEEP) ventilation in patients (which is a recognized treatment of pulmonary edema) is known to increase circulating norepinephrine and plasma renin activity, and to induce acute antidiuresis without attendant plasma vasopressin level increase[48]. Additionally, it increases intrathoracic pressure with decreased venous return and thus decreases cardiac output, while increasing right atrial pressure and right-sided congestion[49].

The achievement of normal left ventricular filling pressures as confirmed with a pulmonary artery catheter (PAC) is associated with greater improvement in functional status and quality of life despite the lack of benefit on mortality (Evaluation Study of Congestive Heart Failure and Pulmonary Artery Catheterization Effectiveness [ESCAPE] trial[50]). Further, use of the inotropic agent milrinone in acute decompensated heart failure without cardiogenic shock demonstrated an increased trend for mortality and significant more adverse events compared to placebo[51]. It can be concluded that peripheral vasodilatation, rather than increased cardiac index, favorably improves outcome in acute heart failure.

After the induction of acute heart failure, there is a generalized increase in peripheral vascular resistance mediated by a combination of vasoconstrictor mechanisms as discussed above. However, there is evidence of regional differences in vascular sensitivity as shown by the preferential increase in blood flow to the brain, kidney, right ventricle, and upper gastrointestinal tract following intravenous administration of the angiotensin-converting enzyme inhibitor enalapril in an acute heart failure model in anesthetized dogs[52]. In nonventilated CHF patients with acute pulmonary edema, a single dose of intravenous enalaprilat improved arterial oxygenation (trend to reduced intrapulmonary shunt Qs/Qt) and musculocutaneous and renal hemodynamics while maintaining cardiac function and cerebral and hepatosplanchnic hemodynamics[25].

Critique of Models

Most of the results and conclusions on regional circulations in AHFS reported above have been performed in animals. The models are numerous: variables include the type of animal species, the use of anesthesia or denervation, the types of ventilation, and finally the mechanism of inducing the heart failure itself. Neurohormonal responses such as baroreflex, sympathetic stimulation, or renin-angiotensin system may be drastically modified by the anesthesia regimen and positive pressure ventilation. Of no less importance, models of heart failure include such different techniques as coronary ligature (for acute ischemic left ventricular failure), pacing-induced heart failure, heart unloading by balloon inflation in vena cava, and mechanical heart constraint to mimic tamponade (and right ventricular failure). The reader thus has to methodically review the literature in order to fully appreciate under what conditions the results have been obtained.

Only a few data on regional circulation during AHFS have been reported in humans. Clinical conditions of the patients, including but not limited to concomitant medications, sedation, and ventilation, have to be carefully reported as they may considerably influence the results.

Conclusion

The patients with AHFS may recover extremely well, depending on the etiology and the underlying pathophysiology. The right heart is as crucial as the left heart in determining organ perfusion. This summary on regional perfusion is aimed at emphasizing the blood flow of various organs that may become crucial to preserve (organ resuscitation) in order to avoid a downward negative spiral for the patient.

References

1. Babaev A, Frederick PD, Pasta DJ, Every N, Sichrovsky T, Hochman JS. Trends in management and outcomes of patients with acute myocardial infarction complicated by cardiogenic shock. JAMA 2005;294:448–54.
2. Lim N, Dubois MJ, De Backer D, Vincent JL. Do all nonsurvivors of cardiogenic shock die with a low cardiac index? Chest 2003;124:1885–91.
3. Gheorghiade M, De Luca L, Fonarow GC, Filippatos G, Metra M, Francis GS. Pathophysiologic targets in the early phase of acute heart failure syndromes. Am J Cardiol 2005;96:11G–17G.
4. Schrier RW, Abraham WT. Hormones and hemodynamics in heart failure. N Engl J Med 1999;341: 577–85.
5. Landry DW, Levin HR, Gallant EM, et al. Vasopressin deficiency contributes to the vasodilation of septic shock [see comments]. Circulation 1997;95: 1122–5.
6. Sivarajan M, Amory DW. Effects of glucagon on regional blood flow during cardiogenic shock. Circ Shock 1979;6:365–73.
7. Viires N, Sillye G, Aubier M, Rassidakis A, Roussos C. Regional blood flow distribution in dog during induced hypotension and low cardiac output. Spontaneous breathing versus artificial ventilation. J Clin Invest 1983;72:935–47.
8. Zelis R, Nellis SH, Longhurst J, Lee G, Mason DT. Abnormalities in the regional circulations accompanying congestive heart failure. Prog Cardiovasc Dis 1975;18:181–99.
9. Gunnes P, Reikeras O. Peripheral distribution of the increased cardiac output by secretin during acute ischemic left ventricular failure. J Pharmacol Exp Ther 1988;244:1057–61.
10. Zelis R, Capone R, Mansour E, Field JM. The effects of short-term venous congestion on forearm venous volume and reactive hyperemia blood flow in human subjects. Circulation 1978;57:1001–3.
11. Kirschenbaum LA, Astiz ME, Rackow EC, Saha DC, Lin R. Microvascular response in patients with cardiogenic shock. Crit Care Med 2000;28:1290–4.
12. Kiuchi K, Sato N, Shannon RP, Vatner DE, Morgan K, Vatner SF. Depressed beta-adrenergic receptor- and endothelium-mediated vasodilation in conscious dogs with heart failure. Circ Res 1993;73: 1013–23.

13. De Backer D, Creteur J, Dubois MJ, Sakr Y, Vincent JL. Microvascular alterations in patients with acute severe heart failure and cardiogenic shock. Am Heart J 2004;147:91–9.
14. Tousoulis D, Antoniades C, Katsi V, et al. The impact of early administration of low-dose atorvastatin treatment on inflammatory process, in patients with unstable angina and low cholesterol level. Int J Cardiol 2005.
15. Maximov MJ, Brody MJ. Changes in regional vascular resistance after myocardial infarction in the dog. Am J Cardiol 1976;37:26–32.
16. Zelis R, Flaim SF. Alterations in vasomotor tone in congestive heart failure. Prog Cardiovasc Dis 1982;24:437–59.
17. Oliver JA, Sciacca RR, Pinto J, Cannon PJ. Participation of the prostaglandins in the control of renal blood flow during acute reduction of cardiac output in the dog. J Clin Invest 1981;67:229–37.
18. Redfield MM, Edwards BS, Heublein DM, Burnett JC Jr: Restoration of renal response to atrial natriuretic factor in experimental low-output heart failure. Am J Physiol 1989;257:R917–23.
19. Lee RW, Raya TE, Michael U, Foster S, Meeks T, Goldman S. Captopril and ANP. changes in renal hemodynamics, glomerular-ANP receptors and guanylate cyclase activity in rats with heart failure. J Pharmacol Exp Ther 1992;260:349–54.
20. Qing G, Garcia R. Characterisation of plasma and tissue atrial natriuretic factor during development of moderate high output heart failure in the rat. Cardiovasc Res 1993;27:464–70.
21. Smiseth OA, Riemersma RA, Steinnes K, Mjos OD. Regional blood flow during acute heart failure in dogs. Role of adipose tissue perfusion in regulating plasma-free fatty acids. Scand J Clin Lab Invest 1983;43:285–92.
22. Arnolda L, McGrath BP, Johnston CI. Systemic and regional effects of vasopressin and angiotensin in acute left ventricular failure. Am J Physiol 1991;260: H499–506.
23. Higgins CB, Vatner SF, Franklin D, Braunwald E. Pattern of differential vasoconstriction in response to acute and chronic low-output states in the conscious dog. Cardiovasc Res 1974;8:92–8.
24. Cody RJ, Ljungman S, Covit AB, et al. Regulation of glomerular filtration rate in chronic congestive heart failure patients. Kidney Int 1988;34: 361–7.
25. Annane D, Bellissant E, Pussard E, et al. Placebo-controlled, randomized, double-blind study of intravenous enalaprilat efficacy and safety in acute cardiogenic pulmonary edema. Circulation 1996; 94:1316–24.
26. Freis ED. Studies in hemodynamics and hypertension. Hypertension 2001;38:1–5.
27. Rose JC, Freis ED. Alterations in systemic vascular volume of the dog in response to hexamethonium and norepinephrine. Am J Physiol 1957;191:283–6.
28. Aubier M, Trippenbach T, Roussos C. Respiratory muscle fatigue during cardiogenic shock. J Appl Physiol 1981;51:499–508.
29. Aubier M. Alteration in diaphragmatic function during cardiac insufficiency: potential pharmacology modulation. J Mol Cell Cardiol 1996;28: 2293–302.
30. Fahey JT, Lister G, Sanfilippo DJ 2nd, Edelstone DI. Hepatic and gastrointestinal oxygen and lactate metabolism during low cardiac output in lambs. Pediatr Res 1997;41:842–51.
31. Hirsch LJ, Glick G. Mesenteric circulation in cardiogenic shock with and without alpha-receptor blockade. Am J Physiol 1973;225:356–9.
32. Burgener D, Laesser M, Treggiari-Venzi M, et al. Endothelin-1 blockade corrects mesenteric hypoperfusion in a porcine low cardiac output model. Crit Care Med 2001;29:1615–20.
33. Bulkley GB, Oshima A, Bailey RW. Pathophysiology of hepatic ischemia in cardiogenic shock. Am J Surg 1986;151:87–97.
34. Reilly PM, MacGowan S, Miyachi M, Schiller HJ, Vickers S, Bulkley GB. Mesenteric vasoconstriction in cardiogenic shock in pigs. Gastroenterology 1992;102:1968–79.
35. Bulkley GB, Oshima A, Bailey RW, Horn SD. Control of gastric vascular resistance in cardiogenic shock. Surgery 1985;98:213–23.
36. Rutlen DL, Welt FG, Ilebekk A. Passive effect of reduced cardiac function on splanchnic intravascular volume. Am J Physiol 1992;262:H1361–4.
37. Risoe C, Hall C, Smiseth OA. Effect of enalaprilat on splanchnic vascular capacitance during acute ischemic heart failure in dogs. Am J Physiol 1994; 266:H2182–9.
38. Gatecel C, Mebazaa A, Kong R, et al. Inhaled nitric oxide improves hepatic tissue oxygenation in right ventricular failure: value of hepatic venous oxygen saturation monitoring. Anesthesiology 1995;82: 588–90.
39. Gruhn N, Larsen FS, Boesgaard S, et al. Cerebral blood flow in patients with chronic heart failure before and after heart transplantation. Stroke 2001; 32:2530–3.
40. Alves TC, Rays J, Fraguas R Jr, et al. Localized cerebral blood flow reductions in patients with heart failure: a study using 99mTc-HMPAO SPECT. J Neuroimaging 2005;15:150–6.

41. Madsen PL, Nielsen HB, Christiansen P. Well-being and cerebral oxygen saturation during acute heart failure in humans. Clin Physiol 2000;20: 158–64.
42. Drexler H. Skeletal muscle failure in heart failure. Circulation 1992;85:1621–3.
43. Drexler H, Lu W. Endothelial dysfunction of hindquarter resistance vessels in experimental heart failure. Am J Physiol 1992;262:H1640–5.
44. Mancini DM, Wilson JR, Bolinger L, et al. In vivo magnetic resonance spectroscopy measurement of deoxymyoglobin during exercise in patients with heart failure. Demonstration of abnormal muscle metabolism despite adequate oxygenation. Circulation 1994;90:500–8.
45. Schiotz Thorud HM, Lunde PK, Nicolaysen G, et al. Muscle dysfunction during exercise of a single skeletal muscle in rats with congestive heart failure is not associated with reduced muscle blood supply. Acta Physiol Scand 2004;181:173–81.
46. Karlsson J, Willerson JT, Leshin SJ, Mullins CB, Mitchell JH. Skeletal muscle metabolites in pat-ients with cardiogenic shock or severe congestive heart failure. Scand J Clin Lab Invest 1975;35:73–9.
47. Fonarow GC. The treatment targets in acute decompensated heart failure. Rev Cardiovasc Med 2001; 2(suppl 2):S7–S12.
48. Payen DM, Farge D, Beloucif S, et al. No involvement of antidiuretic hormone in acute antidiuresis during PEEP ventilation in humans. Anesthesiology 1987;66:17–23.
49. Payen DM, Brun-Buisson CJ, Carli PA, et al. Hemodynamic, gas exchange, and hormonal consequences of LBPP during PEEP ventilation. J Appl Physiol 1987;62:61–70.
50. Shah MR, O'Connor CM, Sopko G, Hasselblad V, Califf RM, Stevenson LW. Evaluation Study of Congestive Heart Failure and Pulmonary Artery Catheterization Effectiveness (ESCAPE): design and rationale. Am Heart J 2001;141:528–35.
51. Cuffe MS, Califf RM, Adams KF Jr, et al. Short-term intravenous milrinone for acute exacerbation of chronic heart failure: a randomized controlled trial. JAMA 2002;287:1541–7.
52. Hall C, Morkrid L, Kjekshus J. Effect of ACE-inhibition on tissue blood flow during acute left ventricular failure in the dog. Res Exp Med (Berl) 1987;187: 59–70.

1.3
Clinical Scenarios

1.3.1
Acute Myocardial Dysfunction

16
Dyspnea: How to Differentiate Between Acute Heart Failure Syndrome and Other Diseases

Clément R. Picard and Abdellatif Tazi

Patient present with acute dyspnea every day in emergency departments (EDs) and intensive care units (ICUs). Acute dyspnea is mostly due to potentially life-threatening cardiac or respiratory conditions, and treating it promptly requires understanding of the underlying mechanisms. A number of disorders cause dyspnea, including acute heart failure syndrome (AHFS), chronic obstructive pulmonary disease (COPD), asthma, pulmonary embolism, pneumonia, metabolic acidosis, neuromuscular weakness, and others. Although the clinical diagnosis of typical acute pulmonary edema or acute severe asthma is readily made, the presentation is less typical in a number of cases, for which consultation among ED physicians and respiratory and cardiology consultants is needed. Because of the prevalence of chronic heart failure (CHF), COPD, and asthma in the general population (2%, 5% to 10%, and 5%, respectively), differentiation among these three disorders is frequently needed[1–3]. Indeed, acute dyspnea in these patients is not necessarily due to an exacerbation of their underlying chronic condition and may have another cause (e.g., pneumothorax in an asthmatic patient). Furthermore, combined cardiopulmonary dysfunction may present with complex or atypical symptoms (e.g., pulmonary edema in a COPD patient). Finally, the differences in the treatment strategies in pulmonary and cardiac diseases and the probability of worsening of the primary disease with the incorrect treatment modality necessitates early and accurate diagnosis.

Depending on the hospital setting, AHFS accounts for 30% to 70% of acute dyspnea in the ED[4]. Quick identification of AHFS remains crucial and lifesaving, and may lead to prompt admission of the patient in a specialized cardiovascular ICU. An early diagnosis of AHFS was also proven to be cost-effective and to reduce the hospital length of stay[5,6]. Thus, a simple and quick way of differentiating cardiac and pulmonary causes of dyspnea is essential in patients admitted to the ED and should be based on routine procedures. In practice, medical history, symptoms, physical examination, chest x-ray (CXR), electrocardiogram (ECG), and, more recently, blood B-type natriuretic peptide (BNP) values are sufficient to recognize AHFS in most patients presenting with acute dyspnea. Other investigations (echocardiography, nuclear scans, or cardiac catheterization) require time and expertise and thus cannot be used as a screening procedure.

Does the Dyspneic Patient have a High Probability of Acute Heart Failure Syndrome?

To address this question, one has to identify among the clinical examination and routine investigations the features that have the highest specificity and the highest positive likelihood ratio (LR) for the diagnosis of AHFS. Few studies have investigated the performance of clinical examination, CXR, and ECG in distinguishing cardiac and noncardiac causes in order to design an evidence-based approach of acute dyspnea in this setting. Since the routine use of blood BNP levels, this question has been revisited, leading to significant progress in the rationale for the diagnosis of dyspnea in ED.

Badgett et al.[7] reviewed the literature to ascertain whether history, physical examination, CXR, and ECG can reliably diagnose left heart failure, that is, decreased left ventricular ejection fraction or increased filling pressure. The overall clinical examination did not yield predictive values that reliably confirmed or excluded an increased filling pressure in typical patients in the ED. Much variability existed in the precision of clinical findings, which was partly attributable to subspecialty training or examiner experience. Nevertheless, the best findings for detecting increased left ventricular filling pressure were jugular venous distention and radiographic vascular redistribution. These results, however, were in patients referred for consideration of cardiac transplant with known severe systolic dysfunction. In patients with less severe systolic dysfunction, these findings may not be useful and their absence cannot exclude the diagnosis. Dependent edema was helpful when present but had a poor sensitivity. The best findings for detecting systolic dysfunction were abnormal apical impulse, radiographic cardiomegaly, and Q waves or left bundle branch block on an ECG. The predictive value of these signs depends on the probability and the severity of left heart dysfunction. Findings that were not significant in a majority of studies to detect decreased ejection fraction were age, orthopnea, left ventricular hypertrophy on ECG, history of hypertension, or congestive heart failure.

In another study on almost 2500 patients with severe heart failure due to systolic dysfunction, an elevated jugular venous pressure and a third heart sound (S3) were found to be diagnostic of AHFS but were present in only 24% and 11%, respectively, of the patients[8]. The use of computerized detection of S3 (Audicor algorithm) improved sensitivity when compared to heart auscultation (41% vs. 18%, respectively) but decreased specificity (87% vs. 98%, respectively) in another study[9]. A small case-control study of eight patients suggested that ultrasonographic examination of the internal jugular vein performed by an ED physician in patients without clinical jugular venous distention could be more sensitive[10].

The clinical focus on dyspneic patients, however, is more useful because not every patient with left ventricular dysfunction or high filling pressures on objective cardiac testing will be subjectively dyspneic, and patients with a reduced ejection fraction may be dyspneic from causes other than heart failure. More recently, Wang et al.[4] selected 22 studies of adult patients presenting with dyspnea at the ED to assess the usefulness of history, symptoms, and signs along with routine diagnostic studies (CXR, ECG, serum BNP) that differentiate heart failure from other causes of dyspnea. Among the features that increased the probability of heart failure, the best feature for each category were a past history of heart failure, the symptoms of paroxysmal nocturnal dyspnea, the sign of the third heart sound (S3) gallop, CXR showing pulmonary venous congestion, and ECG showing atrial fibrillation. The sensitivity, specificity, and positive and negative LRs of these findings for the diagnosis of AHFS are shown in Table 16.1. The presence of new T-wave changes or abnormal ECG findings increased the LR of heart failure but was evaluated in fewer studies. The overall clinical impression of the physician initially treating the patient in the ED was also important to consider and had a high positive LR for the diagnosis of AHFS.

Other tests have been evaluated for the distinction between cardiac and noncardiac causes of

TABLE 16.1. Accuracy of most suggestive features for the diagnosis of AHFS in dyspneic patient presenting to the emergency department

Finding	Sensitivity	Specificity	Positive LR	Negative LR
Past history of AHFS	0.6	0.9	5.8	0.45
Paroxysmal nocturnal dyspnea	0.41	0.84	2.6	0.7
Third heart sound gallop	0.13	0.99	11	0.88
Pulmonary venous congestion on CXR	0.54	0.96	12	0.48
Atrial fibrillation on ECG	0.26	0.93	3.8	0.79

CXR, chest x-ray; ECG, electrocardiogram; LR, likelihood ratio.
Source: Based on date from Wang et al.[4]

dyspnea. Impedance cardiography can be performed by less experienced clinicians than echocardiography and has shown promising performance in the identification of AHFS in the ED[11]. Among different biologic tests, BNP and N-terminal (NT) proBNP are the more helpful tests[12,13]. As the BNP cutoff increased, the positive LR generally increased for heart failure. However, no BNP threshold indicated the presence of heart failure with certainty. The BNP levels must be interpreted differently in patients with renal insufficiency (increasing the threshold values over 100 pg/mL when glomerular filtration is under 60 mL/min/1.73 m^2) and the utility of BNP levels in patients with advanced renal insufficiency glomerular filtration rate (<15 mL/min) is unclear.

One study has examined the accuracy of symptoms, signs, ECG, and serum BNP in diagnosing heart failure in dyspneic ED patients with a prior history of asthma or COPD[14]. A high initial clinical suspicion by the emergency physician was associated with a high LR of heart failure but intermediate or low suspicion (probability ≤20%) did not exclude it. A history of atrial fibrillation or coronary bypass surgery was the most useful finding that increased the likelihood of heart failure. A third heart sound (S3), jugular venous distention, lower extremity edema, pulmonary rales, and hepatic congestion were the clinical features that most predicted AHFS. Pulmonary edema, cardiomegaly, pleural effusion on CXR, atrial fibrillation, and ischemic ST-T waves or Q waves on ECG were all helpful in suggesting a diagnosis of heart failure in the dyspneic ED patient with a history of pulmonary disease. The BNP levels can rise with chronic pulmonary diseases due to right ventricular strain. Nevertheless, BNP appears to be still useful in these patients, but it was more powerful for excluding heart failure when low (BNP <100 pg/mL) (see below). Additional studies are needed to confirm these results and define the optimal cutoff for BNP to diagnose or exclude heart failure in dyspneic patients with various chronic lung diseases.

In the future, other simple sensitive and noninvasive tests could be developed. As an example, impedance cardiography has a sensitivity of 92% and a negative predictive value of 96% and could become another screening test if performed routinely[11]. The sensitivity of ultrasonography of the internal jugular vein suggested in a preliminary study remains to be confirmed in a larger population[10].

Does the Dyspneic Patient Have a High Probability of Absence of Acute Heart Failure Syndrome?

To answer this question, one has to identify among the clinical examination and routine investigations the features that have the lowest negative LR for the diagnosis of AHFS. In their meta-analysis, Wang et al.[4] found that the features that best decreased the probability of heart failure were the absence of the following: a past history of heart failure, dyspnea on exertion, pulmonary rales, cardiomegaly on CXR, and any ECG abnormality. The sensitivity, specificity, and positive and negative LRs of these findings for exclusion of AHFS are shown in Table 16.2. A blood BNP value ≤100 pg/mL, however, was by far the most useful test to eliminate AHFS. The combined criteria of initial judgment and a BNP level ≤100 pg/mL have a similar sensitivity and negative LR. Taken together, BNP may not contribute much more in patients for whom the initial clinical suspicion of heart failure was already high, but when the initial

Table 16.2. Accuracy of most suggestive features of absence of AHFS in dyspneic patient presenting to the emergency department

Finding	Sensitivity	Specificity	Positive LR	Negative LR
Past history of AHFS	0.6	0.9	5.8	0.45
Dyspnea on exertion	0.84	0.34	1.3	0.38
Rales	0.6	0.78	2.8	0.51
Cardiomegaly on CXR	0.74	0.78	3.3	0.33
Any ECG abnormality	0.5	0.78	2.2	0.64

CXR, chest x-ray; ECG, electrocardiogram; LR, likelihood ratio.
Source: Wang et al.[4]

clinical suspicion was not high, BNP was useful particularly for excluding patients without heart failure in the absence of renal insufficiency. Furthermore, in a recent multicentric study including 1586 patients, a normal blood BNP level was a better test than the echocardiographic left ventricular ejection fraction for ruling out the diagnosis of AHFS[15].

In dyspneic patients with a prior history of asthma or COPD, the diagnosis accuracy of the initial clinical judgment was lower than for the non-COPD/asthma patients[4]. The absence of orthopnea, pulmonary rales, lower extremity edema, or jugular venous distention decreased the likelihood of heart failure. Similarly, a normal CXR, absence of cardiomegaly, or absence of edema on CXR also refuted the diagnosis of AHFS. No single ECG result had clinically useful outcomes for lowering the likelihood of heart failure. In this population, the BNP level was particularly useful for excluding AHFS[4].

What Are the Alternative Diagnoses in the Dyspneic Patient in the Emergency Department?

The comprehensive list of etiologies of acute dyspnea in the ED is beyond the scope of this chapter. Precise data on the proportion of the different causes are missing and depend on the hospital setting. In the Breathing Not Properly multinational study, among 1586 patients, 47% had AHFS, 49% had dyspnea due to other diseases, and 4% had dyspnea due to another cause with a past history of heart failure[12]. Here, we briefly discuss only the most frequent alternative diagnoses of AHFS.

Chronic Obstructive Pulmonary Disease

Exacerbation of COPD is the one of the most frequent and challenging differential diagnoses. In a study including 452 patients, it accounted for 17% of cases of acute dyspnea at the ED[5]. The diagnosis of COPD is based on the demonstration of airflow limitation on pulmonary function tests, which are not reliable in an emergency setting. The patient's smoking history is important to consider since the absence of tobacco use is a strong argument against this diagnosis, whereas a smoking history of ≥70 pack-years strongly increases the likelihood of COPD[16]. Measurement of peak expiratory flow (PEF) is a useful adjunct to clinical assessment of patients with dyspnea to differentiate cardiac and pulmonary patients[17–19]. A reduced PEF (<170 to 200 L/min) suggests airflow obstruction, but may also be related to a nonmaximal expiration effort due to dyspnea. It may also be slightly decreased in AHFS because pulmonary edema begins in the peribronchovascular space, resulting in a mild obstructive syndrome[20,21]. Since dyspneic patients with pulmonary diseases are usually more hypoxemic than patients with AHFS, a Dyspnea Differentiation Index (DDI), defined as ($PaO_2 \times PEF$)/1000 has been proposed to differentiate between pulmonary and cardiac dyspnea[18,19]. The DDI, however, does not have the ability to predict combined (cardiac and pulmonary) disease, and that is a significant limitation of the utility of the test.

Acute Asthma

Most patients with acute asthma in the ED have a known history of asthma sometimes since childhood, with previous exacerbation and are younger than patients with AHFS[22]. They are frequently atopic with other allergic manifestations such as rhinitis. The distinction between asthma and AHFS in the elderly and nonallergic patients, however, may be extremely difficult. Although to our knowledge no study has addressed this particular question, PEF and BNP measurements are probably the most relevant features for the differential diagnosis.

Other Chronic Respiratory Conditions

Exacerbation of other chronic respiratory conditions (tuberculosis sequelae, interstitial lung diseases, cystic fibrosis, and others) is a less frequent cause of acute dyspnea in the ED. A meticulous review of the patient medical history, previous treatments, physical examination (e.g., finger clubbing for pulmonary fibrosis), and analysis of lung abnormalities on the CXR are helpful for the diagnosis. The BNP analysis is probably useful to exclude AHFS, although few patients with respiratory conditions other than COPD and asthma were included in large studies evaluating the accuracy of BNP to differentiate pulmonary and cardiac dyspneic patients[12].

Pulmonary Embolism

Pulmonary embolism may be misleading, and patients may present several signs of AHFS, especially if the emboli is located in the proximal artery (jugular venous distention, orthopnea, cardiomegaly on CXR, atrial fibrillation on ECG, and elevated BNP levels). Practical scores for the diagnosis of pulmonary embolism have been elaborated[23,24]. Regarding clinical data, age >65 years old, and the presence of previous episodes of thromboembolism, surgery, fracture within 1 month, active malignancy, unilateral lower limb pain, hemoptysis, cardiac rhythm more than 75 bpm, or painful unilateral calf edema were features useful to classify patients as having low, intermediate, or high probability of pulmonary embolism[24]. In low-probability patients a negative D-dimer testing result using the enzyme-linked immunosorbent assay (ELISA) test is usually sufficient to rule out the diagnosis. In the remaining patients, computed tomography (CT) helicoidal pulmonary angiography combined with lower limb Doppler ultrasonography or CT angiography are currently the recommended investigations.

Pulmonary Infection

Community-acquired pneumonia by itself is a rare cause of acute respiratory failure in the ED as compared with exacerbation of COPD and asthma. In a study among 64 cases of noncardiac acute dyspnea, pneumonia was present in only six cases, compared with 31 and 21 cases of COPD and asthma, respectively[19]. Acute dyspnea in patients with pneumonia is usually associated with other underlying chronic condition (both cardiac and respiratory) or is secondary to noncardiogenic pulmonary edema.

Acute Respiratory Distress Syndrome and Noncardiogenic Pulmonary Edema

The distinction between protein-poor (as a consequence of AHFS) and protein-rich pulmonary edema (secondary to acute lung injury) may be difficult to make. The following criteria have been suggested as favoring the diagnosis of noncardiogenic pulmonary edema: evidence of pulmonary or nonpulmonary infection, history of aspiration, evidence of pancreatitis or peritonitis, hyperdynamic state, normal cardiac silhouette, vascular pedicle width ≤70 mm, peripheral topography of infiltrates and absence of Kerley's B lines on CXR, and a blood BNP level <100 pg/mL. In complex cases, prompt bedside echocardiography and sometimes Swan-Ganz catheterization should be performed to determine precisely the mechanisms of pulmonary edema.

Spontaneous Pneumothorax

Spontaneous pneumothorax involves in most cases young smokers, is a rare cause of acute dyspnea, and is diagnosed on CXR.

Pericardial Effusion

In a study of 103 patients with unexplained dyspnea after discharge from ED, systematic echocardiography revealed a pericardial effusion in 14 cases, and was abundant in four patients[25]. The authors suggest performing an echocardiography when no evident cause of dyspnea is identified.

Cardiac Arrhythmia

In a subgroup of 165 patients from the Breathing Not Properly study with BNP levels between 100 and 500 pg/mL and without heart failure, cardiac arrhythmia was considered to be the cause of dyspnea in 8.5%[26]. The authors suggested that heart failure could have been underestimated, as the reference standard for the diagnosis of heart failure in this study was the concordant opinion of two independent cardiologists. It remains unclear whether cardiac arrhythmia without AHFS can be a satisfying diagnosis for acute dyspnea.

Other Causes

Several other infrequent diagnoses may be discussed such as metabolic acidosis, anemia, abundant pleural effusion, neuromuscular disease, and anxiety. However, AHFS is usually not a differential diagnosis in this context.

Conclusion

For dyspneic adult patients in the ED, a directed history, physical examination, CXR, and ECG should be performed. If the suspicion of heart failure remains, a serum BNP level may be helpful especially for excluding heart failure. Using this approach, the clinician in the ED will miss only 6% of AHFS[4]. A schematic diagnostic approach for dyspneic patients presenting at the ED is proposed in Figure 16.1. More specialized investigations of cardiac function (echocardiography, cardiac catheterization, nuclear scans, cardiac CT

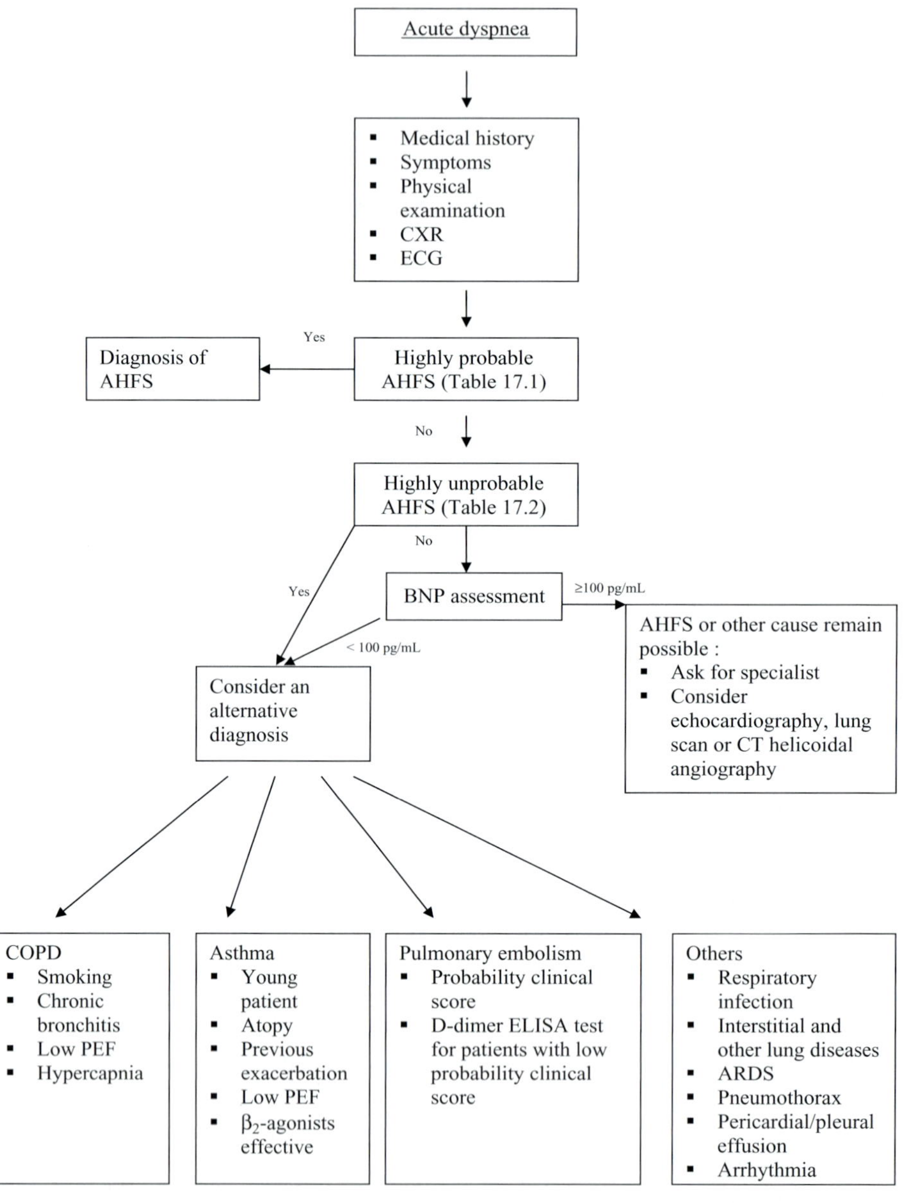

FIGURE 16.1. Example of algorithm for the diagnosis of acute dyspnea in the emergency department. AHFS, acute heart foilum syndrome; ARDS, acute respiratory distress syndrome; BNP, B-type natriuretic peptide; COPD, chronic obstructive pulmonary disease; CT, computed tomography; CXR, chest x-ray; ECG, electrocardiogram; ELISA, enzyme-linked immunosorbent assay; PEF, peak expiratory flow.

scan, or magnetic resonance imaging) are reserved for select patients to identify atypical cardiac failure or to determine precisely the underlying mechanisms of heart failure.

References

1. McMurray JJ, Pfeffer MA. Heart failure. Lancet 2005;365:1877–89.
2. Pauwels RA, Rabe KF. Burden and clinical features of chronic obstructive pulmonary disease (COPD). Lancet 2004;364:613–20.
3. Rees J. ABC of asthma. Prevalence. BMJ 2005;331: 443–5.
4. Wang CS, FitzGerald JM, Schulzer M, et al. Does this dyspneic patient in the emergency department have congestive heart failure? JAMA 2005;294: 1944–56.
5. Mueller C, Scholer A, Laule-Kilian K, et al. Use of B-type natriuretic peptide in the evaluation and management of acute dyspnea. N Engl J Med 2004;350:647–54.
6. Milzman DP, Barbaccia J, Davis G, et al. ED presentation of dyspnea in HF patients results in increased hospital stay and medication costs. Ann Emerg Med 2005;46:S38–S39.
7. Badgett RG, Lucey CR, Mulrow CD. Can the clinical examination diagnose left-sided heart failure in adults? JAMA 1997;277:1712–9.
8. Drazner MH, Rame JE, Stevenson LW, et al. Prognostic importance of elevated jugular venous pressure and a third heart sound in patients with heart failure. N Engl J Med 2001;345:574–81.
9. Storrow AB, Lindsell CJ, Peacock W, et al. Computerized detection of third heart sounds improves sensitivity for the emergency department diagnosis of heart failure. Ann Emerg Med 2004;44:S5.
10. Jang T, Aubin C, Naunheim R, et al. Ultrasonography of the internal jugular vein in patients with dyspnea without jugular venous distention on physical examination. Ann Emerg Med 2004;44: 160–8.
11. Springfield CL, Sebat F, Johnson D, et al. Utility of impedance cardiography to determine cardiac vs. noncardiac cause of dyspnea in the emergency department. Congest Heart Fail 2004;10:14–6.
12. Maisel AS, Krishnaswamy P, Nowak RM, et al. Rapid measurement of B-type natriuretic peptide in the emergency diagnosis of heart failure. N Engl J Med 2002;347:161–7.
13. Taboulet P, Feugeas JP. [Acute dyspnea in the emergency room: the utility of troponin, natriuretic, procalcitonin and D-dimers]. Ann Biol Clin (Paris) 2005;63:377–84.
14. McCullough PA, Hollander JE, Nowak RM, et al. Uncovering heart failure in patients with a history of pulmonary disease: rationale for the early use of B-type natriuretic peptide in the emergency department. Acad Emerg Med 2003;10:198–204.
15. Steg PG, Joubin L, McCord J, et al. B-type natriuretic peptide and echocardiographic determination of ejection fraction in the diagnosis of congestive heart failure in patients with acute dyspnea. Chest 2005;128:21–9.
16. Holleman DR Jr, Simel DL. Does the clinical examination predict airflow limitation? JAMA 1995;273: 313–9.
17. McNamara RM, Cionni DJ. Utility of the peak expiratory flow rate in the differentiation of acute dyspnea. Cardiac vs pulmonary origin. Chest 1992;101:129–32.
18. Ailani RK, Ravakhah K, DiGiovine B, et al. Dyspnea differentiation index: A new method for the rapid separation of cardiac vs pulmonary dyspnea. Chest 1999;116:1100–4.
19. Malas O, Caglayan B, Fidan A, et al. Cardiac or pulmonary dyspnea in patients admitted to the emergency department. Respir Med 2003;97:1277–81.
20. Light RW, George RB. Serial pulmonary function in patients with acute heart failure. Arch Intern Med 1983;143:429–33.
21. Ware LB, Matthay MA. Clinical practice. Acute pulmonary edema. N Engl J Med 2005;353:2788–96.
22. Lahn M, Bijur P, Gallagher EJ. Randomized clinical trial of intramuscular vs oral methylprednisolone in the treatment of asthma exacerbations following discharge from an emergency department. Chest 2004;126:362–8.
23. Wells PS, Anderson DR, Rodger M, et al. Derivation of a simple clinical model to categorize patients probability of pulmonary embolism: increasing the models utility with the SimpliRED D-dimer. Thromb Haemost 2000;83:416–20.
24. Le Gal G, Righini M, Roy PM, et al. Prediction of pulmonary embolism in the emergency department: the revised Geneva score. Ann Intern Med 2006;144:165–71.
25. Blaivas M. Incidence of pericardial effusion in patients presenting to the emergency department with unexplained dyspnea. Acad Emerg Med 2001;8: 1143–6.
26. Knudsen CW, Clopton P, Westheim A, et al. Predictors of elevated B-type natriuretic peptide concentrations in dyspneic patients without heart failure: an analysis from the breathing not properly multinational study. Ann Emerg Med 2005;45:573–80.

17
Acute Heart Failure in the Setting of Acute Coronary Syndromes

José López-Sendón and Esteban López de Sá

Acute heart failure in the setting of acute coronary syndromes (ACS) is a life-threatening situation that requires early identification and treatment. It may occur as the first manifestation of heart failure or in patients with previous heart disease, left ventricular dysfunction, and chronic symptoms of heart failure. In the majority of the patients, ischemic symptoms are clearly identified, but in others the symptoms may be subtle and the clinical picture is dominated by heart failure manifestations. Acute heart failure may present in several forms: forward failure (low output and cardiogenic shock), pulmonary congestion (including pulmonary edema), and right heart failure. Treatment should focus not only on improving the hemodynamics but also in the treatment of ischemia. A significant number of patients present left ventricular dysfunction with reduced left ventricular ejection fraction and only mild or transient symptoms.

Incidence and Prognosis

In contemporary studies, heart failure remains the most severe and frequent complication in patients with ACS. In patients with ST elevation myocardial infarction (STEMI) the incidence of cardiogenic shock, the most severe form of heart failure, varies from 5% to 15%, other forms of heart failure from 15% to 30%, and asymptomatic left ventricular dysfunction from 25% to 40% (1,2). Heart failure is also frequent in patients presenting with other forms of acute coronary syndromes, including non-STEMI and unstable angina (2) (Fig. 17.1). Risk factors for heart failure in the setting of ACS include previous left ventricular dysfunction and failure, age, transmural myocardial infarction, anterior location, infarct size, and absence of reperfusion therapy.

Heart failure has been identified as the single most important factor associated with outcome in patients with ACS (1–4). Mortality is highest during the first days of evolution, decreasing after the first month (Fig. 17.2). Hospital mortality in patients with cardiogenic shock may be as high as 80% to 90%. Excluding shock at admission, mortality at 1 month is around 20% (2,4). Several factors are related to poorer prognosis, including advanced age, hypotension diabetes, increased creatinine, no revascularization, and the presence of comorbidities.

Pathophysiology

Myocardial ischemia may induce ventricular dysfunction and heart failure through several mechanisms (Fig. 17.3). Loss of contractile muscle, myocardial stunning and hibernation, and increased stiffness of the ischemic myocardium are the most important physiopathology factors related to heart failure, producing two distinct alterations in central hemodynamics: an increase in left ventricular filling pressure (responsible for pulmonary congestion), and a decrease in stroke volume and cardiac output (responsible for tissue hypoperfusion).

Mechanical complications, especially interventricular septal rupture and mitral regurgitation,

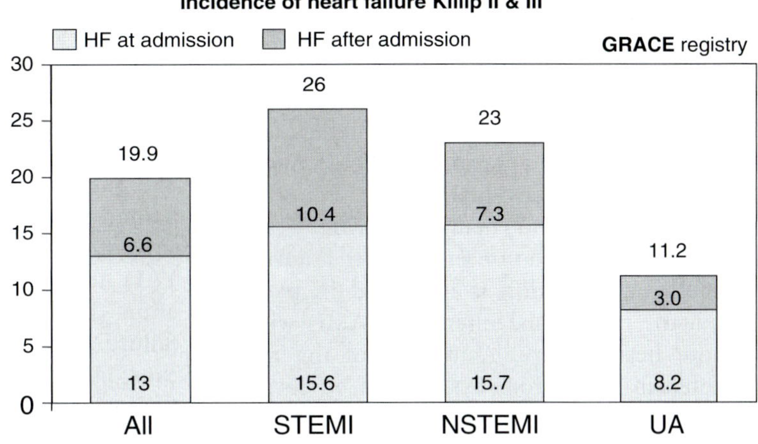

Figure 17.1. Incidence of heart failure (HF) for Killop classes I and II in acute coronary syndromes. NSTEMI, non–ST elevation myocardial infarction; STEMI, ST elevation myocardial infarction; UA, unstable angina. (Data from the Global Registry of Acute Coronary Events [GRACE] registry [2].)

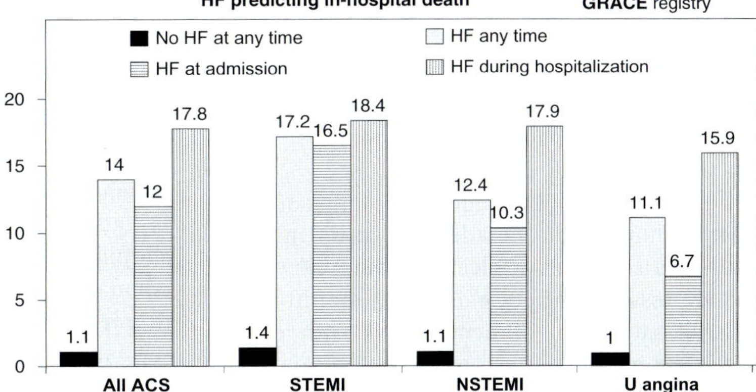

Figure 17.2. In-hospital mortality in patients with acute coronary syndrome (ACS) according to the presence or absence of heart failure. U, unstable. (Data from the Global Registry of Acute Coronary Events [GRACE] registry [2].)

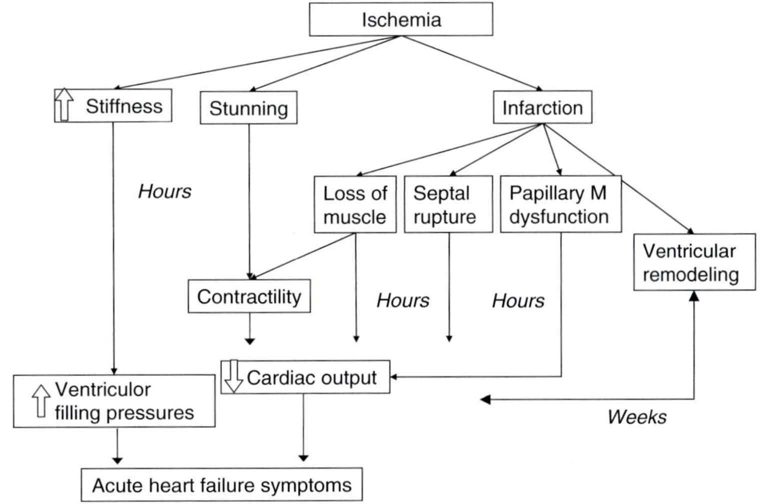

Figure 17.3. Factors contributing to heart failure in acute coronary syndromes. Loss of contractile tissue is the main determinant for heart failure after acute myocardial infarction. Other factors include diastolic dysfunction secondary to ischemia and edema, mechanical complications that impair the performance of the heart as a pump, stunning and hibernation and activation of the neurohormonal system. Increase left ventricular filling pressure and reduction in cardiac output are the main hemodynamic abnormalities responsible for symptoms of pulmonary congestion and hypoperfusion. M, muscle.

when present, may be the major determinants of hemodynamic abnormalities and symptoms. A number of other conditions may contribute or trigger symptoms: previous heart disease, arrhythmias, anemia, hypertension, hypovolemia, acidosis, hypoxia, and inappropriate use of negative inotropic drugs or vasodilators.

Activation of the neuroendocrine systems occurs early after the onset of heart failure (5). Sympathetic activation is increased in patients with acute myocardial infarction (AMI) with or without heart failure. Activation of the renin-angiotensin-aldosterone system can be observed hours or days later, triggered mainly by hypotension or low output. Early neurohormonal activations may contribute to the initial clinical manifestations, but are especially involved in the remodeling of the ventricles and progressive functional and anatomic deterioration characteristic of chronic heart failure.

Clinical Evaluation

All patients with ACS and symptoms of acute heart failure should be admitted to an intensive cardiac care unit. An electrocardiogram (ECG), blood pressure and pulse oximeter monitoring of arterial saturation of hemoglobin with oxygen (SaO_2), complete clinical examination, and basic blood analysis including glycemia, creatinine, ions, hemoglobin. and red blood cell count should be routinely performed (6,7). A chest x-ray is indicated in all patients but should be interpreted with caution as the quick hemodynamic changes of acute heart failure prevents a good correlation with the radiologic abnormalities.

Echocardiography offers functional and anatomic information of great value and should be obtained as soon as possible, specially in severely ill patients and in the presence of hypotension or lack of response to treatment (6,7). Echocardiography has a primary role in the diagnosis of mechanical complications after AMI. It also helps in the distinction of cardiogenic and noncardiogenic shock and provides an estimation of ventricular filling pressure and cardiac output. Left ventricular ejection fraction can be properly assessed with echocardiography, and it provides important prognosis information.

Hemodynamic Monitoring

Right heart catheterization with a flow-directed thermodilution pulmonary artery catheter (Swan-Ganz catheter) may be performed at the bed side and allows the precise evaluation of cardiac output and pulmonary capillary pressure as well as other hemodynamic parameters to further define the severity of the hemodynamic compromise (Table 17.1). It also is helpful in establishing the differential diagnosis of several causes of acute heart failure (6–8). It is useful for distinguishing between cardiogenic and noncardiogenic shock, and cardiogenic and noncardiogenic pulmonary edema, and it identifies different conditions associated with acute heart failure, such as ischemic right ventricular dysfunction, pulmonary embolism, severe mitral regurgitation, cardiac tamponade, and left to right shunts secondary to interventricular septal rupture. It also provides prognostic information and is useful for the efficient titration of potent vasoactive drugs. However, hemodynamic monitoring is not necessary in many patients without severe symptoms of heart failure or when a rapid improvement is observed after initiation of therapy. The following indications should be considered (6–8): (1) acute pulmonary edema, when a trial of diuretic or vasodilator therapy has failed or is associated with high risk; (2) patients with shock in whom a trial of vascular volume expansion has failed; and (3) suspected mechanical complications when echocardiography is unavailable, technically inadequate, or nondiagnostic.

Cardiac Catheterization and Coronary Angiography

Cardiac catheterization and coronary angiography must be strongly considered in all patients with heart failure in the setting of ACS. If possible, in patients with STEMI coronary angiography and percutaneous revascularization must be performed immediately (7,8). After the first 24 hours of evolution, coronary angiography is indicated in patients with residual ischemia or persistent hemodynamic instability. Although there is a lack of prospective studies in patients with ACS and heart failure, indirect data suggest that coronary angiography and revascularization should be con-

TABLE 17.1. Diagnostic information obtained during right heart catheterization in patients with severe heart failure/shock

	BP	RAP	PCP	CI	Observations
Normal	110–140	0–10	5–12	2.7	70–85
Shock Hypovolemic	↓↓	↓	↓	↓↓	Improves with fluid administration
Shock Cardiogenic	↓↓	↑↑	↑↑	↓↓	Does not improve with fluids Consider cardiac catheterization
Right ventricular infarction	↓	↑↑	=	↓	RAP = PCP RAP morphology: y >x May improve with fluids
Cardiac Tamponade	↓↓	↑↑	=	↓	RAP = PCP RAP morphology: y >x Direct diagnosis with echocardiogram Pericardiocentesis Surgery
Interventricular septal rupture	↓	↑	↑	↑↑	Systolic murmur Direct diagnosis with echocardiogram Surgery
Mitral papillary muscle rupture	↓	↑	↑↑	↓	Direct diagnosis with echocardiogram Surgery
Pulmonary embolism	↓	↑↑	=	↓	Diastolic PAP/PCP gradient Anticoagulation. Thrombolysis

BP, blood pressure; CI, cardiac index; PAP, pulmonary artery pressure; PCP, pulmonary capillary pressure; RAP, right atrial pressure.

sidered in patients with heart failure or left ventricular dysfunction (7–9). Conversely, coronary angiography should not be performed in patients with extensive comorbidities in whom the risk of revascularization is likely to outweigh the benefit and in patients with previously known coronary lesion unsuitable for revascularization (8).

Clinical Classifications

Several classifications are currently used to define the main clinical and hemodynamic abnormalities and to stratify the severity of ventricular dysfunction. Forty years ago Killip and Kimball (10) proposed the stratification of patients with AMI in four functional subsets, and this classification is still in use today. Class I corresponds to patients without clinical heart failure; class II is defined physical signs of heart failure, rales, or third heart sound; class III identifies severe pulmonary congestion (acute pulmonary edema); and class IV corresponds to cardiogenic shock. The main pitfall of this simple clinical classification is that hypoperfusion without pulmonary congestion is not considered.

Forrester et al. (11) proposed another clinical and hemodynamic classification that was also initially designed for patients with AMI and describes four groups according to the clinical (C) or hemodynamic (H) status, considering pulmonary congestion and peripheral perfusion (Fig. 17.4). Subset C-I identifies patients without signs of pulmonary congestion and normal peripheral perfusion; subset C-II corresponds to patients with clinical pulmonary congestion (rales, abnormal chest x-ray) and normal peripheral perfusion; subset C-III includes patients without pulmonary congestion but with peripheral hypoperfusion (hypotension, confusion, oliguria); and subset C-IV includes patients with both pulmonary congestion and peripheral hypoperfusion. A parallel hemodynamic classification was also described considering cardiac output and pulmonary capillary pressure (PCP). In subset H-I, both PCP and cardiac index (CI) are normal; subset H-II corresponds to patients with elevated PCP (>18 mm Hg) and normal CI ($\geq$2.2 L/min/m^2); subset III is characterized by normal PCP and low CI; and in subset H-IV both PCP and CI are abnormal.

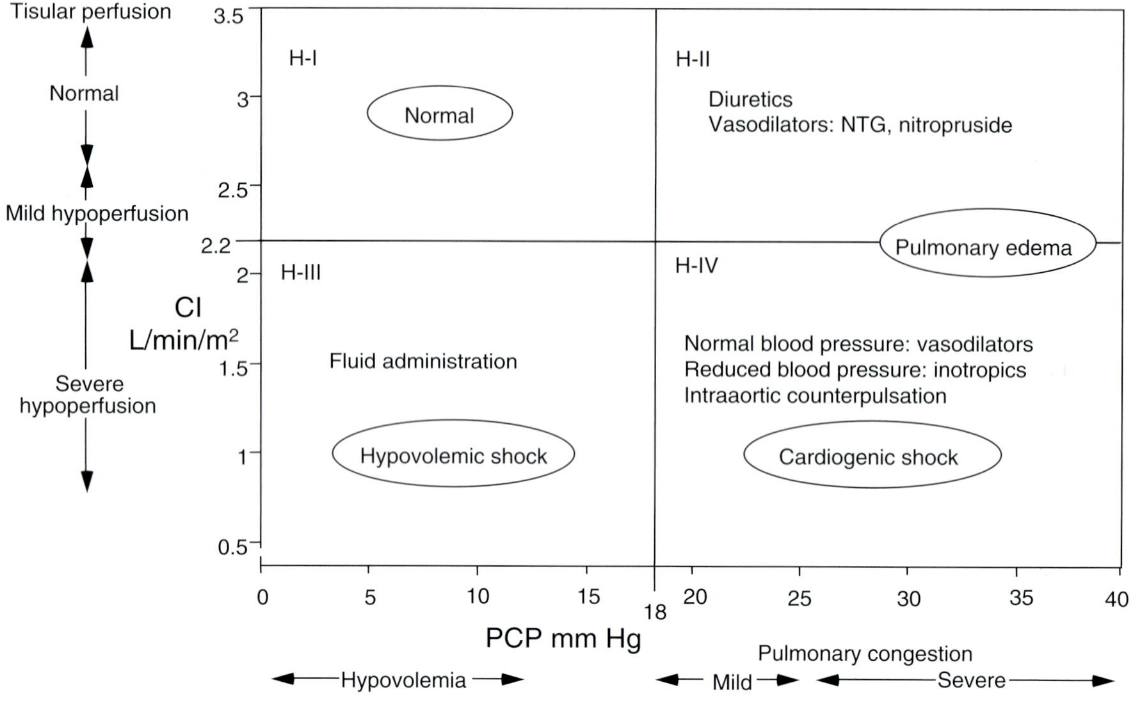

FIGURE 17.4. Clinical and hemodynamic subsets in Forrester classification and indications for vasoactive drugs according to tissular perfusion/cardiac index (CI) and pulmonary congestion/pulmonary capillary pressure (PCP). NTG, nitroglycerin.

A similar but more recent and popular classification stratifies patients according to observation of the peripheral circulation and auscultation of the lungs for congestion. The patients can be classified as class I (dry and warm), class II (wet and cold), class III (cold and dry), and class IV (cold and wet). This classification has been validated prognostically in a cardiomyopathy service (12) but can also be used in acute ischemic heart failure.

Early Treatment

Prevention of Heart Failure

In patients with STEMI early and complete reperfusion either with thrombolysis or primary percutaneous intervention reduces infarct size, preserves regional and global ventricular function, and reduces the incidence of heart failure (8,13,14). In general, if immediately available, primary percutaneous intervention should be preferred to thrombolysis.

General Measures

In the critically ill patient, therapeutic interventions must be started as soon as possible and must not be delayed by any diagnostic procedure other than obtaining an ECG, although early identification of correctable associated factors and causes that need a special therapeutic approach can be made at the same time as treatment is initiated (7,8). Any therapeutic effort may be useless without correction of ischemia, and contributing factors including anemia, arrhythmias, hypovolemia, and acidosis (8).

Myocardial Revascularization

Early reperfusion therapy plays a central role in the treatment of heart failure in the setting of ACS. In general, primary percutaneous coronary intervention (PCI) should be the preferred reperfusion strategy. However, except in patients with cardiogenic shock and younger that 75 years, there is no direct evidence that primary PCI is superior to thrombolysis in patients with acute ischemic heart failure, but the timely use of some reperfusion therapy is likely more important than the choice of reperfusion therapy (8).

After the first 12 hours of evolution of STEMI, myocardial revascularization should still be strongly considered in patients with cardiogenic shock (8,15) and in those with hemodynamic instability (8). Indirect but strong evidence supports an invasive strategy in patients with heart failure after acute coronary syndromes. In the Global Registry of Acute Coronary Events (GRACE) registry, in patients with heart failure after STEMI, non-STEMI, and unstable angina, myocardial revascularization was identified as a strong independent variable related with survival (2). In the InTime (intravenous nPA for treatment of infracting myocardium early) trial in patients with STEMI and thrombolytic therapy, coronary angiography and myocardial revascularization was also an independent predictor of survival (16) (Fig. 17.5). Similar observations were obtained in other registries and clinical trials in patients with ACS without ST elevation (17).

Treatment of Hemodynamic Alterations

Pharmacologic Treatment

The objectives of drug therapy in acute heart failure are to rapidly relieve symptoms, reverse hemodynamic derangement, and preserve myocardial blood flow. Inotropic and vasopressor therapy, venous and arterial vasodilators, and diuretics constitute the basic pharmacologic support in patients with acute heart failure. They are usually administered intravenously to allow for rapid titration of the hemodynamic effect, and they have a short plasma half-life so that any untoward effect can be quickly terminated. Table 17.2 and Figures 17.4 and 17.6 illustrate the appropriate indications for their use. However, it should be mentioned that an improvement in outcome has not been demonstrated with any of these drugs in acute heart failure secondary to ischemia or other etiologies (7,8).

Vasodilators

Venous dilation decreases the preload, thus reducing pulmonary congestion without major changes in cardiac output. Arterial dilation reduces afterload facilitating ventricular emptying and increasing cardiac output.

Nitroglycerin and other nitrates cause nonspecific relaxation of smooth muscle, decreasing right atrial and pulmonary pressures (9), and improving pulmonary congestion. High doses may induce hypotension. Nitrates can also produce coronary vasodilatation, as much through reducing preload as through a direct effect on the vascular endothelium. Nitroglycerin is effective in the treatment of symptoms of pulmonary congestion and edema (18). Sublingual nitroglycerin is highly effective, and can be given in repeated doses (0.4 mg) until

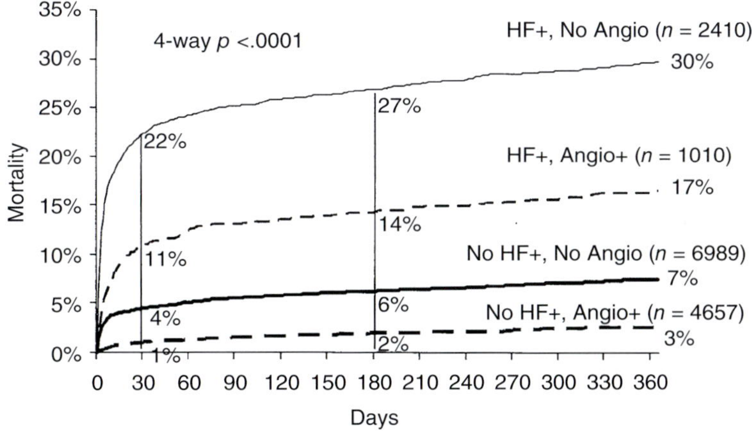

FIGURE 17.5. Short- and long-term mortality in patients with and without heart failure (HF) after myocardial infarction receiving fibrinolytics. Mortality is lower in the groups of patients with coronary arteriography. Revascularization treatment was NOT randomized in this study with coronary angiography (Angio +). (Data from the InTIME trial [16].)

TABLE 17.2. Common drugs in the treatment of patients with severe acute heart failure/shock

Drug	Effects	Indications	Dose	Secondary effects
Dopamine	Low dose: DA stimulant; vasodilatation	Oliguria	0.5–2 μg/kg/min	
	Medium dose: β-stimulant; + inotropy	Hypotension	2–5 μg/kg/min	Tachycardia
	High dose: α-stimulant; vasoconstrictor	Hypotension	5–20 μg/kg/min	Arrhythmias, ischemia
Dobutamine	β stimulant; + inotropy	Hypotension ↑ Cardiac output	1–20 μg/kg/min	Arrhythmias, less than dopamine Tachycardia
Noradrenaline	α and β stimulant vasoconstriction + inotropy	Severe hypotension Failure of dobutamine	0.01–0.1 μg/kg/min	Vasoconstriction Arrhythmias, tachycardia
Other + inotropic agents				
Milrinone	Phosphodiesterase inhibitor; + inotropy Venous and arterial vasodilator	Failure of dobutamine	0.5–1 μg/kg/min	Thrombocytopenia
Amrinone	Phosphodiesterase inhibitor; + inotropy	Failure of dobutamine	5–10 μg/kg/min	Thrombocytopenia
Digital	Venous and arterial vasodilator + inotropy; vagal stimulation	Atrial fibrillation	initial: 0.50 mg maintenance 0.25 mg/24h	AV block, arrhythmias
Vasodilators				
Nitroglycerin	Direct venous vasodilator Antiischemic	= ↑ blood pressure ↑ PCP	0.01–1 μg/kg/min	Hypotension
Nitroprusside	Direct arterial and venous vasodilator	myocardial ischemia = ↑↑ blood pressure ↑ PCP	0.1–5 μg/kg/min	Hypotension

PCP, pulmonary capillary pressure.

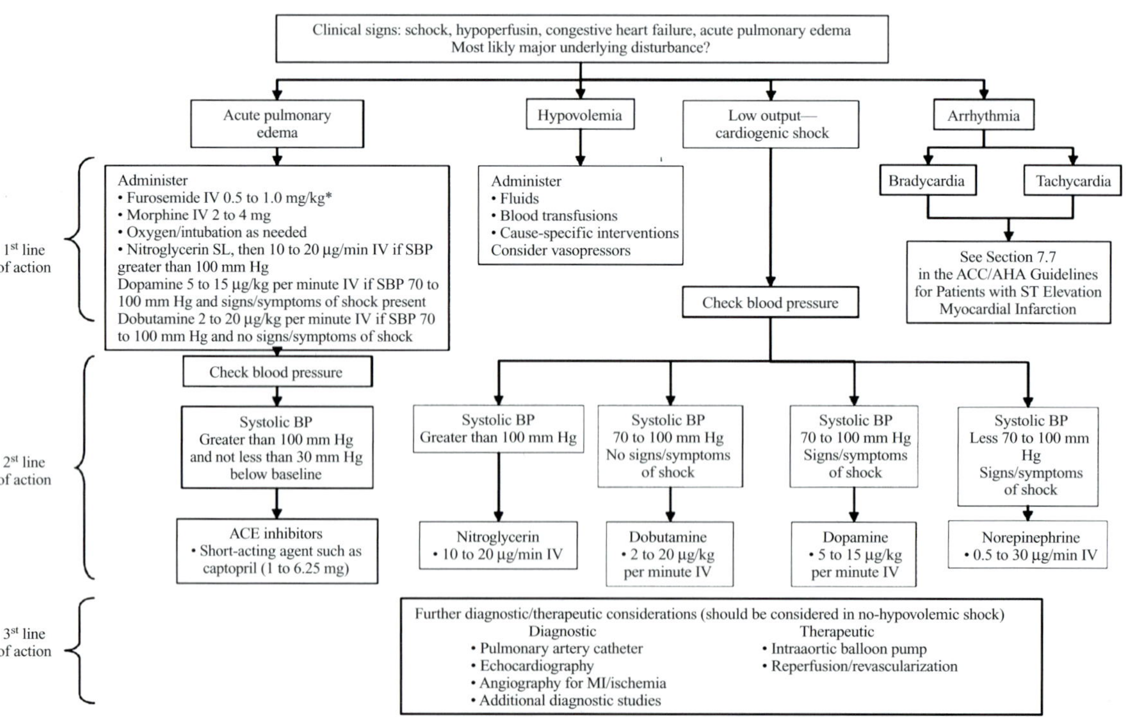

FIGURE 17.6. Management outline of heart failure complicating ST-elevation myocardial infarction. IV, intravenous; SL, sublingual; SBP, systolic BP; BP, blood pressure; ACE, angiotensin-converting enzyme; MI, myocardial infarction.

an intravenous [IV]) preparation is available to be infused. The initial dose of IV nitroglycerin should be low (0.1 μg/kg/min) and may be rapidly titrated upward by 0.1 to 0.2 μg/kg/min increments until congestive symptoms improve, ventricular filling pressures normalize, or the patient becomes hypotensive. Hypotension usually reverts rapidly once the infusion is reduced or stopped. Some patients may be resistant to nitroglycerin and yet others present pharmacodynamic tolerance during continuous IV infusions, necessitating an intermittent increase in dose to maintain the desired hemodynamic effect.

Nitroprusside

Nitroprusside is a powerful venous and arterial vasodilator that induces a reduction both in preload and afterload, with the corresponding decrease in pulmonary pressures and increase in cardiac output. Arterial blood pressure not necessarily decreases, although nitroprusside may have a very strong hypotensive effect. In the only randomized study in 812 men with heart failure after AMI, nitroprusside failed to demonstrate an improvement in outcome as compared with placebo, but it increased mortality at 13 weeks when administered within 9 hours of the onset of pain, although it decreased mortality when used later (19). However, the routine use of nitroprusside to treat heart failure in acute coronary syndromes is not recommended. Nitroprusside should be administered with caution and the optimal dose is quite variable and may vary with time. Therapy should be initiated at a low dose (e.g., 0.1 μg/kg/min) and progressively increased until the desired hemodynamic effect is achieved. Its hemodynamic effects are evident within seconds and are also usually reversible seconds after the infusion has been stopped, as nitroprusside is rapidly degraded. Care should be taken in avoiding sudden changes in the infusion rate (such as when flushing the system) or severe hypotension may occur. In cases of nitroprusside intolerance due to hypotension, the addition of a positive inotropic agent such as dobutamine is often advantageous and may allow for the continuation of nitroprusside. Such a combination may be used while stabilizing particularly severe, low-output heart failure. When systemic hypotension and poor peripheral perfusion are present at the outset, nitroprusside should be started only after initial treatment with dopamine or dobutamine in order to avoid hypotension.

Inotropic Therapy

Inotropic therapy may increase cardiac output and blood pressure, but no benefit in outcome was demonstrated.

Dobutamine

Dobutamine is a synthetic catecholamine that stimulates β_1-receptors in the myocardium and henceforth exerts a positive inotropic activity, improving the hemodynamics in patients with hypotension and systemic hypoperfusion (20). Dobutamine also exerts a mild α_1- and β_2-stimulation on the peripheral vasculature. Dobutamine increases stroke volume and cardiac output and slightly lowers pulmonary pressures. At high doses dobutamine increases blood pressure and heart rate and may induce arrhythmias and ischemia. In a meta-analysis of clinical trials comparing dobutamine or high-dose dopamine against placebo in patients with acute heart failure, inotropic therapy improved symptoms compared to control or placebo, but was associated with a small, nonsignificant increase in mortality (odds ratio [OR], 1.6; 95% confidence interval, 0.7–3.5) (21). Dobutamine is indicated in the presence of hypotension and symptoms of hypoperfusion and can safely be associated with vasodilators. Dobutamine is not indicated (and henceforth should not be used) in the presence of normal cardiac output and normal blood pressure, not to mention hypertension. It has a short half-life (<5 minutes), and the hemodynamic response is obtained within minutes. The initial dose can be progressively increased until the desired effect, mainly an increase in blood pressure, is obtained.

Milrinone and Amrinone

Milrinone and amrinone are phosphodiesterase inhibitors with direct inotropic and vasodilator properties (20), reducing right and left ventricular filling pressures and increasing cardiac output. However, milrinone may worsen preexisting hypotension. Milrinone was compared with placebo in 949 patients with acutely decompensated heart failure (22). No clinical benefit was observed with milrinone; symptoms and severity of heart failure through the study were identical in both treatment groups, treatment failure was less frequent in the placebo group, there was a trend toward higher mortality in patients receiving milrinone, and death or readmission at 60 days was identical. However, milrinone was associated with a higher incidence of hypotension, atrial fibrillation, and ventricular arrhythmias. Based on this single study, milrinone should not be recommended.

Levosimendan

Levosimendan is an inotropic agent with vasodilating properties. The main mechanism of action is through Ca^{2+} sensitization of the contractile proteins responsible for a positive inotropic action and smooth muscle K^+ channel opening responsible for peripheral vasodilation (23). The half-life is very long (80 hours). Levosimendan increases cardiac output, reduces pulmonary pressures, and may induce hypotension. Levosimendan has been compared with placebo and other inotropic agents in several randomized clinical trials (23–25). In the RUSSLAN trial (25) 504 patients with decompensated heart failure after AMI received one of four different doses of IV levosimendan or placebo. During the first 24 hours there was a significant, dose-related decrease in the combined risk of worsening heart failure or death in patients treated with levosimendan. At 14 days, overall mortality was lower in patients treated with levosimendan than in placebo recipients. In the SURVIVE trial (23), the first prospective randomized mortality trial comparing levosimendan with dobutamine in 1327 patients with severe acute heart failure of different etiologies, no differences were observed in mortality at 180 days (primary end point), although a trend of benefit for levosimendan was observed in the first days of evolution. Secondary effects were similar between groups. In the REVIVE trial levosimendan was compared with placebo in 600 patients with acute or acutely decompensated heart failure receiving stable doses of dobutamine, nesiritide, or nitroglycerin (23). Worsening heart failure was less frequent in the levosimendan group, but hypotension, atrial fibrillation, and ventricular arrhythmias were more frequent in the levosimendan group. No survival differences were observed at the prespecified time points of 31 and 90 days.

Levosimendan is indicated in patients with symptomatic low cardiac output heart failure secondary to cardiac systolic dysfunction without severe hypotension (7). Levosimendan is administered in IV infusion in doses ranging from 0.05 to 0.1 µg/kg/min, and the infusion should be continued for 6 to 24 hours.

Vasopressor Therapy

Vasopressor therapy may be considered in patients with hypotension.

Dopamine

Dopamine mediates its effects through activation of dopaminergic (DA) α and β receptors (20). At low doses (0.5 to 2 µg/kg/min) stimulates specific dopaminergic receptors located on vascular smooth muscle cells (mainly in renal and mesenteric vascular beds), inducing renal vasodilatation and increasing renal blood flow and diuresis. With doses up to 5 µg/kg/min, dopamine also stimulates myocardial β_1-receptors, inducing an inotropic and chronotropic effect. As the dose is progressively increased above 5 µg/kg/min, α_1- and α_2-receptors are activated, inducing vasoconstriction and elevation of blood pressure. As indicated previously, high doses of dopamine are not associated with a significant benefit in outcome as compared with placebo in patients with acute heart failure (21). Dopamine may be used in patients with low output and hypotension.

Norepinephrine

Norepinephrine is a potent α-adrenergic and β_1-agonist, and the main elicited hemodynamic response is vasoconstriction (20). Because of the frequent secondary effects (tachycardia, arrhythmias, and myocardial ischemia), norepinephrine use is mostly restricted to severe cases of hypotension when there is no response to dopamine and dobutamine (7). Starting dose is 0.01 µg/kg, which can be progressively increased until a minimal level of desired blood pressure is achieved.

Diuretics

Diuretics are indicated in patients with pulmonary congestion or edema. Diuretics (loop, thiazides, and potassium-sparing) eliminate Na^+ and water by acting directly on the kidney. Eliminating excessive lung water, diuretics decrease acute symptoms that result from pulmonary congestion or edema) (26). No clinical trials have been conducted to evaluate the impact of diuretic therapy on outcomes in patients with acute heart failure. Intravenous or oral furosemide is the loop diuretic most commonly used. The initial dose is 20 to 40 mg IV and it may be increased according to the obtained response. Excessive diuresis can result in hypotension and a decrease in cardiac output.

Drug Selection

The relative severity of pulmonary congestion, peripheral hypoperfusion, and blood pressure are the main determinants for drug selection (Fig. 17.4). When reduction of pulmonary congestion is the first goal of therapy, nitroglycerin, along with diuretics, is probably the first choice. Nitroprusside is a better choice if there is hypoperfusion and in the presence of severe mitral regurgitation or hypertension. On the other hand, the use of these drugs is very difficult in cases of hypotension, and when blood pressure is very low treatment is initiated with dobutamine or dopamine. Fluids are indicated in Forrester class III and if no satisfactory response is obtained, dopamine or dobutamine is the first drugs of choice.

Ventilatory Assistance

Endotracheal intubation is indicated in patients with hypoxemia that is not improving with oxygen therapy and noninvasive ventilatory support (7). Ventilatory support without endotracheal intubations improves oxygen saturation and tissue oxygenation. Two different techniques may be used: continuous positive airway pressure (CPAP) and noninvasive positive pressure ventilation (NIPPV). Both have been associated with a reduction in the need for endotracheal intubation in small randomized trials in patients with acute pulmonary edema, but the studies were too small to demonstrate an effect on mortality or an improvement in long-term outcomes (27,28).

Circulatory Support Devices

Circulatory support devices may dramatically improve hemodynamics, but their use is restricted to patients whose underlying condition may be corrected (e.g., coronary revascularization, candidates for heart transplant) or may recover spontaneously (e.g., myocardial stunning very early after AMI). Several new devices are readily available for use in the acute coronary or intensive care unit (7), but intraaortic balloon counterpulsation remains the only system for routine use in patients with ACS and heart failure.

Intraaortic Balloon Counterpulsation Pump

Synchronized intraaortic balloon counterpulsation (IABC) is performed, inflating and deflating a 30- to 50-mL balloon placed in the thoracic aorta through a femoral artery. The inflation of the balloon in diastole increases aortic diastolic pressure and coronary flow while the deflation during systole decreases afterload and facilitates left ventricular emptying (29). In many hospitals IABC has become a standard component of treatment in patients with cardiogenic shock or severe acute heart failure (6–8) that (1) does not respond rapidly to fluid administration and inotropic support; (2) is complicated by significant mitral regurgitation or rupture of the interventricular septum, to obtain hemodynamic stabilization for definitive treatment; (3) presents as recurrent chest pain or large myocardium at risk in preparation for coronary angiography and revascularization; or (4) presents as recurrent ventricular tachycardia. However, the hemodynamic improvement is not associated with a better survival if the underlying condition is not amenable to correction (revascularization) or spontaneous improvement (in patients with myocardial stunning after revascularization for acute ischemia) is not expected. Intraaortic balloon counterpulsation is contraindicated in patients with aortic dissection or significant aortic insufficiency.

Clinical Scenarios

Severe Pulmonary Congestions and Acute Pulmonary Edema

Acute pulmonary edema is the most severe form of dyspnea and is characterized by a rapid onset of symptoms with severe respiratory distress with orthopnea, crackles over the lungs, and O_2 saturation usually below 90%. Characteristic chest x-ray signs could be delayed and persist hours or days after clinical improvement. Pulmonary edema may be of noncardiogenic origin, as in patients with increased alveolar capillary permeability or decreased oncotic pressure (30). In patients with ACS, severe pulmonary congestion and acute pulmonary edema result from acute systolic or diastolic dysfunction, often associated with severe mitral regurgitation. Transient myocardial ischemia may produce dynamic mitral regurgitation and should be ruled out in all patients (31). Rupture of the interventricular septum should be also ruled out in the setting of AMI. Pulmonary edema in acute coronary syndromes presents a high mortality (20% to 40%) in spite of modern treatments, especially when associated with hypotension (32). Treatment includes adequate oxygenation and preload reduction with morphine, diuretics, and vasodilators to relieve pulmonary congestion. Fluids should be managed with care, as severe pulmonary congestion may be the result of excessive fluid loading. Mechanical ventilation should be considered in patients without a quick response to therapy and who have maintained their hypoxemia and respiratory distress. By this time, the complete evaluation of the patient would have offered information about the possible causes and precipitating factors, the correction of which is a major determinant of prognosis. Special therapeutic interventions such as IABC, revascularization in the presence of ischemia, and surgery in the presence of correctable lesions should be considered on an individual basis.

Severe Hypotension, Low-Output Syndrome, and Cardiogenic Shock

Severe hypotension can result from hypovolemia, arrhythmias, right or left ventricular failure, mechanical complications of AMI, vasodilating drugs, fibrinolysis, or superimposed complications, such as sepsis or pulmonary embolism. Volume loading is recommended as the initial therapeutic strategy in all patients without clinical evidence for volume overload. Persistent hypotension should be evaluated by echocardiography and eventually hemodynamic monitoring. Intraaortic vasopressor therapy and IABC should be considered in severely ill patients not responding to other interventions.

Cardiogenic shock is the most serious form of heart failure and is characterized by a severe decrease in global tissue perfusion (15). The clinical syndrome includes systolic blood pressure <90 mm Hg, or in hypertensive patients a decrease of 30%, signs of tissular hypoperfusion (e.g., lactic acidosis, depressed sensorium/agitation, diaphoresis, cyanosis, or urine output <20 mL/hour with low urinary Na^+). Hemodynamic monitoring provides indicators of cardiogenic shock: decreased cardiac output (CI <2 L/min/m^2) and increased PCP (>20 mm Hg) or hypovolemic shock (CI <2 L/min/m^2) and normal PCP. The primary cause of cardiogenic shock is loss of myocardial contractile function, but hypovolemia, pain, arrhythmias, rupture of the interventricular septum, severe mitral regurgitation, and tamponade may significantly contribute to the shock and must be quickly identified and corrected. Strictly speaking, cardiogenic shock refers to a primary loss of myocardial contractility, and all contributing factors should be excluded (7,8).

Treatment of shock should be individualized, and priority is given to the immediate correction of the aforementioned contributing factors. Early revascularization is recommended for all patients less than 75 years old who develop shock within 36 hours of AMI except when further support is considered futile (8,15). If revascularization is not possible fibrinolysis is indicated in patients with STEMI or left bundle branch block (LBBB). Echocardiography is indicated in all cases, and hemodynamic monitoring and IABC is recommended when there is not rapid improvement after initiation of treatment. Intravenous, brisk fluid administration is the first therapeutic measure in the absence of obvious evidence of pulmonary congestion. If there is not a quick and satisfactory hemodynamic and clinical response, IV administration of inotropic drugs should be started and an indwelling arterial cannula placed for continuous blood pressure monitoring. Hemodynamic monitoring allows a better titration of fluids as well as vasoactive drugs, and refractory heart failure with hypotension requires the simultaneous use of inotropics, fluids, diuretics, and vasodilators. An optimal PCP, associated with an increase of CI above 2.2 L/min/m^2, is around 18 to 20 mm Hg. Blood pressure should be maintained at levels associated with a satisfactory urine output.

Right Ventricular Infarction

In patients with inferior infarction, severe hypotension or shock may be secondary to right ventricular infarction (33). Right ventricular infarction can easily be diagnosed in the presence of ST segment elevation in right precordial leads, and echocardiography shows a dilated right ventricle with segmental contraction abnormalities (34,35). Interestingly, right ventricular dysfunction can be transient, improving after days or weeks (35,36), especially after successful reperfusion with thrombolysis or percutaneous coronary intervention (37). Ischemic right ventricular dysfunction has certain therapeutic implications. Fluid depletion and bradycardia are poorly tolerated. Accordingly, volume loading, temporal right ventricular, atrial or synchronous atrioventricular (AV) pacing, and administration of inotropic agents are the therapeutical measures considered as the initial treatment, although the response is not uniform in all patients (38,39). Dopamine or dobutamine should be used in the presence of hypotension and low output, and probably is more effective than in left ventricular dysfunction because nonnecrotic stunned myocardium is more common in acute ischemic right ventricular dysfunction (38,39). Vasodilators in patients with severe ischemic right ventricular dysfunction should be used with care but may be useful in biventricular failure and in some patients with active ischemia (38,39).

Severe Mitral Regurgitation

Mitral regurgitation is frequently found in echocardiographic studies after AMI. However, moderate or severe regurgitation is a rare complication of acute ischemia. The most frequent cause is ventricular dilatation secondary to left ventricular dysfunction and heart failure. Papillary muscle ischemia or necrosis with or without rupture is uncommon but can result in severe mitral regurgitation complicated with pulmonary edema or shock (40), and in these patients severe mitral regurgitation and rupture of the mitral subvalvular apparatus should be ruled out as soon as possible. Medical treatment should be directed to reduce afterload, but the use of vasodilators may be limited by hypotension. Intraaortic balloon counterpulsation is indicated in the absence of a quick response to therapy and in preparation for surgical revascularization.

With total rupture of a papillary muscle, medical treatment alone is associated with 75% mortality within the first 24 hours, and urgent cardiac surgical repair is indicated unless further support is considered futile because of the patient's comorbidity (8). Coronary revascularization should be considered at the same time as mitral valve surgery (8); conversely, mitral valve surgery, usually annuloplasty, should be undertaken at the same time as CABG for patients with ischemic mitral regurgitation (MR) greater than 2+ (41).

Interventricular Septal Rupture

Rupture of the ventricular septum complicates less than 1% of STEMI. This lethal complication should be suspected in the presence of a new systolic murmur. The diagnosis could be confirmed using several techniques, including the determination of an oximetric gradient at the level of the right ventricle, or the identification of a left to right shunt by angiography or Doppler echocardiography. In most patients, the direct identification of the septal defect is possible using imaging techniques (8). In the majority of the patients rupture of the ventricular septum is complicated with heart failure, often with pulmonary edema and shock. Medical therapy should be directed to afterload reduction; intraaortic balloon pumping is indicated except when surgical correction has been rejected. Urgent surgery should be considered for all patients unless further support is considered futile because of the patient's comorbidity. Surgical mortality is high but mortality may be as high as 90% in absence of surgery (15). Coronary revascularization should be undertaken at the same time as repair of the ventricular septal defect. Transcatheter closure with a septal occluding device still remains an experimental procedure.

Heart Rupture and Cardiac Tamponade

Rupture of the ventricular free wall of the left ventricle is a relatively frequent complication of STEMI, and its incidence has decreased in the reperfusion era (8). In the majority of the cases ventricular rupture is followed by electromechanical dissociation and sudden death. However, some patients survive hours or days after the initial episode of bleeding into the pericardial cavity. Diagnosis of ventricular wall rupture should be suspected in all patients with hypotension. Large pericardial effusions with echocardiographic signs indicative of cardiac tamponade (atrial and right ventricular wall compression) during the first 2 days of STEMI evolution are highly specific of ventricular rupture, but the number of false-positive findings increases in subsequent days of evolution (42,43). Cardiac tamponade may mimic cardiogenic shock, and in all patients with hypotension an echocardiogram should be performed to rule out this and other mechanical complications. Pericardiocentesis may be used to relieve severe, life-threatening cardiac tamponade before surgery, but patients with cardiac tamponade should be considered for urgent cardiac surgical repair that may be lifesaving (8,42,43).

Long-Term Treatment

In patients with ACS, secondary prevention should be initiated as soon as possible. In addition, in patients recovering from acute heart failure, oral treatment with angiotensin-converting enzyme (ACE) inhibitors or diuretics should be initiated soon, in order to weaning (reduce the dose, discontinue) IV vasoactive drugs. Also, in several studies, prehospital initiation of long-term heart failure therapy following the guidelines has been associated with a better clinical outcome (44), and prescription of ACE inhibitors or angiotensin receptor blockers, beta-blockers, and aldosterone antagonists must be considered in all patients (45–47).

Angiotensin-converting enzyme inhibitors should be initiated in patients with signs or symptoms of heart failure, even if transient, after AMI, to improve survival and to reduce reinfarctions and hospitalizations for heart failure. In AMI with signs of heart failure or left ventricular dysfunction, angiotensin receptors blockers and ACE inhibitors have similar or equivalent effects on mortality.

Beta-blockers are recommended to reduce mortality in all patients with left ventricular systolic dysfunction, with or without symptomatic heart failure, following AMI.

Aldosterone antagonists are recommended in addition to ACE inhibitors and beta-blockers in heart failure after AMI with left ventricular systolic dysfunction and signs of heart failure or diabetes to reduce mortality and morbidity.

Implantable cardiac defibrillator (ICD) implantation is reasonable in selected patients with a left ventricular ejection fraction <30% to 35%, who are not within 40 days of AMI, on an optimal background therapy including ACE inhibitor, beta-blockers, and an aldosterone antagonist, where appropriate, to reduce the risk of sudden death.

References

1. Goldberg RJ, Samad NA, Yarzebski J, Gurtwitz J, Bigelow C, Gore JM. Temporal trends in cardiogenic shock complicating acute myocardial infarction. N Engl J Med 1999;340:1162–1268.
2. Steg G, Dabbous OH, Feldman LJ, et al., for the GRACE Investigators. Determinants and prognostic impact of heart failure complicating acute coronary syndromes: Observations from the Global Registry of Acute Coronary Events (GRACE). Circulation 2004;109:494:499.
3. Brener SJ, Lincoff, A, Bates ER, for the GUSTO V Investigators. The relationship between baseline risk and mortality in ST-elevation acute myocardial infarction treated with pharmacological reperfusion: Insights from the Global Utilization of Strategies To open Occluded arteries (GUSTO) V trial. Am Heart J 2005;150:89–93.
4. Kashani A, Gibson M, Murphy SA, for the InTIME investigators. Angiography and revascularization in patients with heart failure following fibrinolytic therapy for ST-elevation acute myocardial infarction. Am J Cardiol 2005;95:228.
5. Sutton MGJ, Norman Sharpe N. Left ventricular remodeling after myocardial infarction pathophysiology and therapy. Circulation 2000;101:2981.
6. Mueller HS, Chatterjee K, Davis KB, et al. Present use of bedside right heart catheterization in patients with cardiac disease. ACC expert consensus document. J Am Coll Cardiol 1998;32:840–864.
7. Nieminen MN, Böhm M, Drexler H, et al. The Task Force on Acute Heart Failure of the European Society of Cardiology. Guidelines for the diagnosis and treatment of acute heart failure. Eur Heart J 2005;26:384–416.
8. Antman E, Amstrong PW, Bates ER, et al. ACC/AHA Guidelines for the Management of Patients UIT ST-Elevation Myocardial Infarction. A Report of the American College of Cardiology/American

Heart Association Task Force on Practice Guidelines (Committee to Revise the 1999 Guidelines for the Management of Patients With Acute Myocardial Infarction) Developed in Collaboration With the Canadian Cardiovascular Society. www.americanheart.org/.

9. Van de Werf F, Ardissino D, Betriu A, et al. For the task force on the management of acute myocardial infarction of the European Society of Cardiology Management of acute myocardial infarction in patients presenting with ST-segment elevation. Eur Heart J 2003;24:28–66.
10. Killip T, Kimball TJ. Treatment of myocardial infarction in a coronary care unit. A two year experience with 250 patients. Am J Cardiol 1967; 20:457–464.
11. Forrester JS, Diamond G, Swan HJC. Correlative classification of clinical and hemodynamic function after acute myocardial infarction. Am J Cardiol 1977;39:137.
12. Nohria A TS, Fang JC, Lewis EF, Jarcho JA, Mudge GH, Stevenson LW. Clinical Assessment identifies hemodynamic profiles that predict outcomes in patients admitted with heart failure. J Am Coll Cardiol 2003;41:1797–1804.
13. Ross AM, Coyne KS, Moreyra E, et al., for the GUSTO-I. Angiographic Investigators. Extended mortality benefit of early postinfarction reperfusion. Global Utilization of Streptokinase and Tissue Plasminogen Activator for Occluded Coronary Arteries Trial. Circulation 1998;97:1549–56.
14. Stone GW, Peterson MA, Lansky AJ, Dangas G, Mehran R, Leon MB. Impact of normalized myocardial perfusion after successful angioplasty in acute myocardial infarction. J Am Coll Cardiol 2002;39:591–597.
15. Hochman JS, Sleeper LA, White HD, et al., for the Should We Emergently Revascularize Occluded Coronaries for Cardiogenic Shock (SHOCK) Investigators. One-year survival following early revascularization for cardiogenic shock. JAMA 2001;285: 190–192.
16. Amir Kashani A, Gibson M, Murphy S, et al., for the InTime investigators. Angiography and revascularization in patients with heart failure following fibrinolytic therapy for ST-elevation acute myocardial infarction. Am J Cardiol 2005;95:228.
17. Gonçalves P de A, Ferreira J, Aguiar C, Seabra-Gomes R. TIMI, PURSUIT, and GRACE risk scores: sustained prognostic value and interaction with revascularization in NSTE-ACS. Eur Heart J 2005; 26:865–872.
18. Bussmann WD, Schupp D. Effects of sublingual nitroglycerin in emergency treatment of severe pulmonary oedema. Am J Cardiol 1978; 41:931–936.
19. Cohn JN, Franciosa JA, GS Francis GS, et al. Effect of short-term infusion of sodium nitroprusside on mortality rate in acute myocardial infarction complicated by left ventricular failure: results of a Veterans Administration cooperative study. N Engl J Med 1982;306:1129–1135.
20. Leier CV. Positive inotropic therapy: An update and new agents. Curr Probl Cardiol 1996; 21:521–581.
21. Thackray S, Easthaugh J, Freemantle N, et al. The effectiveness and relative effectiveness of intravenous inotropic drugs acting through the adrenergic pathway in patients with heart failure-a meta-regression analysis. Eur J Heart Fail 2002;4:515–529.
22. Gheorghiade M, Gattis WA, Klein L. OPTIME in CHF trial: rethinking the use of inotropes in the management of worsening chronic heart failure resulting in hospitalization. Eur J Heart Fail 2003;5:9–12.
23. De Luca L, Colucci WS, Nieminen MS, Barry M. Massie BM, Gheorghiade M. Evidence-based use of levosimendan in different clinical settings. Eur Heart J 2006;27:1908–1920. www:eurheartj.oxfordjournals.org.
24. Follath F, Cleland JG, Just H, et al. Efficacy and safety of intravenous levosimendan compared with dobutamine in severe low-output heart failure (the LIDO study): a randomised double-blind trial. Lancet 2002;360:196–202.
25. Moiseyev VS, Poder P, Andrejevs N, et al. Safety and efficacy of a novel calcium sensitizer, levosimendan, in patients with left ventricular failure due to an acute myocardial infarction. A randomized, placebo-controlled, double-blind study (RUSSLAN). Eur Heart J 2002;23(18):1422–1432.
26. Cody RJ. Clinical trials of diuretic therapy in heart failure: research directions and clinical considerations. J Am Coll Cardiol 1993;22(suppl A):165A–171A.
27. Kelly CA, Newby DE, McDonagh TA et al. Randomised controlled trial of continuous positive airway pressure and standard oxygen therapy in acute pulmonary oedema; effects on plasma brain natriuretic peptide concentrations. Eur Heart J 2002;23:1379–1386.
28. Masip J, Betbese AJ, Paez J et al. Non-invasive pressure support ventilation versus conventional oxygen therapy in acute cardiogenic pulmonary oedema: a randomised trial. Lancet 2000;356: 2126–2132.
29. López-Sendón J, López de Sa E. Acute left ventricular failure. In: Sharpe N, ed. Heart failure 2000. London: Martin Dunitz, 1999:165–182.
30. Colucci W, Braunwald E. Pathophysiology of heart failure. In: Braunwald E, ed. Heart Disease. A Text-

book on Cardiovascular Medicine. Philadelphia: WB Saunders, 1997;394–420.

31. Levine RA. Dynamic mitral regurgitation. More than meets the eye. N Engl J Med 2004;351:1681–1684.
32. Morrow DA, Antman EM, Charlesworth A, et al. TIMI risk score for ST-elevation myocardial infarction: a convenient, bedside, clinical score for risk assessment at presentation: an intravenous nPA for treatment of infarcting myocardium early II trial substudy. Circulation 2000;102:2031–2037.
33. López-Sendón J, Coma-Canella I, Gamallo C. Sensitivity and specificity of hemodynamic criteria in the diagnosis of acute right ventricular infarction. Circulation 1981;64:515–552.
34. López-Sendón J, Coma-Canella I, Alcasena M, Seoane J, Gamallo C. Electrocardiographic findings in acute right ventricular infarction. Sensitivity and specificity of electrocardiographic alterations in leads V4R, V3R, V1, V2, V3. J Am Coll Cardiol 1985;6:1273–1285.
35. López-Sendón J, García Fernandez MA, Coma-Canella I, Moreno Yangüela M, Bañuelos F. Segmental right ventricular function after acute myocardial infarction: Two-dimensional echocardiographic study in 63 patients. Am J Cardiol 1983;51:390–396.
36. López-Sendón J, Coma-Canella I, Gonzalez Maqueda I, Martín Jadraque L. Inverted interatrial septum convexity. A new echocardiographic alteration after right ventricular infarction. J Am Coll Cardiol 1990;15;801–805.
37. Zehender M, Kasper W, Kauder E, et al. Right ventricular infarction as an independent predictor of prognosis after acute inferior myocardial infarction. N Engl J Med 1993;328:981–988.
38. López-Sendón J, Coma-Canella I, Viñuelas Adanez J. Volume loading in patients with ischemic right ventricular dysfunction. Eur Heart J 1981;2:329–338.
39. López-Sendón J, López de Sá E, Delcán JL. Ischemic right ventricular dysfunction. Cardiovasc Drugs and Therap 1994;8:393–406.
40. Hochman JS, Buller CE, Sleeper LA, et al. Cardiogenic shock complicating acute myocardial infarction: etiologies, management and outcome: a report from the SHOCK Trial Registry. Should we emergently revascularize occluded coronaries for cardiogenic shock? J Am Coll Cardiol 2000;36:1063–1070.
41. Adams DH, Filsoufi F, Aklog L. Surgical treatment of the ischemic mitral valve. J Heart Valve Dis 2002;11:S21–S25.
42. López-Sendón J, Gonzalez A, Coma-Canella I, et al. Diagnosis of subacute ventricular wall rupture after acute myocardial infarction: sensitivity and specificity of clinical, hemodynamic and echocardiographic criteria. J Am Coll Cardiol 1992;19:1145–1153.
43. López-Sendón J, López de Sá E, García Fernandez MA, Moreno Yangüela M. Echocardiographic assessment of myocardial rupture to direct a successful repair. Cor Art Dis 1996;7:217–223.
44. Granger CB, Steg PG, Peterson E, et al., for the GRACE Investigators. Medication performance measures and mortality following acute coronary syndromes Am J Med 2005;118:858–865.
45. Swedberg K, Cleland J, Dargie H, et al. Guidelines for the diagnosis and treatment of chronic heart failure: executive summary (update 2005) The Task Force for the Diagnosis and Treatment of Chronic Heart Failure of the European Society of Cardiology. Eur Heart J 2005;26:1115–1140.
46. López-Sendón J, Swedberg K, McMurray J, et al. Expert consensus document on angiotensin converting enzyme inhibitors in cardiovascular disease. The task Force on ACE-inhibitors of the European Society of Cardiology. Eur Heart J 2004;25:1454–1470.
47. López-Sendón J, Swedberg K, McMurray J, et al. Expert consensus document on beta-adrenergic receptor blockers. The task Force on ACE-inhibitors of the European Society of Cardiology. European Society of Cardiology consensus statement. Eur Heart J 2004;25:1341–1362.

18
Acute Heart Failure and Myocarditis

Fredric Ginsberg and Joseph E. Parrillo

Myocarditis is defined as inflammation of heart muscle (1). The study of myocarditis has been made difficult by a number of factors. The clinical picture of myocarditis varies widely, from asymptomatic patients who suffer no long-term sequelae, to critically ill patients with heart failure and cardiogenic shock. Because of the variable clinical picture, a true incidence is difficult to determine. In addition, there are no standardized specific criteria for making the diagnosis of myocarditis or in determining an etiology in individual patients (2). Many different etiologic agents have been implicated in this disease. Also, there has been controversy regarding the most appropriate medical therapy for this condition.

On pathologic examination of myocardial biopsy specimens, or on autopsy series, myocarditis is usually apparent as infiltration of myocardium with lymphocytes and fibroblasts, accompanied by myocyte necrosis (myocytolysis) (2). Other types of inflammatory reactions can be seen less frequently, with giant cells, eosinophils, or granulomas. Myocarditis can also be associated with specific systemic illnesses (Table 18.1).

In most patients with myocarditis, a specific etiology is not found (3). It is presumed, however, that in North America and Europe the most common etiologic agent is viral (1). Enteroviruses, specifically Coxsackie B, are most commonly implicated. Other viruses have been associated with myocarditis, including adenoviruses, hepatitis C, influenza virus, human herpes virus 6, and parvovirus B (4). Myocarditis is a common finding in patients infected with human immunodeficiency virus (HIV); 20% to 45% of HIV-infected patients have pathologic evidence of myocarditis, which is clinically apparent in 10% (5). However, the causative agent responsible in these cases is more likely to be a secondary viral or other infectious agent occurring in these immunocompromised hosts, rather than HIV itself (1). Therapies given for HIV may also lead to myocarditis, and myocarditis occurring in HIV patients has a poorer prognosis than other types of myocarditis (6). Infectious illnesses such as Lyme disease, acute rheumatic fever, and diphtheria often have myocarditis as a prominent feature. In Central and South America, the most common cause of myocarditis is the protozoan *Trypanosoma cruzi,* the cause of Chagas' disease. Systemic diseases such as systemic lupus erythematosus, polymyositis, progressive systemic sclerosis, mixed connective tissue disease, thrombotic thrombocytopenic purpura, and sarcoidosis can be complicated by myocarditis, and myocarditis can be a feature of the infiltrative cardiomyopathies seen in hemochromatosis or amyloidosis (7). Lastly, myocarditis can be associated with doxorubicin cardiomyopathy, peripartum cardiomyopathy, or can be a manifestation of a hypersensitivity reaction to medications (1, 3, 7) (Table 18.2).

Unfortunately, it is difficult to make a rapid clinical diagnosis of a specific viral etiology of myocarditis. This usually requires the measurement of antiviral antibody titers in acute and convalescent phase sera. Viral cultures of tissue specimens are unreliable (3). The identification of viral genomes incorporated in myocyte DNA may specifically indicate a virus as the etiologic agent.

Table 18.1. Distinct forms of myocarditis

Active viral
Postviral (lymphocytic): common form of acute myocarditis
Hypersensitivity
Autoimmune
Infectious
Giant cell myocarditis

Source: Reprinted, with permission, from Haas (3).

The diagnosis of myocarditis is based on clinical presentation, evidence of myocardial dysfunction or heart failure on examination, and abnormalities on laboratory and cardiac imaging tests such as echocardiography and magnetic resonance imaging (MRI). Myocardial biopsy has been considered the "gold standard" for diagnosis of myocarditis, although there are controversies regarding its utility.

Pathogenesis

Based on observations of human myocarditis, as well as murine models of the disease caused by Coxsackie B3, the pathogenesis of viral myocarditis can be described in three stages. The first stage is initiated by viral infection and replication within myocytes. Viral proteases and activation of cytokines may produce myocyte damage and apoptosis (4). The presence of this viral replication phase is difficult to demonstrate clinically, as patients may be asymptomatic during this phase or may have only nonspecific viremic symptoms.

Table 18.2. Causes of myocarditis*

Infectious	Immune-mediated	Toxic myocarditis
Bacterial: brucella, ***Corynebacterium diphtheriae***, gonococcus, ***Haemophilus influenzae***, meningococcus, mycobacterium, ***Mycoplasma pneumoniae***, pneumococcus, salmonella, ***Serratin marcescens***, staphylococcus, ***Streptococcus pneumoniae***, ***S. pyogenes***, ***Treponema pallidum***, ***Tropheryma whippelii***, and ***Vibrio cholerae***	Allergens: acetazolamide, amitriptyline, cefaclor, colchicine, furosemide, isoniazid, lidocaine, methyldopa, penicillin, phenylbutazone, phenytoin, reserpine, streptomycin, tetanus toxoid, tetracycline, and thiazides	Drugs: amphetamines, **anthracyclines**, catecholamines, cocaine, cyclophosphamide, **ethanol**, fluorouracil, hemetine, interleukin-2, lithium, and trastuzumab
Spirocletal: borrelia and leptospira	Alloantigens: heart-transplant rejection	Heavy metals: copper, iron, and lead
Fungal: actinomyces, aspergillus, blastomyces, candida, coccidioides, cryptococcus, histoplasma, mucormycoses, nocardia, and sporothrix	Autoantigens: **Chagas' *disease***, ***Chlamydia pneumoniae***, Churg–Strauss syndrome, inflammatory bowel disease, giant cell myocarditis, insulin–dependent diabetes mellitus, Kawasaki's disease, myasthenia gravis, polymyositis, **sarcoidosis**, **scleroderma**, **systemic lupus erythematosus**, thyrotoxicosis, and Wegener's granulomatosis	Physical agents: electric shock, hyperpyrexia, and radiation
Protozoal: ***Toxoplasma gondii*** and ***Trypanosoma cruzi***		Miscellaneous: arsenic, azides, bee and wasp stings, carbon monoxide, inhalants, phosphorus, scorpion bites, snake bites, and spider bites
Parasitic: ascaris, ***Echinococcus granulosus***, ***Paragonimus westermani***, schistosoma, ***Taenia solium***, ***Trichinella spiralis***, visceral larva migrans, and ***Wuhbereria bancrofti***		
Rickettsial: ***Coxiella burnetii***, ***Rickettsia rickettsii***, and ***R. tsutsugamushi***		
Viral: **Coxsackievirus**, cytomegalovirus, dengue virus, echovirus, encephalomyocarditis, Epstein–Barr virus, hepatitis A virus, hepatitis C virus, herpes simplex virus, herpes zoster, **human immunodeficiency virus**, influenza A virus, influenza B virus, Junin virus, lymphocytic choriomeningitis, measles virus, mumps virus, parvovirus, poliovirus, rabies virus, respiratory syncytial virus, rubella virus, rubeola, vaccinia virus, varicella-zoster virus, variola virus, and yellow fever virus		

*The most common causes are shown in boldface type.
Source: Feldman and McNamara (1).

In addition, there is no rapid screening test to confirm viral infection.

The second stage involves human host immune activation. Stimulation of cellular immunity as well as humoral responses attenuate viral proliferation and can result in recovery from the illness. However, unabated immune activation can result in activated T cells targeting myocardial antigens that cross-react with viral peptides. This leads to release of cytokines such as tumor necrosis factor-α (TNF-α), interleukin-1, and interleukin-6, resulting in further myocyte damage (1, 4). Activation of CD4 cells, leading to clonal expansion of B cells and antibody production, plays a pathogenetic role (8). It is thought that this secondary immune response to viral infection plays a greater role in disease pathogenesis than the primary infection (4).

Evidence supporting these mechanisms includes the following: Myocardial biopsy with recombinant DNA techniques can detect viral genomes in 20% to 35% of patients. Tissue-specific autoantibodies have been detected in 25% to 73% of patients with evidence of myocarditis on biopsy, and inappropriate expression of the major histocompatibility complex can frequently be demonstrated on biopsy specimens (1). A viral genome has been identified on biopsy specimens in up to 38% of myocarditis patients (9) and 10% to 34% of idiopathic dilated cardiomyopathy patients. Elevated levels of inflammatory cytokines are detected in patients with active myocarditis.

Either persistent overactivation of cellular immune activity or incomplete clearing and persistent or recurrent viral replication and host response can lead to the third stage, the occurrence of significant myocardial damage. This in turn leads to left ventricular dilatation and remodeling, left ventricular systolic dysfunction, and manifestations of heart failure (4). These processes can then abate, with reduction in left ventricular size and improvement in left ventricular function, or can continue to progress with development of chronic dilated cardiomyopathy and chronic heart failure.

Activation of similar immune mechanisms have also been implicated in nonviral causes of myocarditis, such as Chagas' Disease, systemic lupus erythematosus, polymyositis, peripartum cardiomyopathy, and giant cell myocarditis. In eosinophilic myocarditis, activation of eosinophils with degranulation and subsequent myocyte damage is a major pathogenetic mechanism.

Clinical Presentation

The clinical presentation of myocarditis varies widely. Patients can be asymptomatic, as myocarditis can be found in 1% to 10% of autopsy specimens of young adults who had no history of cardiac illness. Myocarditis can be found at autopsy in up to 20% of cases of young and apparently healthy adults who die suddenly and unexpectedly (1, 3, 4).

Patients ill with myocarditis most often present with chest pain, fatigue, dyspnea, palpitations, or syncope. Chest pain may be pleuritic or may mimic the pain of angina or acute myocardial infarction. Frequently there have been recent symptoms of a viral infection, including fever, malaise, and arthralgias. Physical examination can show fever, tachycardia, and S_3 and S_4 gallop sounds. A pericardial rub may be heard, as one quarter of patients will have associated pericarditis. Signs of heart failure can be present, including pulmonary rales and wheezes, hepatomegaly, ascites, elevated jugular venous pulse, and peripheral edema. Murmurs of mitral regurgitation and tricuspid regurgitation may be heard. Infrequently, patients can present with a fulminant course, with severe acute heart failure, pulmonary edema, and cardiogenic shock with circulatory collapse (3, 10).

The differential diagnosis includes acute myocardial infarction, pericarditis, or chest pain from pulmonary causes such as pulmonary embolism or pneumonia. Generalized sepsis may also be a consideration.

Laboratory findings can include leukocytosis, eosinophilia, and an elevated erythrocyte sedimentation rate. Elevation of creatine phosphokinase (CPK) is a very insensitive marker and offers low predictive value for diagnosing myocarditis. Troponin T and troponin I are variably elevated, depending in part on the chronicity of the process (1). Recent data suggest that troponin T may be useful in diagnosing myocarditis. In one reported series, the sensitivity of troponin T elevation for the diagnosis of myocarditis was 53%, specificity was 94%, positive predictive value was 93%, and negative predictive value was 56% (11). Elevation of troponin T in patients suspected of having myocarditis reflects ongoing myocyte injury rather than recent completed infarction, as seen in patients with acute coronary syndromes. Rheumatologic serologic markers and HIV status should also be evaluated.

The 12-lead electrocardiogram (ECG) shows sinus tachycardia and ST segment and T-wave changes most often. T-wave inversion, diffuse ST-segment depression, and pathologic Q waves may be seen. Patients may present with chest pain and ST segment elevation in a picture mimicking acute myocardial infarction. Myocarditis should be suspected when ECG leads showing ST-segment elevation do not correspond to a coronary artery distribution or if the ST segment elevation on ECG does not correspond to the location of wall motion abnormalities seen on echocardiography (5). More severe cases of myocarditis can be associated with supraventricular or ventricular arrhythmias, conduction disturbances, and heart block (1).

Echocardiography is essential to diagnose and quantitate regional or global left ventricular wall motion abnormalities, left ventricular wall thickness, left ventricular and right ventricular size and function, and valvular regurgitation. In one series, patients with acute severe myocarditis had greater dilation of left ventricular cavities and lower ejection fractions, whereas patients with fulminant myocarditis had low ejection fractions, less severe cavity dilatation, and increased septal thickness, presumed due to more extensive myocardial edema (12).

Myocardial nuclear scintigraphy is frequently abnormal but is an insensitive test for the diagnosis of myocarditis. Combined thallium 201 with antimyosin antibody cardiac scanning was reported to be compatible with myocarditis in 82% of 45 patients who presented with acute myocardial infarction and normal coronary angiography (13). However, standard nuclear scanning is an insensitive method to diagnosis myocarditis.

Cardiac MRI (cardiac magnetic resonance, CMR) is currently being evaluated as a tool for diagnosing myocarditis as well as guiding endomyocardial biopsy. It can easily visualize all of the myocardium and can detect changes in tissue composition (14). Both early and late enhancement with gadolinium has been seen, likely related to the degree of inflammation and necrosis. In one study, global myocardial enhancement, late enhancement, or abnormal T2-weighted imaging were observed in cases of myocarditis. If any two were abnormal, the sensitivity, specificity and predictive accuracy were 76%, 95.5%, and 85%, respectively (15). Contrast-enhanced CMR was used to guide endomyocardial biopsy in cases of myocarditis based on clinical criteria (16). Myocardial contrast enhancement tended to be patchy, more prominent in the epicardium, and most frequently seen in the lateral free wall of the left ventricle in cases where enhancement was not global or diffuse. If endomyocardial biopsy sampling was taken from areas of enhancement, criteria for myocarditis were found in 90% of patients (19 of 21 patients), whereas biopsy was positive in only one of seven patients if biopsies were taken from areas that did not enhance (16).

Lastly, cardiac catheterization and coronary angiography are often necessary to exclude severe coronary artery disease as the etiology of chest pain, acute heart failure, and ECG and echocardiographic abnormalities.

Diagnosis

Myocarditis is a difficult diagnosis to make, as there are no specific clinical diagnostic criteria. Even though clinical and laboratory features of this illness, as described above, are insensitive and nonspecific (2), myocarditis remains a diagnosis made on clinical grounds. Percutaneous endomyocardial right ventricular biopsy is currently used to aid in the diagnosis of myocarditis and is considered the most definitive diagnostic technique.

Endomyocardial biopsy (EMB) specimens in patients with myocarditis may show infiltration with lymphocytes. The Dallas criteria have been accepted as the standard for histopathologic diagnosis. These criteria define myocarditis as the presence of an active inflammatory myocardial infiltrate, >5 lymphocytes per high power field, accompanied by myocytes necrosis. The term *borderline myocarditis* is defined as active inflammation without myocyte necrosis (8). However, having active or borderline myocarditis tends not to correlate with the clinical course or prognosis

(17). The degree of inflammation seen is variable, depending on the virulence of the causative agent, host factors, and timing of the biopsy in the course of the patient's illness.

Although EMB is useful for diagnostic purposes, there are several significant limitations. A high frequency of interobserver variation has been noted among pathologists in applying the Dallas criteria. Biopsies are not sensitive in diagnosing myocarditis as various series have reported positive biopsy results in only 10% to 67% of patients with myocarditis suspected on clinical grounds or in patients with the recent onset of idiopathic dilated cardiomyopathy. In addition, the presence of standard histopathologic criteria for myocarditis does not correlate well with the presence of viral genomes in biopsy specimens when assessed by molecular techniques. Important clinical variables that affect the sensitivity of EMB include the timing of the biopsy in relation to the course of the patient's illness, and the fact that the myocardial inflammation may be patchy with skip areas, or may predominantly involve the left ventricle, so that random right ventricular biopsies may miss affected myocardium (18). One postmortem analysis of myocarditis patients demonstrated that more than 17 biopsy samples were necessary in order to diagnosis myocarditis in 80% of cases (19).

Therefore, performing EMB earlier in a patient's clinical course, taking multiple biopsy specimens, and taking a biopsy of the left ventricle have been suggested as ways of improving the diagnostic yield of EMB. Biopsies should also be done in centers with a high volume of experience, with proven safety, and that have appropriate pathologic techniques available (18, 20). Lastly, it is important to emphasize that a negative biopsy does not preclude the diagnosis of myocarditis.

Advances in molecular biology techniques have resulted in assays that are sensitive for the detection of viral genome in myocardial biopsy specimens. In-situ hybridization allows visualization of viral genome at the cellular level. Polymerase chain reaction (PCR) allows for rapid detection of viral genome in patients with myocarditis (21). Evidence of viral pathogens may be detected in biopsy specimens that do not show evidence of myocarditis by standard criteria. One study showed evidence of viral genome in EMB specimens of 38% of 624 patients with myocarditis (10). Other studies have found that evidence for viral persistence in biopsy specimens is associated with a worse prognosis (19). Other analyses, such as immunohistochemistry technology to identify upregulated human leukocyte antigen (HLA) proteins may also offer improved diagnostic sensitivity and specificity. Thus, these techniques may establish a new standard for the diagnosis of myocarditis, augmenting or replacing the Dallas criteria (19).

Although EMB is an insensitive test with a number of problems, a positive biopsy has a high positive predictive value (7). Although some authors question the benefits of performing biopsy with standard staining techniques as a routine in suspected myocarditis cases, this remains the best test presently available. Endomyocardial biopsy should be strongly considered in cases of suspected myocarditis when pathology results will affect management decisions, especially in patients with acute refractory heart failure or continued clinical deterioration despite appropriate aggressive heart failure therapy. Biopsy should be considered in patients with worsening ventricular arrhythmias, heart block, or with suspected etiologies such as sarcoidosis, collagen vascular disease, infiltrative cardiomyopathy, giant cell myocarditis, or eosinophilic myocarditis (22) (Table 18.3). Endomyocardial biopsy should

Table 18.3. Indications for endomyocardial biopsy

Exclusion of potential common etiologies of dilated cardiomyopathy (familial, ischemic, alcohol, postpartum, cardiotoxic exposures) and the following:
Subacute or acute symptoms of heart failure refractory to standard management
Substantial worsening of EF despite optimized pharmacologic therapy
Development of hemodynamically significant arrhythmias, particularly progressive heart block and ventricular tachycardia
Heart failure with concurrent rash, fever, or peripheral eosinophilia
History of collagen vascular disease such as systemic lupus erythematosus, scleroderma, or polyarteritis nodosum
New-onset cardiomyopathy in the presence of known amyloidosis, sarcoidosis, or hemachromatosis
Suspicion for giant cell myocarditis (young age, new subacute heart failure, or progressive arrhythmia without apparent etiology)

EF, ejection fraction.
Source: Magnani and Dec (8).

Table 18.4. Comparison of efficacy of various diagnostic modalities for myocarditis

Diagnostic modality	Sensitivity range (%)	Specificity range (%)
ECG changes (AV block, Q, ST changes)	47	Unknown
Troponin	34	89
CK-MB	6	100
Antibodies to virus or myosin	25–32	40
Indium-111 antimyosin scintigraphy	85–91	34–53
Myocardial biopsy (Dallas criteria of pathology)	35–50	78–89
Myocardial biopsy (viral genome by PCR) (9)	38	80–100

The gold standard used in each modality consisted of clinical composites of presentation, natural history, and myocardial biopsy or autopsy.

AV atrioventricular; CK-MB, creatine kinase–myocardial band; ECG, electrocardiography; PCR, polymerase chain reaction.

Source: Liu and Yan (14).

always be performed prior to initiating immunosuppressive therapy. In summary, the diagnosis of myocarditis should take into account the clinical presentation, imaging studies, histopathology, and immunohistochemistry and PCR results of EMB (19) (Table 18.4).

Clinical Course and Prognosis

The clinical course and prognosis of acute myocarditis is quite variable. Patients who are asymptomatic, with self-limited disease, or who present with a flu-like illness, most often recover without complications. It is thought that some of these patients will progress to chronic dilated cardiomyopathy with manifestations of systolic heart failure (2), although a precise incidence is not known. The majority of patients who present with manifestations of myocarditis will improve. Patients with heart failure and left ventricular dysfunction experience spontaneous resolution of their illness in 6 to 12 months in up to 50% of cases, without long-term sequelae (23). This recovery is more likely to occur in patients with less severe reductions in left ventricular systolic function. In one series of 112 patients seen at a tertiary medical center, overall 1-year survival was 79% and 5-year survival was 56%. This reflects a patient population with more severe manifestations of the disease, evaluated at a referral center. Elevated pulmonary capillary wedge pressure (PCWP) at presentation, prolonged QRS duration >0.120 ms, and left ventricular ejection fraction <40% were the only predictors of mortality in a multivariate analysis (24). Other reports indicate a 4-year survival of 87% in patients without heart failure, but a 4-year survival of only 54% in patients with heart failure (23). In addition, a significant percentage of young, apparently healthy, adults who die suddenly are found to have myocarditis at autopsy, suggesting that patients even with apparently mild illness can suffer fatal arrhythmias.

Another series of 21 patients with active myocarditis on biopsy was analyzed for predictors of disease course. In this series there was a 37% in-hospital mortality rate, with death occurring at 27.6 ± 6.9 days. Factors predicting a worse prognosis in this series included hypotension, higher PCWP, and use of mechanical ventilation. Factors that were not predictive of mortality included sex, age, heart rate, cardiac index, peak CPK, or the use of the intraaortic balloon pump for circulatory support (25).

Patients with heart failure and myocarditis can recover normal left ventricular function or can progress to chronic dilated cardiomyopathy; 15% to 25% of patients who present with new-onset dilated cardiomyopathy have evidence of antecedent myocarditis (2). In patients with myocarditis, severe heart failure, and ejection fractions of <35%, roughly one quarter will improve, one half will develop chronic cardiomyopathy and heart failure, and one quarter will deteriorate and may be candidates for cardiac transplantation (5). It is always important to examine the characteristics of the patient population under study and the criteria used for diagnosing myocarditis in any series assessing prognosis and mortality. No clinical markers reliably predict which patients with myocarditis are more likely to recover or worsen.

Fulminant Myocarditis

A small percentage of patients with acute myocarditis present critically ill with acute severe heart failure and cardiogenic shock. This presentation, termed fulminant myocarditis, is important to recognize because although these patients are critically ill, they very often demonstrate recovery of left ventricular function after a period of aggressive therapy and hemodynamic support. Most often these patients give a history of recent onset of symptoms, with fever and other symptoms of a viral illness, and with a distinct time of onset of heart failure symptoms. This presentation can be contrasted with those patients with active myocarditis who have heart failure but not cardiogenic shock, who demonstrate a less distinct time of onset of heart failure symptoms and less severe circulatory compromise.

In a study of 147 patients presenting with heart failure due to biopsy positive active myocarditis, with ejection fraction <40%, 10% of these patients were thought to have fulminant myocarditis. The patients with fulminant myocarditis needed hemodynamic support with high-dose vasopressor therapy or left ventricular assist devices (LVADs). The acute myocarditis patients had more stable hemodynamics, and did not require vasopressors, or received them at low doses. Patients with fulminant myocarditis tended to be younger and have higher heart rates and lower systemic blood pressure. There was no difference between the groups in mean capillary wedge pressure or cardiac index. With aggressive treatment, patients with fulminant myocarditis actually had better survival, 93% at 1 year and 93% at 11 years. Patients with acute but not fulminant myocarditis had a worse prognosis, with 1-year survival of 85% and 11-year survival of 45%. Patients with lower PCWP or higher cardiac index at presentation also had better survival (10).

In another series, patients with fulminant myocarditis had improvement of left ventricular ejection fraction to normal in 57% of cases at 6 months, whereas of patients with acute myocarditis, only 20% had improvement of ejection fraction to normal (12).

Thus, it is thought that fulminant myocarditis has a distinct clinical course, with critical illness at presentation but with excellent long-term survival once patients recover from the acute phase of their illness. Healing of myocardial injury and significant improvement of left ventricular systolic function can be expected. Therefore, a very aggressive approach to therapy is warranted, including the use of ventricular assist devices or other mechanical assist devices, without resorting to early cardiac transplantation (10) (Fig. 18.1).

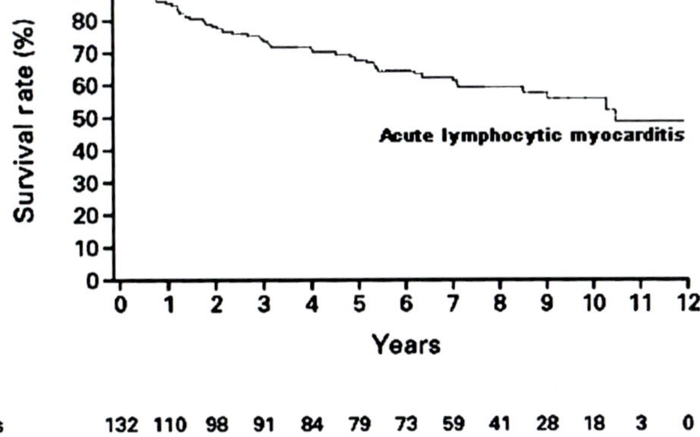

No. at risk													
Acute myocarditis	132	110	98	91	84	79	73	59	41	28	18	3	0
Fulminant myocarditis	15	12	12	10	10	9	7	5	4	3	2	0	0

Figure 18.1. Unadjusted transplantation-free survival according to clinicopathologic classification. Patients with fulminant myocarditis were significantly less likely to die or require heart transplantation during follow-up than were patients with acute myocarditis ($p = .05$ by the log-rank test). (Reprinted, with permission, from McCarthy et al. [10].)

Giant Cell Myocarditis

Giant cell myocarditis is a distinct form of myocarditis, generally with a rapidly progressive course, without significant likelihood of spontaneous resolution. On endomyocardial biopsy, infiltration with inflammatory giant cells is seen. Although the pathogenesis is not clear, it is thought to be an autoimmune disorder, and CD4 T-lymphocytes are thought to play an important role. A total of 63 patients with biopsy confirmed giant cell myocarditis were studied retrospectively (26). Heart failure was the presentation in 75% of cases, 14% presented with ventricular arrhythmias, and 11% presented with chest pain, an abnormal ECG, or heart block. There was an association with inflammatory bowel disease in 8% of cases. Survival was poor, with a median time of 5.5 months to death or cardiac transplantation (Fig. 18.2). In this uncontrolled series, immunosuppressive therapy was associated with prolonged survival from 3 months in 30 patients not given immunosuppressives and 3.8 months in patients treated with prednisone, to 11.5 months in patients given prednisone plus azathioprine and 12.6 months in patients who were given cyclosporine as part of their regimen. Prognosis after cardiac transplantation was also worse when compared with other forms of heart disease, with a 30-day mortality of 15%, and a 26% mortality during the 3.7-year posttransplant follow-up. Twenty-six percent of patients have giant cell infiltrates seen in their transplanted heart at an average time of 3 years posttransplant.

Eosinophilic Myocarditis

Eosinophilic myocarditis, sometimes termed hypersensitivity myocarditis, is a rare form of myocarditis characterized by eosinophilic infiltration and degranulation seen on endomyocardial

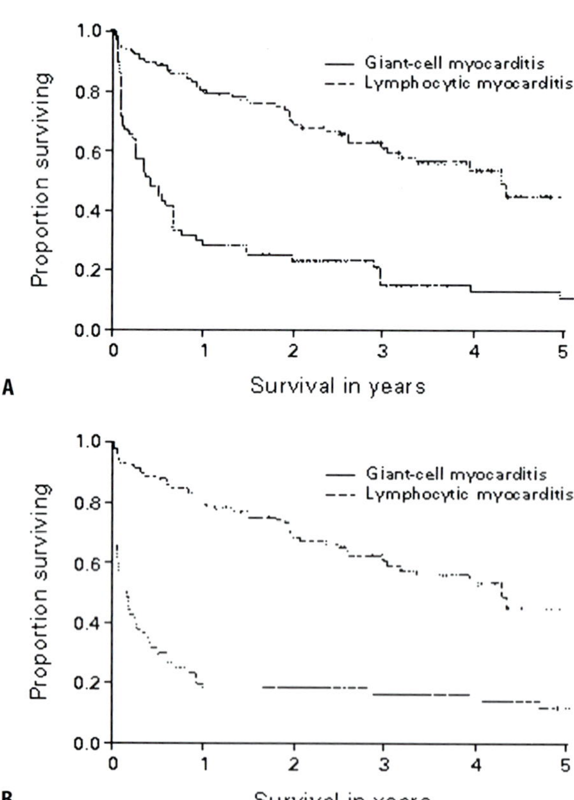

FIGURE 18.2. Line graphs showing the Kaplan–Meier survival curves for patients with giant cell myocarditis and lymphocytic myocarditis from the onset of symptoms (A) and from time of presentation to the referring center (B). In each case, survival was significantly shorter among those with giant-cell myocarditis. (From Cooper et al. [26].)

biopsy. It is thought that pathogenesis involves a direct role of eosinophil-mediated myocyte damage. There can be associated coronary arteritis. This entity is distinct from eosinophilic endocarditis (Loffler's endocarditis). The clinical manifestations are not specific, aside from a high incidence of eosinophilia in peripheral blood. Patients usually present with heart failure due to left ventricular systolic dysfunction. Fever and rash may be present. Untreated, the disease is often rapidly fatal (27).

The etiology is thought to be a hypersensitivity reaction, usually to medication or rarely in association with parasitic infections. Drugs most often implicated are sulfonamides, diuretics, angiotensin-converting enzyme (ACE) inhibitors, cephalosporins, digoxin, or dobutamine (27). Eosinophilic myocarditis has been reported to occur weeks after smallpox vaccination, with an incidence of 1 in 16,000 vaccinated (28). The clinical course is unfavorable, often with rapidly worsening heart failure and sudden death due to ventricular arrhythmia. Treatment involves the discontinuation of all potentially offending medications and the use of high-dose corticosteroids. Excellent responses to corticosteroids, as well as some spontaneously resolving illness, have been reported (29, 30).

Eosinophilic myocardial infiltration has been reported in 2% to 7% of myocardial biopsy specimens of patients awaiting cardiac transplantation, or in the explanted heart posttransplant. The etiology is unclear, and dobutamine therapy, sodium bisulfate used as a preservative in dobutamine solutions, or the use of LVADs has been implicated. The presence of eosinophilic myocarditis in this setting did not have an adverse affect on posttransplant survival and did not recur in the transplanted heart (31, 32).

Relation Between Myocarditis and Idiopathic Dilated Cardiomyopathy

There are much data from animal models indicating that acute myocarditis often leads to chronic idiopathic dilated cardiomyopathy (DCM). An important question in humans is the incidence of unrecognized antecedent myocarditis in patients who present with heart failure and idiopathic DCM. The frequency of myocarditis as the etiology of DCM is unknown, as it is difficult to identify subclinical episodes of myocarditis that may have preceded the presentation of DCM. The relevance of immune-mediated mechanisms in the pathogenesis of DCM also needs to be defined. Polymerase chain reaction (PCR) has been used to identify EMB specimens for the presence of viral genomes, which have been found in 20% of patients with DCM in one series (9). Adenovirus and enterovirus were most commonly found. In another series, 245 patients with DCM, without Dallas criteria for myocarditis on EMB, showed evidence for viral genome by PCR in 67.4% of cases (33). Parvovirus B, human herpes virus-6, and enteroviruses were most common, with multiple viral genomes found in 27%. This high prevalence of viral genome in cardiac tissue of patients with DCM strongly suggests that viral infection and unrecognized myocarditis play roles in the pathogenesis of many cases of DCM.

In another series, 172 patients with DCM and no evidence of myocarditis on routine histopathology had viral genomes detected on biopsy at a mean time of 5 months after symptom onset. Six months after the initial biopsy, repeat EMB showed clearance of viral genome in 36% of patients who had a single viral genome detected initially, and clearance of one of two genomes in 43% with dual infections. This had prognostic significance, as patients who cleared viral genome had significant improvement in left ventricular ejection fraction at 6 months, whereas patients who did not showed no improvement (34).

Circulating autoantibodies to myocyte proteins and myocyte surface receptors have also been described in patients with DCM (35, 36), although these have also been described in a small number of patients (5%) with ischemic cardiomyopathy. It is possible that these antibodies may be a secondary phenomenon and do not necessarily indicate a primary pathogenetic role of antibody-mediated injury.

General Management of Heart Failure

The management of myocarditis is based on the clinical presentation. Patients with mild disease can be treated expectantly, with dietary sodium restriction, and avoidance of strenuous exercise for several weeks or months (2). Animal models indicate that strenuous exercise can worsen myocarditis. Elimination of unnecessary medications is important in patients with eosinophilia.

Nonsteroidal antiinflammatory drugs should be avoided as they may worsen myocarditis (6). The routine use of anticoagulants for prophylaxis of systemic emboli is controversial. Patients who present with symptoms of arrhythmia or heart failure should be hospitalized, with continuous cardiac rhythm monitoring performed for evaluation of possibly serious or life-threatening arrhythmias or conduction abnormalities. If these are diagnosed, they are treated in a similar matter as in patients with other etiologies of heart disease, utilizing antiarrhythmic drugs or pacemakers. However, patients should be observed over a period of time to see if improvement or resolu-tion of the disease takes place prior to implantation of an implantable cardioverter-defibrillator (ICD).

There are no controlled trials in humans that have evaluated standard heart failure medications in patients with myocarditis. However, there are data in murine models of myocarditis supporting the use of captopril (2). There is a large amount of data in humans supporting the use of ACE inhibitors, angiotensin-receptor blockers, beta-blockers, and aldosterone antagonists in patients with dilated cardiomyopathy and heart failure. Since myocarditis often causes left ventricular systolic dysfunction and heart failure, the use of standard multidrug medical therapy for heart failure is indicated (2, 8). These medications have been shown to improve symptoms, prolong life, and cause regression of the adverse left ventricular remodeling, which occurs in patients with dilated cardiomyopathy of various etiologies such as coronary artery disease, hypertension, and idiopathic dilated cardiomyopathy.

Angiotensin-converting enzyme inhibitors (ACEIs) should be initiated in all patients with left ventricular systolic dysfunction (37–39). Treatment should begin at low doses, with upward titration to maximally tolerated doses. Patients should be closely monitored for potential side effects, including renal insufficiency, hyperkalemia, and angioedema. Relative contraindications to the use of ACEIs include renal failure, hyperkalemia, bilateral renal artery stenosis, and hepatic failure. Patients with hypotension should be treated with parenteral vasopressors or circulatory assist devices prior to initiation of low-dose ACEI therapy.

β-adrenergic blockers have not been studied in humans with myocarditis, and their effects in the murine model have been mixed (2). Nevertheless, beta-blocker therapy in large series of patients, which included patients with idiopathic dilated cardiomyopathy, have unequivocally shown benefit in patients with left ventricular systolic dysfunction (40–44), and these agents should also be used in patients with heart failure due to myocarditis. Beta-blockers should be initiated after patients are on a stable dose of ACE inhibitors, and when signs of fluid overload have resolved. Contraindications to beta-blocker therapy include bronchospastic disease or severe chronic obstructive lung disease, heart block, or significant underlying bradycardia. Hypotension should be corrected prior to initiating beta-blockers.

Digoxin has been shown in animal models to decrease levels of cytokines, but digoxin was associated with adverse outcomes in one murine model of myocarditis. Digoxin can be useful in helping to control ventricular rates in patients with atrial fibrillation. The use of digoxin should be considered in patients with significant left ventricular systolic dysfunction, after ACEIs and beta-blockers have been initiated. However, no mortality benefit for digoxin has ever been shown in patients with heart failure due to dilated cardiomyopathy (45). Contraindications to the use of digoxin include renal failure or heart block.

Lastly, the use of the aldosterone antagonist spironolactone has been shown to have symptomatic and survival benefit in patients with class III to IV systolic heart failure (46). In experimental models, these agents can reverse the progressive myocardial fibrosis that occurs in the remodeling process of dilated cardiomyopathy. These agents have not been studied in patients with myocarditis, but their use should be strongly considered in patients with severe left ventricular dysfunction (ejection fraction <35%) and symptomatic heart failure (2). Contraindications to the use of aldosterone antagonists include renal insufficiency, with serum creatinine levels above 2.0 mg/dL, or hyperkalemia. Serum potassium levels needs to be carefully monitored during initiation and dose titration.

In critically ill patients with severe heart failure and low cardiac index, parenteral vasodilators should be used. Intravenous nitroprusside is a powerful venous and arterial dilator, which significantly reduces systemic vascular resistance, mean systemic arterial pressure, and pulmonary capillary wedge pressure, raising cardiac index. It must be administered in the intensive care unit (ICU) with invasive hemodynamic monitoring with a pulmonary artery catheter, in order to best gauge the appropriate dose of medication and to accurately assess response to therapy. Prolonged use of nitroprusside is associated with accumulation of the toxic metabolites thiocyanate and cyanide, and serum levels of these compounds must be monitored. Intravenous nitroglycerin is also an effective vasodilator and coronary vasodilator, with less arterial dilating property than nitroprusside. The use of nitroglycerin in myocarditis has not been studied. Patients often develop tolerance to this drug (47–49).

Patients with severe myocarditis may develop cardiogenic shock, with hypotension, respiratory failure, and signs of end-organ hypoperfusion. In these instances, initial treatment with inotropic agents or vasopressors is indicated. Dobutamine is a potent β_1-agonist with less β_2- and α-agonist properties. Dobutamine has favorable short-term hemodynamic effects with increased myocardial contractility and reduced systemic vascular resistance and reduced pulmonary capillary wedge pressure. However, dobutamine can be proarrhythmic, and patients can develop tolerance to the drug. Long-term mortality can actually be worsened by courses of intravenous dobutamine therapy in patients with ischemic dilated cardiomyopathy (50).

Milrinone is another parenteral inotropic agent that works by inhibiting phosphodiesterase. This drug leads to increased inotropy and decreased systemic vascular resistance and pulmonary capillary wedge pressure, with resultant increased stroke volume and cardiac index. Milrinone may cause hypotension. It is less proarrhythmic than dobutamine and it does not induce tolerance (51, 52).

Arterial vasoconstrictors such as norepinephrine and dopamine can be used in patients with refractory hypotension for short-term urgent blood pressure support. However, these agents cause increased myocardial oxygen consumption and can have deleterious effects on myocardial function.

In patients with fulminant myocarditis or cardiogenic shock, the use of mechanical ventricular assist devices should be strongly considered. These devices offer hemodynamic support and left ventricular afterload reduction and may provide time for spontaneous improvement or recovery of normal left ventricular function. Ventricular assist devices (VADs) are mechanical pumps that take over the function of the failing ventricle, providing normal cardiac output. They are usually univentricular but can be biventricular, supporting both right and left ventricular function. They have been inserted via a mid-line sternotomy, with the inflow conduit to the pump inserted via the left ventricular apex. With improved technology, these devices are being made smaller, and are being implanted through smaller incisions. Newer VADs can be inserted percutaneously. Ventricular assist devices are connected to an external power pack via a drive line through the skin. The power pack is now small enough that it can be portable and thus patients have freedom of movement and can participate in rehabilitation efforts during VAD use. Current devices have textured blood-contacting surfaces so routine anticoagulation therapy is not required. Complications of VADs include local site infection, sepsis, thromboemboli, right ventricular failure, and device failure (53, 54).

In patients with myocarditis, VADs can be used to provide circulatory needs and improve coronary flow during the time necessary for spontaneous resolution of myocarditis to occur. Beneficial reverse remodeling may occur while patients are on VAD support, resulting in improved myocyte structure and function. Ventricular assist devices can provide support for months or even years.

A retrospective study analyzed 22 patients with nonischemic cardiomyopathy who were successfully weaned from left ventricular or biventricular assist devices (55). Patients had either myocarditis or idiopathic dilated cardiomyopathy. The average age of patients was 32 years, and the average duration of VAD support was 57 days (range, 12 to 190 days). Twenty of 22 patients were discharged alive with their native heart, at an average of 22 days after VAD removal. Two patients received cardiac transplants 1 year after VAD removal. Seventeen of these 22 patients remained alive and well with their native hearts at an average of 3.2 years after VAD removal. Sixteen patients were functional class I and one was functional class II. Thus, the survival of native hearts in this series after being weaned successfully from VAD support was 86% at 1 year and 77% at 5 years. This survival was indistinguishable from the survival of patients who received cardiac transplantation after a period of VAD support. These authors thus thought that patients with fulminant myocarditis should be given every opportunity to recover ventricular function, and that cardiac transplantation should be used only as a last resort, when severe heart damage is irreversible (55).

In another series, 6.5% of all adults implanted with VAD recovered left ventricular function so that the device could be removed. The most common underlying diagnoses in this group were myocarditis and peripartum cardiomyopathy (56).

There are several unresolved issues regarding VAD usage in patients with myocarditis. These include appropriate patient selection, the timing of VAD placement, the best medical therapy during VAD support, and the optimal duration of VAD support. A 50-day course of VAD support in the above study allowed identification of 50% of those patients who ultimately recovered, and a 90-day course identified 80% of patients who recovered (55). The optimal means of serial assessment of native heart function while on VAD support needs to be delineated, and the best weaning protocol also needs definition.

Cardiac transplantation is the final option for treating critically ill patients with myocarditis. However, these patients have a higher rate of transplant rejection, and a lower survival when compared with patients transplanted for ischemic or other etiologies of cardiomyopathy. Myocarditis has been reported to recur in the transplanted heart (10) (Fig. 18.3).

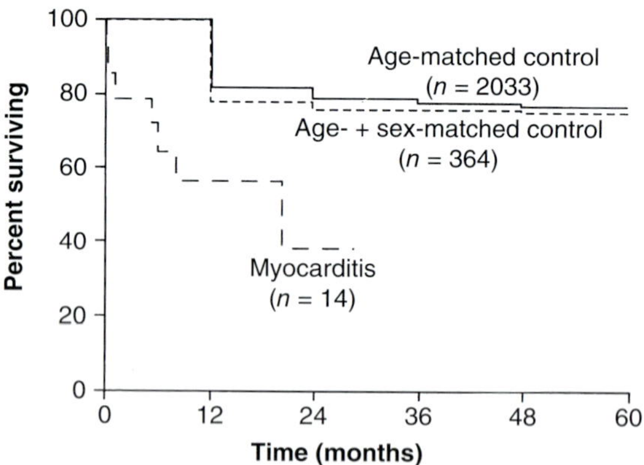

FIGURE 18.3. Graph showing the actuarial survival duration of heart transplant recipients with active lymphocytic myocarditis (– – –) as compared with that of age-matched (—) and age- and sex-matched (- - -) control patients. (Reprinted, with permission, from Haas [3].)

Immunosuppressive Therapy

Immune mechanisms are thought to be responsible for the clinical manifestations of myocarditis and the development of myocardial necrosis and left ventricular dysfunction. Therefore, therapy with immunosuppressive drugs has been used. However, given the high rate of spontaneous recovery of left ventricular function (up to 40% of patients in some series), small trials are limited in their ability to demonstrate significant improvement with therapies (8), and placebo-controlled trials are essential to properly evaluate effects of therapy. In addition, heterogeneous patient populations, consisting of both acute myocarditis and chronic dilated cardiomyopathy patients, have made it difficult to evaluate effective immunosuppressive regimens.

High-dose daily prednisone therapy was used for a 3-month course in 102 patients with dilated cardiomyopathy, 59% of whom were classified as having "reactive" myocarditis on endomyocardial biopsy (57). The authors found a significant improvement in left ventricular ejection fraction at 3 months in treated patients with reactive myocarditis, but this improvement was not sustained at 9 months using alternate-day prednisone maintenance therapy. Improvement did not occur in nonreactive patients. No significant mortality benefit from immunosuppressive treatment was noted, although this was not a prespecified primary end point (Fig. 18.4).

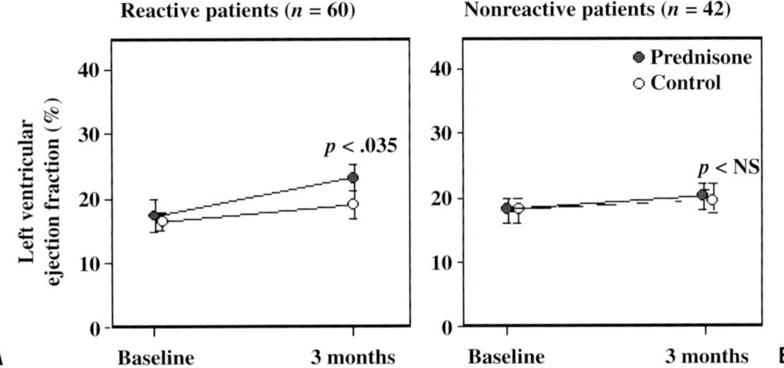

FIGURE 18.4. (A) Ejection fraction in reactive dilated cardiomyopathy (CMP) patients at 3 months. (B) Prednisone does not change ejection fraction in nonreactive patients in 3 months. (From Parrillo et al. [57].)

The Myocarditis Treatment Trial enrolled 111 patients with a positive endomyocardial biopsy and left ventricular ejection fraction <45%, with a duration of illness under 2 years (58). Three treatment groups were compared: daily prednisone plus azathioprine, prednisone plus cyclosporine, and placebo. Overall these patients had a 20% 1-year mortality and 56% 3-year mortality. These investigators found no difference in ejection fraction at week 28 or week 52, no change in left ventricular size at week 28, and no difference in 1-year mortality between treated and untreated groups. Their conclusion was that these immunosuppressive strategies were not beneficial. Significant limitations of this study include a 30% dropout rate, and significant intraobserver variability among pathologists' diagnoses of biopsy specimens despite utilizing the Dallas criteria (Fig. 18.5).

In view of the limitations of histopathologic diagnosis using the Dallas criteria, another group of investigators utilized immunohistologic markers of inflammation, for example upregulation of HLA, to diagnose active myocarditis as an indication for immunosuppressive therapy (59). This criterion has the advantage of indicating that autoimmunity is playing a role in pathogenesis. Also, since HLA is distributed throughout the entire myocardium, biopsy sampling error is eliminated as a confounding variable in assessing response to therapy. In this study, 94 of 202 patients with chronic (<6 months) idiopathic DCM (ejection fraction <40%) were found to have strong expression of HLA in biopsy specimens, and were randomized to receive placebo or prednisone plus azathioprine for 3 months. At 3-month follow-up, a significant improvement in the prespecified secondary end points of left ventricular ejection fraction, left ventricular volumes, and functional capacity was seen in the treated group, and this improvement was maintained at 2 years (71.8% improvement in treated group vs. 30.8% in nontreated group). However, there was no improvement in the prespecified composite primary end point of death, cardiac transplant, or

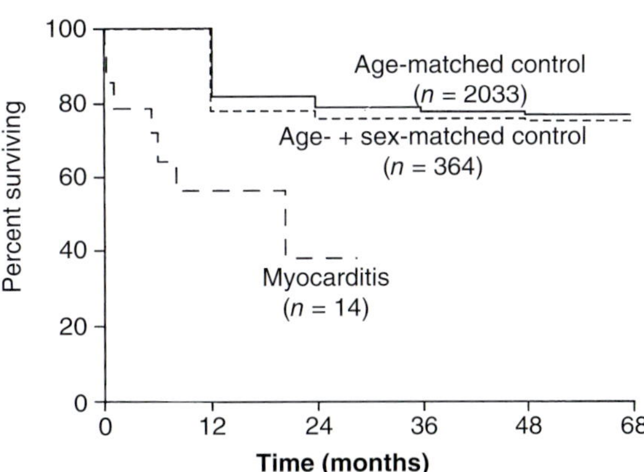

FIGURE 18.5. Actuarial mortality (defined as deaths and cardiac transplantations) in the immunosuppression and control groups. The numbers of patients at risk are shown. There was no significant difference in mortality between the two groups. (From Mason et al. [58].)

hospital readmission. This study was limited by a 31% dropout rate.

In another study, patients with positive endomyocardial biopsy specimens and progressive heart failure who responded to 6 months of therapy with prednisone and azathioprine were more likely to have circulating cardiac autoantibodies and no viral genome in their myocardium as compared with nonresponders (60).

Studies have suggested that in patients with heart failure and low ejection fraction, intravenous immune globulin has a pronounced antiinflammatory effect as measured by circulating levels of inflammatory markers (61). Uncontrolled studies suggested benefit in patients with myocarditis from treatment with intravenous immune globulin (62, 63). However, a placebo-controlled double-blind trial of intravenous immune globulin in patients with myocarditis or idiopathic dilated cardiomyopathy of less than 6 months' duration showed no significant improvement with therapy as assessed by ejection fraction or functional capacity at 6 to 12 months (64). In this study, average left ventricular ejection fraction improved from 25% ± 8% at baseline to 41% ± 17% at 6 months in both treated and untreated groups. One-year event-free survival was 91.9% in both groups. Another study suggested benefit with intravenous immune globulin as measured by improvement in ejection fraction in patients with chronic cardiomyopathy of greater than 6 months' duration (61).

In summary, there is no evidence that patients with lymphocytic myocarditis or idiopathic dilated cardiomyopathy benefit from the routine use of immunosuppressive therapy. However, this treatment approach should be considered in patients with myocarditis and positive endomyocardial biopsies who develop early signs of severe heart failure, or who are shown to have persistent myocardial inflammation or immune activation, or who experience progressive worsening of left ventricular function and symptoms of heart failure. In patients with idiopathic dilated cardiomyopathy who show worsening left ventricular function on short-term follow-up, immunosuppressive therapy should be strongly considered (18). Lastly, immunosuppressive therapy should be used in patients with myocarditis associated with connective tissue diseases, eosinophilic or granulomatous forms of the disease, or in giant cell myocarditis (Fig. 18.6).

Current investigations are evaluating antiviral therapies in the acute stage of myocarditis as well

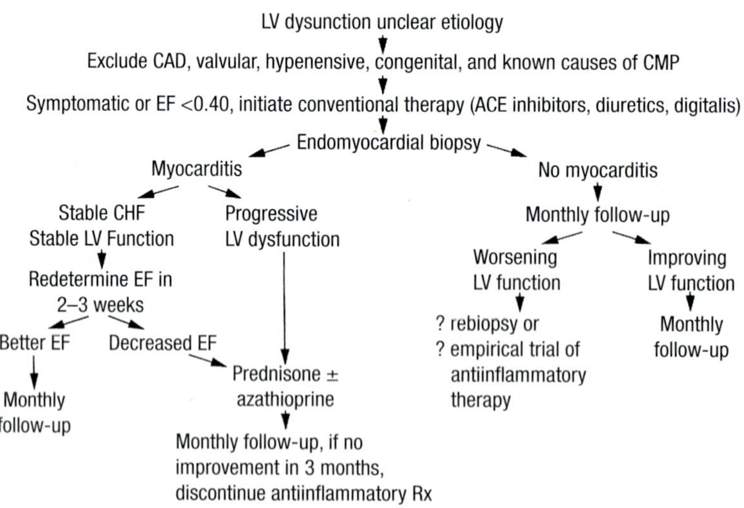

Figure 18.6. Algorithm describing a reasonable approach to myocarditis management based on currently available data. CAD, coronary artery disease; CMP, cardiomyopathy; ACE, angiotensin-converting enzyme; CHF, congestive heart failure; EF, ejection fraction. (From Parrillo [22].)

as the use of antiviral vaccine in the prevention of disease. Appropriately powered, controlled prospective studies of homogeneous patient groups utilizing immunosuppressive therapy are still needed. Evaluating the mechanisms of myocardial recovery during VAD support also may help direct research toward other novel approaches to the treatment of myocarditis.

Conclusion

Among many diverse causes, the most common etiology of myocarditis is thought to be viral, with autoimmune mechanisms prominently involved in pathogenesis. Patients with myocarditis can present with acute chest pain, mimicking acute ischemic heart disease or other cardiopulmonary illnesses, or can present with heart failure due to severe left ventricular systolic dysfunction. Oral and parenteral heart failure pharmacologic therapies that are used in the more common causes of heart failure are also used in these patients. Patients can also present with fulminant myocarditis, characterized by severe heart failure and cardiogenic shock. These patients need intensive, aggressive pharmacologic therapy, often utilizing ventricular assist devices, as they very often show recovery of left ventricular function so that pharmacologic and VAD support can be weaned and discontinued, without needing to resort to cardiac transplantation.

Endomyocardial biopsy is used in the diagnosis of myocarditis and for directing therapy, although it is limited by sampling error and by current histopathologic techniques for assessing disease activity. Newer immunohistologic methods may better define those patients who will respond to immunosuppressive therapy. Patients with myocarditis and progressive myocardial failure, despite conventional heart failure therapy, should be considered for immunosuppressive therapy on a case-by-case basis. Such patients should be followed with serial measures of left ventricular performance and endomyocardial biopsies.

References

1. Feldman A, McNamara D. Myocarditis. N Engl J Med 2000;343:1388–1398.
2. Winkel E, Costanzo M, Parrillo JE. Myocarditis. Curr Treat Options Cardiovasc Med 2000;2:407–419.
3. Haas G. Etiology, evaluation, and management of acute myocarditis. Cardiol Rev 2001;9:88–95.
4. Kavinsky CJ, Parrillo JE. Rheumatic fever and cardiovascular diseases. Samter's Immunol Dis 1995;5: 823–840.
5. Dec GW. Introduction to clinical myocarditis. In: Cooper LT, ed. Myocarditis: From Bench to Bedside. Totowa, NJ: Humana Press; 2003:257–281.
6. Pulerwitz TC, Cappola TP, Felker GM, et al. Mortality in primary and secondary myocarditis. Am Heart J 2004;147:746–750.
7. Liu P, Mason J. Advances in the understanding of myocarditis. Circulation 2001;104:1076–1082.
8. Magnani JW, Dec GW. Myocarditis. Current trends in diagnosis and treatment. Circulation 2006;113: 876–890.
9. Bowles NE, Ni JN, Kearney DL, et al. Detection of viruses in myocardial tissues by polymerase chain reaction: evidence of adenovirus as a common cause of myocarditis in children and adults. J Am Coll Cardiol 2003;42:466–472.
10. McCarthy R, Boehmer J, Hruban F, et al. Long term outcome of fulminant myocarditis as compared with acute (nonfulminant) myocarditis. N Engl J Med 2000;342:690–695.
11. Lauer B, Niederau C, Kuhl U, et al. Cardiac troponin T in patients with clinically suspected myocarditis. J Am Coll Cardiol 1997;30:1354–1359.
12. Felker GM, Boehmer JP, Hruban RH, et al. Echocardiographic findings in fulminant and acute myocarditis. J Am Coll Cardiol 2000;36:227–232.
13. Sarda L, Colin P, Boccara F, et al. Myocarditis in patients with clinical presentation of myocardial infarction and normal coronary angiograms. J Am Coll Cardiol 2001;37:786–792.
14. Liu PP, Yan AT. Cardiovascular magnetic resonance for the diagnosis of acute myocarditis: prospects for detecting myocardial inflammation. J Am Coll Cardiol 2005;45:1823–1825.
15. Abdel-Aty H, Boye P, Zagrosek A, et al. Diagnostic performance of cardiovascular magnetic resonance in patients with suspected acute myocarditis. J Am Coll Cardiol 2005;45:1815–1822.
16. Mahrholdt H, Goedecke C, Wagner A, et al. Cardiovascular magnetic resonance assessment of human myocarditis. Circulation 2004;109:1250–1258.
17. Angelini A, Crosato M, Boffa GM, et al. Active versus borderline myocarditis: clinicopathological correlates and prognostic implications. Heart 2002;87:210–215.

18. Parrillo JE. Inflammatory cardiomyopathy (myocarditis): which patients should be treated with anti-inflammatory therapy? Circulation 2001; 104:4–6.
19. Baughman K. Diagnosis of myocarditis. Death of Dallas criteria. Circulation 2006;113:593–595.
20. McKenna W. Davies M. Immunosuppression for myocarditis. N Engl J Med 1995; 333: 312–313.
21. Klingel K. Molecular biologic detection of virus infection in myocarditis and dilated cardiomyopathy. In: Cooper LT, ed. Myocarditis: From Bench to Bedside. Totowa, NJ: Humana Press; 2003:295–324.
22. Parrillo JE. Myocarditis: how should we treat in 1998? J Heart Lung Transplant 1998;17:941–944.
23. D'Ambrosio A, Patti G, Manzoli A, et al. The fate of acute myocarditis between spontaneous improvement and evolution to dilated cardiomyopathy: a review. Heart 2001;85:499–504.
24. Magnani JW, Danik HJS, Dec GW, DiSalvo TG. Survival in biopsy-proven myocarditis: a long-term retrospective analysis of the histopathologic, clinical and hemodynamic predictors. Am Heart J 2006;151:463–470.
25. Fuse K, Kodama M, Okura Y, et al. Predictors of disease course in patients with acute myocarditis. Circulation 2000;102:2829–2835.
26. Cooper L, Berry G, Shabetai R. Idiopathic giant cell myocarditis-natural history and treatment. N Engl J Med 1997;336:1860–1866.
27. Ginsberg F, Parrillo J. Eosinophilic myocarditis. In: Dec GW, ed. Heart Failure Clinics. Myocarditis. Philadelphia: WB Saunders; 2005;1(3):419–429.
28. Murphy J, Wright S, Bruce K. Eosinophilic-lymphocytic myocarditis after smallpox vaccination. Lancet 2003;362:1378–1380.
29. Galiuto L, Enriquez-Sarano M, Reeder G, et al. Eosinophilic myocarditis manifesting as myocardial infarction: early diagnosis and successful treatment. Mayo Clin Proc 1997;72(7):603–610.
30. Wu L, Lapeyre A, Cooper L. Current role of endomyocardial biopsy in the management of dilated cardiomyopathy and myocarditis. Mayo Clin Proc 2001;76(10):1030–1038.
31. Takkenberg J, Czer L, Fishbein M. Eosinophilic myocarditis in patients awaiting heart transplantation. Crit Care Med 2004;32:714–721.
32. Johnson M. Eosinophilic myocarditis in the explanted hearts of cardiac transplant recipients: interesting pathologic finding or pathophysiologic entity of clinical significance? Crit Care Med 2004;32(3):888–890.
33. Kuhl U, Pauschinger M, Noutsias M, et al. High prevalence of viral genomes and multiple viral infections in the myocardium of adults with "idiopathic" left ventricular dysfunction. Circulation 2005;111:887–893.
34. Kuhl U, Pauschinger M, Seeberg B, et al. Viral persistence in the myocardium is associated with progressive cardiac dysfunction. Circulation 2005; 112:1965–1970.
35. Mason J. myocarditis and dilated cardiomyopathy: an inflammatory link. Cardiovasc Res 2003;60:5–10.
36. Limas C. Cardiac auto-antibodies in dilated cardiomyopathy: a pathogenetic role? Circulation 1997; 95:1979–1980.
37. Pfeffer M, Braunwald E, Moye L, et al. Effect of captopril on mortality and morbidity in patients with left ventricular dysfunction after myocardial infarction. N Engl J Med 1992;327:669–677.
38. The SOLVD investigators. Effect of enalapril on survival in patients with reduced left ventricular ejection fractions and congestive heart failure. N Engl J Med 1991;325:293–302.
39. Garg R, Yusuf S. Overview of randomized trials of angiotensin converting enzyme inhibitors on mortality and morbidity in patients with heart failure. JAMA 1995;273:1450–1456.
40. Packer M. Current role of beta-adrenergic blockers in the management of chronic heart failure. Am J Med 2001;110(7A);81S–84S.
41. CIBIS II Investigators. The cardiac insufficiency bisoprolol study ii: a randomized trial. Lancet 1999;353:9–13.
42. The MERIT-HF Study Group. Effects of controlled release metoprolol on total mortality, hospitalizations and well-being in patients with heart failure. JAMA 2000;283:1295–1302.
43. Bristow M, Gilbert E, Abraham W, et al. Carvedilol produces dose related improvements in left ventricular function and survival in subjects with chronic heart failure. Circulation 1996;94:2807–2816.
44. Packer M, Coats A, Fowler M, et al. Effects of carvedilol on survival in severe chronic heart failure. N Engl J Med 2001;344:1651–1658.
45. The Digitals Investigation Group. The effect of digoxin on mortality and morbidity in patients with heart failure. N Engl J Med 1997;336:525–533.
46. Pitt B, Zannad F, Remme W, et al. The effects of spironolactone on morbidity and mortality in patients with severe heart failure. N Engl J Med 1999;341:709–717.
47. Steimle A, Stevenson L, Chelimsky-Fallick C, et al. Sustained hemodynamic efficacy of therapy tailored to reduce the filling pressures in survivors

with advanced heart failure. Circulation 1997;96: 1165–1172.
48. Stevenson L. Tailored therapy for hemodynamic goals for advanced heart failure. Eur J Heart Fail 1999;1:251–527.
49. Stevenson L, Tillisch J. Maintenance of cardiac output with normal filling pressures in patients with dilated heart failure. Circulation 1986;74: 1303–1308.
50. Jain P, Massie B, Gattis W, et al. Current medical treatment for the exacerbation of chronic heart failure resulting in hospitalization. Am Heart J 2003;145:S3–S17.
51. Jaski B, Fifer M, Wright R, et al. Positive inotropic and vasodilator actions of milrinone in patients with severe congestive heart failure. J Clin Invest 1985;75:643–649.
52. Cuffe M, Califf R, Adams K, et al. Short-term intravenous milrinone for acute exacerbation of chronic heart failure: a randomized controlled trial. JAMA 2002;287:1541–1547.
53. Goldstein G, Oz M, Rose E. Medical progress: implantable left ventricular assist devices. N Engl J Med 1998;339:1522–1533.
54. Nemeh H, Smedira N. Mechanical treatment of heart failure: the growing role of LVADs and ARTIFICIAL HEARTS. Cleve Clin J Med 2003;70:223–234.
55. Farrar D, Holman W, McBride L, et al. Long-term follow-up of thoratec ventricular assist device bridge-to-recovery patients successfully removed from support after recovery of ventricular function. J Heart Lung Transplant 2002;21:516–521.
56. Simon MA, Kormos RL, Murali S, et al. Myocardial recovery using ventricular assist devices. prevalence, clinical characteristics and outcomes. Circulation 2005;112(suppl I): I32–I36.
57. Parrillo JE, Cunnion R, Epstein S, et al. A prospective randomized controlled trail of prednisone for dilated cardiomyopathy. N Engl J Med 1989;321: 1061–1068.
58. Mason J, O'Connell J, Herskowitz A, et al. A clinical trial of immunosuppressive therapy for myocarditis. N Engl J Med 1995;333:269–275.
59. Wojnicz R, Nowalany-Kozielska E, Wojciechowska C, et al. Randomized placebo controlled study for immunosuppressive treatment of inflammatory dilated cardiomyopathy. Two year follow-up results. Circulation 2001;104:39–45.
60. Frustaci A, Chimenti C, Calabrese F, et al. Immunosuppressive therapy for active lymphocytic myocarditis. Virological and immunologic profile of responders versus non-responders. Circulation 2003;107:857–863.
61. Gullestad L, Aass H, Fjeld J, et al. Immunomodulating therapy with intravenous immunoglobulin in patients with chronic heart failure. Circulation 2001;103:220–225.
62. McNamara D, Rosenblum W, Janosko K, et al. Intravenous immune globulin in the therapy of myocarditis and acute cardiomyopathy. Circulation 1997;95:2476–2478.
63. Patel P, Lenihan D. The current status of immune modulating therapy for myocarditis: a case of acute parvovirus myocarditis treated with intravenous immunoglobulin. Am J Med Sci 2003;326(6):369–374.
64. McNamara D, Holubkov R, Starling R, et al. Controlled trail of intravenous immune globulin in recent onset dilated cardiomyopathy. Circulation 2001;103:2254–2259.

19
Management of Severe Acute Heart Failure

Markku S. Nieminen

Definition

Severe acute heart failure (AHF) patients are class IV patients hospitalized due to dyspnea on worsening chronic heart failure or for acute new-onset heart failure with signs and symptoms of severe lung congestion with pulmonary edema, low output syndrome, or cardiogenic shock. It is characterized at the emergency department as heavy dyspnea, with SpO_2 less than 90%, and with physical and psychological stress.

Patients with severe acute heart failure frequently present to the emergency department. The frequency is difficult to assess, as the hospital discharge registers do not differentiate patients by severity.

If we assume that annually there are about 4000 heart failure hospitalizations per 1 million inhabitants, and that the frequency of pulmonary edema or cardiogenic shock, including low-output syndrome, is about 20%, then there are about 800 to 1000 hospitalization due to severe AHF, which corresponds in the United States population to about 200,000 to 250,000 hospitalizations and in the European Union population to almost twice as many. The cost is immense, because in Europe the mean cost for a pulmonary edema patient and a cardiogenic shock patient is 8000 € and 24,000 €, respectively, not including the immediate costs of interventions or any pacemaker or defibrillator implantation. The cause of hospitalization in severe AHF is often related to coronary heart disease and especially acute coronary syndrome. These patients require expensive treatment in coronary care units or intensive care units, and the length of hospitalization is prolonged, thus resulting in high costs for the hospitals. Furthermore, adverse events and outcomes are frequent.

In the recent Euroheart survey, which focused on acute heart failure (AHF), the in-hospital mortality was 8% in pulmonary edema patients and 40% in cardiogenic shock patients.

Many of these patients are elderly, the mean age being 70 to 75 years. Young patients with severe AHF have rare etiologies, such as dilating cardiomyopathy or complicated endocarditis. In young patients the diagnosis is often delayed, as dyspnea is misleadingly associated with respiratory problems, especially bronchial asthma.

The most important background disease is coronary heart disease. In the Euroheart survey coronary artery disease (CAD) was reported as the background disease in 63% of patients. Acute coronary syndrome was the cause of AHF in 42% of acute de-novo patients compared to chronic hospitalized AHF patients (23%). Hypertension and thus diastolic dysfunction is in the history of 50% of AHF patients. Atrial fibrillation is frequent and observed in 30% of patients. The heart failure may also be aggravated by accompanying diseases, such as decreased renal function and anemia, and often by infection. In particular, atrioventricular valvular regurgitation may aggravate the situation as the backflow adversely affects the pulmonary congestion or peripheral edema. The increased preload in turn may adversely affect the regurgitant fraction due to wall stress and dilatation. The causes of worsening heart failure are listed in Table 19.1.

Table 19.1. Precipitating causes and background diseases of worsening heart failure in Euroheart failure survey II

	Chronic decompensated heart failure	Acute onset of new heart failure
Precipitation causes		
Acute coronary syndrome	24.0	43.1
Valvular disease	30.9	20.0
Atrial fibrillation	28.4	27.2
Life-threatening arrhythmia	3.1	3.6
Infection	19.5	14.3
Noncompliance	32.9	5.5
Background/ complicating diseases		
Coronary artery disease	62.9	40.9
Valvular	41.7	18.2
DCMP	22.1	9.4
Atrial fibrillation	48.3	24.7
Hypertension	64.3	59.7
Diabetes	33.4	30.3
Stroke	15.2	11.9
Renal failure	20.0	11.5
Chronic obstructive pulmonary disease	21.4	14.9
Anemia	16.8	10.7

DCMP, dilating cardiomyopathy.

Pathophysiology

Severe heart failure is characterized by volume overload and a decrease in contractility. The role of afterload is less apparent as the blood pressure in these patients is low. Volume overload is caused by fluid retention, which is induced by the enhanced neuroendocrine activation and or by renal dysfunction.

The volume overload can be exacerbated or caused by valvular regurgitation, which may be due to independent valvular heart disease or dysfunction or secondarily related to negative remodeling and no captation of the atrioventricular valve leaflets, leading to mitral regurgitation or tricuspid regurgitation.

Constant volume overload causes constant myocardial stress and leads to ventricular and atrial enlargement and remodeling. The ventricular enlargement may adversely affect the valvular regurgitation. These mechanisms and ventricular dilatation activate a negative vicious circle.

The major cause of myocardial dysfunction is ischemia associated with coronary heart disease, often related to postmyocardial infarction. Ischemia causes not only systolic dysfunction but also diastolic dysfunction. The negative remodeling is well known after myocardial infarction and is especially indicated by the presence of border area ischemia and volume overload in the presence of mitral regurgitation.

Another problem that adversely affects cardiac function is arrhythmias, and especially atrial fibrillation, in the presence of which the atrial support is lacking, the mitral regurgitation may deteriorate further, and the high heart rate may further increase the severity of the case. High ventricular rate can cause rapidly pulmonary congestion or even edema, especially when the right ventricle is relatively intact. The vigorous right ventricular function causes strong pulmonary filling, if the left ventricle cannot adapt to the increased volume load according to the Starling mechanism. The severe imbalance between right and left ventricular function in the presence of diastolic dysfunction is often difficult to address.

These physiologic factors cause volume overload and an increase in filling pressure, which can be evaluated clinically, or measured by echocardiography or by cardiac catheterization. Optimizing wedge pressure, the index of volume overload is important.

When the left ventricular filing pressure increases over 18 mm Hg, accumulation of fluids into interstitial lung tissue occurs and thus congestion. This is true especially in de novo acute heart failure patients, in which the still existing low vascular permeability associated with high intravascular capillary pressure fluid causes interstitial congestion and further may lead to alveolar edema, and rarely florid pulmonary edema is induced.

The atrial volume overload may induce through a reflex mechanisms high heart rate, which again exacerbates the pulmonary congestion. Thus reduction of the heart rate when it is abnormally high is important. It is also important to reduce the volume overload by vasodilatation and by improving diuresis, which both decrease right ventricular filling and, on the other hand, reduce pressure overload and thus help forward flow. If systolic blood pressure is over 100 mm Hg, beta-blockers can be tried and intravenous digitalis given to control the heart rate, especially in the presence of atrial fibrillation. In the failing heart, contractility decreases if the heart rate is high (>120 bpm).

The volume overload, ischemia, and afterload cause extreme stress on myocyte biochemistry and biomechanisms. As contractility is dependent on energy storage, energy substrates, and oxidative breathing, ischemia adversely affects these processes and decreases high-energy phosphate stores, thus also impairing the contractile function. This may also take place even in healthier myocardium, when the stress due volume overload is excessive. Energy depletion also causes accumulation of intracellular calcium and a decrease in sarcoendoplasmic reticulum Ca^{2+}–adenosine triphosphatase (SERCA) function. Continuous calcium overload in myocytes and with inflammatory cytokines induces apoptosis and ultimately fibrosis.

Both systolic and diastolic function are affected in the presence of energy depletion, which further deteriorates the condition and causes a restrictive pattern in ventricular filling, which is easily measured by echocardiography.

The most striking form of acute severe heart failure is the stunned myocardium caused by acute coronary syndromes (ACS) and especially after intervention, when the temporary occlusion of the interventional artery and the contrast agents severely compromises myocardial function and causes stunning of the myocardium.

Components of severe congestive heart failure include the following:

- Myocardial dysfunction
- Heart rate
- Volume overload
- Neuroendocrine activation, sympathetic tone, renin-angiotensin-aldosterone system (RAAS), cytokines
- Valvular dysfunction, stenotic or more often regurgitant components, especially mitral and tricuspid valves
- Systolic and diastolic dysfunction
- Energy depletion, stunning
- Inflammation
- Myocyte intracellular calcium accumulation
- Apoptosis

Figure 19.1 describes in details the vicious cycle of severe heart failure.

The de novo patients are usually in more critical condition, as the hemodynamic system is not adapted to the acute overload, including the heart itself. Before the acute incidence the volume had been normal, and now during acute heart failure the ventricles are not able to remodel to meet the volume or pressure overload. The atria are distended and the heart rate is increased. These patients have severe pulmonary edema or go into cardiogenic shock due to compromised ventricular function, valvular regurgitations, and pulmonary circulation. The situation is similar in cases with hypertrophic heart disease; that is, hypertensive crisis or aortic stenosis occurs, as the noncompliant ventricle and the increased pressure overload lead to pulmonary congestion and edema. In all cases concomitant underlying ischemia and the excess ischemia caused by overload condition aggravates the situation, and then the hemodynamic complications are more severe. Susceptibility to serious arrhythmias or rapid atrial or ventricular function is increased. The presence of moderate mitral regurgitation may make the situation difficult to treat.

The medical response must be immediate, as these patients may be partly volume depleted due to the general shock and due to the transudation from the intravascular to the extravascular compartment. Thus monitoring of these patients is important, and hypotension may require testing the fluid filling.

Severe acute heart failure also may be due to worsening chronic heart failure with congestion and peripheral edema. In these patients the cardiovascular system is more adapted to the situation. The ventricles and atria are remodeled, and pulmonary circulation is also adapted by physiologic changes that enable the lungs to tolerate increased intravascular pressures. The pulmonary arterial pressure can be significantly elevated.

The renin-aldosterone system is activated, and these patients have high angiotensin II levels, the

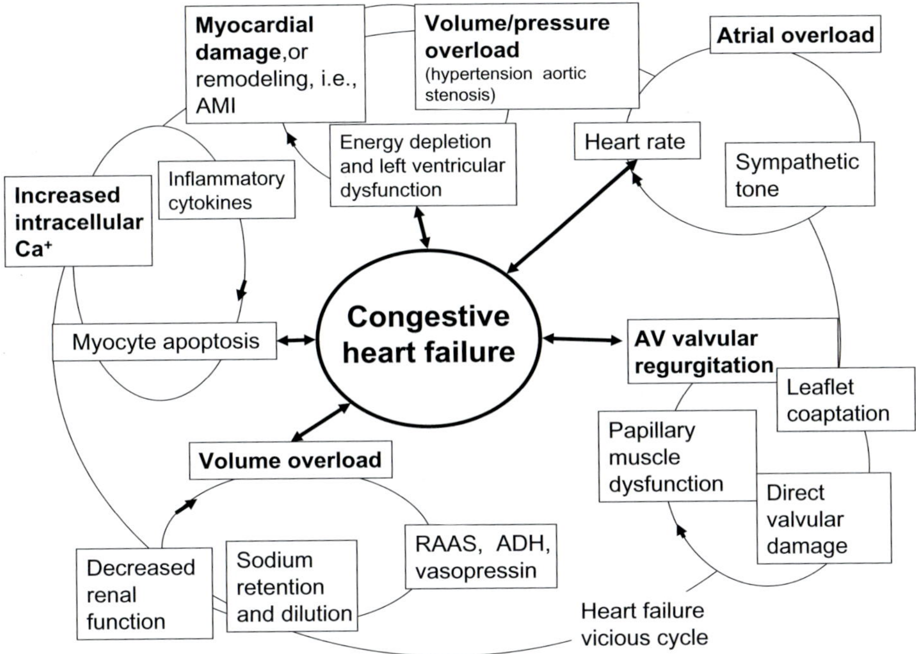

FIGURE 19.1. Vicious pathophysiological cycle in severe heart failure. ADH, antidiuretic hormone; AMI, acute myocardial infarction; AV, atrioventricular; RAAS, renin-angiotensin-aldosterone system.

serum aldosterone levels may be even over 1000 pmol/L, and the norepinephrine and adrenaline levels are elevated. The natriuretic peptide and cytokine levels also are high in these patients.

Due to shock and vasoconstriction, some patients may have relative hypovolemia.

Management

The management is targeted to improving tissue oxygenation and perfusion. Patients are managed on an individual basis, with the therapy tailored to address the patient's condition. It is important to monitor the patient's blood pressure.

The first measures are to improve tissue oxygenation, which is done by high inflow oxygen concentration, usually with 30% to 35% oxygen ventilation, or by continuous positive airway pressure (CPAP) or bi-level positive airway pressure (BiPAP) ventilation to keep the airway open, and to enhance pulmonary carbon dioxide and oxygen exchange and oxygenation of the blood.

The other key issues are to manage heart rate, myocardial function, and pressure. The optimal heart rate should be in the range of 70 to 90 bpm; the systolic blood pressure should be maintained over 90 mm Hg, and the mean blood pressure should be maintained at between 60 and 70 mm Hg, but in coronary patients over 70 mm Hg, as coronary perfusion is dependent on diastolic pressure.

If the systolic blood pressure is over 100 mm Hg and there is pulmonary congestion, the patient can be started on vasodilator, nitrate, nesiritide or sodium nitroprusside, and intravenous diuretics. Close monitoring of HR and blood pressure is required. Usually diuretics are prescribed concomitantly. If hypotension occurs, the vasodilators can be stopped and fluid testing done by 250 mL saline or colloid given intravenously. Fluid testing is sometimes a good way to ensure adequate filling pressure, as the effect is then seen by widening of blood pressure difference and increased systolic blood pressure.

If the patient is volume overloaded and systolic blood pressure is in the range of 90 to 100 mm Hg, treatment again can be initiated with diuretics and by physician consideration with vasodilator, but often some inotropic support is often required to improve the contractility. Levosimendan, which is a vasodilator and calcium sensitizer, increases contractility without increasing myocardial oxygen consumption; it often is ideal in these cases, but close monitoring is required. Levosimendan can be used also in patients with severe congestion and systolic blood pressure over 100 mm Hg, as indicated in the SURVIVE and LIDO trials. Treatment can be started with a loading dose of 6 g/kg/min, and then administering an infusion of 0.2 g/kg/min for 24 hours. Hypotension is the main adverse effect and is usually well treated without loss in efficacy by interrupting the infusion and by giving intravenous saline. If the clinical examination and follow-up indicate that the patient is unstable, the levosimendan treatment is initiated without bolus dosing.

If the systolic blood pressure is less than 85 or 90 mm Hg, the tissue and myocardial perfusion is endangered and will cause even more severe heart failure, as the patient falls into low-output syndrome or cardiogenic shock. The low systolic pressure is increased by ensuring adequate right-sided filling and by increasing vasoconstriction by norepinephrine, and thereafter improving myocardial function by inotropic agents, such as dobutamine, and if the systolic blood pressure is adequately over 85 to 90 mm HG, also by adding levosimendan. The problem with inotropes is that they are associated with increased adverse effects, but in cardiac emergencies these effects must be accepted until other proven therapies are available.

Diuresis is often diminished in heart failure patients, due to serious activation of the neuroendocrine system, with increases in angiotensin II, aldosterone, norepinephrine, and epinephrine levels, often together with chronic changes in renal tissue.

Administration of loop diuretics (furosemide, bumetanide, torsemide) usually is effective and the diuresis increases. The dose is titrated according to the diuretic response and the relief of congestive symptoms. Therapy is usually initiated by giving intravenous boluses of furosemide of 10, 20, or 40 mg, which is repeated if no response is seen. If volume status and pressure are ensured and still diuresis is low, the diuretic effect may be enhanced by a continuous furosemide infusion of 5 to 40 mg/h and by adding thiazide to the therapy. Hypokalemia is a good sign of RAAS activation, and adding spironolactone may significantly improve diuresis. If creatinine values are high, >2 mg/L, adding of spironolactone or eplerone may further decrease renal function. Adding levosimendan or low-dose dobutamine may improve the efficacy of the diuretic agents. In the presence of serious diuretic resistance, ultrafiltration may be initiated.

Ultrafiltration

Especially in chronic severe decompensated heart failure, diuretic resistance may occur, associated with extremely disturbed neuroendocrine activation, sodium retention, increased vasopressin activity, decreased renal function, and vasoconstriction. In cases with fluid retention, renal dysfunction and diluting hyponatremia ultrafiltration is a possibility. New ultrafiltration techniques may even be used on a regular ward. The advantage of ultrafiltration is that at the same time of volume withdrawal, hyponatremia can be corrected, the osmotic pressure may be improved, and thus homeostasis improved. Often repeated ultrafiltration is needed to fulfill the volume depletion needs.

Minipumps

In desperate situations with low cardiac output and cardiogenic shock, new minipumps, temporary flow pumps, or intraaortic balloon pumps can be lifesaving. These techniques improve cardiac output and the unloading of the ventricle. They enhance diuresis and thus allow positive remodeling of the distended ventricle. They are costly. The duration of use is short, 3 to 7 days.

In severe heart failure, acute or chronic, with cardiogenic shock, low output syndrome, and other organ failures, left ventricular assist devices should be considered, according to local practice.

Conclusion

Severe AHF is complex and often challenging problems to treat. The clinical picture varies from severily decompensated chronic volume overloaded patients to cardiogenic shock. The pathophysiology is a spectrum of different problems, such as myocardial damage, stunning, weaning, remodeling and valvular dysfunction, renal dysfunction, anemia, water retention, and neuroendocrine activation. Treating these patients is often complicated by their comorbid respiratory infections and diseases. Treatment is individualized, and tailored based on the patient's response.

Suggested Readings

Assist Devices and Minipumps

Henriques JP, Remmelink M, Baan J Jr, et al. Safety and feasibility of elective high-risk percutaneous coronary intervention procedures with left ventricular support of the Impella Recover LP 2.5. Am J Cardiol 97(7):990–2, 2006

Konstam MA, Czerska B, Bohm M, et al. continuous aortic flow augmentation: a pilot study of hemodynamic and renal responses to a novel percutaneous intervention in decompensated heart failure. Circulation 112(20):3107–14, 2005

Lietz K, Miller LW. Will left-ventricular assist device therapy replace heart transplantation in the foreseeable future? Curr Opin Cardiol 20(2):132–7, 2005

Thiele H, Sick P, Boudriot E, et al. Randomized comparison of intra-aortic balloon support with a percutaneous left ventricular assist device in patients with revascularized acute myocardial infarction complicated by cardiogenic shock. Eur Heart J 26:1276–83, 2005

Levosimendan

Follath F, Cleland JG, Just H, et al. Efficacy and safety of intravenous levosimendan compared with dobutamine in severe low-output heart failure (the LIDO study): a randomised double-blind trial. Lancet 360:196–202, 2002

De Luca L, Sardella G, Proietti P, et al. Effects of levosimendan on left ventricular diastolic function after primary angioplasty for acute anterior myocardial infarction: a Doppler echocardiographic study. J Am Soc Echocardiogr 19(2):172–7, 2006

Mebazaa A, Nieminen MS, Packer M, Cohen-Solal A, Kleber FX, Pocock SJ, Thakkar R, Padley RJ, Poder P, Kivikko M; SURVIVE Investigators. Levosimendan vs dobutamine for patients with acute decompensated heart failure: the SURVIVE Randomized Trial. JAMA 297:1883–91, 2007

Toller WG, Stranz C. Levosimendan, a new inotropic and vasodilator agent. Anesthesiology 104(3):556–69, 2006

Ultrafiltration

Bart BA, Boyle A, Bank AJ, et al. Ultrafiltration versus usual care for hospitalized patients with heart failure: the Relief for Acutely Fluid-Overloaded Patients With Decompensated Congestive Heart Failure (RAPID-CHF) trial. J Am Coll Cardiol 46(11):2043–6, 2005

Continuous Positive Airway Pressure

Bersten AD, Holt AW, Vedig AE, et al. Treatment of severe cardiogenic pulmonary edema with continuous positive airway pressure delivered by face mask. N Engl J Med 325:1825–30, 1991

Masip J, Betbese AJ, Paez J, et al. Non-invasive pressure support ventilation versus conventional oxygen therapy in acute cardiogenic pulmonary oedema: a randomised trial. Lancet 356(9248):2126–32, 2000

Therapy

Fonarow GC, Abraham WT, Albert NM, et al. Organized Program to Initiate Lifesaving Treatment in Hospitalized Patients with Heart Failure (OPTIMIZE-HF): rationale and design. Am Heart J 148(1):43–51, 2004

Heart Failure Society of America. Executive summary: HFSA 2006 comprehensive heart failure practice guideline. J Cardiac Failure 12(1):10–38, 2006

Hunt SA. ACC/AHA 2005 guideline update for the diagnosis and management of chronic heart failure in the adult: a report of the American College of Cardiology/American Heart Association Task Force on Practice Guidelines (Writing Committee to Update the 2001 Guidelines for the Evaluation and Management of Heart Failure). J Am Coll Cardiol 46:e1–e82, 2005. Erratum in J Am Coll Cardiol 47:1503–5, 2006

Stevenson LW. Design of therapy for advanced heart failure. Eur J Heart Failure 7(3):323–31, 2005

Swedberg K, Cleland J, Dargie H, et al., Task Force for the Diagnosis and Treatment of Chronic Heart Failure of the European Society of Cardiology.

Guidelines for the diagnosis and treatment of chronic heart failure: executive summary (update 2005). Eur Heart J 26:1115–40, 2005

Task Force on Acute Heart Failure of the European Society of Cardiology. Executive summary of the guidelines on the diagnosis and treatment of acute heart failure. Eur Heart J 26(4):384–416, 2005

van Meyel JJ, Smits P, Dormans T et al. Continuous infusion of furosemide in the treatment of patients with congestive heart failure and diuretic resistance. J Intern Med 235:329–34, 1994

20
Cardiogenic Shock

Steven M. Hollenberg

Cardiogenic shock, the syndrome that ensues when the heart is unable to deliver enough blood to maintain adequate tissue perfusion, is one of the most challenging emergencies for the practicing intensivist. The leading cause of cardiogenic shock is acute myocardial infarction.(1) Despite advances in management of heart failure and acute myocardial infarction, the mortality of patients with cardiogenic shock has remained high, with reported mortality rates ranging from 50% to 80%.(1, 2) Recently, however, there has been some cause for optimism. Tremendous progress has been made in averting shock in the course of myocardial infarction and in treating cardiogenic shock once it develops. Progress has resulted from the interplay of increased understanding of pathogenesis, more rapid and aggressive institution of supportive measures, and, most importantly, application of a strategy of early revascularization. Data suggest that these measures have increased survival over the last decade.(3) Cardiogenic shock, however, remains the most common cause of death in hospitalized patients with acute myocardial infarction.

Definition

The diagnosis of cardiogenic shock is often made on clinical grounds, by the presence of systemic arterial hypotension along with clinical signs indicative of poor tissue perfusion, including oliguria, clouded sensorium, and cool, mottled extremities—all in the setting of myocardial dysfunction. A rigorous determination requires hemodynamic confirmation, with sustained systemic hypotension (systolic arterial pressure <90 mm Hg or mean arterial pressure 30 mm Hg or more below basal levels), adequate or elevated left ventricular filling pressures (pulmonary artery wedge pressure >15 mm Hg), and a reduced cardiac output (cardiac index <2.2 L/min/m^2).(4) It is important to document myocardial dysfunction and to exclude or correct factors such as hypovolemia, hypoxia, and acidosis.

Epidemiology

The predominant cause of cardiogenic shock is left ventricular failure in the setting of acute myocardial infarction.(1) Cardiogenic shock usually results from an extensive acute infarction, although a smaller infarction in a patient with previously compromised left ventricular function may also precipitate shock. Cardiogenic shock can also be caused by mechanical complications of infarction such as acute mitral regurgitation, rupture of the interventricular septum, or rupture of the free wall—or by large right ventricular infarctions. The distribution of causes of cardiogenic shock in the prospective Should We Emergently Revascularize Occluded Coronaries for Cardiogenic Shock (SHOCK) trial registry is shown in Figure 20.1. Other important etiologies include end-stage cardiomyopathy, prolonged cardiopulmonary bypass, valvular disease, myocardial contusion, sepsis with unusually profound myocardial depression, and fulminant myocarditis.(1, 4) Concurrent conditions such as

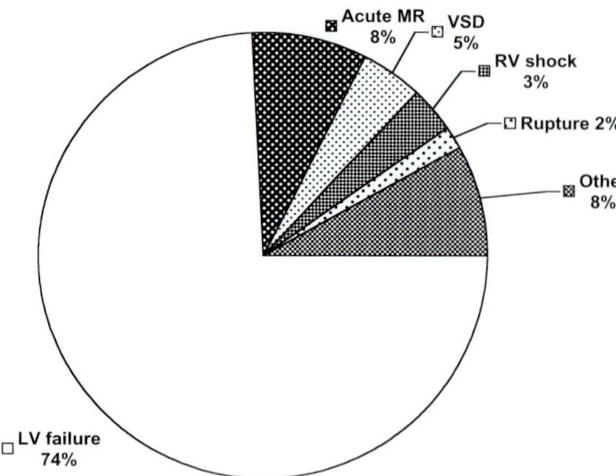

Figure 20.1. Causes of cardiogenic shock in patients with myocardial infarction in the Should We Emergently Revascularize Occluded Coronaries for Cardiogenic Shock (SHOCK) trial registry. LV, left ventricular; RV, right ventricular; MR, mitral regurgitation; VSD, ventricular septal defect. (From Hochman et al. [1].)

hemorrhage or infection may also contribute to shock.

Patients may have cardiogenic shock at initial presentation to the hospital, but most do not; shock usually evolves over several hours,(1, 5) suggesting that early treatment may potentially prevent shock. In fact, some recent data indicate that early thrombolytic therapy may decrease the incidence of cardiogenic shock.(6) Comparison of the clinical characteristics of patients with early and late shock in this registry revealed similar demographic, historical, clinical, and hemodynamic characteristics, but shock tended to develop earlier in patients with single-vessel disease than in patients with triple-vessel disease.(7) This distinction may have clinical implications, since it suggests that early shock in the setting of acute myocardial infarction (MI) may be more amenable to revascularization of the culprit vessel via thrombolysis or angioplasty, whereas shock developing later may require more complete revascularization with multivessel angioplasty or bypass surgery.

Risk factors for the development of cardiogenic shock in MI generally parallel those for left ventricular dysfunction and the severity of coronary artery disease. Shock is more likely to develop in patients who are elderly; diabetic; those who have histories of previous infarction, peripheral vascular disease, and cerebrovascular disease; and those who have anterior infarction.(8–11) Decreased ejection fractions and larger infarctions are also predictors of the development of cardiogenic shock.(10, 11) Recent analysis from the Global Utilization of Streptokinase and Tissue Plasminogen Activator for Occluded Coronary Arteries (GUSTO-3) trial has identified age, lower systolic blood pressure, heart rate, and Killip class as significant predictors of the risk for development of cardiogenic shock after presentation with acute MI.(12) The predictive scoring system derived from this study may be useful in identifying patients at high risk for the development of cardiogenic shock and in targeting such patients for closer monitoring.

Coronary angiography most often demonstrates multivessel disease. In the SHOCK trial, 29% of patients had left main occlusion, 58% had three-vessel disease, and only 22% had one-vessel disease.(13) The high prevalence of multivessel coronary artery disease (CAD) is germane because myocardial segments not involved in an acute MI normally develop compensatory hyperkinesis, a response that helps maintain cardiac output. Failure to develop such a response, either because of previous infarction or because of high-grade coronary stenoses, is an important risk factor for cardiogenic shock and death.(14)

Pathophysiology

Cardiac dysfunction in patients with cardiogenic shock is usually initiated by MI or ischemia. The myocardial dysfunction resulting from ischemia worsens that ischemia, creating a downward spiral (Fig. 20.2). Once a critical mass of ischemic or necrotic left ventricular myocardium (usually about 40%) (15) loses pumping capability, stroke volume and cardiac output can begin to decrease significantly. Myocardial perfusion, which depends on the pressure gradient between the coronary arterial system and the left ventricle and on the duration of diastole, is compromised by hypotension and tachycardia, exacerbating ischemia. The increased ventricular diastolic pressures caused by pump failure further reduce coronary perfusion pressure, and the additional wall stress elevates myocardial oxygen require-

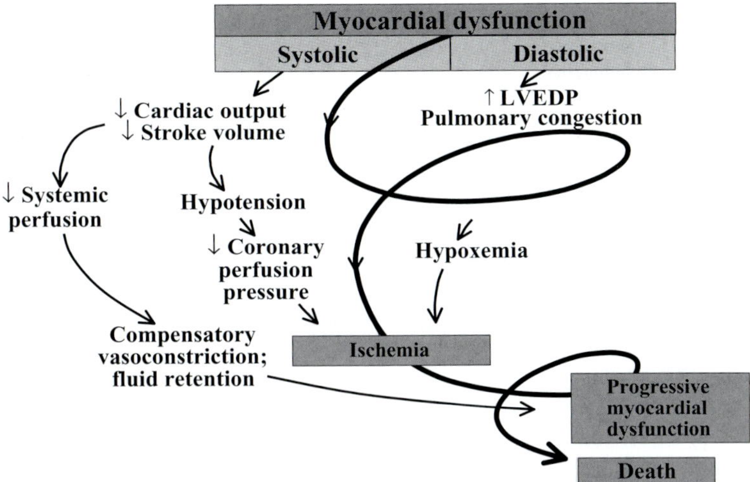

Figure 20.2. The downward spiral in cardiogenic shock. Stroke volume and cardiac output fall with left ventricle (LV) dysfunction, producing hypotension and tachycardia that reduce coronary blood flow. Increasing ventricular diastolic pressure reduces coronary blood flow, and increased wall stress elevates myocardial oxygen requirements. All of these factors combine to worsen ischemia. The falling cardiac output also compromises systemic perfusion. Compensatory mechanisms include sympathetic stimulation and fluid retention to increase preload. These mechanisms can actually worsen cardiogenic shock by increasing myocardial oxygen demand and afterload. Thus, a vicious circle can be established. LVEDP, left ventricular end-diastolic pressure. (Adapted from Hollenberg et al. [4], with permission.)

ments, further worsening ischemia. Decreased cardiac output also compromises systemic perfusion, which can lead to lactic acidosis and further compromise of systolic performance.

Compensatory mechanisms activated when cardiac output is reduced include sympathetic stimulation to increase heart rate and contractility and renal fluid retention to increase preload. These compensatory mechanisms may become maladaptive and can create a vicious cycle that further worsens systolic dysfunction. Vasoconstriction to maintain blood pressure increases myocardial afterload, further impairing cardiac performance and increasing myocardial oxygen demand. Myocardial ischemia increases myocardial stiffness, increasing left ventricular end-diastolic pressure and thus myocardial wall stress at a given end-diastolic volume. The increased left ventricular stiffness limits diastolic filling and may result in pulmonary congestion, causing hypoxemia and worsening the imbalance of oxygen delivery and oxygen demand in the myocardium, resulting in further ischemia and myocardial dysfunction.(4) The interruption of this cycle of myocardial dysfunction and ischemia forms the basis for the therapeutic regimens for cardiogenic shock.

Recent data suggest that not all patients fit into this classic paradigm. In the SHOCK trial, the average systemic vascular resistance (SVR) was not elevated, and the range of values was wide, suggesting that compensatory vasoconstriction is not universal. Some patients had fever and elevated white blood cell counts along with decreased SVR, suggesting a systemic inflammatory response syndrome.(16) This has led to an expansion of the classic paradigm to include the possibility of the contribution of inflammatory responses to vasodilation and myocardial stunning, leading clinically to persistence of shock (Fig. 20.3).(16) Supporting this notion is the fact that the mean ejection fraction in the SHOCK trial was only moderately decreased (30%), suggesting that mechanisms other than pump failure were operative.(16) Immune activation appears to be common to a number of different forms of shock. Activation of inducible nitric oxide synthase (iNOS) with production of nitric oxide and peroxynitrate has been proposed as one potential mechanism.

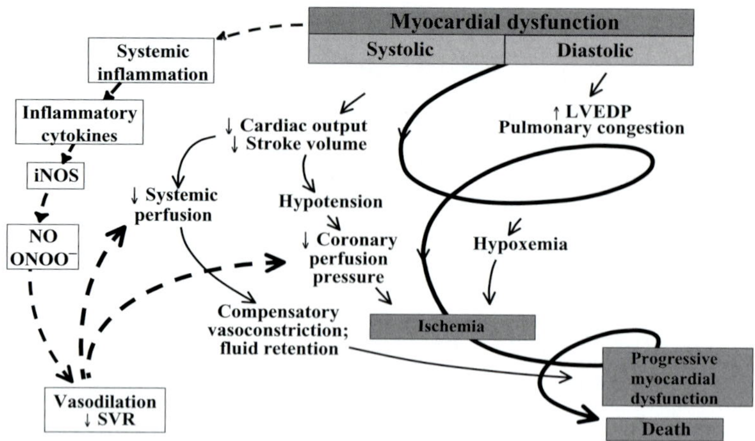

Figure 20.3. Expansion of the pathophysiologic paradigm of cardiogenic shock to include the potential contribution of inflammatory mediators. LVEDP, left ventricular end-diastolic pressure; NO, nitric oxide; iNOS, inducible nitric oxide synthase; $ONOO^-$, peroxynitrite; SVR, systemic vascular resistance. (Adapted from Hochman [16], with permission.)

Reversible Myocardial Dysfunction

A key to understanding the pathophysiology and treatment of cardiogenic shock is to realize that areas of nonfunctional but viable myocardium can also cause or contribute to the development of cardiogenic shock after MI. This reversible dysfunction can be described in two main categories: stunning and hibernation.

Myocardial stunning represents postischemic dysfunction that persists despite restoration of normal blood flow; myocardial performance eventually recovers completely.(17) Direct evidence for myocardial stunning in humans has recently been obtained by demonstrating normal perfusion using positron emission tomography (PET) scanning and ^{13}N-ammonia in patients with persistent wall motion abnormalities after angioplasty for acute coronary syndromes.(18) The pathogenesis of stunning has not been conclusively established but appears to involve a combination of oxidative stress, perturbation of calcium homeostasis, and decreased myofilament responsiveness to calcium.(17) The intensity of stunning is determined primarily by the severity of the antecedent ischemic insult.(17)

Myocardial hibernation can be seen as an adaptive response in which segments with severely reduced coronary blood flow reduce their contractile function to restore equilibrium between flow and function, minimizing the potential for ischemia or necrosis.(19) Function in such segments can be normalized by improving blood flow. Repetitive episodes of myocardial stunning can coexist with or mimic myocardial hibernation.(19)

Consideration of myocardial stunning and hibernation is important in patients with cardiogenic shock because of their therapeutic implications. Both stunned and hibernating myocardium retain inotropic reserve and can respond to catecholamines.(17) Function of hibernating myocardium can improve with revascularization, and function of stunned myocardium can improve with time. The notion that some myocardial tissue may recover function has underscored the importance of expeditious initiation of supportive measures, including both medications and intraaortic balloon counterpulsation, to maintain blood pressure and cardiac output in patients with cardiogenic shock. The presence of reversible myocardial dysfunction also has prognostic implications, and this is supported by data from the SHOCK trial, in which most survivors had only class I or class II heart failure.(16)

General Approach to the Patient with Cardiogenic Shock

After recognizing the presence of cardiogenic shock, the clinician must perform the clinical assessment required to understand its cause while initiating supportive therapy before shock causes irreversible damage to vital organs. The challenge is that since speed is important to achieve a good outcome, evaluation and therapy must begin simultaneously. While the evaluation must be thorough, neither overzealous pursuit of a diagnosis before stabilization has been achieved nor overzealous empiric treatment without establishing the underlying pathophysiology is desirable.(20)

A practical approach is to make a rapid initial evaluation on the basis of a focused history, physical examination, and specific diagnostic procedures (Fig. 20.4). Patients with shock are usually ashen or cyanotic, and can have cool skin and mottled extremities. Cerebral hypoperfusion may cloud the sensorium. Pulses are rapid and faint, and may be irregular in the presence of arrhythmias. Jugular venous distention and pulmonary rales are usually present, although their absence does not exclude the diagnosis. A precordial heave resulting from left ventricular dyskinesis may be palpable. The heart sounds may be distant, and third or fourth heart sounds are usually present. A systolic murmur of mitral regurgitation or ventricular septal defect may be heard, but these complications may occur without an audible murmur. Documentation of myocardial dysfunction and exclusion of alternative causes of hypotension allows for the diagnosis of cardiogenic shock.

An electrocardiogram should be performed immediately. Other initial diagnostic tests should include a chest radiograph and measurement of

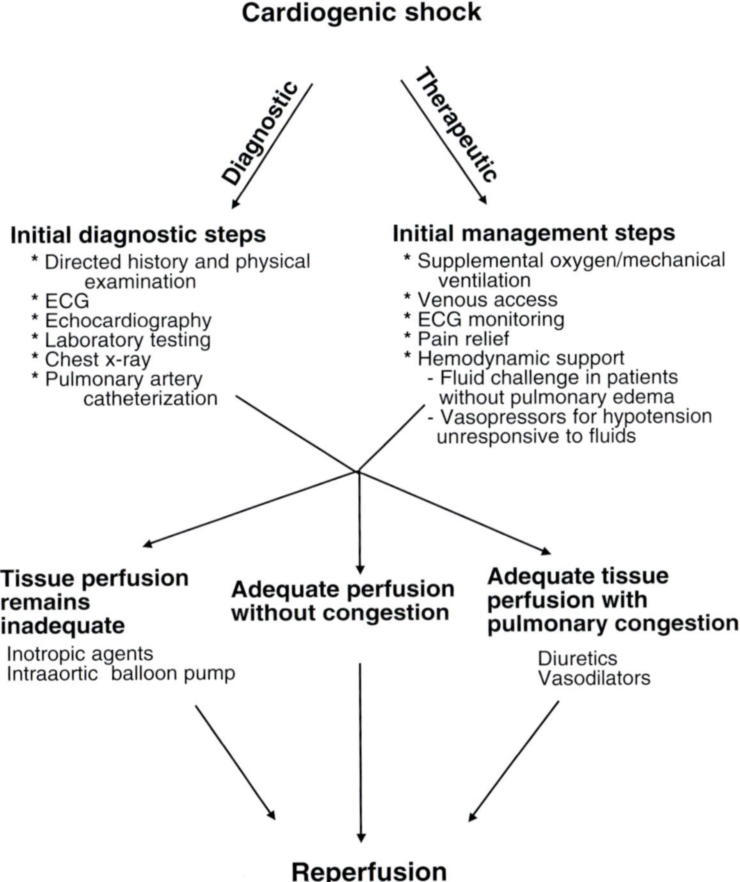

FIGURE 20.4. An approach to the diagnosis and treatment of cardiogenic shock caused by myocardial infarction. Right ventricular infarction and mechanical complications are discussed in the text. CABG, coronary artery bypass grafting; IABP, intraaortic balloon pumping. (Modified from Hollenberg et al. [4], with permission.)

arterial blood gases, electrolytes, complete blood count, and cardiac enzymes.

Echocardiography is an excellent tool for confirming the diagnosis of cardiogenic shock and for sorting through the differential diagnosis, and should be performed as early as possible. Echocardiography is simple, safe, and permits systemic interrogation of cardiac chamber size, left and right ventricular function, valvular structure and motion, atrial size, and the anatomy of the pericardial space. Echocardiography allows for expeditious evaluation of overall and regional left ventricular performance, and can rapidly diagnose mechanical causes of shock such as acute mitral regurgitation resulting from papillary muscle rupture, acute ventricular septal defect, and free wall rupture.(21) In some cases, echocardiography may reveal findings compatible with right ventricular infarction, or suggest alternative diagnoses such as pericardial tamponade. Acute right heart failure, manifested by a dilated and hypokinetic right ventricle without hypertrophy suggestive of chronic pulmonary hypertension, can suggest pulmonary embolism.(22) Transthoracic echocardiographic images may be suboptimal due to a poor acoustic window in critically ill patients, particularly those who are obese, have chronic lung disease, or are on positive pressure ventilation. Contrast echocardiography may be used to improve image quality.(23) Transesophageal echocardiography (TEE) can also provide better visualization, particularly of valvular structures, and can be performed safely at the bedside.

Invasive hemodynamic monitoring can confirm the diagnosis and can exclude volume depletion, right ventricular infarction, and mechanical complications.(24, 25) Right heart catheterization may reveal an oxygen step-up diagnostic of ventricular septal rupture or a large V wave that suggests severe mitral regurgitation. The hemodynamic profile of right ventricular infarction includes high right-sided filling pressures in the presence of normal or low occlusion pressures.(26) Right heart catheterization is most useful, however, to optimize therapy in unstable patients, because clinical estimates of filling pressure can be unreliable,(27) and because changes in myocardial performance and compliance and therapeutic interventions can change cardiac output and filling pressures precipitously.(28) Although patients with low cardiac index (less than 2.2 L/min/m^2) and a pulmonary capillary wedge pressure greater than 15 mm Hg meet the definition of cardiogenic shock, optimal filling pressures may be higher than this in individual patients due to left ventricular diastolic dysfunction.

Initial Management

Maintenance of adequate oxygenation and ventilation is critical. Many patients require intubation and mechanical ventilation, if only to reduce the work of breathing and facilitate sedation and stabilization before cardiac catheterization. Some small studies have suggested that use of continuous positive airway pressure (CPAP) in patients with cardiogenic pulmonary edema can decrease the need for intubation,(29) but these studies need to be evaluated with some caution, as noninvasive ventilation failed at least half of the time, and some data suggest that CPAP can be harmful in this setting. If patients do not manifest rapid clinical improvement with noninvasive ventilation, the strategy should be reconsidered.

Electrolyte abnormalities should be corrected, and morphine (or fentanyl if systolic pressure is compromised) used to relieve pain and anxiety, thus reducing excessive sympathetic activity and decreasing oxygen demand, preload, and afterload. Arrhythmias that alter heart rate or eliminate atrioventricular synchrony can impact cardiac output, and should be corrected promptly with antiarrhythmic drugs, cardioversion, or pacing. Some therapies routinely employed in acute MI (such as nitrates, beta-blockers, and angiotensin-converting enzyme inhibitors) have the potential to exacerbate hypotension in cardiogenic shock, and should be withheld until the patient stabilizes.

Following initial stabilization and restoration of adequate blood pressure, tissue perfusion should be assessed (Fig. 20.4). If tissue perfusion remains inadequate, inotropic support or intraaortic balloon pumping should be initiated. If tissue perfusion is adequate but significant pulmonary congestion remains, diuretics may be employed. Vasodilators can be considered as well, depending on the blood pressure.

The initial approach to the hypotensive patient should include fluid resuscitation unless frank pulmonary edema is present. Patients are commonly diaphoretic, and relative hypovolemia may be present. In the original description of hemodynamic subsets in MI, approximately 20% of patients had a low cardiac index and low pulmonary capillary wedge pressure; most had reduced stroke volume and compensatory tachycardia.(30) Some of these patients would be expected to respond to fluid infusion with an increase in stroke volume, although the magnitude of such a response depends on the degree of ischemia and cardiac reserve.

Fluid infusion is best initiated with predetermined boluses titrated to clinical end points of heart rate, urine output, and blood pressure. Ischemia produces diastolic as well as systolic dysfunction, and thus elevated filling pressures may be necessary to maintain stroke volume in patients with cardiogenic shock. Patients who do not respond rapidly to initial fluid boluses or those with poor physiologic reserve should be considered for invasive hemodynamic monitoring. Optimal filling pressures vary from patient to patient; hemodynamic monitoring can be used to construct a Starling curve at the bedside, identifying the filling pressure at which cardiac output is maximized. Maintenance of adequate preload is particularly important in patients with right ventricular infarction.

When arterial pressure remains inadequate, therapy with vasopressor agents may be required to maintain coronary perfusion pressure. Maintenance of adequate blood pressure is essential to break the vicious cycle of progressive hypotension with further myocardial ischemia. Dopamine increases both blood pressure and cardiac output, and is usually the first choice in patients with systolic pressures less than 90 mm Hg. When hypotension remains refractory, norepinephrine may be necessary to maintain organ perfusion pressure. Phenylephrine, a selective α_1-adrenergic agonist, may be employed to support blood pressure when tachyarrhythmias limit therapy with other vasopressors, although it does not improve cardiac output. Vasopressor infusions need to be titrated carefully in patients with cardiogenic shock to maximize coronary perfusion pressure with the least possible increase in myocardial oxygen demand. Hemodynamic monitoring, with serial measurements of cardiac output, filling pressures, and other parameters, such as mixed venous oxygen saturation, allows for titration of the dosage of vasoactive agents to the minimum dosage required to achieve the chosen therapeutic goals.(28)

In patients with inadequate tissue perfusion and adequate intravascular volume, cardiovascular support with inotropic agents should be initiated. Dobutamine, a selective β_1-adrenergic receptor agonist, can improve myocardial contractility and increase cardiac output, and is the initial agent of choice in patients with systolic pressures greater than 90 mm Hg. Dobutamine may exacerbate hypotension in some patients, and can precipitate tachyarrhythmias. In some situations, a combination of dopamine and dobutamine can be more effective than either agent alone.

Phosphodiesterase inhibitors such as milrinone increase intracellular cyclic adenosine monophosphate (cAMP) by mechanisms not involving adrenergic receptors, producing both positive inotropic and vasodilatory actions. Milrinone has fewer chronotropic and arrhythmogenic effects than catecholamines. In addition, because milrinone does not stimulate adrenergic receptors directly, its effects may be additive to those of the catecholamines. Milrinone, however, has the potential to cause hypotension and has a long half-life; in patients with tenuous clinical status, its use is often reserved for situations in which other agents have proven ineffective.(24) Standard administration of milrinone calls for a bolus loading dose followed by an infusion, but many clinicians eschew the loading dose (or halve it) in patients with marginal blood pressure.

Levosimendan is a novel agent that increases cardiac myocyte calcium responsiveness and also opens adenosine triphosphate (ATP)-dependent potassium channels, giving the drug both inotropic and vasodilatory properties. Levosimendan does not increase myocardial oxygen consumption, and its calcium-sensitizing effect does not appear to impair diastolic filling. The SURVIVE study compared levosimendan to dobutamine in patients with acute heart failure and ejection fraction <30%, who had symptoms and clinical signs of low cardiac output despite intravenous diuretics and vasodilators. Although levosimendan showed some early benefit, with a reduction in worsening heart failure (from 17% to 12.3%, $p = .02$) and a trend toward reduced 30-day mortality (from 6.0% to 4.4%, hazard ratio [HR] = 0.72; 95% confidence interval [CI], 0.55–1.16), the primary outcome, all-cause mortality at 6 months, was not different (26.0% vs. 27.9%, HR = 0.91; 95% CI, 0.74–1.13).(31) Levosimendan is not currently available in the United States, but has been approved for use in some countries in Europe and South America. Levosimendan has the potential to cause hypotension and thus should be used with some caution in patients with cardiogenic shock, but the current data suggest that it is no worse than dobutamine, and there is as much or more evidence of its safety and efficacy as for any other intravenous inotropic or vasodilator agent.

Intraaortic balloon counterpulsation (IABP) reduces systolic afterload and augments diastolic perfusion pressure, increasing cardiac output and improving coronary blood flow.(32) In contrast to those of inotropic or vasopressor agents, these beneficial effects occur without an increase in oxygen demand. Intraaortic balloon counterpulsation does not, however, produce a significant improvement in blood flow distal to a critical coronary stenosis,(33) and has not been shown to improve mortality when used alone without reperfusion therapy or revascularization. In patients with cardiogenic shock and compromised tissue perfusion, IABP can be an essential support mechanism to stabilize patients and allow time for definitive therapeutic measures to be undertaken.(32, 34) In appropriate settings, more intensive support with mechanical assist devices may also be implemented.

Myocardial Reperfusion

As previously noted, pathophysiologic considerations favor interventions to restore flow to occluded arteries in patients with cardiogenic shock due to MI. Fibrinolytic therapy has been shown to restore infarct artery patency, reduce infarct size, preserve left ventricular function, and decrease mortality in patients with acute infarction. (35–37) Although fibrinolytic therapy reduces the likelihood of subsequent development of shock after initial presentation, (5, 36, 38) its role in the management of patients who have already developed shock is less certain. The number of patients in randomized trials is small since most fibrinolytic trials have excluded patients with cardiogenic shock at presentation, (39) but the available data from randomized trials (GISSI, ISIS-2, and GUSTO-1) (36, 40, 41) have not shown decreased mortality with fibrinolytic therapy in patients with established cardiogenic shock. On the other hand, in the SHOCK registry, (42) patients treated with fibrinolytic therapy had a lower in-hospital mortality rate than those who were not (54% vs. 64%, $p = .005$), even after adjustment for age and revascularization status (odds ratio [OR], 0.70; p = .027).

Fibrinolytic therapy is clearly less effective in patients with cardiogenic shock than in those without. The explanation for this lack of efficacy appears to be the low reperfusion rate achieved in this subset of patients. The reasons for decreased thrombolytic efficacy in patients with cardiogenic shock probably include hemodynamic, mechanical, and metabolic factors that prevent achievement and maintenance of infarct-related artery patency.(43) Attempts to increase reperfusion rates by increasing blood pressure with aggressive inotropic and vasopressor therapy and IABP make theoretic sense, and two small studies support the notion that vasopressor therapy to increase aortic pressure improves thrombolytic efficacy.(43, 44) The use of intraaortic balloon pumping to augment aortic diastolic pressure may increase the effectiveness of thrombolytics as well.

To date, emergency percutaneous revascularization is the only intervention that has been shown to consistently reduce mortality rates in patients with cardiogenic shock. Use of angioplasty in patients with cardiogenic shock grew out of its use as primary therapy in patients with MI. An analysis of the first 1000 patients treated with primary angioplasty at the Mid-America Heart Institute showed a mortality of 44% in the subgroup of 79 patients presenting with cardiogenic shock, substantially lower than the mortality in historical controls, which was 80% to 90%.(45) Most other reported case series also showed results with percutaneous intervention superior to those with either fibrinolytic therapy or conservative medical management, with mortality rates of approximately 40% to 50%.(4) Observational studies from registries of randomized trials have also reported improved outcomes in patients with cardiogenic shock selected for revascularization. Notable among these are the GUSTO-1 trial, in which patients treated with an aggressive strategy (coronary angiography performed within 24 hours of shock onset with revascularization by percutaneous transluminal coronary angioplasty [PTCA] or bypass surgery) had significantly lower mortality (38% compared with 62%).(46) This benefit was present even after adjustment for baseline characteristics (46) and persisted out to 1 year.(47)

Reports from the National Registry of Myocardial Infarction–2 (NRMI-2), which collected 26,280 shock patients with cardiogenic shock in the setting of MI between 1994 and 1997, similarly supported the association between revascularization and survival.(48) Improved short-term mortality was noted in those who then underwent revascularization during the reference hospitalization, either via PTCA (12.8% mortality versus 43.9%) or coronary artery bypass graft (CABG) (6.5% vs. 23.9%).(48) These data complement the GUSTO-1 substudy data and are important, not only because of the sheer number of patients from whom these values are derived, but also because NRMI-2 was a national cross-sectional study that more closely represented general clinical practice than carefully selected trial populations.

This extensive body of observational and registry studies showed consistent benefits from revascularization, but could not be regarded as definitive due to their retrospective design. Two randomized controlled trials have now evaluated revascularization for patients with MI.

The SHOCK study (13, 49) was a randomized, multicenter international trial that assigned patients with cardiogenic shock to receive optimal medical management—including IABP and thrombolytic therapy—or cardiac catheterization with revascularization using PTCA or CABG. The trial enrolled 302 patients and was powered to detect a 20% absolute decrease in 30-day all-cause mortality rates. Mortality at 30 days was 46.7% in patients treated with early intervention and 56% in patients treated with initial medical stabilization, but this difference did not quite reach statistical significance ($p = .11$).(13) It is important to note that the control group (patients who received medical management) had a lower mortality rate than that reported in previous studies; this may reflect the aggressive use of thrombolytic therapy (64%) and balloon pumping (86%) in these controls. These data provide indirect evidence that the combination of thrombolysis and IABP may produce the best outcomes when cardiac catheterization is not immediately available. At 6 months, mortality in the SHOCK trial was reduced significantly (50.3% compared with 63.1%, $p = .027$) (13), and this risk reduction was maintained at 12 months (mortality 53.3% vs, 66.4%, $p < .03$) (Fig. 20.5).(49) Subgroup analysis showed a substantial improvement in mortality rates in patients younger than 75 years of age at both 30 days (41.4% vs. 56.8%, $p = .01$) and 6 months (44.9% vs. 65.0%, $p = .003$). (13)

The Swiss Multicenter Trial of Angioplasty Shock (SMASH) trial was independently conceived and had a very similar design, although a more rigid definition of cardiogenic shock resulted in enrollment of sicker patients and a higher mortality.(50) The trial was terminated early due to difficulties in patient recruitment, for two different reasons: early on, several centers declined to participate because it was felt that it would not be ethical to undertake early invasive evaluation in such extremely ill patients, and then, after publication of several encouraging studies

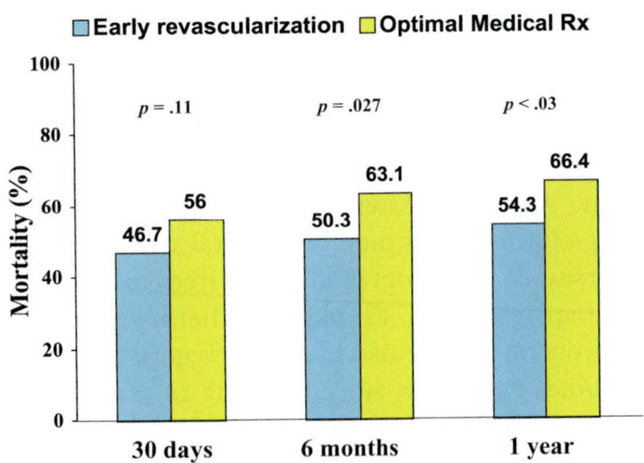

FIGURE 20.5. Mortality in the randomized SHOCK trial at 30 days, 6 months, and 1 year in the early revascularization and optimal medical management groups. (Data from Hochman et al. [13, 49].)

documenting the superiority of PCI over thrombolysis for acute MI, many centers felt that it had become unethical not to proceed to early evaluation and revascularization.(51) In the SMASH trial, an absolute reduction in 30-day mortality similar to that seen in the SHOCK trial was observed (69% mortality in the invasive group vs. 78% in the medically managed group; relative risk [RR], 0.88; 95% CI, 0.6–1.2; p = NS).(50) This benefit was also maintained at 1 year.

When the results of both the SHOCK and SMASH trials are put into perspective with results from other randomized, controlled trials of patients with acute MI, an important point emerges: despite the moderate *relative* risk reduction (for the SHOCK trial 0.72; 95% CI, 0.54–0.95; for the SMASH trial, 0.88; 95% CI, 0.60–1.20), the *absolute* benefit is important, with nine lives saved for 100 patients treated at 30 days in both trials, and 13.2 lives saved for 100 patients treated at 1 year in the SHOCK trial. This latter figure corresponds to a number needed to treat of 7.6, one of the lowest figures ever observed in a randomized controlled trial of cardiovascular disease.

Newer Developments

New approaches to revascularization for patients with acute MI and cardiogenic shock are evolving. Coronary artery stenting is becoming routine, both in elective cases and as a component of primary angioplasty for acute MI. Although data in patients with cardiogenic shock are relatively sparse, case series have reported successful results with direct stenting in this setting.(52, 53) Another consideration is whether to deploy a drug-eluting stent. Although restenosis rates are lower with drug-eluting stents than bare-metal stents, longer courses of clopidogrel are required to prevent in-stent restenosis. Clopidogrel therapy presents a problem if coronary artery bypass surgery becomes necessary, since bleeding rates are substantially higher. One alternative if percutaneous intervention with stenting is employed acutely to stabilize the patient before planned bypass surgery is to use intravenous glycoprotein IIb/IIIa inhibitors to prevent stent thrombosis before surgery and then initiate clopidogrel afterward.

Techniques of surgical revascularization are improving as well, particularly with respect to strategies to minimize post-bypass myocardial dysfunction, and this will likely translate into improved outcomes for patients with cardiogenic shock taken emergently to the operating room.

Other Settings

For patients who present in settings without the capability to perform cardiac catheterization and revascularization, the available data suggest that stabilization with intraaortic balloon counterpulsation and thrombolysis followed by transfer to a tertiary care facility may be the best management option. Intraaortic balloon counterpulsation may be a useful adjunct to thrombolysis in this setting by increasing drug delivery to the thrombus, improving coronary flow to other regions, preventing hypotensive events, or by supporting blood pressure and ventricular function until areas of stunned myocardium can recover. In the NRMI-2 study of 21,718 patients with MI and cardiogenic shock, 32% (6992) received IABP.(54) When patients treated with fibrinolytic therapy were analyzed, those also treated with IABP had a significantly lower mortality rate than those who were not so treated (49% vs. 69%, $p < .001$). Similar results were obtained in the SHOCK trial registry; patients treated with combined IABP and fibrinolytic therapy had a lower mortality rate (47%) than those given fibrinolytic therapy alone (63%, $p = .007$).(42) Although selection bias is clearly a confounding factor in these studies, two retrospective studies (55, 56) have found that patients with cardiogenic shock treated in a community hospital with IABP placement followed by thrombolysis had improved in-hospital survival and improved outcomes after subsequent transfer for revascularization.

Case Presentation

A 58-year-old man with hypertension, a previous smoking history, and a history of inferior wall MI 2 years prior presents to the emergency department with a 2-hour history of oppressive chest discomfort and shortness of breath. His electrocardiogram (ECG) is shown in Figure 20.6.

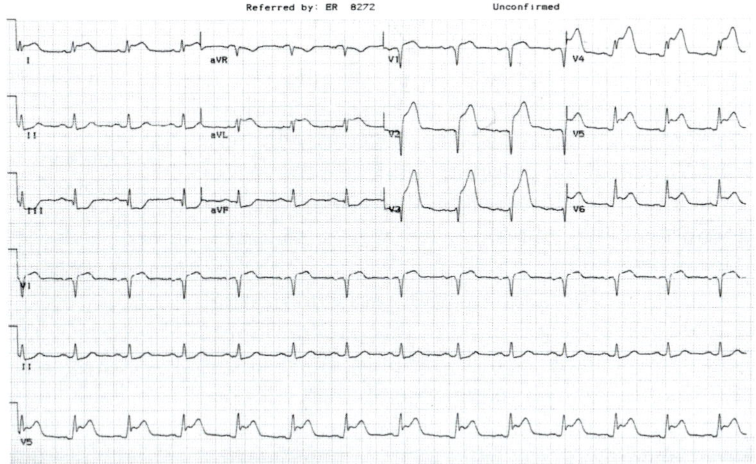

FIGURE 20.6. Electrocardiogram of a 58-year-old man with hypertension, a previous smoking history, and a history of inferior wall myocardial infarction 2 years prior, presenting with a 2-hour history of oppressive chest discomfort and shortness of breath.

Examination reveals him to be ashen and in acute distress, with pulse 130 per minute, blood pressure 90/60 mm Hg, and respiratory rate of 36 per minute. Physical examination shows wheezing and bilateral rales, a diffuse and laterally displaced PMI, an S_3 gallop, a holosystolic apical murmur, and cool extremities.

His arterial blood gas is 7.12/44/61 on a 100% face mask, and he is intubated and mechanically ventilated for hypoxia and to decrease work of breathing. Despite a fluid challenge his hypotension worsens and he requires dopamine 8 mcg/kg/min to maintain a mean arterial blood pressure of 60 mm Hg. His chest x-ray (CXR) shows pulmonary edema.

Urgent echocardiography shows an akinetic and fibrotic inferior wall indicative of old infarction, anteroapical akinesis, and severely depressed overall left ventricular systolic function. There is mild mitral regurgitation but no evidence of papillary muscle rupture.

He is taken to the cardiac catheterization laboratory. An intraaortic balloon pump is inserted. Right heart catheterization reveals RAP 10, RVP 50/12, PAP 50/34, PAOP 32, cardiac index 1.9. Dobutamine is added to dopamine. Left heart catheterization reveals a totally occluded left anterior descending (LAD) artery, and an 80% obstruction in the mid-right coronary artery. A stent is placed in the LAD with a good angiographic result.

The patient still requires vasopressor and inotropic support with dopamine and dobutamine after the procedure, but has slow improvement in hemodynamic parameters, as well as improvement in oxygenation. He is able to be extubated the next day, and the balloon pump is removed the day after that. His blood pressure is improved, and his dopamine is weaned and he is started on angiotensin-converting enzyme inhibition as well as aldosterone receptor blockade. Just prior to discharge, a low dose of beta-blockers is initiated. He is ambulating without symptoms of angina or heart failure.

This case illustrates a number of salient points concerning cardiogenic shock. Cardiogenic shock is most often associated with anterior MI and multivessel coronary disease. Compensatory hyperkinesis normally in myocardial segments not involved in an acute MI normally helps maintain cardiac output. In this case, previous inferior infarction limited the patient's ability to compensate in the setting of acute anterior infarction.

Early intubation and mechanical ventilation is usually a good idea, if only to reduce work of breathing and facilitate sedation. Patients marginally compensated when sitting erect in the emergency department may decompensate rapidly when lying prone for cardiac catheterization.

Echocardiography is an excellent initial tool for confirming the diagnosis of cardiogenic shock and ruling out other causes of shock; therefore, early echocardiography should be routine. Invasive hemodynamic monitoring can be useful diagnostically to help to exclude volume depletion, right ventricular infarction and mechanical complications, but is even more useful to guide vasoactive therapy, allowing for titration of medications to optimize their hemodynamic effects while minimizing potential increases in myocardial oxygen utilization and tachyarrhythmias. Intraaortic balloon pumping is particularly useful for hemodynamic support in this setting because it improves hemodynamics without a concomitant increase in oxygen demand.

Cardiac catheterization with revascularization if appropriate was essential in this patient. Emergency revascularization is the only intervention that has been shown to consistently reduce mortality rates in patients with cardiogenic shock. It is not uncommon for patients to require continued hemodynamic support even after the infarct-related artery has been opened; both myocardial stunning and vasodilation induced by release of inflammatory mediators may play a role. Most patients that do recover, however, have good functional status.

Conclusion

Treatment of patients with cardiogenic shock has advanced in leaps and bounds. A condition once regarded as uniformly fatal is now proving treatable. The potential for reversal of myocardial dysfunction with revascularization provides the rationale for supportive therapy to maintain coronary and tissue perfusion until more definitive measures can be undertaken. Those definitive measures entail revascularization achieved as early as possible. Application of these findings should serve to counteract the tendency, often self-fulfilling, to be fatalistic when treating patients with severe shock. The intensity of research and the recent pace of advances in interventional cardiology and in the treatment of MI hold out the promise of further insights that will translate into even more significant reductions in morbidity and mortality from cardiogenic shock.

References

1. Hochman JS, Boland J, Sleeper LA, et al. Current spectrum of cardiogenic shock and effect of early revascularization on mortality. Results of an International Registry. Circulation. 1995;91:873–81.
2. Goldberg RJ, Gore JM, Alpert JS, et al. Cardiogenic shock after acute myocardial infarction. Incidence and mortality from a community-wide perspective, 1975 to 1988. N Engl J Med. 1991;325:1117–22.
3. Goldberg RJ, Samad NA, Yarzebski J, Gurwitz J, Bigelow C, Gore JM. Temporal trends in cardiogenic shock complicating acute myocardial infarction. N Engl J Med. 1999;340:1162–68.
4. Hollenberg SM, Kavinsky CJ, Parrillo JE. Cardiogenic shock. Ann Intern Med. 1999;131:47–59.
5. Holmes DR Jr, Bates ER, Kleiman NS, et al. Contemporary reperfusion therapy for cardiogenic shock: the GUSTO-I trial experience. The GUSTO-I Investigators. Global Utilization of Streptokinase and Tissue Plasminogen Activator for Occluded Coronary Arteries. J Am Coll Cardiol. 1995;26:668–74.
6. Bonnefoy E, Lapostolle F, Leizorovicz A, et al. Primary angioplasty versus prehospital fibrinolysis in acute myocardial infarction: a randomised study. Lancet. 2002;360:825–29.
7. Webb JG, Sleeper LA, Buller CE, et al. Implications of the timing of onset of cardiogenic shock after acute myocardial infarction: a report from the SHOCK Trial Registry. SHould we emergently revascularize Occluded Coronaries for cardiogenic shocK? J Am Coll Cardiol. 2000;36(3 suppl A): 1084–90.
8. Scheidt S, Ascheim R, Killip T. Shock after acute myocardial infarction. A clinical and hemodynamic profile. Am J Cardiol. 1970;26:556–64.
9. Killip T, Kimball JT. Treatment of myocardial infarction in a coronary care unit. A two year experience with 250 patients. Am J Cardiol. 1967;20: 457–64.
10. Hands ME, Rutherford JD, Muller JE, et al. The in-hospital development of cardiogenic shock after myocardial infarction: incidence, predictors of occurrence, outcome and prognostic factors. The MILIS Study Group. J Am Coll Cardiol. 1989;14: 40–6.
11. Leor J, Goldbourt U, Reicher-Reiss H, Kaplinsky E, Behar S. Cardiogenic shock complicating acute myocardial infarction in patients without heart failure on admission: incidence, risk factors, and outcome. SPRINT Study Group. Am J Med. 1993; 94:265–73.
12. Hasdai D, Califf RM, Thompson TD, et al. Predictors of cardiogenic shock after thrombolytic therapy for acute myocardial infarction. J Am Coll Cardiol. 2000;35:136–43.
13. Hochman JS, Sleeper LA, Webb JG, et al. Early revascularization in acute myocardial infarction

complicated by cardiogenic shock. N Engl J Med. 1999;341:625–34.

14. Grines CL, Topol EJ, Califf RM, et al. Prognostic implications and predictors of enhanced regional wall motion of the noninfarct zone after thrombolysis and angioplasty therapy of acute myocardial infarction. The TAMI Study Groups. Circulation. 1989;80:245–53.
15. Alonso DR, Scheidt S, Post M, Killip T. Pathophysiology of cardiogenic shock. Quantification of myocardial necrosis, clinical, pathologic and electrocardiographic correlations. Circulation. 1973;48: 588–96.
16. Hochman JS. Cardiogenic shock complicating acute myocardial infarction: expanding the paradigm. Circulation. 2003;107:2998–3002.
17. Bolli R. Basic and clinical aspects of myocardial stunning. Prog Cardiovasc Dis. 1998;40:477–516.
18. Gerber BL, Wijns W, Vanoverschelde JL, et al. Myocardial perfusion and oxygen consumption in reperfused noninfarcted dysfunctional myocardium after unstable angina: direct evidence for myocardial stunning in humans. J Am Coll Cardiol. 1999;34:1939–46.
19. Wijns W, Vatner SF, Camici PG. Hibernating myocardium. N Engl J Med. 1998;339:173–81.
20. Hollenberg SM. Clinical assessment and initial management of cardiogenic shock. In: Hollenberg SM, Bates ER, eds. Cardiogenic Shock. Armonk, NY: Futura; 2002:45–62.
21. Nishimura RA, Tajik AJ, Shub C, Miller FA Jr, Ilstrup DM, Harrison CE. Role of two-dimensional echocardiography in the prediction of in-hospital complications after acute myocardial infarction. J Am Coll Cardiol. 1984;4:1080–87.
22. Ribeiro A, Lindmarker P, Juhlin-Dannfelt A, Johnsson H, Jorfeldt L. Echocardiography Doppler in pulmonary embolism: right ventricular dysfunction as a predictor of mortality rate. Am Heart J. 1997;134(3):479–87.
23. Reilly JP, Tunick PA, Timmermans RJ, Stein B, Rosenzweig BP, Kronzon I. Contrast echocardiography clarifies uninterpretable wall motion in intensive care unit patients. J Am Coll Cardiol. 2000;35:485–90.
24. Califf RM, Bengtson JR. Cardiogenic shock. N Engl J Med. 1994;330:1724–30.
25. Hollenberg SM, Parrillo JE. Shock. In: Fauci AS, Braunwald E, Isselbacher KJ, et al., eds. Harrison's Principles of Internal Medicine, 14th ed. New York: McGraw-Hill; 1997:214–22.
26. Nedeljkovic ZS, Ryan TJ. Right ventricular infarction. In: Hollenberg SM, Bates ER, eds. Cardiogenic Shock. Armonk, NY: Futura; 2002:161–86.
27. Mimoz O, Rauss A, Rekei N, Brun-Buisson C, Lemaire F, Brochard L. Pulmonary artery catheterization in critically ill patients: a prospective analysis of outcome changes associated with catheter-prompted changes in therapy. Crit Care Med. 1994;22:573–79.
28. Hollenberg SM, Hoyt JW. Pulmonary artery catheters in cardiovascular disease. New Horizons. 1997;5:207–13.
29. Pang D, Keenan SP, Cook DJ, Sibbald WJ. The effect of positive pressure airway support on mortality and the need for intubation in cardiogenic pulmonary edema: a systematic review. Chest. 1998;114(4): 1185–92.
30. Forrester JS, Diamond G, Chatterjee K, Swan HJC. Medical therapy of acute myocardial infarction by application of hemodynamic subsets. N Engl J Med. 1976;295:1404–13.
31. Mebazaa A, Nieminen MS, Packer M, et al. Levosimendan vs dobutamine for patients with acute decompensated heart failure: the SURVIVE Randomized Trial. JAMA 2007;292:1883–91.
32. Willerson JT, Curry GC, Watson JT, et al. Intraaortic balloon counterpulsation in patients in cardiogenic shock, medically refractory left ventricular failure and/or recurrent ventricular tachycardia. Am J Med. 1975;58:183–91.
33. Kern MJ, Aguirre F, Bach R, Donohue T, Siegel R, Segal J. Augmentation of coronary blood flow by intra-aortic balloon pumping in patients after coronary angioplasty. Circulation. 1993;87:500–11.
34. Bates ER, Stomel RJ, Hochman JS, Ohman EM. The use of intraaortic balloon counterpulsation as an adjunct to reperfusion therapy in cardiogenic shock. Int J Cardiol. 1998;65(suppl 1): S37–42.
35. Fibrinolytic Therapy Trialists' (FTT) Collaborative Group. Indications for fibrinolytic therapy in suspected acute myocardial infarction: collaborative overview of early mortality and major morbidity results from all randomised trials of more than 1000 patients. Lancet. 1994;343:311–22.
36. GUSTO Investigators. An international randomized trial comparing four thrombolytic strategies for acute myocardial infarction. N Engl J Med. 1993;329:673–82.
37. Ryan TJ, Antman EM, Brooks NH, et al. 1999 update: ACC/AHA guidelines for the management of patients with acute myocardial infarction. A report of the American College of Cardiology/ American Heart Association Task Force on Practice Guidelines (Committee on Management of

Acute Myocardial Infarction). J Am Coll Cardiol. 1999;34(3):890–911.

38. AIMS Trial Study Group. Effect of intravenous APSAC on mortality after acute myocardial infarction: preliminary report of a placebo-controlled clinical trial. Lancet. 1988;1:545–49.
39. Col NF, Gurwitz JH, Alpert JS, Goldberg RJ. Frequency of inclusion of patients with cardiogenic shock in trials of thrombolytic therapy. Am J Cardiol. 1994;73:149–57.
40. Gruppo Italiano per lo Studio Della Streptochinasi Nell'Infarto Miocardico (GISSI). Effectiveness of intravenous thrombolytic treatment in acute myocardial infarction. Lancet. 1986;2:397–402.
41. ISIS-2 Collaborative Group. Randomised trial of intravenous streptokinase, oral aspirin, both, or neither among 17 187 cases of suspected acute myocardial infarction: ISIS-2. Lancet. 1988;2:349–60.
42. Sanborn TA, Sleeper LA, Bates ER, et al. Impact of thrombolysis, intra-aortic balloon pump counterpulsation, and their combination in cardiogenic shock complicating acute myocardial infarction: a report from the SHOCK Trial Registry. SHould we emergently revascularize Occluded Coronaries for cardiogenic shocK? J Am Coll Cardiol. 2000;36(3 suppl A):1123–9.
43. Becker RC. Hemodynamic, mechanical, and metabolic determinants of thrombolytic efficacy: a theoretic framework for assessing the limitations of thrombolysis in patients with cardiogenic shock. Am Heart J. 1993;125:919–29.
44. Garber PJ, Mathieson AL, Ducas J, Patton JN, Geddes JS, Prewitt RM. Thrombolytic therapy in cardiogenic shock: effect of increased aortic pressure and rapid tPA administration. Can J Cardiol. 1995;11:30–6.
45. O'Keefe JH Jr, Bailey WL, Rutherford BD, Hartzler GO. Primary angioplasty for acute myocardial infarction in 1,000 consecutive patients. Results in an unselected population and high-risk subgroups. Am J Cardiol. 1993;72(19):107G-15G.
46. Berger PB, Holmes DR Jr, Stebbins AL, Bates ER, Califf RM, Topol EJ. Impact of an aggressive invasive catheterization and revascularization strategy on mortality in patients with cardiogenic shock in the Global Utilization of Streptokinase and Tissue Plasminogen Activator for Occluded Coronary Arteries (GUSTO-I) trial. An observational study. Circulation. 1997;96:122–27.
47. Berger PB, Tuttle RH, Holmes DR Jr, et al. One-year survival among patients with acute myocardial infarction complicated by cardiogenic shock, and its relation to early revascularization: results from the GUSTO-I trial. Circulation. 1999;99(7): 873–78.
48. Rogers WJ, Canto JG, Lambrew CT, et al. Temporal trends in the treatment of over 1.5 million patients with myocardial infarction in the US from 1990 through 1999: the National Registry of Myocardial Infarction 1, 2 and 3. J Am Coll Cardiol. 2000;36: 2056–63.
49. Hochman JS, Sleeper LA, White HD, et al. One-year survival following early revascularization for cardiogenic shock. JAMA 2001;285(2):190–2.
50. Urban P, Stauffer JC, Bleed D, et al. A randomized evaluation of early revascularization to treat shock complicating acute myocardial infarction. The (Swiss) Multicenter Trial of Angioplasty for Shock-(S)MASH. Eur Heart J. 1999;20:1030–8.
51. Urban P, Stauffer J-C. Randomized trials of revascularization therapy for cardiogenic shock. In: Hollenberg SM, Bates ER, eds. Cardiogenic Shock. Armonk, NY: Futura; 2002:135–44.
52. Antoniucci D, Valenti R, Santoro GM, et al. Systematic direct angioplasty and stent-supported direct angioplasty therapy for cardiogenic shock complicating acute myocardial infarction: in-hospital and long-term survival. J Am Coll Cardiol. 1998;31: 294–300.
53. Webb JG, Carere RG, Hilton JD, et al. Usefulness of coronary stenting for cardiogenic shock. Am J Cardiol. 1997;79:81–4.
54. Barron HV, Every NR, Parsons LS, et al. Use of intra-aortic balloon counterpulsation in patients with cardiogenic shock complicating acute myocardial infarction: data from the National Registry of Myocardial Infarction 2. Am Heart J. 2001;141: 933–9.
55. Kovack PJ, Rasak MA, Bates ER, Ohman EM, Stomel RJ. Thrombolysis plus aortic counterpulsation: improved survival in patients who present to community hospitals with cardiogenic shock. J Am Coll Cardiol. 1997;29:1454–58.
56. Stomel RJ, Rasak M, Bates ER. Treatment strategies for acute myocardial infarction complicated by cardiogenic shock in a community hospital. Chest. 1994;105:997–1002.

21
Arrhythmia in Acute Heart Failure

Alexandru B. Chicos and Alan H. Kadish

The ubiquity of arrhythmias, both atrial and ventricular, in chronic heart failure (HF) is well established, and their significance and treatment have been studied quite extensively. The prevalence, significance, and treatment of arrhythmias in acutely decompensated heart failure have been less studied.

Rhythm disturbances may cause symptoms, may cause or worsen the HF decompensation, may make treatment difficult or prevent its success, or may cause death[1]. In other cases arrhythmias may be a simple consequence of HF, or may be a benign "bystander." This chapter discusses the epidemiology, prognostic significance, mechanisms, and treatment of arrhythmias in acute heart failure.

Supraventricular Arrhythmias

Many types of supraventricular rhythm disturbances can be encountered in acute heart failure (AHF), but atrial fibrillation (AF) and flutter are of particular importance. In reports on 150,000 hospitalized heart failure patients, 31% of patients had a history of AF[2,3]. Among 949 patients with AHF decompensation without significant (unstable) arrhythmia on enrollment who were randomized to receive intravenous milrinone or placebo in the Outcomes of a Prospective Trial of Intravenous Milrinone for Exacerbations of Chronic Heart Failure (OPTIME-CHF) trial, only 6% developed new arrhythmias, of which 49% were classified as AF/flutter[1]. The prevalence of AF increases with the New York Heart Association (NYHA) class, and in chronic heart failure trials it ranged from 10% to 50%[4]. Atrial fibrillation with rapid ventricular rate is a common trigger for HF exacerbations, and HF exacerbations are commonly complicated by new or recurrent AF. It is frequently difficult to identify the cause and the effect. Atrial fibrillation may cause or exacerbate heart failure by impairing the ventricular filling via rapid ventricular rate and loss of atrial pump function, especially in hearts with preexisting diastolic dysfunction; it may also directly impair the systolic function through tachycardia-induced cardiomyopathy. A number of studies suggest AF is associated with a significantly increased mortality in the setting of HF[4].

Ventricular Arrhythmias

Ventricular arrhythmias include ventricular premature beats (VPBs), nonsustained ventricular tachycardia (NSVT), accelerated idioventricular rhythm (AIVR), sustained ventricular tachycardia (VT), and ventricular fibrillation (VF). They may present as asymptomatic findings on electrocardiogram (ECG) monitoring, or with a spectrum of symptoms that includes syncope and death. These have been found in about 90% of patients with chronic HF, in both ischemic and nonischemic cardiomyopathy[5–7]. The prevalence of NSVT alone, as determined by ambulatory electrocardiographic recordings, was reported to be 54% in these patients[5]. While limited data are available regarding the prognostic effects of NSVT in AHF, several studies have examined NSVT in chronic heart failure (CHF)[8–10], with findings suggesting that NSVT does not predict a higher risk of sudden death. The relationship of ventricular arrhythmias to overall mortality and sudden death in CHF was examined in 1080 patients with NYHA class III/IV symptoms and a left ventricular ejection fraction ≤35% enrolled in the Prospective Randomized Milrinone Survival Evaluation (PROMISE) trial, about half of whom had coronary artery disease (CAD)[10]. Baseline 24-hour ambulatory ECG recordings showed >30 VPBs/hour, NSVT, and NSVT longer than 10 beats in 60%, 61%, and 10% of the patients, respectively. In multiple logistic analysis with models including the clinical variables with and without the NSVT variable, the frequency of NSVT did not add significant information beyond the clinical variables, and the authors concluded that ventricular arrhythmias do not specifically predict sudden death in patients with moderate-to-severe heart failure.

The epidemiologic information on arrhythmia and its prognosis in AHF is limited. Several data sets on AHF are available in the literature[1–3, 11–22]. Data from published AHF registries and selected trials is summarized in Tables 21.1 and 21.2 and Figure 21.1.

The Acute Decompensated Heart Failure National Registry (ADHERE)[2] enrolled patients that had heart failure as a primary or secondary

Table 21.1. Epidemiology of arrhythmia in acute heart failure: data from the acute heart failure registries

Registry	First author and year of publication	Number of patients	Arrhythmia in the history or at presentation: Afib/Flutter (%)	NSVT (%)	VT (%)	VF (%)	Other
EPICAL[22]	Zannad, 1999	499	25.6 in "nonsinus rhythm"				
EuroHeart[13]	Cleland, 2003	11,327	42 (9% of patients presented with rapid AF)		VT + VF = 8		→Syncope 15%
Swiss Registry (two centers)[20]	Rudiger, 2005	312	29.2 (in 15% of cases AF was new and triggered the AHF)				→7% of cases triggered by symptomatic bradycardia
OPTIMIZE-HF[3]	Fonarow, (initial pub 2004	48,000	31				
IMPACT-HF[19]	O'Connor, 2005	567	35.4 (in 8% of cases AF caused the AHF)		VT + VF = 11.5		→50% on beta-blocker, 36% on ACEI on admission →12.5% arrhythmic death by 60 days
ADHERE[2]	Adams, 2005	110,000	31		8	1	

NSVT, nonsustained ventricular tachycardia; Sust. VT, sustained ventricular tachycardia; VF, ventricular fibrillation; blank box, no data available. ACEI, angiotensin-converting enzyme inhibitor; AF, atrial fibrillation; AHF, acute heart failure.

Table 21.2. Epidemiology of arrhythmia in acute heart failure: data from selected acute heart failure trials

Trial	First author and year of publication	Intervention	No. of patients	Arrhythmia in the history or at presentation				New arrhythmias during hospitalization				Other
				Afib/flutter (%)	NSVT (%)	Sust. VT (%)	VF (%)	Afib/flutter (%)	NSVT (%)	Sust. VT (%)	VF (%)	
OPTIME-CHF[1]	Benza, 2004	Milrinone vs. placebo	949	32		10	3	M-1.5 P-4.6		2.1	1.2	
VMAC[11]	2002	Nesiritide vs. NTG vs. placebo	489	35		13	6					34% had frequent PVSs
LIDO[14]	Follath, 2002	Levosimendan vs. dobutamine	203	13		7	1	D-2 L-4	D-2 L-1	D-2 L-1		
RITZ-2[21]	Torre-Amione, 2003	Tezosentan vs. placebo	285	24.6								
RITZ-4[18]	O'Connor, 2003	Tezosentan vs. placebo	192					P-2.1 T-5.2		P-6.3 T-5.2		Patients excluded if HR >130/min
RITZ-5[17]	Kaluski, 2003	Tezosentan vs. placebo	84	21.4								
PRECEDENT[12]	Burger, 2002	N1 vs. N2 vs. dobutamine	255	27	26	7.5			N1-6 N2-5 D-13			
IMPACT-HF[15]	Gattis, 2004	Start carvedilol predischarge	363	22		VT + VF = 9						

M, milrinone; P, placebo; NTG, nitroglycerin; N1, nesiritide 0.015 µg/kg/min; N2, nesiritide 0.03 µg/kg/min; D, dobutamine; T, tezosentan; L, levosimendan. NSVT, nonsustained ventricular tachycardia; Sust. VT, sustained ventricular tachycardia; VF, ventricular fibrillation; blank box, no data available.

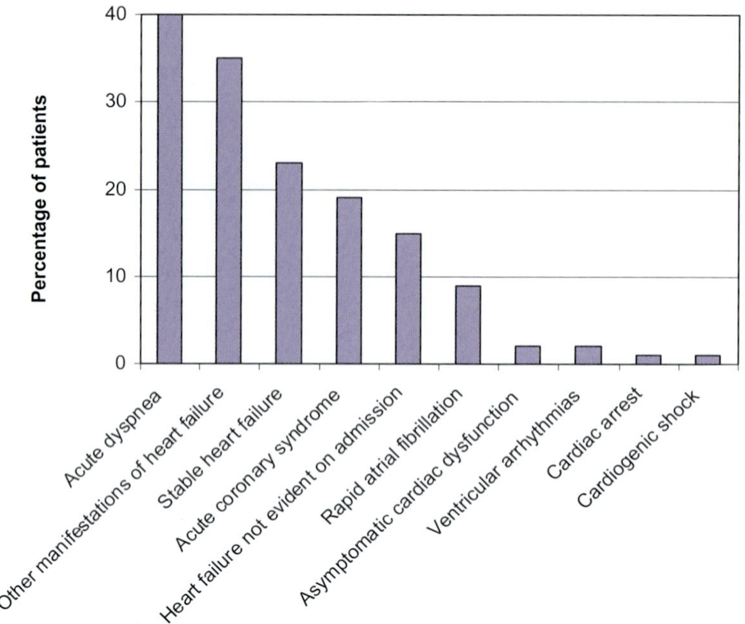

FIGURE 21.1. Cardiovascular status at the time of admission for patients enrolled in the EuroHeart Failure survey. More than one status may apply at the time of admission. (Modified from Cleland et al.[13])

hospitalization diagnosis. Among 105,388 patients reported in 2004, the incidence of VT, VF, and AF on presentation was 8%, 1%, and 31%, respectively, and 4% had electrophysiologic study during hospitalization.

Is Outcome of Acute Heart Failure Related to Arrhythmia?

OPTIME-CHF[1] randomized 949 patients with decompensated heart failure to receive intravenous milrinone or placebo. The impact of arrhythmia in AHF was assessed in a post-hoc analysis of outcomes and their association with the occurrence of a new arrhythmic event during their index hospitalization. Arrhythmic events occurred in a surprisingly low 6% of the study population. Ventricular arrhythmias accounted for half of the episodes. The primary end point of days hospitalized for cardiovascular causes within 60 days after randomization was markedly higher for those in the arrhythmia group. Mortality during index hospitalization was 26% in the arrhythmia group and 1.8% in the no-arrhythmia group ($p = .001$). Death or hospitalization at 60 days was also significantly worse in the arrhythmia group, and new arrhythmias appeared to be an independent risk factor for the primary end point and for death at 60 days. The authors concluded that new arrhythmia (defined as AF, atrial flutter, sustained VT, or VF) during an exacerbation of heart failure identifies a high-risk group with higher intrahospital and 60-day morbidity and mortality. The arrhythmia group was more likely to be treated with milrinone, was heavier, had a lower initial blood pressure, and had more ischemic events during the hospitalization. Whether the observations made would still hold true if patients not treated with milrinone were evaluated alone was not established with certainty.

Mechanisms

A variety of factors may contribute to arrhythmogenesis in acute heart failure syndromes. Some of these factors pertain to the atrial or ventricular myocardial substrate, and include the complex aspects of remodeling at structural, mechanical, and electrical levels. Other factors pertain to the neurohumoral, biochemical, and biophysical environment. This is further compounded by the time course of each process and the superimposition of acute and chronic processes, frequently with different effects, to ultimately generate a picture of tremendous complexity that has yet to be completely understood.

Reentry Versus Focal Activity

In general, multiple mechanisms may participate in arrhythmogenesis in AHF, including reentry and abnormal impulse formation (which includes abnormal automaticity and triggered activity). Ventricular tachycardia in ischemic cardiomyopathy is often sustained by reentry around and within areas of scar. The initiation of VT in nonischemic cardiomyopathy is multifactorial, but in some cases has been shown to be due to triggered activity, primarily from delayed afterdepolarizations that arise from altered cellular Ca dynamics.

We will address here arrhythmogenic factors and mechanisms that are particular to the situation of acutely decompensated HF.

Stretch: Mechanoelectric Coupling[23,24]

Mechanoelectric feedback (or coupling) refers to the ability of mechanical stimuli, such as stretch or stress, to generate immediate and chronic electric responses. This is thought to be largely mediated by mechanosensitive ion channels in cellular and subcellular membranes, but protein stretching and other factors may be involved. In the heart, this can lead to arrhythmia. Mechanosensitive ion channels include voltage-dependent K- and Na-selective, adenosine triphosphate (ATP)-sensitive, and K,Cl-selective and nonselective ion channels. Experimental work in whole hearts and single myocytes has shown rapid and slow responses in the shape and amplitude of intracellular calcium transients[25]. Stretch may increase heart rate within <10 ms[26] and appears not to require metabolism or innervation. Acute stretch during systole leads to shortening of the action potential and, in turn, to shortening of the effective refractory period (ERP) and of the wavelength, favoring reentry. A prolongation of the action potential with occurrence of early after depolarizations has also been described[27].

Acute stretch during diastole may induce inward currents leading to late afterdepolarizations, and, if threshold is reached, premature beats occur. Sustained acute stretch has been shown to depolarize the membrane resting potential, which may lead to abnormal automaticity. In addition, as a result of the three-dimensional shape and structure of the heart, including areas of different local radius, thickness, fiber direction, and mechanical properties, the distribution of mechanical stress in the myocardium is not uniform, and the electrical changes induced through mechanoelectric feedback will be heterogeneous as well[28].

Agents that block stretch-activated channels (including gadolinium, streptomycin, GsMtx-4 peptide) have been shown to suppress stretch-related transient depolarizations and extrasystoles in the dog heart[29] and spontaneous afterdepolarizations in ventricular cells from a rabbit CHF model[24]. In rabbit hearts, acute atrial dilatation facilitated AF, and stretch-activated channel (SAC) blockers (gadolinium and GsMTx-4) suppressed this phenomenon[30].

Chronic stretch activates gene expression, and induces cardiomyocyte dedifferentiation[31], hypertrophy, cardiac cavity enlargement, and fibrosis, which may be mediated by increased expression of angiotensin-converting enzyme[32].

Thus, stretch likely plays an arrhythmogenic role in AHF, through mechanisms that may be reentrant, related to heterogeneous shortening of refractoriness, or slowing of conduction and enlargement of the cardiac chamber; or focal, caused by abnormal automaticity or triggered activity. Both mechanisms may play a role in the different stages of initiation and sustaining of arrhythmia.

Neurohormonal Activation

Acute heart failure is associated with sympathoadrenergic activation and parasympathetic withdrawal. Catecholamines released at the myocardial and systemic levels are arrhythmogenic through β-receptor–mediated effects, which result in spontaneous calcium release from the sarcoplasmic reticulum and delayed afterdepolarizations[33]. Norepinephrine has also been implicated in the occurrence of early afterdepolarizations and abnormal automaticity in heart failure[34–36]. Adrenergic stimulation may also potentiate reentry.

It has been suggested that patients with diabetes mellitus may have a blunted sympathetic response to acutely decompensated heart failure, reflected by a lower norepinephrine level and markedly lower measures of ventricular ectopy in patients with diabetes mellitus. In a study of 207 patients with severe heart failure, of which 48% were diabetic, the risk of developing ventricular tachycardia (as assessed by 24-hour Holter monitoring) was markedly lower in patients with diabetes, with an adjusted odds ratio of 0.41 (95% confidence interval [CI], 0.22–0.75, $p = .004$)[12,37].

Other factors, such as endothelin-1 may be associated with arrhythmia in AHF[38]. However, the mechanism is unclear and endothelin may simply be a marker of HF severity. In fact, tezosentan, an endothelin antagonist, did not seem to have a significant effect on incidence of arrhythmia[18].

Proarrhythmia and Antiarrhythmic Effects of Drugs Used to Treat Acute Heart Failure

Inotropic Agents

Catecholamines (including dobutamine, dopamine, norepinephrine, and epinephrine) have proarrhythmic effects that derive from their β-receptor–mediated physiologic actions, as discussed above. In the Prospective Randomized Evaluation of Cardiac Ectopy with Dobutamine or Natrecor Therapy trial (PRECEDENT), dobutamine was associated with substantial proarrhythmic and chronotropic effects in patients with decompensated CHF[12]. Phosphodiesterase inhibitors are similarly proarrhythmic, causing an increase in cyclic adenosine monophosphate (AMP) concentration leading to enhanced calcium influx into the cell and a rise in cell calcium concentration. Milrinone has been associated with an increased risk of cardiac death, sudden death and arrhythmias in a meta-analysis of 21 trials and 8408 patients[39]. In the OPTIME-CHF trial in AHF patients, it was associated with an increased risk of atrial, but not ventricular arrhythmias[1]. In the Digitalis Investigation Group (DIG) trial, although digoxin significantly reduced mortality from heart failure, overall mortality was not changed. The benefit appeared to be offset by an increase in mortality from arrhythmia[40].

Beta-Blockers

Beta-blocking agents prolong life in patients with CHF. They reduce the incidence of heart failure–related death, a category that, in most trials, includes the arrhythmic deaths occurred during AHF decompensation. They also reduce the incidence of sudden cardiac death (SCD), thought to be arrhythmic in most instances[41,42]. A post-hoc analysis of the Multicenter Automatic Defibrillator Implantation Trial-II (MADIT-II) population showed that patients receiving the higher doses of beta-blockers (those in the top quartile of doses) had a significant reduction in the risk for VT or VF requiring implantable cardioverter-defibrillator (ICD) therapy compared with patients not receiving beta-blockers (hazard ratio 0.48, $p = 0.02$)[43].

The Initiation Management Predischarge: Process for Assessment of Carvedilol Therapy in Heart Failure (IMPACT-HF) trial showed that predischarge initiation of carvedilol in stabilized patients hospitalized for HF was well tolerated and resulted in increased beta-blocker use at 60 days[15]. There is little data regarding the role and impact of beta-blockers on arrhythmia and arrhythmic mortality during AHF. A study of 236 patients admitted for decompensated CHF, 50 of whom were receiving beta-blockers, suggested that concomitant beta-blocker therapy during heart failure decompensation is associated with a marked reduction in complex ventricular ectopy and episodes of ventricular tachycardia[44]. This is consistent with the proarrhythmic role thought to be played by the sympathoadrenergic activation. There has been no randomized study with beta-blockers in AHF. Recently published European guidelines suggest caution in the use of beta-blockers in AHF, and that intravenous metoprolol may be considered for treatment of arrhythmia. If the patient is chronically on beta-blocker, continuation is recommended, unless inotropic support is required, and the dose may be reduced if hypotension or bradycardia is present[45].

Statins

In the Antiarrhythmics Versus Implantable Defibrillators (AVID) trial, patients with arteriosclerotic heart disease (ASHD) who have received an ICD, lipid-lowering therapy was associated with reduction in the probability of VT/VF recurrence[46]. In the MADIT-II patients, the time-dependent statin/no statin therapy hazard ratio was 0.72 ($p = .046$) for VT/VF after adjusting for relevant covariates[47]. While this evidence from post-hoc analyses of patients from AVID and MADIT-II suggests that statins may have antiarrhythmic effects, there are no data on their effects on arrhythmia in AHF.

Other Drugs

Nesiritide, levosimendan, and tolvaptan have not been associated with arrhythmogenic effects.

Diuretics do not have direct proarrhythmic effects, but they can cause electrolyte abnormalities such as hypokalemia and hypomagnesemia, which are associated with atrial and ventricular arrhythmias. They may also contribute to improving or worsening of the autonomic profile via volume and blood pressure changes, and may decrease the mechanical myocardial stress. Rigorous clinical trials are not available, and may not be feasible.

A small retrospective study suggested that concomitant hypoglycemic sulfonylurea therapy, which blocks cardiac ATP-sensitive potassium channels (K_{ATP}), may reduce the occurrence of complex ventricular ectopy in the setting of severe CHF in diabetic patients[38]. Angiotensin-converting enzyme (ACE) inhibitors improve survival in all stages of HF. However, there are conflicting data as to whether ACE inhibitors reduce SCD, and no evidence of ventricular arrhythmia suppression is available. There is evidence suggesting that these agents may help prevent AF via antifibrotic or other effects, but it is difficult to distinguish potential direct effects from their hemodynamic effects. Aldosterone antagonists spironolactone and eplerenone significantly reduced overall mortality and sudden death mortality in patients with advanced HF[48,49]. They may also reduce the frequency of VPBs and NSVT, as suggested by this small randomized trial in 35 patients with NYHA class III CHF[50]. These agents may act by preventing the aldosterone effect on the heart or by elevating the serum potassium level. However, there are no data on their role in AHF.

Ischemia

Ischemia is likely to occur in AHF, as a consequence of an imbalance between oxygen supply and demand. Demand is increased in AHF due to sympathetic activation leading to tachycardia and increased contractility, and increased wall stress due to increased intrachamber pressure and increased chamber size [following Laplace's law: σ = (pressure × radius)/(2 × wall thickness)]. Hypotension, coronary disease or spasm, or severe hypoxemia may lead to a decrease in oxygen supply. Transient ischemia may cause reduced resting membrane potentials and abnormal automaticity, which may cause ectopic beats and tachycardias; it may also impair conduction, leading to unidirectional block and conditions for reentry. The prolongation of repolarization and its heterogeneity generates spatial dispersion and conditions for phase 2 reentry, and leads to susceptibility to drug-induced torsades de pointes tachycardia.

In the setting of acute myocardial infarction (MI), multiple mechanisms mentioned above are believed to be involved, including stretch and electrophysiologic alterations at the border zone of the infarct.

Scar

Ventricular tachycardias in the setting of chronic coronary disease and healed MI are sustained by reentry around the infarcted area[51]. Subendocardial or patchy scarring is found at autopsy or magnetic resonance imaging (MRI) in many patients thought to have nonischemic dilated cardiomyopathy, and reentry around these areas likely contributes to sustained VT in many of these patients. Scarred areas also contain areas of slow, "zigzag" conduction, which are important in sustaining the reentry.

At the atrial level, extensive atrial fibrosis has been found in patients or animal models with CHF or elevated left atrial pressure, creating areas of block and slow conduction, thus providing a substrate for AF or flutter.

Treatment of Arrhythmias in Acute Heart Failure

While many of the deaths in AHF occur through an arrhythmic mechanism, in many studies these deaths have been classified as heart failure–related.

There is a need for better definitions and identification of arrhythmias in AHF, which would help better characterize the impact of different therapeutic measures on arrhythmia incidence and outcomes. However, arrhythmias are common in AHF and it does appear that they may cause significant morbidity and mortality.

Several aspects of the treatment of arrhythmias in AHF differ from the treatment of arrhythmias in CHF: a need for faster achievement of rate or rhythm control; the presence of proarrhythmia from frequent concomitant use of inotropic agents; the presence of electrolyte abnormalities associated with aggressive diuresis or acute renal failure; arterial oxygen desaturation due to respiratory or circulatory failure; and the presence of mechanical factors that are correctable (such as central venous catheters, which may be placed in the right atrium, or pulmonary artery catheters, which may cause ventricular or supraventricular tachycardias). Although stretch-related arrhythmogenic mechanisms are thought to be important in causing arrhythmias in AHF, currently there is no specific treatment to address them, other than common heart failure therapies like diuresis and vasodilatation. Thus, the treatment of arrhythmias in AHF may not always be mechanism specific.

Bradyarrhythmias

Sinus bradycardia or atrioventricular block with escape rhythms, may be a consequence of terminal events in AHF such as respiratory failure, hypoxemia, and severe acidosis, or they may be a result of electrolyte abnormalities (hyperkalemia, hypercalcemia), drugs (beta-blockers, calcium channel blockers, digitalis intoxication, etc.), or ischemia (inferior MI). In addition to addressing the etiologic factors, treatment may include intravenous atropine or temporary transvenous or transcutaneous pacing. Catecholamines should be avoided if possible since they may provoke supraventricular and ventricular tachyarrhythmia.

Atrial Fibrillation and Flutter

The main objectives of management include rate control, prevention of thromboembolism, and correction of the rhythm disturbance; however, the priorities are dictated by the acute clinical situation.

Ventricular rate control is often the first and main intervention required acutely. Rapid control requires intravenous therapy with atrioventricular node blocking agents. Intravenous (IV) beta-blockers such as esmolol or metoprolol are often effective, but they have adverse effects that include negative inotropic activity, hypotension, and worsening of heart failure, which should be balanced against the benefit that comes from rate control.

Nondihydropyridine calcium-channel blockers such as verapamil and diltiazem should be used with caution, since they may also cause hypotension or worsen heart failure via negative inotropic effects.

In the patient with predominantly diastolic dysfunction or hypertensive crisis, the blood pressure-lowering and negative inotropic effects of beta-blockers and calcium channel blockers are beneficial.

Digoxin does not cause hypotension or have negative inotropic effects, but is less effective acutely. It may be used mostly as an adjunct to other agents, and rapid IV loading is most helpful, with 0.25 mg IV every 2 hours up to a total of 1.5 mg[52].

Amiodarone IV is effective for rapid rate control. In approximately 20% to 25% of cases it can produce cardioversion to sinus rhythm, and thus it should be avoided in patients at risk for thromboembolic events. An exception can be made in patients who have frequent episodes of paroxysmal AF and convert spontaneously multiple times, and in whom amiodarone should not introduce additional thromboembolic risk. Because of its prominent vasodilatory effect, amiodarone has modest effects on hemodynamics, but it can cause hypotension either because of its negative inotropic effect or because the Tween80 diluent can provoke hypotension.

The hypotensive patient with rapid AF poses a particular challenge. Immediate electric cardioversion may be necessary if the arrhythmia is causing the hypotension, since rate control may be impossible without the drugs causing a worsening of the hypotension. This strategy should balance the benefits and need for cardioversion against the thromboembolic risk and the likelihood of immediate or early AF recurrence.

Atrial flutter and fibrillation may also need urgent cardioversion when they cause severe AHF or in the setting of acute ischemia.

Electrical cardioversion should be performed under deep conscious sedation or general anesthesia. High initial energy should be used (360 J monophasic and 200 J biphasic waveforms), since studies show that this results in fewer shocks and less cumulative energy[53,54].

Cardioversion can be attempted, when less urgent, using chemical means, with ibutilide, amiodarone, or dofetilide. If it is successful, the drug may be continued. If sinus rhythm is not achieved, electrical cardioversion can be performed with more chances of success and maintenance of sinus rhythm after drug loading.

In general, cardioversion is desirable when the AF or flutter is poorly tolerated and highly symptomatic, as described above. It is also desirable when AF is paroxysmal and when a long-term rhythm control strategy is adopted, according to published guidelines[52]. In addition, we suggest that although the exact time course for the development of irreversible atrial remodeling as a result of fibrillation itself (apart from heart failure) is not known, allowing fibrillation to persist may provide time for these irreversible changes to take place[55]. This could make sinus rhythm more difficult to attain and maintain. The thromboembolic risk depends on the duration of AF and other clinical and echocardiographic factors[52]. Current recommendations of antithrombotic therapy in patients with AF undergoing cardioversion are based on case-control studies, since there are no randomized studies[52].

If AF duration is less than 48 hours, the need for anticoagulation before cardioversion is not clear. For AF lasting longer than 48 hours or of uncertain duration, patients should be anticoagulated with heparin followed by warfarin. If cardioversion is planned, anticoagulation is recommended for at least 3 weeks prior and 4 weeks after the cardioversion unless transesophageal echocardiography is performed. Anticoagulation is required after cardioversion to prevent late events due to thrombus formation in the stunned, hypocontractile atrium, which may take several weeks to recover.

If cardioversion is required immediately, IV or subcutaneous heparin should be given, if possible without delay, before the procedure. Transesophageal echocardiogram to exclude atrial thrombus may be considered if there is time.

Supraventricular Tachycardias

Reentrant supraventricular tachycardias (SVTs) without preexcitation can be treated with adenosine, verapamil, or beta-blockers. Atrial arrhythmias, particularly atrial tachycardia, may be a result of digoxin toxicity, requiring specific therapy. In rare cases of frequent, protracted recurrences of SVT, culprits such as proarrhythmic drugs have to be identified and eliminated, and continuous IV drips may be effective. Amiodarone IV is also very effective, and is recommended in arrhythmias with hemodynamic compromise[56]. In the presence of preexcitation, IV amiodarone, procainamide, or cardioversion should be used. Vagotonic maneuvers are generally not effective in AHF. If the arrhythmia causes hemodynamic instability, synchronized cardioversion with 50 to 100 J biphasic waveform is recommended (Table 21.3)[56].

Ventricular Arrhythmias

The treatment of patients with repetitive episodes of nonsustained or even sustained VT in the presence of AHF represents an important and extraordinarily difficult challenge. While nonsustained VT and sustained VT can exacerbate CHF and produce hypotension, acute treatments directed for VT such as IV amiodarone or procainamide may exacerbate hypotension. In addition, patients with hypotension who require IV inotropic agents may develop ventricular proarrhythmia due to treatment with IV dobutamine, dopamine, or milrinone. However, if these treatments are withheld, hypotension may worsen and exacerbate the clinical situation. Thus, treatment of patients with AHF and frequent episodes of ventricular arrhythmias represent a delicate balancing act.

A few general principles can be suggested. While IV amiodarone can produce hypotension as described above, it is generally better tolerated and more effective overall than IV procainamide or lidocaine. Treatment of hypotension in the

TABLE 21.3. Management of atrial fibrillation/flutter in acute heart failure

Intervention	Examples	Details
Rate control		
	Diltiazem IV	Cautious administration
	Esmolol IV	Cautious administration
	Digoxin IV	Rapid IV loading
	Amiodarone IV	May be preferred in many situations
Chemical cardioversion		
	Amiodarone	Low efficiency rates
	Procainamide	Low efficiency rates
Electrical cardioversion		Start at 200 J biphasic for AF
Adjunctive treatments		
	Optimize electrolytes	Mg, K, Ca
	Minimize inotropic agents	Lowest dose possible
	Anticoagulation	See text
	Add ARB/ACE inhibitors	May have some anti-AF effects

ACE, angiotensin-converting enzyme; AF, atrial fibrillation; ARB, angiotensin receptor blockers.

presence of ventricular arrhythmias should be undertaken with the lowest possible doses of inotropic agents. Occasionally, the addition of α-agonists to maintain blood pressure, while they may be deleterious because they increase afterload, may result in less ventricular proarrhythmia than higher dose β-adrenergic agents or phosphodiesterase inhibitors. Supplementation with magnesium or potassium may help suppress arrhythmias in the presence of inotropic agents even if frank hypokalemia or hypomagnesemia is not present (Table 21.4).

In patients with cardiogenic shock or severe hypotension in whom inotropic agents reproducibly exacerbate ventricular arrhythmias, intravenous balloon pump or left ventricular assist devices may improve hemodynamics. When fluid overload is a primary factor, ultrafiltration or diuresis, rather than additional inotropic agents, may be helpful (Tables 21.3 and 21.4).

Premature Ventricular Beats and Nonsustained Ventricular Tachycardia

Asymptomatic NSVT should not be treated with antiarrhythmic medications. Most of the available evidence does not support NSVT as a predictive factor for mortality, and there is no evidence that

TABLE 21.4. Management of ventricular arrhythmia in acute heart failure

Intervention	Examples	Details
Categorize severity		Most patients will not need treatment for PVCs, NSVT
Pharmacologic control	Amiodarone IV	
	Procainamide IV	
	Lidocaine IV	Less effective except in acute ischemia
Electrical cardioversion		See ACLS protocols
Adjunctive treatments	Optimize electrolytes	
	Minimize inotropic agents	
	Add ARB/ACE inhibitors	May have some anti-AF effects
IABP/LVAD		Possible proarrhythmia
General anesthesia/intubation		

ACLS, advanced cardiac life support; IABP, intraaortic balloon pump; LVAD, left ventricular assist device; PVC, premature ventricular contraction; NSVT, nonsustained ventricular tachycardia.

suppressing NSVT in CHF is beneficial. Symptomatic NSVT may benefit from addressing the AHF, correcting electrolyte abnormalities, and, if it requires specific treatment, amiodarone is probably the safest agent[56,57].

Polymorphic Ventricular Tachycardia

Polymorphic VT may be associated with proarrhythmic drugs or with electrolyte abnormalities (hypokalemia, hypomagnesemia) and QT prolongation. Addressing these factors may be sufficient, together with treatment of the AHF.

Sustained Ventricular Tachycardia and Ventricular Fibrillation

In the setting of AHF, sustained ventricular arrhythmias are poorly tolerated and immediate cardioversion should be the first line of therapy. Pharmacologic intervention with amiodarone, procainamide, or beta-blocking agents should be reserved for maintenance therapy, to prevent recurrences, and for patients who specifically refuse electrical therapy. The initial treatment of pulseless VT and VF should be performed in accordance with published guidelines[58], using biphasic defibrillation with a maximum of 200 J, and, if initial shocks do not terminate the arrhythmia, epinephrine 1 mg, vasopressin 40 IU, or amiodarone IV bolus 300 mg may be used, in conjunction with repeat shocks and with cardiopulmonary resuscitation (CPR). Subsequent suppression of the arrhythmia is attempted with amiodarone and/or beta-blockers, in addition to addressing all possible contributing factors. Correcting causal factors such as electrolyte abnormalities and certain drugs may be sufficient to eliminate polymorphic VT. However, if monomorphic VT is present, it should not be ascribed only to these factors, and specific therapy is required.

Ablation therapy can be very effective for selected patients with recurrent monomorphic VT. Bundle branch reentry may be cured with high success rate, but myocardial VT is also amenable to curative ablation.

Left ventricular assist devices (LVADs) may be helpful for circulatory support in case of intractable, persistent VT or VF, according to anecdotal reports. However, it has been reported that the early period after initiation of LVAD support is associated with a markedly higher incidence of new-onset monomorphic VT, which may be related to myocardial inflammation and wound healing, as well as early postoperative increases in the QTc interval after cardiac unloading[59,60].

The ICDs have not been used specifically for arrhythmia in AHF. While resynchronization therapy may alleviate chronic heart failure, there are little data to support its use in the treatment of AHF.

Case Presentation

A 43-year-old woman with a 1-year history of postpartum cardiomyopathy presents with increasing shortness of breath. Prior cardiac catheterizations have shown no coronary disease. Left ventricular ejection fraction has been 10%. New York Heart Association class III CHF has been present for 6 months, but recently she has complained of increasing light-headedness and shortness of breath. On admission, blood pressure is 80/50 mm Hg, central venous pressure 15 cm H_2O, pulse 110/minute, and rales and an S_3 are present. Repetitive bursts of nonsustained VT that is slightly polymorphic in nature are present on telemetry monitoring. A 12-lead ECG shows left bundle branch block. Potassium is 3.7 mEq/L, magnesium 1.6 mEq/L, blood urea nitrogen (BUN) is 35 mg/dL and creatinine is 1.2 mg/dL. Lasix, dopamine, and milrinone are administered with an increase in systolic blood pressure to 90 mm Hg. However, ventricular arrhythmias have become more frequent and cardiac output has subsequently decreased. What is the next appropriate management?

Discussion

In this patient, magnesium and potassium replacement should be useful. In her case, intravenous inotropic agents are causing a worsening of the ventricular arrhythmia, which is polymorphic and nonsustained at this point, but appears symptomatic, and potentially a harbinger of more serious arrhythmia, if no intervention is initiated. A decrease in the dose of dobutamine, milrinone, or both, or eliminating one of these agents, would probably be useful. If the inotropic agents are considered necessary, we suggest using a pulmonary artery catheter for hemodynamic monitoring, which would allow optimizing inotropic and diuretic management while trying to minimize proarrhythmia.

Conclusion

Arrhythmias in AHF are common, involve complex, multifactorial mechanisms, and have important prognostic and therapeutic implications. There are several therapies that are currently available, and their application has to be tailored to each individual patient. Further research is needed into the mechanisms involved and the epidemiology, prognostic significance, and treatment, including development of mechanism-specific interventions. It is hoped that this will lead to a better understanding and better treatment, and ultimately to better patient outcomes.

References

1. Benza R, Tallaj J, Felker G, et al. The impact of arrhythmias in acute heart failure. J Card Fail 2004;10:279–84.
2. Adams K Jr, Fonarow G, Emerman C, et al. Characteristics and outcomes of patients hospitalized for heart failure in the United States: rationale, design, and preliminary observations from the first 100,000 cases in the Acute Decompensated Heart Failure National Registry (ADHERE). Am Heart J 2005;149:209–16.
3. Fonarow G, Abraham W, Albert N, et al. Organized Program to Initiate Lifesaving Treatment in Hospitalized Patients with Heart Failure (OPTIMIZE-HF): rationale and design. Am Heart J 2004;148: 43–51.
4. Ehrlich J, Nattel S, Hohnloser S. Atrial fibrillation and congestive heart failure: specific considerations at the intersection of two common and important cardiac disease sets. J Cardiovasc Electrophysiol 2002;13:399–405.
5. Francis G. Development of arrhythmias in the patient with congestive heart failure: pathophysiology, prevalence and prognosis. Am J Cardiol 1986;57:3B–7B.
6. Holmes J, Kubo S, Cody R, et al. Milrinone in congestive heart failure: observations on ambulatory ventricular arrhythmias. Am Heart J 1985;110: 800–6.
7. Meinertz T, Hofmann T, Kasper W, et al. Significance of ventricular arrhythmias in idiopathic dilated cardiomyopathy. Am J Cardiol 1984;53: 902–7.
8. Doval H, Nul D, Grancelli H, et al. Nonsustained ventricular tachycardia in severe heart failure. Independent marker of increased mortality due to sudden death. GESICA-GEMA Investigators. Circulation 1996;94:3198–203.
9. Singh S, Fisher S, Carson P, et al. Prevalence and significance of nonsustained ventricular tachycardia in patients with premature ventricular contractions and heart failure treated with vasodilator therapy. Department of Veterans Affairs CHF STAT Investigators. J Am Coll Cardiol 1998;32:942–7.
10. Teerlink J, Jalaluddin M, Anderson S, et al. Ambulatory ventricular arrhythmias in patients with heart failure do not specifically predict an increased risk of sudden death. PROMISE (Prospective Randomized Milrinone Survival Evaluation) Investigators. Circulation 2000;101:40–6.
11. Intravenous nesiritide vs nitroglycerin for treatment of decompensated congestive heart failure: a randomized controlled trial. JAMA 2002;287: 1531–40.
12. Burger A, Horton D, LeJemtel T, et al. Effect of nesiritide (B-type natriuretic peptide) and dobutamine on ventricular arrhythmias in the treatment of patients with acutely decompensated congestive heart failure: the PRECEDENT study. Am Heart J 2002;144:1102–8.
13. Cleland J, Swedberg K, Follath F, et al. The EuroHeart Failure survey programme—a survey on the quality of care among patients with heart failure in Europe. Part 1: patient characteristics and diagnosis. Eur Heart J 2003;24: 442–63.
14. Follath F, Cleland J, Just H, et al. Efficacy and safety of intravenous levosimendan compared with dobutamine in severe low-output heart failure (the LIDO study): a randomised double-blind trial. Lancet 2002;360:196–202.
15. Gattis W, O'connor C, Gallup D, et al. Predischarge initiation of carvedilol in patients hospitalized for decompensated heart failure: results of the Initiation Management Predischarge: Process for Assessment of Carvedilol Therapy in Heart Failure (IMPACT-HF) trial. J Am Coll Cardiol 2004; 43:1534–41.
16. Hasdai D, Topol E, Kilaru R, et al. Frequency, patient characteristics, and outcomes of mild-to-moderate heart failure complicating ST-segment

elevation acute myocardial infarction: lessons from 4 international fibrinolytic therapy trials. Am Heart J 2003;145:73–9.
17. Kaluski E, Kobrin I, Zimlichman R, et al. RITZ-5: randomized intravenous TeZosentan (an endothelin-A/B antagonist) for the treatment of pulmonary edema: a prospective, multicenter, double-blind, placebo-controlled study. J Am Coll Cardiol 2003; 41:204–10.
18. O'Connor C, Gattis W, Adams K Jr, et al. Tezosentan in patients with acute heart failure and acute coronary syndromes: results of the Randomized Intravenous TeZosentan Study (RITZ-4). J Am Coll Cardiol 2003;41:1452–7.
19. O'Connor C, Stough W, Gallup DS. Demographics, clinical characteristics, and outcomes of patients hospitalized for decompensated heart failure: observations from the IMPACT-HF registry. J Card Fail 2005;11:200–5.
20. Rudiger A, Harjola V, Muller A, et al. Acute heart failure: clinical presentation, one-year mortality and prognostic factors. Eur J Heart Fail 2005;7:662–70.
21. Torre-Amione G, Young J, Colucci Wet al. Hemodynamic and clinical effects of tezosentan, an intravenous dual endothelin receptor antagonist, in patients hospitalized for acute decompensated heart failure. J Am Coll Cardiol 2003;42:140–7.
22. Zannad F, Briancon S, Juilliere Y, et al. Incidence, clinical and etiologic features, and outcomes of advanced chronic heart failure: the EPICAL Study. Epidemiologie de l'Insuffisance Cardiaque Avancee en Lorraine. J Am Coll Cardiol 1999;33:734–42.
23. Ravens U. Mechano-electric feedback and arrhythmias. Prog Biophys Mol Biol 2003;82:255–66.
24. Sachs F. Mechanoelectric transduction. In: Zipes D, Jalife J, eds. Cardiac Electrophysiology: From Cell to Bedside. Philadelphia: Saunders; 2004:96–102.
25. Calaghan S, Belus A, White E. Do stretch-induced changes in intracellular calcium modify the electrical activity of cardiac muscle? Prog Biophys Mol Biol 2002;82:81–95.
26. Zabel M, Koller B, Sachs F, et al. Stretch-induced voltage changes in the isolated beating heart: importance of the timing of stretch and implications for stretch-activated ion channels. Cardiovasc Res 1996;32:120–30.
27. Janse M, Coronel R, Wilms-Schopman F, et al. Mechanical effects on arrhythmogenesis: from pipette to patient. Prog Biophys Mol Biol 2003;82: 187–95.
28. Chen R, Penny D, Greve G, et al. Stretch-induced regional mechanoelectric dispersion and arrhythmia in the right ventricle of anesthetized lambs. Am J Physiol Heart Circ Physiol 2004;286:H1008–14.
29. Hansen D, Borganelli M, Stacy GP, Jr, et al. Dose-dependent inhibition of stretch-induced arrhythmias by gadolinium in isolated canine ventricles. Evidence for a unique mode of antiarrhythmic action. Circ Res 1991;69:820–31.
30. Bode F, Sachs F, Franz M. Tarantula peptide inhibits atrial fibrillation. Nature 2001;409:35–6.
31. Ausma J, Borgers M. Dedifferentiation of atrial cardiomyocytes: from in vivo to in vitro. Cardiovasc Res 2002;55(9–12).
32. Shi Y, Li D, Tardif J,, et al. Enalapril effects on atrial remodeling and atrial fibrillation in experimental congestive heart failure. Cardiovasc Res 2002;54: 456–61.
33. Pogwizd S, Schlotthauer K, Li L, et al. Arrhythmogenesis and contractile dysfunction in heart failure: roles of sodium-calcium exchange, inward rectifier potassium current, and residual beta-adrenergic responsiveness. Circ Res 2001;88:1159–554.
34. Janse M. Electrophysiological changes in heart failure and their relationship to arrhythmogenesis. Cardiovasc Res 2004;61:208–17.
35. Nuss H, Kaab S, Kass D, et al. Cellular basis of ventricular arrhythmias and abnormal automaticity in heart failure. Am J Physiol 1999;277: H80–H91.
36. Vermeulen J, McGuire M, Opthof T, et al. Triggered activity and automaticity in ventricular trabeculae of failing human and rabbit hearts. Cardiovasc Res 1994;28:1547–54.
37. Aronson D, Burger A. Diabetes and the occurrence of ventricular arrhythmic events in patients with severe left ventricular dysfunction. Diabetologia 2002;45:1440–5.
38. Aronson D, Burger A. Neurohumoral activation and ventricular arrhythmias in patients with decompensated congestive heart failure: role of endothelin. Pacing Clin Electrophysio 2003;26: 703–10.
39. Amsallem E, Kasparian C, Haddour G, et al. Phosphodiesterase III inhibitors for heart failure. Cochrane Database Syst Rev 2005;CD00:2230.
40. The effect of digoxin on mortality and morbidity in patients with heart failure. The Digitalis Investigation Group. N Engl J Med 1997;336:525–33.
41. Effect of metoprolol CR/XL in chronic heart failure: Metoprolol CR/XL Randomised Intervention Trial in Congestive Heart Failure (MERIT-HF). Lancet 1999;353:2001–7.
42. Packer M, Bristow M, Cohn J, et al. The effect of carvedilol on morbidity and mortality in patients with chronic heart failure. U.S. Carvedilol Heart Failure Study Group. N Engl J Med 1996;334: 1349–55.

43. Brodine W, Tung R, Lee J, et al. Effects of beta-blockers on implantable cardioverter defibrillator therapy and survival in the patients with ischemic cardiomyopathy (from the Multicenter Automatic Defibrillator Implantation Trial-II). Am J Cardiol 2005;96:691–5.
44. Aronson D, Burger A. Concomitant beta-blocker therapy is associated with a lower occurrence of ventricular arrhythmias in patients with decompensated heart failure. J Card Fail 2002;8:79–85.
45. Nieminen M, Bohm M, Cowie M, et al. Executive summary of the guidelines on the diagnosis and treatment of acute heart failure: the Task Force on Acute Heart Failure of the European Society of Cardiology. Eur Heart J 2005;26:384–416.
46. Mitchell L, Powell J, Gillis A, et al. Are lipid-lowering drugs also antiarrhythmic drugs? An analysis of the Antiarrhythmics versus Implantable Defibrillators (AVID) trial. J Am Coll Cardiol 2003;42: 81–7.
47. Vyas A, Guo H, Moss Aet al. Reduction in ventricular tachyarrhythmias with statins in the Multicenter Automatic Defibrillator Implantation Trial (MADIT)-II. J Am Coll Cardiol 2006;47:769–73.
48. Pitt B, Remme W, Zannad F, et al. Eplerenone, a selective aldosterone blocker, in patients with left ventricular dysfunction after myocardial infarction. N Engl J Med 2003;348:1309–21.
49. Pitt B, Zannad F, Remme W, et al. The effect of spironolactone on morbidity and mortality in patients with severe heart failure. Randomized Aldactone Evaluation Study Investigators. N Engl J Med 1999;341:709–17.
50. Ramires F, Mansur A, Coelho O, et al. Effect of spironolactone on ventricular arrhythmias in congestive heart failure secondary to idiopathic dilated or to ischemic cardiomyopathy. Am J Cardiol 2000;85:1207–11.
51. Callans DJ, Josephson ME. Ventricular tachycardia in patients with coronary artery disease. In: Zipes D, Jalife J, eds. Cardiac Electrophysiology: From Cell to Bedside. Philadelphia: Saunders; 2004:569–74.
52. Fuster V, Ryden L, Cannom D, et al. ACC/AHA/ESC 2006 guidelines for the management of patients with atrial fibrillation—executive summary: a report of the American College of Cardiology/ American Heart Association Task Force on Practice Guidelines and the European Society of Cardiology Committee for Practice Guidelines (Writing Committee to Revise the 2001 Guidelines for the Management of Patients With Atrial Fibrillation). J Am Coll Cardiol 2006;48:854–906.
53. Joglar J, Hamdan M, Ramaswamy K, et al. Initial energy for elective external cardioversion of persistent atrial fibrillation. Am J Cardiol 2000;86:348–50.
54. Wozakowska-Kaplon B, Janion M, Sielski J, et al. Efficacy of biphasic shock for transthoracic cardioversion of persistent atrial fibrillation: can we predict energy requirements? Pacing Clin Electrophysiol 2004;27:764–8.
55. Chicos A, Mykytsey A, Lavi N, Avitall B. Atrial remodeling in an atrial fibrillation model without left ventricular systolic dysfunction. Heart Rhythm 2006;3(1S):S306.
56. Zipes D, Camm A, Borggrefe M, et al. ACC/AHA/ ESC 2006 guidelines for management of patients with ventricular arrhythmias and the prevention of sudden cardiac death: a report of the American College of Cardiology/American Heart Association Task Force and the European Society of Cardiology Committee for Practice Guidelines (Writing Committee to Develop Guidelines for Management of Patients With Ventricular Arrhythmias and the Prevention of Sudden Cardiac Death). J Am Coll Cardiol 2006;48:e247–346.
57. Cleland J, Ghosh J, Freemantle N, et al. Clinical trials update and cumulative meta-analyses from the American College of Cardiology: WATCH, SCD-HeFT, DINAMIT, CASINO, INSPIRE, STRATUS-US, RIO-Lipids and cardiac resynchronisation therapy in heart failure. Eur J Heart Fail 2004;6:501–8.
58. 2005 American Heart Association guidelines for cardiopulmonary resuscitation and emergency cardiovascular care. Circulation 2005;112:IV1–203.
59. Harding J, Piacentino V III, Rothman S, et al. Prolonged repolarization after ventricular assist device support is associated with arrhythmias in humans with congestive heart failure. J Card Fail 2005;11: 227–32.
60. Ziv O, Dizon J, Thosani A, et al. Effects of left ventricular assist device therapy on ventricular arrhythmias. J Am Coll Cardiol 2005;45:1428–34.

1.3.2
Right Ventricular Dysfunction

22 Right Ventricular Dysfunction in the Intensive Care Unit

Vincent Caille, Cyril Charron, François Jardin, and Antoine Vieillard-Baron

Assessing right ventricular (RV) function in acute conditions, such as circulatory and respiratory failure, is of great importance for hemodynamic monitoring and therapeutic adaptation (1, 2). Right ventricular function is responsible for the back-pressure of systemic venous return (3), and for the amount of blood that reaches the pulmonary circulation, which is one of the main determinants of left ventricular (LV) stroke volume (4). Right ventricular failure in septic shock may explain why blood volume expansion is unable to increase cardiac output (5). In certain conditions, such as massive pulmonary embolism (PE) and acute respiratory distress syndrome (ARDS), RV failure may be the main cause of shock, leading to specific therapeutic interventions such as thrombolysis or limitation of airway pressures. Before considering the main causes of RV dysfunction, it is essential to understand the specific features of RV physiology.

Right Ventricular Physiology

Three characteristics of the right ventricle are essential: (1) the right ventricle ejects blood into the pulmonary circulation; (2) the right ventricle shares a wall, that is, the interventricular septum, with the left ventricle, and (3) the left and right ventricles are both enclosed in a stiff envelope, the pericardium. The first characteristic explains why changes in pulmonary circulation may alter RV function, while the second and the third characteristics explain why acute RV enlargement may impair LV function (Fig. 22.1).

Right ventricular diastolic function is tolerant. This means that, unlike the left ventricle, the right ventricle dilates acutely under pathophysiologic conditions, such as RV overload, because of a significantly lower diastolic elastance (6). The right ventricle also ejects blood into a low-resistance, high-compliance circuit, that is, the pulmonary circulation. Under acute conditions, it may develop a maximal systolic pressure of only 30 cm H_2O. It can be argued that RV systolic function is sensitive: even a slight increase in pulmonary vascular resistance can overload a normal right ventricle, thereby impairing its systolic function. Unlike the left ventricle, and whatever its origin, acute RV dysfunction is especially reflected in RV dilatation.

Effects of Mechanical Ventilation on Right Ventricular Function

Because mechanical ventilation may alter pulmonary circulation, and because any change in pulmonary circulation may alter RV function (7), RV function should always be assessed according to parameters of mechanical ventilation. Effects of mechanical ventilation on RV function result from increases in pleural pressure and transpulmonary pressure, that is, the distending pressure of the lung. They lead to a decrease in RV stroke volume. Such a decrease is cyclic, related to tidal ventilation (Fig. 22.2), or continuous, by application of a positive end-expiratory pressure (PEEP) (8).

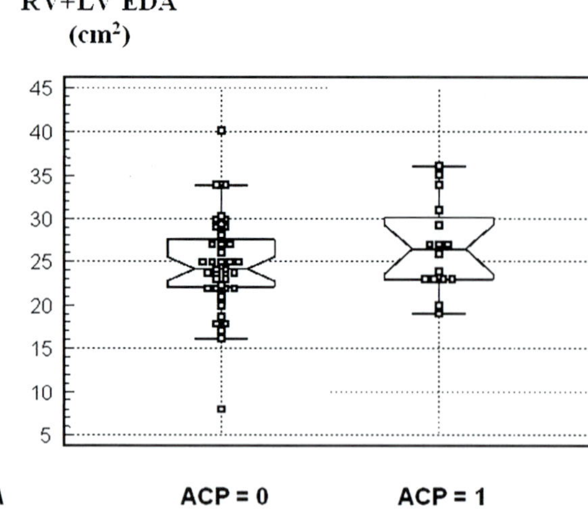

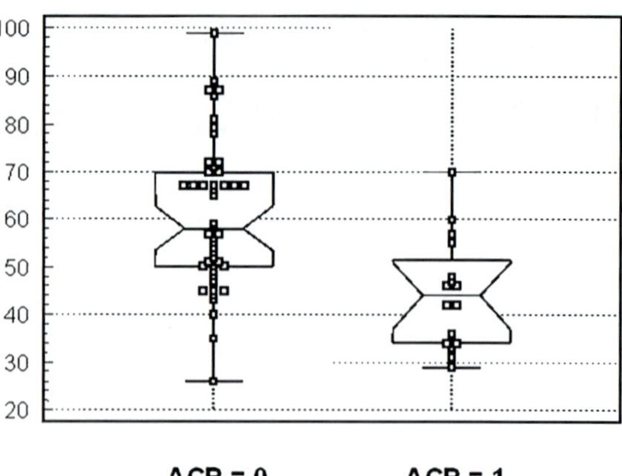

Figure 22.1. Box and Whisker plot analysis (median: horizontal line inside the box) of right and left ventricular size measured on a long-axis view in 75 patients ventilated for acute respiratory distress syndrome (ARDS), according to the presence or absence of acute cor pulmonale (ACP). Whereas the sum of the cardiac chambers did not differ significantly between the two groups (A), left ventricular end-diastolic volume (LVEDV) was significantly lower in patients with ACP (B). RV LV EDA, right and left ventricular end-diastolic area.

Pleural pressure is transmitted to the pericardial space and to the right atrium (9). Any increase in pleural pressure thus leads to an increase in intravascular right atrial pressure and so to a decrease in systemic venous return (3). Indeed, the venous return is promoted by a forward pressure, the mean systemic pressure, and impaired by a backward pressure, the right atrial pressure (3). It has also been demonstrated that increased pleural pressure reduces venous conductance (or increases venous resistance) (10), a consequence of the interposition of a collapsible vascular zone between the periphery and the right atrium. We have recently identified such a collapsible zone as the superior vena cava (SVC). This vessel is able to collapse during tidal ventilation in certain conditions as hypovolemia (11).

An increase in transpulmonary pressure, also resulting from tidal ventilation or application of PEEP, directly affects RV outflow impedance (12) by crushing the pulmonary capillaries (13). This effect on RV function especially predominates in ARDS patients in whom lung compliance is severely depressed (14).

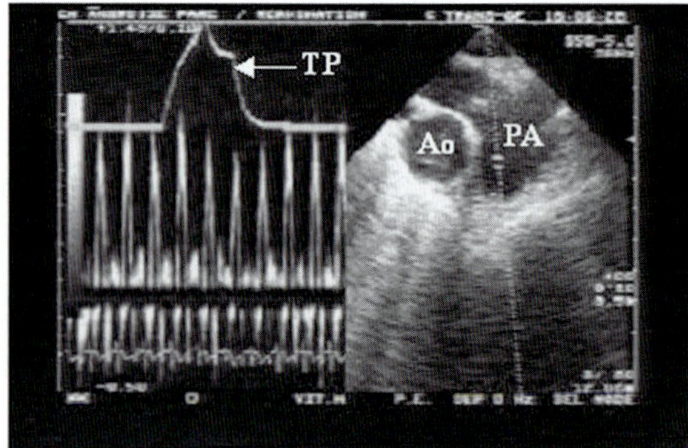

Figure 22.2. Pulsed Doppler in the pulmonary artery using a transesophageal approach in a mechanically ventilated patient. Tidal ventilation induces a cyclic decrease in right ventricular stroke volume, as shown by cyclic alterations in the velocity time integral of the flow.
TP, tracheal pressure; Ao, aorta; PA, pulmonary artery.

Diagnosis of Right Ventricular Dysfunction in the Intensive Care Unit

Numerous methods have been proposed to evaluate RV function in the ICU. In this review, we consider only two: right heart catheterization, because it was for a long time the only method available; and echocardiography, which is, in our

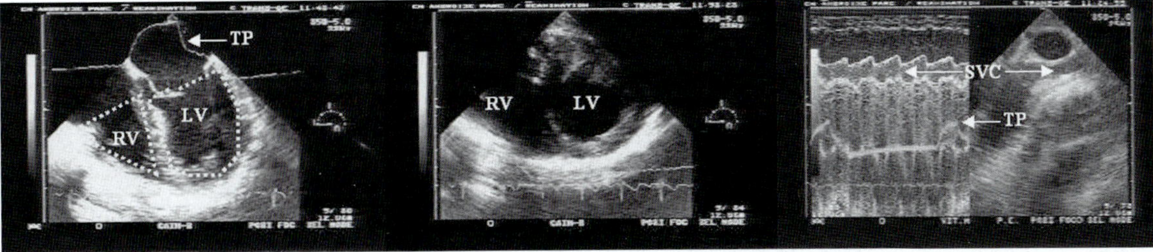

FIGURE 22.3. Three main views by transesophageal echocardiography permitting evaluation of right ventricular function. (A) Measurement of right and left ventricular end-diastolic areas from a long-axis view of the left ventricle (dotted lines). (B) Movements of the interventricular septum seen on a short-axis view of the left ventricle. (C) Long-axis view of the superior vena cava. Two-dimensional M-mode used to evaluate respiratory variations in SVC diameter. RV, right ventricle; LV, left ventricle; SVC, superior vena cava; TP, tracheal pressure.

opinion, the most suitable method of assessing RV function in the ICU (1). Echocardiography allows quick and noninvasive detection of the three main causes of RV dysfunction: preload defect, as in hypovolemia and cardiac tamponade; acute increase in afterload, as in massive PE and ARDS, leading to acute cor pulmonale (ACP); and depressed intrinsic contractility, as in severe sepsis and infarction. Echocardiography is an especially qualitative procedure that is appropriate in the ICU because simple indices are required in an emergency. A transthoracic approach can be used, although a transesophageal approach is preferred in mechanically ventilated patients and because it visualizes the SVC. The airway pressure signal on the screen of echocardiograph is absolutely required to localize cardiac events in the respiratory cycle (14). Only three views are essential (Fig. 22.3): (1) a long-axis view of the left ventricle to evaluate the size of the right ventricle, (2) a short-axis view of the left ventricle by a transgastric approach to evaluate septal kinetics and visualize a paradoxical septal motion, and (3) a long-axis view of the SVC to evaluate respiratory changes in SVC diameter.

Right Ventricular Dysfunction by Preload Insufficiency

Right atrial pressure (RAP), such as RV volumes measured using fast-response thermodilution, has been reported to be inaccurate in detecting RV preload insufficiency (15). In particular, RAP depends not only on RV preload but also on pleural pressure transmitted to the right atrium. So assessment of RV preload requires evaluation of pleural pressure to calculate the transmural RAP, that is, the distending pressure of the right atrium. This is not available in clinical practice. Clinical situations where intravascular RAP overestimates transmural RAP are frequent in the ICU (Fig. 22.4), such as positive pressure ventilation,

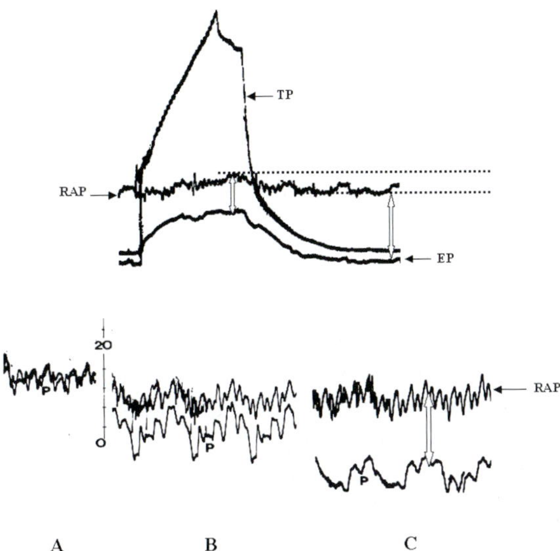

FIGURE 22.4. Differences between intravascular right atrial pressure (RAP) and its transmural pressure during mechanical ventilation (top), and in a patient with cardiac tamponade (bottom). In the first situation (top), tidal ventilation induces an increase in RAP (dotted lines), whereas the transmural pressure significantly decreases (vertical arrows). In the second situation (bottom), progressive drainage of pericardial effusion (B,C) induces a decrease in RAP when compared to baseline (A), whereas the transmural pressure increases (vertical arrows). TP, tracheal pressure; EP, esophageal pressure, reflecting pleural pressure.

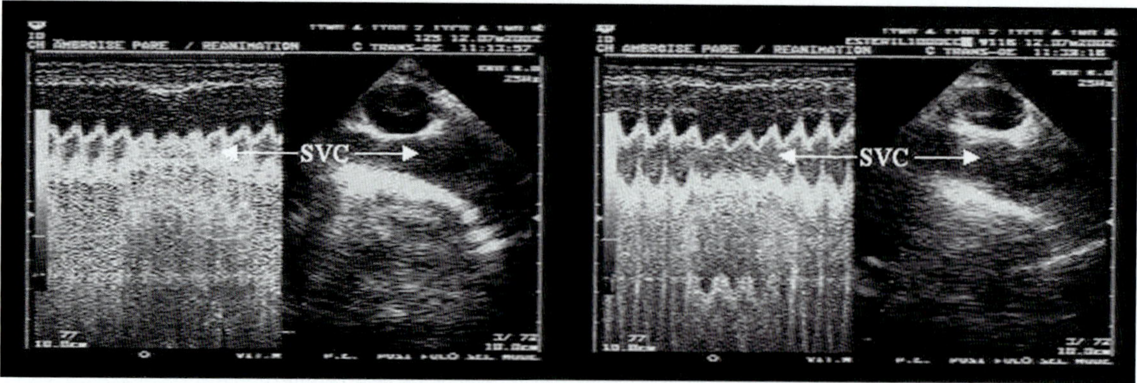

FIGURE 22.5. Respiratory variations in superior vena cava (SVC) diameter in a hypovolemic patient, visualized by two-dimensional M-mode. At baseline (A), SVC exhibited a complete collapse at each insufflation. After volume infusion (B), the collapse disappeared.

cardiac tamponade, and intrinsic PEEP. Although echocardiography may evaluate RAP from the inferior vena cava (IVC) diameter at end-expiration (16) and measure RV size, these limitations mean that such measurements are useless.

In our opinion, the most accurate index is the collapsibility index of the SVC, recorded by echocardiography. We have reported that the SVC can be visualized by a transesophageal approach and that its collapsibility index can be calculated from a long-axis view as its maximal diameter (during expiration) minus minimal diameter (during inspiration) divided by the maximal diameter (17). We have also reported that the SVC collapsibility index is very accurate in detecting hypovolemia; whereas a partial or complete collapse of the vessel during tidal ventilation suggests the need for blood volume expansion (Fig. 22.5), no or minimal respiratory variations in SVC diameter suggests an adequate RV preload (18). We and others have also proposed measuring respiratory variations in IVC diameter (19, 20). Unlike the SVC, the IVC dilates during tidal ventilation (20). The higher the distensibility index of the vessel, the higher the RV preload insufficiency (20). Importantly, the accuracy of these indices requires patients to be perfectly adapted to their respirator.

Right Ventricular Dysfunction by Increased Afterload

Because of its properties, any acute significant increase in RV afterload may induce RV dysfunction. This is responsible for a special condition called acute cor pulmonale. The term *cor pulmonale* was first used to describe the concept of cardiopulmonary interactions (21). Acute cor pulmonale occurs under pathophysiologic conditions in which the right ventricle is suddenly subject to large afterload, as in massive PE and ARDS (22, 23). Echocardiographic definition combines RV dilatation, reflecting RV diastolic overload, paradoxical septal motion, reflecting RV systolic overload, and LV relaxation impairment (24) (Fig. 22.6). Right ventricular dilatation is defined from the long-axis view of the left ventricle by a ratio of RV end-diastolic area to LV end-diastolic area that is above 0.6 (25). When this ratio is above 1, RV dilatation is severe (24). The paradoxical septal motion is visualized from a short-axis view of the left ventricle, such as a movement of the septum toward the center of the left ventricle at end-systole onset of diastole. It can also be diagnosed from a short-axis view by measuring at end-systole the eccentricity index of the left ventricle as the ratio of the anteroposterior diameter of the left ventricle to the septolateral diameter (26). In this case, this index is above 1; the normal value is about 1 (26). Finally, impairment in LV relaxation, induced by RV dilatation, is diagnosed using pulsed Doppler at the mitral annulus by an inverted E over A ratio, where E is the maximal velocity of mitral inflow at early diastole and A the maximal velocity at end-diastole.

Using right heart catheterization to diagnose ACP is problematic. Pulmonary artery pressures and pulmonary vascular resistances are unable to evaluate the tolerance of the right ventricle to overload. We have demonstrated in ARDS a large overlap of pulmonary artery pressures between patients with and without ACP (23). In this study, pulmonary artery pressures were calculated at echocardiography, using Doppler recording of the tricuspid regurgitation flow. Zapol and Snider (27) have reported in ARDS that pulmonary vascular resistances were modified according to cardiac output. Some authors have proposed defining ACP as an RAP greater than the pulmonary capillary wedge pressure (28). Finally, the least incorrect index is probably the presence of a significant gradient between the diastolic pulmonary artery pressure and the pulmonary capillary wedge pressure (29). This is illustrated in Figure 22.6.

Acute cor pulmonale is not rare in the ICU and should have a significant impact on treatment. We found an ACP incidence of 61% in a large population of patients with massive PE, affecting more than two lobar arteries (22). Association of ACP with shock and tissue hypoperfusion resulted in a high mortality rate (22), suggesting the use of thrombolysis in this population. In a large

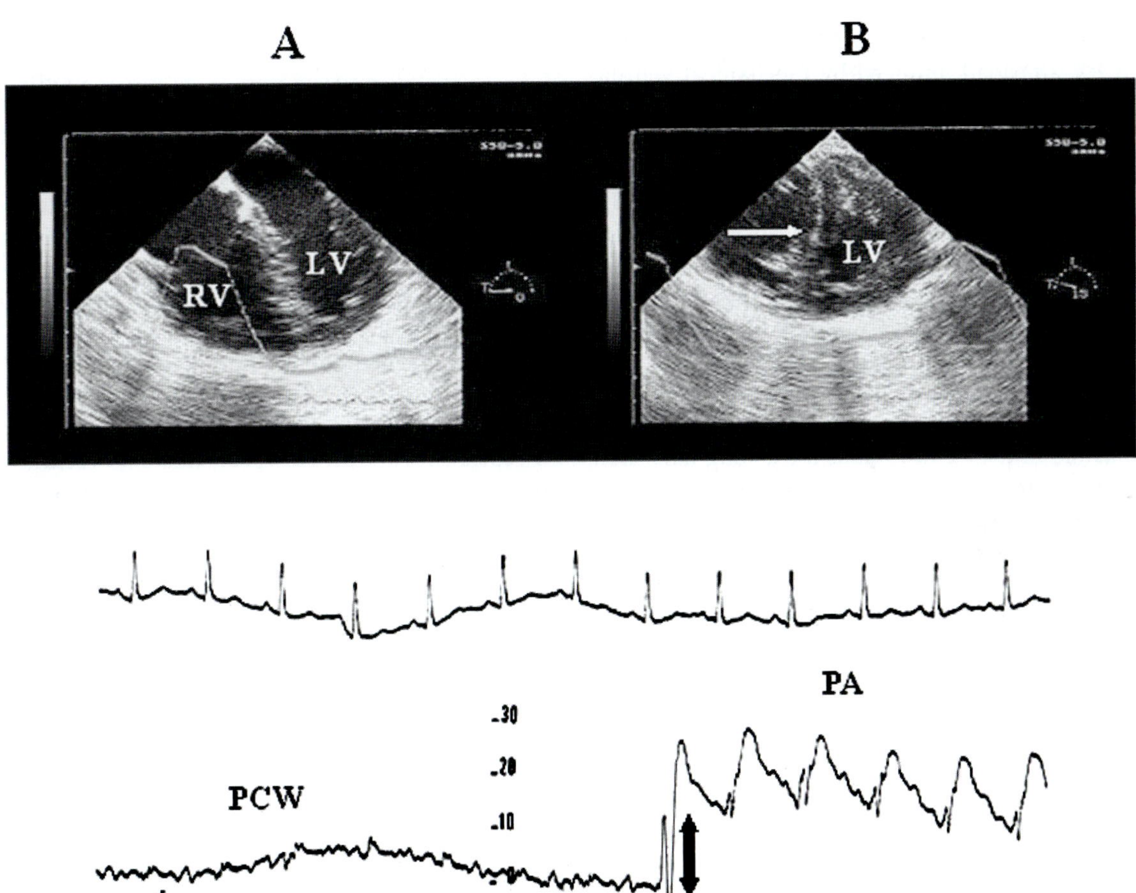

FIGURE 22.6. Top: Transesophageal echocardiography in a patient ventilated for ARDS and who exhibited acute cor pulmonale. The long-axis view demonstrated right ventricular dilatation (A) and the short-axis view paradoxical septal motion (B, arrow). Bottom: Right heart catheterization in a patient ventilated for ARDS. Note the importance of the pressure gradient (vertical arrow) between the pulmonary capillary wedge pressure (PCW) and the diastolic pulmonary artery pressure (PA). RV, right ventricle; LV, left ventricle.

population of 75 ARDS patients, we also reported a 25% incidence of ACP after 3 days under protective mechanical ventilation (23). In our opinion, this strictly limits plateau pressure, decreases PEEP, and controls hypercapnia (30). It is interesting to note that in a previous study performed in ARDS patients ventilated without plateau pressure limitation, the ACP incidence was 60% (31).

Right Ventricular Dysfunction by Depressed Intrinsic Contractility

This situation is especially present in acute infarction affecting the right ventricle, which is described in another chapter, and in severe sepsis. It is also important to reemphasize that mechanical ventilation of a patient with moderately depressed RV contractility may induce ACP. The small increase in RV afterload, induced by mechanical ventilation, is enough to be poorly tolerated by an abnormal right ventricle (2).

When evaluating RV contractility, it seems natural to measure RV ejection fraction (RVEF). This was proposed in severe sepsis using fast-response thermodilution (5, 32), leading to an incidence of RV dysfunction over 50% (32). Right ventricular volume measurement by echocardiography is not accurate in clinical practice, because of the complex geometric form of the right ventricle. We prefer to measure the RV area at end-diastole and at end-systole on a long-axis view and thus to calculate the RV fractional area contraction (RVFAC), which is close to RVEF. Using such an index, we previously reported an over 30% incidence of depressed RV contractility in severe sepsis (33). This largely explains why in some cases blood volume infusion is unable to increase cardiac output significantly, despite relatively low LV filling pressures (5).

However, RVEF and RVFAC have a few limitations. In a population of healthy volunteers, we reported normal values of RVFAC as low as 38% (Fig. 22.7). Furthermore, in a population of ARDS patients, we did not find any difference in RVFAC between presence and absence of ACP (23) (Fig. 22.7). In measuring RVEF by fast-response thermodilution, technical limitations are added to this physiologic limitation. First, the RVEF value largely depends on when it is measured during the respiratory cycle (34). Tidal ventilation underestimates RVEF (34). Second, RV volumes are overestimated in the case of significant pulmonary hypertension, a quite frequent situation in the ICU (35). Finally, the best index of significantly depressed RV contractility is probably RV dilatation, because of the ability of the right ventricle to dilate acutely in pathophysiologic conditions. Using such an index, we previously demonstrated a 33% incidence of RV dysfunction in septic shock (36). However, this also includes ACP related to ARDS, a situation frequently encountered in sepsis.

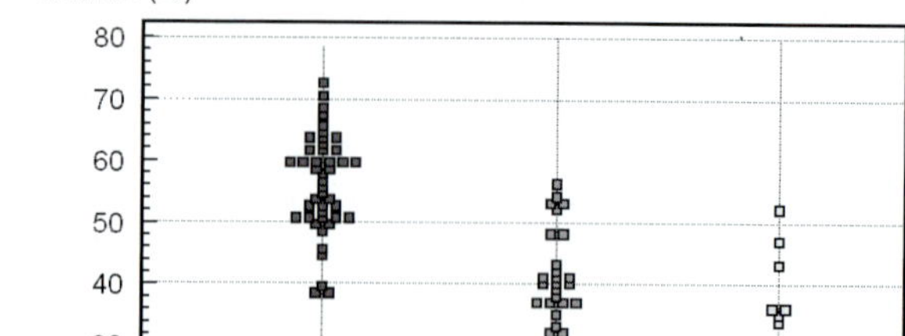
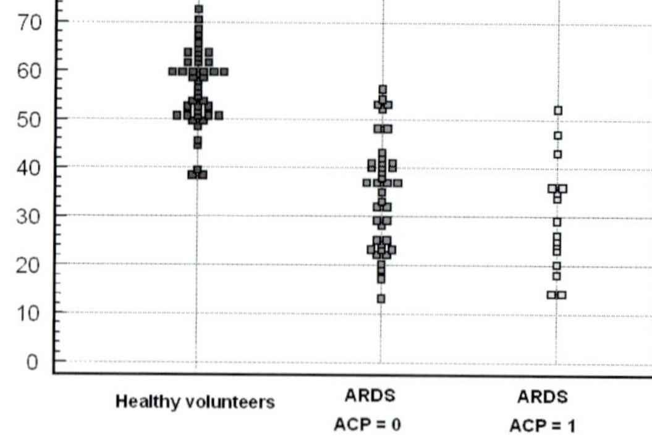

FIGURE 22.7. Distribution of right ventricular fractional area contraction (RVFAC) measured by echocardiography in three groups: healthy volunteers and ARDS patients with and without acute cor pulmonale (ACP).

Case Report 1

This case demonstrates how echocardiography at the bedside can quickly correct misdiagnosis in a setting of circulatory failure.

A 49-year-old woman was admitted to the emergency room for shock. Recent history revealed an ankle sprain. Clinical presentation included hyperthermia (38.5°C), hypotension (systolic blood pressure 89 mm Hg), tachycardia (heart rate 120 beats/min), peripheral vasoconstriction, and encephalopathy. Urine was purulent. Initial laboratory findings were as follows: white blood cell (WBC) count = 18.3×10^9 cells/L, pH = 7.29, PaO_2 = 50 mm Hg, $PaCO_2$ = 70 mm Hg, base excess = −15 mEq/L. The chest x-ray was normal. After initial oxygen therapy and fluid challenge, the patient was quickly admitted to our ICU with a diagnosis of severe sepsis of urinary origin. The patient was sedated and mechanical ventilation was started. Two minutes after mechanical ventilation, sudden cardiac arrest was observed and required cardiac resuscitation. Transesophageal echocardiography (TEE) demonstrated acute cor pulmonale (Fig. 22.8), and visualized thrombi in the right atrium and pulmonary artery (Fig. 22.8), leading to a diagnosis of massive pulmonary embolism. Thrombolysis was immediately started without radiologic exams. Unfortunately, the patient died of multiple organ failure on the fifth day of intensive care hospitalization.

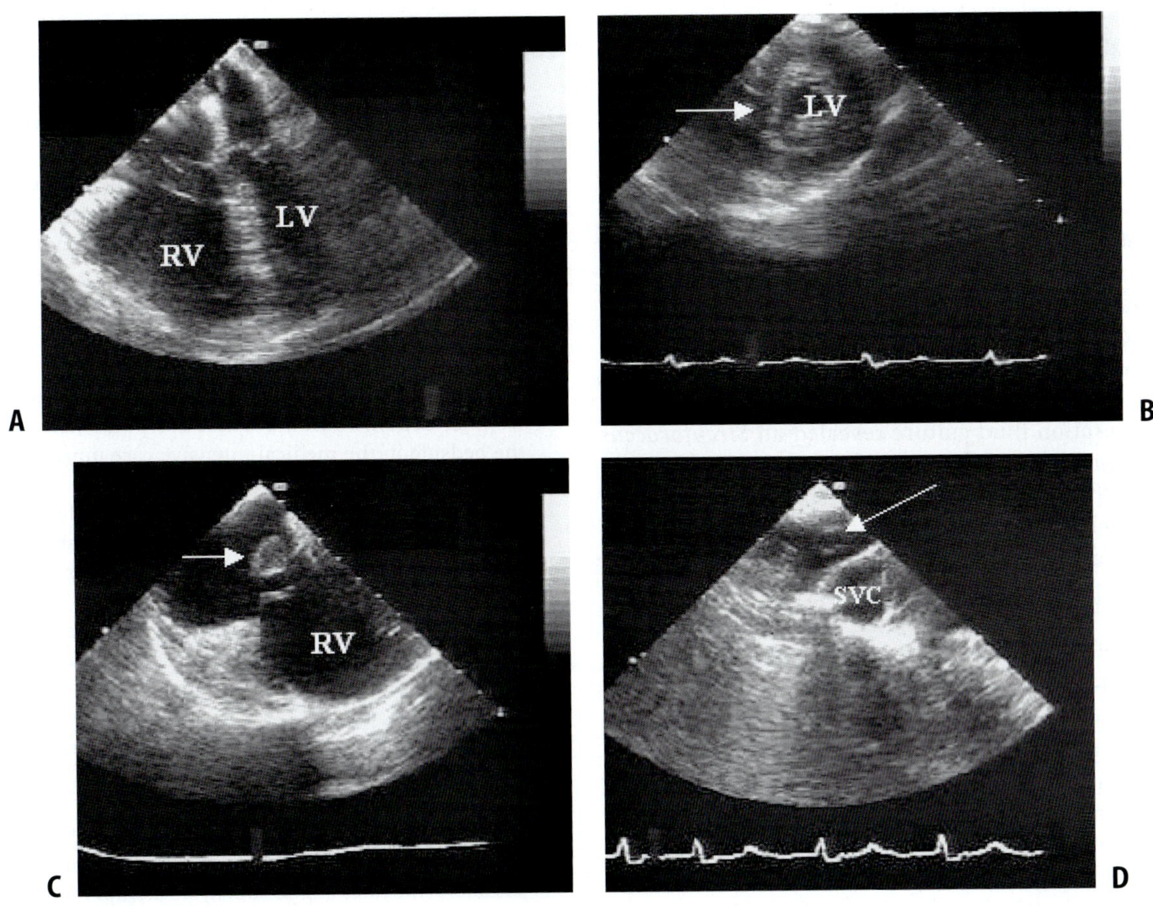

FIGURE 22.8. Case report 1: transesophageal echocardiography (TEE), from A to D, demonstrated acute cor pulmonale.

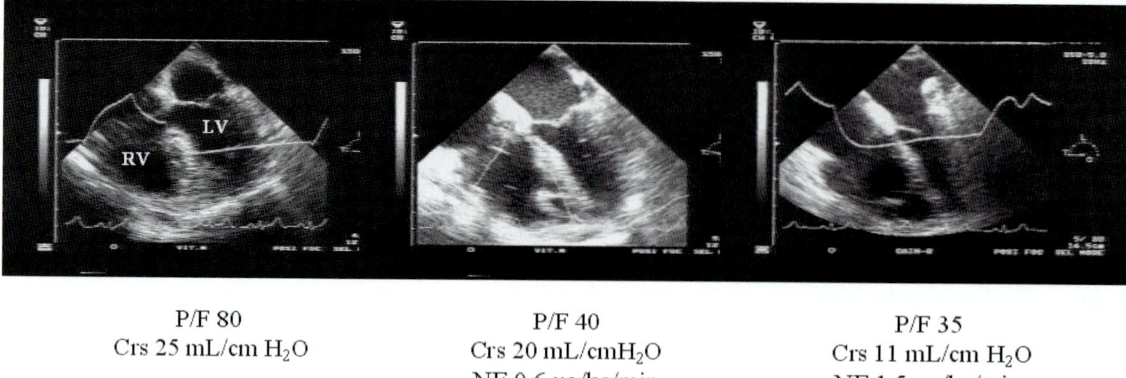

FIGURE 22.9. Case report 2: Transesophageal echocardiography was performed after 2, 5, and 9 days of mechanical ventilation. P/E, PaO_2/FiO_2 ratio; Crs, compliance of the respiratory system; NE, norepinephrine.

Case Report 2

In this case, daily TEE detected progressive RV failure in an ARDS patient.

A 60-year-old woman was admitted to our intensive care unit for extensive pneumonia. No past medical conditions were noted. She presented a 1-day history of fever and cough productive of thick yellow sputum. The physical examination noted hyperthermia, tachycardia (100/min), dyspnea (40/min), and cyanosis associated with x-ray bilateral chest infiltrates. Initial broncho-aspiration fluid culture revealed an *Streptococcus pneumoniae* strain. Mechanical ventilatory support was quickly needed. The patient rapidly developed ARDS. Cardiocirculatory status was initially preserved, but the patient exhibited acute cor pulmonale. Transesophageal echocardiography was performed after 2, 5, and 9 days of mechanical ventilation (Fig. 22.9). We demonstrated that progressive impairment of respiratory mechanics and of oxygenation was responsible for progressive right ventricular enlargement, leading to progressive left ventricular restriction, which caused shock (Fig. 22.9). In our opinion, it was necessary to strictly limit plateau pressure and positive end-expiratory pressure to relieve right ventricular function. After 21 days, the patient recovered and right function was completely normalized.

Conclusion

Diagnosing RV dysfunction is of great importance in the ICU because it frequently contributes to shock, especially in mechanically ventilated patients. In this situation, echocardiography is clearly the best diagnostic technique.

References

1. Vieillard-Baron A, Prin S, Chergui K, et al. Echo-Doppler demonstration of acute cor pulmonale at the bedside in the medical intensive care unit. Am J Respir Crit Care Med 2002;166:1310–1319.
2. Vieillard-Baron A, Prin S, Chergui K, et al. Hemodynamic instability in sepsis: bedside assessment by Doppler echocardiography. Am J Respir Crit Care Med 2003;168:1270–1276.
3. Guyton A, Lindsey A, Abernathy B, et al. Venous return at various right atrial pressures and the normal venous return curve. Am J Physiol 1957; 189:609–615.
4. Milnor W, Jose A, McGaff C. Pulmonary vascular volume, resistance and compliance in man. Circulation 1960;22:130.
5. Schneider A, Teule G, Groeneveld A, et al. Biventricular performance during volume loading in patients with early septic shock, with emphasis on the right ventricle: a combined hemodynamic and radionuclide study. Am Heart J 1988;116: 103–112.

6. Laks M, Garner D, Swan H. Volumes and compliances measured simultaneously in the right and left ventricles of the dog. Circ Res 1967;20:565–569.
7. Jardin F, Vieillard-Baron A. Right ventricular function and positive pressure ventilation in clinical practice: from hemodynamic subsets to respirator settings. Intensive Care Med 2003;29: 1426–1434.
8. Jardin F, Brun-Ney D, Cazaux P, et al. Relation between transpulmonary isovolumetric pressure change during respiratory support. Cathet Cardiovasc Diagn 1989;16:215–220.
9. Morgan B, Guntherot W, Dillard D. Relationship of pericardial to pleural pressure during quiet respiration and cardiac tamponade. Circ Res 1965;16: 493–498.
10. Fessler H, Brower R, Wise R, Permutt S. Effects of positive end-expiratory pressure on the canine venous return curve. Am Rev Respir Dis 1992;146: 4–10.
11. Vieillard-Baron A, Augarde R, Prin S, et al. Influence of superior vena caval zone condition on cyclic changes in right ventricular outflow during respiratory support. Anesthesiology 2001;95: 1083–1088.
12. Whittenberger J, McGregor M, Berglund E, et al. Influence of state of inflation of the lung on pulmonary vascular resistance. J Appl Physiol 1960;15: 878–882.
13. West J, Dollery C, Naimark A. Distribution of blood flow in isolated lung; relation to vascular and alveolar pressures. J Appl Physiol 1964;19:713–724.
14. Vieillard-Baron A, Loubières A, Schmitt JM, et al. Cyclic changes in right ventricular output impedance during mechanical ventilation. J Appl Physiol 1999;87:1644–1650.
15. Michard F, Teboul JL. Predicting fluid responsiveness in ICU patients. A critical analysis of the evidence. Chest 2002;121:2000–2008.
16. Barbier C, Loubières Y, Jardin F, et al. Author's reply to the comment by Dr. Bendjelid. Intensive Care Med 2004;30:1848.
17. Vieillard-Baron A, Chergui K, Augarde R, et al. Cyclic changes in arterial pulse during respiratory support revisited by Doppler echocardiography. Am J Respir Crit Care Med 2003;168:671–676.
18. Vieillard-Baron A, Chergui K, Rabiller A, et al. Superior vena caval collapsibility as a gauge of volume status in ventilated septic patients. Intensive Care Med 2004;30:1734–1739.
19. Feissel M, Michard F, Faller JP, et al. The respiratory variation in inferior vena cava diameter as a guide to fluid therapy. Intensive Care Med 2004;30: 1834–1837.
20. Barbier C, Loubières Y, Schmit C, et al. Respiratory changes in inferior vena cava diameter are helpful in predicting fluid responsiveness in ventilated septic patients. Intensive Care Med 2004;30: 1740–1746.
21. Testa AG: Delle malattie del cuore: loro cagioni, specie, segni e cura. Nuova edition. Schieppati, Truffi e Fusi, ed. Milano: 1831.
22. Vieillard-Baron A, Page B, Augarde R, et al. Acute cor pulmonale in massive pulmonary embolism: incidence, echocardiographic pattern, clinical implications and recovery rate. Intensive Care Med 2001;27:1481–1486.
23. Vieillard-Baron A, Schmitt JM, Augarde R, et al. Acute cor pulmonale in acute respiratory distress syndrome submitted to protective ventilation: incidence, clinical implications, and prognosis. Crit Care Med 2001;29:1551–1555.
24. Jardin F, Dubourg O, Bourdarias JP. Echocardiographic pattern of acute cor pulmonale. Chest 1997; 111:209–217.
25. Weyman AE. Cross-Sectionnal Echocardiography. In: Lea & Febiger, ed. Philadelphia, PA:1982:501–502.
26. Ryan T, Petrovic O, Dillon J, et al. An echocardiographic index for separation of right ventricular volume and pressure overload. J Am Coll Cardiol 1985;5:918–924.
27. Zapol W, Snider M. Pulmonary hypertension in severe acute respiratory failure. N Engl J Med 1977; 296:476–480.
28. Monchi M, Bellenfant F, Cariou A, et al. Early predictive factors of survival in the acute respiratory distress syndrome. A multivariate analysis. Am J Respir Crit Care Med 1998;158:1076–1081.
29. Her C, Mandy S, Bairamian M. Increased pulmonary venous resistance contributes to increased pulmonary artery diastolic-pulmonary wedge pressure gradient in acute respiratory distress syndrome. Anesthesiology 2005;102:574–580.
30. Vieillard-Baron A, Jardin F. Why protect the right ventricle in patients with acute respiratory distress syndrome? Curr Opin Crit Care 2003;9:15–21.
31. Jardin F, Gueret P, Dubourg O, et al. Two-dimensional echocardiographic evaluation of right ventricular size and contractility in acute respiratory failure. Crit Care Med 1985;13:952–956.
32. Kimchi A, Ellrodt G, Berman D, et al. Right ventricular performance in septic shock: a combined radionuclide and hemodynamic study. J Am Coll Cardiol 1984;4:945–951.
33. Jardin F, Brun-Ney D, Auvert B, et al. Sepsis-related cardiogenic shock. Crit Care Med 1990;110:402–409.

34. Groeneveld J, Berendsen R, Schneider A, et al. Effect of the mechanical ventilatory cycle on thermodilution right ventricular volumes and cardiac output. J Appl Physiol 2000;89:89–96.
35. Hoeper M, Tongers J, Leppert A, et al. Evaluation of right ventricular performance with right ventricular ejection fraction thermodilution catheter and MRI in patients with pulmonary hypertension. Chest 2001;120:502–507.
36. Vieillard-Baron A, Schmitt JM, Beauchet A, et al. Early preload adaptation in septic shock? A transesophageal echocardiographic study. Anesthesiology 2001;94:400–406.

23 Acute Pericardial Disease

Gorazd Voga

Acute pericardial diseases include acute pericarditis and cardiac tamponade. Both conditions can be associated with acute hemodynamic instability or cardiac failure and require immediate diagnostic workup and treatment.

The pericardium surrounds the heart with two layers. The outer fibrous layer is called the parietal pericardium; the inner layer, which covers the cardiac surface, is the serous visceral pericardium. The pericardium is attached to the sternum and diaphragm by ligamentous bindings. Up to 50 mL of fluid produced by visceral pericardial cells is normally present in the pericardial space (1).

The pericardium can be affected by a wide variety of microorganisms, a nonspecific inflammatory process, and various heart and systemic diseases. Irrespective of the etiology, clinical manifestations of the pericardial diseases correspond the pericardial inflammation, pericardial effusion with cardiac tamponade, and pericardial constriction due to calcifications (2).

Acute Pericarditis

A number of diseases, syndromes, and agents can produce a clinical syndrome termed acute pericarditis, which is the consequence of the inflammation of the pericardial layers. In a majority of cases the histopathologic changes show hyperemia, increased microvasculature, accumulation of leukocytes, deposition of fibrin, and adhesions that can be formed between layers or pericardium and adjacent structures. If an acute pericarditis is accompanied by myocarditis or pericardial effusion it can present with symptoms of acute heart failure. The etiologic causes are listed in Table 23.1.

Clinical Picture

Acute pericarditis is characterized by progressive central chest pain, pericardial friction rub, and repolarization changes in the electrocardiogram. The chest pain occurs rapidly and is usually sharp, pleuritic, and postural, being worse while lying supine and by coughing, and frequently reduced by sitting up. It can radiate to the neck, trapezius ridge, or shoulder, and can mimic angina pectoris, making the differentiation from acute coronary syndrome more difficult. On the other hand, acute pericarditis can present with only vague precordial distress, or it may be asymptomatic. Fever and cough can also occur, and some patients report breathing problems, but true dyspnea is present only in patients with cardiac tamponade or coexisting pulmonary and cardiac diseases. Pleural effusion may also be present.

The most typical physical sign is the pericardial friction rub, which can be heard in approximately three fourths of patients. It has classically three components related to atrial systole, ventricular systole, and ventricular diastole. Since the rub usually waxes and wanes, a repeated auscultation in various positions is mandatory. Cardiac sounds can be distant or muted due to development of pericardial effusion.

Diagnosis

The basic diagnostic workup requires a history, physical examination, electrocardiography,

TABLE 23.1. Etiology of pericarditis

Infectious pericarditis
Pericarditis in systemic autoimmune diseases
Pericarditis and effusion in diseases of surrounding organs
Pericarditis in metabolic disorders
Traumatic pericarditis
Neoplastic pericardial disease
Idiopathic pericarditis

Source: Adapted from Maisch et al. (3).

laboratory tests, and chest x-ray. Electrocardiogram (ECG) is abnormal in most patients with pericarditis. Changes are present in the majority of limb and precordial leads with four characteristic phases: ST segment elevation with J point elevation and upright T waves (phase I), normalization of ECG (phase II), T-wave inversion (phase III), and normal ECG tracing (phase IV) (4). In more than 40% of patients atypical ECG changes are found. ST elevation in only a few leads can be confusing and may suggest myocardial infarction. However, in patients with pericarditis, reciprocal ST depression is usually absent.

Laboratory tests can show changes in white blood cell count, sedimentation rate, and other acute-phase reactants. Serum troponin level can be elevated, especially when pericarditis is accompanied with myocarditis (5).

Cardiomegaly on chest radiography is usually not evident, unless more than 250 mL of pericardial fluid is present.

Radionuclide studies with indium 111 or gallium 67 can be useful for confirmation of pericardial inflammation (6, 7).

Idiopathic pericarditis is the most common form of the acute pericarditis, but in fact most cases are due to viral infection. Specific etiologic diagnosis can be confirmed by tuberculin skin testing, viral studies, rheumatoid factor, and antinuclear antibodies. Renal failure, neoplastic diseases, cardiac surgery, and secondary to chest radiotherapy should be considered as causes of secondary pericarditis. The term *autoreactive pericarditis* is characterized by elements of autoimmune response (8). Considering that idiopathic pericarditis resolves spontaneously in most patients, the tests for diagnosis of viral and autoimmune etiology (immunoglobulins, complements in pericardial fluid, virologic and immunohistologic studies) are too complex and expensive for routine practice (2). On the other hand, suspected purulent pericarditis in the presence of bacterial chest infections should be confirmed or excluded as soon as possible (9).

Echocardiography, which should be performed in all patients, is not specific for the diagnosis of pericarditis, but it shows pericardial effusion in approximately 10% of patients. Cardiac tamponade occurs more frequently in patients with specific etiology (tuberculosis, neoplastic and purulent pericarditis) than in patients with idiopathic pericarditis (10).

In the differential diagnosis acute coronary syndrome, dissecting aortic aneurysm, and pleuritis should be considered.

In the diagnostic workup of acute pericarditis, the three-stage approach seems to be appropriate:

Stage 1 is a history, physical examination, ECG, chest x-ray, general blood analysis, and echocardiography. In patients with tamponade or prolonged pericardial effusion (more than 1 week), tuberculosis should be excluded and antinuclear antibodies should me measured. Stage 2 is pericardiocentesis and proper examination of the pericardial fluid, which should be performed in patients with suspected purulent or neoplastic pericarditis and in patients with cardiac tamponade (therapeutic indication). Stage 3 is a pericardial biopsy, which is indicated only in patients with recurrent tamponade and in patients with persistent clinical effusion and clinical symptoms without etiologic diagnosis for more than 3 weeks (2). Other authors advocate an early invasive approach with pericardioscopy and pericardial biopsy for establishing the specific etiologic diagnosis (11–13).

Treatment

Despite the fact that most patients with acute pericarditis are hospitalized, hospital admission and treatment are absolutely necessary only for patients with idiopathic or viral pericarditis, who have large effusion or cardiac tamponade, concomitant myocarditis, high fever, or subacute clinical course, and for immunocompromised patients and those with anticoagulant treatment (14).

Patients are treated with aspirin (initial dose of 500 to 1000 mg every 6 hours) or with nonsteroidal antiinflammatory agents (ibuprofen 1800 to 2400 mg/day, indomethacin 75 to 225 mg/day, or paracetamol 3 to 4 g/day) for at least 3 weeks (2, 3). Indomethacin should not be used in elderly patients and in patients with coronary artery disease. Corticosteroids should be avoided and considered only in patients in whom tuberculosis is excluded and who are resistant to treatment and have persistent symptoms for more than 1 week. Corticosteroids can be used also in patients with connective tissue diseases or autoreactive and uremic pericarditis. Intrapericardial application of corticosteroids is effective and avoids systemic side effects (8).

Recurrent pericarditis occurs in around 24% of patients, usually in the first weeks after the first episode of acute pericarditis (15). The treatment of recurrences is basically the same as for the first episode, but in patients with two or more recurrences, treatment with colchicine may be successful (16). Intrapericardial treatment with cisplatin appeared to prevent recurrences of neoplastic pericardial effusion (17).

Table 23.2. Etiology of cardiac tamponade

Medical diseases
Common
Malignant diseases
Renal failure
Viral pericarditis
Less common
Radiation therapy, anticoagulant therapy
Hypothyrosis
Rheumatoid arthritis, systemic lupus erythematosus
Tuberculosis, AIDS
Acute myocardial infarction (thrombolysis, rupture)
Purulent pericarditis
Surgical conditions
Invasive cardiac procedures with perforation
Cardiovascular surgery and postpericardiotomy syndrome
Chest trauma
Aortic dissection

Source: Adapted from Davies et al. (18).

Cardiac Tamponade

Cardiac tamponade is the pathologic restraint of cardiac filling due to increased pericardial pressure, caused by the excess of fluid in the pericardial cavity. Typical characteristics of tamponade are equalization of left and right ventricular filling pressure, restricted diastolic filling of both ventricles, and decreased cardiac output with development of shock (1). Cardiac tamponade can occur in any disease with pericardial effusion, but it is most common in patients with pericardial effusion due to malignant diseases, renal failure, and viral pericarditis. Other medical diseases and surgical conditions that can provoke tamponade are listed in Table 23.2. Parietal pericardium can exert an important radial stress on the heart and can significantly limit the cardiac volume even in normal conditions. Pericardial restrain becomes very important under pathologic conditions. Cardiac chambers compliance is markedly decreased and diastolic ventricular interaction is augmented. The compressive effect of pericardial pressure is exerted primarily on the right heart and caval vessels. The left ventricular function becomes compromised later on as a consequence of inadequate filling. The different effect on the right and left ventricle is probably related to high right ventricular compliance, the extrapericardial part of the left atrium, and the long intrapericardial segment of the caval vessels (18). In patients with classic findings of tamponade without pericardial effusion, a tension pneumopericardium must be suspected (19).

Clinical Picture

The clinical picture depends on the underlying etiology, preexistent heart and lung diseases, and the rapidity of fluid accumulation. Accumulation of the intrapericardial fluid is associated with initial small increase of the intrapericardial pressure and followed by a steep rise. Once pericardium can no longer stretch, a tamponade is typically produced with very little accumulated fluid (Fig. 23.1) (20). In acute severe hemorrhage tamponade can occur with accumulation of 100 to 300 mL. It is typically clinically presented as an obstructive shock with systemic hypotension and elevated central venous pressure (distended neck veins!) without pulmonary congestion. The diagnosis of cardiac tamponade must always be considered as a possible etiology of unexplained

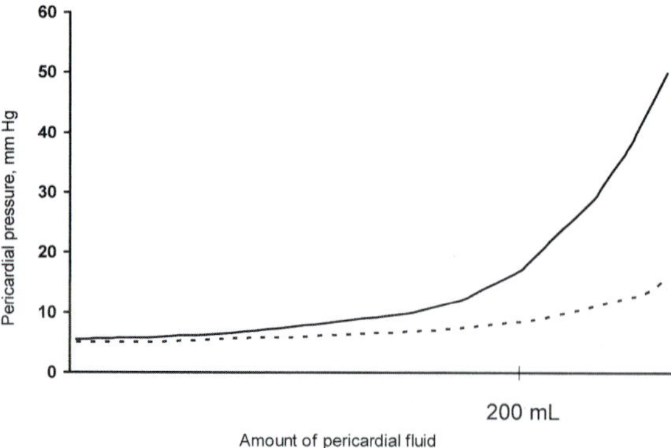

FIGURE 23.1. Schematic drawing representing the relation between amount of the accumulated pericardial fluid and pericardial pressure in acute (solid line) and subacute (dotted line) tamponade.

obstructive shock. If the pericardial fluid accumulates slowly, much larger amounts (2 L or more) can be accommodated. Dyspnea with orthopnea and signs of low output syndromes or mechanical compression of adjacent organs are the most common patient complaints (21, 22).

Acute tamponade, which is usually associated with severe hemodynamic compromise, is most frequently caused by trauma and rupture of the heart or aorta. Subacute tamponade has a less dramatic clinical presentation and is associated with idiopathic, uremic, or neoplastic pericarditis. Regional tamponade (loculated pericardial effusion or localized hematoma) occurs usually after pericardiectomy or myocardial infarction.

On physical examination, signs of elevated jugular venous pressure, tachycardia, tachypnea, and paradox arterial pulse can be found. However, pulsus paradoxus can be absent in patients with cardiac tamponade and preexistent elevation of left ventricle filling pressure, right-to-left cardiac shunt, aortic stenosis, and severe chest trauma.

Heart sounds are usually very silent or even absent; pericardial friction rub is heard in only one third of patients.

Electrocardiographic changes are nonspecific and include reduced voltage, electrical alternans, and electrical changes, which are typical for pericarditis (23).

The chest x-ray can show an enlarged cardiac silhouette (shaped like a water bottle) and oligemic lungs. In patients with acute tamponade, cardiac size and shape may be quite normal (24).

Definitive diagnosis of pericardial effusion and severity of cardiac tamponade can easily be accomplished by transthoracic echocardiography in almost all patients. A transesophageal approach is occasionally necessary in patients with localized tamponade or poor visibility. The size of the effusion can be graded according to the echo-free space in diastole as small (<10 mm), moderate (10 mm to <20 mm), large (≥20 mm), or very large (≥20 mm with compression of chambers). In patients with large effusions the heart is moving free in the pericardium ("swinging heart") (3).

Echocardiographic signs of tamponade are diastolic or early systolic collapse of the right atrium, diastolic collapse of the right ventricle, respiratory variation of ventricular volumes, decreased collapsibility index of the inferior vena cava, and exaggerated respiratory variation of mitral and tricuspid inflow velocity (25–27). Ninety percent of patients with typical clinical signs of tamponade had collapse of one or both right cardiac chambers, which was found also in 38% of patients without clinical tamponade. Abnormal pulmonary venous flow has a good correlation with clinical features of tamponade, with a higher sensitivity than right ventricular collapse and a much higher specificity than right atrial collapse (28). In patients after cardiac surgery, localized posterior pericardial effusion with left ventricular diastolic collapse may be responsible for cardiac tamponade (29).

Hemodynamic variables show equalization of right atrial, right ventricular diastolic, pulmonary diastolic, and pulmonary artery occlusion pressures, and inspiratory increase of right-sided pressures with a decrease of left-sided cardiac pressures. The latter is responsible for pulsus paradoxus, which is defined as inspiratory drop in systolic pressure more than 10 mm Hg.

In the differential diagnosis of obstructive shock pulmonary embolism, right ventricular infarction and tension pneumothorax should be considered. On the other hand, in patients with large pericardial effusion, congestive heart failure is the most common differential diagnostic problem.

Treatment

Medical therapy of cardiac tamponade is only a temporizing measure and includes volume expansion and inotropic support. Plasma expanders or saline infusion may be useful in hypovolemic patients, but inotropic support is usually not effective for initial hemodynamic stabilization (20). All anticoagulant medication should be discontinued, and treatment with vitamin K or protamine sulfate should be considered. Patient who absolutely need anticoagulation should received heparin instead of warfarin. Positive pressure mechanical ventilation should be avoided before pericardiocentesis, since it further decreases the venous return.

The only effective treatment of cardiac tamponade is pericardiocentesis and evacuation of accumulated fluid. Pericardiocentesis should be done immediately in hemodynamically compromised patients. A blind subxiphoid approach may be indicated as a lifesaving procedure, but pericardiocentesis under echocardiographic guidance is preferred. Echocardiography identifies the best place and shortest approach for the puncture, which is frequently at atypical sites of the chest (30, 31). After drainage, all patients should be monitored for possible cardiac failure due to increased venous return. A pericardial catheter can be left in place for 2 to 3 days until secretion is reduced to <25 mL/day (3). It allows a reliable control of the pericardial fluid reaccumulation and reduces the need for repetitive pericardiocentesis.

Pericardiocentesis is contraindicated in patients with aortic dissection; further relative contraindications are severe uncorrected coagulopathy, thrombocytopenia, and small or loculated effusion (32).

Examination of pericardial fluid includes complete laboratory assessment, and culture and stains for bacteria, tuberculosis, and fungi, and it should be done as soon as possible to obtain an etiologic diagnosis.

If no safe access for pericardiocentesis is possible, surgical drainage may be indicated. A subxiphoid surgical approach is commonly applied, but a thoracotomy has to be done occasionally. Surgical drainage is preferable in patients with acute traumatic and purulent pericardial effusion (1).

After drainage of the pericardial fluid, the treatment depends on the etiology. In patients with inflammatory diseases, aspirin, antiinflammatory drugs, and rarely steroids are used. In patients with uremic pericarditis, hemodialysis must be intensified. In purulent pericarditis rinsing of pericardial cavity together with systemic antibiotic treatment is mandatory. Instillation and irrigation with streptokinase or urokinase can liquefy the pericardial effusion and allow better drainage (33). Intrapericardial installation of chemotherapeutic drugs or tetracycline may be useful in patients with malignant pericardial effusion (34). Cardiac perforation or rupture and purulent pericarditis require immediate surgical management.

Clinical Case

A 37-year-old man who is an alcoholic and has insulin-dependent diabetes was admitted to the pulmonary department because of fever and abdominal and lower back pain. During hospitalization (12 days) he was hemodynamically stable, without respiratory or renal failure. Electrocardiogram was normal and no infiltrations were found on the chest x-ray. Abdominal ultrasound was normal. Laboratory findings show mild anemia (Hb 110 g/L), leukocytosis (19.7×10^9/L), and slightly pathologic liver tests. C-reactive protein (CRP) was elevated (156 mg/L). He was treated with ciprofloxacin 400 mg b.i.d., and after 1 week became afebrile.

Neuropathy was suspected and the patient was transferred to the neurology department. Neuropathy was excluded, but after 3 days the fever returned and he became hypotensive (95/70 mm Hg). An ECG was reported as normal, but cardiac enlargement without pulmonary infiltration or congestion was found on the chest x-ray. The laboratory tests revealed anemia (Hb 95 g/L), leukocytosis (18.6×10^9/L), progressive liver failure, and elevated CRP (335 mg/L).

The patient was transferred to the gastroenterology department. The next day, clinical signs of shock with distended jugular veins developed. On abdominal ultrasound a liver congestion with small amount of ascites was found, and cardiac tamponade as a reason for shock was suspected.

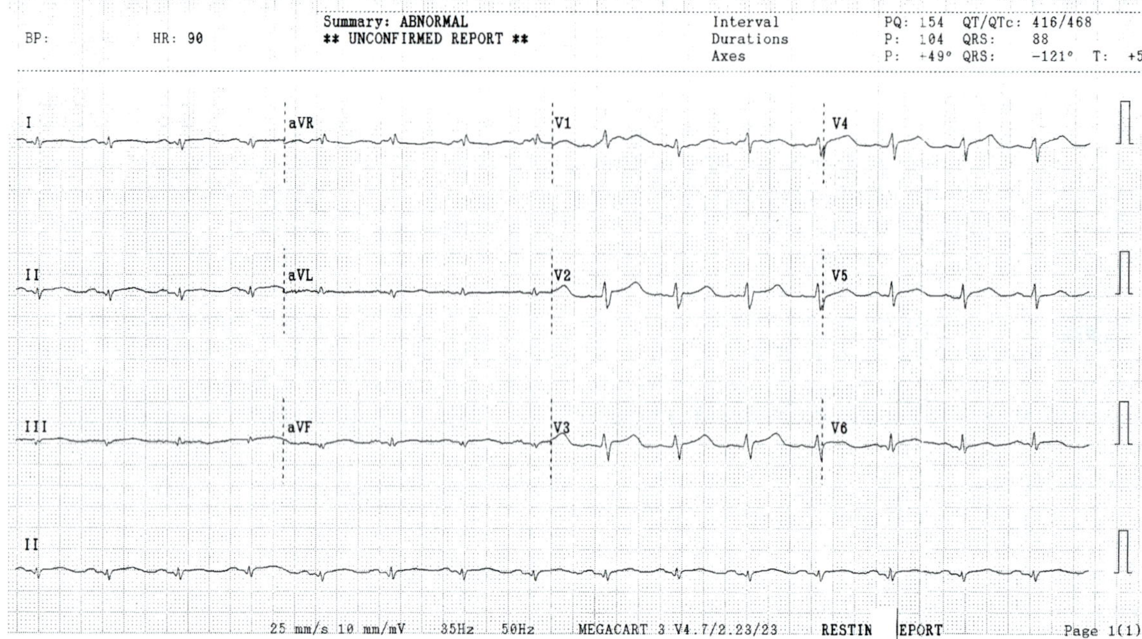

FIGURE 23.2. Electrocardiogram shows normal sinus rhythm and only discrete ST segment elevation in standard and precordial leads.

The patient was transferred to the intensive care unit. On admission he was hypotensive (90/70 mm Hg), with distended neck veins (CVP + 27.5 cm of water); his skin was pale, cool, and clammy; breathing sounds were normal; heart sounds were distant with no friction rub; and abdominal palpation was slightly tender, but no muscular defense was present. Saturation with pulse oximetry was 92% while breathing 60% oxygen. Laboratory tests showed anemia (Hb 92 g/L, Ht 0.29), leukocytosis (17.9×10^9/L), mild renal failure (urea 20.8 mmol/L, creatinine 125 μmol/L), liver failure (bilirubin 75 μmol/L, alanine aminotransferase [ALT] 3.4 μcat/L, aspartate aminotransferase [AST] 1.28 μcat/L, gamma GT 4.21 μcat/L, NH_3 103 μmol/L, prothrombin time 2.6 international normalized ratio [INR]), elevated serum lactate (4.39 mmol/L), CRP (361 mg/L), and PCT (6.6 μg/L). The ECG showed sinus rhythm 90/min and ST segment elevation in standard and precordial leads (Fig. 23.2). On chest x-ray the heart was enlarged and the lungs were clear (Fig. 23.3). Transthoracic and transesophageal echocardiograms showed localized pericardial effusion with a cauliflower-like appearance of the fluid and compression of the right heart chambers (Fig. 23.4).

The patient received 2 L of crystalloids for hemodynamic stabilization and four units of fresh froze plasma for correction of coagulopathy. Afterward, pericardiocentesis was performed with an anterior approach, and 920 mL of purulent

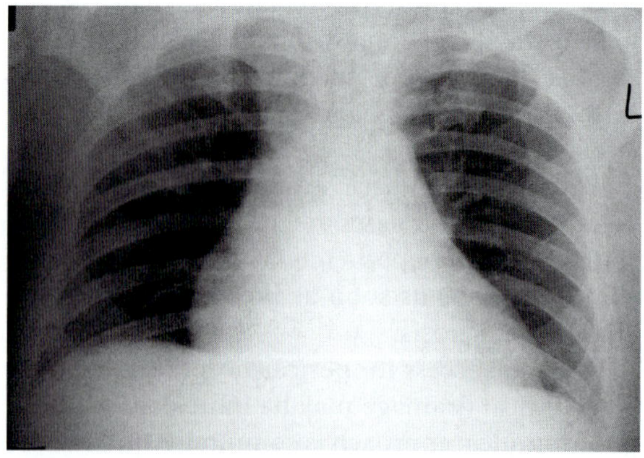

FIGURE 23.3. Chest x-ray showing enlarged cardiac silhouette with clear lungs.

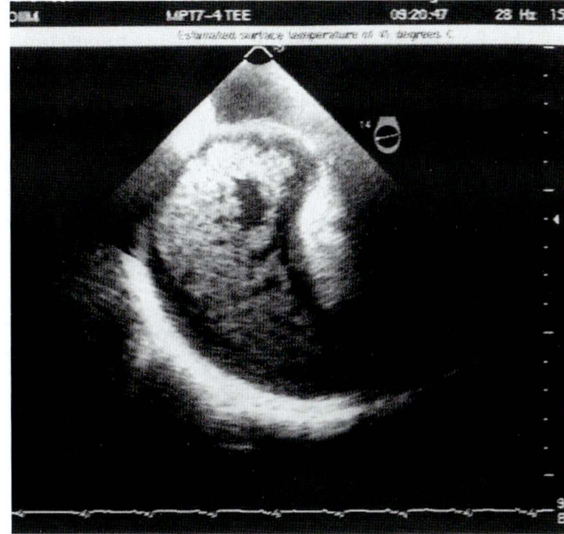

FIGURE 23.4. Large cauliflower-like pericardial effusion in front of right ventricle on transesophageal echocardiography.

effusion with pH of 6.42 was evacuated. Immediately after drainage the cardiac silhouette was smaller on chest x-ray and marked hemodynamic improvement was observed (heart rate 107/min, arterial blood pressure 135/75 mm Hg, CVP +11 cm of water, $SatO_2$ 96%). Direct examination of pericardial fluid showed granulocytes and grampositive cocci. *Enterococcus faecalis* and *Acinetobacter baumani* were isolated in the culture. Drainage was left in place and the pericardium was irrigated every 6 hours with netilmicin and vancomycin. Systemic antibiotic treatment was started as well.

In the next 2 days the patient improved, but septic shock developed again on day 3 after pericardiocentesis. Diffuse purulent peritonitis was diagnosed with abdominal fluid examination and gastric ulcer by endoscopy. He was treated with repetitive surgical intervention, and perforatio tecta contained perforation of the gastric ulcer with peritonitis was confirmed. The gastric ulcer perforation was also the cause of the purulent pericarditis, which was the first manifestation of the disease. He needed prolonged intensive care because of septic multiple organ failure.

After 4 weeks he was discharged to the ward and after 8 weeks from the hospital. No recurrent pericardial effusion or signs of constriction occurred 1 year after discharge.

References

1. Spodick DH. The Pericardium. A Comprehensive Textbook. New York: Marcel Dekker; 1997.
2. Sagrista Sauleda J, Permanyer Miralda G, Soler Soler J. Diagnosis and management of acute pericardial syndromes. Rev Esp Cardiol 2005;58: 830–841.
3. Maisch B, Seferović PM, Ristić AD, et al. Guidelines on the diagnosis and management of pericardial diseases executive summary. The Task Force on the Diagnosis and Management of Pericardial Diseases of the European Society of Cardiology. Eur Heart J 2004;25:587–610.
4. Spodick DH. Electrocardiogram in acute pericarditis. Distribution of morphologic and axial changes by stages. Am J Cardiol 1974;33:470–474.
5. Bonnefoy E, Godon P, Kirkorian G, et al. Serum cardiac troponin I and ST-segment elevation in patients with acute pericarditis. Eur Heart J 2000; 21:832–836.
6. Coupland DB, Teriff B, Fung AY, et al. The "hot halo" sign. Pyogenic pericarditis on In 111 leukocyte scintigraphy. Clin Nucl Med 1992;17:579–580.
7. Parry R Akhtar N, Hartnell GG. Case report: unsuspected pericarditis diagnosed with gallium 67 scan. Clin Radiol 1994;48:332–333.
8. Maisch D, Ristić AD, Pankuweit S. Intrapericardial treatment of autoreactive pericardial effusion with triamcinolone: the way to avoid side effects of systemic corticosteroid therapy. Eur Heart J 2002;19: 1503–1508.
9. Sagrista Sauleda J, Barrabes JA, Permanyer Miralda G, Soler Soler J. Purulent pericarditis: a twenty years experience in a general hospital. J Am Coll Cardiol 1993;22:1661–1665.
10. Permanyer Miralda G, Sagrista Sauleda J, Soler Soler J. Primary acute pericardial disease: a prospective series of 231 consecutive patients. Am J Cardiol 1985;56:623–630.
11. Maisch B, Bethge C, Drude L, Hufnagel G, Herzum M, Schoenlan U. Pericardioscopy and epicardial biopsy: new diagnostic tool in pericardial and perimyocardial diseases. Eur Heart J 1994;15(suppl C):68–73.
12. Nugue O, Milliare A, Porte H, et al. Pericardioscopy in the etiologic diagnosis of pericardial effusion in 141 consecutive patients. Circulation 1996;94:1635–1641.
13. Seferović PM, Ristić AD, Maksimović R, et al. Diagnostic value of pericardial biopsy: improvement with extensive sample enabled by pericardioscopy. Circulation 2003;107:978–983.

14. Imazio M, Demichelis B, Parrini I, et al. Day-hospital treatment of acute pericarditis. A management program for outpatient therapy. J Am Coll Cardiol 2004;43:1042–1046.
15. Soler Soler J, Sagrista Soleda J, Permanyer, Miralda G. Relapsing pericarditis. Heart 2004;90:1364–1368.
16. Adler Y, Finkelstein Y, Guindo J, et al. Colchicine treatment for acute pericarditis: a decade of experience. Circulation 1998;97:2183–2185.
17. Maisch B, Ristić AD, Pankuweit S, Neubauer A, Moll R. Neoplastic pericardial effusion. Efficacy and safety of intrapericardial treatment with cisplatin. Eur Heart J 2002;23:1625–1631.
18. Davies WM, LeWinter M. Cardiac tamponade. In: Pinsky MR, Dhainaut JFA, eds. Pathophysiologic Foundations of Critical Care, 1st ed. Baltimore: Williams & Wilkins; 1993:337–347.
19. Levin S, Maldonado I, Rehm C, et al. Cardiac tamponade without pericardial effusion after blunt chest trauma. Am Heart J 1996;131:198–200.
20. Spodick DH. Acute pericardial tamponade. N Engl J Med 2003;349:684–690.
21. Reddy PS, Curtiss EI, O'Toole JD, Shaver JA. Cardiac tamponade: hemodynamic observation in man. Circulation 1978;58:265–272.
22. Reddy PS, Curtiss EI, Uretsky BF, et al. Spectrum of hemodynamic changes in cardiac tamponade. Am J Cardiol 1990;66:1487–1491.
23. Horowitz MS, Shultz CS, Stinson SB, et al. Sensitivity and specificity of echocardiographic diagnosis of pericardial effusion. Circulation 19974;50:239–247.
24. Eisenberg MJ, Dunn MM, Kanth N, et al. Diagnostic value of chest radiography for pericardial effusion. J Am Coll Cardiol 1993;22:588–593.
25. Singh S, Wann LS, Schuchard GH, et al. Right ventricular and right atrial collapse in patients with cardiac tamponade: a combined echocardiographic and hemodynamic study. Circulation 1984;70:966–971.
26. Bommer WJ, Follette D, Pollock M, Arena F, Bognar M, Berkoff H. Tamponade in patients undergoing cardiac surgery: a clinical-echocardiographic diagnosis. Am Heart J 1995;130:1216–1223.
27. Appleton CP, Hatle LK, Popp RL. Cardiac tamponade and pericardial effusion: respiratory variation in transvalvular flow velocities studied by Doppler echocardiography. J Am Coll Cardiol 1988;11:120–130.
28. Merce J, Sagrista Sauleda J, Permanyer Miralda G, Evangelista A, Soler Soler J. Correlation between clinical and Doppler echocardiographic findings in patients with moderate and large pericardial effusion: implications for the diagnosis of cardiac tamponade. Am Heart J 1999;138:759–764.
29. Chuttani K, Tischler MD, Pandian NG, Lee RT, Mohanty PK. Diagnosis of cardiac tamponade after cardiac surgery: relative value of clinical, echocardiographic, and hemodynamic signs. Am Heart J 1994;127:913–918.
30. Tsang TS, Freeman WK, Barnes ME, Reeder GS, Packer DL, Seward JB. Rescue echocardiographically guided pericardiocentesis for cardiac perforation complicating catheter-based procedures. J Am Coll Cardiol 1998;32:1345–1350.
31. Tsang TS, Enriquez-Sarano M, Freeman WK, et al. Consecutive 1127 therapeutic echocardiographically guided pericardiocentesis: clinical profile, practice pattern, and outcomes spanning 21 years. Mayo Clin Proc 2002;77:429–436.
32. Isselbacher EM, Ciggaroa JE, Eagle KA. Cardiac tamponade complicated proximal aortic dissection: is pericardiocentesis harmful? Circulation 1994;90:2375–2379.
33. Defouilloy C, Meyer G, Slama M, et al. Intrapericardial fibrinolysis: a useful treatment in the management of purulent pericarditis. Intensive Care Med 1997;23:117–118.
34. Shepherd FA, Morgan C, Evans WK, et al. Medical management of malignant pericardial effusion by tetracycline sclerosis. Am J Cardiol 1987;60:1161–1166.

24
Acute Pericardial Disease: Pericardiocentesis and Percutaneous Pericardiotomy

Hani Jneid, Andrew O. Maree, and Igor F. Palacios

Pericardial diseases can present with a myriad of clinical manifestations including pericarditis, pericardial effusion, and tamponade. While pericarditis is often a self-limiting disorder that is responsive to nonsteroidal antiinflammatory agents, pericardial tamponade is a life-threatening condition requiring immediate therapy. Echocardiography and cardiac catheterization are important diagnostic tools and helpful in guiding therapies. Percutaneous catheter-based therapies, including pericardiocentesis and percutaneous balloon pericardiotomy, are safe and effective therapeutic modalities. Percutaneous balloon pericardiotomy is a relatively novel catheter-based technique that is gradually replacing the more invasive surgical pericardial window procedures. Pericardiectomy, on the other hand, remains the definitive therapy for certain conditions such as constrictive pericardial disease. This chapter presents an overview of acute pericardial disorders, with an emphasis on catheter-based techniques for pericardial space decompression.

Etiology of Pericardial Effusion and Tamponade

Pericardial effusion occurs as a result of a variety of clinical conditions including infectious, metabolic, inflammatory, autoimmune, and neoplastic processes[1–3] (Table 24.1).

The frequency of specific etiologies of pericardial effusion is highly dependent on the geographic location, time period, and characteristics of the populations studied. For example, in a European series of 322 patients presenting with moderate and severe pericardial effusions, acute idiopathic pericarditis and iatrogenic causes accounted for the majority of cases (20% and 16%, respectively)[1]. On the other hand, in a smaller series in the United States involving patients presenting to a tertiary medical center with large pericardial effusions, malignancy was the most etiology cause and accounted for 23% of all 75 cases[4]. Pericardial effusions occurring after radiation therapy, myocardial infarction, and surgical and interventional cardiac procedures are progressively increasing in incidence. Uremia and hypothyroidism remain important etiologies but are becoming less frequent given the prompt diagnosis and treatment of these metabolic disorders.

Pericardial fluid can be a transudate or an exudate, with the latter characterized by a high concentration of proteins and fibrin. While transudative effusions typically occur in patients with congestive heart failure, exudative effusions may occur with most types of pericarditis. Pericardial effusions may be serous (or serosanguineous), suppurative, or hemorrhagic. While the presence of suppurative effusion is usually pathognomonic for an acute infectious etiology, usually bacterial, hemorrhagic pericardial effusion is not uncommonly related to chronic infections, with tuberculosis standing as the classic example, particularly in developing countries. However, in developed countries, hemorrhagic pericardial effusions are likely to be iatrogenic or malignant in etiology. In a retrospectives analysis of 150 patients in the United States who underwent pericardiocentesis

Table 24.1. Etiology of pericardial effusion/tamponade

Idiopathic
Infectious
Viral
Bacteria
Fungal
Others
Metabolic
Uremia
Myxedema
Collagen and other autoimmune disorders
Systemic lupus erythematosus
Rheumatoid arthritis
Rheumatic fever
Dressler syndrome
Others
Neoplastic
Primary
Pericardial metastasis
Local invasion
Volume overload
Chronic heart failure
Miscellaneous
Chest wall irradiation
Cardiotomy or thoracic surgery
Adverse drug reaction
Aortic dissection
Postmyocardial infarction
Traumatic

for relieving cardiac tamponade, 64% of patients had a hemorrhagic pericardial effusion[5]. In this analysis, iatrogenic diseases (related to invasive cardiac procedures) and malignancy accounted for the majority of cases (31% and 26%, respectively)[5].

Clinical Presentation

The clinical presentation of patients with pericardial effusion is highly variable, with some being completely asymptomatic while others develop pericardial tamponade and cardiovascular collapse.

The normal pericardium is a fibroelastic sac composed of visceral and parietal layers separated by the pericardial cavity and containing a thin layer (20 to 50 mL) of straw-colored fluid surrounding the heart[3]. The normal pericardium has a steep pressure-volume curve. It is distensible when the total intrapericardial volume is small, but becomes gradually inextensible when the volume increases. In the presence of pericardial effusion, the intrapericardial pressure depends on the relationship among the absolute volume of the effusion, the speed of fluid accumulation, and pericardial elasticity. While the rapid accumulation of small amounts of fluid (150 to 200 mL) can result in cardiac tamponade, the slow accumulation of larger effusions (>1 L, as in uremic pericardial effusions) is usually well tolerated[6,7]. The clinical presentation is thus related not only to the size of the effusion but also and more importantly to the rapidity of fluid accumulation.

Pericardial tamponade is a clinical syndrome with defined hemodynamic and echocardiographic abnormalities, which results from the accumulation of intrapericardial fluid and impairment of ventricular diastolic filling[7,8]. The ultimate mechanism of hemodynamic compromise is the compression of cardiac chambers secondary to increased intrapericardial pressure[8]. In the majority of patients, pericardial tamponade can be diagnosed clinically. Patients with cardiac tamponade have elevated systemic venous pressure, tachycardia, dyspnea, and arterial pulsus paradoxus[3]. Their heart sounds are muffled[3]. Pulsus paradoxus, which describes the exaggerated inspiratory decline in arterial blood pressure (>10 mm Hg), is largely attributed to interventricular dependence within the confined pericardial space. Although its diagnostic utility was recognized many decades earlier[9], various conditions may lead to its absence in patients with cardiac tamponade (such as in those with concomitant aortic regurgitation, atrial septal defects, severe left ventricular dysfunction, aortic regurgitation, severe hypotension, pericardial adhesions, or pulmonary artery obstruction, and in patients on positive-pressure ventilation)[8].

The electrocardiogram (ECG) shows sinus tachycardia and low voltage. Electrical alternans, which describes the beat-to-beat alterations in the QRS complex reflecting cardiac swinging in the pericardial fluid, is a relatively specific sign for tamponade and is rarely seen with very large pericardial effusions alone[10]. Patients with pericardial effusions have an enlarged cardiac silhouette with clear lung fields on chest x-ray. The pericardial effusion has to reach 200 mL in volume to appear on chest x-ray, which occurs usually in slowly accumulating pericardial effusions (which are less likely to cause tamponade)[11]. Rapidly accumulating small pericardial effusions may cause tamponade while presenting with a normal chest x-ray.

The diagnosis of pericardial tamponade is best confirmed by a two-dimensional echocardiogram that demonstrates a pericardial effusion, right atrial compression, and abnormal respiratory variations in the right and left ventricular dimensions and in the tricuspid and mitral valves flow velocities[12]. The classic hemodynamic findings of pericardial tamponade include arterial pulsus paradoxus, elevation, diastolic equalization of right and left ventricular diastolic pressures with pericardial pressure, and depression of cardiac output[8]. Since patients with critical tamponade operate on the steep portion of the pericardial pressure-volume curve, drainage of even small pericardial volume results in a drastic fall in intrapericardial pressure and rapid clinical and hemodynamic improvement (by shifting the stretched pericardium back to the flat portion of the pericardium pressure-volume curve)[8].

The Role of Echocardiography

A few decades ago, echocardiography was recognized as a particularly useful imaging modality for pericardial disease[13,14]. Currently, two-dimensional echocardiography has become the gold standard diagnostic modality, as it provides a highly sensitive and specific noninvasive imaging technique for pericardial pathology[12,15]. It is also an important tool for the longitudinal follow-up of pericardial effusions over time (given a class IIa recommendation in the American Heart Association [AHA]/American College of Cardiology [ACC] guidelines for the clinical application of echocardiography)[12]. Classically, a persistent echo-free space throughout the cardiac cycle between the parietal pericardium and the epicardium is pathognomonic for pericardial effusion by M-mode echocardiography[13].

Two-dimensional echocardiography allows delineation of the size and distribution of the effusion, including loculated effusions, and helps assess the success of pericardiocentesis. The echocardiogram can also provide a reasonable estimate of the total volume of the effusion[16]. Circumferential effusions >1 cm in width are considered large (>500 mL). Moderate effusions (100 to 500 mL) are usually circumferential but <1 cm in effusion, while small effusions (<100 mL) are usually localized posterior to the left ventricle and measure <1 cm. These classification criteria differ significantly among various echocardiographers and institutions. The typical echocardiographic signs of pericardial tamponade are shown in Table 24.2.

The nature of the pericardial fluid is difficult to identify by echocardiography. However, increased echogenicity is suspicious for the presence of proteins or cells in the pericardial fluid. Fibrin deposits localized in the epicardial surface can be identified as echogenic masses. In one study of 42 patients with tuberculous and viral/idiopathic pericardial effusions, the presence of intrapericardial echo abnormalities, such as a greater degree of pericardial thickening, frequency and thickness of exudative coating or deposits, and strands crossing the pericardial space, was a useful criterion in the diagnosis of tuberculous pericardial effusion and in differentiating it from chronic idiopathic pericardial effusion[17].

The classic echocardiographic signs of cardiac tamponade are right atrial and right ventricular diastolic collapse. Both the right atrium and right ventricle are compliant structures. As a result, increased intrapericardial pressure leads to their collapse when intracavitary pressures are only slightly exceeded by those in the pericardium. At end-diastole (i.e., during atrial relaxation), right atrial volume is minimal, but pericardial pressure is maximal, causing the right atrium to buckle. Right atrial collapse, especially when it persists for more than one third of the cardiac cycle, is a

Table 24.2. Echocardiographic findings

1. Abnormal inspiratory increase of right ventricle dimensions and abnormal inspiratory decrease of left ventricle dimensions
2. Right atrium collapse (>30% of the cardiac cycle)
3. Right ventricular early diastolic collapse
4. Abnormal inspiratory increase in blood flow velocity through the tricuspid valve and pulmonic valves and abnormal inspiratory decrease of mitral and aortic valves flow velocity
5. Respiratory variations of pulmonary and hepatic venous flow
6. Dilated inferior vena cava with lack of inspiratory collapse
7. Swinging heart

highly sensitive but less specific sign for tamponade. Early diastolic collapse of the right ventricle (usually occurs in early diastole when the ventricular volume is still low) is present when the intrapericardial pressure exceeds the right ventricular pressure and is a highly specific sign for tamponade. Right ventricular collapse may not occur when the right ventricle is hypertrophied or its diastolic pressure is greatly elevated. Left atrial collapse is seen in nearly 25% of patients and is a very specific for tamponade. Left ventricular collapse is less common, since the wall of the left ventricle is more muscular.

Dilatation of the inferior vena cava with lack of inspiratory collapse (usually <50% reduction in its diameter) and swinging of the heart are also seen in patients with pericardial tamponade. Doppler echocardiography provides direct assessment of the ventricular filling patterns in pericardial tamponade[11,12,15,18]. Patients with pericardial tamponade have both a marked increase in tricuspid and pulmonic flow velocities and a marked decrease in mitral and aortic valve flow velocities during inspiration when compared with normal subjects and patients with effusions but not tamponade. Changes in left atrial inflow pattern and exaggerated respiratory variations in pulmonary venous flow velocity are also observed. In one study aiming to correlate clinical and echocardiographic findings prospectively, the highest specificity (98%) was seen in patients with right atrial and right ventricular collapse plus abnormal venous flow[19]. The sensitivity and specificity of any chamber collapse were 90% and 65%, respectively[19].

In addition to echocardiography, computed tomography and magnetic resonance imaging are useful techniques in the evaluation of patients with pericardial disease. Their high resolution is useful in the assessment of pericardial thickness (particularly important in constrictive-effusive pericarditis) and in the detection of pericardial effusion, masses and cysts.

The Role of Cardiac Catheterization

Cardiac catheterization has been historically the standard diagnostic modality for cardiac tamponade. Right heart catheterization can confirm the significance of a pericardial effusion and allows evaluation of hemodynamic changes occurring after pericardiocentesis. It usually demonstrates two major findings in patients with pericardial tamponade: (1) elevation and equilibration of intracardiac diastolic pressures (usually between 10 and 30 mm Hg); and (2) inspiratory increase in right-sided pressures with reduction in left-sided pressures, which are responsible for the presence of a pulsus paradoxus[8] (Table 24.3). With equalization of intrapericardial pressures, the mean right atrial, left atrial, diastolic pulmonary artery, and right and left ventricular end diastolic pressures are all within 5 mm Hg of each other.

In addition to producing elevation in the central venous pressure, cardiac tamponade produces characteristic changes in the waveforms of the hemodynamic tracings. With increasing severity of cardiac tamponade, the "Y descent" and the early diastolic dip in the ventricular pressure tracings are gradually obliterated and eventually disappear. The absence of the Y descent in the right atrial tracing is a hemodynamic hallmark of pericardial tamponade. As pericardial fluid is removed, the intrapericardial pressure usually returns to the intrapleural pressure level and the right atrial waveform normalizes with reappearance of the diastolic Y descent. However, when the right atrial pressure remains elevated after the pericardiocentesis and a prominent Y descent appears, the diagnosis of effusive-constrictive disease must be considered[20]. Although the latter is an infrequent pericardial pathology, it may be missed in some patients presenting with tamponade in whom it usually causes significant morbidity until they undergo surgical epicardiectomy.

Pulsus paradoxus is another hallmark of pericardial tamponade. As previously stated, it is an exaggeration of the normal physiologic decrease

Table 24.3. Cardiac catheterization findings

1. Elevated filling pressures
2. Diastolic equalization of pressures
3. Absence or blunted "Y" descent in the right atrium pressure tracing
4. Absence or blunted early diastolic dip in the right ventricular pressure tracing
5. Arterial pulsus paradoxus

in systolic arterial blood pressure during inspiration (usually >10 mm Hg). Although arterial pulsus paradoxus is an important sign of pericardial tamponade, it may be absent in many conditions (see above) or alternatively may be present in patients without cardiac tamponade, as in those with severe chronic obstructive pulmonary disease.

Pericardiocentesis

Indications

Pericardiocentesis is the technique of catheter-based aspiration of pericardial fluid. It serves as a diagnostic and therapeutic modality in patients with pericarditis with pericardial effusion, pericardial effusion with pericardial tamponade, and effusive-constrictive pericarditis.

Once the diagnosis of pericardial effusion has been made, it is important to determine whether the effusion is creating significant hemodynamic compromise. Many asymptomatic patients with large effusions do not require pericardiocentesis if they have no hemodynamic compromise, unless there is a need for fluid analysis for diagnostic purposes. In a prospective long-term follow-up of large idiopathic chronic pericardial effusion (up to 20 years), Sagrista-Sauleda et al.[21] concluded that large idiopathic chronic pericardial effusions were usually well tolerated for long periods in most patients with severe tamponade; however, they developed unexpectedly at any time. Although pericardiocentesis was effective in resolving these effusions, recurrences were common, prompting the authors to recommend referral of these patients for pericardiectomy when recurrence occurs[21]. When cardiac tamponade occurs, the emergency drainage of pericardial fluid by pericardiocentesis is a lifesaving therapy in a patient who would otherwise develop pulseless electrical activity and cardiac arrest.

When performed, pericardiocentesis should achieve several objectives: (1) relieving tamponade, when present; (2) obtaining fluid for appropriate analyses; and (3) assessing hemodynamics after pericardial fluid evacuation to exclude effusive-constrictive pericardial effusion.

Elective pericardiocentesis is contraindicated in patients receiving anticoagulation, and in patients with bleeding disorders or thrombocytopenia with platelet count <50,000/mm^3. Pericardiocentesis is also ill-advised when the presence of pericardial fluid is not confirmed, and when the effusion is very small or loculated.

The Pericardiocentesis Technique

Pericardiocentesis is most commonly performed via a subxiphoid approach under ECG and fluoroscopy guidance (Fig. 24.1A). Traditionally, pericardiocentesis has been performed in the cardiac catheterization laboratory with arterial and right heart pressure monitoring. However, nowadays the procedure is also performed in the noninvasive laboratory, intensive care units, or even at the bedside under echocardiographic guidance[22,23]. Whichever modality is utilized, it is a safe procedure when performed by appropriately trained personnel.

Pericardiocentesis is a procedure based on the Seldinger technique of percutaneous catheter insertion. After the administration of local anesthesia (1% to 2% lidocaine) to the skin and deeper tissues of the left xiphocostal area, the pericardial needle is connected to an ECG lead. The needle is advanced from the left of the subxiphoid area while aiming toward the left shoulder (usually under fluoroscopic or echocardiographic guidance; however, blinded procedures are undertaken in cases of extreme emergencies). Often, a discrete pop is felt as the needle enters the pericardial space. ST-segment elevation is seen on the ECG lead tracing when the needle touches the epicardium and helps confirm the needle position (Fig. 24.1B). The needle should be withdrawn slightly until the ST segment elevation disappears. Once the pericardial space is entered, a stiff guidewire is introduced into the pericardial space through the needle, which is thereafter removed and a catheter is inserted into the pericardial sac over the guidewire (Fig. 24.2). The drainage catheter utilized (often a pigtail catheter, denoting its shape), has an end hole and multiple side holes. Intrapericardial pressure is measured by connecting a pressure transducer system to the intrapericardial catheter. Pericardial fluid is then removed. Samples of pericardial fluid should be sent for

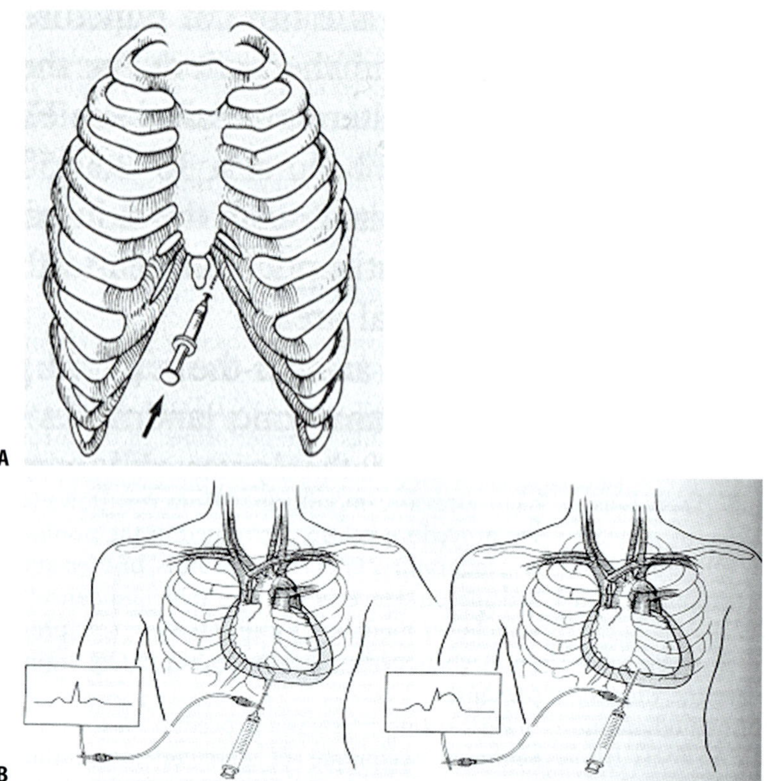

FIGURE 24.1. (A) Diagrammatic representation of a pericardiocentesis procedure using the subxiphoid approach. (B) The pericardial needle is connected to an electrocardiogram (ECG) lead. The needle is advanced from the left of the subxiphoid area aiming toward the left shoulder. ST-segment elevation is seen on the ECG lead tracing when the needle touches the epicardium. The needle should be retracted slightly until the ST segment elevation disappears.

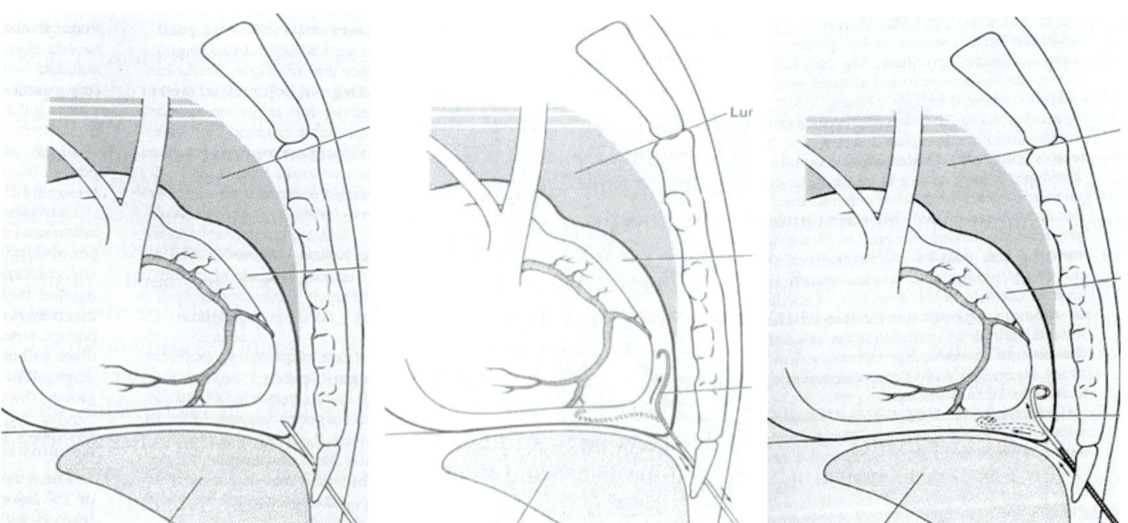

FIGURE 24.2. Diagrammatic representation of a pericardiocentesis procedure using the subxiphoid approach. Once the pericardial space is entered with the pericardial needle, a guidewire is introduced in the pericardial space through the needle. The needle is removed and a catheter is inserted in the pericardial sac over the guidewire. As shown in the figure the guidewire and pericardial catheter can be placed anteriorly or inferiorly in the pericardial sac.

appropriate biochemical, cytologic, bacteriologic, and immunologic analyses to assist in the diagnosis of the etiology of the effusion (the first sample is usually reserved for microbiologic studies).

In the presence of pericardial tamponade, aspiration of fluid should be continued until a clinical and hemodynamic improvement occurs. The catheter is frequently left in place for continuous drainage and as a route to instill sclerosing or chemotherapeutic agents if needed. The catheter is secured to the skin with sterile sutures and covered with a sterile dressing. The success rate of pericardiocentesis increases and the incidence of complications decreases with the increasing size of the effusion.

Complications of Pericardiocentesis

The potential complications of pericardiocentesis include the laceration of the heart or a coronary vessel, sometimes causing fatal consequences. Puncture of the right atrium or the right ventricle with hemopericardial fluid accumulation, arrhythmias, air embolism, pneumothorax, and puncture of the peritoneal cavity or abdominal viscera have all been reported. Acute pulmonary edema may infrequently occur when the pericardial tamponade is decompressed too rapidly.

Other approaches of pericardiocentesis include the right xiphocostal, apical, right-sided, and parasternal approaches. Although these may be useful under certain circumstances, they are associated with a greater incidence of complications. The right xiphocostal approach is associated with higher incidence of right atrium and inferior vena cava injury. Puncture of the left pleura and the lingula is more frequent with the apical approach, while puncture of the left anterior descending and the internal mammary artery is more frequent with the parasternal approach.

Echocardiographically guided pericardiocentesis is a safe and effective technique[23,24]. In a series of 1127 therapeutic echocardiograph-guided pericardiocenteses performed in 977 patients at the Mayo Clinic between 1979 and 1998, the procedural success rate was 97% overall, with a total complication rate of 4.7%[24]. Echocardiography enables identification of the ideal site of needle entry and trajectory, and is especially useful in patients with loculated effusions. Unlike pericardiocenteses performed in the cardiac catheterization lab, the left chest wall rather than the subcostal approach is often utilized with echocardiographically guided pericardiocenteses.

Management After Pericardiocentesis

Pericardiocentesis does not completely evacuate the effusion in most cases, given particularly that active secretion and bleeding into the pericardial space may continue. Therefore, it is best to leave the pericardial catheter in place for 24 to 72 hours after the initial fluid evacuation. The patient is admitted for continuous ECG monitoring, and for assessment of the rate of pericardial drainage. The pericardial space should be drained every 8 hours and the catheter flushed with heparinized solution and systemic antibiotics (usually first-generation cephalosporin for empirical coverage of gram-positive bacteria) are administered for the duration of the catheter stay. Based on the etiology of the effusion, the patient's clinical and hemodynamic condition, and the amount drained, the pericardial catheter is removed usually within 72 hours and decisions about additional therapy are made.

No special care is required after an uncomplicated pericardiocentesis. If pericardiocentesis is performed for cardiac tamponade, the patient is watched for signs of recurrent tamponade, and a follow-up echocardiogram is useful to monitor the resolution of the pericardial effusion and for signs of cardiac compression.

Prevention of Recurrent Tamponade

For many patients with pericardial effusion and tamponade, standard percutaneous pericardial drainage with an indwelling pericardial catheter is sufficient to avoid recurrence of pericardial effusion and tamponade. Patients who continue to drain more than 100 ml per 24 hours 3 days after standard catheter drainage should be considered for more aggressive therapy. Reaccumulation of the pericardial fluid is particularly common in patients with malignant pericardial effusions. Additional therapeutic approaches are available to prevent pericardial fluid reaccumulation. They include intrapericardial instillation of sclerosing agents, and the use of chemotherapy, radiotherapy, percutaneous balloon pericardial window, and surgical intervention[25–28]. Reaccumulation of fluid with recurrence of cardiac tamponade has been considered a definitive indication for a pericardial window[29].

Percutaneous Balloon Pericardiotomy (Percutaneous Balloon Pericardial Window)

Patients with a malignant pericardial effusion and tamponade are likely to be suboptimal surgical candidates because of their overall poor health conditions and limited life expectancies. Palacios and colleagues[29,30] pioneered at Massachusetts General Hospital in Boston the technique of percutaneous balloon pericardial window (also called percutaneous balloon pericardiotomy) as an alternative to, and less invasive technique than, the surgical pericardial window. With this modality, adequate drainage of pericardial effusion is performed and a pericardial window is created percutaneously under fluoroscopic guidance utilizing a balloon-dilation catheter. The technique of percutaneous pericardial window is relatively simple and safe, and is performed in the catheterization laboratory under local anesthesia with minimal patient discomfort. Conscious sedation with intravenous narcotics and a short-acting benzodiazepine are generally used.

The Percutaneous Balloon Pericardiotomy Technique

The percutaneous balloon pericardial window is offered as an alternative technique to the surgical pericardial window procedure for those patients with persistent drainage from their indwelling intrapericardial catheter (3 days or more of >100 mL/24-hour drainage) or as primary therapy at the time of initial pericardiocentesis.

The subxiphoid area around the indwelling pigtail pericardial catheter is infiltrated with local anesthesia (1% to 2% lidocaine). A small amount (5 to 10 mL) of iodinated contrast agent is injected in the pericardial space to help outline the parietal pericardium (Fig. 24.3A). A 0.038-inch stiff guidewire with a preshaped curve at the tip is advanced through the pigtail catheter into the pericardial space. The catheter is then removed, leaving the guidewire in the pericardial space. After predilation of the skin and subcutaneous tissue along the track of the wire utilizing a 10-French dilator, a 20 mm-diameter by 3 cm-long balloon dilating catheter (Boston Scientific, Watertown, MA) is advanced over the guidewire and positioned to straddle the parietal pericardium. Care should be taken to advance the proximal end of the balloon beyond the skin and the subcutaneous tissue to avoid dilation of the skin and subcutaneous tissue (and the resultant formation of a pericardial-cutaneous fistula) (Fig. 24.3B). The balloon is inflated manually until the waist produced by the

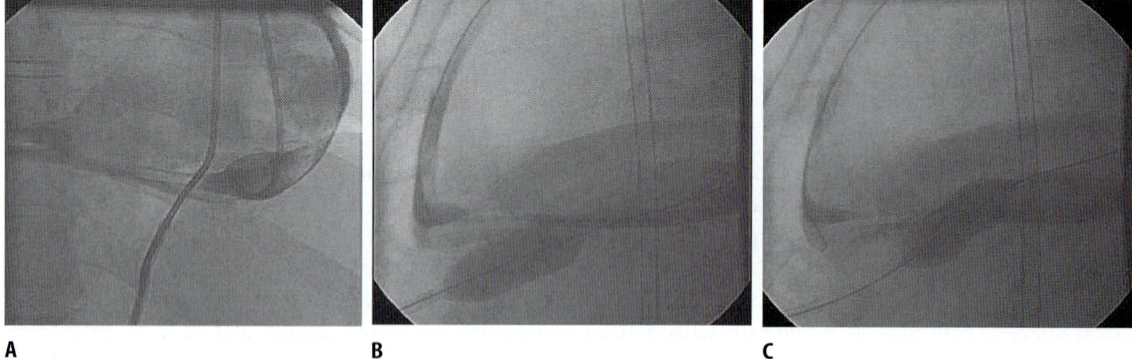

Figure 24.3. Percutaneous balloon pericardiotomy procedure. (A) Injection of a small amount of iodinated contrast confirms the intrapericardial location of the catheter. (B) A left lateral projection showed an inflated dilating balloon catheter without a waist indicating the need to reposition the balloon catheter to straddle the parietal pericardium. (C) The balloon catheter is in the correct position and appears straddling the parietal pericardium in the left lateral projection.

parietal pericardium disappears (Fig. 24.3C). Biplane fluoroscopy is helpful to ascertain the correct position of the balloon straddling the parietal pericardium, with the left lateral projection being particularly useful (Fig. 24.3B,C). Two to three inflations are usually performed to have adequate opening of the parietal pericardium. The balloon-dilation catheter is removed, leaving the stiff guidewire in the pericardial space, where a new pigtail catheter is then advanced over it and left indwelling the pericardial space.

Management After Percutaneous Balloon Pericardiotomy

Patients are admitted to a regular medical ward unit after a percutaneous balloon pericardiotomy procedure and do not require a coronary unit admission. The pericardial catheter is aspirated every 6 to 8 hours and flushed with heparinized solution (5 mL, 100 U/mL). Pericardial drainage volumes are recorded and the catheter removed when there is less than 50 to 75 mL of pericardial drainage in 24 hours. Chest x-rays are performed to check for the development of pleural effusion resulting from drainage of the pericardial fluid.

Outcomes Data of Percutaneous Balloon Pericardiotomy

Palacios and colleagues[29] reported the first human experience with the technique of percutaneous balloon pericardiotomy in eight patients with malignant pericardial effusion and tamponade. The technique was successful in all patients with no immediate or late procedure-related complications. The mean time to radiologic development of a new or a significantly increased pleural effusion was 2.9 ± 0.4 days (range, 2 to 5 days). No patient developed recurrence of the pericardial effusion or tamponade at a mean follow-up of 6 ± 2 months (range, 1 to 11 months). Five patients died from their primary malignancy at 1, 4, 9, 10, and 11 months, respectively. On the other hand, a success rate of 87% was reported in the multicenter percutaneous balloon pericardial window registry, which enrolled 130 patients between 1987 and 1994 in 16 centers[31,32]. In this registry, three patients sustained pericardial bleeding and were considered to have a failed procedure and ended up undergoing surgical window procedures. Eight patients had recurrence of pericardial effusion (mean time to recurrence 54 ± 65 days), of whom seven ended up having surgical window procedures (with recurrence occurring in four of those patients).

Complications of Percutaneous Balloon Pericardiotomy

Minor complications occurred in 13% of the patients[31,32]. The development of large pleural effusion remains the major concern following percutaneous balloon pericardial window. Most patients develop a left pleural effusion within 24 to 48 hours of the procedure, which in most cases resolves spontaneously (presumably due to the greater resorption capacity of the pleural surface). Thoracocentesis or chest tube placement was required in 15% of patients with preexisting pleural effusions compared to 9% of patients without preexisting pleural effusions[31,32]. It is desirable to aspirate most of the pericardial fluid before creating the window in order to limit the potential volume of fluid that can immediately leak to the pleural space. When the preprocedure chest x-ray reveals a large pleural effusion, the chance of requiring thoracentesis subsequent to the percutaneous pericardial window is higher, and the procedure should be performed only when its benefits outweigh the risks of thoracentesis or chest tube placement. It is ill-advised to perform the procedure in patients with marginal pulmonary reserve, as in postpneumonectomy patients, since the development of a pleural effusion may significantly compromise their respiratory function. Finally, an increased risk of bleeding from the pericardiotomy site occurs in patients with either platelet or coagulation abnormalities. In these patients a surgical procedure under direct visualization may be safer. Thoracoscopic techniques were developed to create a larger pericardial window with low morbidity compared to open surgical techniques[33]. This technique allows adequate long-term drainage and the ability to obtain specimens for pathologic analysis[33].

References

1. Sagrista-Sauleda J, Merce J, Permanyer-Miralda G, Soler-Soler J. Clinical clues to the causes of large pericardial effusions. Am J Med. 2000;109:95–101.

2. Troughton RW, Asher CR, Klein AL. Pericarditis. Lancet. 2004;363:717–27.
3. Lange RA, Hillis LD. Clinical practice. Acute pericarditis. N Engl J Med. 2004;351:2195–202.
4. Corey GR, Campbell PT, Van Trigt P, et al. Etiology of large pericardial effusions. Am J Med. 1993;95: 209–13.
5. Atar S, Chiu J, Forrester JS, Siegel RJ. Bloody pericardial effusion in patients with cardiac tamponade: is the cause cancerous, tuberculous, or iatrogenic in the 1990s. Chest. 1999;116:1564–9.
6. Spodick DH. Pathophysiology of cardiac tamponade. Chest. 1998;113:1372–8.
7. Fowler NO. Cardiac tamponade. A clinical or an echocardiographic diagnosis? Circulation. 1993;87: 1738–41.
8. Spodick DH. Acute cardiac tamponade. N Engl J Med. 2003;349:684–90.
9. Shabetai R, Fowler NO, Fenton JC, Masangkay M. Pulsus paradoxus. J Clin Invest. 1965;44:1882–98.
10. Bruch C, Schmermund A, Dagres N, Bartel T, Caspari G, Sack S, Erbel R. Changes in QRS voltage in cardiac tamponade and pericardial effusion: reversibility after pericardiocentesis and after anti-inflammatory drug treatment. J Am Coll Cardiol. 2001;38:219–26.
11. Maisch B, Seferovic PM, Ristic AD, et al. Guidelines on the diagnosis and management of pericardial diseases executive summary; The Task force on the diagnosis and management of pericardial diseases of the European society of cardiology. Eur Heart J. 2004;25:587–610.
12. Cheitlin MD, Armstrong WF, Aurigemma GP, et al. ACC/AHA/ASE 2003 guideline update for the clinical application of echocardiography: summary article: a report of the American College of Cardiology/American Heart Association Task Force on Practice Guidelines (ACC/AHA/ASE Committee to Update the 1997 Guidelines for the Clinical Application of Echocardiography). Circulation. 2003;108: 1146–62.
13. Feigenbaum H, Waldhausen JA, Hyde LP. Ultrasound Diagnosis of Pericardial Effusion. JAMA. 1965;191:711–4.
14. Moss AJ, Bruhn F. The echocardiogram. An ultrasound technic for the detection of pericardial effusion. N Engl J Med. 1966;274:380–4.
15. Appleton CP, Hatle LK, Popp RL. Cardiac tamponade and pericardial effusion: respiratory variation in transvalvular flow velocities studied by Doppler echocardiography. J Am Coll Cardiol. 1988;11: 1020–30.
16. Prakash AM, Sun Y, Chiaramida SA, Wu J, Lucariello RJ. Quantitative assessment of pericardial effusion volume by two-dimensional echocardiography. J Am Soc Echocardiogr. 2003;16:147–53.
17. George S, Salama AL, Uthaman B, Cherian G. Echocardiography in differentiating tuberculous from chronic idiopathic pericardial effusion. Heart. 2004;90:1338–9.
18. Schutzman JJ, Obarski TP, Pearce GL, Klein AL. Comparison of Doppler and two-dimensional echocardiography for assessment of pericardial effusion. Am J Cardiol. 1992;70:1353–7.
19. Merce J, Sagrista-Sauleda J, Permanyer-Miralda G, Evangelista A, Soler-Soler J. Correlation between clinical and Doppler echocardiographic findings in patients with moderate and large pericardial effusion: implications for the diagnosis of cardiac tamponade. Am Heart J. 1999;138:759–64.
20. Sagrista-Sauleda J, Angel J, Sanchez A, Permanyer-Miralda G, Soler-Soler J. Effusive-constrictive pericarditis. N Engl J Med. 2004;350:469–75.
21. Sagrista-Sauleda J, Angel J, Permanyer-Miralda G, Soler-Soler J. Long-term follow-up of idiopathic chronic pericardial effusion. N Engl J Med. 1999;341: 2054–9.
22. Ristic AD, Seferovic PM, Maisch B. Management of pericardial effusion the role of echocardiography in establishing the indications and the selection of the approach for drainage. Herz. 2005;30: 144–50.
23. Lindenberger M, Kjellberg M, Karlsson E, Wranne B. Pericardiocentesis guided by 2-D echocardiography: the method of choice for treatment of pericardial effusion. J Intern Med. 2003;253:411–7.
24. Tsang TS, Enriquez-Sarano M, Freeman WK, et al. Consecutive 1127 therapeutic echocardiographically guided pericardiocenteses: clinical profile, practice patterns, and outcomes spanning 21 years. Mayo Clin Proc. 2002;77:429–36.
25. Shepherd FA, Morgan C, Evans WK, Ginsberg JF, Watt D, Murphy K. Medical management of malignant pericardial effusion by tetracycline sclerosis. Am J Cardiol. 1987;60:1161–6.
26. Davis S, Sharma SM, Blumberg ED, Kim CS. Intrapericardial tetracycline for the management of cardiac tamponade secondary to malignant pericardial effusion. N Engl J Med. 1978;299:1113–4.
27. Vaitkus PT, Herrmann HC, LeWinter MM. Treatment of malignant pericardial effusion. JAMA. 1994;272:59–64.
28. Palatianos GM, Thurer RJ, Kaiser GA. Comparison of effectiveness and safety of operations on the pericardium. Chest. 1985;88:30–3.
29. Palacios IF, Tuzcu EM, Ziskind AA, Younger J, Block PC. Percutaneous balloon pericardial window

for patients with malignant pericardial effusion and tamponade. Cathet Cardiovasc Diagn. 1991;22: 244–9.
30. Ziskind AA, Pearce AC, Lemmon CC, et al. Percutaneous balloon pericardiotomy for the treatment of cardiac tamponade and large pericardial effusions: description of technique and report of the first 50 cases. J Am Coll Cardiol. 1993;21:1–5.
31. Ziskind AA. Final report of the percutaneous balloon pericardiotomy registry for the treatment of effusive pericardial disease. Circulation. 1994;90: I-121.
32. Ziskind AA, Rodriguez S, Lemmon C, Burstein S. Percutaneous pericardial biopsy as an adjunctive technique for the diagnosis of pericardial disease. Am J Cardiol. 1994;74:288–91.
33. Ozuner G, Davidson PG, Isenberg JS, McGinn JT, Jr. Creation of a pericardial window using thoracoscopic techniques. Surg Gynecol Obstet. 1992;175: 69–71.

1.3.3
Acute Heart Failure Syndromes and Coexisting Disease

25
Severe Cardiac Disease in Pregnancy

Walther N.K.A. van Mook and Louis Peeters

Clinically significant cardiac disease during pregnancy occurs in 0.1% to 4% of pregnancies (1–4), and this incidence has remained more or less unchanged. The relative contribution of the different causes of heart disease preceding or diagnosed during pregnancy varies with the study population and study period (5). While rheumatic heart disease remains a major problem in developing countries (6), its prevalence in developed countries displays a decline. This implies that congenital heart disease, ischemic heart disease, and arrhythmias have become more common in the developed world (5, 7). However, in developed countries with high immigration rates, "foreign" patterns of disease cause shifts in the incidence and distribution of the different causes of heart disease in pregnancy. Examples are Chagas' disease, syphilis, rheumatic valvular disease, and beriberi cardiomyopathy (5, 8). Nevertheless, in these countries the group of patients with congenital heart disease currently comprises 70% to 80% due to improved pediatric surgery outcomes, and medical therapy, followed by the group of women with rheumatic heart disease, which has decreased due to the decrease in the incidence of rheumatic fever (7, 9, 10). Whereas the incidence of cardiac disease in pregnancy is unchanged, maternal mortality has decreased from 6% in the 1930s (11), to 0.5% to 2.7% now (1–3, 12). Currently cardiac disease in pregnancy accounts for 15% of pregnancy-related maternal mortality (13), emphasizing its importance as nonobstetric cause of maternal death (10, 13, 14). Pregnancy in cardiac patients increases the maternal mortality risk as compared to the general population (4), and actual risk depends on the underlying cardiac disease. With the exception of patients with Eisenmenger syndrome (ES), pulmonary vascular obstructive disease, and Marfan syndrome with aortopathy, maternal death during pregnancy is rare in women with heart disease (2, 15–18). Although maternal mortality is low, pregnant women with heart disease are at risk for serious morbidity like heart failure, arrhythmias, and stroke (7, 19). Since the hemodynamic changes of normal pregnancy per se have profound effects on preexisting cardiac function, counseling of and care for this subset of patients to optimize maternal and neonatal survival is challenging (20). For a detailed discussion of the hemodynamic changes during normal pregnancy, the reader is referred to a recent extensive review article on this topic (21).

The Approach to the Pregnant Patient with Complaints

It can be difficult to differentiate between patients with complaints attributable to pregnancy and those with complaints related to heart disease. Shortness of breath, palpitations, dizziness, edema, and limited exercise capacity are common complaints during pregnancy. Pregnancy can also alter results of commonly used diagnostic tools, thereby complicating the workup of these patients (5). These findings are summarized in Table 25.1. Nevertheless, chest pain, syncope or near-syncope, paroxysmal nocturnal dyspnea, hemoptysis, and progressive edema are not normal in pregnancy and should be carefully evaluated (5). Acute

Table 25.1. Findings on physical examination and variants encountered using common additional investigation tools

Physical examination
Inspection
Jugular venous distention and prominent pulsation
Brisk and diffuse apex pulsation
Right ventricular impulse
Auscultation
Mitral component S_1 increased, S_1 widely split
Pulmonary component S_2 increased, S_2 split
Occasional S_3
Aortic or pulmonary middiastolic flow murmurs
Systolic brachiocephalic trunk murmur
Continuous venous hum over jugulum
Systolic or continuous mammary souffle audible
Chest x-ray
Apparent cardiomegaly
Enlarged left atrium
Increased vascular marking
Straightening of left-sided heart border
Postpartum pleural effusion (right sided)
Electrocardiography
Rhythm, rate and intervals
Increased rate, sinus tachycardia
Small decreases of PR and QT (heart rate dependent)
Right bundle-branch block
Axis
15 degrees axis rotation
Deviation of electrical axis to the left
Depolarization/repolarization changes
Q waves in III
T-wave inversion in III, V2, V3
Echocardiogram
Trivial tricuspid regurgitation
Pulmonary regurgitation
Increased left atrial size (12–14%)
Increased left ventricular end-diastolic dimensions (6–10%)
Inconsistent increase in left ventricular thickness
Mitral regurgitation
Pericardial effusions

Source: Modified from Gei and Hankins (5), with permission.

pulmonary edema in pregnancy is frequently caused by cardiac disease (25.5%) (22), and 15% to 52% of cardiac abnormalities are diagnosed during pregnancy (2, 5, 22).

Management of Cardiac Disease in Pregnancy

Risk stratification and counseling is best performed before conception. The information required for this purpose comes from cardiovascular history taking and physical examination, along with a 12-lead electrocardiogram (ECG), echocardiography, and, in some cases, arterial oxygen saturation. In counseling, six areas should be considered: the underlying cardiac lesion; maternal functional status; the possibility/necessity of further palliative or corrective surgery; the presence of additional associated risk factors; maternal life expectancy and ability to care for a child; and, in cases of congenital heart disease (CHD), the risk of congenital heart disease in offspring (7).

The underlying cardiac lesion is important, as almost all patients can be stratified into low-, intermediate-, and high-risk groups (Table 25.2). Maternal functional status is an important predictor of maternal and neonatal complications (17). Further palliative or corrective surgery should be undertaken before pregnancy if necessary and if possible, and is indicated, for example, in cyanotic heart disease patients and in other symptomatic patients. The additional risk factors for a complicated pregnancy include a history of arrhythmia, presence of prosthetic heart valves, and the use of (necessary) potentially teratogenic medication. Maternal life expectancy and ability to care for a child are important considerations. A consequence of limited maternal physical capacity or the birth of an infant with a handicap is the risk that the mother will not be able to care for her child. The risk of congenital CHD in offspring in cases of familial CHD is also relevant. If a first-degree relative is affected, the risk increases 10-fold, and reaches 50% in autosomal dominant diseases (7). Patients with pulmonary hypertension (PH) (systolic pulmonary artery pressure >50 mm Hg), either primary or in ES; dilated cardiomyopathy; Marfan syndrome with cardiovascular involvement; pulmonary arteriovenous fistulas; or any uncorrectable cardiac lesion in patients with New York Heart Association (NYHA) functional class III or IV should be strongly advised against pregnancy, and in case of pregnancy, these conditions can be considered indications for pregnancy termination (5). Some authors advise that counseling about termination of pregnancy should include the advice of a woman, preferably one who has experience of pregnancy and child care (10). Pregnant women with uncomplicated cardiac disease should receive their prenatal care at similar intervals as is common practice for other women with a preexistent risk condition. Admission to hospital is recommended when

TABLE 25.2. Mortality risk in groups of patients with cardiac disease in pregnancy

Group	Cardiac disease	Risk of cardiac complications	Mortality
I	Small left-right shunt (atrial septal defect, ventricular septal defect, patent ductus arteriosus) Mild pulmonic/tricuspid valve abnormalities Corrected tetralogy of Fallot Bioprosthetic valve Repaired lesions without residual cardiac dysfunction Isolated mitral valve prolapse without significant regurgitation Bicuspid aortic valve without stenosis Valvular regurgitation with normal ventricular systolic function	Low risk	<1%
II	Mitral stenosis Large left-to-right shunt Mechanical prosthetic heart valve Severe pulmonic stenosis Aortic stenosis Uncorrected coarctation of aorta Uncorrected tetralogy of Fallot and other unrepaired cyanotic congenital heart disease Previous myocardial infarction Moderate to severe systemic ventricular dysfunction History of peripartum cardiomyopathy without residual dysfunction	Intermediate risk	5–15%
III	Marfan syndrome with aortic or valvular involvement Severe pulmonary hypertension NYHA class III and IV symptoms Severe aortic stenosis History of peripartum cardiomyopathy with residual ventricular dysfunction	High risk	25–50%

Source: Adapted from Gei and Hankins (5) and Siu and Colman (7), with permission.

signs of congestive heart failure (CHF), infection, or anemia are present (5). Women with PH (in case of continuation of pregnancy) should be hospitalized at around week 20, and patients in functional class IV should be hospitalized throughout pregnancy (23, 24). All other patients seem to benefit from a policy of liberal hospital admission based on maternal functional status, fetal growth and well-being, and standard prenatal care (5, 8). Further management and planning requires a multidisciplinary approach. Timing and mode of delivery, intrapartum hemodynamic monitoring, peripartum medication management including endocarditis prophylaxis, anticoagulation, and inotropic and vasopressor support, should all be discussed (5). In the following subsections, characteristics of specific cardiac diseases are discussed in more detail.

Congenital Heart Disease

The majority of women with heart disease during pregnancy have a congenital heart disease (CHD), since the number of women in this group reaching reproductive age has increased markedly over the last decades, and the desire to become pregnant is strong (25). Atrial septal defect is the most common CHD in adults, and tetralogy of Fallot is the most common cyanotic CHD (18). Maternal risks consist of atrial arrhythmias, cardiac failure, increasing cyanosis, and thromboembolic events (25).

Left-to-Right Shunts

Atrial and ventricular septal defects (ASD, VSD), and patent ductus arteriosus (PDA), when operated on early in infancy, do not require any special treatment (25). Left-to-right shunts in these CHDs are usually well tolerated and asymptomatic, and volume overload is counteracted by a decrease in pulmonary vascular resistance (PVR). Pregnancy is usually uneventful if PH is absent, maternal functional class is I or II, and systemic ventricular function is normal (4, 25, 26). Problems like arrhythmias, ventricular dysfunction, and progression of PH occur in patients with large shunts or preexisting PH(4). Therefore, repeated echocardiography should be performed during pregnancy. The preexisting left-to-right shunt can be reversed due to elevation in PVR, or secondary to systemic vasodilatation (4). Sometimes paradoxical embolization (with right to left shunting) may occur (7). Because pregnancy is a hypercoagulable state some authors recommend prophylaxis with low-dose aspirin (80 mg daily) from the 10th week of pregnancy onward (11, 27). In patients with (residual) shunts and valvular regurgitation endocarditis, prophylaxis is essential.

Stenotic Valvular Lesions

Aortic valve stenosis (AVS) is usually a consequence of congenital bicuspid aortic valve (28). The severity of AVS can be described as the average valve area or the peak pressure gradient across the valve. Severe AVS is defined by the American Heart Association (AHA) as a peak gradient greater than 50 mm Hg. Severe or symptomatic aortic stenosis should be corrected before pregnancy (29). Absence of symptoms does not rule out complications (7). A review of multiple small studies yielded a maternal mortality rate of 11% and a perinatal mortality of 4% (7). One study reported no maternal mortality and overall satisfactory outcome with deterioration of functional status in 20% of patients (30). A study in 49 AVS pregnant patients reported that 10% suffered complications, but they occurred only in the women who had severe AVS and not in women known to have mild or moderate AVS. Fetal morbidity was observed in 12% (31). Therefore, management of mild to moderate AVS should be conservative. Open valve replacement during pregnancy in severe AVS is possible but associated with 30% fetal mortality (32) (see Cardiac Surgery During Pregnancy, below). Use of balloon valvuloplasty during pregnancy or peripartum has been reported sporadically (33, 34), but is contraindicated in the presence of significant aortic regurgitation.

When pulmonic stenosis is mild or treated by valve replacement or valvuloplasty, it is well tolerated in pregnancy, and maternal and fetal outcome are favorable. In severe or symptomatic stenosis, right heart failure and arrhythmias may occur and if possible, should be treated before pregnancy (7). In cases of deteriorating cardiac function, valvuloplasty may be the treatment of choice in pregnancy. Details on mitral valve stenosis are described in valvular heart disease, including rheumatic heart disease.

Cyanotic Heart Disease

The most common form of cyanotic heart disease is tetralogy of Fallot. After successful correction of tetralogy, the pregnancy risk is low (16, 17), but remaining abnormalities increase the complication risk. In uncorrected cyanotic CHD such as tetralogy of Fallot and single ventricle, the increase in cardiac output (CO) and decrease in systemic vascular resistance (SVR) in pregnancy enhance the right-to-left shunt, thus increasing the degree of hypoxemia and cyanosis. In these patients the risk of maternal and fetal complications is high (7, 18, 25, 35), as indicated by the high rate of maternal thromboembolic disease (32%), prematurity (37%), low birth weight, and low live-birth rate (43%). One death occurred 2 months after delivery due to endocarditis (35). Severity of maternal cyanosis and functional class correlate inversely with neonatal outcome (4, 35).

Coarctation of the Aorta

Uncorrected coarctation of the aorta is associated with a maternal mortality risk of 3%, but is higher in the presence of associated cardiac defects, aortic abnormalities, or preexisting longstanding hypertension (7). Aortic rupture in the third trimester is the most frequent cause of death (36), but its incidence had declined in a recent study, in which maternal and perinatal mortality were low (37). Management of hypertension is challenging and difficult at the same time since control of hypertension proximal to the coarctation may compromise distal blood flow and with it, uteroplacental perfusion (7).

Marfan Syndrome

Cardiovascular complications in Marfan syndrome are hallmarked by aortopathy resulting in increased risk of dilation, dissection, and valvular regurgitation. Pregnancy predisposes to rapid aortic dilatation and dissection, perhaps due to the combined effects of hemodynamic stress and hormonal changes. With increasing aortic root diameter the risk of maternal mortality increases (38, 39). Replacement of the ascending aorta in asymptomatic patients is recommended when the root diameter exceeds 5.5 cm (40). Pregnant women with Marfan syndrome should have echocardiograms at regular intervals to follow the aortic root diameter. Prophylactic beta-blockade is advised (7), and hypertension should be aggressively treated to minimize the risk of aortic dissection. If the diameter of the aortic root is normal and has been stable for some time, pregnancy is likely to develop normally, although the risk of dissection is always present (7). Patients with an aortic root diameter of less than 4.5 cm without cardiovascular complications may deliver vaginally with epidural anesthesia, with low threshold for assistance in the second stage. Maternal mortality has decreased from 30% to 1%, with a fetal mortality rate of 22% (7).

Transposition of Great Vessels

Although most adults have had surgical corrections, theoretically problems can still arise in pregnancy, and the rates of fetal loss and maternal cardiovascular morbidity are raised (41). No maternal mortality was reported in two studies addressing this subject; seven of 41 patients (with 105 pregnancies) developed heart failure, endocarditis, stroke, or myocardial infarction, and there was a 27% fetal mortality rate (7, 41, 42).

Eisenmenger Syndrome and Pulmonary Hypertension

The most common cause of Eisenmenger syndrome and pulmonary hypertension is a large VSD, followed by a large PDA and ASD (11). Once the increased pulmonary vascular blood flow has given rise to increased pulmonary resistance that exceeds the SVR, reversal of flow and cyanosis will develop. Surgical correction of the defect does not influence the PH at this stage (11). Eisenmenger syndrome, therefore, is defined as PH (PVR >800 dynes $\cdot$ $sec^{-1} \cdot cm^{-5}$, or systolic pulmonary artery pressure >30 mm Hg, or mean pulmonary artery pressure >25 mm Hg at rest [4]) coupled with a reversed or bidirectional shunting of blood flow in patients with CHD and initial left-to-right shunt. Eisenmenger syndrome carries a 30% risk of maternal mortality in each pregnancy, with most complications occurring at term or the first week postpartum (43, 44). Counseling should include sterilization and other contraceptive measures, as well as the possibility of terminating a pregnancy. All patients with pulmonary vascular disease who decide against termination of pregnancy should be hospitalized in the second trimester (4). Medical treatment consists of avoiding increases in PVR, maintaining right ventricular preload, and left and right ventricular contractility. This includes vasodilation by calcium antagonists, angiotensin-converting enzyme inhibitors, AT-1–receptor blockers, and the use of inotropic agents, anticoagulation, diuretics, and supplemental oxygen. The use of newer drugs such as intravenous epoprostenol or aerosolized iloprost are promising in reducing PVR (45–47). Inhaled nitric oxide induces selective vasodilatation of the pulmonary vascular bed (45, 46, 48). Apart from the maternal risks, there are enormous risks for the fetus. Spontaneous abortion and fetal growth restriction are seen in 30%, whereas perinatal mortality mostly due to extreme prematurity amounts to 28% (43). In a recent review of patients with pulmonary vascular disease, including ES, and primary and secondary PH, maternal mortality rates were high in all groups (36%, 30%, and 56%, respectively), with neonatal survival rates of 87%, 89%, and 88% (49). The severity of preconceptional PH correlates with the risk of heart failure developing in pregnancy (4). It follows that patients with CHD and PH, ES, and primary or secondary PH are to be counseled before pregnancy, and often be advised to refrain from pregnancy (49).

Valvular Heart Disease, Including Rheumatic Heart Disease

Regurgitant valvular abnormalities are better tolerated than stenotic lesions (5). Even severe aortic and mitral regurgitations are generally well tolerated during pregnancy, although worsening of maternal functional class has been observed. However, pregnancy does affect stenotic lesions profoundly as emphasized by deterioration of their NYHA functional class, the development of CHF, and adverse perinatal outcome in as many as 62%, 38%, and 23% of the cases, respectively (50). Although the adverse impact of pregnancy increases with the functional impairment of the lesion being larger, maternal mortality is rare (50).

Rheumatic Mitral Valve Stenosis

Mitral valve stenosis (MVS) is the most common rheumatic valvular lesion (28). The severity of MVS is classified on the basis of valve area: a valve area of $>1.5\,cm^2$ is mild, 1.1 to $1.5\,cm^2$ moderate, and $\leq 1\,cm^2$ is severe (29). The severity of MVS assessed by the echo-Doppler measurement of the mitral valve area was the most powerful predictor of maternal pulmonary edema (51, 52). Pregnancy-induced hypervolemia and tachycardia magnifies the negative impact of MVS on cardiac function, leading to a higher left atrial pressure, and with it, an increased risk of atrial fibrillation and heart failure (51). In several recent studies no mortality was reported, but substantial morbidity persists (17, 50–52). Nevertheless, a 5% to 7% maternal mortality has been reported in women categorized in an unfavorable functional class before pregnancy (2, 53) and was accompanied by a perinatal mortality rate of 12% to 31% (11, 53). Indications for invasive intervention with mitral valve commissurotomy, balloon valvuloplasty, or valve replacement are a valve area smaller than $1.2\,cm^2$, poor response to medical therapy, and absence of valvular calcifications (4, 51). Invasive intervention preferably should be performed before pregnancy, although balloon mitral valvuloplasty can be performed relatively safely during pregnancy (54–56). As compared to open mitral-valve commissurotomy, percutaneous balloon mitral valvuloplasty is safe and effective and appears to be preferable in pregnancy (57). Theoretically, patients with MVS may deliver vaginally (1, 5). However, primary cesarean section should be considered if cardiac reserves are reduced, which implies compromised maternal and fetal tolerance of labor stress (4).

Rheumatic Aortic Valve Stenosis

With rheumatic involvement of the aortic valve, outcome is comparable to congenital aortic stenosis, as described above.

Mitral Valve Prolapse

Mitral valve prolapse (MVP) is the most common cardiac abnormality observed in obstetrics, affecting 12% to 17% of women in the childbearing years (58). It can be primary (idiopathic) or secondary (and associated with ASD, endocarditis, MVS, or a calcified mitral annulus). In pregnancy, MVP seldomly gives rise to cardiovascular complications (59).

Ischemic Heart Disease

The prevalence of acute myocardial infarction (MI) during pregnancy and in the puerperium is low, but associated with significant maternal, fetal, and neonatal morbidity and mortality. In the first days postpartum, women have a sixfold higher rate of MI than age-matched nonpregnant women (60). A recent study reported 151 cases with an incidence of 1 in 35,700 deliveries and a maternal mortality rate of 7.3% confined to the peripartum period and entirely due to acute myocardial infarction (AMI) (61). Mortality risk is highest at the time of infarction and the first 2 weeks afterward. Delivery within 2 weeks of AMI was associated with up to 50% maternal mortality (62, 63), and therefore delivery should be delayed, if possible, for at least 2 weeks after AMI. Chronic hypertension, diabetes, advanced maternal age, eclampsia, and severe preeclampsia were identified as independent risk factors for AMI (61). The classic risk factors for vascular disease (e.g., familial hypercholesterolemia [64–66]) have all been associated with an elevated risk for cardiac events in pregnant women (67). With an increasing proportion of first mothers being aged over 30 years (68), an increase in ischemic heart disease in pregnancy can be expected (67).

Often MI results from coronary spasms as suggested by a study in 136 cases with 47% having no appreciable abnormality at angiography (69). Myocardial ischemia (secondary to coronary spasm) may occur after the use of prostaglandin E_1 (70), prostaglandin E_2 (71) (both for abortion), ergonovine (for postpartum hemorrhage) (72), and ritodrine and nifedipine (for preterm labor) (73). Perhaps their use in patients with risk factors for cardiac ischemia should be avoided. Isolated cases of dissection or plaque disruption with normal findings at angiography have been described. Spontaneous coronary artery dissection has been demonstrated in up to 16% of patients (74–78). Atherosclerotic coronary artery disease is also commonly seen in as many as 43% of cases (74). Rare causes include congenital coronary abnormalities, Kawasaki disease, vasculitis, cocaine abuse, pheochromocytoma, sickle cell disease, collagen vascular disease, and abnormal hemostasis (67, 79).

Beta-blockers, nitrates, and low-dose aspirin are treatment options for cardiac ischemia in pregnancy. Treatment of myocardial infarction in pregnancy is comparable to that in the nonpregnant patient. Successful use of thrombolytics has been reported (80, 81), although the occurrence of placental abruption and neonatal intracranial hemorrhage have been reported (74). Angioplasty and stent placement have been carried out successfully during pregnancy (67). The (relatively low) radiation exposure during diagnostic and interventional procedures (60 minutes of fluoroscopy exposes the fetus to 1300 mrad) is a concern (67, 69, 74, 82). Protecting the pregnant uterus from exposure to radiation using a lead shield and avoiding pelvic fluoroscopy can keep the dose to the fetus below 100 mrad. The currently accepted maximum limit for fetal exposure during pregnancy is 5 rad, and the risk of malformations is significantly increased above 15 rad (67).

In the past, the coexistence of myocardial ischemic heart disease and diabetes has been considered a absolute contraindication for pregnancy (83), and still the presence of an ischemic heart disease should be considered a high-risk condition. Nevertheless, adequate ventricular performance and normal coronary vasculature warrant a satisfactory prognosis for women with diabetes who conceive after an MI (64). Morbidity during subsequent pregnancy in patients with a history of MI ranges between 20% and 50%, including CHF, and unstable angina, but the reported risk for maternal mortality is low (12, 84, 85).

Arrhythmias

During labor and delivery, almost all women have resting abnormalities in their ECG, including premature atrial, ventricular, or nodal complexes; sinoatrial arrest; wandering atrial pacemaker; sinus tachycardia; and paroxysmal ventricular tachycardia (86). Atrial and ventricular premature beats are usually benign. Supraventricular tachycardia and ventricular tachyarrhythmia occur less frequent. Pregnancy may increase the incidence and hemodynamic severity of preexisting arrhythmias (87), and even induce de novo arrhythmias. It is conceivable that these effects are related to the change in circulatory function in pregnancy. The latter consists of a primary fall in systemic cardiovascular tone, inducing the institution of a high flow/low resistance circulation, as well as changes in volume homeostasis and autonomic circulatory control. The direct cardiac effects of pregnancy consist of increases in cardiac compliance, stroke volume, and heart rate, and a change in its autonomic control (21). These changes together with direct hormonal effects can be expected to act in concert to modulate the sequence of pulse generation, subsequent conduction, excitation of cardiac muscle tissue, and ultimately myocardial contraction. Obviously, these pregnancy-related cardiac effects may unmask occult cardiac disorders and aggravate existing underlying heart disease (88), but most arrhythmias in young women are not associated with structural heart disease (88). The risk of arrhythmias in pregnancy is highest during labor and delivery (88). Pregnancy in patients with long QT syndrome can be complicated by torsades de pointes in the postpartum period when heart rate decreases (88).

Treatment of Arrhythmias During Pregnancy

Management of arrhythmias in pregnant women is similar to that in nonpregnant women, but it is essential to avoid adverse effects on the fetus. Removal of potential stimuli of (supra)ventricular premature beats like smoking, caffeine, and alcohol is usually sufficient, and drug therapy is usually not needed (88). Although no drug is completely safe, most are well tolerated and can be given with relatively low risk. Drug therapy should be avoided during the first trimester if possible, and drugs that are least likely to have adverse effects should be used as first-line therapy (88, 89). Electrical cardioversion is safe during pregnancy. In paroxysmal supraventricular tachycardia, vagal stimulation maneuvers should be attempted, and adenosine or a cardioselective beta-blocker can be used if this attempt is unsuccessful (88). Drug treatment is indicated when arrhythmias result in severe symptoms or in patients with ventricular hypertrophy, ventricular dysfunction, or valvular obstruction. Sustained

Table 25.3. Maternal and fetal effects of commonly used cardiac medications

Medication	Potential adverse fetal and maternal effects	U.S. Food and Drug Administration (FDA) category*	Compatible with breast-feeding
ACE inhibitors	Teratogenesis, skull ossification defects like hypocalvaria, renal defects, oligohydramnios, Potter syndrome; fetal growth retardation and death, preterm birth, neonatal hypotension and anuria, neonatal death, anemia, patent ductus arteriosus	C (1st trimester) D (2nd and 3rd trimesters)	Enalapril, captopril compatible; others unknown
Adenosine	None reported except for one case of fetal bradycardia; use during first trimester limited to few patients; dyspnea	C	Yes
Amiodarone	Hypothyroidism, growth retardation, prematurity	D	No
Atenolol	Hypospadias?; lower birth weight; possible neonatal bradycardia	D	Yes, use with caution
Azathioprine	Potential for skeletal and visceral anomalies in animals, not in humans; intrauterine growth restriction	D	Not recommended by manufacturer
Coumadin	Warfarin embryopathy; central nervous system abnormalities; spontaneous abortion; stillbirth; hemorrhage	D (X, according to manufacturer)	Yes
Cyclosporine	No apparent teratogenesis; preterm birth; intrauterine growth restriction; fetal loss	C	No
Digoxin	Accelerated labor reported; low birth weight	C	Yes
Diltiazem	No fetal effects reported; fetal stress due to maternal hypotension; fetal bradycardia and heart block	C	Yes
Disopyramide	Uterine contraction	C	Yes
Diuretics	Placental hypoperfusion, thrombocytopenia, jaundice, hyponatremia, bradycardia	Furosemide C Hydrochlorothiazide B	Unknown Compatible, may suppress lactation
Heparin	No teratogenesis (does not cross placenta); maternal hemorrhage; maternal osteoporosis	C	Yes
Lidocaine	Central nervous system depression due to high blood levels and fetal acidosis, bradycardia	B	Yes
Metoprolol	No teratogenesis; possible neonatal bradycardia	B	Yes
Propranolol	No teratogenesis; intrauterine growth restriction; neonatal hypoglycemia; possible respiratory depression	C	Yes
Quinidine	Maternal and fetal thrombocytopenia; toxic dose may induce preterm labor and eighth cranial nerve damage, torsades de pointes	C	Yes, caution advised
Sotalol	Growth retardation; bradycardia; hyperbilirubinemia; hypoglycemia; uterine contractions	B	Yes
Sodium nitroprusside	Potential thiocyanate toxicity, fetal mortality in animal studies	C	Unknown

ACE, angiotensin-converting enzyme.

*Definition of FDA pregnancy categories: Category A: Controlled studies shown no risk. Adequate, well-controlled studies in pregnant women have failed to demonstrate risk to the fetus in any trimester of pregnancy. Category B: No evidence of risk in humans. Adequate, well-controlled studies in pregnant women have not shown increased risk of fetal abnormalities despite adverse findings in animals; or in the absence of adequate human studies, animal studies have shown no fetal risk. The chance of fetal harm is remote but remains a possibility. Category C: Risk cannot be ruled out. Adequate, well-controlled human studies are lacking, and animal studies have shown a risk to the fetus or are lacking as well. There is chance of fetal harm if the drug administered during pregnancy, but the potential benefits outweigh the risk. Category D: Positive evidence of risk. Studies in humans have shown evidence of fetal risk. Nevertheless, the potential benefits from the use of the drug in pregnant women outweigh the risk. Category X: Contraindicated in pregnancy. Studies in animals or humans have shown fetal risk, which clearly outweighs any possible future benefit to the patient.

Source: Modified from Gei and Hankins (5), Klein and Galan (11), Gowda et al., (88), and Joglar and Page (89), with permission.

tachyarrhythmias should be treated promptly, preferably using nonteratogenic medication. In patients with atrial fibrillation conversion to sinus rhythm is the primary goal. The use of amiodarone is contraindicated, although case reports mention successful use with adequate (neonatal) follow-up. Termination of ventricular arrhythmias can usually be achieved by intravenous lidocaine or procainamide or by electrical cardioversion (88). Beta-blocker therapy must be continued during pregnancy and in the postpartum period in women with long QT syndrome and torsades de pointes (88). Pregnancy in patients with implantable cardioverter defibrillators (ICDs) neither increases the risk of major ICD-related complications nor results in a high number of ICD discharges, and is associated with favorable maternal and fetal outcomes (90). An overview of antiarrhythmic medication and their effects on the fetus is listed in Table 25.3.

Cardiomyopathy During Pregnancy Including Peripartum Cardiomyopathy

Cardiomyopathy during pregnancy can be divided into two groups: peripartum cardiomyopathy (PP-CMP) and all other forms of cardiomyopathy. The latter group consists of the dilated, restrictive, and hypertrophic cardiomyopathies and can be idiopathic or due to a specific cause with known time of onset. A recent study reported that 70% of cardiomyopathy-related mortality during 1991 and 1997 in the United States was due to PP-CMP, and that cardiomyopathy accounts for an increasing proportion of pregnancy-related deaths (91). Still PP-CMP constitutes less than 1% of all cardiovascular events related to pregnancy (92, 93) and is most often seen in the last month of pregnancy or after delivery. It is a diagnosis of exclusion. Currently used criteria are summarized in Table 25.4. The reported incidence of PP-CMP varies between 1 in 100 and 1 in 15,000 pregnancies (92–101), with a currently accepted incidence in the U.S. of 1 in 3000 to 1 per 4000 live births (102). Table 25.5 summarizes the reported and postulated associations and risk factors. Usually (87% of cases) symptomatic PP-CMP develops between the 36th week of pregnancy and 4 months postpartum, with most cases (78%) presenting postpartum (94). Clinical signs are often those of heart failure. Other late complications of pregnancy such as massive pulmonary embolism and amniotic fluid embolism may resemble heart failure, and thus lead to misdiagnosis (103).

Normal pregnancy is often accompanied by fatigue and shortness of breath. Therefore, the NYHA classification to estimate the severity of heart failure is only partly applicable in pregnancy (92, 94, 104). Myocarditis is proposed to be a causal factor (105–110), with a reported incidence ranging from 9% (108) to 78% (106). Also, an infectious (111, 112) or an autoimmune etiology has been suggested (102, 106, 108, 113), more so as pregnancy increases the susceptibility to either (105, 108). Peripartum cardiomyopathy is indeed associated with high titers of auto-antibodies against certain cardiac tissue proteins (102, 113). With respect to an infectious etiology, patients

Table 25.4. Criteria for peripartum cardiomyopathy

Criteria for peripartum cardiomyopathy (all four of the following)	Reference
1. Cardiac failure occurring in the last month of pregnancy, or within 5 months postpartum	95
2. Absence of an identifiable cause for the cardiac failure	95
3. Absence of heart disease prior to the last month of pregnancy	95
4. Left ventricular systolic dysfunction by echographic criteria: —Left ventricular ejection fraction <45% or —Decreased fractional shortening <30% —End diastolic dimension >2.7 cm/m^2	92, 94, 103

Table 25.5. Peripartum cardiomyopathy: reported associations

Associated condition	Reference
Older maternal age (>30 years)	94
Multiparity	94
Twin pregnancy	94
Preeclampsia/gestational hypertension	93, 182
Black race	94, 183
Living in a tropical or subtropical region	184
Familial occurrence	185, 186
Malnutrition	18, 94
Cocaine use by mother	187
Long-term tocolytic therapy	188
Selenium deficiency	116, 189
Chlamydia infection	190
Enterovirus infection	111

who died of PP-CMP had higher peripheral levels of inflammatory cytokines than their surviving counterparts (114), although this response could also be a secondary effect of splanchnic hypoperfusion. Other postulated etiologic factors include abnormalities of relaxin (115) and selenium deficiency (116). But the exact cause of this disorder is still unknown. The most important complication of PP-CMP is thromboembolism (117–122), occurring in up to 50% of cases (94, 123, 124).

Medical treatment of PP-CMP is mainly supportive and thus similar to that of other forms of CHF (94). Immunosuppressive therapy has been used in patients with PP-CMP with biopsy-proven myocarditis, resulting in improvement of clinical features coinciding with loss of the inflammatory infiltrate on repeated biopsies (105), and improvement of left ventricular (LV) function and prognosis (109). The use of immunosuppressive therapy (prednisone and azathioprine) remains controversial until the precise role of myocarditis is clarified (94). Its use may be considered in patients with myocarditis on biopsy who fail to improve spontaneously within 2 weeks of initiation of standard heart failure therapy (102). In a retrospective study LV ejection was found to have improved more after intravenous immunoglobulins (2 g/kg, $n = 6$) than previously observed in 11 historical control subjects (125). An intraaortic balloon pump (IABP) or insertion of a left ventricular or biventricular assist device (LVAD, BVAD) can be used as a bridge until transplantation or recovery (92, 96, 126–128). Cases of transplantation for PP-CMP (129–131) and successful next pregnancy have been reported (132, 133). Some authors state that only myocarditis-negative patients should be offered transplantation (129). Women with PP-CMP requiring a cardiac transplant have an 88% survival rate after 2 years. However, as compared to patients who had a cardiac transplant for idiopathic cardiomyopathy, they had 30% more often early rejection, required more immunosuppressive therapy, and had higher infection rates (131). It has been suggested that for patients with PP-CMP developing in late pregnancy, a trial of labor is allowed provided invasive hemodynamic monitoring is warranted throughout all stages of labor (134).

Mortality ranges from 25% to 50%, with nearly half of the mortality occurring in the first 3 months postpartum (92, 94, 95, 97, 117–123, 135). Causes of death include chronic progressive CHF, fatal arrhythmias, or thromboembolic complications. Currently, there is no consensus regarding recommendations for future pregnancy after PP-CMP (102). Most authors agree that the next pregnancy carries a very high risk and therefore should be discouraged and avoided in cases of persisting LV dysfunction. Whether those patients recovering with normal LV function can safely undergo a next pregnancy is still unsettled. Elkayam et al. (136) reported that a next pregnancy in women with a history of PP-CMP was associated with a significant fall in LV function regardless of whether LV function had returned to normal after the previous pregnancy. If LV function had completely recovered, heart failure developed in 21% of next pregnancies. However, an incompletely recovered LV function predisposed to 44% recurrent heart failure in the subsequent pregnancy. Maternal mortality was seen in 0% and 19%, and preterm labor in 11% and 37% of subsequent pregnancies, respectively (136). Obviously, all subsequent pregnancies should be managed in a high-risk perinatal center (102).

Case Report of Peripartum Cardiomyopathy

At gestational age of 36 weeks ± 1 week, a 34-year-old African woman (gravida 5, para 3) was admitted to hospital with preeclampsia (blood pressure 140/100 mm Hg, peripheral edema, and proteinuria of 0.3 g/L). After stimulation with prostaglandin E_2 gel, a healthy girl weighing 2.66 kg was born 5 days later. Initial postpartum recovery was uneventful, but 4 days after discharge she was readmitted with dyspnea (30 shallow breaths/min), a blood pressure of 140/100 mm Hg, tachycardia (130 bpm), and pyrexia (38.2°C), but no peripheral edema. Auscultation of the chest revealed normal breath sounds and a gallop rhythm. The patient now reported that her second pregnancy 10 years previously was complicated by dyspnea and heart failure. Details subsequently obtained led to a clinical diagnosis of CHF and PP-CMP with a normal ejection fraction 1 month after delivery. Her third pregnancy 4 years later was uncomplicated. A fourth pregnancy was an ectopic requiring surgical management at 8 weeks.

Laboratory investigations revealed a hemoglobin level of 9.0 g/dL with normal leukocyte and thrombocyte counts. Electrolytes, renal function, thyroid function, glucose-6-phosphate dehydrogenase, vitamin B_{12}, folic acid, and iron levels were also normal. Liver enzymes were slightly elevated (although lactate dehydrogenase was 948 U/L), and the total bilirubin level was 9.9 μmol/L. Chest radiography showed an enlarged heart and a dubious infiltrate in the left lower lobe. Despite initial treatment with antibiotics her condition deteriorated with progressive dyspnea. Blood pressure (175/115 mm Hg) and heart rate (145 bpm) remained elevated, bilateral crepitations were now heard on auscultation, and repeat chest radiography now showed pulmonary edema. Electrocardiographic ST depression with T-wave inversion was present in the anterior chest leads with flat ST segments inferiorly. The patient was treated with intravenous furosemide, subcutaneous morphine, and continuous positive airway pressure without improvement. After subsequent intubation and initiation of pressure-regulated volume controlled mechanical ventilation, echocardiography revealed an enlarged left ventricle, a global decrease in contractility with a left ventricular ejection fraction (LVEF) of 28%, moderate mitral valve insufficiency, and an estimated stroke volume of 30 mL. Dobutamine and nitroglycerin were started. Swan-Ganz catheter measurements subsequently revealed central venous, pulmonary artery, and pulmonary artery wedge pressures of 12, 41/29, and 20 mm Hg, respectively, and a cardiac output of 6.28 L/min (cardiac index 3.27 $L\,min^{-1}\,m^{-2}$). After cessation of the antibiotics bronchoalveolar lavage revealed no abnormalities and no microbial growth. Serology for respiratory viral infections remained negative, serum selenium was normal, and an autoimmune screen (antinuclear factor, antineutrophil cytoplasmic antibody, anti–double-stranded DNA, anticardiolipin antibody, and antibodies against cardiac muscle) also proved negative. A diagnosis of PPCMP was thus made. A continuous furosemide infusion and angiotensin-converting enzyme (ACE) inhibitors were added to the nitrate and dobutamine therapy.

After 6 days the patient was extubated; however, repeat echocardiography showed worsening of cardiac function (LVEF 17%, mitral insufficiency grade 2 to 3, right ventricular pressure 55 to 60 mm Hg). The patient was transferred to the coronary care unit for IABP counterpulsation. Five days later the nitrates were stopped. Repeat echocardiography showed a LVEF of 35%, with grade I mitral insufficiency. Two days later the IABP was removed. Her condition gradually improved, and almost 1 month after admission she was discharged on bumetanide, carvedilol, and quinapril. Discharge echocardiography showed a LVEF of 50% and normal electrocardiography. Another pregnancy was strongly discouraged. In the outpatient clinic 10 months later, echocardiography showed further normalization (LVEF of 62%, normal dimensions, and no evidence of valvular insufficiency).

Pregnancy in Patients with Prosthetic Heart Valves

Pregnancy is usually well tolerated in patients with bioprosthetic valves. Pregnancy affects neither the structural and functional state of the valves (137) nor the maternal outcome (138, 139). Pregnancy in women with mechanical valve prosthesis carries an increased risk (3% to 14%) of valve thrombosis (140, 141) and is more pronounced, when subcutaneous unfractionated heparin (UFH) instead of warfarin is used as anticoagulant agent (29, 142). The risk of thrombosis is markedly raised in the puerperium with an additional rise after cesarean section to a level 25-fold that of the general population (35% as compared to 1.25–5.4%) (143, 144). The 1998 guidelines from the American College of Cardiology (ACC)/AHA recommended the use of warfarin throughout pregnancy with the exception of the period with highest risk of teratogenicity (weeks 6 to 12 of gestation) and before anticipated delivery after 36 weeks, when it is to be substituted by heparin (1, 29, 139). The latter approach was adopted as various reports claim embryopathy of oral anticoagulant (OA) drugs, with the embryonic/fetal skeleton formation being most vulnerable to defects (145, 146). Substituting OA by heparin between 6 and 12 weeks reduces the risk of fetopathic effects, but with an increased risk of thromboembolic complications in this period (risk of valve thrombosis with OA throughout [3.9%; 95% confidence interval (CI), 2.9–5.9%]; risk of valve thrombosis using heparin only between 6 and 12 weeks' gestation [9.2%; 95% CI, 5.9%–13.9%]) (141). The use of adjusted-dose heparin warrants aggressive monitoring and appropriate dose adjustment (141).

Obviously, low-molecular-weight heparins (LMWHs) also appear most appropriate for obstetric thromboprophylaxis (147, 148). These agents are safe to both the embryo and the fetus as they do not cross the placenta. The latter feature implies negligible risk for teratogenicity, a supposition supported by a number of studies (140, 149). For these obvious reasons many physicians now use these agents during pregnancy in patients with mechanical valves (150). Although cases of valve thrombosis using LMWH have been reported (144, 151–153), and a trial comparing enoxaparin with warfarin and unfractionated heparin was stopped due to two deaths from valve thrombosis in the enoxaparin group (154, 155), further data on the effectiveness of LMWHs in pregnant women with mechanical heart prostheses were lacking (141). No definite recommendations on the use of LMWHs can be made until the availability of more data (29, 156). But since all anticoagulant strategies used in the situation of a pregnant women with one or more prosthetic heart valves are associated with increased risks, coumarin is contraindicated, and unfractionated heparins have significant maternal side effects. The LMWHs (with a good safety profile for mother and child) should not be discarded until there are better comparative data (150). The most recent, 2004 American College of Chest Physicians (ACCP) conference guidelines therefore recommend one of the following strategies in pregnant patients with prosthetic heart valves: LMWH b.i.d. throughout pregnancy in doses adjusted either to keep a 4-hour postinjection anti-Xa heparin level at approximately 1.0 to 1.2 U/mL (preferable) or according to weight, or aggressive unfractionated heparin throughout pregnancy, administered subcutaneously q12 hours in doses adjusted to keep the mid-interval activated partial thromboplastin time (aPTT) at least twice that of control or to attain an anti-Xa heparin level of 0.35 to 0.70 U/mL, or LMWH or UFH (as above) until the 13th week, change to warfarin until the middle of the third trimester, and then restart UFH or LMWH (despite medicolegal concerns since the package insert of warfarin states that it is contraindicated in pregnancy). If warfarin is used, the target international normalized ratio (INR) is 3.0 (range 2.5–3.5), and a lower therapeutic range of 2.0 to 3.0 can be used in patients with bileaflet aortic valves (provided that they do not have atrial fibrillation or left ventricular dysfunction). All the above recommendations are grade 1C, meaning that experts are very certain that benefits do outweigh risks, burdens, and costs, and that the evidence comes from observational studies) (150). In high-risk women with prosthetic heart valves, the addition of low-dose aspirin (75 to 162 mg/day) is suggested. The latter is a grade 2C recommendation, meaning that experts are less certain of the magnitude of the benefits and risks, burdens, and costs, and their relative impact, and that the evidence comes from observational studies) (150).

Cardiac Surgery During Pregnancy

Cardiopulmonary bypass (CPB) during pregnancy was first performed in 1958 (157). It creates a high-risk condition as it activates the coagulation and complement systems, and increases the chance for the formation of particulate or air emboli. In addition, it promotes the release of vasoactive substances, and carries the risks associated with nonpulsatile flow, hypotension, and hypothermia (158, 159). Since uterine flow is not autoregulated, high flow rates and maintenance of blood pressure are necessary for optimal placental perfusion. The reported effects of hypothermia are conflicting with inconsistent data on the occurrence of fetal loss. Mild hypothermia (32°C) is considered safe (11). The phase of rewarming is associated with uterine contractions (158). Maternal mortality rate ranges from 1.5% to 8.6% with an average of 2.5%, and fetal mortality ranges from 16% to 33% (32, 158, 160). The maternal risk is now similar to that for nonpregnant female patients (161), although a high maternal mortality could result from the emergency nature of the surgical intervention (162) or the severity of the presurgical maternal condition at surgery (160). Cardiac surgery is relatively contraindicated in the first two trimesters (except in life-threatening emergencies), as the incidence of teratogenesis is high. Irrespective of the time of surgery in pregnancy, fetal mortality will be high. During the

Table 25.6. Guidelines for the use of cardiopulmonary bypass (CPB) during pregnancy

Open-heart surgery should be avoided, if at all possible, during the first trimester since the incidence of teratogenesis is high.
High-flow, high-pressure, normothermic bypass offers the least risk for the fetus.
Hyperoxygenation and hematocrit higher than 25% should be maintained.
Fetal heart and uterine monitoring should be used to allow adjustments to the flow and pharmacologic manipulations to ensure adequate placental perfusion.
When the fetus is more than 28 weeks' gestation, it is a safe option to deliver the child by cesarean section immediately before, and at the same operation as, the cardiac operation.

Source: Modified from Parry and Westaby (161), with permission.

third trimester, and also as a result of improved neonatal outcome with modern neonatal care, delivery by cesarean section prior to CPB has been reported a safe procedure (161). If intervention during pregnancy is indicated, high-flow, high-pressure, normothermic bypass is to be used for as brief a period as possible. Experimental evidence in animal studies suggests that uteroplacental circulation is better preserved with pulsatile perfusion (163). Its benefit in humans remains to be confirmed. Fetal monitoring during surgery is essential to minimize fetal loss (161). Table 25.6 summarizes the guidelines for CPB in pregnancy.

Eclampsia and Hypertensive Crisis During Pregnancy

Eclampsia is the most severe hypertensive disorder of pregnancy, complicating 0.04% to 0.1% and up to 15% of all pregnancies in the developed and developing countries, respectively. It is associated with a high rate of maternal and perinatal mortality and morbidity (164). Although preeclampsia often precedes eclampsia, in about 20% of the cases it develops suddenly with blood pressures prior to the eclamptic fit being below 140/90 mm Hg (165). Although eclampsia is difficult to predict, rapidly progressing maternal complaints as well as acutely developing severe hypertension are generally considered predisposing conditions (166). Between 3% and 10% of women with eclampsia develop severe cardiovascular complications, such as aortic dissection, intracranial bleeding, disseminated intravascular coagulation, and renal failure (167). The incidence of severe cardiovascular complications in (pre)eclampsia is particularly high in conditions where systolic blood pressure increases rapidly to values over 200 mm Hg (166, 167). In this context the management of unstable preeclampsia is important. In unstable preeclampsia, clinical symptoms and abnormal laboratory findings evolve rapidly and are accompanied by progressive hypertension.

In the management of this condition, prophylactic administration of magnesium sulfate to prevent eclamptic fits should always accompanied by the timely and adequate control of the hypertension (166). A rapid rise in diastolic pressure to values over 130 mm Hg, presumably triggered by excess placental release of reactive oxygen species and placental villous debris (168, 169), may lead to a hypertensive crisis, which is defined as a condition of acutely developing severe hypertension requiring immediate (within 1 hour) blood pressure lowering to prevent permanent organ damage (170). Organ damage in these cases results from the uncontrolled rise in capillary perfusion pressure causing an unbalance in the microcirculatory Starling pressures and with it, uncontrolled edema formation. This condition not only undermines tissue exchange. The higher pressure in the capillaries also implies a higher likelihood of microvessel damage giving rise to microbleedings. The associated structural abnormalities seen in the brain of eclamptics indicates that eclampsia resembles the encephalopathy of hypertensive crises unrelated to eclampsia (166). In general, antihypertensive treatment is initiated at systolic blood pressure >170 mm Hg or diastolic blood pressure >110 mm Hg. In cases of preexistent vascular disease or rapid clinical progression, treatment should be considered at systolic blood pressure >140 mm Hg or diastolic blood pressure >90 mm Hg. The risk that the intravenous administration of antihypertensives will induce an abrupt fall in blood pressure is particularly increased in unstable (pre)eclampsia, as the intravascular compartment tends to be constricted in response to sympathetic overactivity. Therefore, gradual increments in the dosage of antihypertensives should be accompanied by the infusion of modest amounts of plasma expanders, to avoid drug-related compromise of the uteroplacental blood flow and oxygenation. Details about managing hypertensive emergencies in obstetrics are reported elsewhere (164, 166, 168, 170).

Endocarditis Prophylaxis During Pregnancy

Bacteremia is found in 1% to 5% of deliveries (171, 172), with possibly an increased risk when the placenta has to be removed manually. The AHA guidelines state that delivery by cesarean section and vaginal delivery (in the absence of infection) do not require endocarditis prophylaxis except in high-risk patients (11, 173). When infection is suspected or documented, prophylaxis for suspected bacteremia is recommended for the high- and moderate-risk groups, but not for the negligible-risk group (11, 171) (Table 25.7). However, in clinical practice endocarditis prophylaxis, when indicated, is often routinely started at the onset of active labor, as complications in the course of labor (with risk of bacteremia) are difficult to predict (7). This liberal policy could theoretically promote bacterial resistance.

Anesthesiologic Management of Patients with Cardiac Disease in Pregnancy

Vaginal delivery is recommended with few exceptions (7), since cesarean section increases the risk of hemorrhage, postpartum infection, pulmonary comorbidity, and puerperal fluid shifts (174–177). When vaginal delivery is pursued, it is less stressful for heart and circulatory function to adopt the left-lateral tilt position. Use of forceps or vacuum extraction may be considered to shorten the second stage of labor (11). The sympathetic stimulation triggered by labor stress and pain increases myocardial work, which can be adequately

TABLE 25.7. America College of Cardiology/American Heart Association recommendations for antibiotic prophylaxis in labor and delivery

Cardiac lesion	Prophylaxis for uncomplicated delivery	Prophylaxis for suspected bacteremia[a]
High-risk category		
Prosthetic cardiac valves (both homograft and bioprosthetic)	Optional	Recommended
Prior bacterial endocarditis	Optional	Recommended
Complex cyanotic congential cardiac malformations	Optional	Recommended
Surgically constructed systemic pulmonary shunts or conduits	Optional	Recommended
Moderate-risk category		
Congenital cardiac malformations (except repaired atrial septal defect, ventricular septal defect, or patent ductus arteriosus, or isolated secundum atrial septal defect)	Not recommended	Recommended
Acquired valvular dysfunction (most commonly rheumatic heart disease)	Not recommended	Recommended
Hypertrophic cardiomyopathy	Not recommended	Recommended
Mitral valve prolapse with valvar regurgitation or thickened leaflets or both	Not recommended	Recommended
Negligible-risk category[b]		
Mitral valve prolapse without valvar regurgitation	Not recommended	Not recommended
Physiologic, functional, or innocent heart murmurs	Not recommended	Not recommended
Previous Kawasaki disease without valvar dysfunction	Not recommended	Not recommended
Previous rheumatic fever without valvar dysfunction	Not recommended	Not recommended
Cardiac pacemakers and implanted defibrillators	Not recommended	Not recommended
Prior coronary bypass graft surgery	Not recommended	Not recommended

[a]For example, intraamniotic infection.
[b]Risk for developing endocarditis is no higher than in the general population.
Source: Adapted from the American College of Obstetrics and Gynecology (171), with permission.

controlled by applying analgesic measures. The resulting lower myocardiac oxygen consumption and work can be expected to prevent an adverse outcome (11). Obstetric indications for cesarean section are the same as those in the general population, and cardiac indications include aortic dilatation or dissection, Marfan syndrome with aortic root involvement, endocarditis necessitating emergency valve replacement near or at term, severe aortic stenosis, a history of recent MI, acute severe CHF during delivery, and failure to switch from warfarin to heparin at least 2 weeks before labor (5, 7). Higher rates of cesarean section (~35%) in patients with heart disease than predicted on the basis of the indications delineated above may reflect excessive concern of the responsible care providers (5, 178). In selected cases, emergency cardiovascular surgery can follow cesarean section (5). There is no consensus on the use of invasive monitoring during labor (7). During emergency cardiovascular surgery, the cardiac condition can be monitored by echocardiography or a pulmonary artery catheter. Echocardiography is readily available and easy to repeat, but has the disadvantage of overdiagnosing pulmonary hypertension in 32% of pregnant patients (179). The postdelivery use of oxytocin may induce hypotension and therefore it should be administered slowly. Obviously, indications for its use should outweigh the risk of postpartum hemorrhage, which is reported to be raised in PH (4) and Marfan syndrome (180). Detailed information on general and anesthesiologic management per disease category is provided in a recent review on this subject (181).

Conclusion

The maternal circulatory adaptation to pregnancy consists almost entirely of adaptive changes in the maternal cardiovascular system in response to a primary systemic vasodilatation. Conversely, hemodynamic maladaptation consists of a combination of the absence of these changes with signs of sympathetic dominance in the autonomic control of the cardiovascular system.

Over the last three decades the prevalence of the different causes of heart disease has shifted toward congenital heart disease. Because diseases like rheumatic fever are still common in developing countries, immigration will lead to the importation of these diseases in developed countries. Therefore, the most common preexistent cardiac disorder in pregnancy is congenital heart disease followed by rheumatic heart disease.

With the exception of patients with Eisenmenger syndrome (ES), pulmonary vascular obstructive disease, and Marfan syndrome with aortopathy, the mortality rate due to pregnancy is extremely low in women with a preexistent heart disease. Although maternal mortality is low, pregnant women are at risk for serious morbidity such as heart failure, arrhythmias, and stroke. Ischemic heart disease is rare, but expected to increase with an increasing proportion of mothers being aged over 30 years.

Subsequent pregnancy in women with a history of peripartum cardiomyopathy is associated with a significant decrease in left ventricular function regardless of whether or not left ventricular function had returned to normal in the prior pregnancy. Therefore, pregnancy should be discouraged in women with a history of peripartum cardiomyopathy.

The best regimen for thromboembolic prophylaxis in pregnant women with prosthetic heart valves is subject of ongoing debate.

Cardiac surgery during pregnancy carries considerable risk, especially for the fetus. The procedure is ill-advised until the 28th week of pregnancy due to the high risk of damage to embryo or fetus, whereas delivery of the infant by cesarean section afterward and just prior to CPB has been reported to be a safe procedure, with improvements in outcome for premature infants with modern neonatal intensive care.

In unstable or rapidly progressive preeclampsia, proper management consists of the swift prophylactic administration of magnesium sulfate in concert with intravenous "titration" of antihypertensives. The latter warrants a gradual decline in blood pressure to levels of 140 to 160 mm Hg systolic and 90 to 110 mm Hg diastolic. The purpose of this approach is to circumvent compromise of the uteroplacental perfusion and with it, acute fetal asphyxia.

Antibiotic prophylaxis during pregnancy in patients with cardiac disease is used more frequently than advised by the AHA guidelines, since it is difficult to predict which deliveries become complicated.

Anesthesiologic management of patients depends on the underlying cardiac disorder. Natural birth is recommended in most cases, except for aortic dilatation or dissection, Marfan syndrome with aortic root involvement, endocarditis necessitating emergency valve replacement near or at term, severe aortic stenosis, history of recent MI, acute CHF during delivery, and failure to switch from warfarin to heparin at least 2 weeks before labor.

There is no consensus regarding the optimal mode of monitoring during labor and delivery.

References

1. Siu SC, Sermer M, Colman JM, et al. Prospective multicenter study of pregnancy outcomes in women with heart disease. Circulation 2001;104(5):515–21.
2. McFaul PB, Dornan JC, Lamki H, Boyle D. Pregnancy complicated by maternal heart disease. A review of 519 women. Br J Obstet Gynaecol 1988;95(9):861–7.
3. Jindal UN, Dhall GI, Vasishta K, Dhall K, Wahi PL. Effect of maternal cardiac disease on perinatal outcome. Aust N Z J Obstet Gynaecol 1988;28(2):113–5.
4. Weiss BM, Hess OM. Pulmonary vascular disease and pregnancy: current controversies, management strategies, and perspectives. Eur Heart J 2000;21(2):104–15.
5. Gei AF, Hankins GD. Cardiac disease and pregnancy. Obstet Gynecol Clin North Am 2001;28(3):465–512.
6. Bhatla N, Lal S, Behera G, et al. Cardiac disease in pregnancy. Int J Gynaecol Obstet 2003;82(2):153–9.
7. Siu SC, Colman JM. Heart disease and pregnancy. Heart 2001;85(6):710–5.
8. Katz M, Pinko A, Lurio S, Pak I. Outcome of pregnancy in 110 patients with organic heart disease. J Reprod Med 1986;31(5):343–7.
9. Somerville J. Grown-up congenital heart disease—medical demands look back, look forward 2000. Thorac Cardiovasc Surg 2001;49(1):21–6.
10. Somerville J. The Denolin Lecture: The woman with congenital heart disease. Eur Heart J 1998;19(12):1766–75.
11. Klein LL, Galan HL. Cardiac disease in pregnancy. Obstet Gynecol Clin North Am 2004;31(2):429–59, viii.
12. Avila WS, Rossi EG, Ramires JA, et al. Pregnancy in patients with heart disease: experience with 1,000 cases. Clin Cardiol 2003;26(3):135–42.
13. Chang J, Elam-Evans LD, Berg CJ, et al. Pregnancy-related mortality surveillance—United States, 1991–1999. MMWR Surveill Summ 2003;52(2):1–8.
14. Oakley CM. Cardiovascular disease in pregnancy. Can J Cardiol 1990;6(suppl B[2]):3B–9B.
15. Whittemore R, Hobbins JC, Engle MA. Pregnancy and its outcome in women with and without surgical treatment of congenital heart disease. Am J Cardiol 1982;50(3):641–51.
16. Shime J, Mocarski EJ, Hastings D, Webb GD, McLaughlin PR. Congenital heart disease in pregnancy: short- and long-term implications. Am J Obstet Gynecol 1987;156(2):313–22.
17. Siu SC, Sermer M, Harrison DA, et al. Risk and predictors for pregnancy-related complications in women with heart disease. Circulation 1997;96(9):2789–94.
18. Ayoub C, Jalbout M, Baraka A. The pregnant cardiac women. Curr Opin Anaesthesiol 2002;15:285–91.
19. Siu SC, Colman JM, Sorensen S, et al. Adverse neonatal and cardiac outcomes are more common in pregnant women with cardiac disease. Circulation 2002;105(18):2179–84.
20. de Beus E, van Mook WN, Ramsay G, Stappers JL, van der Putten HW. Peripartum cardiomyopathy: a condition intensivists should be aware of. Intensive Care Med 2003;29(2):167–74.
21. van Mook WNKA, Peeters L. Severe cardiac disease in pregnancy, part I: hemodynamic changes and complaints during pregnancy, and general management of cardiac disease in pregnancy. Curr Opin Crit Care 2005;11:430–34.
22. Sciscione AC, Ivester T, Largoza M, Manley J, Shlossman P, Colmorgen GH. Acute pulmonary edema in pregnancy. Obstet Gynecol 2003;101(3):511–5.
23. Oakley CM. Pregnancy and heart disease. Br J Hosp Med 1996;55(7):423–6.
24. Pitkin RM, Perloff JK, Koos BJ, Beall MH. Pregnancy and congenital heart disease. Ann Intern Med 1990;112(6):445–54.
25. Iserin L. Management of pregnancy in women with congenital heart disease. Heart 2001;85(5):493–4.
26. Zuber M, Gautschi N, Oechslin E, Widmer V, Kiowski W, Jenni R. Outcome of pregnancy in women with congenital shunt lesions. Heart 1999;81(3):271–5.

27. Poppas A. Congenital and acquired heart disease. In: Lee RV, Rosene-Montella K, Barbour LA, Garner PR, Keely E, eds. Medical Care of the Pregnant Patient. Philadelphia, PA. Am Coll Physicians. 2000:359–60.
28. Reimold SC, Rutherford JD. Clinical practice. Valvular heart disease in pregnancy. N Engl J Med 2003;349(1):52–9.
29. Bonow RO, Carabello B, de Leon AC Jr, et al. Guidelines for the management of patients with valvular heart disease: executive summary. A report of the American College of Cardiology/ American Heart Association Task Force on Practice Guidelines (Committee on Management of Patients with Valvular Heart Disease). Circulation 1998;98(18):1949–84.
30. Lao TT, Sermer M, MaGee L, Farine D, Colman JM. Congenital aortic stenosis and pregnancy—a reappraisal. Am J Obstet Gynecol 1993;169(3): 540–5.
31. Silversides CK, Colman JM, Sermer M, Farine D, Siu SC. Early and intermediate-term outcomes of pregnancy with congenital aortic stenosis. Am J Cardiol 2003;91(11):1386–9.
32. Chambers CE, Clark SL. Cardiac surgery during pregnancy. Clin Obstet Gynecol 1994;37(2):316–23.
33. Lao TT, Adelman AG, Sermer M, Colman JM. Balloon valvuloplasty for congenital aortic stenosis in pregnancy. Br J Obstet Gynaecol 1993; 100(12):1141–2.
34. Presbitero P, Prever SB, Brusca A. Interventional cardiology in pregnancy. Eur Heart J 1996;17(2): 182–8.
35. Presbitero P, Somerville J, Stone S, Aruta E, Spiegelhalter D, Rabajoli F. Pregnancy in cyanotic congenital heart disease. Outcome of mother and fetus. Circulation 1994;89(6):2673–6.
36. Deal K, Wooley CF. Coarctation of the aorta and pregnancy. Ann Intern Med 1973;78(5):706–10.
37. Beauchesne LM, Connolly HM, Ammash NM, Warnes CA. Coarctation of the aorta: outcome of pregnancy. J Am Coll Cardiol 2001;38(6):1728–33.
38. Rossiter JP, Repke JT, Morales AJ, Murphy EA, Pyeritz RE. A prospective longitudinal evaluation of pregnancy in the Marfan syndrome. Am J Obstet Gynecol 1995;173(5):1599–606.
39. Pyeritz RE. Maternal and fetal complications of pregnancy in the Marfan syndrome. Am J Med 1981;71(5):784–90.
40. Lipscomb KJ, Smith JC, Clarke B, Donnai P, Harris R. Outcome of pregnancy in women with Marfan's syndrome. Br J Obstet Gynaecol 1997;104(2): 201–6.
41. Connolly HM, Grogan M, Warnes CA. Pregnancy among women with congenitally corrected transposition of great arteries. J Am Coll Cardiol 1999; 33(6):1692–5.
42. Therrien J, Barnes I, Somerville J. Outcome of pregnancy in patients with congenitally corrected transposition of the great arteries. Am J Cardiol 1999;84(7):820–4.
43. Gleicher N, Midwall J, Hochberger D, Jaffin H. Eisenmenger's syndrome and pregnancy. Obstet Gynecol Surv 1979;34(10):721–41.
44. Lieber S, Dewilde P, Huyghens L, Traey E, Gepts E. Eisenmenger's syndrome and pregnancy. Acta Cardiol 1985;40(4):421–4.
45. Monnery L, Nanson J, Charlton G. Primary pulmonary hypertension in pregnancy: a role for novel vasodilators. Br J Anaesth 2001;87(2): 295–8.
46. Decoene C, Bourzoufi K, Moreau D, Narducci F, Crepin F, Krivosic-Horber R. Use of inhaled nitric oxide for emergency cesarean section in a woman with unexpected primary pulmonary hypertension. Can J Anaesth 2001;48(6):584–7.
47. Stewart R, Tuazon D, Olson G, Duarte AG. Pregnancy and primary pulmonary hypertension: successful outcome with epoprostenol therapy. Chest 2001;119(3):973–5.
48. Lust KM, Boots RJ, Dooris M, Wilson J. Management of labor in Eisenmenger syndrome with inhaled nitric oxide. Am J Obstet Gynecol 1999; 181(2):419–23.
49. Weiss BM, Zemp L, Seifert B, Hess OM. Outcome of pulmonary vascular disease in pregnancy: a systematic overview from 1978 through 1996. J Am Coll Cardiol 1998;31(7):1650–7.
50. Hameed A, Karaalp IS, Tummala PP, et al. The effect of valvular heart disease on maternal and fetal outcome of pregnancy. J Am Coll Cardiol 2001;37(3):893–9.
51. Desai DK, Adanlawo M, Naidoo DP, Moodley J, Kleinschmidt I. Mitral stenosis in pregnancy: a four-year experience at King Edward VIII Hospital, Durban, South Africa. Br J Obstet Gynaecol 2000;107(8):953–8.
52. Silversides CK, Colman JM, Sermer M, Siu SC. Cardiac risk in pregnant women with rheumatic mitral stenosis. Am J Cardiol 2003;91(11):1382–5.
53. Sawhney H, Aggarwal N, Suri V, Vasishta K, Sharma Y, Grover A. Maternal and perinatal outcome in rheumatic heart disease. Int J Gynaecol Obstet 2003;80(1):9–14.
54. Onderoglu L, Tuncer ZS, Oto A, Durukan T. Balloon valvuloplasty during pregnancy. Int J Gynaecol Obstet 1995;49(2):181–3.

55. Gupta A, Lokhandwala YY, Satoskar PR, Salvi VS. Balloon mitral valvotomy in pregnancy: maternal and fetal outcomes. J Am Coll Surg 1998;187(4): 409–15.
56. Kinsara AJ, Ismail O, Fawzi ME. Effect of balloon mitral valvoplasty during pregnancy on childhood development. Cardiology 2002;97(3):155–8.
57. de Souza JA, Martinez EE Jr, Ambrose JA, et al. Percutaneous balloon mitral valvuloplasty in comparison with open mitral valve commissurotomy for mitral stenosis during pregnancy. J Am Coll Cardiol 2001;37(3):900–3.
58. Savage DD, Garrison RJ, Devereux RB, et al. Mitral valve prolapse in the general population. 1. Epidemiologic features: the Framingham Study. Am Heart J 1983;106(3):571–6.
59. Chia YT, Yeoh SC, Lim MC, Viegas OA, Ratnam SS. Pregnancy outcome and mitral valve prolapse. Asia Oceania J Obstet Gynaecol 1994;20(4):383–8.
60. Salonen Ros H, Lichtenstein P, Bellocco R, Petersson G, Cnattingius S. Increased risks of circulatory diseases in late pregnancy and puerperium. Epidemiology 2001;12(4):456–60.
61. Ladner HE, Danielsen B, Gilbert WM. Acute myocardial infarction in pregnancy and the puerperium: a population-based study. Obstet Gynecol 2005;105(3):480–4.
62. Ramsey PS, Ramin KD, Ramin SM. Cardiac disease in pregnancy. Am J Perinatol 2001;18(5):245–66.
63. Hankins GD, Wendel GD, Jr, Leveno KJ, Stoneham J. Myocardial infarction during pregnancy: a review. Obstet Gynecol 1985;65(1):139–46.
64. Darias R, Herranz L, Garcia-Ingelmo MT, Pallardo LF. Pregnancy in a patient with type 1 diabetes mellitus and prior ischaemic heart disease. Eur J Endocrinol 2001;144(3):309–10.
65. Hameed AB, Tummala PP, Goodwin TM, et al. Unstable angina during pregnancy in two patients with premature coronary atherosclerosis and aortic stenosis in association with familial hypercholesterolemia. Am J Obstet Gynecol 2000;182(5): 1152–5.
66. Frenkel Y, Etchin A, Barkai G, Reisin L, Mashiach S, Battler A. Myocardial infarction during pregnancy: a case report. Cardiology 1991;78(4):363–8.
67. Sullebarger JT, Fontanet HL, Matar FA, Singh SS. Percutaneous coronary intervention for myocardial infarction during pregnancy: a new trend? J Invasive Cardiol 2003;15(12):725–8.
68. Heck KE, Schoendorf KC, Ventura SJ, Kiely JL. Delayed childbearing by education level in the United States, 1969–1994. Matern Child Health J 1997;1(2):81–8.
69. Kulka PJ, Scheu C, Tryba M, Grunewald R, Wiebalck A, Oberheiden R. [Myocardial infarction during pregnancy]. Anaesthesist 2001;50(4): 280–4.
70. Schulte-Sasse U. Life threatening myocardial ischaemia associated with the use of prostaglandin E1 to induce abortion. Br J Obstet Gynaecol 2000;107(5):700–2.
71. Meyer WJ, Benton SL, Hoon TJ, Gauthier DW, Whiteman VE. Acute myocardial infarction associated with prostaglandin E2. Am J Obstet Gynecol 1991;165(2):359–60.
72. Tsui BC, Stewart B, Fitzmaurice A, Williams R. Cardiac arrest and myocardial infarction induced by postpartum intravenous ergonovine administration. Anesthesiology 2001;94(2):363–4.
73. Oei SG, Oei SK, Brolmann HA. Myocardial infarction during nifedipine therapy for preterm labor. N Engl J Med 1999;340(2):154.
74. Roth A, Elkayam U. Acute myocardial infarction associated with pregnancy. Ann Intern Med 1996; 125(9):751–62.
75. Klutstein MW, Tzivoni D, Bitran D, Mendzelevski B, Ilan M, Almagor Y. Treatment of spontaneous coronary artery dissection: report of three cases. Cathet Cardiovasc Diagn 1997;40(4):372–6.
76. Badui E, Enciso R. Acute myocardial infarction during pregnancy and puerperium: a review. Angiology 1996;47(8):739–56.
77. Koul AK, Hollander G, Moskovits N, Frankel R, Herrera L, Shani J. Coronary artery dissection during pregnancy and the postpartum period: two case reports and review of literature. Catheter Cardiovasc Intervent 2001;52(1):88–94.
78. Nishikawa H, Nakanishi S, Nishiyama S, et al. Primary coronary artery dissection: its incidence, mode of the onset and prognostic evaluation. J Cardiol 1988;18(2):307–17.
79. Chaithiraphan V, Gowda RM, Khan IA, Reimers CD. Peripartum acute myocardial infarction: management perspective. Am J Ther 2003;10(1): 75–7.
80. Webber MD, Halligan RE, Schumacher JA. Acute infarction, intracoronary thrombolysis, and primary PTCA in pregnancy. Cathet Cardiovasc Diagn 1997;42(1):38–43.
81. Schumacher B, Belfort MA, Card RJ. Successful treatment of acute myocardial infarction during pregnancy with tissue plasminogen activator. Am J Obstet Gynecol 1997;176(3):716–9.
82. Kulka PJ, Scheu C, Tryba M, Oberheiden R, Zenz M. Coronary artery plaque disruption as cause of

acute myocardial infarction during cesarean section with spinal anesthesia. J Clin Anesth 2000; 12(4):335–8.
83. Gordon MC, Landon MB, Boyle J, Stewart KS, Gabbe SG. Coronary artery disease in insulin-dependent diabetes mellitus of pregnancy (class H): a review of the literature. Obstet Gynecol Surv 1996;51(7):437–44.
84. Frenkel Y, Barkai G, Reisin L, Rath S, Mashiach S, Battler A. Pregnancy after myocardial infarction: are we playing safe? Obstet Gynecol 1991;77(6): 822–5.
85. Dawson PJ, Ross AW. Pre-eclampsia in a parturient with a history of myocardial infarction. A case report and literature review. Anaesthesia 1988; 43(8):659–63.
86. Upshaw CB Jr. A study of maternal electrocardiograms recorded during labor and delivery. Am J Obstet Gynecol 1970;107(1):17–27.
87. Tawam M, Levine J, Mendelson M, Goldberger J, Dyer A, Kadish A. Effect of pregnancy on paroxysmal supraventricular tachycardia. Am J Cardiol 1993;72(11):838–40.
88. Gowda RM, Khan IA, Mehta NJ, Vasavada BC, Sacchi TJ. Cardiac arrhythmias in pregnancy: clinical and therapeutic considerations. Int J Cardiol 2003;88(2–3):129–33.
89. Joglar JA, Page RL. Antiarrhythmic drugs in pregnancy. Curr Opin Cardiol 2001;16(1):40–5.
90. Natale A, Davidson T, Geiger MJ, Newby K. Implantable cardioverter-defibrillators and pregnancy: a safe combination? Circulation 1997;96(9): 2808–12.
91. Whitehead SJ, Berg CJ, Chang J. Pregnancy-related mortality due to cardiomyopathy: United States, 1991–1997. Obstet Gynecol 2003;102(6):1326–31.
92. Heider AL, Kuller JA, Strauss RA, Wells SR. Peripartum cardiomyopathy: a review of the literature. Obstet Gynecol Surv 1999;54(8):526–31.
93. Cunningham FG, Pritchard JA, Hankins GD, Anderson PL, Lucas MJ, Armstrong KF. Peripartum heart failure: idiopathic cardiomyopathy or compounding cardiovascular events? Obstet Gynecol 1986;67(2):157–68.
94. Lampert MB, Lang RM. Peripartum cardiomyopathy. Am Heart J 1995;130(4):860–70.
95. Demakis JG, Rahimtoola SH. Peripartum cardiomyopathy. Circulation 1971;44(5):964–8.
96. Brown CS, Bertolet BD. Peripartum cardiomyopathy: a comprehensive review. Am J Obstet Gynecol 1998;178(2):409–14.
97. Davidson NM, Parry EH. Peri-partum cardiac failure. Q J Med 1978;47(188):431–61.
98. Hsieh CC, Chiang CW, Hsieh TT, Soong YK. Peripartum cardiomyopathy. Jpn Heart J 1992;33(3): 343–9.
99. Seftel H, Susser M. Maternity and myocardial failure in African women. Br Heart J 1961;23: 43–52.
100. Woolford R. Postpartum myocarditis. Ohio State Med 1952;48:924–30.
101. Pierce J, Brice B, Joyce J. Familial occurrence of postpartal heart failure. Arch Int Med 1963;111:651–6.
102. Pearson GD, Veille JC, Rahimtoola S, et al. Peripartum cardiomyopathy: National Heart, Lung, and Blood Institute and Office of Rare Diseases (National Institutes of Health) workshop recommendations and review. JAMA 2000;283(9): 1183–8.
103. Hibbard JU, Lindheimer M, Lang RM. A modified definition for peripartum cardiomyopathy and prognosis based on echocardiography. Obstet Gynecol 1999;94(2):311–6.
104. Lee W. Clinical management of gravid women with peripartum cardiomyopathy. Obstet Gynecol Clin North Am 1991;18(2):257–71.
105. Melvin KR, Richardson PJ, Olsen EG, Daly K, Jackson G. Peripartum cardiomyopathy due to myocarditis. N Engl J Med 1982;307(12):731–4.
106. Sanderson JE, Olsen EG, Gatei D. Peripartum heart disease: an endomyocardial biopsy study. Br Heart J 1986;56(3):285–91.
107. O'Connell JB, Costanzo-Nordin MR, Subramanian R, et al. Peripartum cardiomyopathy: clinical, hemodynamic, histologic and prognostic characteristics. J Am Coll Cardiol 1986;8(1):52–6.
108. Rizeq MN, Rickenbacher PR, Fowler MB, Billingham ME. Incidence of myocarditis in peripartum cardiomyopathy. Am J Cardiol 1994;74(5): 474–7.
109. Midei MG, DeMent SH, Feldman AM, Hutchins GM, Baughman KL. Peripartum myocarditis and cardiomyopathy. Circulation 1990;81(3):922–8.
110. Felker GM, Jaeger CJ, Klodas E, et al. Myocarditis and long-term survival in peripartum cardiomyopathy. Am Heart J 2000;140(5):785–91.
111. Cenac A, Gaultier Y, Devillechabrolle A, Moulias R. Enterovirus infection in peripartum cardiomyopathy. Lancet 1988;2(8617):968–9.
112. Sainani GS, Dekate MP, Rao CP. Heart disease caused by Coxsackie virus B infection. Br Heart J 1975;37(8):819–23.
113. Ansari A, Neckelmann N, Wang Y, Gravanis M, Sell K, Herskowitz A. Immunologic dialogue between cardiac myocytes, endothelial cells, and mononuclear cells. Clin Immunol Immunopathol 1993;68:208–14.

114. Sliwa K, Skudicky D, Bergemann A, Candy G, Puren A, Sareli P. Peripartum cardiomyopathy: analysis of clinical outcome, left ventricular function, plasma levels of cytokines and Fas/APO-1. J Am Coll Cardiol 2000;35(3):701–5.
115. Coulson CC, Thorp JM, Mayer DC, Cefalo RC. Central hemodynamic effects of recombinant human relaxin in the isolated, perfused rat heart model. Obstet Gynecol 1996;87(4):610–2.
116. Cenac A, Simonoff M, Moretto P, Djibo A. A low plasma selenium is a risk factor for peripartum cardiomyopathy. A comparative study in Sahelian Africa. Int J Cardiol 1992;36(1):57–9.
117. Aroney C, Khafagi F, Boyle C, Bett N. Peripartum cardiomyopathy: echocardiographic features in five cases. Am J Obstet Gynecol 1986;155(1):103–6.
118. Janssens U, Klues HG, Hanrath P. Successful thrombolysis of right atrial and ventricle thrombi in a patient with peripartum cardiomyopathy and extensive thromboembolism. Heart 1997;78(5):515–6.
119. Bassaw B, Ariyanayagam DC, Roopnarinesingh S. Peripartum cardiomyopathy and arterial embolism. West Indian Med J 1992;41(2):79–80.
120. Hodgman M, Pessin M, Homans D, et al. Cerebral embolism as the initial manifestation of peripartum cardiomyopathy. Neurology 1982;32:668–71.
121. Chan F, Ngan Kee WD. Idiopathic dilated cardiomyopathy presenting in pregnancy. Can J Anaesth 1999;46(12):1146–9.
122. Ford RF, Barton JR, O'Brien JM, Hollingsworth PW. Demographics, management, and outcome of peripartum cardiomyopathy in a community hospital. Am J Obstet Gynecol 2000;182(5):1036–8.
123. Walsh J, Burch G, Black W, Ferrans V, Hibbs R. Idiopathic myocardiopathy of the puerperium (postpartal heart disease). Circulation 1965;32:19–31.
124. Walsh J, Burch G. Postpartal heart disease. Arch Intern Med 1961;108:817–23.
125. Bozkurt B, Villaneuva FS, Holubkov R, et al. Intravenous immune globulin in the therapy of peripartum cardiomyopathy. J Am Coll Cardiol 1999;34(1):177–80.
126. Deng M, Tjan T, Asfour B, Scheld H. Left ventricular assist devices—reasons to be enthusiastic. Eur J Heart Fail 1999;1(3):289–91.
127. Lewis R, Mabie W, Burlew B, Sibai B. Biventricular assist device as a bridge to cardiac transplantation in the treatment of peripartum cardiomyopathy. South Med J 1997;90(9):955–8.
128. Tandler R, Schmid C, Weyand M, Scheld H. Novacor LVAD bridge to transplantation in peripartum cardiomyopathy. Eur J Cardiothorac 1997;11(2):394–6.
129. Aziz TM, Burgess MI, Acladious NN, et al. Heart transplantation for peripartum cardiomyopathy: a report of three cases and a literature review. Cardiovasc Surg 1999;7(5):565–7.
130. Aravot DJ, Banner NR, Dhalla N, et al. Heart transplantation for peripartum cardiomyopathy. Lancet 1987;2(8566):1024.
131. Keogh A, Macdonald P, Spratt P, Marshman D, Larbalestier R, Kaan A. Outcome in peripartum cardiomyopathy after heart transplantation. J Heart Lung Transplant 1994;13(2):202–7.
132. Kreitmann B, D'Ercole C, Yao JG, Ambrosi P, Metras D. Successful pregnancy 5 years after cardiac transplantation for peripartum cardiomyopathy. Transplant Proc 1997;29(5):2457.
133. Carvalho AC, Almeida D, Cohen M, et al. Successful pregnancy, delivery and puerperium in a heart transplant patient with previous peripartum cardiomyopathy. Eur Heart J 1992;13(11):1589–91.
134. Lee W, Cotton DB. Peripartum cardiomyopathy: current concepts and clinical management. Clin Obstet Gynecol 1989;32(1):54–67.
135. Meadows W. Idiopathic myocardial failure in the last trimester of pregnancy and the puerperium. Circulation 1957;15:903–14.
136. Elkayam U, Tummala PP, Rao K, et al. Maternal and fetal outcomes of subsequent pregnancies in women with peripartum cardiomyopathy. N Engl J Med 2001;344(21):1567–71.
137. North RA, Sadler L, Stewart AW, McCowan LM, Kerr AR, White HD. Long-term survival and valve-related complications in young women with cardiac valve replacements. Circulation 1999;99(20):2669–76.
138. Dore A, Somerville J. Pregnancy in patients with pulmonary autograft valve replacement. Eur Heart J 1997;18(10):1659–62.
139. Sadler L, McCowan L, White H, Stewart A, Bracken M, North R. Pregnancy outcomes and cardiac complications in women with mechanical, bioprosthetic and homograft valves. Br J Obstet Gynaecol 2000;107(2):245–53.
140. Ginsberg JS, Chan WS, Bates SM, Kaatz S. Anticoagulation of pregnant women with mechanical heart valves. Arch Intern Med 2003;163(6):694–8.
141. Chan WS, Anand S, Ginsberg JS. Anticoagulation of pregnant women with mechanical heart valves: a systematic review of the literature. Arch Intern Med 2000;160(2):191–6.
142. Vitale N, De Feo M, De Santo LS, Pollice A, Tedesco N, Cotrufo M. Dose-dependent fetal complica-

tions of warfarin in pregnant women with mechanical heart valves. J Am Coll Cardiol 1999;33(6): 1637–41.
143. Nelson-Piercy C, Rosenthal E, Harding K, Bewley S. Routine elective cesarean section is not justified for women with mechanical heart valves. J Am Coll Cardiol 2000;35(5):1365–6.
144. Roberts N, Ross D, Flint SK, Arya R, Blott M. Thromboembolism in pregnant women with mechanical prosthetic heart valves anticoagulated with low molecular weight heparin. Br J Obstet Gynaecol 2001;108(3):327–9.
145. Hall JG. Embryopathy associated with oral anticoagulant therapy. Birth Defects Orig Artic Ser 1976;12(5):33–7.
146. Wesseling J, Van Driel D, Heymans HS, et al. Coumarins during pregnancy: long-term effects on growth and development of school-age children. Thromb Haemost 2001;85(4):609–13.
147. Nelson-Piercy C, Letsky EA, de Swiet M. Low-molecular-weight heparin for obstetric thromboprophylaxis: experience of sixty-nine pregnancies in sixty-one women at high risk. Am J Obstet Gynecol 1997;176(5):1062–8.
148. Ginsberg JS, Hirsh J. Use of antithrombotic agents during pregnancy. Chest 1998;114(5 suppl):524S–30S.
149. Sanson BJ, Lensing AW, Prins MH, et al. Safety of low-molecular-weight heparin in pregnancy: a systematic review. Thromb Haemost 1999;81(5): 668–72.
150. Bates SM, Greer IA, Hirsh J, Ginsberg JS. Use of antithrombotic agents during pregnancy: the Seventh ACCP Conference on Antithrombotic and Thrombolytic Therapy. Chest 2004;126(3 suppl): 627S–44S.
151. Leyh RG, Fischer S, Ruhparwar A, Haverich A. Anticoagulation for prosthetic heart valves during pregnancy: is low-molecular-weight heparin an alternative? Eur J Cardiothorac Surg 2002;21(3): 577–9.
152. Mahesh B, Evans S, Bryan AJ. Failure of low molecular-weight heparin in the prevention of prosthetic mitral valve thrombosis during pregnancy: case report and a review of options for anticoagulation. J Heart Valve Dis 2002;11(5): 745–50.
153. Lev-Ran O, Kramer A, Gurevitch J, Shapira I, Mohr R. Low-molecular-weight heparin for prosthetic heart valves: treatment failure. Ann Thorac Surg 2000;69(1):264–5; discussion 265–6.
154. Danik S, Fuster V. Anticoagulation in pregnant women with prosthetic heart valves. Mt Sinai J Med 2004;71(5):322–9.
155. Brennand JE, Walker ID, Greer IA. Anti-activated factor X profiles in pregnant women receiving antenatal thromboprophylaxis with enoxaparin. Acta Haematol 1999;101(1):53–5.
156. Groce JB 3rd. "Bridging" therapy with low molecular weight heparin in pregnant patients and patients with mechanical prosthetic heart valves. J Thromb Thrombolysis 2003;16(1–2):79–82.
157. Leyse R, Ofstun M, Dillard DH, Merendino KA. Congenital aortic stenosis in pregnancy, corrected by extracorporeal circulation, offering a viable male infant at term but with anomalies eventuating in his death at four months of age—report of a case. JAMA 1961;176:1009–12.
158. Mahli A, Izdes S, Coskun D. Cardiac operations during pregnancy: review of factors influencing fetal outcome. Ann Thorac Surg 2000;69(5):1622–6.
159. Strickland RA, Oliver WC Jr, Chantigian RC, Ney JA, Danielson GK. Anesthesia, cardiopulmonary bypass, and the pregnant patient. Mayo Clin Proc 1991;66(4):411–29.
160. Arnoni RT, Arnoni AS, Bonini RC, et al. Risk factors associated with cardiac surgery during pregnancy. Ann Thorac Surg 2003;76(5):1605–8.
161. Parry AJ, Westaby S. Cardiopulmonary bypass during pregnancy. Ann Thorac Surg 1996;61(6): 1865–9.
162. Salazar E, Espinola N, Molina FJ, Reyes A, Barragan R. Heart surgery with cardiopulmonary bypass in pregnant women. Arch Cardiol Mex 2001; 71(1):20–7.
163. Jahangiri M, Clarke J, Prefumo F, Pumphrey C, Ward D. Cardiac surgery during pregnancy: pulsatile or nonpulsatile perfusion? J Thorac Cardiovasc Surg 2003;126(3):894–5.
164. Aagaard-Tillery KM, Belfort MA. Eclampsia: morbidity, mortality, and management. Clin Obstet Gynecol 2005;48(1):12–23.
165. Sibai BM, Abdella TN, Spinnato JA, Anderson GD, Eclampsia V. The incidence of nonpreventable eclampsia. Am J Obstet Gynecol 1986;154(3): 581–6.
166. Sibai BM. Diagnosis, prevention, and management of eclampsia. Obstet Gynecol 2005;105(2): 402–10.
167. Douglas KA, Redman CW. Eclampsia in the United Kingdom. B Med J 1994;309(6966):1395–400.
168. Patel HP, Mitsnefes M. Advances in the pathogenesis and management of hypertensive crisis. Curr Opin Pediatr 2005;17(2):210–4.
169. Redman CW, Sargent IL. The pathogenesis of preeclampsia. Gynecol Obstet Fertil 2001;29(7–8): 518–22.

170. The sixth report of the Joint National Committee on prevention, detection, evaluation, and treatment of high blood pressure. Arch Intern Med 1997;157(21):2413–46.
171. American College of Obstetrics and Gynecology (ACOG) practice bulletin number 47, October 2003. Prophylactic antibiotics in labor and delivery. Obstet Gynecol 2003;102(4):875–82.
172. Sugrue D, Blake S, Troy P, MacDonald D. Antibiotic prophylaxis against infective endocarditis after normal delivery—is it necessary? Br Heart J 1980;44(5):499–502.
173. Dajani AS, Taubert KA, Wilson W, et al. Prevention of bacterial endocarditis: recommendations by the American Heart Association. Clin Infect Dis 1997;25(6):1448–58.
174. Mabie WC, Anderson GD, Addington MB, Reed CM Jr, Peeden PZ, Sibai BM. The benefit of cesarean section in acute myocardial infarction complicated by premature labor. Obstet Gynecol 1988;71(3 pt 2):503–6.
175. Mendelson MA. Pregnancy in the woman with congenital heart disease. Am J Card Imaging 1995;9(1):44–52.
176. Mendelson MA. Congenital cardiac disease and pregnancy. Clin Perinatol 1997;24(2):467–82.
177. Nolan TE, Hess LW, Hess DB, Morrison JC. Severe medical illness complicating cesarean section. Obstet Gynecol Clin North Am 1988;15(4):697–717.
178. Thilen U, Olsson SB. Pregnancy and heart disease: a review. Eur J Obstet Gynecol Reprod Biol 1997;75(1):43–50.
179. Penning S, Robinson KD, Major CA, Garite TJ. A comparison of echocardiography and pulmonary artery catheterization for evaluation of pulmonary artery pressures in pregnant patients with suspected pulmonary hypertension. Am J Obstet Gynecol 2001;184(7):1568–70.
180. Elkayam U, Ostrzega E, Shotan A, Mehra A. Cardiovascular problems in pregnant women with the Marfan syndrome. Ann Intern Med 1995;123(2): 117–22.
181. Ray P, Murphy GJ, Shutt LE. Recognition and management of maternal cardiac disease in pregnancy. Br J Anaesth 2004;93(3):428–39.
182. Witlin AG, Mabie WC, Sibai BM. Peripartum cardiomyopathy: an ominous diagnosis. Am J Obstet Gynecol 1997;176(1 Pt 1):182–8.
183. Julian DG, Szekely P. Peripartum cardiomyopathy. Prog Cardiovasc Dis 1985;27(4):223–40.
184. Veille JC, Zaccaro D. Peripartum cardiomyopathy: summary of an international survey on peripartum cardiomyopathy. Am J Obstet Gynecol 1999; 181(2):315–9.
185. Massad LS, Reiss CK, Mutch DG, Haskel EJ. Familial peripartum cardiomyopathy after molar pregnancy. Obstet Gynecol 1993;81(5 (Pt 2)):886–8.
186. Pearl W. Familial occurrence of peripartum cardiomyopathy. Am Heart J 1995;129(2):421–2.
187. Mendelson MA, Chandler J. Postpartum cardiomyopathy associated with maternal cocaine abuse. Am J Cardiol 1992;70(11):1092–4.
188. Lampert MB, Hibbard J, Weinert L, Briller J, Lindheimer M, Lang RM. Peripartum heart failure associated with prolonged tocolytic therapy. Am J Obstet Gynecol 1993;168(2):493–5.
189. Kothari S. Aetiopathogenesis of peripartum cardiomyopathy: prolactin-selenium interaction? Int J Cardiol 1977;60:111–4.
190. Cenac A, Djibo A, Sueur JM, Chaigneau C, Orfila J. [Chlamydia infection and peripartum dilated cardiomyopathy in Niger]. Med Trop (Mars) 2000;60(2):137–40.

26 Acute Heart Failure Syndromes and Endocrine Disorders

Ioannis Ilias, Ioanna Dimopoulou, and Stylianos Tsagarakis

Common and uncommon endocrine abnormalities may be found or be associated with or even cause acute heart failure syndrome (AHFS). Nevertheless, the frequency of endocrine abnormalities in AHFS is mostly unknown, since the vast majority of the relevant medical literature is based on sporadic case reports. Clinicians should bear this caveat in mind, and particularly seek the factors from the past medical history that are associated with endocrine disease.

Acromegaly

Definition

Acromegaly is caused by excess secretion of growth hormone (GH) by micro- or macroadenomas of anterior pituitary.

Epidemiology

The annual incidence is 3 per 1 million.

Clinical Presentation

Symptoms

Symptoms include arthralgias, fatigue, headaches, and perspiration.

Signs

Signs include skeletal overgrowth and soft tissue enlargement (particularly facial tissues and skin). Acromegaly is associated with cardiomegaly and cardiomyopathy of insidious onset. Fibrosis is prominent. Inadequate filling capacity leads to diastolic heart failure. Arrhythmias are noted: ectopic beats, paroxysmal atrial fibrillation, paroxysmal supraventricular tachycardia, sick sinus syndrome, ventricular tachycardia, and bundle branch blocks.

Diagnosis

Diagnosis is made by baseline GH, GH after glucose loading, and insulin-like growth factor-I (IGF-I).

Treatment

Transsphenoidal pituitary surgery provides cure in 90% of microadenomas but less than 50% of macroadenomas. The GH antagonists and somatostatin receptor agonists (SRS-A) are prescribed for inoperable disease or after failure of surgery; SRS-A can also be given before surgery. Radiotherapy is considered only in patients who cannot undergo surgery or in patients with large residual tumors following surgery.

Cushing's Syndrome

Definition

Endogenous Cushing's syndrome (vis-à-vis exogenous caused by glucocorticoid administration) is the result of excessive cortisol secretion by adrenal tumors (15%), excessive corticotropin (ACTH) secretion from the anterior pituitary (Cushing's disease; 70%), or nonpituitary tumors (ectopic ACTH secretion; 15%) that leads to excess cortisol production from the adrenals.

Epidemiology

It is a rare disorder; the incidence is reported to be about $2.5/10^6$ population.

Clinical Presentation

Symptoms

Symptoms include headaches, muscle weakness, and depression.

Signs

Specific features (centripetal obesity with increased supraclavicular fat, proximal muscle weakness, and purple striae wider than 1 cm) occur in patients. Patients with sustained hypercortisolism may have hypertension, hypercoagulability, ventricular hypertrophy, and concentric remodeling that increase cardiovascular risk.

Diagnosis

When glucocorticoid excess is suspected, screening should be done with measurements of urine cortisol or dexamethasone suppression testing. When the diagnosis of Cushing's syndrome is established, it should be followed by the measurement of plasma ACTH to determine whether hypercortisolism is ACTH-dependent or -independent (caused by adrenal tumors). In patients with ACTH-dependent hypercortisolism the high-dose dexamethasone test, the corticotropin-releasing hormone (CRH) test, pituitary magnetic resonance imaging (MRI), and bilateral inferior petrosal sinus sampling are performed to distinguish pituitary from ectopic ACTH secretion.

Treatment

Surgical resection of the tumor causing Cushing's syndrome is the optimal treatment for all its forms. The prognosis is better for Cushing's disease (transsphenoidal resection has postoperative cure rates of 78% to 97% for microadenomas and 50% to 80% for macroadenomas) and benign

Table 26.1. Emergency medical treatment of endocrine abnormalities in acute heart failure syndrome (AHFS)

Cushing syndrome	Hyperthyroidism (thyroid storm)	Hypothyroidism (myxedema coma)	Hyperparathyroidism (hypercalcemia)	Hypocalcemia	Pheochromocytoma
Ketoconazole p.o. 200–1200 mg/day in 2–3 divided doses	Propylthiouracil p.o.* 200–300 mg every 4–8 hours. Lugol's solution p.o.* or SSKI p.o.* 2–8 drops every 6–12 hours	Thyroxine 7 µg/kg (total dose 150–500 µg) bolus i.v. followed by 100 µg/day	Hydration and furosemide i.v. 20–80 mg every 2–4 hours	Calcium gluconate OR calcium chloride (10% w/v) i.v. 10–20 mL over 10 minutes (faster administration may compromise cardiac function) followed by infusion at 1 mg/kg/hour	Phenoxybenzamine p.o. 10–240 mg/day in 2–4 doses OR prazosin p.o. 1–5 mg every 8 hours
Etomidate i.v.	Propranolol p.o. 40–60 mg every 6 hours OR i.v. slowly 2 mg every 4 hours Hydration, cooling and analgesics	± Hydrocortisone 50–100 mg every 6–8 hours with gradual tapering	Pamidronate i.v. 30–90 mg over 4 hours OR zoledronate i.v. 4 mg over 15 minutes	Switch to oral supplementation and add vitamin D for chronic therapy.	In extreme hypertensive situations nitroprusside, phentolamine, urapidil, magnesium or α-methyl-p-tyrosine can be administered

SSKI, saturated solution of potassium iodide.

*Can also be given with nasogastric tube and has also been administered rectally.

adrenal causes of Cushing's syndrome than for adrenocortical cancer (5-year survival rate of 20% to 58%) and malignant ACTH-producing tumors. Bilateral adrenalectomy, medical treatment (with ketoconazole; Table 26.1) or radiotherapy are options for inoperable or recurrent cases.

Hyperthyroidism

Definition

Hyperthyroidism is excess thyroid hormones in the plasma.

Epidemiology

The lifetime prevalence is 2% in women and 0.2% in men.

Causes

Hyperthyroidism is caused by Graves' disease (80%) or toxic multinodular goiter or single hyperfunctioning nodule (20%). It is rarely attributed to amiodarone use (particularly type I amiodarone-induced hyperthyroidism, as seen in patients with a history of Graves' disease or goiter).

Clinical Presentation

Symptoms

Symptoms include hyperactivity, palpitations, dyspnea, weight loss, and muscular weakness.

Signs

Signs include sinus tachycardia, atrial fibrillation, congestive (high-output) heart failure, and exacerbation of coronary artery disease (particularly in thyrotoxic crisis, thyroid storm with tachycardia, fever, arrhythmias, nausea, vomiting and diarrhea precipitated by surgery, infections, postparturition, diabetic ketoacidosis, and patients with previously untreated hyperthyroidism).

Diagnosis

Diagnosis is made by thyrotropin (thyroid-stimulating hormone, TSH), free thyroxine (FT_4), and occasionally thyroid scintigraphy (with iodine-123 or technetium-99m) to delineate Graves' disease from nodular disease.

Treatment

Beta-blockers are prescribed for symptomatic relief (verapamil if these are contraindicated), as are antithyroid medications (thioamides). Definitive treatment is with radioactive iodine-131 or surgery. In thyrotoxic crisis (Table 26.1) propylthiouracil, SSKI, beta-blockers, or verapamil and glucocorticoids (in extremis and if available: plasmapheresis or dialysis) are prescribed. The prognosis is poor (mortality of 25% to 60%).

Hypothyroidism

Definition

Hypothyroidism is the deficient production of thyroid hormones.

Epidemiology

Clinical hypothyroidism affects 2% of adult women and 0.2% of adult men. Subclinical disease may affect 7% to 15% of adults (see below for definitions of clinical/subclinical disease).

Causes

In 99%, the cause is primary thyroid gland failure. It is rarely attributed to drugs such as amiodarone, lithium, interferon-α, or interleukin-2.

Clinical Presentation

Symptoms

Symptoms include lethargy, weight gain, and constipation.

Signs

Signs include dry skin, bradycardia, diastolic hypertension, pleural and pericardial effusions, and coma (myxedema coma).

Diagnosis

Diagnosis is made by TSH, FT_4, and possibly thyroid autoantibodies. Clinical hypothyroidism is diagnosed if TSH is high and FT_4 is low, and subclinical hypothyroidism is diagnosed if TSH is high and FT_4 is normal. Cardiac tamponade is very rare in hypothyroidism but should be taken into consideration in patients with pericardial effusion.

Treatment

Treatment entails replacement with levothyroxine (plus glucocorticoids and appropriate supportive measures if myxedema coma; the latter can have approximately a 50% mortality rate) (Table 26.1).

Nonthyroidal Illness (Euthyroid Sick Syndrome)

Acutely ill patients may show transient abnormalities in thyroid function testing such as low serum triiodothyronine (T_3), low T_4, high reverse T_3, and elevated TSH (particularly during recovery). The interpretation of TSH levels in acutely ill patients can be hampered if dobutamine is administered, since it decreases TSH in serum. Usually no treatment is needed; furthermore, the beneficial effects of T_3 supplementation have not been scrutinized adequately.

Hyperparathyroidism

Definition

Hyperparathyroidism is excess parathyroid hormone (PTH) secretion, usually with accompanying hypercalcemia.

Epidemiology

Hypercalcemia affects 0.4% to 2.0% of the general population (primary hyperparathyroidism and malignancies account for 90% of cases).

Causes

In 80% of cases the cause is adenoma of a single parathyroid gland; the remaining cases are due to benign hyperplasia of the parathyroids, which in some patients may be part of multiple endocrine neoplasia (MEN) syndromes (MEN-1 and less often MEN-2). Critical illness provokes a transient PTH secretion. In patients recovering from multiple organ failure, but having the added burden of acute oliguric renal failure, serum ionized calcium may be high with PTH secretion remaining accordingly high (tertiary hyperparathyroidism).

Clinical Presentation

Symptoms

Symptoms include constipation and fatigue.

Signs

Signs include nephrolithiasis, skeletal complications, shortened QT interval, bradycardia, and first-degree atrioventricular block.

Diagnosis

Diagnosis is made by serum ionized calcium, PTH, and renal calcium clearance.

Treatment

Definitive treatment of hyperparathyroidism is surgical. In cases of tertiary hyperparathyroidism after multiple organ failure, if the calcium/PTH disturbances are left unattended, serious life-threatening bradycardia may ensue. Medical treatment is with hydration, calciuresis (loop diuretics), and administration of bisphosphonates (Table 26.1).

Hypocalcemia

Definition

Hypocalcemia is caused by hypoparathyroidism (usually after neck surgery), in recovering from hyperparathyroidism (hungry bone syndrome), or by high phosphate load (tumor lysis or overuse of phosphate-containing enemas or laxatives).

Epidemiology

Low total calcium is common (up to 90%) in patients hospitalized in intensive care units. Ionized calcium is a more reliable marker, if available.

Clinical Presentation

Symptoms

Symptoms include numbness and tingling.

Signs

Signs include tetany, stridor, seizures, Chvostek's sign, Trousseau's sign, papilledema (in the subacute setting), decreased myocardial contraction, and QT prolongation.

Diagnosis

Diagnosis is made by ionized calcium, phosphate, and parathormone levels, and if possible by 25-vitamin D and 1,25-vitamin D levels.

Treatment

Treatment entails supplementation with calcium and vitamin D derivatives (after correction of acute calcium disturbance) (Table 26.1). Caution must be applied when administering beta-blockers and calcium channel blockers in patients with suspected hypocalcemia; these medications may exacerbate cardiac failure.

Pheochromocytoma

Definition

Pheochromocytoma is a catecholamine-producing chromaffin-cell tumor; extraadrenal chromaffin-cell tumors are termed paragangliomas. Prolonged and repetitive catecholamine surges provoke necrosis of myocardial cells and fibrosis.

Epidemiology

The annual incidence of pheochromocytoma is approximately 1.5 to 2.0 per 1 million.

Clinical Presentation

Symptoms

Symptoms include headache, palpitations, and flushing.

Signs

Signs include diaphoresis, hypertension, tachycardia, supraventricular, nodal or ventricular tachycardia, atrial or ventricular fibrillation, torsades de pointes, and Wolff-Parkinson-White syndrome. Both hypertrophic and dilated forms of cardiomyopathy have been described with pheochromocytoma.

Diagnosis

Diagnosis is made by measurement of plasma free metanephrines (first choice, if available), or urinary metanephrines (second choice). Anatomic imaging studies with computed tomography or magnetic resonance imaging and if possible functional imaging (scintigraphy with iodine-123 metaiodobenzylguanidine or other radionuclides) are also used.

Treatment

Surgical removal may be the definitive treatment. For preparation, blood pressure control is imperative with α-adrenergic blockers; beta-blockers may be added only after adequate α-blocking (Table 26.1). Since partial or complete reversibility of cardiomyopathy may be achieved in a patient presenting with unexplained systolic heart failure the assessment of possible catecholamine excess/pheochromocytoma is crucial. The prognosis of patients with acute heart failure syndrome and overlooked catecholamine-induced myocarditis/cardiomyopathy is not good.

Suggested Readings

Brilakis ES, Young WF Jr, Wilson JW, Thompson GB, Munger TM. Reversible catecholamine-induced cardiomyopathy in a heart transplant candidate without persistent or paroxysmal hypertension. J Heart Lung Transplant 1999;18:376–80.

Brouwers F, Lenders JWM, Eisenhofer G, Pacak K. Pheochromocytoma as an endocrine emergency. Rev Endocr Metab Dis 2003;4:121–8.

Colao AM, Ferone D, Marzullo P, Lombardi G. Systemic complications of acromegaly: epidemiology, pathogenesis, and management. Endocr Rev 2004;25:102-52.

Henderson KE, Baranski TJ, Bickel PE. The Washington Manual Endocrinology Subspecialty Consult. Philadelphia: Lippincott Williams & Wilkins, 2005.

Jeffries CC, Ledgerwood AM, Lucas CE. Life-threatening tertiary hyperparathyroidism in the critically ill. Am J Surg 2005;189:369–72.

Klemperer JD. Thyroid hormone and cardiac surgery. Thyroid 2002;12:517–21.

Nieman LK, Ilias I. Evaluation and treatment of Cushing's syndrome. Am J Med 2005;118:1340–6.

Shane E. Hypocalcemia: pathogenesis, differential diagnosis and management. In: Favus MJ, ed. Primer on the Metabolic Bone Diseases and Disorders of Mineral Metabolism. Philadelphia: Lippincott Williams & Wilkins 1999:223–6.

Wartofsky L. Myxedema coma. In: Braverman LE, Utiger RD, eds. The Thyroid: A Fundamental and Clinical Text, 9th ed. Philadelphia: Lippincott Williams & Wilkins 2005:850–7.

Wartofsky L. Thyrotoxic storm. In: Braverman LE, Utiger RD, eds. The Thyroid: A Fundamental and Clinical Text, 9th ed. Philadelphia: Lippincott Williams & Wilkins 2005:651–9.

27
Acute Heart Failure Syndromes in β-Thalassemia

Dimitrios Th. Kremastinos, John T. Parissis, and Gerasimos S. Filippatos

β-thalassemia is a hereditary disorder that causes anemia as a result of the decrease in the production of β-globin chains. This disorder is caused by more than 200 point mutations, and more rarely deletions seem to be related with increased long-term morbidity and mortality, affecting the structure and function of many human organs (1). Although the disease has been characterized as a Mediterranean anemia, it seems to spread well beyond its traditional locations (Greece, Southern Italy, and France). Thus, it also appears in India and Africa, and affects certain populations in Asia and South Pacific, as well as black Americans.

Hemolysis and inadequate erythropoiesis are the predominant causes of anemia in β-thalassemia. Depending on clinical severity, two forms of the disease have been recognized: thalassemia major and thalassemia intermedia. The homozygous form of the disease is known as thalassemia major or Cooley's anemia, and leads to severe congenital hemolytic syndrome (2). Clinical manifestations of the syndrome are usually present during the first 6 months of life, and patients need frequent transfusions to survive until the second decade of life. The thalassemia intermedia has a later clinical onset with milder anemia and longer life expectancy, requiring no frequent blood transfusions (3).

In thalassemia major, the correction of anemia by blood transfusions increases the survival rate but causes significant hemosiderosis combined with excessive extravascular hemolysis and inappropriate absorption of intestinal iron. The multiorgan abnormal iron deposition leads to tissue damage and to altered cardiac, hepatic, and endocrine functions (1,2).

Cardiac complications, such as heart failure and arrhythmias, are very frequent and still remain the major cause of patient mortality. However, the pathophysiology of cardiac dysfunction in thalassemia major is poorly understood and seems to have a multifactorial etiology. Left-sided and, progressively, biventricular heart failure are the most common forms of cardiac dysfunction in younger patients, expressed by systolic left ventricular dysfunction and dilatation (4,5). In older patients, chronic myocardial iron deposition causes directly excessive left ventricular diastolic dysfunction characterized by restriction and elevated pulmonary pressures. In this mode of cardiac dysfunction, symptoms and signs of right-sided heart failure are the predominant clinical features of β-thalassemic patients (6,7). This chapter summarizes the current knowledge regarding the implication of various forms of β-thalassemic heart in the appearance of acute heart failure syndromes as well as the thalassemia-related aggravating factors that lead to worsening or decompensation of heart failure of β-thalassemic patients.

Pathophysiology of Heart Failure

Histopathology and Structural Abnormalities

The iron overload and tissue deposition created by the increased plasma iron turnover and by the subsequent saturation of iron storage and transporting proteins are key pathophysiologic factors of cardiovascular complications in β-thalassemias (1,2). This activated biochemical pathway is a powerful stimulus for the overproduction of oxygen free radicals and promotes myocardial injury through the increased oxidative stress (8,9). More specifically, iron-mediated oxidative stress leads to lipid peroxidation and disruption of cell membranes, mitochondrial dysfunction, abnormal cell metabolism, and excessive cardiomyocyte loss through apoptosis and necrosis (9). In vivo studies have also confirmed that endothelial dysfunction and abnormal vascular remodeling are associated with iron overload and increased oxidative stress in the circulation of thalassemic patients (10). This vascular dysfunction leads to increased afterload as well as to further worsening of cardiac function and impaired exercise capacity of thalassemic patients, while it seems to be reversible by various iron chelation treatment modalities. Figure 27.1 provides a proposed pathophysiologic mechanism of iron overload-induced accelerated cardiovascular injury in major thalassemia.

Histopathologic findings indicate that advanced iron overload in β-thalassemias is characterized by a rust-brown myocardial appearance in the subepicardial layers and, more rarely, in the conduction system (11). Furthermore, extensive areas of extracellular fibrosis as well as disruption of sarcomeres in myofibrils in the presence of intracellular iron-containing granules have been detected by electron microscopy in the failing hearts of patients with thalassemia major (12). Macroscopic findings also include cardiac muscle hypertrophy, chamber dilatation, pericardial effusion, and focal myocardial degeneration (11,12). These abnormalities appear as a result of the combined effects on cardiac structure and function of anemia-induced volume overloading and abnormal iron metabolism.

Finally, abnormal remodeling of the pulmonary vascular bed, similar to that observed in idiopathic pulmonary hypertension, as well as secondary pulmonary abnormalities created by chronic embolic disease, are predominant pathophysiologic features in older patients with thalassemia major (13). Iron infiltration also may be present in the coronary artery wall, pericardium, and heart valves, leading to degenerative conditions (11).

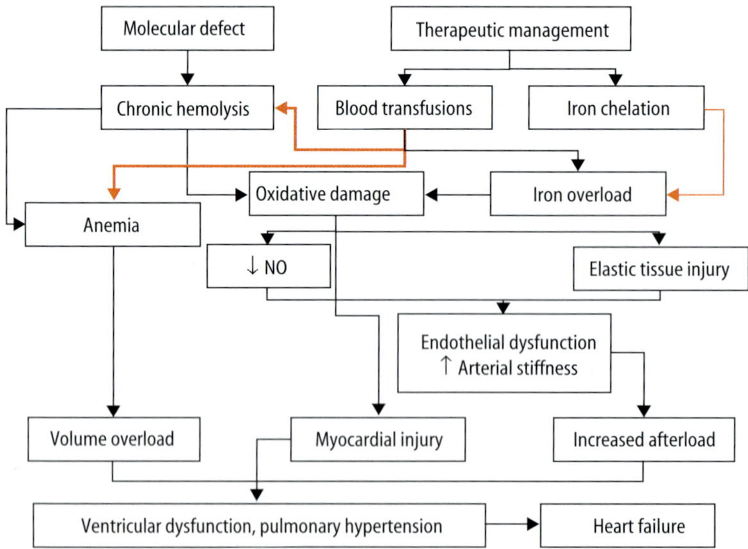

FIGURE 27.1. A proposed pathophysiologic mechanism of iron overload-induced accelerated cardiovascular injury leading to heart failure in thalassemia major. NO, nitric oxide. Red arrows represent inhibitory pathways.

Cardiac Involvement in Thalassemia Major

Dilated Cardiomyopathy

Left-sided and subsequently biventricular dysfunction and failure are the most common clinical conditions in younger patients. This type of cardiac dysfunction in thalassemia major seems to be multifactorial and leads progressively to symptoms of heart failure such as dyspnea, fatigue, and impaired exercise capacity. High cardiac output and volume overloading secondary to anemia as well as multiendocrinopathies, genetic predisposition, infectious agents, and unknown factors are underlying pathophysiologic mechanisms of heart failure in β-thalassemic patients. Secondary mediators such as neurohormonal activation, increased oxidative stress, and overexpression of proinflammatory cytokines create vicious circles of cardiovascular injury through cardiac hypertrophy, dilatation (adverse cardiac remodeling), and dysfunction of vascular endothelium, and lead to worsening of the syndrome. Figure 27.2 describes the pathophysiologic process that leads to heart failure progression in young patients with thalassemia major and left-sided cardiac dysfunction.

Myocarditis/Pericarditis

Acute infectious myocarditis is a frequent cause of acute heart failure in young patients with thalassemia major, causing symptoms of pulmonary congestion and peripheral hypoperfusion, and having a dismal prognosis (13). Accumulating evidence also suggests that proven myocarditis confirmed by biopsy findings leads to left-sided chronic heart failure in about 4.5% of this patient population. Myocarditis may predispose to the development of a dilated cardiomyopathy phenotype through the chronic activation of immune/inflammatory mechanisms rather than viral infection and replication (13). This process seems to be related with a genetic dysregulation of biochemical pathways that control the immune response to infection and tissue injury. Thus, it has been shown that human leukocyte antigen (HLA)-DQA1*0501 allele frequency is significantly higher in β-thalassemic patients with left-sided heart failure and may be actively implicated in the development and clinical deterioration of the syndrome (14,15). However, more studies using novel molecular biology techniques need to identify the exact immunogenetic background of heart failure pathogenesis in thalassemia major.

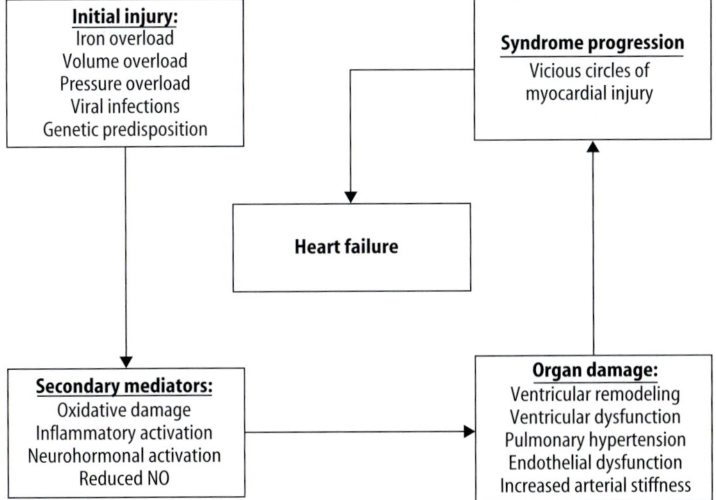

FIGURE 27.2. A schematic pathophysiologic process that leads to heart failure progression in young patients with thalassemia major and left-sided cardiac dysfunction. NO: nitric oxide.

Pericarditis, a very frequent clinical entity in the past, seems to be a very rare complication in the modern era of intensive chelation treatment.

Restrictive Form of Left Ventricular Cardiomyopathy

In elderly β-thalassemic patients, chronic iron deposition into heart tissue causes left ventricular myocardial restriction, with highly elevated intracardiac filling pressures and pulmonary arteriolar resistance (6,7). This condition leads progressively to right heart dilatation and failure, while left ventricular dimensions and contractility remain within or near normal limits. Right-sided heart failure symptoms and signs are the most common clinical features in this patient population (6,7). Figure 27.3 describes echocardiographically the various forms of cardiac dysfunction in thalassemia major.

Pulmonary Arterial Hypertension

Accumulating evidence suggests that pulmonary arterial hypertension (PAH) is an essential feature of the clinical spectrum of both thalassemia major and intermedia. It occurs in about 10% of patients with thalassemia major, while in thalassemia intermedia it is the predominant heart complication (3,16). However, the development of PAH in two forms of disease seems to be related to the underlying genetic defect as well as the effects of applied therapies. A variety of thalassemia-related factors that result in both increased cardiac output and pulmonary vascular resistance are implicated in the pathogenesis of PAH in β-thalassemic patients.

A potential mechanism that leads to a high-output state in β-thalassemia is tissue hypoxia that is derived from the chronically low hemoglobin concentrations or the abnormal hemoglobin types that are characterized by reduced oxygen delivery to peripheral tissues. Liver injury, caused by viral infections, iron deposition, and extramedullary hematopoiesis, also contributes to the cardiac output elevation through the development of peripheral arterial-venous shunts (17).

On the other hand, the hemolytic syndrome through its detrimental effects on nitric oxide production and L-arginine availability leads to pulmonary artery vasoconstriction and increased pulmonary artery resistance. Red cell membrane elements and other hemolytic products as well as iron overload also induce oxidative tissue damage that in turn causes endothelial dysfunction, elastic tissue injury, and adverse vascular remodeling with increased tone and reduced compliance of the pulmonary vascular bed (18). Finally, iron overload promotes interstitial pulmonary fibrosis, while left ventricular systolic or diastolic dysfunction are additional factors that may increase pulmonary vascular resistance (16).

Hypercoagulability associated with abnormalities of erythrocyte membrane phospholipids as well as with coexistent thrombocytosis in splenectomized patients leads in many cases to silent or clinically manifested thrombolic events, reducing the active vascular pulmonary bed and predisposing to further deterioration of PAH (18). Lung damage because of recurrent respiratory track infections or extramedullar intrathoracic hemopoietic masses secondary to bone marrow expansion, may also be implicated in the development and progression of PAH in β-thalassemia (16).

Consequently, PAH is a common condition in both forms of β-thalassemia, which seems to have multifactorial etiology and requires special attention and management in order to prevent the clinical worsening of syndrome.

Factors Linking β-Thalassemia with Acute Heart Failure

Anemia Exacerbation

This condition is an important factor that predisposes to heart failure decompensation and worsening of congestion through peripheral tissue hypoxia, vasodilatation, sympathetic and angiotensin–renin–aldosterone system activation, and volume overloading. Thus, a rational approach to prevent heart failure exacerbations because of anemia is to give red cell transfusions at regular intervals to keep the hemoglobin levels ≥9 to 9.5 g/dL.

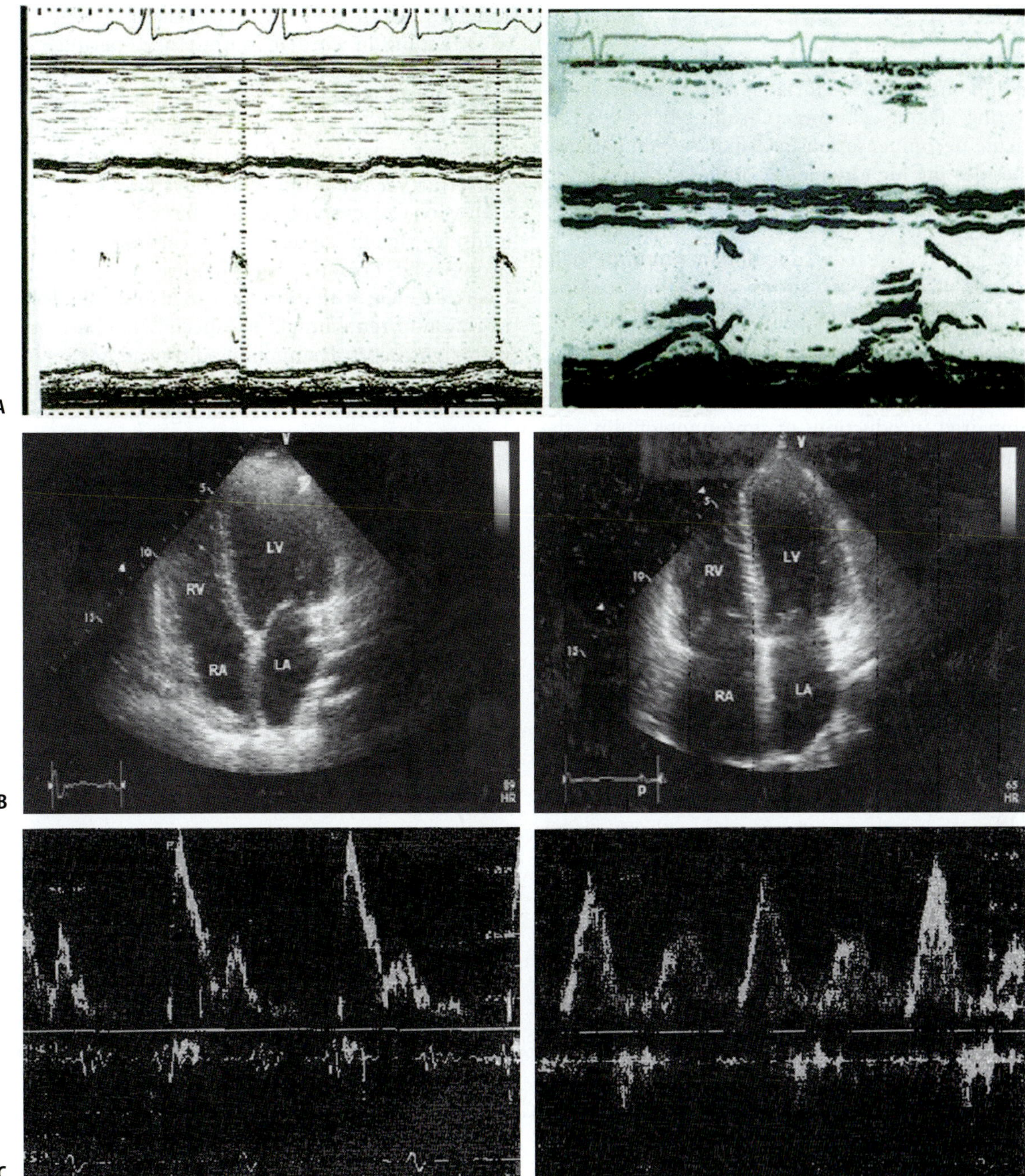

Figure 27.3. (A) M-mode tracings (parasternal long axis) showing left-sided (left panel: left ventricular dilatation) and right-sided (right panel: nondilated hypokinetic left ventricle with right ventricular dilatation) heart dysfunction in thalassemia major. (B) Two-dimensional echocardiogram (apical four-chamber view) demonstrating left ventricular dilatation (left panel: left-sided heat dysfunction) in younger patients versus right ventricular dilatation (right panel: right-sided heart dysfunction) in elderly with thalassemia major. LV, left ventricle; RV, right ventricle; LA, left atrium; RA, right atrium. (C) Left: Transmitral restrictive diastolic flow pattern in a thalassemic patient with dilated-right/restrictive-left cardiomyopathy. Right: Pulmonary vein flow velocity pattern of the same patient demonstrating increased diastolic, decreased systolic velocity and prominent atrial reversal flow.

Infections

Infectious complications are the second most common cause of mortality and a main aggravating factor causing chronic heart failure acute decompensation in β-thalassemic patients. Besides the high incidence of blood-borne infections related with multiple transfusions, the high susceptibility of these patients to infections has been attributed to a concomitant immune deficiency. Recent observations on immune competence in β-thalassemia have described a variety of quantitative and functional abnormalities of immune system components, including the abnormal properties of T and B lymphocytes, the impaired production of immunoglobulin, the functional defects of neutrophils and macrophages related to chemotaxis and phagocytosis, and the dysfunction of complement system (19). From the wide spectrum of thalassemia-related infectious diseases, respiratory track infections seems to play the most important role in the acute decompensated episodes of heart failure by increasing pulmonary vascular resistance and right heart dysfunction, by promoting tissue hypoxia, and by activation secondary inflammatory mediators (interleukin-6, tumor necrosis factor-α, etc.) that depress cardiac contractile function and enhance pulmonary congestion (19).

Current prevention strategies are numerous. Detailed health information should be made available to patients, who should be encouraged to maintain scrupulous personal hygiene and to avoid specific environments (e.g., abrupt variations in temperature, unhealthy air). Moreover, prophylaxis (pneumonococcal vaccination in splenectomized patients or immunization against influenza) plays a role, as does the search for the management and monitoring of infective foci.

Deterioration of Renal Failure

Renal dysfunction predicts a poor prognosis in β-thalassemic patients with heart failure, and is more powerful adverse prognostic factor than other clinical variables such as left ventricular ejection fraction or New York Heart Association (NYHA) class (20). Although impaired cardiac function can directly influence renal function by a reduction in cardiac output and peripheral hypoperfusion, or elevated venous pressures, it is likely that in this patient population, activation of various neurohormonal and oxidative molecules with vasoconstricting and deleterious effects can cause further renal injury and dysfunction. This activation causes sodium and water retention, and leads to vicious circles of the cardiorenal syndrome that promote heart failure progression. Overtreatment with diuretics can also cause deterioration of renal function, especially, in patients with right heart dysfunction who need adequate preload. Additionally, the hepatorenal syndrome secondary to extensive liver damage by iron deposition is another clinical condition that leads to worsening of renal function in β-thalassemic patients (1).

Although it is not clear which management strategy is best for thalassemic patients with heart failure exacerbation because of renal dysfunction, administration of inotropes (dobutamine, dopamine) and ultrafiltration are useful therapeutic approaches in many cases. Novel drugs such as vasopressin antagonists or neseritide may be promising treatment modalities in this field.

Arrhythmias

Paroxysmal supraventricular arrhythmias and, especially, atrial fibrillation are also common causes of heart failure decompensation in thalassemic patients (21). In cases with hemodynamic instability, electric cardioversion should be applied, while digoxin and beta-blockers are acceptable therapeutic interventions in order to control heart rate. Amiodarone can also be used for the restoration of sinus rhythm or the prevention of recurrent episodes. Anticoagulation is indicated in patients with atrial fibrillation, although due to concomitant hepatic dysfunction, a lower-than-average dose of warfarin is required.

Endocrinopathies

Thyroid disorders due to abnormal iron deposition or infections are rare complications associated with heat failure deterioration in thalassemic patients (22). These disorders accelerate myocardial injury through the abnormalities in cardiomyocyte metabolism, the enhancement of cardiotoxic effects of circulating catecholamines, and the high output state. Management of these disorders by endocrinologists should be considered in order to avoid heart failure exacerbations.

Therapeutic Considerations and Treatment Algorithm

β-Thalassemia Major

The timing of heart failure onset in this patient population depends on the background anemia and chelation therapies as well as the genetic susceptibility. Pump failure is the principal mode of death, while sudden death is a relatively rare complication. The medical advances as well as the better understanding of the molecular basis of the disease have led to improved patient prognosis during the last two decades. In general, the long-term survival of patients on optimal chelation therapy is very satisfactory. In heart failure patients, the long-term prognosis has also been improved in the modern era compared with that of patients in the prechelation era. Our group found that thalassemic patients with heart failure had a 5-year survival of about 48%, while older series demonstrated a 3-month mortality rate of about 58% and all patients died within 1 year of the onset of symptoms (23–25). Potential explanations for this improvement were the intensification of chelation treatment, the frequent blood transfusions to increase the hemoglobin levels, and the use of neurohormonal antagonists that prevent deterioration of left ventricular remodeling such as angiotensin-converting enzyme (ACE) inhibitors (23). According to these observations, the natural course of heart failure in well-treated thalassemia major seems to be similar to that of heart failure in the general population.

Intensification of chelation therapy (desferrioxamine administration) as well as early identification and treatment of aggravating factors should be considered if the patients have asymptomatic left ventricular dysfunction or symptoms of heart failure. Furthermore, neurohormonal antagonists (ACE inhibitors, angiotensin II receptor I antagonists if there is intolerance to ACE inhibitors, aldosterone antagonists) should be used in patients with systolic dysfunction (26). Beta-blockers are recommended only in cases with stable disease, while diuretics and digoxin should be preferred in patients with congestion and excessive dyspnea. Finally, intravenous inotropes and diuretics are useful in alleviating the symptoms during the episodes of acute decompensation, while interventional procedures (biventricular pacing, automatic implantable cardioverter-defibrillators [AICDs], heart transplantation) may be considered in selected cases (26).

Echocardiography or left ventricular radionuclide ventriculography are valuable tools for the early detection of myocardial dysfunction as well as for the assessment of cardiac disease progression. Finally, cardiovascular T2-star magnetic resonance technique (T2*) is a very promising approach for the noninvasive quantification of iron overload and can be used periodically for the monitoring of chelation treatment effectiveness (27).

β-Thalassemia Intermedia

In thalassemia intermedia, age-related PAH and, rarely, high-output state with left ventricular remodeling are frequent clinical conditions that may adversely affect patient clinical outcomes (3). However, the optimal therapeutic approach of disease cardiac complications as well as the exact mechanisms of disease worsening and death remain poorly understood. In this context, further studies are needed to clarify the optimal medical management of these patients, including more accurate criteria of transfusion and chelation therapies.

At the present time, treatment should be individualized based on hemoglobin levels (≥8.5 g/dL), clinical and laboratory findings of iron overload (serum ferritin levels ≥1000 ng/mL, or hepatic iron concentration >3.2 mg/g), and the existence of PAH or left-sided heart failure documented by echocardiography (28). In the cases of PAH, lifelong treatment with vasodilators (calcium channel blockers, sildenafil, prostacyclin [PGI_2] agonists) should be used with careful monitoring of

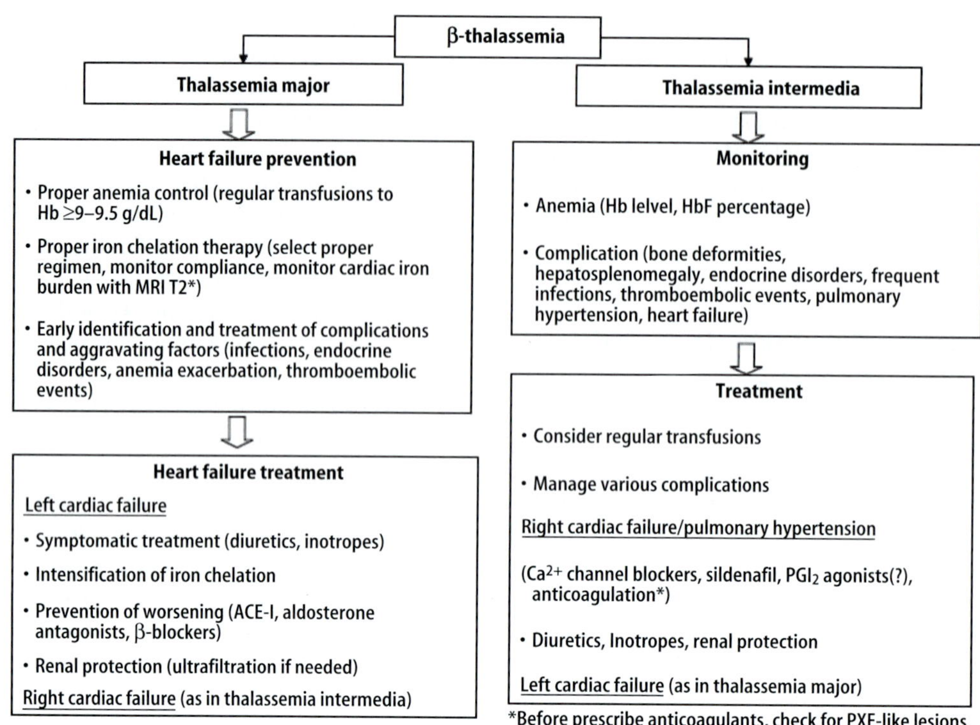

FIGURE 27.4. A treatment algorithm that summarizes current recommendations for the management of heart failure in thalassemia major and thalassemia intermedia. Hb, hemoglobin; MRI, magnetic resonance imaging: ACE-I, angiotensin-converting enzyme inhibitor; PGI, prostacyclin; PXE, pseudoxanthoma.

systemic blood pressure levels. In left-sided heart failure cases, oxygen administration, diuretics, and digoxin for symptomatic improvement as well as neurohormonal antagonists (ACE inhibitors, aldosterone antagonists, and possibly beta-blockers) for attenuation of heart failure progression should be considered according to NYHA class and renal function. Anticoagulants should be given in splenectomized patients or those with a history of thromboembolic events or atrial fibrillation. Serial echocardiographic studies seem to be useful to detect patients at high risk for the development of heart failure or to monitor the efficacy of various therapies (28). A treatment algorithm summarizes all these considerations in thalassemia intermedia as well as the current recommendations for the management of heart failure in thalassemia major (Fig. 27.4).

Conclusion

Heart failure is a frequent complication of β-thalassemia syndromes and leads to increased mortality and morbidity. A variety of aggravating factors (anemia exacerbation, infections, renal dysfunction, arrhythmias, and endocrinopathies) lead to episodes of acute decompensation requiring specialist care (cardiologists, hematologists, and endocrinologists). Correction of anemia, intensive chelation therapy, and recent advances in medical treatment of heart failure have dramatically improved the prognosis of patients, especially, in those with thalassemia major. Novel oral chelators (deferiprone), allogenic bone arrow transplantation, and gene therapy are future strategies targeting to the prevention or more effective treatment of the syndromes (26,29).

References

1. Rund D, Rachmilewitz E. β-thalassemia. N Engl J Med 2005;353:1135–46.
2. Old JM, Olivieri NF, Thein SL. Diagnosis and management of thalassemia. In: Weatherall DJ, Clegg B, eds. The Thalassemia Syndromes, 4th ed. Oxford, England: Blackwell Science 2001:630–85.
3. Aessopos A, Farmakis D, Karagiorga M, et al. Cardiac involvement in thalassemia intermedia: a multicenter study. Blood 2001;97:3411–16.
4. Kremastinos D. Heart failure in β-thalassemia. Congestive Heart Fail 2001;7:312–14.
5. Kremastinos D, Toutouzas P, Vyssoulis G, et al. Global and segmental left ventricular function in β-thalassemia. Cardiology 1985;72:129–39.
6. Kremastinos D, Tsiapras D, Tsetsos G, et al. Left ventricular diastolic Doppler characteristics in β-thalassemia major. Circulation 1993;88:1127–35.
7. Kremastinos D, Rentoukas E, Mavrogeni S, et al. Left ventricular filling pattern in β-thalassemia major-a Doppler echocardiographic study. Eur Heart J 1993;14:351–7.
8. Livrea MA, Tesoriere L, Pintaudi AM, et al. Oxidative stress and antioxidant status in β-thalassemia: iron overload and depletion of lipid-soluble antioxidants. Blood 1996;88:3608–14.
9. Gutteridge JMC, Halliwell B. Iron toxicity and oxygen radicals. Baillieres Clin Hematol 1989;2:195–256.
10. Cheung YF, Chan GC, Ha SY, et al. Arterial stiffness and endothelial function in patients with beta-thalassemia major. Circulation 2002;106:2561–66.
11. Lewis BS, Rachmilewitz EA, Amitai N, Halon DA, Gotsman MS. Left ventricular function in beta-thalassemia and the effect of multiple transfusions. Am Heart J 1978;96(5):636–45.
12. Iancu TC, Shiloh H. Morphologic observations in iron overload: an update. Adv Exp Med Biol 1994:356:255–65.
13. Kremastinos D, Tiniakos G, Theodorakis G, et al. Myocarditis in β-thalassemia major. A cause of heart failure. Circulation 1995;91:66–71.
14. Kremastinos D, Flevari P, Spyropoulou M, et al. Association of heart failure in homozygous beta-thalassemia with the major histocompatibility complex. Circulation 1999;100:2074–78.
15. Economou-Petersen E, Aessopos A, Kladi A, et al. Apolipoprotein E e4 allele as a genetic risk factor for left ventricular failure in homozygous β-thalassemia. Blood 1998;92:3455–59.
16. Hahalis G, Manolis A, Apostolopoulos D, et al. Right ventricular cardiomyopathy in beta-thalassemia major. Eur Heart J 2002;23:147–56.
17. Du ZD, Roguin N, Milgram E, et al. Pulmonary hypertension in patients with thalassemia major. Am Heart J 1997;134:532–7.
18. Eldor A, Rachmilewitz EA. The hypercoagulable state in thalassemia. Blood 2002;99:36–43.
19. De Sousa M. Immune cell functions in iron overload. Clin Exp Immunol 1989;75:1–6.
20. Gheorghiade M, De Luka L, Fonarow GC, et al. Pathophysiologic targets in the early phase of acute heart failure syndromes. Am J Cardiol 2005; 96(suppl):11G–17G.
21. Moratelli S, De Sanctis V, Gemmati D, et al. Thrombotic risk in thalassemic patients. J Pediatr Endorinol Metab 1998;11(suppl 3):915–21.
22. Jensen CE, Tuck SM, Old J, et al. Incidence of endocrine complications and clinical disease severity related to genotype analysis and iron overload in patients with beta-thalassaemia. Eur J Haematol 1997;59:76–81.
23. Kremastinos D, Tsetsos GA, Tsiapras D, et al. Heart failure in β-thalassemia: a 5-year follow-up study. Am J Med 2001;111:349–54.
24. Zurlo MG, De Stefano P, Borgna-Pignatti C, et al. Survival and causes of death in thalassemia major. Lancet 1989;2:27–30.
25. Engle MA, Erlandson M, Smith CH. Late cardiac complications of chronic, severe, refractory anemia with hemochromatosis. Circulation 1964;30:698–705.
26. Hahalis G, Alexopoulos D, Kremastinos D, et al. Heart failure in beta-thalassemia syndromes: a decade of progress. Am J Med 2005;118:957–67.
27. Jonston DL, Rice L, Vick III GK, et al. Assessment of tissue iron overload by nuclear magnetic resonance imaging. Am J Med 1989;87:40–7.
28. Aessopos A, Farmakis D, Deftereos S, et al. Thalassemia heart disease: a comparative evaluation of thalassemia major and thalassemia intermedia. Chest 2005;127:1523–30.
29. Nienhuis AW, Hanawa H, Sawai N, et al. Development of gene therapy for hemoglobin disorders. Ann N Y Acad Sci 2003;996:101–11.

28 Acute Heart Failure and Systemic Diseases

Iris Cohen, Nadia Benyounes-Iglesias, Nadia Belmatoug, and Ariel A. Cohen

Systemic Lupus Erythematosus

Acute heart failure in systemic lupus erythematosus (SLE) may result from myocarditis, endocarditis, systemic hypertension, coronary artery disease, and left ventricular dysfunction secondary to drug toxicity. Pericarditis is an early and common cardiac manifestation of active lupus. Moderate to severe pericardial disease is infrequent (1), and constrictive pericarditis is rare. Pericardial fluid is usually exudative (1), and may contain anti-DNA antibodies, with low complement levels. Treatment includes nonsteroidal antiinflammatory drugs (NSAIDs) or corticosteroids in mild pericarditis (2). In cardiac tamponade, higher corticosteroid doses are needed, and often intravenous bolus and invasive procedures (pericardiocentesis, pericardial window, or pericardial stripping) are considered. In patients with relapsing pericarditis, methotrexate, azathioprine, and intravenous immunoglobulins (IVIGs) may be beneficial.

Myocardial involvement may be due to different mechanisms. Clinically overt myocarditis is uncommon (1). The diagnosis should be considered in patients with unexplained tachycardia, third heart sound, new murmur, or abnormal electrocardiogram (ECG) (1). Echocardiography shows nonspecific left ventricular (LV) global or segmental wall motion abnormalities, decreased left ventricular ejection fraction (LVEF), and/or increased chamber size (2). Magnetic resonance imaging (MRI) may detect asymptomatic myocardial involvement in active SLE (3).

Myocarditis is treated with high doses of corticosteroids. Cyclophosphamide or azathioprine and IVIG are used in refractory cases (2, 4). Conventional treatment of heart failure may be necessary. Response to treatment is monitored by serial transthoracic echocardiography (TTE) and sometimes by endomyocardial biopsies. In echocardiographic studies, LV systolic and diastolic dysfunctions are common, often determined by SLE duration and activity. Coronary arteritis is rare, seen in the young with active disease of short duration (2), and not receiving corticosteroids. The most common clinical presentation is angina or myocardial infarction. Arteritis is suspected when coronary aneurysms or smooth focal lesions are found, or if there are rapidly developing stenoses (5). The differential diagnosis with coronary atherosclerosis is important for treatment considerations. Arteritis is treated with high doses of corticosteroids (2), and angiographic improvement has been documented under treatment on serial angiographies.

Coronary artery disease (CAD) prevalence ranges from 6% to 20% (6, 7). Systemic lupus erythematosus patients have an increased risk for developing CAD and myocardial infarction. Presenting symptoms are angina pectoris, myocardial infarction, and sudden death. Atherosclerosis affects older SLE patients, with long-standing disease and longer corticosteroids intake. Thallium-201 scintigraphy allows the detection of asymptomatic CAD. Carotid color Doppler ultrasonography (6) and electron beam computed tomography have been used to screen for coronary artery calcification (7). For treatment in the setting of SLE, statins should be considered when the low-density lipoprotein (LDL) cholesterol is greater than 3.4 mmol/L with or without other risk factors (8). Antimalarial treatments such as hydroxychloroquine exert a beneficial effect on lipids. Anticoagulation with warfarin is indicated in SLE patients with antiphospholipid antibody syndrome. Aspirin is recommended in patients with antiphospholipid antibodies, cardiovascular events, or risk factors for CAD (9, 10).

Chloroquine-induced cardiomyopathy is seen with high drug doses and long durations of treatment. It is usually reversible after drug discontinuation (11). Patients receiving chloroquine should be evaluated with serial TTE.

Valvular disease is very common in SLE patients, ranging from valve thickening to vegetations (Libman-Sacks endocarditis). Anatomic lesions have been reported in 40% to 50% of patients in TTE studies and 50% to 60% using transesophageal echocardiography (TEE) (12, 13). Embolic events (13%), heart failure (13%), infective endocarditis (7%), and valve replacement (9%) are more prevalent in SLE patients with valvular involvement (12). Treatment entails anticoagulation for sterile vegetations (4), infective endocarditis prophylaxis, and close follow-up for hemodynamically significant lesions. In the early active phase, corticosteroids are recommended. When valve replacement is indicated, mechanical valve may be the best choice.

Case Report 1 (14)

A 23-year-old man presented with complaints of dyspnea, symmetrical arthritis, and facial exanthema. Cardiac auscultation revealed a loud systolic murmur at the apex. Laboratory evaluation was positive for antinuclear and antibodies to double-stranded DNA (dsDNA) antibodies. Lupus anticoagulants and anticardiolipin antibodies were negative. The TTE and TEE showed severe mitral regurgitation (MR). A LV thrombus was present, embedding the posterior leaflet, with valve destruction. Libman-Sacks endocarditis was diagnosed, along with SLE. Immunosuppressive treatment with high doses of prednisolone and five cycles of cyclophosphamide decreased LV thrombus size, and mitral valve repair was performed.

Antiphospholipid Syndrome and Heart Failure

The antiphospholipid syndrome (APS) is defined by pregnancy morbidity, occurring in the presence of antiphospholipid (aPL) antibodies, anticardiolipin (aCL) antibodies, or positive lupus anticoagulant (LAC) test (15).

Heart failure may result from valvular abnormalities (regurgitant lesions, infective and noninfective endocarditis), myocardial infarction (MI) with intact coronary arteries (thrombotic or embolic), in the context of primary or secondary APS, or in the rare catastrophic antiphospholipid (CAPL) syndrome, CAD, and LV dysfunction (ongoing chronic thrombotic events, or CAPL) (16, 17).

Table 28.1 summarizes the findings and recommendations for the various cardiac manifestations in APS (16, 18, 19).

Case Report 2 (20)

A 17-year-old boy was hospitalized with cardiogenic shock. Three days prior to admission, he had fever (38.3°C), pain in the upper abdomen, and painless hematuria. The urinary protein level was 100 mg/dL. Laboratory data: hematocrit of 33%, white blood cell count of 23,500/dL, erythrocyte sedimentation rate (ESR) of 135 mm/h, prothrombin time of 14.7 seconds, partial thromboplastin time <100 seconds, positive D-dimer test, and aspartate aminotransferase of 209 U/L.

At admission, there was a grade 3/6 holosystolic apical murmur. The TTE disclosed severe mitral regurgitation. On TEE, there was a bivalvular prolapse, resulting in severe mitral regurgitation. There was no ruptured chordae or vegetations. The posteromedial papillary muscle appeared echodense, thinned, and elongated. The LV size was normal, but LVEF was mildly impaired. Coronary arteries were normal.

Diagnostic hypotheses for this acute onset of severe MR with fever, hematuria, hemolysis, and coagulopathy were inflammatory or rheumatologic disease, infectious disease, or MI. The mitral valve was replaced by a mechanical St. Jude Medical prosthesis. On gross pathologic

TABLE 28.1. Cardiac involvement in antiphospholipid syndrome (APS)

Abnormality	Prevalence in APS	Prevalence of antiphospholipid (aPL)	Strength of data	Panel treatment consensus
Valve disease	35–50% (6% in TTE study, 82% in TEE)	35–50%	Many TEE and TTE population studies	Anticoagulation for *symptomatic* patients with valvulopathy Prophylactic antiplatelet therapy may be appropriate for hemodynamically stable *asymptomatic* patients (no history of vascular or pregnancy events) Corticosteroids?? Distinguishing among valvulitis, valve alterations, and vegetations is important as treatment implications may differ
Coronary occlusion	5%	5.9%	Population studies, primarily of SLE patients	Aggressive treatment of all risk factors for atherosclerosis, consider hydroxychloroquine and statins Anticoagulation for nonatherosclerotic thrombosis (antiplatelet agents instead?)
Ventricular dysfunction	No reliable figures	23–32% in SLE No reliable figures in APS	Case studies not segregated by APS status; SLE population studies	No known effective treatment and no recommendations
Intracardiac thrombi	No reliable figures	No reliable figures	Case reports	Anticoagulation ± surgical excision
Pulmonary hypertension	1–3%	4% (symptomatic) Up to 14% (asymptomatic)	Population studies using TTE	Anticoagulation, consider endothelial antagonists epoprostenol

SLE, systemic lupus erythematosus; TEE, transesophageal echocardiography; TTE, transthoracic echocardiography.

examination, the papillary muscle was ruptured at the base, and there were areas of focal hemorrhage consistent with infarction. Within the myocardium, arterioles were occluded by thrombi with fibrin and platelets.

Additional laboratory results were as follows: LAC was negative but became positive during follow-up and aCL (immunoglobulin G [IgG] and IgM) were high at 1:64 (normal is <1:15). Later, a high titer of IgG antibodies against β_2-glycoprotein I confirmed the diagnosis APS. Antinuclear antibodies (ANAs) were positive (1:320), with a speckled pattern. Antibodies to dsDNA were absent, but elevated titers of antibodies against ribonucleoprotein (RNP) antigens (anti-RNP, anti-Sm, anti-La, and anti-Ro) were detected by enzyme-linked immunosorbent assay (ELISA).

This case report illustrates primary APS. The prevalence of aPL is 2–5% in the general population. The prevalence of LAC and Acl in SLE patients is 15–34% and 12–30% respectively. Primary APS as opposed to secondary is not related to any connective tissue disease, or other diseases. In this case report SLE was suspected, but only three out of four needed were met at that point of the disease course (arthritis, antiphospholpid antibodies and ANA).

The criteria for the diagnosis of SLE is that four or more of the following must be met either simultaneously or sequentially: malar rash, discoid rash, photosensitivity, oral ulcers, arthritis (tenderness or swelling, involving two or more peripheral joints), serositis (pleuritis or pericarditis), renal disorder (indicated by persistent proteinuria or the presence of cellular casts), nephrotic syndrome (seizures or psychosis), Hematologic disorder (indicated by the presence of anti DNA, anti-Sm, or antiphospholipid antibodies), and antinuclear antibodies (ANA).

Catastrophic Antiphospholipid Syndrome

The catastrophic antiphospholipid (CAPL) syndrome is an extreme example of the thrombotic effects, affecting less than 1% of APS patients (16, 17). It is characterized by a widespread coagulopathy, affecting predominantly the small vessels. The thrombotic process may be spontaneous or triggered (21). Thrombocytopenia and microangiopathic anemia are frequent.

Clinical symptomatology is related to the extent of thrombotic process. Kidneys are involved in up to 70% (16, 17). Hypertension is often malignant and accelerated, and is the main feature. Acute respiratory distress syndrome (ARDS) dominates pulmonary involvement. Initial confusion and disorientation or coma may be seen, as well as focal signs, mononeuritis multiplex, and retinal vascular involvement. Skin manifestations of microvascular occlusive disease include livedo reticularis, gangrene, and superficial skin necrosis. Cardiac manifestations of the microangiopathy include a reduction in LVEF and MI.

Usually the clinical evidence of vessel occlusion is confirmed by imaging techniques when appropriate. Renal involvement is defined by a 50% rise in serum creatinine, severe systemic hypertension (>180/100 mm Hg), or proteinuria (>500 mg/24 hours). For histopathologic confirmation, significant thrombosis must be present, although vasculitis may coexist occasionally. If the patient had not been previously diagnosed as having APS, laboratory confirmation requires the presence of aPL, detected on two or more occasions at least 6 weeks apart (not necessarily at the time of the event), according to the proposed preliminary criteria for the classification of definite APS (15).

Despite appropriate treatment, mortality reaches 50% (21). First-line therapies include anticoagulation with intravenous heparin and high doses of steroids. Intravenous immunoglobulin (IVIG), plasma exchange (PE), and fresh frozen plasma (FFP) are indicated in the extensive clotting process. Cyclophosphamide, prostacyclin, ancrod (a powerful fibrinolytic), and defibrotide (a potent inhibitor of endothelin I, thrombin-induced platelet aggregation, and thromboxane synthesis) are considered as third-line therapies. Fibrinolytics may be used in life-threatening situations of ongoing clotting (21).

Prophylaxis in APS patients should include parenteral anticoagulation before any surgical procedure, and prompt treatment of infections is mandatory.

Rheumatoid Arthritis and Heart Failure

The cardiovascular system can be the site of extraarticular manifestations of rheumatoid arthritis (RA). All cardiac structures may be involved. Cardiovascular diseases (CVDs) represent 35% to 50% of total mortality in RA. Classic risk factors do not explain this excess of CVD (22–24). Heart failure is either due to cardiac involvement of RA or may result from treatment side effects. Table 28.2 summarizes the potential cardiovascular side effects of RA medications.

Adverse event reports to the U.S. Food and Drug Administration's (FDA) Med Watch system were examined (25) for evidence that tumor necrosis factor (TNF) antagonists may exacerbate heart failure or promote new-onset congestive heart failure (CHF). Accordingly, the following recommendations were formulated (26):

Rheumatoid arthritis patients with no history of CHF and concomitant indication for anti–TNF-α do not need a baseline cardiac evaluation.

Patients with well-compensated mild CHF (New York Heart Association [NYHA] class I and II) and concomitant indications for anti–TNF-α should be evaluated at baseline and then closely monitored.

Patients with NYHA class III or IV heart failure should not be treated with TNF-α blockers.

TABLE 28.2. Potential cardiovascular side effects of rheumatoid arthritis (RA) medications (28)

Medication	Potential cardiovascular side effects
Conventional nonsteroidal antiinflammatory drugs	Fluid retention Hypertension
Selective COX-2 inhibitors	Fluid retention Hypertension Prothrombotic?
Steroids	Dyslipidemia? Hyperglycemia Hypertension
Gold	Increase in LDL and HDL cholesterol
Sulfasalazine	Hyperhomocystinemia?
TNF-α antagonists	Exacerbate heart failure?

COX, cyclooxygenase; TNF, tumor necrosis factor; HDL, high-density lipoprotein; LDL, low-density lipoprotein.

Case Report 3 (27)

A 60-year-old man was admitted for dyspnea. His medical history included hypertension treated with verapamil, and RA managed with prednisone (5 mg daily) and methotrexate. Six months before admission, etanercept was substituted for methotrexate. Physical examination demonstrated inspiratory crackles at lung bases, a trace of pedal edema, and rheumatoid deformities prominent in the hands. The ECG showed atrial flutter with high-degree atrioventricular block and ventricular ectopic beats, while thorax x-ray showed bilateral pleural effusions but no pericardial calcifications. At TTE he had normal LV size and systolic function. Abrupt cessation of diastolic relaxation, septal bounce (ventricular interdependence), and slight left atrial enlargement were described. Mitral and tricuspid inflows varied by approximately 25% with respiration suggesting a diastolic syndrome. Right ventricular (RV) size and function were normal. The estimated RV systolic pressure was 35 mm Hg. Right atrial pressure was elevated (dilated inferior vena cava and hepatic veins). Cardiac catheterization showed a hemodynamics profile consistent with constriction, and coronary angiography revealed minimal coronary atherosclerosis. The MRI revealed regional pericardial thickening. Endomyocardial biopsy was negative for myocarditis, vasculitis, and amyloidosis.

Pericardiectomy was performed. The pericardial specimen was thickened, with focal calcification. Multiple rheumatoid nodules were found within the pericardium.

Pericardial involvement is the most prevalent feature of cardiac involvement in RA. It is often asymptomatic. Recent echocardiographic studies report pericardial effusion in 1% to 30% (28), usually associated with an increased disease activity. The fluid is exudative, containing leukocytes, lactate dehydrogenase, and a low concentration of glucose. Chronic inflammation may lead to constrictive pericarditis. Pericardial calcification is rare.

Treatment includes NSAID and sometimes a short course of steroids. The need for invasive procedures such as pericardiocentesis depends on the hemodynamic tolerance.

Endocardial involvement is frequent but usually asymptomatic. Nonspecific diffuse thickening and calcification at the base of the valve (the mitral valve more than the aortic valve) and valve ring (5–30%), usually asymptomatic (29), have been reported.

Sarcoidosis and Heart Failure

Myocardial involvement occurs in at least 25% of patients and accounts for 13 to 25% of deaths from sarcoidosis in the U.S. (30). In Japan, sarcoid heart disease is more common. Pathologic features are noncaseating granulomas. The myocardium is by far the most frequently involved, followed by the pericardium and endocardium. The predominant sites of involvement in decreasing order of frequency are the LV free wall and papillary muscles, the basal septum, the RV free wall, and the atrial walls (31, 32).

Cardiac involvement includes conduction abnormalities (atrioventricular and bundle branch blocks), mitral regurgitation, congestive heart failure, ventricular aneurysms, pericarditis, pericardial effusion and tamponade, supraventricular and ventricular arrhythmias, and sudden death (31).

Conduction abnormalities are common manifestations in cardiac sarcoidosis (31). Complete heart block occurs in 23% to 30% of patients. Right bundle branch block (RBBB) is more common than left bundle branch block. Sustained and nonsustained ventricular tachycardia (VT) and frequent ventricular ectopy are detected in 23% of patients (32). Antiarrhythmic drug therapy of VT remains associated with a high rate of arrhythmia recurrence and sudden death (33).

Small pericardial effusion has been described on TTE in 3% to 19% of sarcoid patients. Symptomatic pericarditis, tamponade, and constrictive pericarditis are rare (32).

Congestive heart failure (CHF) is the second most frequent cause of sarcoid-related mortality after sudden death. Progressive CHF causes death in 25% of case (32). Cardiac infiltration by sarcoid granulomas may result in restrictive or dilated cardiomyopathy.

Mitral regurgitation is the most common valvular abnormality. Valvular dysfunction due to papillary muscle involvement is more frequent than direct destruction of valvular leaflets. Aortic, tricuspid, and pulmonic valve involvement are rare (31).

Cardiac involvement is associated with a poor prognosis. Mortality rates may exceed 40% at 5 years and 55% at 10 years (34). Due to steroid therapy and devices (pacemakers), the main cause of mortality has shifted from sudden death to CHF. Predictors of mortality are the absence of steroid treatment, NHYA functional class, LV end diastolic diameter, and sustained VT. Survival is shortened in comparison with idiopathic dilated cardiomyopathy patients (35).

Hiraga et al. (36) published guidelines for the diagnosis of cardiac sarcoidosis (Table 28.3). Endomyocardial biopsy is highly specific but lacks sensitivity and is invasive. Biopsy findings of non-caseating granulomas were reported in 20% to 50% of patients with clinically diagnosed cardiac sarcoidosis (37).

Transthoracic echocardiography should be routinely performed in all systemic sarcoidosis. Asymptomatic LV anomalies exist in 24% to 31% of cases. Transthoracic echocardiography abnormalities correlate well with the histologic indications of cardiac sarcoidosis: interventricular septal thickening, global left ventricular hypertrophy (LVH), diminished LVEF, LV dilatation, anomalies of mitral papillary muscle, and diastolic dysfunction (38).

Table 28.3. Guidelines for diagnosing cardiac sarcoidosis (36)

1. Histologic diagnosis group
   Cardiac sarcoidosis is confirmed when histologic analysis of operative or endomyocardial biopsy specimens demonstrates epithelioid granuloma without caseating granuloma
2. Clinical diagnosis group
   In patients with a histologic diagnosis of extracardiac sarcoidosis, cardiac sarcoidosis is suspected when item (a), below, and one or more items from (b) through (e) are present:
   (a) Complete right bundle branch block, left axis deviation, atrioventricular block, ventricular tachycardia, premature ventricular contractions or abnormal Q or ST-T changes on ECG or ambulatory ECG
   (b) Abnormal wall motion, regional wall thinning or dilatation of the left ventricle (LV) on TTE
   (c) Perfusion defect on thallium-201 myocardial scintigraphy or abnormal accumulation on gallium-67 or technetium-99m myocardial scintigraphy
   (d) Abnormal intracardiac pressures, low cardiac output or depressed left ventricular ejection fraction (LVEF)
   (e) Interstitial fibrosis or cellular infiltration over moderate grade (even these findings are nonspecific)

Resting thallium-201 scintigraphy typically shows segmental areas of decreased uptake in ventricular myocardium. Reverse distribution may help in differentiating cardiac sarcoidosis from ischemic heart disease and improve specificity. Thallium-201 scintigraphy sensibility in detecting cardiac sarcoidosis ranges from 32% to 58% (39–41). Gallium-67 accumulates in areas of active inflammation and is positive in active disease. Positron emission tomography with ^{18}F-fluorodeoxyglucose (FDG) shows a sensitivity of 100% for the detection of cardiac sarcoidosis (41).

Contrast magnetic resonance (CMR) is useful in the early detection of cardiac sarcoidosis (39, 42). The sensitivity of CMR approaches 100% for the diagnosis, and specificity is nearly 78%. Treatment initially includes 60 to 80 mg of prednisone daily. The dose is tapered gradually to a maintenance level of 10 to 15 mg per day over a period of 6 months (34, 39). Alternative agents such as methotrexate and azathioprine may be given to nonresponders. Antiarrhythmic drugs are sometimes needed, but beta-blockers may exacerbate heart blocks and amiodarone may exacerbate restrictive lung disease (39). Thus, pacemaker implantation is common. In refractory ventricular arrhythmias, an implantable cardioverter defibrillator (ICD) is mandatory (39). Cardiac transplantation is considered in refractory CHF or resistant VT (43).

Case Report 4 (44)

A 58-year-old African woman was admitted with NYHA III dyspnea and lower extremity edema. A TTE performed 2 years prior showed LVEF of 65%. Physical examination at admission revealed bibasilar lung rales and a 4/6 holosystolic murmur at the apex. On TTE, concentric LVH, moderate right ventricular dysfunction, severe MR and tricuspid regurgitation (TR), and LVEF of 60% were noted. The TEE showed a structurally normal mitral valve, with papillary muscle dysfunction.

Mitral valve replacement and tricuspid annuloplasty were performed. Biopsies from the pericardium and papillary muscles were obtained, revealing noncaseating granulomas consistent with sarcoidosis. Postoperatively, the patient developed numerous episodes of non-sustained

VT, for which amiodarone was started. Complete heart block followed, with dual-chamber pacemaker implantation. High doses of corticosteroids were initiated. Treatment led to dramatic clinical and TTE improvement.

Hypereosinophilic Syndrome and Heart Failure

Hypereosinophilic syndrome (HES) is defined as persistent eosinophilia of 1.5×10^9/L (1500/mm^3) for longer than 6 months, lack of evidence of parasitic, allergic, or other known causes of hypereosinophilia, and signs and symptoms of organ involvement (45). Cardiovascular system is involved in 58% (46).

Cardiac involvement generally evolves in three stages:

In the first or necrotic stage, eosinophilic myocarditis develops due to eosinophilic myocardial and endocardial infiltration, leading to microabscesses.

The second or thrombotic stage is characterized by the formation of thrombi along the damaged endocardium of either or both ventricles and occasionally the atria. Thrombi may also form on the atrioventricular valve leaflets.

The third or fibrotic stage includes mural thrombi and fibrous thickening of the endocardium. Entrapment of leaflets and chordae tendineae cordis may cause MR, TR, or both (47).

Clinical manifestations include CHF (18%), atrioventricular valve regurgitation, arrhythmias, restrictive cardiomyopathy, embolic events (16%), and nonspecific T wave inversion on ECG (48). The frequency of death reaches 33% (48).

The most common findings on echocardiography are ventricular apical obliteration, posterior mitral valve thickening with absent or markedly limited motion leading to mitral regurgitation (48), and atrial enlargement (Table 28.4). Pericardial effusion is seen in CHF, and RV and LV end-diastolic pressures are usually elevated (49).

Magnetic resonance imaging and computed tomography may add information on the presence of LV thrombi and the extent of the subendocardial infiltration, and may localize the site for endomyocardial biopsy (47). Endomyocardial biopsy is the gold standard for diagnosing eosinophilic endomyocardial disease. However, RV biopsy sampling may miss the left-sided disease (48, 49).

Table 28.4. Differential echocardiographic features of hypereosinophilic syndrome (HES)

Chronic parietal endocarditis
Chronic parietal endocarditis and endomyocardial fibrosis (EMF):
• Infiltration of the LV apex, papillary muscle involvement
• No LV dilatation
• Biatrial dilatation
• Normal LV systolic function
• Valvular abnormalities related to papillary muscles infiltration
• Atrioventricular regurgitation or stenosis
• LV apical thrombus
• Restrictive inflow pattern of the mitral and tricuspid valves
EMF is left sided, right sided, or biventricular.
Eosinophilic myocarditis
• LV systolic dysfunction
• LV dilatation
• Myocardial infiltration
• Equalization of RV pressures
• Restrictive inflow pattern of the mitral and tricuspid valves

LV, left ventricular; RV, right ventricular.

In advanced HES with CHF, a median survival of 9 months and a 3-year survival of 12% have been reported (46). In later HES reports, the 5-year survival rate was 80%, decreasing to 42% at 15 years (45). Poor prognostic factors were a concurrent myeloproliferative syndrome, lack of response to corticosteroids, cardiac involvement, male sex, and the importance of eosinophilia. First-line treatment includes corticosteroids and hydroxyurea (50). Vincristine, pulsed chlorambucil, cyclophosphamide, and etoposide are proposed as second-line agents. Interferon-α is used when HES is resistant to other therapies (46). Imatinib mesylate (46, 51) has shown promising results. Allogenic bone marrow transplantation may be necessary (46).

Cardiac surgery may be performed in extensive endomyocardial fibrosis (EMF) with valvular insufficiency. Operative mortality (endomyocardectomy or endocardial decortication) reaches 16% to 20% in univentricular disease and 40% in biventricular. Anticoagulants and antiplatelet agents have shown variable success in preventing recurrent thromboembolism (46).

Scleroderma and Heart Failure

Systemic sclerosis (SSc) or scleroderma is a generalized disorder of connective tissue, characterized by thickening and fibrosis of the skin and the involvement of internal organs, such as the heart, lungs, kidneys, and gastrointestinal tract (52–59).

Heart involvement is either primary or secondary to lung or kidney involvement and has serious implications on the prognosis of the disease.

The clinical symptoms of heart involvement may be difficult to distinguish from other SSc complications symptoms. Congestive heart failure is rare (59). Table 28.5 summarizes the clinical symptoms of heart involvement.

Clinically symptomatic pericardial disease (5% to 16%) is less frequent than that reported in autopsy studies (53, 54). The presence of small (<50 mL) pericardial effusions does not affect prognosis, while a large effusion (>200 mL) is associated with poor prognosis (55). Tamponade is rare.

Myocardial fibrosis of both ventricles is the hallmark of cardiac involvement. Subsets of patients with SSc have features of polymyositis, such as proximal muscle weakness, elevations of creatine phosphokinase (CPK), aldolase, and an abnormal electromyogram. Muscle biopsy reveals fibrosis and inflammation. Patients with an elevated CPK at any time have an increased frequency of cardiac dysfunction, CHF, and cardiac death (56).

Thallium perfusion defects, suggesting coronary artery disease, are reported in 71% to 100% of patients, despite normal coronary arteries (57). The effects of vasodilators on thallium perfusion abnormalities have been studied (57). Most of the defects did not improve, due to fibrosis. The reversible component may imply vasospasm.

Decreased coronary vasodilator reserve has been documented in SSc at catheterization (58). Valvular disease in uncommon. Nodular thickening (54) is seen in the mitral valve. Mitral (and tricuspid) valve vegetations have been described. Aortic valve involvement is rare.

Nearly half SSc patients have abnormal resting ECG (59). Only conduction defects and septal Q waves appear to be more frequent in scleroderma population after adjustment for sex and age. The frequency of conduction and rhythm abnormalities increases when ambulatory 24-hour ECG is used. Reduced heart rate variability on ambulatory 24-hour ECG suggests autonomic cardiac neuropathy and may represent an important prognostic feature (59). Exercise-induced atrial and ventricular arrhythmias were reported in more advanced myocardial disease, acting as a substrate for ectopy (59). Ventricular ectopy on 24-hour ambulatory monitoring is associated with increased total and sudden mortality (60). Abnormal signal-averaged ECG does not seem to be a good predictor of threatening VT.

TABLE 28.5. Clinical symptoms in scleroderma heart involvement (53, 59)

Physiopathologic alterations	Clinical symptoms	Treatments
Right–left ventricular dysfunction	Fatigue	ACE inhibitors, Ca-channel blockers
Pulmonary hypertension	Dyspnea	Prostanoids, sildenafil, bosentan
Congestive heart failure (rare)	Edema Venous congestion	Diuretics
Pericarditis	Chest pain	Steroids
Angina pectoris (rare)	Chest pain	Ca-channel blockers
Autonomic cardiac neuropathy	Palpitations	Antiarrhythmics
Rhythm disturbances	Dizziness Sudden death	Radiofrequency ablation Implantable cardioverter defibrillator
Conduction defects	Syncope	Pacemaker

ACE, angiotensin-converting enzyme; Ca, calcium.

Pulmonary hypertension (PH) is either secondary to pulmonary fibrosis or a pure manifestation of pulmonary arterial vascular disease. It occurs as an isolated event in the CREST syndrome (calcinosis cutis, Raynaud's phenomenon, esophageal motility disorder, sclerodactyly, and telangiectasia), and complicates pulmonary fibrosis in diffuse SSc. The prevalence of PH varies from 8% to 18% (61) and depends on diagnostic tools (Doppler echocardiography versus catheterization). It carries a particularly adverse prognosis (62, 63).

Left ventricular hypertrophy has been reported in the absence of systemic hypertension (64). The videodensitometric parameters, in particular those of the septum and posterior wall, are significantly lower in SSc patients, in relation to the fibrotic process (64). Left ventricular systolic dysfunction is not frequent (64). Segmental LV abnormalities have been reported in about 32% of limited scleroderma patients and about 22% of patients with diffuse SSc. The transmitral flow observed is that of impaired relaxation. On stress tests, a reduction in LVEF has been documented in 80% of SSc patients with impaired relaxation on TTE (64). Diastolic dysfunction depends on the severity of the disease and may precede the anatomic remodeling changes. On tissue Doppler imaging (TDI), an alteration of longitudinal myocardial fibers deformation was reported.

A decrease in RV ejection fraction has been reported (65). Pulsed tissue Doppler imaging applied to the tricuspid annulus enables evaluation of RV systolic function and filling pressures. Adverse prognostic factors in SSc are related to the extent of cutaneous sclerosis; the presence of one or more visceral organ involvement, mainly lungs, heart, or kidneys; male gender; diffuse cutaneous involvement; serum anti-Scl 70 antibodies (while anticentromere antibodies seem to be "protective" for severe visceral involvement); PH; right heart failure; and rhythm and conduction disturbances (66).

Mixed Connective Tissue Disease (Overlap Syndrome) and Heart Failure

Mixed connective tissue disease (MCTD) combines clinical features of SLE, polymyositis-dermatomyositis (PM/DM), and scleroderma. The characteristic laboratory abnormalities are high titer (>1:1000), speckled ANAs, high levels of anti RNAse-sensitive extractable nuclear antigen antibodies, and the presence of autoantibodies against small nuclear RNP (snRNP) (67).

Cardiac involvement has been reported in 11% to 85% of MCTD patients (68).

Acute symptomatic pericarditis, paucisymptomatic pericardial effusions (10–30% in TTE studies), and chronic pericarditis have been reported (69). Tamponade is rare. Mild pericarditis is treated with NSAIDs (indomethacin). If symptoms persist, corticosteroids are added. Percutaneous or surgical drainage is performed in the rare cases of tamponade (70).

Myocardial involvement results either from inflammatory myocarditis or from coronary vasculitis. The first may account for 13% of deaths in MCTD. Acute myocarditis is treated with corticosteroids, in association with CHF conventional therapy. Cyclophosphamide may be added in severe cases (70).

Mitral valve prolapse and regurgitation have been reported in 26% of cases (68), as have aortic calcifications. Pulmonary hypertension is more prevalent in MCTD when diffusing capacity on pulmonary function tests is altered. It is associated with higher morbidity and mortality (71). Mortality rates range from 4% to 36% in patients with disease duration of 6 to 12 years. Death results mainly from PH and severe infections (72).

Amyloidosis and Heart Failure

Amyloidosis is classified as primary, secondary, hereditary, and age related (73, 74). Primary (idiopathic, systemic) amyloidosis appears with no coexistent disease and involves the cardiovascular system (73). Secondary (reactive) amyloidosis is associated with chronic diseases. Heart involvement is rare (73). Hereditary amyloidosis has mostly an autosomal dominant inheritance. Cardiac involvement is rare and occurs late in the disease (73). Age-related (elderly) amyloidosis includes the isolated atrial form and the systemic senile type.

Primary Amyloidosis

Symptoms of amyloidosis are nonspecific. The prevalence of cardiac involvement ranges from

45% to 80% and carries a poor prognosis. Clinical signs include dyspnea, fatigue or weakness, chest pain, orthopnea or paroxysmal nocturne dyspnea, syncope, palpitations, peripheral arterial thrombosis, hypotension, hypertension, atrial fibrillation, tachycardia, peripheral edema, and third heart sound (75).

The ECG is abnormal in 90% of cases (Table 28.6). A TTE is crucial in the detection of myocardial involvement, even in the absence of any clinical sign. Table 28.7 summarizes TTE findings in amyloidosis (75). Parietal wall thickness has prognostic implications (76). An impaired relaxation pattern was noted when LV wall thickness was 12 to 15 mm. Restrictive transmitral pattern was noted when the mean parietal wall thickness was >15 mm (78). Increased left atrial pressures are documented in advanced disease (77), using transmitral and pulmonary venous flows in association with TDI at the mitral annulus. Transmitral flow and the Tei index (80) are powerful mortality predictors in histologically proven cardiac amyloidosis.

The RV free wall thickness may increase over 7 mm in advanced cardiac amyloidosis (79). Right ventricular dilatation is a strong predictor of mortality (80,81). Transtricuspid flow reflects diastolic RV function (79). Pulmonary insufficiency flow shows a dip plateau aspect in restrictive cardiomyopathy.

Tissue Doppler and strain imaging have been used for early detection of cardiac involvement in familial amyloidotic polyneuropathy (FAP) (82, 83), before morphologic changes occur.

Table 28.6. Electrocardiogram modifications in amyloidosis AL according to Dubrey et al. (75)

Electrocardiographic (ECG) findings	$n = 232$	%
Abnormal ECG	223	96
Left axis deviation	82	35
Right axis deviation	35	15
Low precordial QRS voltage*	164	71
Pseudoinfarct pattern	171	75
—Inferior leads	46	20
—Anteroseptal leads	125	55
—Inferior and anteroseptal leads	29	13
Conduction abnormalities**	82	36

*Low voltage is defined as QRS amplitude ≤0.5 mV in all limb leads or ≤1 mV in all precordial leads.

**Ventricular and supraventricular arrhythmias are also seen.

Table 28.7. Echocardiographic findings in AL amyloidosis

Echocardiographic criteria	%
Thickened interventricular septum	87
Sparkling appearance of the myocardium	64
Thickened right ventricular free wall	44
Pericardial effusion	44
Left atrial enlargement	46
Biatrial enlargement	47
Thickened interatrial septum	39
Thickened valve leaflets with minimal regurgitation	66
Atrial and ventricular thrombi	26

Source: modified from Dubrey et al. (75).

Moderate pericardial effusion is seen in 44% of AL amyloidosis (75). Cardiac tamponade and constrictive pericarditis are rare.

If performed, radionuclide cardiac imaging with technetium-99m is usually abnormal and correlates with the degree of amyloidal infiltration (83). Imaging with antimyosine antibodies is positive in patients with cardiac amyloidosis (84). Imaging with radiolabeled amyloid P protein allows the localization and the quantification of the amyloid infiltration.

Magnetic resonance imaging localizes the amyloidal infiltration (85) and improves the differentiation between amyloidosis and hypertrophic cardiomyopathy. The standard methods for demonstrating amyloid deposition are rectal, abdominal fat, gingival, and salivary glands biopsies (74). In the presence of extracardiac amyloidosis (positive biopsy), endomyocardial biopsy is not essential when cardiac amyloidosis is suspected on clinical, ECG, and TTE signs (86). Endomyocardial biopsy remains the gold standard for the diagnosis of cardiac amyloidosis when noninvasive tests are not contributive (86).

Cardiac Involvement in Other Forms of Amyloidosis

AA amyloidosis (AAA) is a secondary amyloidosis, complicating chronic inflammation such as rheumatic diseases, Crohn's disease, and infections. Cardiac involvement is rare (87–89), and cardiac symptoms are usually related to systemic hypertension, occurring in 20% to 40%, as a complication of renal injury.

In age-related amyloidosis, cardiac involvement does not carry a grave prognosis (74, 90). Age-related amyloidosis is a common postmortem finding in the elderly. Atrial natriuretic peptide is the major protein subunit of the amyloid fibril. Patients are more likely to develop atrial fibrillation.

The prevalence of senile systemic amyloidosis reaches 25% over the age of 80 years. The major constituent of the amyloid fibrils is derived from normal transthyretin (TTR). In hereditary (familial) amyloidosis, several variants with cardiac involvement have been described, characterized by severe heart failure and arrhythmias (74, 90, 91).

Prognosis

Prognosis varies according to the type of amyloidosis, the stage of the disease, and the age of the patient at the time of diagnosis. Primary amyloidosis has the worst prognosis, with cardiac and multisystem involvement (92, 93).

Serum levels of N-terminal (NT)-pro–B-type natriuretic peptide (pro-BNP) >152 pmol/L demonstrate 93% sensitivity for the detection of significant cardiac involvement in AL amyloidosis and represent a powerful prognostic factor (94). Table 28.8 summarizes the clinical and echocardiographic prognostic parameters in AL amyloidosis.

Treatment depends on amyloidosis classification. Digoxin, verapamil, and nifedipine should be avoided (74). Primary AL amyloidosis is treated with chemotherapy or stem-cell transplantation. Melphalan and prednisone have proven benefit from randomized trials (95). Further alternative drugs under consideration are vincristine and interferon-α.

Secondary amyloidosis requires aggressive treatment of the underlying cause. Stem cell transplantation produces dramatic results in carefully selected AL amyloidosis, but cardiac involvement seems to be an exclusion criterion (96). The familial form of amyloidosis (FAP) can be managed successfully with liver transplantation (97). Combined heart and liver transplantation appears promising when the heart is involved.

Cardiac transplantation in cardiac AL amyloidosis remains controversial (98). Recurrence of amyloidosis in the cardiac allograft (99) and the progression in other organs have been reported. Patients transplanted for cardiac amyloidosis have reduced survival compared with those transplanted for other conditions.

Human Leukocyte Antigen B27 and Heart Failure

The association between human leukocyte antigen (HLA) B27 and ankylosing spondylitis (AS) is strong, about 90%, and the primary cause of death

TABLE 28.8. Clinical and echocardiographic prognostic parameters in AL amyloidosis

Prognostic markers	Author, year	No. of patients	Mean survival (months)
Clinical			
Cardiac localization	Kyle, 1995 (92)	474	13.2
Heart failure	Kyle, 1995 (92)	80	4
Cardiac localization	Dubrey, 1998 (75)	258	13
Heart failure	Dubrey, 1998 (75)	161	9
Doppler echocardiography			
Wall thickness >15 mm	Cueto-Garcia, 1985 (76)	132	5
Wall thickness <12 mm	Cueto-Garcia, 1985 (76)		28
Wall thickness >15 mm	Kyle, 1995 (92)	121 (57)	7
Wall thickness <15 mm	Kyle, 1995 (92)	121 (64)	26
Deceleration time <150 ms	Klein, 1991 (78)	60 (3)	11
E/A >2	Klein, 1991 (78)	60 (15)	–
RV dilatation	Patel, 1997 (81)	37 (25)	4
Tei index	Kim, 2004 (80)	30	–

E/A on transmitral flow >2. E, left ventricular filling during early diastole; A, left ventricular filling during atrial contraction.

TABLE 28.9. Diseases associated with human leukocyte antigen (HLA) B27

Disease	Frequency
Ankylosing spondylitis (AS)	>90%
Reiter's syndrome	70–90%
Psoriatic spondylitis	60–70%
Peripheral psoriatic arthritis	25%
Guttate psoriasis	
Psoriasis vulgaris	6–8%
IBD with spondylitis	50–60%
IBD with sacroiliitis	6–8%
IBD with peripheral arthritis	6–8%
IBD	6–8%
Acute anterior uveitis	70%
Cardiac conduction defects (requiring pacemaker)	15–20%
Isolated* aortic insufficiency (with concomitant aortic stenosis)	15%

IBD, inflammatory bowel disease.
*Not related to an arthropathy.

in AS remains cardiovascular (100). Table 28.9 outlines the diseases associated with HLA B27 (100). HLA B27–associated cardiac abnormalities are aortic root dilatation, valvular regurgitation (aortic more than mitral), atrioventricular blocks, myocardial disease, and rarely pericarditis (101, 102). Most AS patients >45 years old with a disease duration >15 years have aortic root or valve disease, with dynamic evolution, related to intermittent, recurrent, or persistent aortitis or valvulitis (103). Young AS patients have a high mortality, due to cardiovascular and cerebral events (104).

Conduction abnormalities are frequent in AS, diagnosed either in asymptomatic or symptomatic patients having dizziness, syncope, or persistent congestive heart failure (105). A pacemaker is indicated in symptomatic patients. Left ventricular systolic dysfunction has been reported in 18% of AS (106), while diastolic dysfunction using transmitral flow profiles has been described in 20% to 53% (107, 108).

Pericardial involvement is common; minimal effusion is reported in 42% of AS patients by TTE (108).

Hemochromatosis and Heart Failure

Hereditary hemochromatosis is characterized by increased iron absorption from the duodenum and upper intestine, with consequent deposition in various parenchymal organs, including the heart (74, 109, 110). Clinical manifestations often occur at the age of 40 to 60 years, and symptomatic disease is 10 times more common in males than in females. *HFE* is the candidate gene. Two missense mutations were initially identified, the *C282Y* and the *H63D* mutations. In 178 phenotypic hereditary hemochromatosis (HH) patients, 83% were homozygous for *C282Y* and 4% were heterozygous *(C282Y/H63D)*. A minority (11%) of compound heterozygous *(C282Y/H63D)* develop clinical symptoms of hemochromatosis. Juvenile hemochromatosis is rare and severe (109, 110).

The diagnosis of hemochromatosis has to be considered in patients with unexplained hepatomegaly, abnormal skin pigmentation, idiopathic cardiomyopathy, arthritis, diabetes, or loss of libido.

Signs and symptoms of heart failure are often the first manifestations of cardiac involvement. It is usually of rapid onset, with predominant right heart failure and less often CHF. The main cause of death is cardiomyopathy. The ECG modifications are not specific but may be observed in 70% of patients with heart failure (109, 110).

At TTE, the left ventricle is usually dilated, without significant increase in wall thickness. Left ventricular systolic dysfunction occurs in the late stages of the disease (111, 112). Restrictive transmitral pattern is predominant in symptomatic patients.

An MRI detects the presence of iron deposition in various tissues. It is a tool for early diagnosis and monitoring of iron-deposition cardiomyopathy (113). Endomyocardial biopsy in patients with unexplained cardiomyopathy has a sensitivity and a specificity of 100% for the diagnosis of hemochromatosis (114). In those with diagnosed hemochromatosis, cardiac involvement is assessed by TTE and MRI.

Treatment aims to remove the iron in excess, using phlebotomy and chelating agents (115). Iron chelation therapy (deferoxamine) for more than 12 months may alter LV systolic function (115). This effect seems to be reversible after vitamin C supplementation.

Liver transplantation can be done in cirrhosis. In the setting of liver transplantation, cyclosporine treatment, blood transfusions, and rapid mobilization of the intramyocardial iron may contribute to CHF (116).

Heart transplantation in end-stage iron overload cardiomyopathy (IOC), refractory to maximal medical therapy, has been exceptionally proposed (117).

References

1. Shearn MA. The heart in systemic lupus erythematosus. Am Heart J. 1959;58:452–66.
2. Doria A, Iaccarino L, Sarzi-Puttini P, et al. Cardiac involvement in systemic lupus erythematosus. Lupus. 2005;14:683–6.
3. Singh JA, Woodard PK, Davila-Roman VG, et al. Cardiac magnetic resonance imaging abnormalities in systemic lupus erythematosus: a preliminary report. Lupus. 2005;14:137–44.
4. Petri M. Cardiovascular systemic lupus erythematosus. In: Lahita RG, ed. Systemic Lupus Erythematosus. Amsterdam: Elsevier Academic Press, 2004:913–942.
5. Heibel RH, O'Toole JD, Curtiss EI, et al. Coronary arteritis in systemic lupus erythematosus. Chest. 1976;69:700–3.
6. Roman MJ, Shanker BA, Davis A, et al. Prevalence and correlates of accelerated atherosclerosis in systemic lupus erythematosus. N Engl J Med. 2003; 349:2399–406.
7. Asanuma Y, Oeser A, Shintani AK, et al. Premature coronary-artery atherosclerosis in systemic lupus erythematosus. N Engl J Med. 2003;349:2407–15.
8. Bruce IN. Cardiovascular disease in lupus patients: should all patients be treated with statins and aspirin? Best Pract Res Clin Rheumatol. 2005; 19:823–38.
9. Wajed J, Ahmad Y, Durrington PN, et al. Prevention of cardiovascular disease in systemic lupus erythematosus—proposed guidelines for risk factor management. Rheumatology (Oxford). 2004;43:7–12.
10. Naqvi TZ, Luthringer D, Marchevsky A, et al. Chloroquine-induced cardiomyopathy-echocardiographic features. J Am Soc Echocardiogr. 2005; 18:383–7.
11. Petri M, Perez-Gutthann S, Spence D, et al. Risk factors for coronary artery disease in patients with systemic lupus erythematosus. Am J Med. 1992; 93:513–9.
12. Roldan CA, Shively BK, Crawford MH. An echocardiographic study of valvular heart disease associated with systemic lupus erythematosus. N Engl J Med. 1996;335:1424–30.
13. Roldan CA, Shively BK, Lau CC, et al. Systemic lupus erythematosus valve disease by transesophageal echocardiography and the role of antiphospholipid antibodies. J Am Coll Cardiol. 1992;20: 1127–34.
14. Schneider C, Bahlmann E, Antz M, et al. Images in cardiovascular medicine. Unusual manifestation of Libman-Sacks endocarditis in systemic lupus erythematosus. Circulation. 2003;107:e202–4.
15. Wilson WA, Gharavi AE, Koike T, et al. International consensus statement on preliminary classification criteria for definite antiphospholipid syndrome: report of an international workshop. Arthritis Rheum. 1999;42:1309–11.
16. Tenedios F, Erkan D, Lockshin MD. Cardiac involvement in the antiphospholipid syndrome. Lupus. 2005;14:691–6.
17. Asherson RA, Cervera R. Unusual manifestations of the antiphospholipid syndrome. Clin Rev Allergy Immunol. 2003;25:61–78.
18. Lockshin M, Tenedios F, Petri M, et al. Cardiac disease in the antiphospholipid syndrome: recommendations for treatment. Committee consensus report. Lupus. 2003;12:518–23.
19. Erkan D, Roman MJ, Tenedios F, et al. Cardiac involvement in antiphospholipid syndrome. In: Doria A, Pauletto P, eds. Handbook of Systemic Autoimmune Diseases, vol 1. The Heart in Systemic Autoimmune Diseases. Amsterdam: Elsevier, 2004:213–225.
20. Bloom BJ, Smith RN. Case records of the Massachusetts General Hospital. Weekly clinicopathological exercises. Case 29-2002. A 17-year-old boy with acute mitral regurgitation and pulmonary edema. N Engl J Med. 2002;347:921–8.
21. Asherson RA. The catastrophic antiphospholipid (Asherson's) syndrome in 2004—a review. Autoimmun Rev. 2005;4:48–54.
22. Nicola PJ, Crowson CS, Maradit-Kremers H, et al. Contribution of congestive heart failure and ischemic heart disease to excess mortality in rheumatoid arthritis. Arthritis Rheum. 2006;54:60–7.
23. Wolfe F, Freundlich B, Straus WL. Increase in cardiovascular and cerebrovascular disease prevalence in rheumatoid arthritis. J Rheumatol. 2003; 30:36–40.
24. del Rincon ID, Williams K, Stern MP, et al. High incidence of cardiovascular events in a rheumatoid arthritis cohort not explained by traditional cardiac risk factors. Arthritis Rheum. 2001;44: 2737–45.
25. Chung ES, Packer M, Lo KH, Fasanmade AA, et al. Anti-TNF Therapy Against Congestive Heart Failure Investigators. Randomized, double-blind,

placebo-controlled, pilot trial of infliximab, a chimeric monoclonal antibody to tumor necrosis factor-alpha, in patients with moderate-to-severe heart failure: results of the anti-TNF Therapy Against Congestive Heart Failure (ATTACH) trial. Circulation. 2003;107:3133–40.

26. Mann DL, McMurray JJ, Packer M, et al. Targeted anticytokine therapy in patients with chronic heart failure: results of the Randomized Etanercept Worldwide Evaluation (RENEWAL). Circulation. 2004;109:1594–602.
27. Kwon HJ, Cote TR, Cuffe MS, et al. Case reports of heart failure after therapy with a tumor necrosis factor antagonist. Ann Intern Med. 2003;138:807–11.
28. Goodson NJ. Cardiac involvement in rheumatoid arthritis. In: Doria A, Pauletto P, eds. Handbook of Systemic Autoimmune Diseases, vol 1. The Heart in Systemic Autoimmune Diseases. Amsterdam: Elsevier, 2004:121–143.
29. Guedes C, Bianchi-Fior P, Cormier B, et al. Cardiac manifestations of rheumatoid arthritis: a case-control transesophageal echocardiography study in 30 patients. Arthritis Rheum. 2001;45:129–35.
30. Silverman KJ, Hutchins GM, Bulkley BH. Cardiac sarcoid: a clinicopathologic study of 84 unselected patients with systemic sarcoidosis. Circulation. 1978;58:1204–11.
31. Bargout R, Kelly RF. Sarcoid heart disease: clinical course and treatment. Int J Cardiol. 2004;97:173–82.
32. Roberts WC, McAllister HA Jr, Ferrans VJ. Sarcoidosis of the heart. A clinicopathologic study of 35 necropsy patients (group 1) and review of 78 previously described necropsy patients (group 11). Am J Med. 1977;63:86–108.
33. Belhassen B, Pines A, Laniado S,et al. Failure of corticosteroid therapy to prevent induction of ventricular tachycardia in sarcoidosis. Chest. 1989;95:918–20.
34. Yazaki Y, Isobe M, Hiroe M, et al. Prognostic determinants of long-term survival in Japanese patients with cardiac sarcoidosis treated with prednisone. Am J Cardiol. 2001;88:1006–10.
35. Yazaki Y, Isobe M, Hiramitsu S, et al. Comparison of clinical features and prognosis of cardiac sarcoidosis and idiopathic dilated cardiomyopathy. Am J Cardiol. 1998;82:537–40.
36. Hiraga H, Yuwai K, Hiroe M, et al. Guideline for Diagnosis of Cardiac Sarcoidosis: Study Report on Diffuse Pulmonary Diseases from the Japanese Ministry of Health and Welfare. Tokyo: Japanese Ministry of Health and Welfare, 1993:23–24.
37. Uemura A, Morimoto S, Hiramitsu S, et al. Histologic diagnostic rate of cardiac sarcoidosis: evaluation of endomyocardial biopsies. Am Heart J. 1999;138:299–302.
38. Fahy GJ, Marwick T, McCreery CJ, et al. Doppler echocardiographic detection of left ventricular diastolic dysfunction in patients with pulmonary sarcoidosis. Chest. 1996;109:62–6.
39. Doughan AR, Williams BR. Cardiac sarcoidosis. Heart. 2006;92:282–8.
40. Okumura W, Iwasaki T, Toyama T, et al. Usefulness of fasting 18F-FDG PET in identification of cardiac sarcoidosis. J Nucl Med. 2004;45:1989–98.
41. Yamagishi H, Shirai N, Takagi M, et al. Identification of cardiac sarcoidosis with (13)N-NH(3)/(18)F-FDG PET. J Nucl Med. 2003;44:1030–6.
42. Vignaux O, Dhote R, Duboc D, et al. Clinical significance of myocardial magnetic resonance abnormalities in patients with sarcoidosis: a 1-year follow-up study. Chest. 2002;122:1895–901.
43. Valantine HA, Tazelaar HD, Macoviak J, et al. Cardiac sarcoidosis: response to steroids and transplantation. J Heart Transplant. 1987;6:244–50.
44. Desai MY, Fallert MA. Rapidly progressing congestive heart failure due to cardiac sarcoidosis involving papillary muscles: a case report and brief review of the literature. Cardiol Rev. 2003;11:163–8.
45. Roufosse F, Cogan E, Goldman M. The hypereosinophilic syndrome revisited. Annu Rev Med. 2003;54:169–84.
46. Gotlib J, Cools J, Malone JM 3rd, et al. The FIP1L1-PDGFRalpha fusion tyrosine kinase in hypereosinophilic syndrome and chronic eosinophilic leukemia: implications for diagnosis, classification, and management. Blood. 2004;103:2879–91.
47. Blauwet LA, Breen JF, Edwards WD, et al. Atypical presentation of eosinophilic endomyocardial disease. Mayo Clin Proc. 2005:1078–84.
48. Ommen SR, Seward JB, Tajik AJ. Clinical and echocardiographic features of hypereosinophilic syndromes. Am J Cardiol. 2000;86:110–3.
49. Hassan WM, Fawzy ME, Al Helaly S, et al. Pitfalls in diagnosis and clinical, echocardiographic, and hemodynamic findings in endomyocardial fibrosis: a 25-year experience. Chest. 2005;128:3985–92.
50. Parrillo JE, Fauci AS, Wolff SM. Therapy of the hypereosinophilic syndrome. Ann Intern Med. 1978;89:167–72.
51. Cortes J, Ault P, Koller C, et al. Efficacy of imatinib mesylate in the treatment of idiopathic hypereosinophilic syndrome. Blood. 2003;101:4714–6.

52. Lonzetti LS, Joyal F, Raynauld JP, et al. Updating the American College of Rheumatology preliminary classification criteria for systemic sclerosis: addition of severe nailfold capillaroscopy abnormalities markedly increases the sensitivity for limited scleroderma. Arthritis Rheum. 2001;44: 735–6.
53. Deswal A, Follansbee WP. Cardiac involvement in scleroderma. Rheum Dis Clin North Am. 1996;22: 841–60.
54. D'Angelo WA, Fries JF, Masi AT, et al. Pathologic observations in systemic sclerosis (scleroderma). A study of fifty-eight autopsy cases and fifty-eight matched controls. Am J Med. 1969;46:428–40.
55. Smith JW, Clements PJ, Levisman J, et al. Echocardiographic features of progressive systemic sclerosis (PSS). Correlation with hemodynamic and postmortem studies. Am J Med. 1979;66:28–33.
56. Follansbee WP, Zerbe TR, Medsger TA Jr. Cardiac and skeletal muscle disease in systemic sclerosis (scleroderma): a high risk association. Am Heart J. 1993;125:194–203.
57. Kahan A, Devaux JY, Amor B, et al. Nifedipine and thallium-201 myocardial perfusion in progressive systemic sclerosis. N Engl J Med. 1986;314:1397–402.
58. Kahan A, Nitenberg A, Foult JM, et al. Decreased coronary reserve in primary scleroderma myocardial disease. Arthritis Rheum. 1985;28:637–46.
59. Ferri C, Giuggioli D, Sebastiani M,et al. Heart involvement and systemic sclerosis. Lupus. 2005; 14:702–7.
60. Kostis JB, Seibold JR, Turkevich D, et al. Prognostic importance of cardiac arrhythmias in systemic sclerosis. Am J Med. 1988;84:1007–15.
61. Hachulla E, Gressin V, Guillevin et al. Early detection of pulmonary arterial hypertension in systemic sclerosis: a French Nationwide Prospective Multicenter Study. Arthritis Rheum 2005;52:3792–800.
62. Mukerjee D, St George D, Coleiro B, et al. Prevalence and outcome in systemic sclerosis associated pulmonary arterial hypertension: application of a registry approach. Ann Rheum Dis. 2003; 62:1088–93.
63. Kawut SM, Taichman DB, Archer-Chicko CL, et al. Hemodynamics and survival in patients with pulmonary arterial hypertension related to systemic sclerosis. Chest. 2003;123:344–50.
64. Ferri C, Di Bello V, Martini A, et al. Heart involvement in systemic sclerosis: an ultrasonic tissue characterisation study. Ann Rheum Dis. 1998; 57:296–302.
65. Lindqvist P, Caidahl K, Neuman-Andersen G, et al. Disturbed right ventricular diastolic function in patients with systemic sclerosis: a Doppler tissue imaging study. Chest. 2005;128:755–63.
66. Ferri C, Valentini G, Cozzi F, et al. Systemic sclerosis: demographic, clinical, and serologic features and survival in 1,012 Italian patients. Medicine (Baltimore). 2002;81:139–53.
67. Sharp GC, Irvin WS, May CM, et al. Association of antibodies to ribonucleoprotein and Sm antigens with mixed connective-tissue disease, systematic lupus erythematosus and other rheumatic diseases. N Engl J Med. 1976;295:1149–54.
68. Alpert MA, Goldberg SH, Singsen BH, et al. Cardiovascular manifestations of mixed connective tissue disease in adults. Circulation. 1983;68:1182–93.
69. Oetgen WJ, Mutter ML, Lawless OJ, et al. Cardiac abnormalities in mixed connective tissue disease. Chest. 1983;83:185–8.
70. Kim P, Grossman JM. Treatment of mixed connective tissue disease. Rheum Dis Clin North Am. 2005;31:549–65.
71. Wiener-Kronish JP, Solinger AM, Warnock ML, et al. Severe pulmonary involvement in mixed connective tissue disease. Am Rev Respir Dis. 1981; 124:499–503.
72. Burdt MA, Hoffman RW, Deutscher SL, et al. Long-term outcome in mixed connective tissue disease: longitudinal clinical and serologic findings. Arthritis Rheum. 1999;42:899–909.
73. Falk RH, Comenzo RL, Skinner M. The systemic amyloidoses. N Engl J Med. 1997;337:898–909.
74. Falk RH. Diagnosis and management of the cardiac amyloidoses. Circulation 2005;112:2047–60.
75. Dubrey SW, Cha K, Anderson J, et al. The clinical features of immunoglobulin light-chain (AL) amyloidosis with heart involvement. QJM. 1998; 91:141–57.
76. Cueto-Garcia L, Reeder GS, Kyle RA, et al. Echocardiographic findings in systemic amyloidosis: spectrum of cardiac involvement and relation to survival. J Am Coll Cardiol. 1985;6:737–43.
77. Palka P, Lange A, Donnelly JE, et al. Doppler tissue echocardiographic features of cardiac amyloidosis. J Am Soc Echocardiogr. 2002;15:1353–60.
78. Klein AL, Hatle LK, Taliercio CP, et al. Prognostic significance of Doppler measures of diastolic function in cardiac amyloidosis. A Doppler echocardiography study. Circulation. 1991;83:808–16.
79. Klein AL, Hatle LK, Burstow DJ, et al. Comprehensive Doppler assessment of right ventricular dia-

stolic function in cardiac amyloidosis. J Am Coll Cardiol. 1990;15:99–108.
80. Kim WH, Otsuji Y, Yuasa T, Minagoe S, Seward JB, Tei C. Evaluation of right ventricular dysfunction in patients with cardiac amyloidosis using Tei index. J Am Soc Echocardiogr 2004;17:45–9.
81. Patel AR, Dubrey SW, Mendes LA, et al. Right ventricular dilation in primary amyloidosis: an independent predictor of survival. Am J Cardiol. 1997 15;80:486–92.
82. Lindqvist P, Olofsson BO, Backman C, et al. Pulsed tissue Doppler and strain imaging discloses early signs of infiltrative cardiac disease: a study on patients with familial amyloidotic polyneuropathy. Eur J Echocardiogr. 2006;7:22–30.
83. Aprile C, Marinone G, Saponaro R, et al. Cardiac and pleuropulmonary AL amyloid imaging with technetium-99m labelled aprotinin. Eur J Nucl Med. 1995;22:1393–401.
84. Lekakis J, Dimopoulos M, Nanas J, et al. Antimyosin scintigraphy for detection of cardiac amyloidosis. Am J Cardiol. 1997;80:963–5.
85. Maceira AM, Joshi J, Prasad SK, et al. Cardiovascular magnetic resonance in cardiac amyloidosis. Circulation 2005;111:186–93.
86. Pellikka PA, Holmes DR Jr, Edwards WD, et al. Endomyocardial biopsy in 30 patients with primary amyloidosis and suspected cardiac involvement. Arch Intern Med. 1988;148:662–6.
87. Hamer JP, Janssen S, van Rijswijk MH, et al. Amyloid cardiomyopathy in systemic non-hereditary amyloidosis. Clinical, echocardiographic and electrocardiographic findings in 30 patients with AA and 24 patients with AL amyloidosis. Eur Heart J. 1992;13:623–7.
88. Nicolosi GL, Pavan D, Lestuzzi C, et al. Prospective identification of patients with amyloid heart disease by two-dimensional echocardiography. Circulation. 1984;70:432–7.
89. Dubrey SW, Cha K, Simms RW, et al. Electrocardiography and Doppler echocardiography in secondary (AA) amyloidosis. Am J Cardiol. 1996; 77:313–5.
90. Kholova I, Niessen HW. Amyloid in the cardiovascular system: a review. J Clin Pathol. 2005;58:125–33.
91. Merlini G, Bellotti V. Molecular mechanisms of amyloidosis. N Engl J Med. 2003;349:583–96.
92. Kyle RA, Gertz MA. Primary systemic amyloidosis: clinical and laboratory features in 474 cases. Semin Hematol. 1995;32:45–59.
93. Felker GM, Thompson RE, Hare JM, et al. Underlying causes and long-term survival in patients with initially unexplained cardiomyopathy. N Engl J Med. 2000;342:1077–84.
94. Palladini G, Campana C, Klersy C, et al. Serum N-terminal pro-brain natriuretic peptide is a sensitive marker of myocardial dysfunction in AL amyloidosis. Circulation. 2003;107:2440–45.
95. Kyle RA, Greipp PR. Primary systemic amyloidosis: comparison of melphalan and prednisone versus placebo. Blood. 1978;52:818–27.
96. Comenzo RL, Gertz MA. Autologous stem cell transplantation for primary systemic amyloidosis. Blood. 2002;99:4276–82.
97. Suhr OB, Svendsen IH, Andersson R, et al. Hereditary transthyretin amyloidosis from a Scandinavian perspective. J Intern Med. 2003;254:225–35.
98. Dubrey SW, Burke MM, Khaghani A, et al. Long term results of heart transplantation in patients with amyloid heart disease. Heart. 2001;85: 202–7.
99. Hosenpud JD, DeMarco T, Frazier OH, et al. Progression of systemic disease and reduced long-term survival in patients with cardiac amyloidosis undergoing heart transplantation. Follow-up results of a multicenter survey. Circulation. 1991; 84(suppl):III338–43.
100. Reveille JD. HLA-B27 and the seronegative spondyloarthropathies. Am J Med Sci. 1998;316: 239–49.
101. Bergfeldt L. HLA-B27–associated cardiac disease. Ann Intern Med. 1997;127:621–9.
102. O'Neill TW, King G, Graham IM, et al. Echocardiographic abnormalities in ankylosing spondylitis. Ann Rheum Dis. 1992;51:652–4.
103. Roldan CA, Chavez J, Wiest PW, et al. Aortic root disease and valve disease associated with ankylosing spondylitis. J Am Coll Cardiol. 1998;32:1397–404.
104. Peters MJ, Van der Horst-Bruinsma IE, Dijkmans BA, Nurmohamed MT. Cardiovascular risk profile of patients with spondylarthropathies, particularly ankylosing spondylitis and psoriatic arthritis. Semin Arthritis Rheum 2004;34:585–92.
105. Brunner F, Kunz A, Weber U, Kissling R. Ankylosing spondylitis and heart abnormalities: do cardiac conduction disorders, valve regurgitation and diastolic dysfunction occur more often in male patients with diagnosed ankylosing spondylitis for over 15 years than in the normal population? Clin Rheumatol 2006;25:24–9.
106. Crowley JJ, Donnelly SM, Tobin M, et al. Doppler echocardiographic evidence of left ventricular diastolic dysfunction in ankylosing spondylitis. Am J Cardiol. 1993;71:1337–40.

107. Gould BA, Turner J, Keeling DH, et al. Myocardial dysfunction in ankylosing spondylitis. Ann Rheum Dis. 1992;51:227–32.
108. Shah A, Askari AD. Pericardial changes and left ventricular function in ankylosing spondylitis. Am Heart J. 1987;113:1529–31.
109. Schmitt B, Golub RM, Green R. Screening primary care patients for hereditary hemochromatosis with transferrin saturation and serum ferritin level: systematic review for the American College of Physicians. Ann Intern Med 2005; 143:522–36.
110. Whitlock EP, Garlitz BA, Harris EL, Beil TL, Smith PR. Screening for hereditary hemochromatosis: a systematic review for the US preventive services task force. Ann Intern Med 2006;145:209–23.
111. Olson LJ, Baldus WP, Tajik AJ. Echocardiographic features of idiopathic hemochromatosis. Am J Cardiol. 1987;60:885–9.
112. Cecchetti G, Binda A, Piperno A, et al. Cardiac alterations in 36 consecutive patients with idiopathic haemochromatosis: polygraphic and echocardiographic evaluation. Eur Heart J. 1991;12:224–30.
113. Anderson LJ, Holden S, Davis B, et al. Cardiovascular T2-star (T2*) magnetic resonance for the early diagnosis of myocardial iron overload. Eur Heart J. 2001;22:2171–9.
114. Ardehali H, Qasim A, Cappola T, et al. Endomyocardial biopsy plays a role in diagnosing patients with unexplained cardiomyopathy. Am Heart J. 2004;147:919–23.
115. Dabestani A, Child JS, Henze E, et al. Primary hemochromatosis: anatomic and physiologic characteristics of the cardiac ventricles and their response to phlebotomy. Am J Cardiol. 1984;54: 153–9.
116. Brandhagen DJ. Liver transplantation for hereditary hemochromatosis. Liver Transpl. 2001;7: 663–72.
117. Caines AE, Kpodonu J, Massad MG, et al. Cardiac transplantation in patients with iron overload cardiomyopathy. J Heart Lung Transplant. 2005;24: 486–8.

29
Acute Heart Failure in the Postoperative Period

Todd A. Watson and Lee A. Fleisher

In the perioperative period, heart failure is one of the most common conditions requiring evaluation and treatment. Furthermore, heart failure is the most frequently encountered postoperative cardiac complication of noncardiac surgery (1, 2). Postoperatively, acute heart failure (AHF), defined as the rapid onset of symptoms and signs secondary to abnormal cardiac function, often presents in patients with underlying chronic heart failure. However, occasionally, it may present acutely in previously healthy patients. With such prevalence, it is vital for clinicians caring for patients in the perioperative period to be skilled in managing AHF. This chapter discusses acute postoperative heart failure.

Prevalence and Mortality

Based on American Heart Association statistics, there are an estimated 550,000 new cases of heart failure each year, with an estimated prevalence of 5 million patients (3). This growing number has yielded an increase in the number of patients with heart failure presenting for surgery. Following major noncardiac surgery, heart failure has been reported in 1% to 6% of patients. In patients with existing cardiac conditions, such as coronary heart disease, prior heart failure, or valvular heart disease, the incidence is higher, between 6% and 25% (4–6). The risk may also be increased for patients with diabetes mellitus or renal insufficiency; in cases of high-risk surgery, such as vascular surgery (5); or when an excessive volume of fluid is administered intraoperatively (7).

Preoperative heart failure is an important risk factor for postoperative cardiac complications. In the American College of Cardiology/American Heart Association guidelines, decompensated heart failure is a major clinical marker, and prior heart failure is an intermediate clinical marker for postoperative cardiac complications (8). In a 2004 study, heart failure patients over age 65 had a greater incidence of operative mortality and readmission rates than patients with coronary artery disease and a control group (9). Along those same lines, whether the patient has chronic, stable heart failure or decompensated heart failure has prognostic implications. Patients undergoing major surgery who have left ventricular (LV) dysfunction or clinical evidence of congestive heart failure (CHF) have a very high risk of developing postoperative pulmonary edema (15%), whereas those with medically controlled CHF have a much lower risk (approximately 5%) (10).

Patients develop acute postoperative heart failure after cardiac surgery. Postcardiotomy cardiogenic shock, defined as the inability to wean from cardiopulmonary bypass or hemodynamic instability post bypass despite maximal inotropic and balloon pump use, has been reported to occur following 2% to 6% of all adult cardiac surgical procedures, and has been associated with a high mortality rate (11). Many of these patients are at greater risk than those undergoing noncardiac surgery because of the higher incidence of preoperative cardiac, vascular, and renal disease. In a 2001 study, heart failure was the most common etiology of death among coronary artery bypass graft (CABG) patients. Of the 8641 patients in the study, there were 387 deaths (4.48%) and of these 249 (64.3%) were attributed to heart failure. In their multivariate analysis, female sex, prior CABG surgery, ejection fraction <40%, urgent or emergency surgery, advanced age, peripheral vascular disease, diabetes, dialysis-dependent renal failure, and three-vessel coronary disease were significant predictors of fatal postoperative heart failure (12).

Patients with acute heart failure have a very poor prognosis. Mortality is especially high in patients with acute myocardial infarction accompanied by severe heart failure, with a 30% 12-month mortality (13). For patients in acute pulmonary edema, a 12% in-hospital and 40% 1-year mortality have been reported (13). While there have been no reports of mortality from acute postoperative heart failure, it would be safe to assume that it would at least approach the previously mentioned statistics, if not exceed them (14).

Definition and Etiology

As with chronic heart failure, acute postoperative heart failure can result from a variety of different conditions (Table 29.1). In general, greater than 70% of the episodes of AHF are the result of worsening chronic heart failure (15). This is paralleled in the postoperative period. In this setting, the majority of postoperative AHF occurs in patients who had decreased cardiovascular reserve and chronic heart failure prior to surgery. In the perioperative period, patients may be faced with numerous triggers of AHF, including withdrawal of heart failure medication, hypertension, inadequate volume management, anemia, tachyarrhythmias, hypercoagulability, and myocardial ischemia. Other potential causes of postoperative AHF include acute or chronic valvular heart disease (also potentially secondary to myocardial ischemia), myocardial contusion in the trauma patient, and aortic dissection. Pulmonary and fat emboli syndromes occur in postoperative patients, which can present as acute right ventricular failure secondary to increased right ventricular (RV) afterload.

Patients recovering from cardiac surgery and who present in AHF have some unique causes of failure particular to their type of surgery. Specifically, these patients may have mechanical complications related to heart surgery. Examples might include spasm or occlusion of a coronary graft, prosthetic valve paravalvular regurgitation, cardiac tamponade or hematoma, and pneumo- or hemothorax. In addition, by the use of cardiopulmonary bypass, they are exposed to prolonged ischemia with resultant reperfusion injury and inflammatory response. Patients with preexisting LV dysfunction are more prone to AHF post-cardiac surgery than those with normal preoperative function.

Table 29.1. Causes of acute postoperative heart failure

1. Exacerbation of chronic heart failure—secondary to withdrawal of heart failure medications, volume overload, ischemia, hypertension, anemia, tachyarrhythmias
2. Acute myocardial infarction
   a. Pump failure
   b. Mechanical complications—papillary muscle rupture, ventricular septal defect, free wall rupture, pericardial tamponade
   c. Right ventricular infarction
3. Postcardiotomy, cardiopulmonary bypass, myocardial stunning
4. Other causes
   a. Type A aortic dissection
   b. Acute/chronic valvular insufficiency
   c. Trauma—myocardial contusion
   d. Left ventricular outflow tract obstruction—systolic anterior motion of the mitral valve, aortic stenosis, hypertrophic obstructive cardiomyopathy
   e. Left ventricular inflow tract obstruction—mitral stenosis, left atrial myxoma
   f. Septic shock
   g. Massive pulmonary/fat/air embolus
   h. Pericardial tamponade

Diagnosis

The diagnosis of AHF during the postoperative period is based on symptoms and clinical findings and supported by appropriate investigations, such as electrocardiogram (ECG), chest x-ray, laboratory investigation and biomarkers, and echocardiography.

In the postoperative setting, the majority of patients present with symptoms of dyspnea secondary to pulmonary congestion. Symptoms of congestion may be related to increased left- or right-sided filling pressures. Dyspnea on minimal exertion, orthopnea, and paroxysmal nocturnal dyspnea can indicate elevated left-sided filling pressures, whereas abdominal discomfort, early satiety (in those patients not NPO), nausea, and vomiting may be caused by right-sided overload. On physical examination, rales and a third heart sound may be noted. Signs of right-sided failure may include hepatic congestion, ascites, and peripheral edema. Many of these signs may also be seen in surgical patients with normal cardiac function, therefore necessitating further workup.

The ECG is an important first-line diagnostic tool and it is rarely normal in AHF. The ECG allows the clinician to identify the rhythm and may help to determine the etiology of the heart failure. It is essential in the diagnosis of acute coronary syndromes. The ECG may also indicate acute right or left ventricular or atrial strain. In addition, signs of left or right ventricular hypertrophy may be seen. Arrhythmias as a cause of heart failure should be evident on ECG.

The chest x-ray should be performed early for all patients with AHF to evaluate heart size and to search for pulmonary congestion. It can be used to confirm the diagnosis of pulmonary edema, and it may also be used to monitor improvement after therapy is initiated. In the setting of possible pulmonary emboli, helical computed tomography (CT) enables visualization of the emboli. When aortic dissection is of concern, transesophageal echocardiography and CT scanning should enable the clinician to make the diagnosis.

There are many laboratory tests that can be utilized in evaluating patients postoperatively. A complete blood count (CBC) and chemistry panel are helpful initially to rule out anemia, infection, electrolyte abnormalities, and worsening renal insufficiency. An arterial blood gas provides information about oxygenation and ventilation status as well as information about acid–base chemistry and base deficit. This peptide is released from the cardiac ventricles in response to increased wall stretch and volume overload and is elevated in patients with left ventricular dysfunction (16). The levels of plasma B-type natriuretic peptide (BNP) correlate with the severity of symptoms and the prognosis (16). Currently, its role in the perioperative period is less clear. Bail et al. (17) demonstrated that BNP levels increased 24 hours after coronary artery bypass graft surgery, and that this peak did not reflect a state of acute perioperative heart failure or myocardial damage. In contrast, Kerbaul et al. (18) investigated levels of BNP before and immediately after off-pump coronary artery bypass and suggested that elevated levels were predictive of postoperative cardiac events. The BNP has the potential to strengthen the diagnosis of AHF when used in conjunction with history, physical exam, and other diagnostic tools.

Echocardiography with Doppler imaging should be used to evaluate global and regional left and right ventricular function. It provides a direct measurement of ejection fraction, and detection of regional wall motion abnormalities correlates well with ischemic territories of myocardium. In addition, it provides data on valvular regurgitation, volume status, and, with the use of Doppler technology, an estimate of pulmonary artery pressures can obtained. Finally, it also can be used for the diagnosis of pericardial diseases such as tamponade, and aortic pathology such as aortic dissection, causing AHF. Echocardiography is an important adjunct for the diagnosis and management of patients with heart failure, and has been shown to provide significant information that can be used for tailoring treatment and altering the prognosis in such patients (19).

Monitoring

In postoperative patients who are at high risk for heart failure, close monitoring is vital. At a minimum, many patients should be on a telemetry unit to evaluate ischemia or rhythm abnormalities. However, most will benefit from monitoring in the intensive care unit (ICU). In patients who are hemodynamically unstable, the use of an intraarterial catheter enables continuous monitoring of blood pressure. Central venous access enables the measurement of right atrial pressure and the direct infusion of medications. Caution must be used in overinterpreting right atrial pressure measurements, as these rarely correlate with left atrial pressures and therefore with left ventricular filling pressures in patients with AHF (13). Central venous pressure (CVP) measurements are also affected in the presence of tricuspid regurgitation and positive end-expiratory pressure (PEEP) (13).

The role of pulmonary artery catheterization is contentious. Direct measurement of hemodynamics can be helpful in patients in whom the physical examination is limited or discordant with symptoms (such as critically ill surgical patients). It can be useful for determining the contribution of heart failure to a complex clinical picture, such as sepsis, acute renal failure, or acute coronary syndrome in the setting of chronic heart failure. In addition, it might be helpful in the evaluation of dyspnea in patients with pulmonary disease as well as cardiac disease. The pulmonary artery catheter also helps in tailoring therapy. Cardiac output and mixed venous saturation are useful for trending general circulatory status and usually improve with reduction of filling pressures.

The role of the pulmonary artery catheter in surgical patients is controversial, with results of studies ranging from beneficial to harmful. One recent study looked at 1994 high-risk patients undergoing urgent or elective major surgery. Entry criteria included patients 60 years of age or older who were American Society of Anesthesiologists (ASA) class III or IV scheduled for urgent or elective major surgery. In both cohorts, 16% of patients had a history of congestive heart failure. The participants were randomly assigned to perioperative management with or without a pulmonary artery catheter. There was no significant difference in in-hospital mortality between the two groups (7.8% vs. 7.7%, respectively), in 6-month mortality (12.6% vs. 11.9%), or in rate of postoperative heart failure (12.9% vs. 11.2%). The only significant difference was a higher rate of pulmonary embolism (PE) in the pulmonary artery catheter group (0.9% vs. 0%) (20). However, with clinicians skilled in interpreting results from the pulmonary artery catheter in patients with heart failure, it could have a beneficial role in managing these patients.

As with the diagnosis of heart failure, echocardiography can play a pivotal role in monitoring. Echocardiography can be used to follow the progress of therapy and to evaluate such factors as recovery of ventricular function, volume status, or improvement after treatment for tamponade.

Management of Postoperative Heart Failure

General Considerations

Management of AHF in the postoperative period requires rapid diagnosis and treatment to prevent further myocardial and end-organ damage. The best initial approach involves prevention by identifying patients at high risk, avoiding known triggers of AHF, maintaining appropriate perioperative cardiac medications, and identifying the appropriate postoperative care setting, such as the ICU, for high-risk patients.

In the postoperative patient presenting in AHF, a differential diagnosis for the etiology must be established as resuscitation measures are initiated. While resuscitation is critical, a differential diagnosis will establish an etiology for the AHF and allow definitive treatment through the use of specific therapies. For example, in the patient with AHF secondary to a large acute myocardial infarction (MI), reperfusion via angioplasty, stenting, or bypass grafting will be necessary. Acute mitral regurgitation from an MI causing AHF might require urgent surgical repair, or acute RV failure from a PE might require anticoagulation if appropriate in the postsurgical patient.

As the etiology of AHF is being identified for definitive treatment, appropriate resuscitation measures must be undertaken. Table 29.2 high-

Table 29.2. A general approach to postoperative acute heart failure (AHF) management

1. Develop differential diagnosis (DDx) for etiology (see Table 29.1); treat repairable lesions
2. While developing DDx, initiate resuscitation measures
   - Maximize oxygenation/ventilation
   - Control postoperative pain/tachycardia
   - Correct acid–base and electrolyte abnormalities
3. Evaluate and optimize preload, afterload, contractility, heart rate, and rhythm
   - Preload—volume load vs. diuresis based on evaluation of volume status
   - Afterload—if high, consider dilation with nitroglycerine (NTG), sodium nitroprusside, or other afterload reducing agent; if low, consider augmentation with alpha agent
   - Contractility—utilize inotropic agent
   - Establish stable heart rate and rhythm
4. Utilize mechanical assistance for patients resistant to above measures

lights the general approach to postoperative AHF management.

Initial Resuscitation Measures

A critical principle of AHF management is the correction of oxygen supply–demand mismatch by increasing the supply of oxygen and decreasing the heart's demand for it. This includes correction of hypoxia, proper positioning, and control of postoperative pain and anxiety. The correction of hypoxia may be through simple measures such as nasal cannula or a nonrebreathing oxygen mask, or may require urgent intubation and mechanical ventilation. Continuous positive airway pressure (CPAP) (21) and bi-level positive pressure support (BiPAP) (22) have been demonstrated to be beneficial in the management of pulmonary edema by providing more rapid symptomatic relief and better oxygenation. The proposed mechanism involves a decreased left ventricular afterload and reduced work of breathing. Control of postoperative pain through the use of intravenous or neuraxial analgesia will help to control tachycardia and will improve ventilation in patients splinting from pain. Morphine is useful in patients with severe AHF because it induces venodilation, mild arterial dilation, and reduces heart rate (23). Finally, correction of electrolyte and acid–base abnormalities should be undertaken, as they can greatly affect contractility and rhythm.

Pharmacologic Management of Postoperative Heart Failure

Following the initial resuscitation measures outlined above, care of the postoperative patient with AHF often involves diuresis, inotropic augmentation, or vasodilator/vasoconstrictor therapy.

Preload

The goal of managing preload is to increase intravascular volume, while avoiding pulmonary edema or a reduction in coronary perfusion pressure. The overall impact of preload augmentation depends on the underlying state of RV and LV contractility. The normal RV is less preload dependent than the normal LV. However, in the presence of increased afterload or impaired RV contraction (such as in an RV infarction), RV preload becomes critical. The factors that govern the preload of each chamber are different. Flow to the RV depends on the pressure difference between the intrathoracic and extrathoracic venous beds, whereas the major determinant of LV preload is pulmonary venous drainage, and is independent of changes in intrathoracic pressure (14). Thus, in managing a low preload state, a first step would be to optimize ventilation in mechanically ventilated patients to allow for adequate venous return. After this, volume loading is appropriate. Depending on the clinical situation, blood, blood components, colloid (such as albumin or hydroxyethylstarch), or crystalloid solutions may be used (14).

The use of diuretics is considered one of the mainstays of AHF management. However, in the postoperative period, patients are often extravascularly edematous but intravascularly dry. Thus, careful evaluation of volume status must be undertaken before beginning diuresis. While diuretics can provide rapid symptomatic relief, the mechanism of action has been attributed to diuretic-induced vasodilation rather than volume diuresis (24). Because of this, the administration of nitrates has been suggested as an alternative to diuretics to induce vasodilation with equal clinical effects (25). A prospective outcome trial comparing diuretics and nitrates as first-line therapy in acute pulmonary edema showed a decreased need for mechanical ventilation, and a reduced incidence of MI within 24 hours of hospital admission and in hospital death in patients treated with nitrates (26).

Afterload

In the postoperative setting, patients with AHF may have either increased or decreased afterload. Excessive postoperative afterload is commonly seen in patients with poorly controlled hypertension or secondary to postoperative pain. Patents with acidosis, hypoxia, hypercarbia, or underlying primary or secondary pulmonary hypertension will have increased pulmonary artery pressures, leading to increased RV afterload. Decreased afterload will not cause AHF per se, but in the failing heart excessive vasodilation may contribute to hypotension. This situation is most common in the cardiac surgical patient. Post-bypass patients may have ventricular dysfunction secondary to multiple possibilities, and may be severely vasodilated from rewarming or preoperative medications such as angiotensin-converting enzyme (ACE) inhibitors.

In the patient with AHF caused or worsened by excessive afterload, vasodilators are often indicated as first-line therapy. In the setting of severe afterload increase, sodium nitroprusside (SNP) can augment cardiac output by unloading the left ventricle. Sodium nitroprusside is extremely potent and should be reserved for severe heart failure associated with high systemic vascular resistance, and afterload reduction during or after surgery for ventricular septal defects, aortic insufficiency, and mitral insufficiency (14). It must be titrated cautiously and requires invasive arterial monitoring and close monitoring in an ICU. In AHF caused by acute coronary syndromes, nitrates are preferred to SNP, as SNP is known to cause coronary steal syndrome (13). Toxicity from prolonged administration is well known, and is associated with its metabolites thiocyanate and cyanide, and should be avoided in patients with severe renal or hepatic failure.

Nitroglycerin (NTG) is similar to SNP in that it has rapid onset, an ultrashort half-life, and easy titratability. Unlike SNP, NTG has a predominant influence on the venous bed such that preload can be reduced without significantly compromising systemic arterial pressure. Thus, the overall benefits of NTG are improvement in stroke volume, reduction in wall tension and myocardial oxygen consumption, increased perfusion to the subendocardium as a result of lower LV end-diastolic pressure, and maintenance of coronary perfusion pressure (14). It is preferable in the setting of elevated pulmonary capillary wedge pressure and pulmonary artery pressure or myocardial ischemia because of the coronary artery dilation and lack of coronary steal (14).

While calcium channel blockers have historically been contraindicated for heart failure, the use of nicardipine for acute hypertensive emergencies has been described. A review article by Burlew et al. (27) suggested that nicardipine may be used safely in the presence of heart failure for the management of surgical hypertension and hypertensive emergencies. As an infusion it is easily titrated, and provides predominantly arterial afterload reduction.

For the patient with perioperative AHF and increased afterload, the use of ACE inhibitors has not been established. In a small, randomized prospective study, the administration of captopril in the early postoperative period to patients with severe postcardiotomy dysfunction has been shown to improve tissue perfusion and decrease mortality, morbidity, and length of hospital stay (28). More randomized trials are necessary before widespread use of ACE inhibitors in postoperative AHF can be recommended.

Neseritide is a human recombinant B-type natriuretic peptide with venous, arterial, and coronary vasodilator properties. It has no intrinsic inotropic properties. In clinical trials, neseritide has been shown to decrease cardiac filling pressures, increase cardiac index, and improve the clinical status of patients with acute decompensated heart failure (24). Several investigators have reported beneficial effects with AHF in various perioperative settings (24). Regardless, much controversy still exists regarding its use. A large randomized control trial enrolled 489 patients with acute decompensated heart failure and randomized patients to neseritide, nitroglycerin, or placebo in addition to standard therapy in a double-blind fashion. The trial failed to demonstrate greater advantages of neseritide over nitroglycerin (29). In addition, recent data have suggested an increased trend in 30-day mortality in patients treated with neseritide (30). There have been recent concerns about neseritide increasing the risk for renal failure (31). Thus, while a potential future role of neseritide in the treatment of perioperative AHF remains to be defined, neseritide has revealed itself as a unique agent in the management of decompensated heart failure. Unlike nitroglycerin, its use has not been associated with tolerance to its hemodynamic effects, and unlike nitroprusside there is no association with toxic metabolites.

As mentioned earlier, reduced afterload states will not create AHF, but postoperatively they may contribute to hypotension from AHF. Common scenarios are decreased afterload from the effects of sedation and anesthesia on the autonomic and central nervous systems and on vascular muscle tone; altered viscosity (hemodilution); vasodilation associated with rewarming in cardiac surgery; and preoperative use of ACE inhibitors, α_2-agonists, calcium channel blockers, and nitrates (14). In these situations, α_1-agonists (phenylephrine or norepinephrine) may be required to maintain adequate perfusion pressure. α-Adrenergic agonists may also benefit patients with circulatory failure refractory to inotropic and fluid therapy (14).

Contractility

Decreased contractility is a common mechanism of postoperative acute heart failure, and is the mechanism seen in perioperative myocardial ischemia leading to cardiogenic shock, and in postcardiotomy syndrome with reperfusion injury. In the setting of the failing ventricle, inotropes often act as one of the first-line agents. Intravenous inotropic therapy usually produces symptomatic and hemodynamic improvement in the short term. In patients with acute postoperative heart failure, the symptoms, clinical course, and prognosis often depend on the initial hemodynamics. Therefore, improvements made in the hemodynamics through the use of inotropes are clearly necessary, help in the short term, and, also in the short term, may be lifesaving in AHF (13).

While the use of inotropes is a mainstay of treatment in AHF, and the improvement in hemodynamics is quite clear, there have been clinical trials suggesting that their effect on overall mortality is questionable, and that they may even be detrimental in the long term. In the Outcomes of Prospective Trial of Intravenous Milrinone for Exacerbations of Chronic Heart Failure (OPTIME-CHF), the investigators randomized 951 patients with an exacerbation of chronic CHF not requiring inotropic support to receive 48-hour therapy with either milrinone or placebo. The milrinone group was associated with a higher incidence of worsening heart failure, symptomatic hypotension, and new atrial arrhythmias. Although not statistically significant, there was an increase in the number of deaths in hospital and after 60 days in the milrinone group (32–34). In another trial, retrospective data from the Flolan International Randomized Survival Trial showed an increased risk of clinical events for patients treated with dobutamine, with 70% of the patients on dobutamine dying compared with 37% in those without dobutamine (32, 35). Other trials have shown that inotropic agents are associated with the development of arrhythmias and sudden cardiac death (35, 36).

The reasons for the negative results of inotropic therapy have been linked to their mechanism of action. All of these agents increase cyclic adenosine monophosphate (cAMP) in myocytes, which promotes the release of calcium. Increases in intracellular calcium will increase inotropy; however, it does so at the expense of an increase in myocardial energy consumption and oxygen demand, which can accelerate myocardial cell death (37). Due to this common mechanism, there has been much work done to identify an intravenous inotrope with a mechanism of action independent of cAMP activation. One newer agent that is meeting this need is levosimendan, which acts to sensitize the myocyte to calcium without actually increasing the intracellular concentration of calcium, the end result being increased inotropy and vasodilation. Levosimendan has proven to increase cardiac output without increasing myocardial oxygen demand and without creating significant arrhythmias. It has been shown to be superior to dobutamine for the treatment of AHF (24). In addition, levosimendan has been successfully used for the management of perioperative AHF, including peripartum cardiomyopathy, AHF in an infant after cardiac surgery, low-output failure after cardiac surgery, and cardiogenic shock (24). Finally, by working through different mechanisms, levosimendan offers the possibility of augmenting contractility when combined with other inotropes and perhaps reducing the dose required of the inotrope.

Heart Rate and Rhythm

Arrhythmias during AHF place patients at high risk (38). Tachycardia is common in patients postoperatively, and is usually secondary to pain or hypovolemia. In this setting, analgesia or gentle volume loading would be appropriate. Post–cardiac surgery, atrial fibrillation is the most common arrhythmia (39). With new-onset atrial fibrillation and AHF, electrical cardioversion should be performed, but atrial thrombus should be ruled out by transesophageal echocardiography.

In AHF patients with chronic atrial fibrillation, an appropriate strategy may involve anticoagulation and rate control when hemodynamically stable. Verapamil and diltiazem should be avoided in AHF, as they may worsen heart failure and potentially cause third-degree heart block (13). Amiodarone and beta-blockers are commonly used for rate control, and are a good choice in AHF patients. Of the two, amiodarone is probably the better choice, as it has the least myocardial depressant effects (40).

Mechanical Assistance

In situations in which the use of pharmacologic therapy alone is insufficient to augment ventricular performance, mechanical modes of assistance are an appropriate option. Currently, three methods employed are (1) the intraaortic balloon pump (IABP), (2) percutaneous cardiopulmonary bypass system (PCPS), and (3) mechanical assist devices. Many of these mechanical devices have been shown to relieve the symptoms of AHF, allow for separation from cardiopulmonary bypass, and act as a bridge to transplantation following an intraoperative myocardial infarction and subsequent AHF (41–43).

The IABP is able to decrease ventricular afterload and augment coronary perfusion pressure, providing an excellent means for treating the elevated filling pressures and decreased contractility accompanying AHF, and potentially reversible ventricular dysfunction (14). Frequently, the IABP is used for acute heart failure in cardiac surgical patients to aid in weaning from cardiopulmonary bypass, or in patients with left main coronary artery stenosis/occlusion to augment diastolic flow. Limitations of the IABP include only a relatively modest increase in cardiac output (15% to 20%), requirement of regular cardiac rhythm, absence of aortic and peripheral vascular disease, and absence of significant aortic insufficiency (14).

The PCPS is a portable bypass system that utilizes the standard components for bypass, including a centrifugal pump, heat exchanger, and membrane oxygenator. It has been used for refractory cardiac arrest and cardiogenic shock, and for myocardial infarction complications (14). It does not salvage patients who do not regain a stable cardiac rhythm, but can stabilize patients who develop cardiogenic shock for possible revascularization. It should be used with IABP assistance and for a maximum of 2 to 3 days (14). In many studies, 75% of patients cannulated were successfully weaned from PCPS, and 25% to 39% were long-term survivors (12). Complications include sepsis, progressive heart failure, and lower leg ischemia.

Ventricular assist devices (VADs) are an option of last resort for patients with refractory heart failure. They are mechanical devices that can be placed extracorporeally or intracorporeally, and they remove blood from the ventricle and, through pulsatile or laminar flow, inject blood back into the systemic or pulmonary vasculature. Left ventricular assist devices (LVADs) have become increasingly used because of a shortage of organs to transplant. The VADs may be used as a bridge to transplant, recovery, or, with newer devices, as destination therapy. Indications for device placement include postcardiotomy shock, acute MI, and myocarditis (44). Clearly, for physicians caring for patients in the perioperative period, the most common indication for VAD placement is in the postcardiotomy shock patient. In this setting VAD placement is often reserved for patients in shock after high-dose inotropy and vasopressors, combined with IABP support.

In the setting of VAD placement, reported discharge rates for patients with postcardiotomy heart failure has been disappointing (45). In one study in which 965 patients with postcardiotomy heart failure were treated with a VAD, only 25% survived to discharge (46). A 1995 New York State database of postcardiotomy heart failure patients treated with VAD support showed a similar 24% survival rate to hospital discharge (47). Finally, another study showed an improved survival rate when patients were managed at dedicated referral centers specializing in the care of this critically ill population. In this study, 44 patients where temporized at outside hospitals with a temporary VAD and transferred to the study center for definitive treatment. Of the 44 patients, 66% survived to hospital discharge, thus suggesting the role of a referral network for this complex patient population (45). Major complications of VAD use include infection, RV failure in LVAD use, and bleeding. Finally, echocardiography is critical to rule out aortic insufficiency and atrial septal defect, all of which need to be corrected for proper VAD function.

Conclusion

Postoperative acute heart failure results in significant morbidity and mortality, and represents a major problem for perioperative physicians. Currently, the best option for patients is prevention through proper preoperative and intraoperative management. For patients who eventually develop AHF, the current mainstay of treatment remains inotropic support with diuresis. There are emerging areas, however. The role of BNP measurements in the early diagnosis of postoperative AHF has yet to be elucidated, along with the role of new pharmacologic agents such as levosimendan and nesiritide. It is hoped that further research in mechanical support of the heart will provide long-term therapy in patients and allow for longer survival to transplantation.

References

1. Lee TH, Marcantonio ER, Mangione CM, et al. Derivation and prospective validation of a simple index for prediction of cardiac risk of major noncardiac surgery. Circulation 1999;100:1043.
2. Mangano DT, Browner WS, Hollenberg M, et al. Long term cardiac prognosis following noncardiac surgery. The study of perioperative ischemia research group. JAMA 1992;268:233.
3. American Heart Association. Heart Disease and Stroke Statistics-2005 Update. Dallas, TX: American Heart Association, 2005.
4. Goldman L, Caldera DL, Nussbaum SR, et al. Multifactorial index of cardiac risk in noncardiac surgical procedures. N Engl J Med 1977;297:845.
5. Charlson ME, MacKenzie CR, Gold JP, et al. Risk for postoperative congestive heart failure. Surg Gynecol Obstet 1991;172:95.
6. Mangano DT, Browner WS, Hollenberg M, et al. Association of perioperative myocardial ischemia with cardiac morbidity and mortality in men undergoing noncardiac surgery. The study of perioperative ischemia research group. N Engl J Med 1990;323:1781.
7. Arieff AI. Fatal postoperative pulmonary edema: Pathogenesis and literature review. Chest 1999;115:1371.
8. Committee to Update the 1996 Guidelines on Perioperative Cardiovascular Evaluation for Noncardiac Surgery. J Am Col Cardiol 2002;39:542.
9. Hernandez AF, Whellan DJ, Stroud S, et al. Outcomes in heart failure patients after major noncardiac surgery. J Am Col Cardiol 2004;44:1446–53.
10. Cole D, Schlunt M. Adult Perioperative Anesthesia: The Requisites in Anesthesiology. New York: Elsevier, 2004:24.
11. Pae WE, Miller CA, Matthews Y, Pierce WS. Ventricular assist devices for postcardiotomy cardiogenic shock. A combined registry experience. J Thorac Cardiovasc Surg 1992;104:541–53.
12. Surgenor SD, et al. Predicting the risk of death from heart failure after coronary artery bypass graft surgery. Anesth Analg 2001;92:596–601.
13. The Task Force on Acute Heart Failure of the European Society of Cardiology. Executive summary of the guidelines on the diagnosis and treatment of acute heart failure. Eur Heart J 2005;26:384–416.
14. Griffin MJ, Hines RL. Management of perioperative ventricular dysfunction. J Cardiothorac Vasc Anesth 2001;15:90–106.
15. Gheorghiade M, Mebasaa A. Introduction to acute heart failure syndromes. Am J Cardiol 2005;96(6A):1–4.
16. Mueller C, Scholer A, Laule-Kilian K, et al. Use of B-type natriuretic peptide in the evaluation and management of acute dyspnea. N Engl J Med 2004;350:647–54.
17. Bail DH, Kofler M, Ziemer G. Brain natriuretic peptide (BNP) in patients undergoing coronary artery bypass grafting. Thorac Cardiovasc Surg 2004;52:135–40.
18. Kerbaul F, Collart F, Giorgi R, et al. Increased plasma levels of pro-brain natriuretic peptide in patients with cardiovascular complications following off-pump coronary artery surgery. Intensive Care Med 2004;30:1799–806.
19. Vitarelli A, Tiukinhoy S, DiLuzio S, Zampino M, Gheorghiade M. The role of echocardiography in the diagnosis and management of acute heart failure. Heart Fail Rev 2003;8:181–9.
20. Sandham JD, Hull RD, Brant RF, et al. A randomized, controlled trial of the use of pulmonary-artery catheters in high-risk surgical patients. N Engl J Med 2003;348:5.
21. Bellone A, Monari A, Cortellaro F, et al. Myocardial infarction rate in acute pulmonary edema: noninvasive pressure support ventilation versus continuous positive airway pressure. Crit Care Med 2004;32:1860–5.
22. Yosefy C, Hay E, Ben-Barak A, et al. BiPAP ventilation as assistance for patients presenting with

respiratory distress in the department of emergency medicine. Am J Respir Med 2003;2:343–7.
23. Lee G, DeMaria AN, Amsterdam EA, et al. Comparative effects of morphine, meperidine and pentazocine on cardiocirculatory dynamics in patients with acute myocardial infarction. Am J Med 1976; 60:949–55.
24. Toller WG, Metzler H. Acute perioperative heart failure Curr Opin Anesthesiol 2005;18:129–35.
25. Northridge D. Furosemide of nitrates for acute heart failure? Lancet 1996;347:667–8.
26. Cotter G, Metzkor E, Kaluski E, et al. Randomized trial of high-dose isosorbide dinitrate plus low-dose furosemide versus high-dose furosemide plus low-dose isosorbide dinitrate in severe pulmonary oedema. Lancet 1998;351:389–93.
27. Burlew BS, Gheorghiade M, Jafri SM, Goldberg AD, Goldstein S. Acute and chronic hemodynamic effects of nicardipine hydrochloride in patients with heart failure. Am Heart J 1987;114:793–804.
28. Sirivella S, Gielchinsky I, Parsonnet V. Angiotensin converting enzyme inhibitor therapy in severe postcardiotomy dysfunction: a prospective randomized study. J Card Surg 1998;13:11–17.
29. Publication Committee for the VMAC Investigators (Vasodilation in the Management of Acute CHF). Intravenous neseritide vs nitroglycerin for treatment of decompensated congestive heart failure: a randomized controlled trial. JAMA 2002; 287:1531–40.
30. Sackner-Bernstein JD, Kowalski M, Fox M, Aaronson K. Short-term risk of death after treatment with neseritide for decompensated heart failure. JAMA 2005;293:1900–5.
31. Sackner-Bernstein JD, Skopicki HA, Aaronson KD. Risk of worsening renal function with neseritide in patients with acutely decompensated heart failure. Circulation 2005;111:1487–91.
32. Sharma M, Teerlink JR. A rational approach for the current treatment of acute heart failure: current strategies and future options. Curr Opin Cardiol 2004;19:254–63.
33. Cuffe MS, Califf RM, Adams KF Jr, et al. Short-term intravenous milrinone for acute exacerbation of chronic heart failure: a randomized controlled trial. JAMA 2002;287:1541–7.
34. Felker GM, Benza RL, Chandler AB, et al. Heart Failure etiology and response to milrinone in decompensated heart failure: results from the OPTIME-CHF study. J Am Coll Cardiol 2003;41:997–1003.
35. O'Connor CM, Gattis WA, Uretsky BF, et al. Continuous intravenous dobutamine is associated with an increased risk of death in patients with advanced heart failure: insights from the Flolan International Randomized Survival Trial (FIRST). Am Heart J 1999;138:78–86.
36. Packer M, Carver JR, Rodeheffer RJ, et al. Effect of oral milrinone on mortality in severe chronic heart failure. The PROMISE Study Research Group. N Engl J Med 1991;325:1468–75.
37. Toller WG, Stranz C. Levosimendan, a new inotropic and vasodilator agent. Anesthesiology 2006;104: 556–69.
38. Benza RL, Tallaj JA, Felker GM, et al. The impact of arrhythmias in acute heart failure. J Cardiac Failure 2004;10(4):279–84.
39. Chung M. Cardiac surgery: postoperative arrhythmias. Crit Care Med 2000;28(10):N136–N144.
40. Bovill J. Anesthesia for patients with impaired ventricular function. Semin Cardiothorac Vasc Anesth 2003;7:49–54.
41. Noon GP, Ball JW Jr, Short HD. Bio-Medicus centrifugal ventricular support for postcardiotomy cardiac failure: a review of 129 cases. Ann Thorac Surg 1996;61:291–5.
42. DeRose JJ Jr, Umana JP, Argenziane M, et al. Improved results for postcardiotomy cardiogenic shock with the use of implantable left ventricular assist devices. Ann Thorac Surg 1997;64:1757–62.
43. Siegenthaler MP, Brehm K, Strecker T, et al. The Impella Recover microaxial left ventricular assist device reduces mortality for postcardiotomy failure: a three-center experience. J Thorac Cardiovasc Surg 2004;127:812–22.
44. Magner JJ, Royston D. Heart failure. Br J Anesth 2004;93:74–85.
45. Helman D, Morales D, Edwards N, et al. Left ventricular assist device bridge-to-transplant network improves survival after failed cardiotomy. Ann Thorac Surg 1999;68:1187–94.
46. Pae WE, Miller CA, Matthews Y, Pierce WS. Ventricular assist devices for postcardiotomy cardiogenic shock. A combined registry experience. J Thorac Cardiovasc Surg 1992;104:541–53.
47. New York State Department of Health Cardiac Surgical Outcomes Database, 1995 Annual Report.

30
Myocardial Dysfunction in Sepsis and Septic Shock

Anand Kumar, Aseem Kumar, and Joseph E. Parrillo

Sepsis and septic shock represent a major cause of mortality and morbidity in the developed world. The most widely accepted estimate of incidence of severe sepsis in the United States is 750,000 cases per year, with 215,000 annual deaths (1). Over the past 40 years, the incidence of sepsis has increased at approximately 8.7% per year (2). During the same time period, total mortality has increased even though the overall mortality rate has fallen from 27.8% to 17.9% (2). Despite major advances in our understanding of the pathophysiology of septic shock, the associated mortality of septic shock per se appears substantially unchanged over the past 40 years (3).

Sepsis has been defined as the systemic inflammatory response to infection (4). The inciting focus of sepsis, via either exotoxins or a structural microbial component (endotoxin, teichoic acid, peptidoglycans, bacterial nucleic acids), causes local and systemic release of a wide variety of endogenous inflammatory mediators like tumor necrosis factor-α (TNFα), interleukin-1β (IL-1β), platelet activating factor (PAF), oxygen free radicals, interferon-γ (IFN-γ), and arachidonic acid metabolites from monocytes/macrophages and other cells. To maintain homeostasis (and likely as part of a feedback mechanism), several antiinflammatory mediators are also released, including IL-10, transforming growth factor-β (TGF-β), and IL-1 receptor antagonist (IL-1ra). If homeostasis cannot be maintained, there can be progressive and sequential dysfunction of various organ systems, termed the multiple organ dysfunction syndrome (MODS). If the inflammatory stimulus is particularly intense or if there is limited cardiovascular reserve, effects on the cardiovascular system as manifested by septic shock may dominate the clinical presentation. Sepsis-associated myocardial depression occurs as one manifestation of cardiovascular dysfunction in septic shock.

Clinical Manifestations of Cardiovascular Dysfunction

Historical Perspectives

Before the introduction of the balloon-tipped pulmonary artery catheter (PAC) to assess cardiovascular performance over 30 years ago, much of our understanding of septic hemodynamics was based on clinical findings. There were two distinct clinical presentations of septic shock: warm shock characterized by high cardiac output (CO), warm dry skin, and bounding pulses; and cold shock characterized by low CO, cold clammy skin, and diminished pulses (5). Clowes et al. (6) described the relationship between warm and cold shock as a continuum in which either recovery or progression to death occurred. A correlation between survival and a high cardiac index (CI) was also supported in other clinical studies (5,7). The concept was further reinforced by experimental animal studies of low-output endotoxic shock (8,9). However, all the clinical studies used central venous pressure (CVP) as a reflection of left ventricular end-diastolic volume (LVEDV) and adequacy of resuscitation. Based on evidence collected over the past 4 decades, we now know that CVP is a poor measure of preload in critically ill patients, particularly septic patients (10). In addition, endotoxic shock was found to be a poor model of the cardiovascular response to clinical infection with live organisms in a defined focus of infection. During this early period of study, the direct linkage between adequacy of intravascular volume and CI and their relationship to survival was suggested in only a handful of studies (11,12).

In addition to allowing the routine measurement of cardiac output, the introduction of the PAC enabled the routine measurement of preload as pulmonary capillary wedge pressure (PCWP). Studies using the PAC and other modern technologies consistently demonstrate that adequately volume resuscitated septic shock patients consistently manifest a hyperdynamic circulatory state with high CO and reduced systemic vascular resistance (SVR) (13,14), with this hyperdynamic profile usually persisting until death in nonsurvivors (Fig. 30.1) (15,16). These findings have now been confirmed in several live infection animals models of sepsis (17,18).

In the years following the introduction of the PAC, radionuclide cineangiography (RNCA) and its application to critically ill patients have offered insight into the relative contribution of decreased contractility and compliance in myocardial depression. More recently, bedside transthoracic and transesophageal echocardiographic techniques have further expanded our understanding of cardiac dysfunction during sepsis and septic shock.

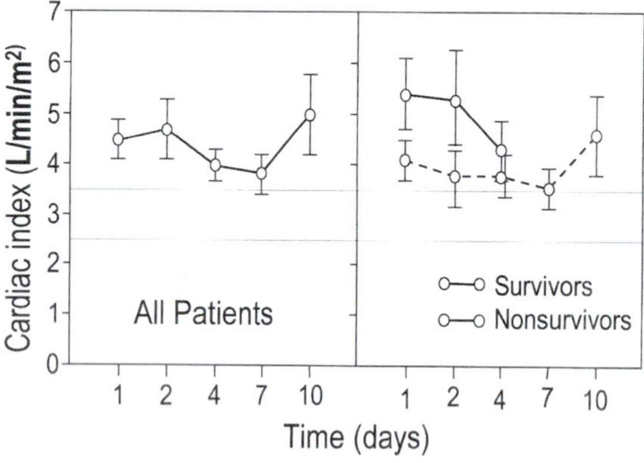

Figure 30.1. The mean (±standard error of the mean [SEM]) cardiac index plotted against time for all patients, survivors, and nonsurvivors. The dotted line shows the normal range. All groups maintained an elevated cardiac index throughout the study period. The difference between the survivors and nonsurvivors was not statistically significant. Open circles, survivors; closed circles, nonsurvivors.

Ventricular Function

MacLean and colleagues (5) were among the first to argue that heart failure remained an issue during septic shock despite elevated CI because metabolic demand exceeds myocardial performance. The concept of septic myocardial depression despite a hyperdynamic circulatory state was reinforced by both Weisel et al. (19) and Rackow et al. (20). They examined responses to fluid resuscitation in septic shock patients using pulmonary artery catheters. Each team demonstrated similar evidence of myocardial depression in septic shock patients, showing decreased stroke work response to fluid resuscitation.

The two studies were hampered by inherent limitations in standard PAC-derived data. Changes in myocardial contractility or compliance can identically produce the depression of the Frank-Starling curve derived from PAC-derived filling pressures. This problem was solved by the application of nuclear cardiology imaging techniques (RNCA) to critically ill patients (21–25).

Left Ventricular Function

Systolic dysfunction has been shown to be impaired in septic patients in a number of studies. Parker et al. (22) demonstrated that septic shock survivors had decreased left ventricular ejection fraction (LVEF) and acute left ventricular (LV) dilatation evidenced by increased LVEDV index (LVEDVI) (Fig. 30.2) using RNCA. These changes in survivors corrected to baseline in 7 to 10 days. Nonsurvivors sustained normal LVEF and LVEDVI until death. Despite systolic dysfunction, septic shock patients maintained a high CO and low SVR as shown by the PAC. In a later study, Ognibene et al. (26) compared left ventricular performance curves (plotting LV stroke work index [LVSWI] vs. LVEDVI) of septic and nonseptic critically ill patients (Fig. 30.3). They showed a flattening of the curve in septic shock patients,

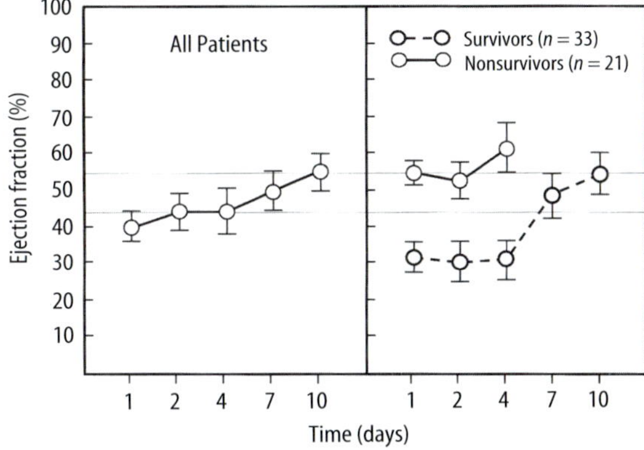

FIGURE 30.2. The mean (± SEM) left ventricular ejection fraction (LVEF) plotted versus time for all patients, survivors, and nonsurvivors. Overall, septic shock patients showed a decreased LVEF at the time of initial assessment. This effect was due to marked early depression of LVEF among survivors that persisted for up to 4 days and returned to normal within 7 to 10 days. Nonsurvivors maintained LVEF in the normal range. The dotted line represents the normal range. Open circles, survivors; closed circles, nonsurvivors.

with significantly smaller LVSWI increments in response to similar LVEDVI increments when compared to nonseptic critically ill controls (26). In the years since these observations, other studies have confirmed the presence of significant left ventricular systolic dysfunction in septic patients using both RNCA and echocardiographic techniques (23,27–31). Raper and colleagues (32) in particular have confirmed myocardial depression in septic patients without shock.

Left ventricular diastolic dysfunction in septic patients is less clearly defined. The acute LV dilatation shown by Parker et al. (22) and a concordant relation between pulmonary arterial wedge pressure (PAWP) and LVEDV do not support the presence of significant diastolic dysfunction. However, Ellrodt and colleagues (23) suggested the possibility of significant variations of diastolic compliance in septic patients, based on a lack of correlation between measured pulmonary wedge pressure (PWP) and any parameter of left ventricular performance or volume. Jafri et al. (33), using Doppler echocardiographic techniques, demonstrated reduced rapidity of ventricular filling and greater reliance on atrial contributions to LVEDV in patients with either normotensive sepsis or septic shock, when compared with controls. Recently, using transesophageal echocardiography (TEE) of vasopressor-dependent septic shock, Poelaert and colleagues (34) demonstrated a continuum of LV pathophysiology ranging from isolated diastolic dysfunction to combined systolic and diastolic abnormalities. This was subsequently confirmed by Munt and colleagues (35), who demonstrated aberrant left ventricular relaxation by Doppler echocardiography in a group of patients with severe sepsis. These investigators have further documented a more severe defect in nonsurvivors than in survivors of severe sepsis.

The concept of preload adaptation by acute left ventricular dilatation in septic shock has been questioned by Jardin and colleagues (36). Transesophageal echocardiography was performed in patients with septic shock following fluid and pressor resuscitation. The LVEDV appeared to remain in the normal range and a low LVEF correlated with stroke index independently of LVEDV. A subsequent longitudinal echocardiographic study found significantly smaller LVEDV in nonsurvivors than in survivors (29).

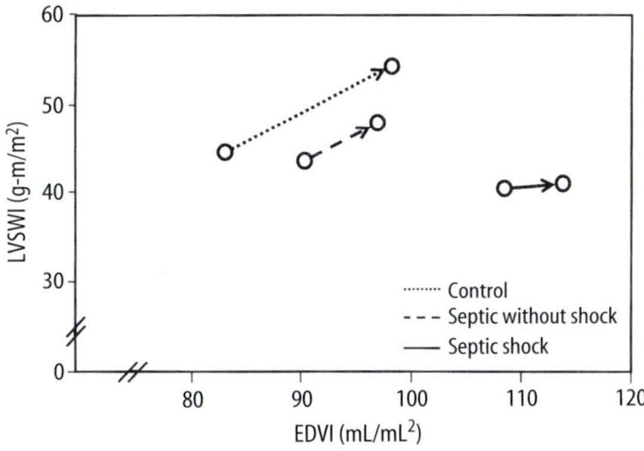

FIGURE 30.3. Frank-Starling ventricular performance relationships for each of the three patient groups. Data points plotted represent the mean prevolume and postvolume infusion values of end-diastolic volume index (EDVI) and left ventricular stroke work index (LVSWI) for each patient group. Control patients showed a normal increase of EDVI and LVSWI in response to volume infusion. The absolute increases of EDVI and LVSWI in patients with sepsis without shock were less than those of control subjects, but the slope of the curve is similar to control patients. Patients with septic shock had a greatly diminished response and showed a marked rightward and downward shift of the Frank-Starling relationship.

Unfortunately, the authors did not utilize PAC monitoring as a measure of fluid loading, so direct comparison with the series of studies by Parker and colleagues is difficult (22,26,30). However, differences in observations in the two groups may potentially be explained by more modest fluid loading in recent echocardiographic studies (29,36).

Right Ventricular Function

Although the output of the ventricles cannot differ in the absence of anatomic cardiopulmonary shunts, the right ventricle may be subject to substantially different influences than the left ventricle, particularly in pathophysiologic conditions such as shock. For that reason, right ventricular (RV) function in sepsis and septic shock cannot be assumed to closely parallel LV function. In the systemic circulation, septic shock is associated with a decreased vascular resistance and blood pressure, almost always resulting in decreased LV afterload, which in turn tends to maintain or elevate CO despite the presence of depressed LV contractility. In contrast, RV afterload is often elevated in sepsis and septic shock due to increases in pulmonary vascular resistance (PVR) associated with acute lung injury and adult respiratory distress syndrome (37), tending to decrease the RV output. Further, it has also been suggested that differentially reduced RV perfusion and contractility could potentially result from a decrease in the RV perfusion gradient during septic shock associated with pulmonary hypertension (38).

Systolic RV dysfunction has been shown by decreased RV ejection fraction (RVEF) and RV dilatation in volume resuscitated patients (39–41). Kimchi et al. (39) and Parker et al. (41) showed that RV dysfunction can occur even in the absence of increased pulmonary artery pressures and pulmonary vascular resistance, suggesting that increased RV afterload may not be the sole explanation for RV dysfunction in septic shock. Parker et al. also showed that RV and LV function paralleled each other in dysfunction and recovery (Fig. 30.4). In this study survivors showed RV dilatation and decreased RVEF and RV stroke work index (RVSWI), which normalized in 7 to 14 days. As with the LV, the RV was only moderately dilated and RVEF marginally decreased; both persisted through their course of sepsis.

Since RV dysfunction occurred independently of PVR and pulmonary arterial pressure (PAP), as also noted by others (32,39), increased RV afterload could not be the dominant cause of RV depression in human septic shock. Another hypothesis suggested that sepsis-associated RV dilation caused septal displacement (due to pericardial constraint), thereby decreasing LV compliance, preload, and performance. Parker et al. (41) also argued against this proposal since biventricular dilation makes that possibility highly unlikely.

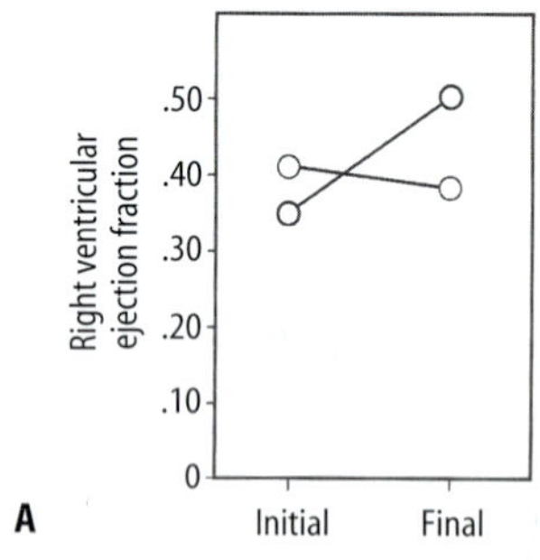

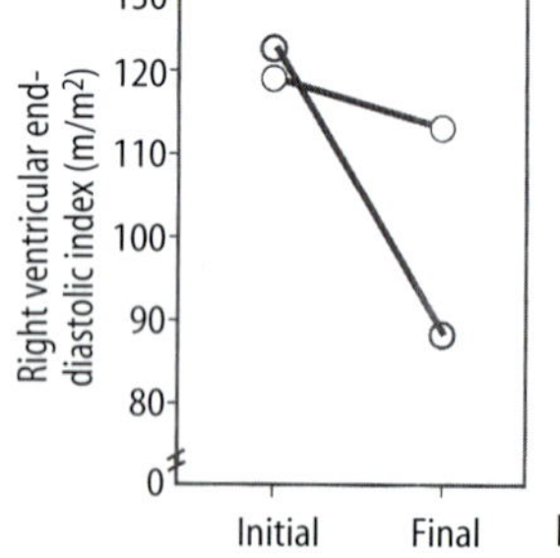

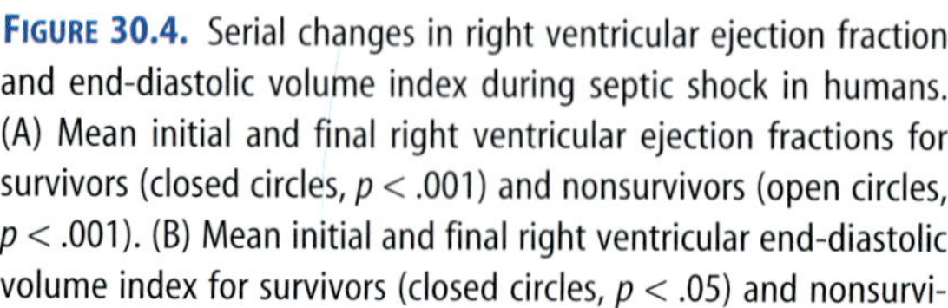

Figure 30.4. Serial changes in right ventricular ejection fraction and end-diastolic volume index during septic shock in humans. (A) Mean initial and final right ventricular ejection fractions for survivors (closed circles, $p < .001$) and nonsurvivors (open circles, $p < .001$). (B) Mean initial and final right ventricular end-diastolic volume index for survivors (closed circles, $p < .05$) and nonsurvivors (open circles, $p =$ not significant). The right ventricle, similar to the left, undergoes dilation with a drop in ejection fraction with the acute onset of septic shock. In 7 to 10 days, right ventricular dilation and decreased ejection fraction revert to normal in survivors.

Newer technologies, using newly developed PACs equipped with fast response thermistors coupled to computerized analytic equipment have generated confirmatory data regarding RV dysfunction in sepsis (42,43). Available evidence suggests that despite the differences between the ventricles in structure and function, RV dysfunction in septic shock closely parallels LV dysfunction. Right ventricular function in both sepsis and septic shock is characterized by ventricular dilation and decreased RVEF, changes that resolve over 7 to 14 days in septic shock survivors. The cardiovascular profiles of nonsurvivors are characterized by persistence of RV dysfunction.

Diastolic (compliance) dysfunction of the RV has also been demonstrated in a number of studies. Kimchi et al. (39) noticed a lack of correlation between right atrial pressure and RVEDV, suggesting altered RV compliance. In another study, a subgroup of patients who were volume loaded demonstrated increase in CVP but not RVEDVI (40). As in the LV, the relative contribution of systolic and diastolic dysfunction in the RV is unknown.

Cardiovascular Prognostic Factors in Septic Shock

Cardiac index appears not to be a reliable predictor of mortality in septic shock. Despite early evidence suggesting low CI as a poor prognostic factor (5–7,11), introduction of the PAC has shown that septic shock patients, when adequately fluid-resuscitated, have a high CI and low SVR among both survivors and nonsurvivors (13,14). Armed with the PAC, other hemodynamic parameters were investigated as prognostic indicators.

Baumgartner et al. (44) recognized that patients with extremely high CI (>7.0 L/min/m^2) and accordingly low SVR had poor outcomes. Groeneveld et al. (45) also found nonsurvivors had lower SVRs than survivors after matching other characteristics, concluding that there may be a link between outcome in septic shock and the degree of peripheral vasodilation.

Parker et al. (15) reviewed hemodynamic data from septic shock patients on presentation and at 24 hours to identify prognostic value. On presentation, only heart rate <106 beats/min suggested a favorable outcome. At 24 hours, heart rate <95 beats/min, SVRI >1529 dynes·sec·cm^5/m^2, a decrease in heart rate >18 beats/min, and a decrease in CI >0.5 L/min/m^2 all predicted survival. In a subsequent study (16), the same authors confirmed previous findings of decreased LVEF and increased LVEDVI in survivors of septic shock but not in nonsurvivors, a finding that has been confirmed by other groups (28,29). Although myocardial depression has been historically linked to increased mortality, these data may imply that depression, at least as manifested by decreased ejection fraction with ventricular dilatation, may actually represent an adaptive to stress rather than a maladaptive manifestation of injury.

From the studies of Parker and Parillo's team (15,16), it is apparent that, despite not developing significant LV dilatation overall, nonsurvivors could be divided into two patterns: those with progressively declining LVEDVI and CI, and those with incremental increases in LVEDVI while maintaining CI. Based on this, Parker et al. described different hemodynamic collapse profiles leading to death in septic shock (15,16). On one pattern, some patients die from refractory hypotension secondary to distributive shock with preserved or elevated CI. The other pattern consists of cardiogenic form of septic shock with decreased CI and mixture of cardiogenic and distributive shock patterns. The explanation of the two patterns came from a study by Parker et al. (16). It appears that patients who cannot dilate their LV (decreasing CI and LVEDVI) die from cardiogenic form of septic shock. The other fatal pattern consists of those patients who can dilate their LV and preserve CI (increase LVEDVI while maintaining CI) but eventually die of distributive shock.

The prognostic value of RV hemodynamic parameters has been debated. A number of studies have shown that RV dilatation and decreased RVEF, if persistent, are associated with poor prognosis (39–41,43). However, Vincent et al. (43) suggested that high initial RVEF portends a good prognosis. On the other hand, Parker et al. (41) found that the survivors had a lower RVEF. The answer to this question requires additional investigation.

The other prognostic parameter is response of hemodynamic parameters to dynamic challenges, namely dobutamine. Nonsurvivors of septic shock have a blunted response to dobutamine (46–48), whereas survivors demonstrated increased stroke work index (SWI), increased mixed venous oxygen saturation, ventricular dilatation, and a decrease in diastolic blood pressure after a dobutamine challenge. The above response to dobutamine predicts survival in patients with septic shock.

Etiology of Myocardial Depression in Sepsis and Septic Shock

The exact sequence of events in the pathophysiology of septic myocardial depression has only begun to be elucidated in recent years. There are likely a multitude of mechanisms and factors that play a role. A number of potential pathogenic mechanisms have been proposed. The two major theories have been myocardial hypoperfusion or a circulating myocardial depressant substance.

Organ Level: Myocardial Hypoperfusion

The potential of myocardial hypoperfusion leading to myocardial depression via global ischemia has been largely dismissed by a number of studies. Cunnion et al. (49) inserted thermodilution catheters into the coronary sinus of septic patients and measured serial coronary flow and metabolism (Fig. 30.5). Flow measurements were stratified into heart rates above and below 100 beats/min. Coronary blood flow in septic shock patients equaled (heart rate <100/min) or exceeded (heart rate >100/min) coronary blood flow in control patients. There was also no difference in myocardial blood flow between septic patients who did and did not developed myocardial dysfunction. There also was no net lactate production.

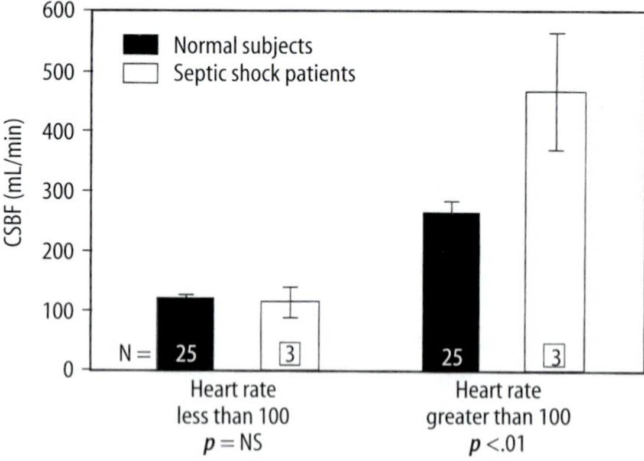

Figure 30.5. Mean coronary sinus blood flow (CSBF) in seven patients with septic shock compared with normal subjects. Flow measurements were stratified into heart rates above and below 100 beats/min. Coronary blood flow in septic shock patients equaled (heart rate < 100/min) or exceeded (heart rate > 100/min) coronary blood flow in control patients.

Dhainaut et al. (50) also confirmed these findings while employing similar methods. In addition to human studies, a canine model of sepsis study (51) showed that myocardial high-energy phosphates and oxygen utilization were preserved in septic shock. Both of these observations argue against neither global myocardial ischemia nor hypoperfusion.

Perfusion aside, there is evidence for myocardial cell injury evidenced by increased troponin I levels in septic shock (52). A study by ver Elst et al. (53) examined levels of troponin I and T in patients with septic shock. A correlation between LV dysfunction and troponin I (TnI) positivity (78% vs. 9% in cTnI-negative (cardiac troponin I, cTnI) patients $p < .001$) existed. They also found that older patients with underlying cardiovascular disease more often had both troponin positivity and LV dysfunction. However, whether the clinically inapparent myocardial cell injury contributes to or is a consequence of septic shock is yet to be determined (53). Although troponin is used as a marker of myocardial injury (particularly in the context of myocardial ischemia), it does not specifically suggest myocardial hypoperfusion in other contexts.

Myocardial Depressant Substances

The theory of a circulating myocardial depressant factor was put forth by Wiggers (54) in 1947 in the context of hemorrhagic shock. The presence of such a factor was confirmed by Brand and by Lefer (55) in 1966. Lefer's work prompted further research into septic myocardial depressant substances. A number of endogenous substances have been implicated as potential causes of septic myocardial depression. These have included estrogenic compounds, histamine, eicosanoids/prostaglandins, and several novel substances that could never be effectively isolated (for review, see

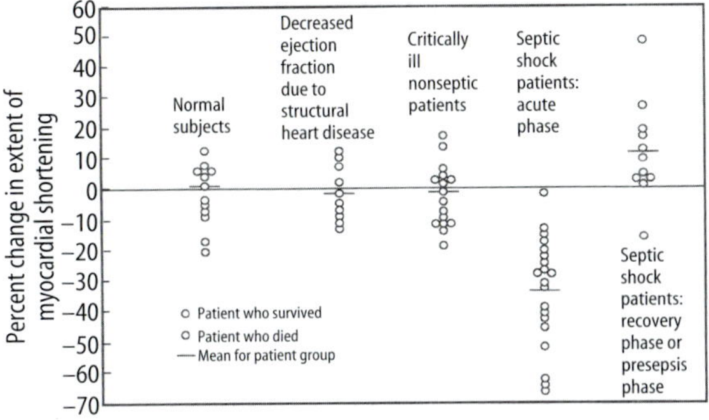

FIGURE 30.6. The effect of serum from septic shock patients and control groups on the extent of myocardial cell shortening of spontaneously beating rat heart cells in vitro. Septic shock patients during the acute phase demonstrated a statistically significant lower extent of shortening ($p < .001$) compared with any other group. Open circles, survivors; closed circles, nonsurvivors; horizontal line, mean for each group.

Kumar et al. [56]). In the last decade, the dominant focus has been on inflammatory cytokines.

In one of the seminal studies in the field, Parillo et al. in 1985 (57) showed a link between myocyte depression and septic serum from a patient with sepsis associated myocardial depression. The serum from patients demonstrated concentration-dependent depression of in vitro myocyte contractility (Fig. 30.6). Septic shock patients during the acute phase demonstrated a statistically significant lower extent of shortening ($p < .001$) compared with any other group. Parrillo et al. were also able to correlate a temporal and qualitative relationship between in vivo myocardial depression (decreased LVEF) and in vitro cardiac myocyte depression induced by serum from corresponding patients.

In another study, investigators noted that higher levels of myocardial depressant activity correlated with higher peak serum lactate, increase ventricular filling pressures, increased LVEDVI, and mortality (36% vs. 10%) when compared with patients with lower or absent activity levels (58). Subsequent work focused on identifying the myocardial depressant substances and thereby investigating potential treatments.

Potential circulating myocardial depressant substances include arachidonic acid metabolites, platelet-activating factor, histamine, and endorphins. Filtration studies (58) found that the substance was water soluble, heat labile, and greater than 10kd. These characteristics pointed toward a protein or polypeptide consistent with cytokines such as TNF-α and IL-1β.

It is likely that TNF-α has a role as a myocardial depressant substance for a number of reasons. It shares the same biochemical profile as myocardial depressant substances (57,59). Clinically, TNF-α is associated with fever, increased lactic acid, disseminated intravascular coagulation, acute lung injury, and death. The hemodynamic effects of TNF-α are similar to sepsis, in particular hypotension, increased cardiac output, and low systemic vascular resistance (60,61).

Healthy human volunteers given TNF-α infusions have similar responses (62,63). Experimentally, TNF-α given to in vitro and ex vivo animal and human myocardial tissue demonstrated a concentration-dependent depression of contractility (64,65). Kumar et al. (66) showed that removal of TNF-α from patients serum with septic shock decreased the myocardial depression. Also, Vincent et al. (67), in a pilot study, showed improved LVSWI with administration of anti–TNF-α monoclonal antibody even though there was no survival benefit.

Interleukin-1β produces similar hemodynamic responses to TNF-α. The IL-1β levels are also elevated in sepsis and septic shock (68). In vitro and ex vivo myocardial contractility is depressed when cardiac tissue is exposed to IL-1β (65,69,70). Removal of IL-1β via immunoabsorption from septic human serum attenuates the depression of cardiac myocytes (66). The effects of IL-1β antagonist on cardiac function and survival are unimpressive (71–73), even though metabolic derangements are attenuated by IL-1β antagonist (72,73).

It is likely that cytokines such as TNF-α and IL-1β, rather than working in isolation, synergize to exert their depressant effects. In isolation, TNF-α and IL-1β require very high concentration to induce in vitro rat myocyte depression (66). However, when combined, they act synergistically and require concentrations 50 to 100 times lower than those required individually (66,74). These concentrations are within the range of those found in septic shock patients.

Another recent series of studies by Pathan and colleagues (75–77) have strongly implicated circulating IL-6 as an important myocardial depressant substance in human septic shock. These investigators have demonstrated that meningococcal sepsis is associated with induction of IL-6 expression in blood mononuclear cells and that the level of serum IL-6 corresponds with the degree of cardiac function in such patients. Further, they have recently shown that IL-6 depresses contractility of myocardial tissue in vitro and that neutralization of IL-6 in serum from patients with meningococcal septic shock neutralizes this effect (75).

Evidence for other potential myocardial depressant substances (MDSs) continue to be developed. Recently, Mink et al. (78) have implicated lysozyme c (consistent with that found in the spleen, and leukocytes in the spleen or other organs) as a potential MDS. In the canine model of *Escherichia coli* sepsis, lysozyme c caused myocardial depression and attenuated the response to β-agonists (78). The potential mechanism proposed was lysozyme binding or hydrolyzing the membrane glycoprotein of cardiac myocytes, thereby affecting signal transduction (linking physiologic excitation with physiologic contraction). The levels of lysozyme c were found to be elevated in the heart and spleen, but not in lymphocytes when compared to preseptic levels (78). Mink et al. (79) went on to show that pretreatment with an inhibitor of lysozyme (N,N′,N″-triacetylglucosamine) prevented myocardial depression in canine sepsis. However, the effect of this lysozyme inhibitor (TAC) was only seen in pretreatment and early treatment groups (1.5 hours after onset of septic shock) and not in late treatment groups (greater than 3.5 hours).

An important microbial factor that has recently been shown to potentially exert hemodynamic and myocardial depressant activity in sepsis and septic shock is bacterial nucleic acid. Several investigators have demonstrated that unique aspects of bacterial nucleic acid structure may allow bacterial DNA to generate a shock state similar to that produced by endotoxin when administered to animals (80). Extending these observations, we have recently demonstrated depression of rat myocyte contraction with bacterial DNA and RNA (81). This effect was more marked when DNA and RNA came from pathogenic strains of *Staphylococcus aureus* and *E. coli.* These effects were not seen when the test solution was pretreated with DNase and RNase.

Other factors may also play a role in septic myocardial depression. Data developed in recent years have suggested that macrophage migration inhibitory factor, a novel neuropeptide and proinflammatory cytokine involved in immune homeostasis, is also a cardiac-derived myocardial depressant substance associated with endotoxin-induced myocardial dysfunction (82,83). Based on the history of the field over the last 30 years, it is likely that other important substances that may play a role in septic myocardial dysfunction remain to be discovered.

Cellular Level

The sequence of mechanisms leading from an MDS to cellular dysfunction remains substantially opaque. There are several potential mechanisms that may play a role at the cellular level. Overproduction of nitric oxide (NO) and derangements of calcium physiology in the myocardial cell are two potential cellular mechanisms.

In vitro, myocyte depression in response to inflammatory cytokines can be divided into early and late phases. Early cardiac myocyte depression occurs within minutes of exposure to either TNF-α or IL-1β, or to TNF-α and IL-1β given together, or to septic serum (66,84). Tumor necrosis factor-α also demonstrates the ability to cause rapid myocardial depression in dogs (61,85). Besides the early effects of TNF-α, IL-1β and supernatants of activated macrophages also have a later, prolonged effect on in vitro myocardial tissue (69,70,85,86). This late phase establishes within hours and lasts for days. This suggests a different mechanism from early myocardial depression.

Production of nitric oxide (NO) may be a potential explanation for both early and late myocardial depression. Nitric oxide is produced from conversion of L-arginine to L-citrulline by nitric oxide synthase (NOS), which has two forms: constitutive (cNOS) and inducible (iNOS). Nitric oxide produced by cNOS appears to have a regulatory role in cardiac contractility (87–89). However, when cardiac myocytes are exposed to supraphysiologic levels of NO or NO donors (nitroprusside and SIN-1), there is a reduction in myocardial contractility (90). Paulus et al. (91) infused nitroprusside into coronary arteries, which decreased intraventricular pressures and improved diastolic function.

Current evidence suggests that early myocyte dysfunction may occur through generation of NO and resultant cyclic guanosine monophosphate (cGMP) via cNOS activation in cardiac myocytes and adjacent endothelium (74,84,92). Late myocardial depression may be secondary to induction of synthesis of iNOS NO (70,84,93,94). In addition, the generation of peroxynitrite via interaction of the free radical NO group and oxygen may also play a role in more prolonged effects (95). We have demonstrated that the early phase may involve both a NO-dependent but β-adrenergic–independent mechanism and a NO-independent defect of β-adrenoreceptor signal transduction (56,92,96,97). Others have shown that IL-6 can cause both early and late NO-mediated myocardial depression in an avian myocardial cell model via sequential activation of cNOS followed by induction of iNOS, a finding that could explain recent human data implicating IL-6 in meningococcal septic myocardial dysfunction (75,76,98–100). This study suggests a role for sequential production of NO from cNOS and iNOS in the pathogenesis of myocardial depression from cytokines.

Potential Therapies of Septic Myocardial Depression

Although there have been tremendous advances in understanding the almost universal presence of myocardial dysfunction in septic shock, there is a startling lack of data on the clinical importance of this phenomenon. The majority of patients maintain a hyperdynamic circulatory state despite the presence of septic myocardial dysfunction. There are no published data on the frequency and survival characteristics of overt myocardial depression with reduced cardiac output in septic shock. In an unpublished data set held by the primary author, 7% of the approximately 1620 unselected septic shock patients in whom a pulmonary artery catheter was placed within 48 hours of presentation had a cardiac index of <2.2. Overall survival was 36%. However, among those with a cardiac index of less than 2.2 L/min/m^2, survival was only 30%. Interestingly, the subgroup with pulmonary wedge pressure of >18 had an even lower survival at 26%. The majority of patients with low cardiac index (>60%) were not known to have significant preexisting ventricular dysfunction. These data suggest that overt myocardial depression with low cardiac output due to sepsis may occur in 4% to 5% of septic shock and appears to be associated with increased mortality.

For patient's with the usual hyperdynamic circulatory state of high cardiac output and low systemic vascular resistance with hypotension, standard therapy with fluid loading followed by vasopressor therapy (dopamine, norepinephrine, phenylephrine ± vasopressin) suffices. One notable aspect of recent findings on therapy of septic shock relates to the demonstration that early augmentation of oxygen delivery (early goal-directed therapy) in a protocolized manner in patients with a central venous (superior vena cava) oxygen saturation of <70% can improve outcome in patients with associated organ failure (Fig. 30.7) (101,102). Augmentation of oxygen delivery in this context can be effected through fluid resuscitation, packed red blood cell transfusion, and dobutamine infusion. The impact of hemodynamic support on survival may imply that despite the usual hyperdynamic, high-output state in septic shock, cardiac output may be inadequate relative to needs due to myocardial dysfunction. Detailed analysis of key aspects of therapy of such patients exists elsewhere (102–104).

In the minority of case where septic myocardial depression may be sufficiently expressed clinically to require treatment, options are available. Epinephrine, dobutamine, milrinone, and digoxin have all been shown to improve cardiac function in low-output septic shock (105–107). In the case of catecholamines, sepsis can clearly be associated with reduced responsiveness. However, with milrinone and digoxin, our clinical experience suggests increased sensitivity. For that reason, initial doses should be at or below the minimum usual starting dose. These modalities are nonspecific and strictly supportive in nature. It is unclear if augmentation of cardiac output in these situations will favorably impact on outcome.

Research into the pathophysiology of sepsis-induced myocardial depression naturally leads to potential specific therapies to reverse septic myocardial dysfunction. Several investigators have examined the use of various hemofiltration modalities in septic shock (108–112). However,

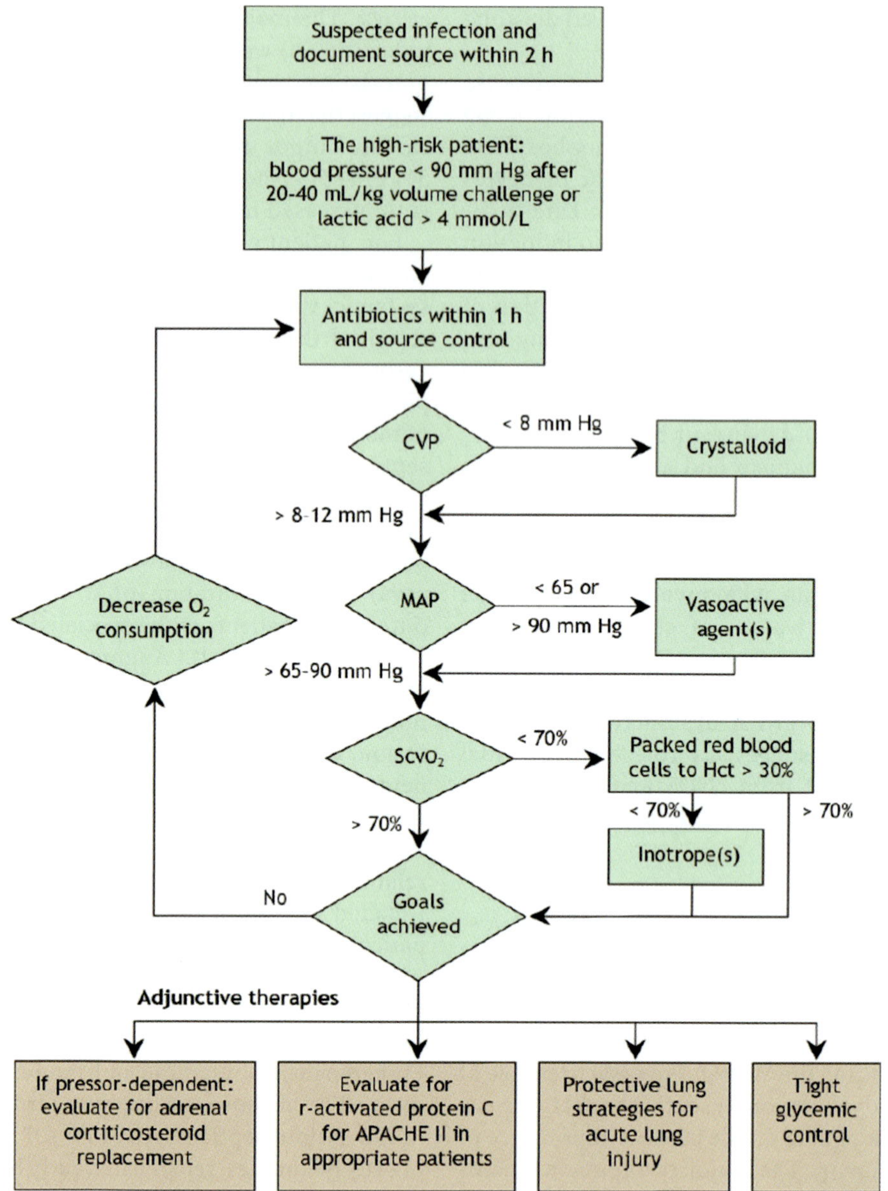

Figure 30.7. Approach to treatment in severe sepsis and septic shock. CVP, central venous pressure; MAP, mean arterial pressure; $ScvO_2$, central venous oxygen saturation; Hct, hematocrit. (From Rivers et al. [102], with permission.)

results have been highly inconsistent. Mink et al. (109) utilized continuous arteriovenous hemofiltration combined with systemic vasopressor therapy to reverse cardiac depression and hypotension in an endotoxicosis-equivalent canine *E. coli* sepsis model. Freeman and colleagues (110), however, were unable to demonstrate such a benefit.

Inflammatory cytokine antagonists are another area of research. As previously mentioned, TNF-α monoclonal antibodies have improved LV function when given to patients in septic shock (67), despite failing to show a survival benefit. The IL-1β antagonists have shown mixed results. Despite the absence of a survival benefit, attenuation of metabolic derangements in septic shock was noted

(72,73), although no hemodynamic benefit was apparent (71).

Further down the sequence of pathogenesis in septic myocardial depression are the therapeutic potential of NO scavengers or NO inhibitors. Methylene blue (NO scavenger) has been shown to attenuate the hemodynamic alterations in a randomized open-label pilot of 20 patients with sepsis (113). Suzuki et al. (114) used an inhibitor of iNOS (L-canavanine) in septic rats, which showed prevention of myocardial contractility depression. However, L-canavanine itself depressed myocardial contractility via decreased coronary blood flow, an effect that was thought to be potentially responsible for the increased mortality in the only randomized double-blinded clinical study of a NOS inhibitor in clinical septic shock (115,116).

Conclusion

Myocardial dysfunction is an important component in the hemodynamic collapse induced by sepsis and septic shock. A series of inflammatory cascades triggered by the inciting infection generate circulatory myocardial depressant substances, including TNF-α, IL-1β, PAF, and lysozyme. Current evidence suggests that septic myocardial depression in humans is characterized by reversible biventricular dilatation, decreased systolic contractile function, and decreased response to both fluid resuscitation and catecholamine stimulation, all in the presence of an overall hyperdynamic circulation. This phenomenon is linked to the presence of a circulating myocardial depressant substance or substances, which probably represent low concentrations of proinflammatory cytokines including TNF-α, IL-1β, and perhaps IL-6 acting in synergy. These effects are mediated through mechanisms that include but are not limited to NO and cGMP generation. The mechanism through which NO depresses cardiac contractility is largely unknown. Recent data suggest that preapoptotic signaling involving the transcription factors signal transducer and activator of transcription (STAT1), interferon regulatory factor (IRF1), and nuclear factor (NF)-κB leading to apoptotic pathways may play a role in septic myocardial depression related to inflammatory cytokines circulating during septic shock. Links between this response and nitric oxide generation are postulated but have not been fully delineated.

References

1. Angus DC, Linde-Zwirble WT, Lidicker J, Clermont G, Carcillo J, Pinsky MR. Epidemiology of severe sepsis in the United States: analysis of incidence, outcome, and associated costs of care. [see comments.]. Crit Care Med 2001;29(7):1303–10.
2. Martin GS, Mannino DM, Eaton S, Moss M. The epidemiology of sepsis in the United States from 1979 through 2000. N Engl J Med 2003;348(16):1546–54.
3. Chaudry IH. Sepsis: lessons learned in the last century and future directions. Arch Surg 1999;134(9):922–9.
4. Bone RC, Balk R, Cerra FB, et al. ACCP/SCCM Consensus Conference: definitions for sepsis and organ failure and guidelines for use of innovative therapies in sepsis. Chest 1992;101:1644–55.
5. MacLean LD, Mulligan WG, McLean APH, Duff JH. Patterns of septic shock in man: a detailed study of 56 patients. Ann Surg 1967;166:543–62.
6. Clowes GHA, Vucinic M, Weidner MG. Circulatory and metabolic alterations associated with survival or death in peritonitis. Ann Surg 1966;163:866–44.
7. Nishijima H, Weil MH, Shubin H, Cavanilles J. Hemodynamic and metabolic studies on shock associated with gram-negative bacteremia. Medicine (Baltimore) 1973;52:287–94.
8. Weil MH, MacLean LD, Visscher MD, Spink W. Studies on the circulatory changes in the dog produced by endotoxin from gram-negative microorganisms. J Clin Invest 1956;35:1191–8.
9. Solis RT, Downing SE. Effects of E. coli endotoxemia on ventricular performance. Am J Physiol 1966;211:307–13.
10. Packman MI, Rackow EC. Optimum left heart filling pressure during fluid resuscitation of patients with hypovolemic and septic shock. Crit Care Med 1983;11:165–9.
11. Weil MH, Nishijima H. Cardiac output in bacterial shock. Am J Med 1978;64:920–2.
12. Blain CM, Anderson TO, Pietras RJ, Gunnar RM. Immediate hemodynamic effects of gram-negative vs gram-positive bacteremia in man. Arch Intern Med 1970;126:260–5.
13. Winslow EJ, Loeb HS, Rahimtoola SH, Kamath S, Gunnar RM. Hemodynamic studies and results of therapy in 50 patients with bacteremic shock. Am J Med 1973;54:421–32.

14. Krausz MM, Perel A, Eimerl D, Cotev S. Cardiopulmonary effects of volume loading in patients with septic shock. Ann Surg 1977;185:429–34.
15. Parker MM, Shelhamer JH, Natanson C, Alling DW, Parrillo JE. Serial cardiovascular variables in survivors and nonsurvivors of human septic shock: Heart rate as an early predictor of prognosis. Crit Care Med 1987;15:923–9.
16. Parker MM, Suffredini AF, Natanson C, Ognibene FP, Shelhamer JH, Parrillo JE. Responses of left ventricular function in survivors and non-survivors of septic shock. J Crit Care 1989;4:19–25.
17. Kumar A, Haery C, Paladugu B, et al. Duration of hypotension prior to antibiotic administration is a critical determinant of outcome in a murine model of E. coli septic shock. J Infect Dis 2006;193:251–8.
18. Natanson C, Fink MP, Ballantyne HK, MacVittie TJ, Conklin JJ, Parrillo JE. Gram-negative bacteremia produces both severe systolic and diastolic cardiac dysfunction in a canine model that simulates human septic shock. J Clin Invest 1986;78:259–70.
19. Weisul RD, Vito L, Dennis RC, Valeri CR, Hechtman HB. Myocardial depression during sepsis. Am J Surg 1977;133:512–21.
20. Rackow EC, Kaufman BS, Falk JL, Astiz ME, Weil MH. Hemodynamic response to fluid repletion in patients with septic shock: evidence for early depression of cardiac performance. Circ Shock 1987;22:11–22.
21. Calvin JE, Driedger AA, Sibbald WJ. An assessment of myocardial function in human sepsis utilizing ECG gated cardiac scintigraphy. Chest 1981;80:579–86.
22. Parker MM, Shelhamer JH, Bacharach SL, et al. Profound but reversible myocardial depression in patients with septic shock. Ann Intern Med 1984;100:483–90.
23. Ellrodt AG, Riedinger MS, Kimchi A, et al. Left ventricular performance in septic shock: Reversible segmental and global abnormalities. Am Heart J 1985;110:402–9.
24. Thomas F, Smith JL, Orme J, et al. Reversible segmental myocardial dysfunction in septic shock. Crit Care Med 1986;14:587–8.
25. Chidiac TA, Salon JE. Left ventricular segmental wall motion abnormality in septic shock. Crit Care Med 1995;23:594–8.
26. Ognibene FP, Parker MM, Natanson C, Shelhamer JH, Parrillo JE. Depressed left ventricular performance. Response to volume infusion in patients with sepsis and septic shock. Chest 1988;93:903–10.
27. Raper R, Sibbald WJ. Misled by the wedge? The Swan-Ganz catheter and left ventricular preload. Chest 1986;89(3):427–34.
28. Vieillard BA, Schmitt JM, Beauchet A, et al. Early preload adaptation in septic shock? A transesophageal echocardiographic study. Anesthesiology 2001;94(3):400–6.
29. Jardin F, Fourme T, Page B, et al. Persistent preload defect in severe sepsis despite fluid loading: A longitudinal echocardiographic study in patients with septic shock. Chest 1999;116(5):1354–9.
30. Mellow E, Parker MM, Cunnion RE, Parrillo JE. Reversible depression and ventricular dilation demonstrated by two dimensional echocardiography in humans with septic shock. Critical Care Medicine 1986;14:342.
31. Monslave F, Rucabado L, Salvador A, Bonastre J, Ruano M. Myocardial depression in septic shock caused by meningococcal infection. Crit Care Med 1984;12:1021–3.
32. Raper RF, Sibbald WJ, Driedger AA, Gerow K. Relative myocardial depression in normotensive sepsis. J Crit Care 1989;4:9–18.
33. Jafri SM, Lavine S, Field BE, Thill-Baharozian MC, Carlson RW. Left ventricular diastolic function in sepsis. Crit Care Med 1991;18:709–14.
34. Poelaert J, Declerck C, Vogelaers D, Colardyn F, Visser CA. Left ventricular systolic and diastolic function in septic shock. Intensive Care Med 1997;23:553–60.
35. Munt B, Jue J, Gin K, Fenwick J, Tweeddale M. Diastolic filling in human severe sepsis: An echocardiographic study. Crit Care Med 1998;26:1829–33.
36. Jardin F, Valtier B, Beauchet A, Dubourg O, Bourdarias JP. Invasive monitoring combined with two-dimensional echocardiographic study in septic shock. Intensive Care Med 1994;20:550–4.
37. Sibbald WJ, Paterson NAM, Holliday RL, Anderson RA, Lobb TR, Duff JH. Pulmonary hypertension in sepsis: measurement by the pulmonary artery diastolic-pulmonary wedge pressure gradient and the influence of passive and active factors. Chest 1978;73:583–91.
38. Calvin JE. Acute right heart failure: Pathophysiology, recognition, and pharmacological management. J Cardiothorac Vasc Anesth 1991;5:507–13.
39. Kimchi A, Ellrodt GA, Berman DS, et al. Right ventricular performance in septic shock: a combined radionuclide and hemodynamic study. J Am Coll Cardiol 1984;4:945–51.
40. Schneider AJ, Teule GJJ, Groenveld ABJ, Nauta J, Heidendal GAK, Thijs LG. Biventricular perform-

ance during volume loading in patients with early septic shock, with emphasis on the right ventricle: a combined hemodynamic and radionuclide study. Am Heart J 1988;116:103–12.

41. Parker MM, McCarthy KE, Ognibene FP, Parrillo JE. Right ventricular dysfunction and dilatation, similar to left ventricular changes, characterize the cardiac depression of septic shock in humans. Chest 1990;97:126–31.
42. Dhainaut JF, Lanore JJ, de Gournay MF, et al. Right ventricular dysfunction in patients with septic shock. Intensive Care Med 1988;14:488–91.
43. Vincent JL, Reuse C, Frank N, Contempre B, Kahn RJ. Right ventricular dysfunction in septic shock: assessment by measurements of right ventricular ejection fraction using the thermodilution technique. Acta Anaesthesiol Scand 1989;33:34–8.
44. Baumgartner J, Vaney C, Perret C. An extreme form of hyperdynamic syndrome in septic shock. Intensive Care Med 1984;10:245–9.
45. Groenveld ABJ, Nauta JJ, Thijs L. Peripheral vascular resistance in septic shock: its relation to outcome. Intensive Care Med 1988;14:141–7.
46. Rhodes A, Lamb FJ, Malagon R, Newman PJ, Grounds M, Bennett D. A prospective study of the use of a dobutamine stress test to identify outcome in patients with sepsis, severe sepsis or septic shock. Crit Care Med 1999;27:2361–6.
47. Vallet B, Chopin C, Curtis SE. Prognostic value of the dobutamine test in patients with sepsis syndrome and normal lactate values: a prospective, multicenter study. Crit Care Med 1993;21:1868–75.
48. Kumar A, Schupp E, Bunnell E, et al. The cardiovascular response to dobutamine in septic shock. Clin Invest Med 1994;17(B18):107.
49. Cunnion RE, Schaer GL, Parker MM, Natanson C, Parrillo JE. The coronary circulation in human septic shock. Circulation 1986;73:637–44.
50. Dhainaut JF, Huyghebaert MF, Monsallier JF, et al. Coronary hemodynamics and myocardial metabolism of lactate, free fatty acids, glucose, and ketones in patients with septic shock. Circulation 1987;75:533–41.
51. Solomon MA, Correa R, Alexander HR, et al. Myocardial energy metabolism and morphology in a canine model of sepsis. Am J Physiol 1994;266: H757–68.
52. Turner A, Tsamitros M, Bellomo R. Myocardial cell injury in septic shock. Crit Care Med 1999; 27(9):1775–80.
53. ver Elst KM, Spapen HD, Nguyen DN, Garbar C, Huyghens LP, Gorus FK. Cardiac troponins I and T are biological markers of left ventricular dysfunction in septic shock. Clin Chem 2000;46(5): 650–7.
54. Wiggers CJ. Myocardial depression in shock. A survey of cardiodynamic studies. Am Heart J 1947;33:633–50.
55. Lefer AM. Mechanisms of cardiodepression in endotoxin shock. Circ Shock 1979;1:1–8.
56. Kumar A, Krieger A, Symeoneides S, Kumar A, Parrillo JE. Myocardial dysfunction in septic shock, Part II: Role of cytokines and nitric oxide. J Cardiovasc Thorac Anesth 2001;15(4):485–511.
57. Parrillo JE, Burch C, Shelhamer JH, Parker MM, Natanson C, Schuette W. A circulating myocardial depressant substance in humans with septic shock. Septic shock patients with a reduced ejection fraction have a circulating factor that depresses in vitro myocardial cell performance. J Clin Invest 1985;76:1539–53.
58. Reilly JM, Cunnion RE, Burch-Whitman C, Parker MM, Shelhamer JH, Parrillo JE. A circulating myocardial depressant substance is associated with cardiac dysfunction and peripheral hypoperfusion (lactic acidemia) in patients with septic shock. Chest 1989;95:1072–80.
59. Seckinger P, Vey E, Turcatti G, Wingfield P, Dayer J. Tumor necrosis factor inhibitor: purification, NH2–terminal amino acid sequence and evidence for anti-inflammatory and immunomodulatory activities. Eur J Immunol 1990;20:1167–74.
60. Eichacker PQ, Hoffman WD, Farese A, et al. TNF but not IL-1 in dogs causes lethal lung injury and multiple organ dysfunction similar to human sepsis. J Appl Physiol 1991;71:1979–89.
61. Eichenholz PW, Eichacker PQ, Hoffman WD, et al. Tumor necrosis factor challenges in canines: Patterns of cardiovascular dysfunction. Am J Physiol 1992;263:H668–75.
62. van der Poll T, van Deventer SJ, Hack CE, et al. Effects on leukocytes following injection of tumor necrosis factor into healthy humans. Blood 1992; 79:693–8.
63. van der Poll T, Romjin JA, Endert E, Borm JJ, Buller HR, Sauerwein HP. Tumor necrosis factor mimics the metabolic response to acute infection in healthy humans. Am J Physiol 1991;261: E457–65.
64. Gu M, Bose R, Bose D, et al. Tumor necrosis factor-a but not septic plasma depresses cardiac myofilament contraction. Can J Anaesth 1998;45: 352–9.
65. Weisensee D, Bereiter-Hahn J, Low-Friedrich I. Effects of cytokines on the contractility of cultured cardiac myocytes. Int J Immunopharmacol 1993; 15:581–7.

66. Kumar A, Thota V, Dee L, Olson J, Uretz E, Parrillo JE. Tumor necrosis factor-alpha and interleukin-1 beta are responsible for depression of in vitro myocardial cell contractility induced by serum from humans with septic shock. J Exp Med 1996;183:949–58.
67. Vincent JL, Bakker J, Marecaux G, Schandene L, Kahn RJ, Dupont E. Administration of anti-TNF antibody improves left ventricular function in septic shock patients: Results of a pilot study. Chest 1992;101:810–5.
68. Hesse DG, Tracey KJ, Fong Y, et al. Cytokine appearance in human endotoxemia and primate bacteremia. Surg Gynecol Obstet 1988;166:147–53.
69. Gulick T, Chung MK, Pieper SJ, Lange LG, Schreiner GF. Interleukin-1 and tumor necrosis factor inhibit cardiac myocyte adrenergic responsiveness. Proc Natl Acad Sci 1989;86:6753–7.
70. Hosenpud JD, Campbell SM, Mendelson DJ. Interleukin-1-induced myocardial depression in an isolated beating heart preparation. J Heart Transplant 1989;8:460–4.
71. Vincent JL, Slotman G, van Leeuwen PAM, et al. IL-1ra administration does not improve cardiac function in patients with severe sepsis. Intensive Care Med 2004;21:S11.
72. Fisher CJ Jr, Dhainaut JF, Opal SM, et al. Recombinant human interleukin 1 receptor antagonist in the treatment of patients with sepsis syndrome. Results from a randomized, double-blind, placebo-controlled trial. Phase III rhIL-1ra Sepsis Syndrome Study Group. JAMA 1994;271(23):1836–43.
73. Fisher CJ Jr, Slotner GJ, Opal SM, et al. Initial evaluation of human recombinant interleukin-1 receptor antagonist in the treatment of sepsis syndrome: a randomized, open-label, placebo-controlled multicenter trial. Crit Care Med 1994;22:12–21.
74. Cain BS, Meldrum DR, Dinarello CA, et al. Tumor necrosis factor-a and interleukin-1b synergistically depress human myocardial function. Crit Care Med 1999;27:1309–18.
75. Pathan N, Hemingway CA, Alizadeh AA, et al. Role of interleukin 6 in myocardial dysfunction of meningococcal septic shock. Lancet 2004;363(9404):203–9.
76. Pathan N, Sandiford C, Harding SE, Levin M. Characterization of a myocardial depressant factor in meningococcal septicemia. Crit Care Med 2002;30(10):2191–8.
77. Thiru Y, Pathan N, Bignall S, Habibi P, Levin M. A myocardial cytotoxic process is involved in the cardiac dysfunction of meningococcal septic shock. Crit Care Med 2000;28(8):2979–83.
78. Mink SN, Jacobs H, Bose D, et al. Lysozyme: a mediator of myocardial depression and adrenergic dysfunction in septic shock in dogs. J Mol Cell Cardiol 2003;35:265–75.
79. Mink SN, Jacobs H, Duke K, Bose D, Cheng ZQ, Light RB. N,N′,N″-triacetylglucosamine, an inhibitor of lysozyme, prevents myocardial depression in Escherichia coli sepsis in dogs. Crit Care Med 2004;32(1):184–93.
80. Sparwasser T, Miethke T, Lipford G, et al. Bacterial DNA causes septic shock. Nature 1997;386(6623):336–7.
81. Paladugu B, Kumar A, Parrillo JE, et al. Bacterial DNA and RNA induce rat cardiac myocyte contraction depression in-vitro. Shock 2004;21(364):369.
82. Garner LB, Willis MS, Carlson DL, et al. Macrophage migration inhibitory factor is a cardiac-derived myocardial depressant factor. Am J Physiol Heart Circ Physiol 2003;285(6):H2500–9.
83. Chagnon F, Metz CN, Bucala R, Lesur O. Endotoxin-induced myocardial dysfunction: effects of macrophage migration inhibitory factor neutralization. Circ Res 2005;96(10):1095–102.
84. Finkel MS, Oddis CV, Jacobs TD, Watkins SC, Hattler BG, Simmons RL. Negative inotropic effects of cytokines on the heart mediated by nitric oxide. Science 1992;257:387–9.
85. Walley KR, Hebert PC, Wakai Y, Wilcox PG, Road JD, Cooper DJ. Decrease in left ventricular contractility after tumor necrosis factor-a infusion in dogs. J Appl Physiol 1994;76:1060–7.
86. DeMeules JE, Pigula FA, Mueller M, Raymond SJ, Gamelli RL. Tumor necrosis factor and cardiac function. J Trauma 1992;32:686–92.
87. Hare JM, Keaney JF, Balligand JL, Loscalzo J, Smith TW, Colucci WS. Role of nitric oxide in parasympathetic modulation of beta-adrenergic myocardial contractility in normal dogs. J Clin Invest 1995;95:360–6.
88. Sawyer DB, Colucci WS. Nitric oxide in the failing myocardium. Cardiol Clin North Am 1998;16:657–4.
89. Balligand JL, Kobzik L, Han X, et al. Nitric oxide-dependent parasympathetic signalling is due to activation of constitutive endothelial (type III) nitric oxide synthase in cardiac myocytes. J Biol Chem 1995;270:14582–6.
90. Brady AJ, Poole-Wilson PA, Harding SE, Warren JB. Nitric oxide production within cardiac myocytes reduces their contractility in endotoxemia. Am J Physiol 1992;263:H1963–6.
91. Paulus WJ, Vantrimpont PJ, Shah AM. Acute effects of nitric oxide on left ventricular relaxation

and diastolic distensability in humans. Assessment by bicoronary sodium nitroprusside infusion. Circulation 1994;89:2070–8.
92. Kumar A, Brar R, Wang P, et al. The role of nitric oxide and cyclic GMP in human septic serum-induced depression of cardiac myocyte contractility. Am J Physiol 1999;276:R265–76.
93. Rozanski GJ, Witt RC. IL-1 inhibits b-adrenergic control of cardiac calcium current: role of L-arginine/nitric oxide pathway. Am J Physiol 1994; 267:H1753–8.
94. Smith JA, Radomski MW, Schulz R, Moncada S, Lewis MJ. Porcine ventricular endocardial cells in culture express the inducible form of nitric oxide synthase. Br J Pharmacol 1993;108:1107–10.
95. Szabo C. The pathophysiological role of peroxynitrite in shock, inflammation, and ischemia-reperfusion injury. Shock 1996;6:79–88.
96. Anel R, Paladugu B, Makkena R, et al. TNFa induces a proximal defect of b-adrenoreceptor signal transduction in cardiac myocytes. Crit Care Med 1999;27:A95.
97. Kumar A, Brar R, Sun E, Olson J, Parrillo JE. Tumor necrosis factor (TNF) impairs isoproterenol-stimulated cardiac myocyte contractility and cyclic AMP production via a nitric oxide-independent mechanism. Crit Care Med 1996;24: A95.
98. Kinugawa K, Takahashi T, Kohmoto O, et al. Nitric oxide-mediated effects of interleukin-6 on [Ca2+]i and cell contraction in cultured chick ventricular myocytes. Circ Res 1994;75:285–95.
99. Kinugawa KI, Kohmoto O, Yao A, Serizawa T, Takahashi T. Cardiac inducible nitric oxide synthase negatively modulates myocardial function in cultured rat myocytes. Am J Physiol 1997; 272(1 pt 2):H35–47.
100. Ishibashi Y, Urabe Y, Tsutsui H, et al. Negative inotropic effect of basic fibroblast growth factor on adult rat cardiac myocyte. Circulation 1997; 96(8):2501–4.
101. Rivers E, Nguyen B, Havstad S, et al. Early goal-directed therapy in the treatment of severe sepsis and septic shock. N Engl J Med 2001;345(19):1368–77.
102. Rivers EP, McIntyre L, Morro DC, Rivers KK. Early and innovative interventions for severe sepsis and septic shock: taking advantage of a window of opportunity. Can Med Assoc J 2005; 173(9):1054–65.
103. Kumar A, Parrillo JE. Shock: pathophysiology, classification and approach to management. In: Parrillo JE, Dellinger RP, eds. Critical Care Medicine: Principles of Diagnosis and Management in the Adult. St. Louis: Mosby, 2001:371–420.
104. Dellinger RP, Carlet JM, Masur H, et al. Surviving sepsis campaign guidelines for management of severe sepsis and septic shock. Crit Care Med 2004;32(3):858–73.
105. Barton P, Garcia J, Kouatli A, et al. Hemodynamic effects of i.v. milrinone lactate in pediatric patients with septic shock. A prospective, double-blinded, randomized, placebo-controlled, interventional study. Chest 1996;109:1302–12.
106. Le Tulzo Y, Seguin P, Gacouin A, et al. Effects of epinephrine on right ventricular function in patients with severe septic shock and right ventricular failure: a preliminary descriptive study. Intensive Care Med 1997;23(6):664–70.
107. Nasraway SA, Rackow EC, Astiz ME, Karras G, Weil MH. Inotropic response to digoxin and dopamine in patients with severe sepsis, cardiac failure, and systemic hypoperfusion. Chest 1989;95:612–5.
108. Gomez A, Wang R, Unruh H, et al. Hemofiltration reverses left ventricular dysfunction during sepsis in dogs. Anesthesiology 1990;73:671–85.
109. Mink SN, Jha P, Wang R, et al. Effect of continuous arteriovenous hemofiltration combined with systemic vasopressor therapy on depressed left ventricular contractility and tissue oxygen delivery in canine Escherichia coli sepsis. Anesthesiology 1995;83(1):178–90.
110. Freeman BD, Yatsiv I, Natanson C, et al. Continuous arteriovenous hemofiltration does not improve survival in a canine model of septic shock. J Am Coll Surg 1995;180(3):286–92.
111. Mink SN, Li X, Bose D, et al. Early but not delayed continuous arteriovenous hemofiltration improves cardiovascular function in sepsis in dogs. Intensive Care Med 1999;25(7):733–43.
112. Lee PA, Matson JR, Pryor RW, Hinshaw LB. Continuous arteriovenous hemofiltration therapy for Staphylococcus aureus-induced septicemia in immature swine. Crit Care Med 1993;21(6):914–24.
113. Kirov MY, Evgenov OV, Evgenov NV, et al. Infusion of methylene blue in human septic shock: a pilot, randomized, controlled study. Crit Care Med 2001;29(10):1860–7.
114. Suzuki N, Sakamoto A, Ogawa R. Effect of L-canavanine, an inhibitor of inducible nitric oxide synthase, on myocardial dysfunction during septic shock. J Nippon Med Sch 2002;69:1–13.
115. Davis JO, Freeman RH. Mechanisms regulating renin release. Physiol Rev 1976;56:1–56.
116. Grover R, Zaccardelli D, Colice G, et al. An open-label dose escalation study of the nitric oxide synthase inhibitor NG-methyl-L-arginine hydrochloride (546C88), in patients with septic shock. Crit Care Med 1999;27:913–22.

31 Acute Heart Failure Syndromes and Drug Intoxication

Bruno Mégarbane, Nicolas Deye, and Frédéric J. Baud

Cardiovascular drugs are responsible for life-threatening poisonings with increasing incidence. Acute heart failure is a potential complication following accidental or intentional overdose with various classes of drugs. The most frequent ones are beta-blockers, calcium-channel antagonists, sodium-channel blocker agents, and cardioglycosides. However, in medical toxicology, the term *cardiotoxic drug* is not limited to the cardiovascular drugs but also include various other toxicants, such as antidepressants, nivaquine, meprobamate, H1-antihistaminic neuroleptics, cocaine, cyanide, organophosphates, and certain plants. In Europe, the incidence and prevalence of acute poisoning–associated heart failure remain unknown. In the United States, cardiovascular drugs account for the fifth toxicant category responsible of death, following analgesics, sedative drugs, antidepressants, and stimulants (1). Calcium-channel blocker poisoning is associated in the U.S. with the highest reported number of fatalities among cardiovascular agents (0.7% of exposures) (1). Membrane-stabilizing agents, such as tricyclic antidepressants, are a well-established cause of increased mortality in acute poisonings (2,3). In contrast, beta-blockers appear safer, with only 64 reported fatalities among 52,156 exposures in a retrospective review of the American Association of Poison Control Centers Toxic Exposure Surveillance System 1985–1995 data (4). However, the global mortality rate of poisonings remains low (about 1%), increasing to about 10% to 20% when cardiotoxic drugs are involved.

Pathophysiology of Drug-Induced Cardiocirculatory Failure

According to Poiseuille's law, ΔP equals $Q \times SVR$, where ΔP denotes the perfusion pressure or the mean arterial pressure, Q the cardiac output, and SVR the systemic vascular resistance. Furthermore, Q equals $V_S \times HR$, where V_S denotes the stroke volume and HR the heart rate. Finally, ΔP equals $V_S \times HR \times SVR$. Thus, perfusion pressure is determined by three main factors. However, in healthy humans, rapidly acting compensation mechanisms preclude any significant modification of the perfusion pressure due to the variation of one parameter. A decrease in HR caused by digitalis is associated with an increase in V_S and in SVR, whereas a decrease in V_S caused by drug-induced hypovolemia is associated with an increase in HR and SVR. Finally, a decrease in SVR caused by arterial vasodilating agents is initially associated with an increase in HR and V_S. Thus, the occurrence of hypotension is always associated with some degree of failure of the compensation mechanisms. In drug-induced cardiovascular disturbances, hypotension only describes some modification of macrocirculation. However, the decision of treatment should take into account the cellular consequences of hypotension, which reflect the degree of impairment of microcirculation related to hypotension. This example emphasizes the importance of considering more than the macrocirculation, which is assessed by a decrease in mean arterial pressure; it is of utmost importance to look at the consequences of the microcirculation level.

The pathogenesis of drug-associated hypotension varies and may include hypovolemia, myocardial depression, cardiac arrhythmias, and systemic vasodilatation. The major mechanism of acute toxic heart failure is related to systolic dysfunction due to decreased myocardial contractility, although other mechanisms may also be involved, including diastolic dysfunction (cardioglycosides), asymmetric cardiac contractility (membrane stabilizing agents, drug-induced ventricular tachycardia), myocarditis (ethylene glycol, organophosphate), anoxia (cyanide), or acute coronary syndrome (cocaine). Calcium-channel blockers, beta-blockers, and membrane-stabilizing agents may induce arterial dilatation and myocardial negative inotropic effects, by various mechanisms (4–6). Calcium-channel blockers inhibit calcium influx by blocking L-type voltage-sensitive calcium channels, while beta-blockers competitively antagonize β-receptors. Verapamil is a more negative inotrope, while nifedipine has more vasodilator effects. Membrane-stabilizing agents inhibit the fast sodium-channel–related entering sodium flux of the 0 phase of the cardiac action potential. At toxic doses, certain beta-blockers, such as propranolol or acebutolol, demonstrate membrane-stabilizing activity that significantly enhances morbidity (7). Drug-induced acute heart failure is generally reversible with the elimination of the toxicant ("functional toxicant"). However, some toxicants may induce injury, resulting in irreversible failure or significant sequelae; for example, colchicine inhibits microtubule polymerization, and cocaine induces ischemia.

Diagnosis and Cardiovascular Failure Assessment

A diagnosis of poisoning is based on the history and on the search for toxic syndromes (8,9). If the patient is comatose, relatives, friends, and ambulance crews can usually provide useful information. All cardiotropic toxicants may cause hypotension, bradycardia, sinus nodal suppression, junctional rhythms, atrioventricular blocks, idioventricular rhythms, congestive heart failure with or without pulmonary edema, and asystole (8,9).

An electrocardiogram (ECG) is essential in the diagnosis of drug-induced heart failure. An increased QRS (>0.12 seconds) is observed with membrane-stabilizing agents, and a narrowed QRS is observed with meprobamate, severe sinusal bradycardia, or high-degree atrioventricular block with beta-blockers or calcium-blocker agents. A Brugada pattern on the ECG is a particular manifestation of the frequently occurring intraventricular conduction disturbances with antidepressants and more generally in membrane-stabilizing agent poisonings (Fig. 31.1). In intoxicated patients in whom the substance is unknown, early recognition of the conduction disturbances is important for suspecting poisoning with an antidepressant (10). Cardiovascular effects generally occur within 6 hours after ingestion. The time gap is very short following antiarrhythmic drug ingestion. Thus, intensive cardiac monitoring, including clinical parameters (blood pressure, heart rate, respiratory rate, SpO_2, and Glasgow Coma Scale score) and ECG are mandatory, and should begin as soon as the patient is admitted in the emergency room. Other manifestations include mental status deterioration, seizures, metabolic acidosis from hyperlactacidemia, and acute respiratory failure. Neurologic features generally occur consecutively after cerebral hypoperfusion. Thus, management focuses on restoring hemodynamic function, and involves multiple additive therapies.

Macrocirculation can be easily assessed using clinical evaluation as well as a large number of devices. Echocardiography coupled with Doppler remains operator-dependent. Right-heart catheterization is performed in most intensive care units (ICUs), but must be completed by the simultaneous measurement of arterial and mixed venous blood gases, providing insight on oxygen transfer, delivery, and consumption as well as the ability of macrocirculation to meet metabolic cellular demand. In some conditions there is evidence of failure of microcirculation, including cardiopulmonary arrest, or a pulseless tachycardic unconscious female patient who has taken flecainide or chloroquine. The need for life support has been clarified in the toxicologic-oriented

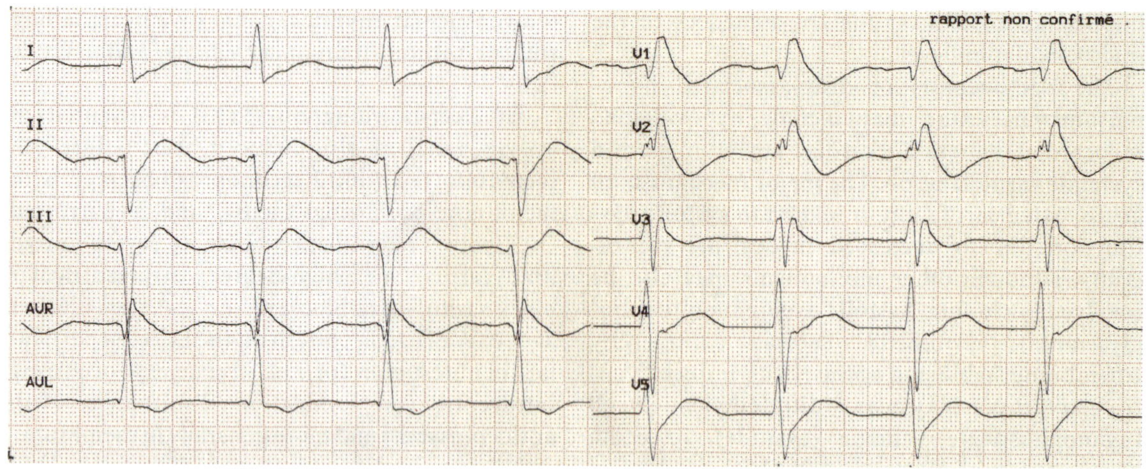

FIGURE 31.1. Brugada electrocardiographic pattern in a carbamazepine severely poisoned patient, with a right bundle branch block, a 200-ms QRS duration, and an unusual ST-segment elevation in the right precordial leads (V_1 to V_3) (35).

advance cardiac life support (TOX-ACLS) protocol (11).

In other conditions it is more difficult to assess whether failure of macrocirculation induces failure in microcirculation. The most common cases we see are patients with a past history of significant hypertension and patients with advanced cardiac disease. In the former, apparently normal values of macrocirculation may be associated with progressive deterioration of microcirculation that would be not noted or would be noted too late if the history of hypertension were unknown; in the latter, abnormal signs of macrocirculation may be still associated with abnormal signs of microcirculation, such as plasma lactate at the upper level of the normal range, low urine output, and increased serum creatinine. However, the concern of the attending physician is to determine whether deterioration is progressing due to the effect of the suspected poisoning or the patient's being in stable but poor condition. We have to assess in the near future new devices allowing the noninvasive or minimally invasive assessment of microcirculation including continuous SVO_2 measurement and near-infrared spectroscopy.

The prognostic factors of cardiotropic drug poisonings have been poorly investigated, except for digitalis, colchicine, theophylline, and antidepressants. Interestingly, the prognostic value of the toxicant blood concentration also needs to be determined. In cardioglycoside poisoning, outcome assessment has shown that mortality increases in patients exhibiting five prognostic factors: advanced age, heart disease, male sex, high-degree atrioventricular block, and hyperkalemia (12). In antidepressant poisoning, determination of the maximal limb-lead QRS duration predicts the risk of seizures and ventricular arrhythmias in an acute overdose of tricyclic antidepressants, whereas serum drug levels are not of predictive value (13). In chloroquine poisoning, poor prognosis factors related to severe cardiocirculatory failure are an ingested dose >4 g, systolic blood pressure <100 mm Hg, and QRS duration >0.10 ms (14,15). In beta-blocker poisoning, the single most important factor associated with the development of cardiovascular morbidity is a history of a cardioactive co-ingestant (7). A history of ingesting a beta-blocker with membrane stabilizing activity is significantly associated with the development of cardiovascular morbidity.

General Management in the Intensive Care Unit

Regional or national poisons centers should be consulted for information on the treatment of poisoned patients. The need for ICU admission should be determined by using the clinical risk factors identified by Brett et al. (16), including systolic blood pressure <80 mm Hg, QRS duration <0.12 seconds, cardiac arrhythmias, second- or third-degree atrioventricular block, unresponsiveness to verbal stimuli, need for endotracheal intubation, Pa_{CO_2} >45 mm Hg, and toxin-induced seizures. In cases of poisoning-induced cardiac arrest, standard basic and advanced life support should be provided (17). With the exception of torsades de pointes, cardioversion is indicated for life-threatening tachyarrhythmias. Nonspecific intensive supportive care aims to correct hypoxia, hypotension, acid–base, and electrolyte disorders. Tracheal intubation and mechanical ventilation are required in cases of coma, severe collapse, or cardiac dysrhythmias. Multidose activated charcoal is not helpful except in sustained-release preparations. Due to large distribution volumes and high protein binding ratios, extracorporeal elimination enhancement techniques are not feasible options.

For hypotension, treatment should be individualized according to each drug class; however, an initial strategy of rapid IV saline infusion is indicated in most circumstances (8,9). Vasopressors are required for refractory hypotension. The vasopressor of choice depends on the type of intoxication. In the emergency room or in the absence of close cardiac monitoring, we think that epinephrine should be the first-line catecholamine. Sodium bicarbonate is required if ventricular conduction is delayed in membrane-stabilizing poisonings. Administration of intravenous sodium bicarbonate to achieve a systemic pH of 7.5 to 7.55 reduces QRS prolongation and reverses hypotension in patients with moderate to severe tricyclic antidepressant poisoning (18). Studies suggest also its benefit in reducing antidepressant-associated ECG Brugada syndromes (10). However, the exact indications and dosing recommendations remain to be clarified. The immediate treatment of arrhythmias involves correcting hypoxia, electrolyte abnormalities, hypotension, and acidosis. Administration of sodium bicarbonate may resolve arrhythmias even in the absence of acidosis, and only if this therapy fails should conventional antiarrhythmic drugs be used. The class 1b agent phenytoin may reverse conduction defects and may be used for resistant ventricular tachycardia. There is also limited evidence for benefit from magnesium infusion. However, class 1a and 1c antiarrhythmic drugs should be avoided since they worsen sodium channel blockade, further slow conduction velocity, and depress contractility. Class II agents (beta-blockers) may also precipitate hypotension and cardiac arrest.

In chloroquine poisonings, combining early mechanical ventilation with the administration of diazepam and epinephrine may be effective in the treatment of severe cardiocirculatory failure (15). For cardioglycoside poisonings, digoxin-specific Fab fragments are the treatment for life-threatening events (12). The prognostic factors of life-threatening events for digitalis poisoning considerably simplify the indication of this antidote. Digoxin-specific Fab fragments are indicated if atropine failed as the first-line antiarrhythmic therapy to correct bradycardia-induced arrhythmia. Thus, digitalis-induced heart failure due to ventricular arrhythmias may only be observed if Fab fragments are not administered early or not available. During digitalis intoxication, a pacemaker has limited preventive and curative effects, is difficult to handle, and exposes patients to severe iatrogenic accidents.

Despite these recommendations, management of cardiotoxic poisonings remains difficult when the usual therapy fails. Ventricular arrhythmia, sudden cardiac arrest, or refractory cardiovascular failure may cause death, despite all aggressive resuscitative measures and high-dose vasopressors (5,7,14,19).

Management of Calcium Channel Poisoning

The first-line drug therapy of calcium channel blocker (CCB) poisoning remains catecholamine-type vasopressors (Fig. 31.2) (11). Despite controversial clinical efficacy, calcium salts are still recommended initially by some authors (8,9,20) or only in refractory shock to conventional vasopressors by others (11). The required dosage and agent (i.e., calcium gluconate or chloride) is undetermined. Repeated 1-g IV boluses every 15 to 20 minutes for a total of four doses is usually recommended, followed by an infusion of 20 to 50 mg/kg/h in patients a with beneficial hemodynamic

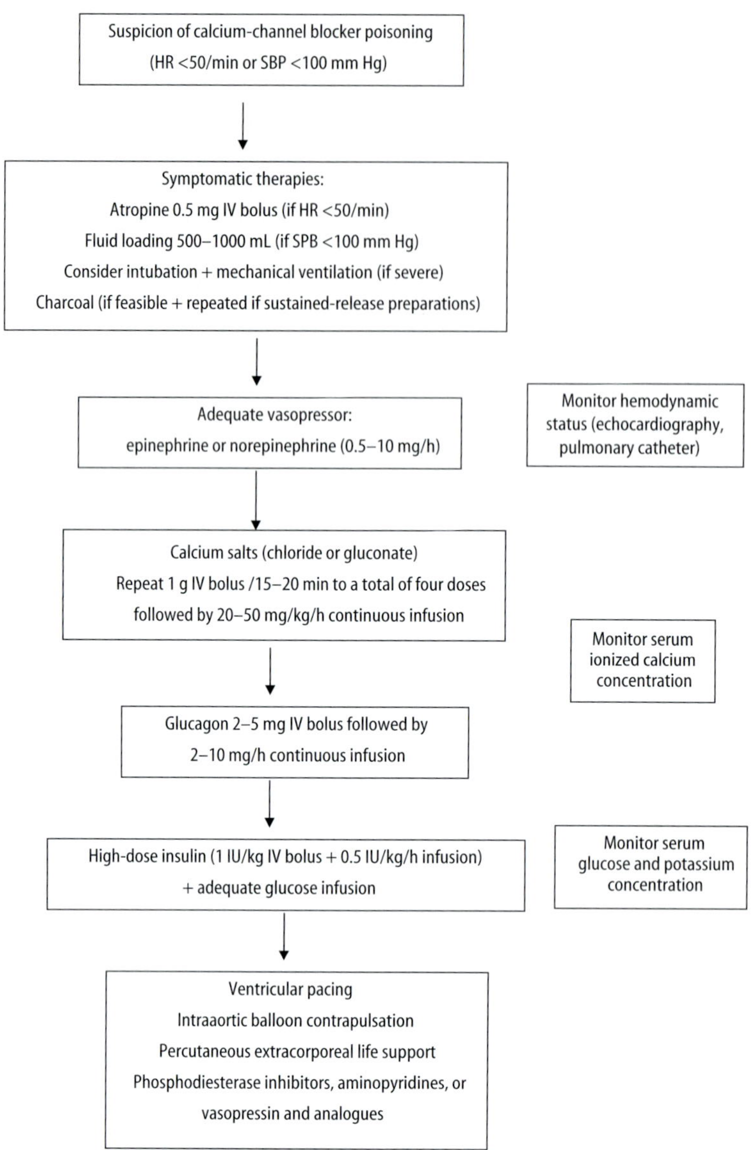

FIGURE 31.2. Proposed algorithm for the treatment of calcium channel blocker poisoning. This algorithm is based on series and case reports. HR, heart rate; SBP, systolic blood pressure.

response to initial calcium infusions. Serum calcium concentration should be measured at least twice daily and maintained at normal levels, given the lack of evidence of benefit at supraphysiologic levels (5,11). Glucagon, administered as a 5- to 10-mg IV bolus over 1 minute followed by an infusion of 1 to 10 mg/h may also have beneficial effects on hemodynamic parameters (21).

Some experts mentioned hyperinsulinemia-euglycemia therapy in the 2001 guidelines for CCB intoxication management, but without further recommendation (11). However, based not only on animal data but also on case reports (22) of its efficacy compared to the other inotropic agents, we think that hyperinsulinemia-euglycemia therapy should be used early as adjunctive treatment (23). The proposed protocol consists of 1 IU/kg IV bolus followed by 0.5 to 1.0 IU/kg/h infusion, mandating high concentrated glucose infusion to maintain euglycemia. Although some authors recommended it as a first-line therapy after initial resuscitation (24), we think, as do others (11,22), that it is indicated only if vasopressors fail to improve hemodynamic function, with persistent refractory shocks, bradyarrhythmias or conduction disturbances (Fig. 31.2).

Management of Beta-Blocker Poisoning

For beta-blocker poisoning, only selected patients may benefit from hyperinsulinemia-euglycemia therapy due to the limited clinical experience, although it may prove to be superior to glucagon alone (23). Despite the lack of clinical studies to support its beneficial effects, glucagon is widely used (21). However, it should not be the first choice, based on the limited clinical data and availability in comparison to other inotropic agents. Indeed, the lack of availability of adequate supplies and the high cost may limit its use as first-line antidote, even though it is safe. In France, for instance, 5 mg/h glucagon regimen costs 95 euros, whereas an equivalent 30 UI/h insulin regimen costs only 0.84 euros. We thus recommend, if initial supportive measures fail, antidote administration in the following order: dobutamine glucagon, and epinephrine (Fig. 31.3). Isoproterenol is lifesaving in sotalol intoxication-associated bradycardia, as drug-related QT interval prolongation may cause torsades de pointes or favor sustained ventricular tachycardia or fibrillation. Sodium bicarbonate is recommended in the presence of QRS-interval widening

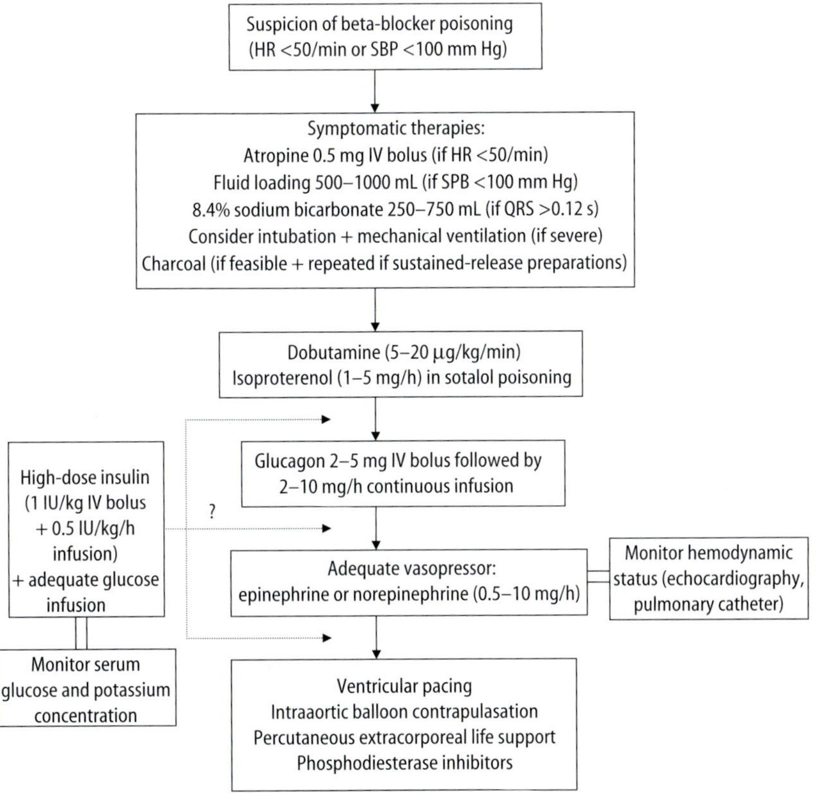

Figure 31.3. Proposed algorithm for treatment of beta-blocker poisoning. This algorithm is based on series and case reports. HR, heart rate; SBP, systolic blood pressure.

on electrocardiogram. Calcium chloride infusion was also reported beneficial in the setting of beta-blocker poisoning, to restore blood pressure and narrow the QRS complexes (25,26). However, this therapy is not recommended for beta-blocker toxicity treatment (11).

Refractory Poisoning-Related Acute Heart Failure

There is no clear definition of drug-induced refractory acute heart failure. In the absence of response to the usual supportive and antidotal treatments including low doses of catecholamines, central hemodynamic monitoring is mandatory (11). Recently, criteria of unresponsive to pharmacological agents were characterized for poisonings with membrane stabilizing activity with elevated sensitivity and specificity rates to predict death, unless cardiopulmonary bypass is considered (Fig. 31.4) (19). In nonresponsive beta-blocker and calcium channel antagonist poisonings, high-dose titrated vasopressor therapy, ventricular pacing (transvenous or transthoracic), intraaortic balloon pump, or percutaneous cardiopulmonary bypass should be considered as lifesaving measures. However, available data analyzing the benefit of these exceptional therapies

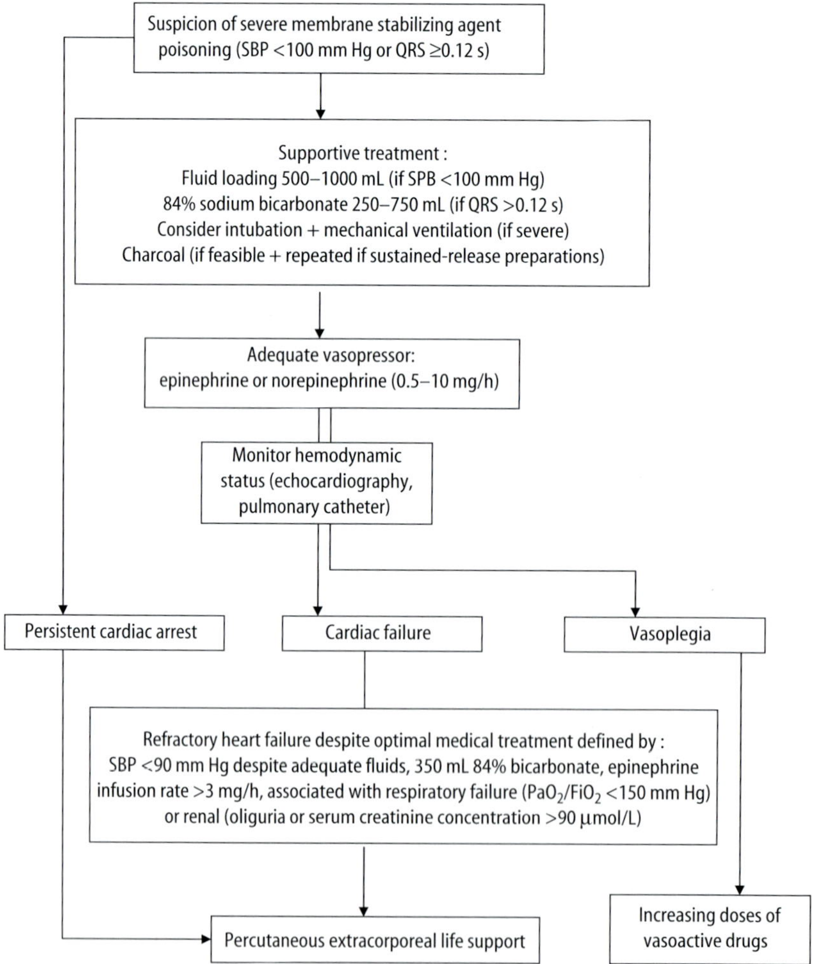

FIGURE 31.4. Proposed algorithm for the treatment of membrane-stabilizing agent poisoning. This algorithm is based on series and case reports. SBP, systolic blood pressure; QRS, QRS duration on ECG.

are limited. Results obtained with these techniques should be interpreted only in regard to severe toxicity. Interest in the intraaortic balloon pump appears to be limited by the need for intrinsic cardiac rhythm for synchronization and diastolic augmentation.

Extracorporeal life support (ECLS) is an arteriovenous method providing circulatory support but requiring bypass of blood from the right to the left system, with extracorporeal blood oxygenation. Extracorporeal membrane oxygenation (ECMO) is a venovenous method improving PaO_2 without providing any support of the circulatory system. In poisoning-related acute heart failure, only ECLS may be indicated (Table 31.1). For reversible cardiac toxicity, ECLS has a sound basis but clinical experience is still limited in toxicology, with insufficient evidence for recommending it (grade C) (27,28). Peripheral circulatory assist devices are particularly useful for poisoning-related heart failure, in comparison to invasive conventional bypass support by sternotomy (29). However, femoral cannulation for ECLS is not lacking in potential severe risks, such as bleeding, cannulated limb ischemia, and mechanical problems. Based on the review of seven case reports from the literature, a recent article concluded that cardiopulmonary bypass may have potential benefit for hemodynamic instability that is not responding to conventional measures, provided that the patient has not sustained hypoxic cerebral damage due to resistant hypotension prior to its use (28). In fact, adequate supportive care remains essential before considering cardiac assistance. The purpose of ECLS is to take over heart function during refractory cardiac shock until recovery can occur, thus minimizing myocardial work, improving organ perfusion, and maintaining the renal and biliary elimination of the toxicant.

Table 31.1. Toxic severe acute heart failure that may indicate extracorporeal life support

Pharmacologic class	Toxicants
Membrane stabilizing agent	
Vaughan Williams class 1 antiarrhythmic drugs	Quinidine, lidocaine, phenytoin, mexiletine, cibenzoline, tocainide, procainamide, disopyramide, flecainide, propafenone
Some beta-blockers	Propranolol, acebutolol, nadoxolol, pindolol, penbutolol, labetalol, metoprolol, oxprenolol
Tricyclic or tetracyclic antidepressants	Amitriptyline, imipramine, clomipramine, dosulepine, maprotiline
Some serotonin-reuptake inhibitors	Venlafaxine, citalopram
Anticonvulsive drugs	Carbamazepine
Neuroleptics	Phenothiazines
Analgesics	Dextropropoxyphene
Antimalarial drugs	Chloroquine, quinine
Festive drugs	Cocaine
Other toxicants	
Calcium channel blockers	Nifedipine, nicardipine, verapamil, diltiazem, nimodipine, amlodipine, nitrendipine, bepridil perhexiline
Other cardiotoxic drugs	Meprobamate, colchicine, beta-blocker without membrane stabilizing activity, H1-antihistaminic drugs, organophosphates, aconite, yew, scombroid fish

Interestingly, in calcium channel blocker poisoning, various antidotes have shown promise, including phosphodiesterase III inhibitors (milrinone), vasopressin analogues, levosimendan, and potassium-channel antagonists used as nondepolarizing neuromuscular blocking agents (4-aminopyridine, and two related potent dihydropyridines—3,4-diaminopyridine and Bay K8664) (30–34). All these agents showed interesting effects in animal studies or if tested in human cases. However, their lack of availability limits their utilization.

Case Report

A 35-year-old woman was admitted to the emergency room, 2 hours after the ingestion of 2.5 g of flecainide in a suicide attempt. She has no remarkable medical past history. She explained that she decided to ingest her husband's medication when he announced that he planned to leave her. On arrival, she was conscious (Glasgow Coma Scale score of 14), with a blood pressure of 110/50 mm Hg, a heart rate of 100/min, and an SpO_2 of 97% when breathing air.

Due to the supposed elevated ingested dose, she was immediately transferred to the ICU. One hour after ICU admission, she presented cardiovascular shock (arterial blood pressure, 82/54 mm Hg; heart rate, 88/min) that was unresponsive to 500 mL of saline infusion. Examination revealed a decrease in her level of consciousness (Glasgow Coma Scale score of 12) with intermittent agitation but no discernible focal neurologic defect. Breathing and thoracic auscultation were normal. Electrocardiogram showed a right bundle branch block with 160-ms QRS and 520-ms QT_c interval durations. Laboratory tests revealed serum potassium concentration at 2.3 mmol/L, serum creatinine concentration at 110 μmol/L, PaO_2/FiO_2 of 350 mm Hg, plasma lactate concentration at 4.4 mmol/L, and prothrombin time (expressed as percentage of normal) at 80%. The usual toxicologic screenings were negative and serum flecainide level was 2.2 mg/L (therapeutic range, 0.4–0.9).

She was promptly intubated and sedated (midazolam + fentanyl), as soon as cardiac monitoring revealed sustained ventricular extrasystoles. A 50-g dose of activated charcoal was administered. Within 2 hours, her hemodynamic status worsened (blood pressure, 67/40 mm Hg; heart rate, 70/min), despite volume expansion (500 mL of gelatin), 250 mL of 84% sodium bicarbonate, and inotropic support (epinephrine, 2 mg/h). She was oliguric with acute renal failure (serum creatinine concentration, 150 μmol/L). Plasma lactate concentration was measured at 5.5 mmol/L. Cardiogenic shock was suggested by a persistent hypotension despite increasing epinephrine requirements, a moderate hypoxemia, and pulmonary edema on chest radiograph. No recurrent arrhythmia occurred following the patient intubation.

Transthoracic echocardiography revealed marked global hypokinesia (left ventricular ejection fraction, 35%) without left ventricular dilatation and signs of hypovolemia. Asymmetric and nonsynergic contractility were observed with a delay between the interventricular septum and lateral wall contractions. Right heart catheterization confirmed severe myocardial dysfunction (SvO_2, 60%; pulmonary artery occlusion pressure, 18 mm Hg; cardiac index, 2.3 L/min/m^2; systemic vascular resistance, 1850 dynes·s^{-1}·cm^{-5}; arteriovenous oxygen difference, 8.1 mL/%). An increase in the epinephrine infusion rate (2.5 mg/h) and a readministration of 175 mL of 84% sodium bicarbonate allowed stabilization of her hemodynamic status 12 hours after her admission. Urine output increased, serum creatinine concentration remained stable (140 μmol/L), and plasma lactate concentration decreased (3 mmol/L). The QRS-complex duration narrowed and the QT_c interval was normalized. Forty hours after ICU admission, the cardiogenic shock completely reversed, with the normalization of the heart contractility on echocardiography.

Recovery was then rapid. Sedation was stopped on day 3 and extubation was performed on day 4. Antibiotic (amoxicillin-clavulanic acid) was administered for aspiration pneumonia, from day 2 to day 7. Laboratory tests and ECG were normalized, except for T negative waves in the precordium. Successive measurements of plasma flecainide concentration showed a progressive decrease until becoming undetectable, with an elimination half-life of 20 hours. The patient left the ICU on day 8. She was transferred to the psychiatry department. At 1-year follow-up, she was healthy and had no symptoms or myocardial sequelae.

In antiarrhythmic drug poisonings, if refractory heart failure is assessed (using the criteria established for membrane stabilizing agent poisoning), the indications for mechanical circulatory support are determined, and ECLS is used with peripheral femorofemoral cannulation. This mechanical assistance provides support until the heart recovers, with the maintenance of renal elimination of the toxicant. Epinephrine is rapidly tapered and withdrawn. During cardiac assistance, complete electromechanical dissociation is often observed. Dobutamine (10 μg/kg/min) with or without vasopressors is often administered until device explantation, when recovery of myocardial function is assessed by successive echocardiography.

Conclusion

Careful management of poisoning-induced acute heart failure is mandatory to reduce fatalities. Usual ICU monitoring and supportive therapies are required. Specialized medical toxicology or poison center advisories are helpful to guide antidotal treatment. Assessment of the mechanism of circulatory failure is essential to choose the appropriate catecholamine and to indicate quickly the necessity of cardiac assistance, in case of refractory heart failure.

References

1. Watson WA, Litovitz TL, Rodgers GC Jr, et al. 2004 Annual report of the American Association of Poison Control Centers Toxic Exposure Surveillance System. Am J Emerg Med 2005;23:589–666.
2. Henry JA, Cassidy SL. Membrane stabilising activity: a major cause of fatal poisoning. Lancet 1986; 1:1414–17.
3. Henry JA, Alexander CA, Sener EK. Relative mortality from overdose of antidepressants. BMJ 1995;310:221–4.
4. Love JN, Litovitz TL, Howell JM, Clancy C. Characterization of fatal beta blocker ingestion: a review of the American Association of Poison Control Centers data from 1985 to 1995. J Toxicol Clin Toxicol 1997;35:353–9.
5. Salhanick SD, Shannon MW. Management of calcium channel antagonist overdose. Drug Saf 2003;26:65–79.
6. Kolecki PF, Curry SC. Poisoning by sodium channel blocking agents. Crit Care Clin 1997;13:829–48.
7. Love JN, Howell JM, Litovitz TL, Klein-Schwartz W. Acute beta blocker overdose: factors associated with the development of cardiovascular morbidity. J Toxicol Clin Toxicol 2000;38:275–81.
8. Zimmerman JL. Poisonings and overdoses in the intensive care unit: general and specific management issues. Crit Care Med 2003;31:2794–801.
9. Mokhlesi B, Leiken JB, Murray P, Corbridge TC. Adult toxicology in critical care: part I: general approach to the intoxicated patient. Chest 2003;123: 577–92.
10. Monteban-Kooistra WE, van den Berg MP, Tulleken JE, Lightenberg JJM, Meertens JHJM, Zijlstra JG. Brugada electrocardiographic pattern elicited by cyclic antidepressants overdose. Intensive Care Med 2006;32:281–5.
11. Albertson TE, Dowson A, de Latorre F, et al. American Heart Association;International Liaison Committee on Resuscitation. TOX-ACLS: toxicologic-oriented advanced cardiac life support. Ann Emerg Med 2001;37:S78–90.
12. Taboulet P, Baud FJ, Bismuth C. Clinical features and management of digitalis poisoning—rationale for immunotherapy. J Toxicol Clin Toxicol 1993;31: 247–60.
13. Boehnert MT, Lovejoy FH Jr. Value of the QRS duration versus the serum drug level in predicting seizures and ventricular arrhythmias after an acute overdose of tricyclic antidepressants. N Engl J Med 1985;313:474–9.
14. Clemessy JL, Taboulet P, Hoffman JR, et al. Treatment of acute chloroquine poisoning: a 5-year experience. Crit Care Med 1996;24:1189–95.
15. Riou B, Barriot P, Rimailho A, Baud FJ. Treatment of severe chloroquine poisoning. N Engl J Med 1988;318:1–6.
16. Brett AS, Rothschild N, Gray R, Perry M. Predicting the clinical course in intentional drug overdose. Implications for use of the intensive care unit. Arch Intern Med 1987;147:133–7.
17. European Resuscitation Council. Part 8: advanced challenges in resuscitation. Section 2: toxicology in ECC. European Resuscitation Council. Resuscitation 2000;46:261–6.
18. Bradberry SM, Thanacoody HK, Watt BE, Thomas SH, Vale JA. Management of the cardiovascular complications of tricyclic antidepressant poisoning: role of sodium bicarbonate. Toxicol Rev 2005; 24:195–204.
19. Mégarbane B, Andujar P, Delahaye A, et al. Acute poisonings with membrane stabilizing agents: analysis of the predictive parameters of non-responsiveness to conventional therapies. J Toxicol Clin Toxicol 2003;41:553–4(abstr).
20. Lam YM, Tse HF, Lau CP. Continuous calcium chloride infusion for massive nifedipine overdose. Chest 2001;119:1280–2.
21. Bailey B. Glucagon in beta-blocker and calcium channel blocker overdoses: a systematic review. J Toxicol Clin Toxicol 2003;4:595–602.
22. Boyer EW, Shannon M. Treatment of calcium-channel-blocker intoxication with insulin infusion. N Engl J Med 2001;344:1721–2.
23. Mégarbane B, Karyo S, Baud FJ. The role of insulin and glucose (hyperinsulinaemia/euglycaemia) therapy in acute calcium channel antagonist and beta-blocker poisoning. Toxicol Rev 2004;23:215–22.
24. Chu J, Wang RY, Hill NS. Update in clinical toxicology. Am J Respir Crit Care Med 2002;166:9–15.
25. Brimacombe JR, Scully M, Swainston R. Propranolol overdose—a dramatic response to calcium chloride. Med J Aust 1991;155:267–8.
26. Pertoldi F, D'Orlando L, Mercante WP. Electromechanical dissociation 48 hours after atenolol overdose: usefulness of calcium chloride. Ann Emerg Med 1998;31:777–81.
27. Banner W Jr. Risks of extracorporeal membrane oxygenation: is there a role for use in the

management of the acutely poisoned patient? J Toxicol Clin Toxicol 1996;34:365–371.

28. Purkayastha S, Bhan,goo P, Athanasiou T, et al. Treatment of poisoning induced cardiac impairment using cardiopulmonary bypass: a review. Emerg Med J 2006;23:246–50.
29. Massetti M, Bruno P, Babatasi G, Neri E, Khayat A. Cardiopulmonary bypass and severe drug intoxication. J Thorac Cardiovasc Surg 2000;120:424–5.
30. Wolf LR, Spadafora MP, Otten EJ. Use of amrinone and glucagon in a case of calcium channel blocker overdose. Ann Emerg Med 1993;22:1225–8.
31. Tuncok Y, Apaydin S, Gelal A, Ates M, Guven H. The effects of 4-aminopyridine and Bay K 8644 on verapamil-induced cardiovascular toxicity in anesthetized rats. J Toxicol Clin Toxicol 1998;36: 301–7.
32. Tuncok Y, Apaydin S, Kalkan S, Ates M, Guven H. The effects of amrinone and glucagon on verapamil-induced cardiovascular toxicity in anaesthetized rats. Int J Exp Pathol 1996;77:207–12.
33. ter Wee PM, Kremer Hovinga TK, Uges DR, van der Geest S. 4-Aminopyridine and haemodialysis in the treatment of verapamil intoxication. Hum Toxicol 1985;4:327–9.
34. Plewa MC, Martin TG, Menegazzi JJ, Seaberg DC, Wolfson AB. Hemodynamic effects of 3,4-diaminopyridine in a swine model of verapamil toxicity. Ann Emerg Med. 1994;23:499–507.
35. Mégarbane B, Pascal Leprince P, Deye N, Guerrier G, Résière D, Bloch V, Baud FJ. Extracorporeal life support in a case of acute carbamazepine poisoning with life-threatening refractory myocardial failure. Intensive Care Med 2006;32:1409–13.

32
Sleep-Related Breathing Disorders and Acute Heart Failure Syndrome

Rami N. Khayat, Martin A. Valdivia-Arenas, and William T. Abraham

An association between severe heart failure and a form of breathing irregularity, Cheyne-Stokes respiration (CSR), has been recognized for well over two centuries. Only in the past three decades, however, has intensive epidemiologic and experimental work uncovered an intriguing and reciprocal relationship between sleep-related breathing disorders (SRBDs) and cardiovascular disease. For example, obstructive sleep apnea hypopnea syndrome (OSAHS, also known more simply as obstructive sleep apnea or OSA) causes hypertension, left ventricular hypertrophy, and early atherosclerosis. Obstructive sleep apnea also worsens ischemic heart disease and cardiac arrhythmias, and it is an independent risk factor for the development of heart failure. That is, in otherwise healthy individuals, OSA can be a cause of cardiac dysfunction, and in patients with existing cardiovascular disorders, OSA can accelerate the progression to heart failure, or induce an exacerbation of underling chronic heart failure (1, 2). Moreover, central sleep apnea (CSA), a rare form of SRBD in the general population, is highly prevalent in patients with systolic heart failure, where it seems to be a result of the heart failure and portends a poor prognosis in these patients. Thus, SRBD may be either a cause or a consequence of heart failure, and in both cases it may contribute to disease progression as well as to acute exacerbations of heart failure.

Definitions

The term *sleep-related breathing disorders* encompasses all types of respiratory disturbance during sleep: obstructive, central, and mixed. Since most patients have a predominance of either central or obstructive events, SRBDs are commonly divided into two main clinical syndromes: central and obstructive sleep disorders. Obstructive sleep apnea syndrome is defined by the presence of compatible clinical symptoms, including excessive daytime sleepiness, and at least five obstructive respiratory events, apneas or hypopneas, per hour of sleep. Obstructive apneas are produced by complete collapse of the upper airway, resulting in cessation of airflow, against which the inspiratory effort persists. Obstructive hypopneas result from a partial collapse of the upper airway, causing reduction in, but not complete cessation of, airflow. Another way to think of obstructive sleep events is that the patient cannot breathe due to either total or partial obstruction of the airway.

In CSA, the respiratory events are secondary to absent or reduced respiratory drive and are characterized by cessation of or reduction in respiratory effort, resulting in a cessation or reduction of airflow. Thus in the circumstance of CSA, the patient does not breathe. Cheyne-Stokes respiration describes a unique morphology of central apnea events, in which a crescendo-decrescendo pattern of ventilation is followed by a central apnea.

The apnea hypopnea index (AHI), the total number of apneas and hypopneas per hour of sleep, indicates the severity of the SRBD, obstructive or central. Polysomnography (PSG), an attended sleep study, is the standard test to establish the diagnosis of SRBD. It includes measurement of the electroencephalogram (EEG), electrocardiogram (ECG), respiratory effort, airway flow, and peripheral oxygen saturation. Thus, the PSG is highly effective at evaluating

SRBD and differentiating OSA from CSA events. However, successful identification of respiratory events on PSG depends on several methodologic considerations, including the technique used to measure effort and flow, and the polygraphic criteria used to define obstructive and central events. The reader is referred to the report by the American Academy of Sleep Medicine for more details on these criteria (3).

Epidemiology of Sleep-Related Breathing Disorder in Heart Failure

Estimates of the prevalence of SRBD in patients with heart failure differ slightly among studies, due to the varying definitions used. These studies agree, however, that a staggering number of patients with chronic systolic heart failure, estimated at 50% to 70% have a significant degree of SRBD (4, 5). This prevalence is even higher in patients with acute heart failure (6). Central sleep apnea appears to affect about 40% of patients with systolic heart failure. Obstructive sleep apnea, the most common form of SRBD in the general population, affecting 4% to 9% of middle-aged adults (7), is reported in about 11% to 37% of patients with stable systolic heart failure (4, 5). The distribution of OSA versus CSA in patients with heart failure may depend on the population studied (8). Patients with advanced or decompensated heart failure might be expected to have predominantly CSA, while stable chronic outpatients may exhibit a predominance of OSA. The association between heart failure and obesity may also favor the occurrence of OSA in patients with high body mass indexes. Many heart failure patients exhibit both obstructive and central events. In any event, heart failure may be considered the most important risk factor for SRBD.

Mechanisms of Sleep-Related Breathing Disorder

Central Sleep Apnea

During sleep, CO_2 level is the main stimulus for ventilation, and respiration ceases if CO_2 falls below a level called the apnea threshold. Patients with heart failure have a pattern of chronic hyperventilation that is characterized by close proximity between their eupneic level of CO_2 and their apnea threshold. This makes it very likely that a slight increase in ventilation during sleep, such as with arousal or changes in airway resistance, will result in a drop in CO_2 below the apnea threshold precipitating apnea. Given the inertia in the respiratory control system, breathing does not resume until an excessive chemical stimulus (hypercapnia or hypoxia) has accumulated, producing excessive ventilation that is likely to drop CO_2 again below the apnea threshold and create periodic breathing and CSR. Furthermore, patients with heart failure have reduced cerebral blood flow response to changes in CO_2, which reduces the ability of the respiratory control center to dampen overshoot and undershoot in the ventilatory response to carbon dioxide (9). The mechanism of this chronic hyperventilation in patients with heart failure is thought to be related to pulmonary interstitial congestion. It is, therefore, possible that the acute decompensation of heart failure may be associated with worsening of CSA. In turn, worsening of sleep apnea may perpetuate the conditions for heart failure decompensation. Thus, a vicious cycle of deleterious cardiorespiratory interactions ensues.

Obstructive Sleep Apnea

A tenuous balance between constrictor and dilator forces maintains the patency of the upper airway during sleep. Obstructive sleep apnea occurs when this balance shifts toward the constricting forces. The two collapsing factors of the upper airway are the intraluminal negative pressure generated by the diaphragm during inspiration and the extraluminal pressure from the tissue surrounding the airway. The dilating forces are those of the tone of the pharyngeal muscles, and the longitudinal traction on the airway from lung inflation during inspiration. The mechanism of OSA in patients with heart failure is similar to that in the general population. Additional influences on the upper airway patency, such as pharyngeal edema or cervical venous congestion, may contribute to the genesis of OSA in patients with heart failure. This latter concept is important in the setting of acute heart failure syndromes, where fluid retention and worsening of the heart failure can worsen the OSA, and, as is the case with CSA, a vicious cycle ensues.

Given that CSA in heart failure is a very common manifestation of respiratory control instability, it is very likely (as noted above) that the two types of apnea, obstructive and central, may exist in the same patient. Furthermore, respiratory control instability may cause changes in the upper airway tone, producing obstruction during central apneas (10). In fact, worsening of systolic heart failure during the course of one night in a patient with severe chronic heart failure and OSA may give rise to central apneas by the end of the same night (11, 12).

Clinical Manifestations and Risk Factors of Sleep-Related Breathing Disorder

Half of all patients with SRBD report no specific symptoms. Combined with the significant overlap between symptoms of SRBD and symptoms of heart failure, this makes it difficult to identify SRBD in patients with chronic heart failure based on history alone. For example, symptoms such as fatigue, tiredness, sleepiness, reduced physical activity level, and poor mentation may be due to either SRBD or heart failure and do not aid in determining which patients to screen for SRBD. Given the severe impact untreated SRBD has on patients with heart failure, it imperative to maintain a very high index of suspicion for this diagnosis. To date, there is no consensus on a cost-effective approach to conduct surveillance of SRBD in heart failure patients. Such an approach will most likely include the use of validated questionnaires and portable screening devices. One such device has recently been validated in a head-to-head comparison to PSG (13).

Risk factors for OSA include obesity, increased neck circumference, male sex, and postmenopause in women. These risk factors remain the same in patients with heart failure. The typical symptoms of OSA—snoring, excessive daytime sleepiness, and poor sleep quality—also occur in patients with heart failure. However, their sensitivity and specificity for the diagnosis of SRBD may be reduced by the heart failure state. Other significant presentations in this population include worsening heat failure, recurrence of atrial fibrillation, ventricular arrhythmia, nocturnal angina, stroke, and recurrence of stroke.

The form of CSA found in the general population, idiopathic central sleep apnea, has no known risk factors. In patients with heart failure, CSA is very common, and several risk factors have been suggested: reduced systolic function, male sex, advanced age, atrial fibrillation, and reduced daytime $Pa{CO_2}$. Usually, these patients present with fatigue, insomnia, and poor sleep continuity. Table 32.1 summarizes the clinical features of the SRBD syndromes and their risk factors.

Table 32.1. Clinical features of the sleep-related breathing disorder (SRBD) syndromes and risk factors

SRBD syndrome	Symptoms in the general population	Additional symptoms in cardiac patients	Risk factors in patients with heart failure
CSA	Excessive daytime sleepiness	Ventricular tachyarrhythmia	Systolic dysfunction
	Insomnia	Atrial fibrillation	Lower awake $P{CO_2}$
		Exacerbation of heart failure	Age greater than 65
		Poor rehabilitation performance or deteriorating functional status	Male sex
			Atrial fibrillation
		Cognitive impairment	Nonobese patients
OSA	Excessive daytime sleepiness	Angina	Obesity
	Snoring	Stroke	Male gender
	Choking or gasping during sleep	Poorly controlled hypertension	Craniofacial abnormalities
	Fatigue	Pulmonary edema	Hypothyroidism
	Impaired concentration		Postmenopausal women
			Family history
			Diastolic dysfunction

Cardiovascular Consequences of Sleep-Related Breathing Disorder

In patients with SRBD, the recurrence, throughout the night, of apnea or hypopnea followed by a recovery phase induces a cyclic pattern of intermittent hypoxia-reoxygenation, arousal, increased inspiratory effort, sympathetic activation, and surges in blood pressure. These perturbations are strikingly similar in both central and obstructive sleep disorders and are associated with the same cardiovascular consequences (Fig. 32.1).

Intermittent Hypoxia

During apnea, in both OSA and CSA, hypoxia stimulates chemoreceptors that mediate an increase in sympathetic activity (14). This sympathetic activation produces vasoconstriction and a surge in blood pressure (15). It may also be toxic to myocytes and worsen the myocardial oxygen supply–demand equation, and promote myocardial ischemia. With the recurrence of apnea-recovery and the associated hypoxia-reoxygenation, a cyclic pattern of sympathetic activation and blood pressure surges recurs throughout the sleep period. Interestingly, the increase in sympathetic activity and blood pressure persists during the daytime (16). This memory effect or plasticity in the neurocirculatory response is unique to the stimulus of intermittent hypoxia and explains the causal link between SRBD and hypertension. It may also explain, in part, the persistently elevated plasma norepinephrine levels seen in some heart failure patients. Furthermore, intermittent hypoxia causes endothelial dysfunction, platelet aggregation, and left ventricular hypertrophy, and induces an inflammatory response. Therefore, intermittent hypoxia is the most important perturbation in SRBD. Other pathophysiologic consequences related to this cycle of hypoxia-reoxygenation may include increases in oxidative stress and decreases in nitric oxide bioavailability.

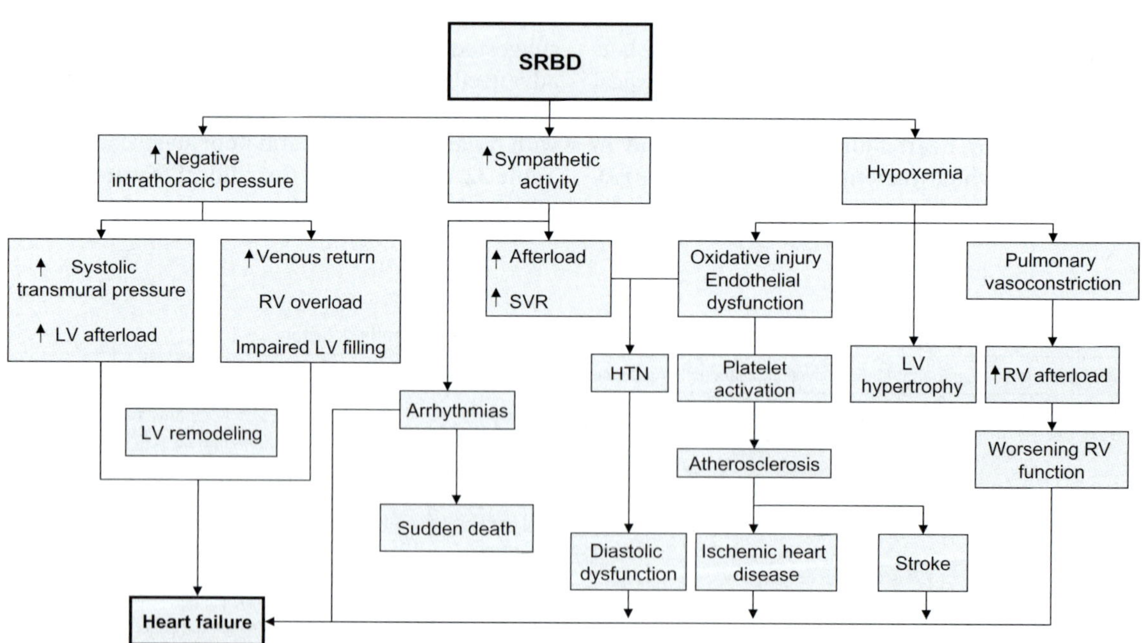

FIGURE 32.1. The chronic cardiovascular consequences of sleep-related breathing disorder (SRBD). HTN, hypertension; LV, left ventricle; RV, right ventricle; SVR, systemic vascular resistance; ↑, increased.

Increased Respiratory Effort

The mechanical perturbations in OSA are more profound than those in CSA, and appear to have more severe implications for patients with heart failure. In patients with OSA, as the balance between the dilating and constricting forces of the upper airway shifts toward the latter, an obstructive event ensues. The resulting hypoxia stimulates the respiratory centers, which generate vigorous inspiratory effort, and the subsequent large respiratory effort against a closed airway causes a profound increase in negative intrathoracic pressure with each inspiration. This negative pressure reaches a value that is severalfold the normal inspiratory negative pressure and can have serious effects on the heart via several mechanisms. First, the negative intrathoracic pressure augments the gradient between the intraventricular pressure and the intrathoracic pressure, resulting in increased left ventricular work and wall stress during systole, thus increasing afterload. Second, while varying effects on central venous pressure during apnea are reported in patients with OSA, an increase in venous return to the right ventricle is likely (17). This may serve to increase right ventricular preload and may cause a shift in the interventricular septum, reducing the left ventricular end diastolic volume. Finally, the negative intrathoracic pressure may affect the balance of forces governing the transudation of fluid into the interstitial space. In fact, pulmonary edema following repeated upper airway obstruction has been reported in humans and reproduced in experimental animals (18).

In central apnea, the large breaths occur during the recovery phase after an arousal terminates the apnea, usually without significant accompanying upper airway obstruction, and, therefore, with less profound negative swings in the intrathoracic pressure. Changes in the venous return and transmural cardiac pressure, however, may still occur. The sympathetic activation associated with CSA (also due to hypoxia) appears to be more important in mediating the cardiovascular effects of CSA than these less profound pressure changes.

Sleep-Related Breathing Disorder in Acute Heart Failure Syndrome

Remarkably, little is known about the acute consequences of SRBD in decompensated heart failure patients. To date, no substantive studies of adequate size have systematically evaluated either the prevalence or the importance of SRBD in this setting. The association of CSR-CSA and poor outcomes in hospitalized patients with decompensation has been observed for many years. The coronary care unit nurse who observes the classic CSR pattern of breathing often is the one to identify these patients and appropriately raise concern. It is likely that the aforementioned cardiovascular consequences of SRBD seen in general and in chronic heart failure patients contribute to the decompensated state and poor outcomes for acute heart failure syndromes. Indeed, prospective epidemiologic data of the cardiovascular outcomes of SRBD (19), while still limited, show increased incidence of fatal and nonfatal cardiovascular events in patients with SRBD, and support a conclusion of a detrimental impact of SRBD on the morbidity and mortality of patients with heart failure.

Figure 32.2 reviews the various mechanisms by which SRBD may contribute to the pathophysiology of acute heart failure syndromes. This scheme is based on known pathways, and its contribution to acute heart failure is biologically plausible on multiple levels. In particular, the interrelationship between obstructive and central sleep apnea and the vicious cycle of acute heart failure and SRBD should be noted. While the figure underscores the question of which comes first, worsening SRBD or heart failure, the point is probably less relevant since effective treatment should target both disorders. In this regard, experience with noninvasive ventilation (e.g., continuous positive airway pressure, bi-level positive airway pressure; see below) in decompensated heart failure has generally been good, and it is recommended in some algorithms of treatment of acute heart failure (20). Thus, while SRBD should be diagnosed and treated in chronic heart failure patients, the imperative to do so may be even greater in patients with acute heart failure since the perturbations caused by

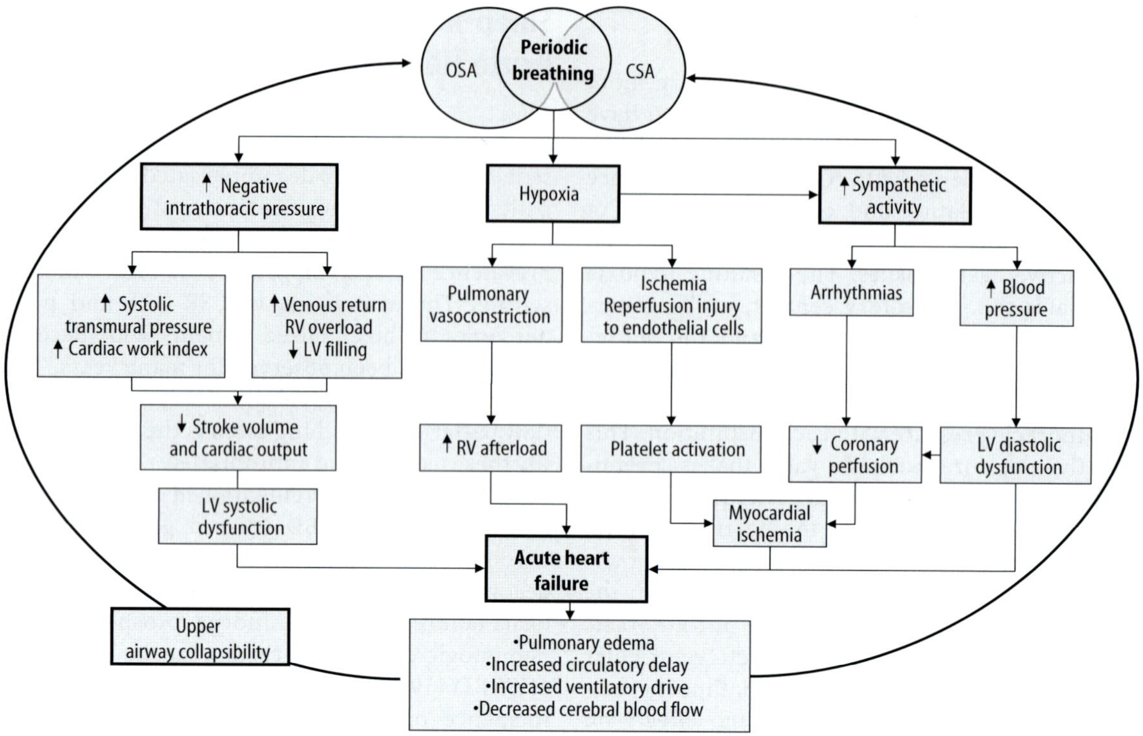

FIGURE 32.2. The effects of SRBD in patients with acute heart failure syndrome. CSA, central sleep apnea; LV, left ventricle; OSA, obstructive sleep apnea; RV, right ventricle; ↑, increased; ↓, decreased.

SRBD may be immediately critical and potentially life threatening.

Treatment of Sleep-Related Breathing Disorder in Patients with Heart Failure

Treatment of Obstructive Sleep Apnea

Nasal continuous positive airway pressure (CPAP) is the standard treatment for OSA in the general population, and its use in patients with heart failure may have additional cardiac benefits. It acts as an "air splint" for the upper airway, preventing collapse and episodes of apnea and hypopnea. Large epidemiologic studies, however, are still needed to confirm the impact of CPAP on mortality in general and in heart failure patients. Continuous positive airway pressure reduces daytime sleepiness, improves cognitive function, and lowers daytime and nocturnal blood pressure in patients with OSA and normal heart function (21). Multiple studies have shown improvement in the ejection fraction after 1 to 3 months in patients with OSA and heart failure treated with CPAP. These benefits of CPAP extend to the biologic markers of heart failure such as atrial natriuretic peptide and sympathetic activity. Continuous positive airway pressure may improve heart failure when added to drug therapy through the following mechanisms: (1) It increases the intrathoracic pressure with subsequent reduction in the left ventricular transmural pressure and improvement in the ejection fraction. (2) It reduces sympathetic activation by improving the apnea driven hypoxia. (3) It abolishes the nocturnal variations of blood pressure triggered by apneic episodes, and has additive benefits in the treatment of patients with established systemic hypertension. These direct benefits to the heart are in addition to eliminating respiratory events and hypoxia, and improving the quality of sleep. Furthermore, the use of positive pressure ventilation reduces the need for intubation in patients with cardiogenic pulmonary edema by improving the oxygenation and cardiac output.

Bilevel positive airway pressure (BiPAP), a modality that allows independent adjustment of inspiratory and expiratory positive airway pressures (rather than a single continuous pressure as with CPAP), is also used to treat OSA. There are no convincing data supporting the superiority of BiPAP over CPAP in the outpatient setting. In fact, there is a concern that the use of BiPAP may promote episodes of central apnea during sleep in patients with mixed CSA-OSA, by increasing ventilation in these patients who have close proximity between eupneic CO_2 and the apnea threshold during sleep (22, 23). It is generally accepted that, in the acutely decompensated heart failure, either CPAP or BiPAP will improve pulmonary edema and reduce the need for intubation and mechanical ventilation.

A patient admitted to the hospital with acute heart failure syndrome and with OSA on CPAP treatment should continue the treatment. Pressure requirements may change during an exacerbation of heart failure. There is no evidence, however, that titrating the pressure again in the hospital is beneficial. In patients with acute heart failure and no diagnosis of OSA in whom the disorder is highly suspected, a sleep medicine consultation or empirical CPAP is strongly advised. The use of portable screening studies or empirical treatment with CPAP can be considered in this setting. Attention to the pressure administered and the patient–device interface is critical in determining immediate acceptance of and long-term compliance with the device.

Possible adverse reactions to nasal CPAP or BiPAP are very mild and include nasal congestion, upper respiratory tract dryness, epistaxis, skin abrasion, conjunctivitis, claustrophobia, chest discomfort, aerophagia, and rarely pneumothorax. The use of humidifiers helps to prevent nasal dryness and epistaxis, and may help to reduce resistance to the airflow. A proper mask fitting is an important step, to avoid leaks that can cause conjunctivitis and to prevent skin abrasion due to excessive pressure from the mask. It is very likely that meticulous attention to patients' initial acceptance of the introduction of CPAP will positively impact their future compliance with the device treatment.

Treatment of Central Sleep Apnea

Optimization of medical therapy for heart failure improves and can eliminate CSA. If CSA persists despite optimal medical therapy, the therapeutic options are noninvasive ventilation or oxygen. In small, single-center randomized trials, CPAP improved central sleep apnea, increased the left ventricular ejection fraction (LVEF), reduced daytime levels of atrial natriuretic peptide and plasma norepinephrine, and improved the quality of life in patients with chronic systolic heart failure after 1 to 3 months of treatment. In a recent randomized, single-blind, multicenter trial, CPAP improved oxygenation and ejection fraction but failed to improve transplantation-free survival or to decrease the number of hospitalizations (24). It should be noted that this latter trial may have been underpowered, and that all these studies apply to outpatients with chronic heart failure and CSA. In patients with acutely decompensated heart failure, and CSA or OSA, CPAP can be beneficial via the mechanisms described above.

Adaptive pressure support servo ventilation (APSSV), a modality that delivers positive expiratory airway pressure and expiratory pressure support based on the detection of CSA-CSR with a backup of respiratory rate, is as effective as CPAP in improving daytime sleepiness, B-type natriuretic peptide levels, and urinary catecholamine excretion. In a small prospective, randomized, multicenter trial, this mode of ventilation significantly improved compliance and left ventricular function after 6 months when compared with CPAP (25). Nocturnal supplemental oxygen also improves central apnea and eliminates apnea-related hypoxia, but it lacks some of the benefits of positive pressure, such as improvement of heart function or water redistribution in the congestive lung. The inability of oxygen to relieve the obstructive events in patients with the mixed form is another disadvantage. Moreover, oxygen therapy has not been adequately studied as a treatment for CSA in heart failure, although its administration to patients presenting with acute heart failure syndromes is empirically encouraged.

Acetazolamide and theophylline have been used to treat central apnea; however, safety data regarding their use in patients with heart failure are not adequately reassuring. With the former agent, urinary potassium wasting leading to hypokalemia and increased arrhythmia risk is a real concern. In the case of theophylline, its stimulatory affect on the heart may produce tachycardia and theoretically increase the risk of life-threatening arrhythmias. Both should be avoided in the setting of heart failure.

Conclusion

In otherwise healthy individuals, SRBDs constitute a significant risk factor for the development of cardiovascular disease or the progression of existent cardiovascular disorders toward heart failure, stroke, or death. Similarly, heart failure is the most important risk factor for developing SRBD, either central or obstructive, or for the worsening of existent SRBD. Understanding this reciprocal relationship between SRBD and heart failure is critical for successful clinical management of both disorders.

The distinction between central and obstructive disorders in patients with heart failure may be difficult due to the complex physiologic interaction between the mechanisms leading to either disorder. A mixed pattern of SRBD is present in many patients with heart failure, resulting in central, obstructive, and mixed apneas and hypopneas during the course of one night. Patients with acute heart failure syndromes with or without SRBD may benefit from treatment with CPAP, which improves pulmonary edema and cardiac output in patients with high preload. Patients with acute heart failure and OSA should certainly be treated with CPAP to eliminate upper airway obstruction. Physiologic evidence supports the use of some form of noninvasive ventilation in patients with acute heart failure and CSA. However, the best way to treat CSA in this setting or in chronic heart failure requires further investigation.

References

1. Nieto FJ, et al., Association of sleep-disordered breathing, sleep apnea, and hypertension in a large community-based study. Sleep Heart Health Study. JAMA, 2000;283(14):1829–36.
2. Parker JD, et al., Acute and chronic effects of airway obstruction on canine left ventricular performance. Am J Respir Crit Care Med, 1999;160(6):1888–96.
3. Sleep-related breathing disorders in adults: recommendations for syndrome definition and measurement techniques in clinical research. The Report of an American Academy of Sleep Medicine Task Force. Sleep, 1999;22(5):667–89.
4. Javaheri S, et al., Sleep apnea in 81 ambulatory male patients with stable heart failure. Types and their prevalences, consequences, and presentations. Circulation, 1998;97(21):2154–9.
5. Sin DD, et al., Risk factors for central and obstructive sleep apnea in 450 men and women with congestive heart failure. Am J Respir Crit Care Med, 1999;160(4):1101–6.
6. Tremel F, et al., High prevalence and persistence of sleep apnoea in patients referred for acute left ventricular failure and medically treated over 2 months. Eur Heart J, 1999;20(16):1201–9.
7. Young T, et al., The occurrence of sleep-disordered breathing among middle-aged adults. N Engl J Med, 1993;328(17):1230–5.
8. Trupp RJ, et al., Prevalence of sleep disordered breathing in a heart failure program. Congest Heart Fail, 2004;10(5):217–20.
9. Xie A, et al., Cerebrovascular response to carbon dioxide in patients with congestive heart failure. Am J Respir Crit Care Med, 2005;172(3):371–8.
10. Badr MS, et al., Pharyngeal narrowing/occlusion during central sleep apnea. J Appl Physiol, 1995; 78(5):1806–15.
11. Shepard JW, Jr., et al., Effects of changes in central venous pressure on upper airway size in patients with obstructive sleep apnea. Am J Respir Crit Care Med, 1996;153(1):250–4.
12. Tkacova R, et al., Overnight shift from obstructive to central apneas in patients with heart failure: role of PCO2 and circulatory delay. Circulation, 2001; 103(2):238–43.
13. Abraham WT, et al., Validation and clinical utility of a simple in-home testing tool for sleep disordered breathing in heart failure: Results of the Sleep Events, Arrhythmias, and Respiratory analysis in Chronic Heart failure (SEARCH) study. Congestive Heart Failure 2006;12:241–7.
14. Morgan BJ, et al., Neurocirculatory consequences of negative intrathoracic pressure vs. asphyxia

during voluntary apnea. J Appl Physiol, 1993;74(6): 2969–75.
15. Katragadda S, et al., Neural mechanism of the pressor response to obstructive and nonobstructive apnea. J Appl Physiol, 1997;83(6):2048–54.
16. Somers VK, et al., Sympathetic neural mechanisms in obstructive sleep apnea. J Clin Invest, 1995;96(4): 1897–904.
17. Bradley TD and Floras JS, Sleep apnea and heart failure: Part I: obstructive sleep apnea. Circulation, 2003;107(12):1671–8.
18. Fletcher EC, et al., Pulmonary edema develops after recurrent obstructive apneas. Am J Respir Crit Care Med, 1999;160(5 pt 1):1688–96.
19. Marin JM, et al., Long-term cardiovascular outcomes in men with obstructive sleep apnoea-hypopnoea with or without treatment with continuous positive airway pressure: an observational study. Lancet, 2005;365(9464):1046–53.
20. Nieminen MS, et al., Executive summary of the guidelines on the diagnosis and treatment of acute heart failure: the Task Force on Acute Heart Failure of the European Society of Cardiology. Eur Heart J, 2005;26(4):384–416.
21. Engleman HM, et al., Effect of continuous positive airway pressure treatment on daytime function in sleep apnoea/hypopnoea syndrome. Lancet, 1994; 343(8897):572–5.
22. Johnson KG and Johnson DC, Bilevel positive airway pressure worsens central apneas during sleep. Chest, 2005;128(4):2141–50.
23. Parthasarathy S and Tobin MJ, Sleep in the intensive care unit. Intensive Care Med, 2004;30(2):197–206.
24. Bradley TD, et al., Continuous positive airway pressure for central sleep apnea and heart failure. N Engl J Med, 2005;353(19):2025–33.
25. Philippe C, et al., Compliance with and efficacy of adaptive servo-ventilation (ASV) versus continuous positive airway pressure (CPAP) in the treatment of Cheyne-Stokes respiration in heart failure over a six month period. Heart, 2005;92:337–42.

1.3.4
Acute Heart Failure Syndromes in the Extreme Ages

33 Acute Heart Failure Syndromes in the Elderly

Michael W. Rich

In the United States, persons 75 years of age or older comprise just 6.2% of the general population, yet they account for well over half of all emergency department visits for acute decompensated heart failure (ADHF),[1] and the median age of patients enrolled in the Acute Decompensated Heart Failure National Registry (ADHERE) is 75.3 years.[2] Moreover, these patients differ substantially from patients typically enrolled in HF clinical trials; not only are they older, but they are more likely to be women, more likely to have preserved left ventricular (LV) ejection fraction, more likely to have hypertension rather than coronary artery disease as the primary etiology, and more likely to have multiple coexisting medical conditions (especially renal insufficiency) that complicate management.[3] Furthermore, hospital mortality rates for ADHF are higher by a factor of three among patients 75 years of age or older compared to patients younger than age 75.[4]

Thus, elderly patients constitute a large and high-risk subgroup of the ADHF population, a subgroup that has been markedly underrepresented in heart failure (HF) clinical trials, and a group for which both the risks and potential benefits of therapeutic interventions may differ considerably from those in younger HF patients. The objective of this chapter, therefore, is to briefly review the pathophysiology, clinical features, and management of ADHF in the very elderly, herein defined as age 75 years of age or older.

Pathophysiology

Cardiovascular Aging

Normal aging is associated with a multitude of changes in the cardiovascular system that predispose to the development of HF (Table 33.1).[5,6] Increased collagen deposition and collagen cross-linking in the arterial walls, coupled with degeneration in elastin fibers, leads to a progressive increase in arterial stiffness with increasing age, resulting in a gradual rise in systolic blood pressure, arterial pulse wave velocity, and impedance to LV ejection (i.e., afterload). The heart itself also becomes stiffer as a result of interstitial collagen deposition and compensatory myocyte hypertrophy related to increased afterload and age-associated apoptosis. These changes result in a characteristic shift in the pattern of LV diastolic filling, with a decline in early diastolic filling rate and volume, and an increase in the contribution of atrial contraction to LV end-diastolic volume.[7] Altered diastolic function also leads to a marked increase in the prevalence of HF with normal LV ejection fraction at older age, as well as a progressive rise in the incidence and prevalence of atrial fibrillation.

Diminished responsiveness to β-adrenergic stimulation with advancing age leads to a progressive decline in maximum attainable heart rate (HR) (often represented by the formula: maximum

TABLE 33.1. Major effects of aging on the cardiovascular system

- Increased arterial stiffness
  - —Progressive rise in systolic blood pressure and pulse pressure
  - —Increased pulse-wave velocity and early pulse-wave reflection
- Increased myocardial stiffness
  - —Altered pattern of left ventricular diastolic filling
  - —Augmentation of atrial contraction
  - —Predisposition to diastolic heart failure and atrial fibrillation
- Impaired responsiveness to β-adrenergic stimulation
  - —Progressive decline in maximum heart rate and contractility
  - —Impaired β_2-mediated peripheral arterial vasodilation
- Diminished capacity of mitochondria to increase adenosine triphosphate production in response to increased demands
- Endothelial dysfunction, especially endothelium dependent vasodilation
  - —Diminished peak coronary blood flow
  - —Accelerated atherosclerosis

HR = 220 − age), peak LV contractility, and peripheral vasodilation (mediated by β_2-adrenergic receptors). Since cardiac output (CO) is the product of heart rate (HR) and stroke volume (SV) (CO = HR × SV), the age-related decline in β-adrenergic responsiveness translates into a progressive decline in maximum cardiac output with increasing age. Decreased capacity of the myocardial mitochondria to increase adenosine triphosphate (ATP) production commensurate with increased demands further impairs the capacity of the aging heart to increase cardiac output in response to stress.

Aging is also associated with endothelial dysfunction, mediated in part by diminished production of nitric oxide. Since nitric oxide plays a vital role in coronary vasodilation and regulation of coronary blood flow, maximum coronary blood flow declines with age, which in turn predisposes the older heart to ischemia under conditions of increased myocardial oxygen demand. In addition, endothelial dysfunction contributes both to the development and progression of atherosclerosis, the presence of which further increases the risk of ischemia in the aging heart.

Taken together, the above changes lead to an accelerating decline in maximum cardiac performance and cardiac reserve capacity with increasing age, even in the absence of subclinical or overt cardiovascular disease.[8] Note in particular that the four primary determinants of cardiac output—preload, afterload, heart rate, and contractility—are all adversely affected by the aging process. This marked decline in cardiovascular reserve predisposes elderly individuals to the development of both acute and chronic HF; that is, the threshold for cardiac decompensation (ADHF) in response to ischemia, volume overload, atrial fibrillation, pneumonia, or a surgical procedure is much lower in an 85-year-old person than in a 55-year-old person. Thus, to a considerable extent, cardiovascular changes associated with normal aging account for both the disproportionately high incidence of ADHF at elderly age, as well as the markedly worse prognosis associated with ADHF in the very elderly.

Coexisting Cardiovascular Disease

A second key factor that predisposes older individuals to ADHF is the increasing prevalence of age-associated cardiovascular diseases, particularly hypertension and coronary artery disease (CAD), but also including valvular heart disease (especially aortic stenosis and mitral regurgitation), rhythm disorders (notably atrial fibrillation and sinoatrial dysfunction), and certain cardiomyopathies (e.g., hypertensive hypertrophic cardiomyopathy of the elderly and "senile" cardiac amyloid).

Hypertension and CAD are the two most common etiologies of HF among older patients, and the prevalence of both of these conditions increases progressively with age, in part due to the age-related changes in the cardiovascular system discussed above. Not only are hypertension and CAD more common in the elderly, but the duration of these conditions tends to be longer, thus increasing the risk for end-organ dysfunction. Moreover, the severity of hypertension, especially systolic hypertension, and the extent and severity of CAD, also tend to be greater in the elderly. Superimposed on the effects of normal cardiovascular aging, the high prevalence of age-associated cardiovascular diseases (and often multiple diseases) greatly increases the risk of older patients for the development of ADHF.

Comorbid Conditions

A third factor impacting the risk of older patients for ADHF is the effect of aging on other organ systems, and the associated increasing prevalence of noncardiovascular comorbid conditions. Most importantly, aging is associated with a progressive decline in renal function, such that a large proportion of persons over 80 years of age have at least mild to moderate chronic kidney disease, defined as a glomerular filtration rate (GFR) of <60 cc/min. The ability of the elderly kidney to excrete a fluid or sodium load is significant impaired, thus increasing the propensity for intravascular volume overload and clinical HF. Pulmonary reserve also declines with age, while the prevalence of chronic pulmonary disease increases, thereby reducing the buffer capacity of the lungs to compensate for the failing heart, and resulting in increased dyspnea and impaired exercise tolerance. The deleterious effects of aging on the gastrointestinal tract, liver, and kidneys also influence the absorption, distribution, and metabolism of most drugs, as a result of which older individuals are at increased risk for toxicity from both cardiac (e.g., digoxin) and noncardiac (e.g., nonsteroidal antiinflammatory drugs) medications.

In summary, multiple overlapping factors contribute to the extraordinarily high incidence of ADHF at elderly age, as well as to an unfavorable prognosis. In addition, these same factors increase the complexity of managing ADHF in the elderly, and may alter the response to specific therapeutic interventions.

Clinical Features

Symptoms and Signs

As in younger individuals, acute dyspnea is the most common symptom associated with ADHF in the elderly. On the other hand, the prevalence of atypical symptoms, including confusion, irritability, somnolence, and anorexia, increases in frequency with advancing age, especially among institutionalized elders. Conversely, acute shortness of breath in the elderly may be attributable to diverse other causes, such as myocardial ischemia or infarction, pneumonia (including aspiration pneumonitis), pulmonary embolism, an exacerbation of chronic lung disease, pleural or pericardial effusion, and anxiety.

The classic physical findings associated with ADHF—pulmonary rales, an S_3 gallop, elevated jugular venous pressure, and dependent pitting edema—are also less reliable markers in the elderly. Thus, rales may be attributable to lung disease or atelectasis, and peripheral edema may be due to venous insufficiency, renal or hepatic disease, or medications (especially calcium channel blockers) rather than HF. Jugular venous distention and an S_3 gallop are less commonly observed in elderly patients with ADHF due to the increased prevalence of HF with preserved LV ejection fraction at older age.

Laboratory Studies

Technical factors, such as patient confusion, poor inspiratory effort, or kyphosis of the thoracic spine, may make it difficult to obtain a high-quality chest radiograph in an acutely ill older patient. Interpretation of the film may be further confounded by the presence of chronic lung disease, scarring, or atelectasis. Heart size may be relatively normal in elderly patients with diastolic HF.

In recent years, plasma levels of B-type natriuretic peptide (BNP) and N-terminal pro-BNP (NT-pro-BNP) have proven to be a useful adjunct for diagnosing ADHF and for distinguishing this condition from acute dyspnea arising from other causes. However, it is important to recognize that levels of both of these peptides increase with age, especially in women (Fig. 33.1), so that the specificity of an elevated BNP or NT-pro-BNP level

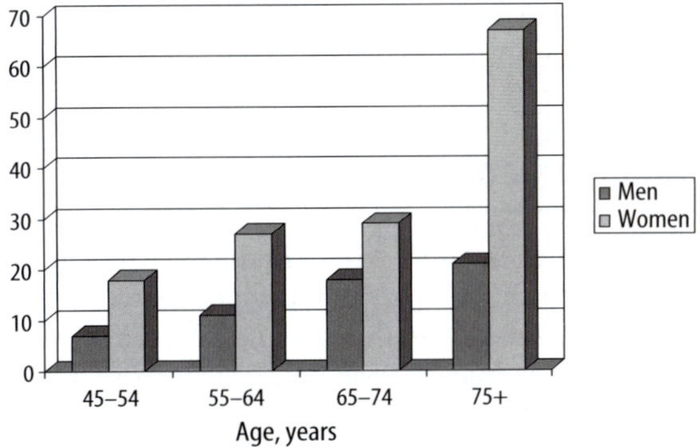

FIGURE 33.1. B-type natriuretic peptide levels by age and gender. (Adapted from Redfield et al.[9])

declines with age.[9] Conversely, a normal BNP or NT-pro-BNP level virtually excludes active HF in an elderly patient presenting with acute dyspnea.

The value of echocardiography and other cardiac imaging procedures in the diagnosis of ADHF in the elderly is limited, in part because over half of elderly HF patients have preserved LV systolic function at rest (i.e., the absence of reduced ejection fraction does not preclude a diagnosis of HF). In addition, diastolic dysfunction, as manifested by a reversal of the amplitudes of the early and late diastolic filling waves on echocardiography, is a hallmark of normal aging and is therefore of little use in diagnosing HF. Despite these limitations, echocardiography remains a valuable tool for diagnosing unsuspected valvular lesions, pericardial disease, or cardiomyopathy, and an assessment of ventricular function is important for determining long-term therapy.

Precipitants

Determination of the proximate cause of ADHF is critical, since identification of a specific cause (or causes) may facilitate treatment, shorten recovery time, and have a favorable impact on long-term outcomes. Common precipitants of ADHF in the elderly include myocardial ischemia or infarction (often in the absence of chest discomfort), uncontrolled hypertension, nonadherence to prescribed medications, new-onset atrial fibrillation or atrial flutter, noncardiac illnesses that impose increased stress on the aged heart's fragile reserve (e.g., pneumonia, sepsis, acute renal insufficiency, anemia), and certain medications (especially nonsteroidal antiinflammatory drugs).

Management

Initial management of ADHF in the elderly is generally similar to that in younger patients as reviewed elsewhere in this volume. The diagnostic evaluation should include an electrocardiogram, chest x-ray, complete blood count, serum electrolytes and routine blood chemistries, at least two sets of cardiac biomarker proteins to exclude acute coronary syndrome, a urinalysis, and either a BNP or NT-pro-BNP level in cases where the diagnosis of HF is uncertain. Potential precipitants of HF should be identified and treated as indicated.

Intravenous diuretic therapy should be initiated to relieve congestion and edema. However, it must be recognized that elderly HF patients, especially those with diastolic HF, may be preload dependent and volume-sensitive; that is, overly vigorous diuresis may result in an abrupt decline in stroke volume and cardiac output, precipitating relative hypotension, impaired cerebral and renal perfusion, and worsening renal function (a potent marker of increased short-term mortality).[10] The addition of small doses of morphine sulfate may aid in relieving dyspnea and reducing anxiety, but caution and close monitoring are essential to avoid oversedation.

The role of intravenous vasodilator therapy in the management of ADHF in the elderly is controversial, in part because few studies have enrolled older patients. Due to the progressive decline in renal function with increasing age, it would seem prudent to avoid nitroprusside and nesiritide in the elderly. On the other hand, intravenous nitroglycerin remains a reasonable therapeutic option, especially in patients with active myocardial ischemia, poorly controlled hypertension, or severe decompensated HF associated with reduced LV ejection fraction.

Intravenous inotropic agents, including dobutamine, dopamine, and milrinone, may be less effective in the elderly and are not recommended for routine use. Occasionally, use of inotropic therapy may be warranted as a temporizing measure in elderly patients with a treatable cause for ADHF, such as myocardial infarction or critical aortic stenosis.

Invasive Procedures

The use of invasive procedures, including pulmonary artery catheterization, cardiac catheterization, percutaneous coronary revascularization, intraaortic balloon counterpulsation, ventricular assist devices, and cardiac surgery, must be individualized. In particular, the patient and the patient's family (or other surrogates) should be provided with a realistic appraisal of the potential benefits and risks of undertaking any invasive procedure, including the likely impact on long-term outcomes. In addition, the patient's preferences (including views on quality of life vs.

duration of survival) should be carefully considered in the decision-making process, and elderly patients should not be pressured to undergo procedures contrary to their wishes.

Clinical Case

An 87-year-old woman nursing home resident is brought to the emergency room because of acute confusion and shortness of breath. She has a history of hypertension, paroxysmal atrial fibrillation, heart failure, mild chronic renal insufficiency (baseline serum creatinine 1.5 mg/dL), mild Alzheimer's disease, gastroesophageal reflux disease, and degenerative joint disease.

On the morning prior to admission the patient was alert, oriented, and apparently free of distress. Shortly after lunch, she was found to be confused, oriented only to name, and breathing heavily and erratically. She was placed in bed, oxygen was administered, and she was given furosemide 20 mg by mouth. Over the course of the afternoon her condition failed to improve and she was transferred to the emergency room by ambulance.

On examination in the emergency room, the patient is lethargic, moans intermittently, and appears mildly short of breath. Her temperature is 35.8°C, heart rate 130–140/minute and irregular, respiratory rate 24/minute with intermittent Cheyne-Stokes breathing, blood pressure 180/74 mm Hg, and oxygen saturation 92% on 5 L by nasal cannula. The jugular venous pressure is about 6 cm H_2O at 45 degrees. There are diffuse crackles throughout both lung fields. Cardiac examination reveals an irregularly irregular rhythm with a II/VI systolic ejection murmur; no gallops or rubs are appreciated. The abdomen is somewhat obese and palpation elicits loud moaning. There is no definite hepatomegaly. Examination of the lower extremities reveals chronic venous stasis changes and trace bilateral edema; no calf tenderness is elicited. The neurologic examination, apart from the altered mental status, appears grossly intact.

Initial Laboratory Data

ECG: atrial fibrillation with rapid ventricular response, left ventricular hypertrophy (LVH) with strain pattern, no definite ischemia.

Chest x-ray: poor quality film, rotated, moderate pulmonary congestion(?).

CBC: hemoglobin 9.7 g/dL, WBC 5600/μL, platelets 214,000/μL.

BMP: Na 135 mmol/L, K 3.2 mmol/L, Cl 97 mmol/L, CO_2 21 mmol/L, creatinine 1.6 mg/dL, BUN 35 mg/dL, Ca 8.7 mg/dL, glucose 137 mg/dL.

Troponin I: 0.3 ng/mL (normal ≤0.1 ng/mL)

BNP: 1160 ng/mL

Prior Cardiac Studies Obtained 6 Months Previously When the Patient Presented with Similar Symptoms

Echocardiogram: Mild LVH with normal LV systolic function, grade I diastolic dysfunction, mild aortic stenosis, mild mitral regurgitation.

Adenosine-thallium stress test: LV ejection fraction 65%, no evidence for ischemia.

How Should This Patient Be Managed?

This patient exhibits many of the features typical of ADHF in the elderly, including atypical symptoms (confusion) and physical findings (absence of a gallop rhythm, normal jugular venous pressure, no hepatomegaly or peripheral edema), a nondiagnostic chest radiograph (albeit suspicious for HF in light of other findings), and preserved LV ejection fraction. However, the markedly elevated BNP level establishes the diagnosis with reasonable certainty (although elderly patients with chronic HF and chronic renal insufficiency may have BNP levels in this range on an ongoing basis), and the presence of atrial fibrillation with rapid ventricular response suggests a possible mechanism for ADHF. Nonetheless, the possibility that the rapid atrial fibrillation itself may have been precipitated by another condition, such as pulmonary embolism, pneumonia, ischemia, poorly controlled hypertension, or even hyperthyroidism must also be considered. The slightly abnormal troponin I level suggests myocardial ischemia, but this could be due to the tachycardia, hypertension, and hypoxemia rather than a primary ischemic event; the normal stress test 6 months previously supports this scenario.

Acute-phase management should include an intravenous diuretic (e.g., furosemide 40 mg) and continuation of supplemental oxygen. An atrioventricular (AV)-nodal blocking agent such as metoprolol or diltiazem should be administered to lower the heart rate to <100/min. If needed, additional antihypertensive therapy should be given to decrease the systolic blood pressure to 140 to 160 mm Hg initially.

The value of heparin in this setting is unclear. Although there is no history of falls, the patient does have altered sensorium, so it may be prudent to obtain a head computed tomography (CT) scan prior to initiating heparin. If there is no evidence of intracranial hemorrhage, heparinization is probably warranted, considering that the patient is at high risk for cardioembolic stroke.

In anticipation of possible clinical deterioration, an effort should be made to obtain a copy of the patient's advance directive, if available. If no advance directive has been executed, a discussion with the patient's next-of-kin should be undertaken to determine her views regarding end-of-life care, especially with respect to endotracheal intubation and cardiopulmonary resuscitation. As soon as the patient's mental status permits, these issues should be discussed directly with the patient.

Once the patient's condition has been stabilized and her end-of-life wishes have been clarified (to the extent possible), the patient should be hospitalized for further evaluation and management, the intensity of which will depend on her initial response to therapy (including the trajectory of her confusion) and her stated preferences regarding the use of aggressive interventions. In all likelihood, a conservative approach to management is appropriate, with the primary objectives being to restore the patient to her previous level of function as quickly as possible, optimize her medical regimen, and transfer her back to the nursing home within a few days.

Conclusion

Aging is associated with a multitude of changes in the heart, vasculature, and other organ systems that predispose to the development of HF. As a result, the incidence and prevalence of HF, including ADHF, increase progressively with age. However, despite the fact that patients 75 years of age or older comprise over half of all cases of ADHF, these patients have been markedly underrepresented in clinical trials, and there is little published information to support an evidence-based approach to diagnosis and treatment. In addition, elderly HF patients differ substantially from younger patients, most notably with respect to the increasing proportion of women, the high prevalence of diastolic HF, and the frequent coexistence of multiple other medical conditions that confound diagnosis and complicate management. As a result, the approach to the elderly patient with ADHF must be individualized, the potential risks and benefits of diagnostic and therapeutic interventions must be carefully balanced, and therapeutic decision making must be undertaken in the context of the patient's stated preferences and lifestyle goals. In addition, it must be recognized that optimal management of the elderly patient with ADHF remains ill-defined, and substantial research is needed to illuminate the best approaches to the diagnosis and treatment of this increasingly important segment of the HF population.

References

1. Hugli O, Braun JE, Kim S, Pelletier AJ, Camargo CA. United Status emergency department visits for acute decompensated heart failure, 1992–2001. Am J Cardiol 2005;96:1537–42.
2. Fonarow GC, for the ADHERE Scientific Advisory Committee. Overview of acutely decompensated congestive heart failure (ADHF): a report from the ADHERE Registry. Heart Failure Rev 2004;9:179–85.
3. Rich MW, Kitzman D. Heart failure in octogenarians: a fundamentally different disease. Am J Geriatr Cardiol 2000;9(suppl):97–104.
4. Goldberg RJ, Spencer FA, Farmer C, Meyer TE, Pezzella S. Incidence and hospital death rates associated with heart failure: a community-wide perspective. Am J Med 2005;118:728–34.
5. Lakatta EG, Levy D. Arterial and cardiac aging: major shareholders in cardiovascular disease enterprises: Part I: aging arteries: a "set-up" for vascular disease. Circulation 2003;107:139–46.

6. Lakatta EG, Levy D. Arterial and cardiac aging: major shareholders in cardiovascular disease enterprises: Part II: the aging heart in health: links to heart disease. Circulation 2003;107:346–54.
7. Kitzman DW, Sheikh KH, Beere PA, Philips JL, Higginbotham MB. Age-related alterations of Doppler left ventricular filling indexes in normal subjects are independent of left ventricular mass, heart rate, contractility and loading conditions. J Am Coll Cardiol 1991;18:1243–50.
8. Fleg JL, Morrell CH, Bos AG, et al. Accelerated longitudinal decline of aerobic capacity in healthy older adults. Circulation 2005;112:674–82.
9. Redfield MM, Rodeheffer RJ, Jacobsen SJ, Mahoney DW, Bailey KR, Burnett JC. Plasma brain natriuretic peptide concentration: impact of age and gender. J Am Coll Cardiol 2002;40:976–82.
10. Forman DE, Butler J, Wang Y, et al. Incidence, predictors at admission, and impact of worsening renal function among patients hospitalized with heart failure. J Am Coll Cardiol 2004;43:61–7.

34
Acute Heart Failure Syndromes in Neonatal and Pediatric Populations

Brian Feingold and Steven A. Webber

The etiologies, presentation, and management of acute heart failure syndromes (AHFSs) in children vary significantly from those in adults. Childhood cardiac disease is a result, primarily, of congenital heart defects and cardiomyopathies, rather than coronary heart disease. Furthermore, the prevalence of cardiac disease in children is far lower than in the adult population. Also, unlike adults, pediatric cardiac arrest is rarely a primary cardiac event (1), but typically occurs secondary to circulatory collapse due to sepsis or from respiratory failure. Appreciation of these differences yields important implications for the diagnostic evaluation and management of a child with suspected acute heart failure. Therapies designed for adults are often not applicable to neonates and children with AHFS.

Unique Features of the Pediatric Heart

From the ultrastructural, physiologic, and anatomic perspectives, the neonatal and pediatric heart differs from that of the adult, with the greatest differences being apparent in the neonate. Studies in experimental animals have shown that diastolic cardiac function is diminished in the neonate as compared to the adult. From a structural perspective, this results in large part from differences in calcium handling by the cardiomyocyte. Because the immature cardiomyocyte has less sarcoplasmic reticulum, intracellular calcium stores are limited (2). The reduced numbers and activities of sarcoplasmic reticulum membrane transport proteins further hamper the flux of calcium. As a result, the immature cardiomyocyte has a greater reliance on extracellular calcium to enable myofibril contraction and relaxation (3). Also contributing to the unique physiologic profile of the neonatal and infant heart are fewer numbers of contractile elements per myocyte and a greater relative proportion of noncardiomyocytes to cardiomyocytes as compared to the mature heart. The former likely impacts the ability to generate systolic tension, whereas the latter is thought to contribute to the relative noncompliance of the neonatal and infant heart.

Many of these structural differences impact the clinical characteristics of the neonatal and infant heart. For example, the neonatal and infant heart is exquisitely sensitive to serum calcium concentration, such that following cardiac surgery, calcium infusions are often used for inotropic support. Also, relatively poor ventricular compliance limits the ability to augment stroke volume as a means of increasing cardiac output. Thus, the neonate and infant rely almost exclusively on increases in heart rate as the primary mechanism to augment cardiac output.

With advanced age, great confidence is placed in the assumption that no significant anatomic cardiac abnormality exists. However, when evaluating a neonate, infant, or young child who presents with acute heart failure, it is mandatory that a thorough assessment of the underlying cardiac anatomy be made. Indeed, congenital heart disease is the commonest cause of acute severe heart failure in infancy.

Presentation of Acute Heart Failure Syndromes

Heart failure in older children often presents somewhat insidiously, after repeated evaluation and medical testing for other, more common pediatric conditions. Neonates and infants often present acutely unwell, yet the diagnosis of a primary cardiac disorder is often not made on initial evaluation. It is not uncommon for cardiac disease to be considered only after initial resuscitative attempts fail to improve the child's condition or ancillary studies fail to corroborate the presumed diagnosis (e.g., shock due to sepsis). While much of the diagnostic difficulty results from the relative infrequency of primary cardiac disease in children, the inability of infants and young children to verbally convey their symptoms also contributes. Also the frequency with which young children experience nasal, respiratory, or gastrointestinal symptoms, particularly during the winter and spring, often results in the initial symptoms of heart failure being attributed to these much more common maladies.

Generally speaking, with advancing age of the child, the symptoms and signs of acute heart failure more closely mirror those of adults. Infants often present with a history of poor feeding, respiratory distress, and listlessness. Irritability may be the only manifestation of an incessant tachyarrhythmia that has resulted in myocardial dysfunction. Common adult symptoms of paroxysmal nocturnal dyspnea and orthopnea are uncommon in pediatric patients. Abdominal pain is often observed with acute severe heart failure in children and likely reflects liver capsule distention from hepatomegaly.

On physical examination, the child may appear anxious, and sinus tachycardia is present. Sweating is often prominent in infants. Elevation of the jugular venous pulse is often present but may be difficult to identify in the infant and toddler. Pallor and cool extremities may be present and is often associated with poor peripheral pulses and prolonged capillary refill. Resting tachypnea (rate >40 for toddlers or >60 for infants) and retractions (suprasternal, intercostal, and subcostal) are common. Unlike in adults, crackles are exceedingly rare in infants and young children with heart failure, even when pulmonary edema is present. Wheezes are more likely to be present. While hepatomegaly is a common finding, it is often overlooked or underappreciated by the inexperienced practitioner. Periorbital edema (infants and young children) with or without ascites (older children) is more common than peripheral edema in children.

Many of the specific etiologies for neonatal and pediatric acute heart failure have "classic" presentations. Given the variety of causes, specific presentations are described with each pathophysiology in the following section.

Etiologies of Acute Heart Failure Syndromes

Although acute heart failure syndromes are rare in infants and children, there are a large number of causes. While myocarditis and cardiomyopathies account for a considerable proportion of cases, congenital abnormalities, in the form of structural intracardiac lesions and coronary anomalies, are also significant contributors. Acquired conditions, such as Kawasaki disease, acute rheumatic fever, and incessant tachyarrhythmias, may also lead to heart failure in children. The causes of AHFS in children are summarized in Table 34.1.

Myocarditis

The clinical distinction between acute myocarditis and the acute presentation of chronic dilated cardiomyopathy (DCM) is often difficult. Many patients have a history of an intercurrent or recent viral illness. However, viral syndromes are so common in early childhood that the etiologic relationship to the onset of acute heart failure is often not clear. Indeed, in one study of children undergoing endomyocardial biopsy for the evaluation of possible myocarditis, only 20% had evidence of cardiac inflammation, most commonly when the history was very short (4). This distinction between DCM and fulminant myocarditis is vital, as many patients with the latter will recover completely if able to be supported, whereas children with severely decompensated heart failure from DCM generally will not recover without

Table 34.1. Etiologies of acute heart failure syndrome (AHFS) in the neonate and child

- Nonstructural disease
  —Myocarditis
  —Acute presentation of chronic idiopathic cardiomyopathy
  —Metabolic cardiomyopathy
  —Acute rheumatic fever
  —Incessant tachyarrhythmia
- Structural disease
  —Left heart obstructive lesions
  - Coarctation of the aorta
  - Hypoplastic left heart syndrome
  - Critical aortic stenosis

  —Large left-to-right shunt lesions (rare to cause AHFS)
  - Unrestrictive ventricular septal defect
  - Atrioventricular septal defect
  - Large patent ductus arteriosus

  —Arteriovenous malformation
  - Hepatic
  - Vein of Galen

  —Pulmonary venous obstruction
  - Obstructed total anomalous pulmonary venous return
  - Cor triatriatum
  - Supravalvar mitral ring
  - Pulmonary vein stenosis
- Coronary arterial disorders
  —Anomalous left coronary artery from the pulmonary artery
  —Myocardial bridging
  —Kawasaki disease with coronary aneurysm and/or stenosis
  —Posttransplant coronary arteriopathy (chronic rejection)
  —Supravalvar aortic stenosis with coronary ostial stenosis (Williams syndrome)

transplantation. The expectations from mechanical support (ECMO or ventricular assist device) and the consideration for listing for cardiac transplantation are directly impacted by the underlying diagnosis.

Viruses are the most common cause of myocarditis in children, with adenovirus and enteroviruses (particularly Coxsackie B) being most frequent (5). A wide variety of other viruses has also been reported, including cytomegalovirus, Epstein-Barr virus, respiratory syncytial virus, parvovirus, HIV, influenza, herpes, and hepatitis C viruses. Other less common causes include bacterial infection, myocarditis associated with autoimmune diseases such as systemic lupus erythematosus, and giant cell myocarditis.

Chest radiography and electrocardiogram may be of some help in the differentiation of myocarditis from DCM. Marked cardiomegaly with left atrial and left ventricular enlargement, and prominent left precordial forces would be expected with long-standing DCM. In contrast, absence of (or mild) cardiomegaly and globally diminished voltages on electrocardiogram are more typical of acute myocarditis. Confirmation of a diagnosis of myocarditis is usually sought by endomyocardial biopsy, except in neonates and infants under 1 year of age in whom the risk of perforation is felt to be too great (6). Viral cultures of stool, urine, and respiratory secretions may contribute to the diagnosis, as may polymerase chain reaction analysis of blood, pericardial effusion, or cerebral spinal fluid. Viral titers (at presentation and during convalescence) are often performed but are generally noncontributory to the diagnosis of childhood myocarditis.

Cardiomyopathies

Pediatric cardiomyopathies have a reported incidence of 1.13 to 1.24 cases per 100,000 population in two recent large studies (7, 8). Dilated (55%) and hypertrophic (35%) cardiomyopathies account for nearly all cases, with the remainder of pediatric cardiomyopathies composed of restrictive (5%) and noncompaction cardiomyopathy (<1%). Up to half of all pediatric cardiomyopathies present in the first year of life.

The presentation of an infant with acute cardiomyopathy necessitates a thorough diagnostic evaluation to exclude potentially reversible causes of myocardial dysfunction (e.g., congenital coronary anomalies, myocarditis, incessant tachyarrhythmias) and assess for the presence of underlying metabolic diseases. In the older child, a number of neuromuscular disorders are also associated with cardiomyopathies (e.g., Friedreich's ataxia, Duchenne and Becker muscular dystrophies, myotonic dystrophy, juvenile progressive spinal muscular atrophy). Patients with cardiomyopathy associated with these conditions most often present outside of infancy.

Acute presentation of chronic cardiomyopathy may occur for several reasons. Suspicion of cardiac disease in children by primary care physicians is low, due to the rarity of heart disease and heart failure in this population. Therefore, symptoms and signs of heart disease are often missed, leading to delayed diagnosis. This is compounded by the problem that young children are poor historians. Acute or chronic arrhythmias may go undiagnosed, and young children often fail to accurately describe palpitations. Sudden onset of tachyarrhythmia such as atrial tachycardia may result in profound cardiovascular collapse in a child with severe undiagnosed cardiomyopathy. This is particularly true of children with restrictive cardiomyopathy if they develop rapid atrial flutter or fibrillation. Finally, intercurrent infections are common in childhood and may precipitate acute heart failure in patients with little cardiac reserve.

Coronary Abnormalities

Congenital coronary abnormalities underlie a small percentage of the total number of infants and children who present with AHFS. However, detection is vital as most are amenable to surgical intervention with resultant normalization, or at the very least stabilization, of cardiac function.

An anomalous left coronary artery arising from the pulmonary artery is a well-described cause of severe left ventricular systolic dysfunction. This rare anomaly (1 in 300,000 live births) typically presents between 6 weeks and 4 months of age, coincident with the normal postnatal decrease in pulmonary vascular resistance. Initially, antegrade perfusion of the left coronary artery (LCA) is from the pulmonary artery with desaturated blood. Collateral vessels from the right coronary artery (RCA) often develop to aid in perfusion of the LCA distribution. Later, as pulmonary vascular resistance falls, flow becomes retrograde from the LCA into the pulmonary artery. This "steal" results in myocardial ischemia of the LCA distribution. Frequently, there is ischemia of the papillary muscles and severe mitral regurgitation. The extent of compromise in part reflects the extent of collateral circulation from the RCA to the left distribution. A high index of suspicion is required to make the diagnosis, as patients have been misdiagnosed as having congenital mitral regurgitation, neonatal myocarditis, or DCM. Diagnosis is often suggested by pathologic Q waves in leads aVR and aVL on electrocardiogram and echogenicity of the papillary muscles of the mitral valve. Mitral regurgitation and dilation of the RCA are often present on echocardiography. Cardiac catheterization may be required if a definitive diagnosis cannot be made by echocardiography. With prompt recognition, surgical reimplantation of the LCA onto the aortic root is curative and often results in complete normalization of left ventricular function and resolution of mitral regurgitation (9).

Other congenital coronary lesions that may predispose to sudden death or acute heart failure include origin of the LCA from the right coronary sinus (or proximal RCA), coronary ostial stenoses, and coronary-to-cardiac (or pulmonary artery) fistulas. Coronary arterial compression is believed to be the pathophysiologic basis of cardiovascular collapse or sudden death associated with origin of LCA from the right coronary sinus since the LCA courses between the aorta and pulmonary artery. Surgical unroofing of the proximal LCA into the aorta or bypass grafting may be curative. Coronary ostial stenoses may occur as isolated congenital lesions but are most commonly observed in patients with Williams syndrome and supravalvar aortic stenosis. Coronary ostial stenoses are often asymptomatic but can result in cardiovascular collapse. This is sometimes observed during hypotension, as may occur with induction of anesthesia for elective surgery. Finally, coronary-to-cardiac or pulmonary artery fistulas result in a low-resistance runoff for coronary flow and potential for myocardial ischemia. Although many children present asymptomatically with a continuous murmur, large lesions may present with congestive heart failure, myocardial infarction, or even sudden death due to acute coronary ischemia.

Acquired coronary lesions that may present with acute heart failure or death occur in homozygous forms of severe familial dyslipidemias, coronary dissection with Marfan's syndrome and other connective tissue diseases, vasospasm from cocaine or inhalant abuse, and complications of Kawasaki disease. While the etiology of Kawasaki disease remains unknown, the acute illness typically occurs in children 2 months to 8 years of age and consists of a constellation of swollen, red extremities, cervical lymphadenopathy, injected sclera, oral mucosal involvement, and high-grade fever. Following the acute phase, children may develop coronary artery ectasia, aneurysms, and stenoses with the potential for thrombus formation, acute myocardial infarction, and death. Treatment with intravenous immunoglobulin at the time of the acute illness is thought to lessen the risk of subsequent coronary complications.

The development of posttransplant coronary artery disease (CAD) also warrants mention as a cause of pediatric acute heart failure. Despite the success of pediatric cardiac transplantation, chronic rejection, which manifests as accelerated graft coronary artery disease, typically presents between 5 and 15 years after transplantation. As well as disease of the epicardial coronary arteries, there is often diffuse disease of small intramyocardial branches, leading to restrictive physiology and associated heart failure. Posttransplant CAD is the leading cause of death long after transplantation.

Congenital Heart Disease

A detailed review of the many circumstances in which congenital heart disease can lead to AHFS is beyond the scope of this chapter. While a brief overview of the mechanisms of heart failure resulting from cyanotic and acyanotic disease is pertinent, the focus of this section is on those specific congenital lesions that characteristically present with severe acute heart failure.

There are several anatomic pathways leading to heart failure in infants and young children; these include simple left to right shunts, severe left heart outflow obstruction, left heart inflow obstruction, and high output states associated with large arteriovenous malformations. In many patients, more than one mechanism may be present. In general, large left-to-right shunts (such as a large ventricular septal defect, atrioventricular septal defect, or patent ductus arteriosus) do not lead to AHFS or shock. In this setting of two ventricles and a large left to right shunt, systemic cardiac output is usually preserved at normal to low-normal levels despite the massive pulmonary overcirculation. Thus, these patients often present with tachypnea, poor feeding, and failure to thrive after the first month of life, but rarely have cool extremities, mottling, or other evidence of poor systemic output. If left unrepaired and the infant survives the acute heart failure, pulmonary vascular resistance will increase, failure will resolve, and eventually cyanosis ensues due to right-to-left shunt in the setting of irreversible pulmonary hypertension (Eisenmenger syndrome).

Acute severe heart failure in neonates is most often due to left heart obstructive disease resulting from severe coarctation of the aorta, hypoplastic left heart syndrome, or critical aortic stenosis. Presentation with cardiogenic shock has become less frequent due to prenatal diagnosis by fetal echocardiography. After delivery, infusion of prostaglandin E_1 maintains ductal patency and prevents the development of compromised systemic output. However, in the undiagnosed neonate, left heart obstructive lesions typically present in the first week of life upon closure of the arterial duct. In the absence of a patent ductus, systemic cardiac output is severely compromised and shock and acidosis quickly ensue. Death follows rapidly, often within hours. The use of prostaglandin E_1 infusion maintains ductal patency, restores systemic blood flow (at the expense of some systemic desaturation), and allows reversal of acidosis and end-organ dysfunction prior to palliation by surgery or catheter intervention techniques.

A third mechanism of infant heart failure is left heart inflow obstruction. When occurring as an isolated lesion (e.g., pulmonary vein stenosis, cor triatriatum, supravalvar mitral ring), presentation is with severe pulmonary edema. When left heart inflow obstruction occurs in the setting of intracardiac mixing or obstruction to pulmonary blood flow, pulmonary edema is associated with severe cyanosis. The most common cause of left heart inflow obstruction is pulmonary venous obstruction associated with total anomalous pulmonary venous return. This may occur either as an isolated lesion or in conjunction with complex congenital heart disease in the heterotaxy syndromes. Presentation usually occurs in the neonatal period and manifests as severe congestive lung disease with cyanosis and respiratory failure. Chest radiography shows severe pulmonary edema often with bilateral "white-out." The diagnosis may be missed and the infant's condition mistakenly attributed to severe neonatal parenchymal lung disease. The anomalous pulmonary venous return can be diagnosed by echocardiography, with exclusive right-to-left shunting at the foramen ovale being an important clue to the diagnosis. Most often, obstruction occurs when the pulmonary venous confluence drains inferiorly to the systemic or portal veins below the diaphragm. Treatment is urgent and comprises surgical anastomosis of the confluence to the left atrium with ligation of the descending vertical vein.

Large arteriovenous malformations (AVMs) most often present with high-output biventricular failure in the neonate. The commonest lesions are vein of Galen aneurysms and large hemangiomas (frequently hepatic). Neonates with vein of Galen aneurysms are often profoundly ill and may have associated pulmonary hypertension, the mechanism of which is poorly understood. These patients often succumb rapidly to severe cardiac failure. The remainder of infants with large AVMs often manifest tachycardia, warm skin, and a widened pulse pressure with bounding pulses. Coil embolization has been utilized in select cases with resolution of heart failure.

Arrhythmia

The role of arrhythmia in causing pediatric heart failure is primarily constrained to neonates, infants, and young children. Incessant tachycardia results in diminished ventricular function and low cardiac output. In infants, unrecognized and sustained reentrant (accessory pathway mediated) tachycardia is most often implicated, with ectopic atrial tachycardias a more common cause in children. Infants often present with poor feeding and irritability. Ventricular dysfunction may be so severe as to cause hypotension or cardiovascular collapse. The differential diagnosis is that of dilated cardiomyopathy with secondary arrhythmia.

Acute Heart Failure Syndromes Therapies

Many of the principles of acute heart failure therapy are the same in the neonatal and pediatric populations as in the adult. However, because of the differing physiologies, varying etiologies, and limitations imposed by the size of the smallest patients, some adaptations are required while other therapies are not appropriate. The critically ill patient who presents on the verge of hemodynamic collapse requires aggressive therapy to augment oxygen delivery while minimizing consumption. As in adults, intubation with mechanical ventilation and sedation (± paralysis) is useful to eliminate the work of breathing while improving pulmonary edema as a result of positive pressure ventilation. Placement of central venous and arterial monitoring lines is also facilitated by these maneuvers. Although subclavian and jugular venous lines are placed, femoral lines are perhaps more common in infants and young children due to the technical ease of placement. In addition to being able to administer medications, these lines allow for monitoring of central venous pressure and arterial blood pressure. They also serve to limit the need for repeated phlebotomy in infants and young children, in whom patient fear, agitation, and site availability are complicating issues. The use of pulmonary arterial catheters is less common in the pediatric age group.

Intravenous diuretics are used to augment diuresis and improve congestive symptoms. Continuous infusions of furosemide have been used with success in pediatric patients when intermittent dosing has failed to result in adequate diuresis. Inotropes are used to augment cardiac function and output. Therapy often consists of low to moderate doses (2 to 5 μg/kg/min) of dopamine for renal perfusion and blood pressure support and milrinone (0.125 to 1 μg/kg/min) to diminish afterload and augment cardiac output. Augmented inotropy can be achieved with dobutamine (1 to 10 μg/kg/min), while further afterload reduction may be achieved with sodium nitroprusside (0.3 to 4 μg/kg/min), if blood pressure tolerates. In contrast to adults, nitroglycerine is uncommonly utilized in pediatrics. Rarely do patients require support with infusions of high doses of epinephrine or norepinephrine. In these cases (except when pathology is believed to be rapidly reversible), serious consideration should be given to early institution of mechanical circulatory support (see below). Caution must also be taken with regard to the arrhythmogenic potential of all inotropes, particularly with escalating doses. Appropriate monitoring is essential and care must be taken to aggressively correct all electrolyte disturbances, particularly hypo/hyperkalemia and hypomagnesemia.

Only limited data exist regarding the use of nesiritide for the treatment of acute heart failure in the pediatric population. Our experience has primarily involved its use in children who were otherwise recalcitrant to diuretics (10). With appropriate monitoring of blood pressure and serum sodium, no complications were noted and some success was achieved in inducing diuresis. Others have reported use of nesiritide immediately after cardiac surgery, reporting no adverse hemodynamic effects or arrhythmias (11).

With stabilization and improvement in end-organ perfusion, gradual weaning of therapies is indicated. When oral medications can be safely tolerated and adequately absorbed, digoxin is often initiated, though of unproven benefit in pediatric patients. Intravenous diuretics are changed to oral forms, and angiotensin-converting enzyme (ACE) inhibitors are begun for afterload reduction while weaning milrinone.

When AHFSs are unresponsive to aggressive medical management, institution of mechanical circulatory support should be considered. Historically, extracorporeal membrane oxygenation (ECMO) has been the mainstay of mechanical circulatory support in infants and young children. Extensive experience with ECMO has been gained in pediatrics since its introduction as a rescue therapy for neonatal respiratory failure in the 1970s. In fact, the number of ECMO cannulations for cardiac indications in neonates and children in the United States is nearly 10-fold the number in adults (12). Extracorporeal membrane oxygenation has the ability to provide rapid hemodynamic stabilization, effective oxygenation, and removal of carbon dioxide in a wide range of patients, from neonates to adults. Cannulation may be achieved peripherally (usually from the neck) or centrally, depending on preexisting access and surgeon preference. Limitations include the need for continuous sedation, systemic anticoagulation, and external cannulation. These result in escalating risk of major complications including infection, bleeding, and thromboembolism (13). Survival after being placed onto ECMO for cardiac failure is exceedingly rare after 14 days. Extracorporeal membrane oxygenation is most appropriately used when recovery from severe cardiac failure is anticipated. Its usefulness as a bridge to transplantation is limited since in most centers the wait times for donor organs exceed the period for which the patient can be successfully sustained on ECMO. Nonetheless, when donor organs can be found, even the most critically sick children supported on ECMO can achieve successful long-term outcomes after transplantation (14).

The role of ventricular assist devices (VADs) in pediatrics continues to expand since the late 1980s, when they were first employed in adolescents and children. Most early pediatric experience in the U.S. was with externally driven centrifugal pumps. These have been used for univentricular or biventricular support in myocarditis or after congenital heart surgery (Norwood stage I, coronary translocations) (15). Since the mid-1990s, there has been growing experience with the use of long-term, pneumatically driven, pulsatile paracorporeal assist devices in children. The most widely available device in the U.S. is the Thoratec® (Pleasanton, CA) system. This device, designed for use in adults, has been used to support children as small as 25 kg. Similar pneumatic pulsatile devices, specifically designed for use in children and infants, have been developed in Europe (Berlin Heart®; Berlin, Germany, MEDOS® Stolberg, Germany). Utilization in the U.S. is currently limited by the Food and Drug Administration to compassionate care only. Because VAD placement is relatively more complex than ECMO, these devices are not considered appropriate as a bridge to recovery in neonates and infants who are anticipated to only require very short-term support (e.g., <7–10 days). The pulsatile, paracorporeal VADs offer distinct advantages over centrifugal pumps and ECMO, allowing the patient to awaken, extubate, ambulate, and even be discharged from the hospital while awaiting transplantation. Fully implantable VADs, including axial-type left-ventricular assist devices, are not available for use in infants and small children at this time. Although most VADs used in children were developed for adult use, a recent multicenter review of North American pediatric VAD experience has shown excellent results with 77% of children successfully bridged to transplant and 5% bridged to recovery. This is superior to the results in most adult programs (16).

Despite the vast experience with intraaortic balloon pumps (IABP) as a means of circulatory support in adults, use in the treatment of severe heart failure in children is rare. Much of the limitation extends from the relatively large size of sheaths required for percutaneous access and the difficulties encountered in synchronizing balloon timing with the faster heart rates of children. Relatively greater aortic compliance in children has also been thought to limit the effectiveness of this therapy. Finally, whereas IABP has proven effective in the setting of left-ventricular dysfunction from ischemia, most pediatric cardiac dysfunction does not result from underlying ischemic disease.

Prognosis

Prognosis is pediatric AHFS is dependent on the underlying pathophysiology, severity of illness at presentation, success of medical management, and potential for definitive surgical or catheterization-based intervention. When recovery is not achieved, mechanical support may be highly effective as a bridge to recovery or transplantation.

Clinical Case

A 5-day-old boy presented with a 1- to 2-day history of fussiness, decreased breast-feeding, and fever. Evaluation revealed rectal temperature of 38.6°C, heart rate 150 bpm, respiratory rate 46, and blood pressure 76/50 mm Hg. The infant appeared well, had clear lung fields, a 2/6 ejection systolic murmur at the left sternal border, no hepatomegaly, and normal brachial and femoral pulses. Evaluation for sepsis was undertaken (including blood, urine, and cerebrospinal fluid [CSF] cultures), and antibiotics were initiated empirically. Echocardiogram for evaluation of the murmur was normal. The child continued to have intermittent fevers for the next 5 days. On the 4th hospital day, the child experienced intermittent episodes of regular, narrow complex tachycardia at 250 bpm and poor oral intake. Repeat echocardiogram showed an ejection fraction (EF) of 40%, severe left ventricular (LV) posterior wall dyskinesis, moderate mitral valve insufficiency, and a small pericardial effusion. However, there was minimal left ventricular and left atrial dilatation. Troponin I was 9.9 ng/mL (normal ≤0.1 ng/mL). Milrinone infusion was begun, and transfer to the tertiary care center was arranged. The patient was also treated with intravenous immune globulin for possible diagnosis of acute myocarditis. Upon transfer, the heart rate was 180, respiratory rate 70, and blood pressure 50/30 mm Hg. There were diffusely poor pulses, poor perfusion, increased work of breathing, a 2/6 blowing pansystolic murmur at the apex, a gallop rhythm, and moderate hepatomegaly. The ECG showed sinus tachycardia, diffusely low voltages, and ST segment depression in leads V_1 and V_2.

How Should This Child Be Managed?

The clinical picture is that of rapidly progressive myocardial dysfunction in a neonate. The associated troponin elevation, regional wall motion abnormality, and ECG findings suggest myocardial ischemia or infarction. Acute viral myocarditis fits the clinical picture best, but congenital coronary anomalies, such as anomalous coronary artery from the left pulmonary artery, must be considered. Thus the patient underwent aortic root angiography, which showed normal coronary origins with antegrade flow in the LCA, ruling out this diagnosis. The regional wall motion abnormalities do not preclude a diagnosis of myocarditis, which may be associated with focal myocardial infarction. Congenital cardiomyopathy is less likely due to the preserved systolic function on the initial echocardiogram and diffusely small voltages on ECG. Based on the clinical picture, a tentative diagnosis of myocarditis was made and the potential for rapid deterioration was anticipated.

Further Course of the Illness

Over the next 24 hours progressive deterioration occurred, culminating in need for support with ECMO. After institution of mechanical support, chest radiograph and echocardiography revealed persistent pulmonary edema, evidence of minimal flow across the aortic valve, and a hypertensive left atrium. Balloon atrial septostomy was performed to decompress the left atrium, thereby relieving pulmonary edema and minimizing left ventricular wall stress. Viral cultures from the referring hospital became positive for enterovirus, adding further support to the diagnosis of acute myocarditis. The infant was successfully removed from ECMO on the 10th day of mechanical support. Follow-up echocardiography showed progressive improvement in systolic function but continued LV posterior wall thinning and dyskinesia with mild mitral regurgitation. The patient was transitioned to oral therapy with furosemide, enalapril, and carvedilol. Discharge occurred at 5 weeks of life. This case demonstrates one of the commoner causes of AHFS in childhood. Acute myocarditis frequently has a fulminant course in the very young, but recovery is common with excellent long-term survival without transplantation, providing the child's circulation can be successfully supported until spontaneous recovery occurs (17).

References

1. Recognition of respiratory failure and shock. In: Chameides L, Hazinski MF, eds. Pediatric Advanced Life Support. Dallas: American Heart Association, 1997:2-1-2-8.
2. Fisher DJ. Basic science of cardiovascular development. In: Garson A, Bricker JT, Fisher DJ, Neish SR, eds. The Science and Practice of Pediatric Cardiology. Baltimore: Williams and Wilkins, 1998:201–9.
3. Ralphe JC. Pathophysiology of chronic myocardial dysfunction. In: Slonim AD, Pollack MM, eds. Pediatric Critical Care Medicine. Baltimore: Lippincott Williams & Wilkins, 2006:230–4.
4. Webber SA, Boyle GJ, Jaffe R, et al. Role of right ventricular endomyocardial biopsy in infants and children with suspected or possible myocarditis. Br Heart J 1994;72:360–3.
5. Martin AB, Webber S, Fricker FJ, et al. Acute myocarditis. Rapid diagnosis by PCR in children. Circulation 1994;90:330–9.
6. Pophal SG, Sigfusson G, Booth KL, et al. Complications of endomyocardial biopsy in children. J Am Coll Cardiol 1999;34:2105–10.
7. Lipshultz SE, Sleeper LA, Towbin JA, et al. The incidence of pediatric cardiomyopathies in two regions of the United States. N Engl J Med 2003;348:1647–55.
8. Nugent AW, Daubeney PE, Chondros P, et al. The epidemiology of childhood cardiomyopathy in Australia. N Engl J Med 2003;348:1639–46.
9. Feingold B, Munoz R, Gandhi SK. Normal ventricular function six days after repair of anomalous left coronary artery. Int J Cardiol 2006;108:393–4.
10. Feingold B, Law YM. Nesiritide use in pediatric patients with congestive heart failure. J Heart Lung Transplant 2004;23:1455–9.
11. Simsic JM, Scheurer M, Tobias JD, et al. Perioperative effects and safety of nesiritide following cardiac surgery in children. J Intensive Care Med 2006;21:22–6.
12. ECMO Registry of the Extracorporeal Life Support Organization (ELSO), Ann Arbor, Michigan, July, 2004.
13. Kulik TJ, Moler FW, Palmisano JM. Outcome-associated factors in pediatric patients treated with extracorporeal membrane oxygenator after cardiac surgery. Circulation 1996;94(9 suppl):II63–8.
14. Gajarski RJ, Mosca RS, Ohye RG, et al. Use of extracorporeal life support as a bridge to pediatric cardiac transplantation. J Heart Lung Transplant 2003;22:28–34.
15. Karl TR. Sano S. Horton S. Centrifugal pump left heart assist in pediatric cardiac operations. Indication, technique, and results. J Thorc Cardiovasc Surg 1991;102:624–30.
16. Blume ED, Naftel DC, Bastardi HJ, Duncan BW, Kirklin JK, Webber SA. Pediatric Heart Transplant Study Investigators. Outcomes of children bridged to heart transplantation with ventricular assist devices: a multi-institutional study. Circulation 2006;113:2313–9.
17. English RF, Janosky JE, Ettedgui JA, Webber SA. Outcomes for children with acute myocarditis. Cardiology in the Young 2004;14:488–93.

2
Diagnostic and Therapeutic Management of Severe Acute Heart Failure Syndromes

2.1
Procedures and Technology

35
Esophageal Doppler: Noninvasive Estimation of Stroke Volume

Bernard P. Cholley

Hemodynamic monitoring is central to intensive care as well as perioperative patient management. For anesthesiologists and intensivists, it is crucial to maintain adequate organ perfusion throughout the body during the time course of critical illness or surgery. Adequate organ perfusion implies (1) a perfusion pressure that is high enough to maintain capillary patency within all organs, and (2) enough flow to deliver oxygen and substrates and to remove carbon dioxide (CO_2) and other metabolic by-products. But in many instances, the only aspect of perfusion that is carefully monitored is pressure, whereas flow is simply ignored. One of the reasons for this may be related to the difficulties encountered in obtaining flow measurements. Esophageal Doppler is one of the alternative devices that facilitate flow measurement by avoiding the placement of a pulmonary artery catheter.

This chapter discusses the principle of stroke volume estimation using esophageal Doppler, as well as the validation and the limitations of the technique.

Principles

The esophageal Doppler technique is based on the measurement of blood flow velocity in the descending aorta by means of a Doppler transducer placed at the tip of a flexible probe. This transducer can be 4-MHz continuous wave (CardioQ®, Deltex; Waki®, Atys medical, Montpellier, France; Arrow, Reading, PA, USA; Deltex, West Sussex, UK), or 5-MHz pulsed-wave (HemoSonic®, Arrow). The probe is either disposable (Deltex) or reusable (Atys Medical and Arrow) and can be introduced orally in anesthetized, mechanically ventilated patients. Following oral introduction, the probe is advanced until its tip is located approximately at the mid-thoracic level, and then rotated so that the transducer faces the aorta and a characteristic aortic velocity signal is obtained (Fig. 35.1). A new generation of probes from Deltex is now available for "awake" patients and requires nasal introduction. However, in our experience it is best to place the probe while the patient is anesthetized and to leave it after recovery and extubation. Probe position is optimized by slow rotation in the long axis (Fig. 35.2) and alteration of the depth of insertion to generate a clear signal with the highest possible peak velocity (Fig. 35.3). Gain setting is adjusted to optimize signal to noise ratio (Fig. 35.4).

The measurement of instantaneous blood flow velocity in the descending aorta enables computing the velocity–time integral representing the stroke distance (i.e., progression of the column of blood in the descending aorta)[1]. Several assumptions are required to transpose stroke distance into systemic stroke volume: (1) an accurate measurement of descending aortic blood flow velocity; (2) a "flat" velocity profile throughout descending aorta; (3) a constant aortic cross-sectional area during systole; (4) a negligible diastolic flow; and (5) a constant division of blood flow between the descending aorta and the brachiocephalic and coronary arteries (Fig. 35.5).

The accuracy of velocity measurement requires a good alignment between the Doppler beam and blood flow and knowledge of the angle at which

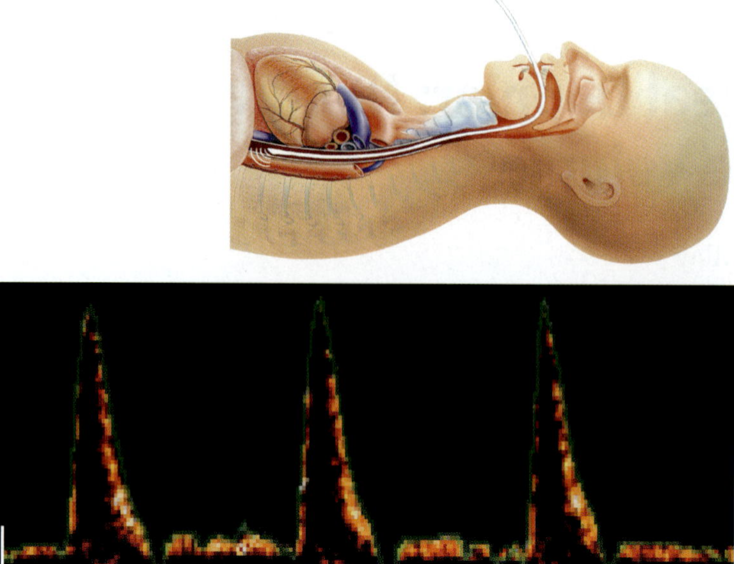

FIGURE 35.1. Top: Schematic representation of esophageal Doppler probe in a patient demonstrating the close relation between esophagus and descending thoracic aorta. Bottom: Characteristic velocity waveform obtained in the descending aorta. The spectral representation shows that most red blood cells (orange-white color) are moving at the maximum velocity (close to the green envelope) during systole, and that diastolic flow is minimal. (From Cholley and Singer[1], with permission.)

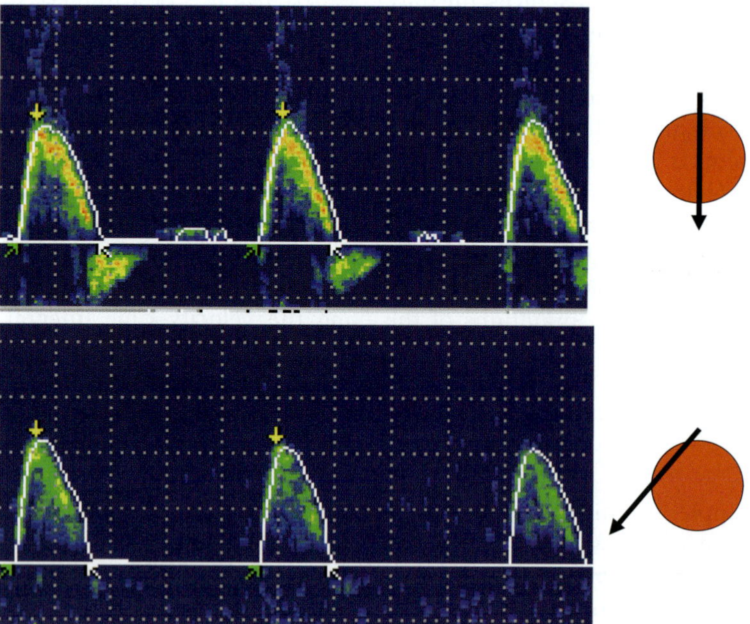

FIGURE 35.2. Probe rotation enables locating the position where the ultrasound beam faces the aorta, corresponding to the brightest spectral representation of aortic flow velocity (upper panel). In contrast, when the ultrasound beam is not facing the aorta, the signal is faint and poorly defined (lower panel).

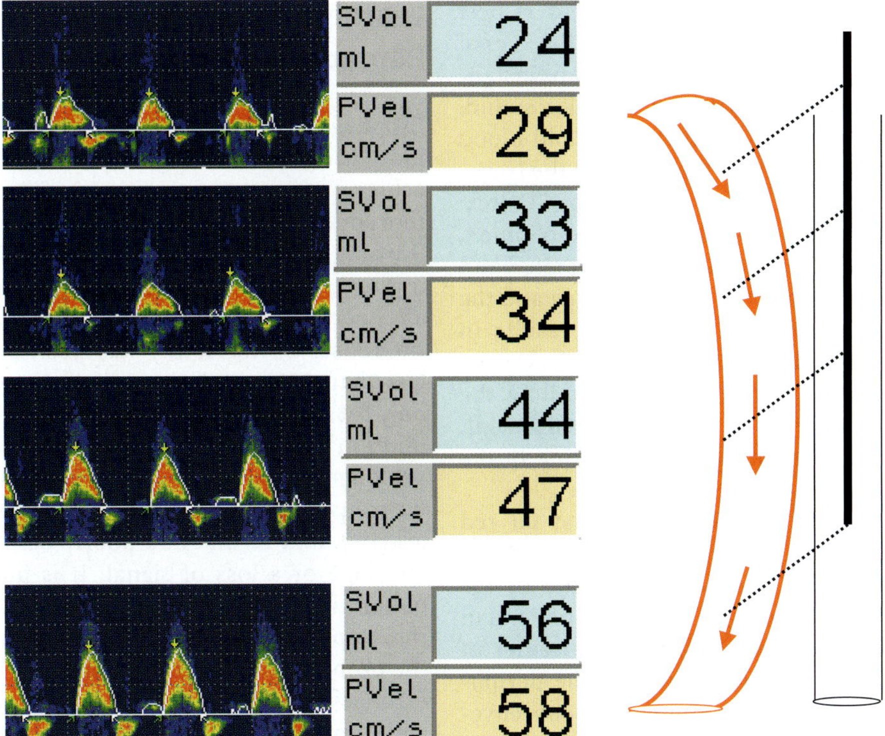

FIGURE 35.3 Changing the depth of insertion of the probe may result in striking differences in velocity measurement and stroke volume estimation when the esophagus and aorta are not parallel in the thorax, as illustrated here. The schematic representation depicts the decreasing angle between ultrasound beam (dotted line) and aortic blood flow (arrows) as the transducer is advanced down in the esophagus. The smallest angle (at the bottom of the picture) yields the highest peak velocity (PVel, cm/s) and the largest stroke volume (SVol, ml), due to the influence of the cosine in the Doppler equation. This corresponds to the best placement of the probe because this position can easily be reproduced.

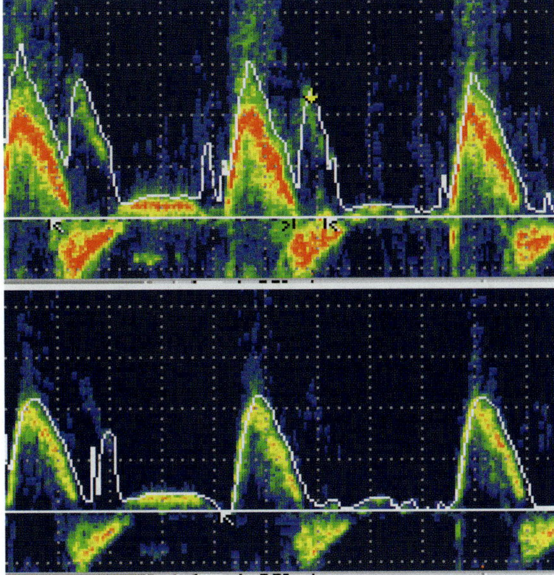

FIGURE 35.4. Gain should be adjusted to obtain a good signal-to-noise ratio. The upper panel demonstrates an excess of gain, while gain setting is correct in the lower panel.

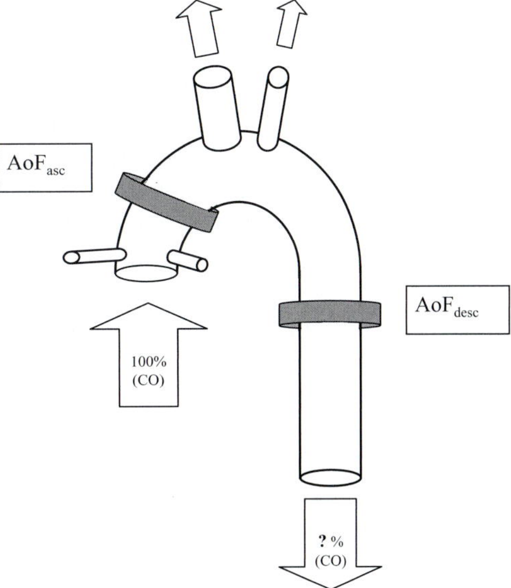

FIGURE 35.5. Experimental setup used to study the proportion of systemic cardiac output (CO) between supraaortic vessels (AoF_{asc})and the descending aorta (AoF_{desc})in sheep. (From Dumans-Nizard[3], with permission.)

the blood flow is insonated. Alignment is best assessed subjectively by optimizing the signal quality with the aid of the visual display of instantaneous velocity waveform and Doppler sound. The angle between the Doppler beam and blood flow is roughly the same as that between the transducer and the probe (45 degrees [CardioQ, Deltex; Waki, Atys Medical] or 60 degrees [HemoSonic®, Arrow]). Any discrepancy between estimated and real angles, for example, if the esophagus and the aorta are not parallel in the thorax, results in errors in calculated blood velocity. The larger the angle between Doppler beam and blood flow, the greater the inaccuracy in velocity measurement, as a consequence of inappropriate cosine in the Doppler equation.

A "flat" velocity profile implies that all red blood cells move at the same speed through the vessel. In fact, the flow velocity profile in the descending thoracic aorta is more parabolic than flat[2], that is, the red blood cells at the center of the vessel move faster than those at the periphery. Hence, use of the maximum velocity envelope to compute stroke distance may result in overestimation of stroke volume. The cross-sectional area of the descending aorta is required to convert stroke distance into stroke volume, but its measurement cannot be obtained routinely at bedside. The manufacturers of esophageal Doppler have solved this problem in two different ways: HemoSonic has an M-mode echo transducer into the probe to measure instantaneous aortic diameter, while CardioQ and Waki provide a nomogram to estimate the cross-sectional area of the descending aorta based on patient's age, weight, and height. Systematic errors due to a discrepancy between the actual area and the nomogram value do not affect the trend of cardiac output variation with time. However, a large variation in cardiac output can be underestimated by not taking into account the concomitant change in aortic diameter, which is necessarily in the same direction. Finally, to provide systemic cardiac output, esophageal monitors multiply descending aortic blood flow by a correcting factor assuming a constant partition of blood between supra-aortic vessels and the descending aorta. The robustness of this assumption was suggested by validation studies and was confirmed experimentally in an hemorrhagic shock model[3].

Learning Curve and Reproducibility

Esophageal Doppler is a simple technique, and most users acknowledge that it is fairly easy to achieve adequate probe positioning and obtain reproducible results[4,5]. Authors studying the learning curve of the technique noted a dramatic improvement in the skills of untrained operators after performing only 10 or 12 probe placements[6,7]. Interobserver variability has been shown to be less than 10%, while intraobserver variability is only 8%, a figure that is closer to 12% for thermodilution[4,8–10]. Probe displacement can occur during prolonged monitoring as a consequence of various causes (e.g., nursing procedures, deglutition, gravity), and results in a poorly defined velocity envelope or a loss of signal. It is mandatory to obtain the best possible signal prior to interpreting Doppler-derived data. Failure to reposition the probe prior to each measurement may lead to erroneous cardiac output values and variation with time.

Validation of Cardiac Output Measurement Using Esophageal Doppler

"Gold standard" techniques for cardiac output measurement, such as aortic electromagnetic or ultrasound transit time flowmeters, are highly invasive and cannot be used routinely in patients. The widespread use of thermodilution in intensive care units has made it a "reference" technique, despite its well-known pitfalls[11]. A meta-analysis by Dark and Singer[12] recently reviewed all validation studies for esophageal Doppler. The CardioQ was the most widely investigated (11 studies), while only two studies reviewed the Hemosonic. The authors concluded that the CardioQ estimates absolute cardiac output values with minimal bias but with limited clinical agreement due to the lack of accuracy of both Doppler and thermodilution. More importantly, they found that this monitor had a high validity (no bias and high clinical agreement) for monitoring changes in cardiac output in critically ill patients.

Limitations of the Technique

Beside the limitations inherent to the various assumptions used by esophageal Doppler monitors to compute stroke volume from descending aortic velocity measurements, there are a number of situations in which this technique cannot be used. Esophageal disease (e.g., diverticulum, cancer, recent variceal bleeding) and recent surgery are contraindications. In addition, the monitor cannot provide reliable estimations of stroke volume in patients with dissection of the descending aorta because flow is no longer laminar in the true lumen. Aortic clamping suppresses flow in the descending aorta and prevents stroke volume estimation. However, esophageal Doppler is perfectly effective after the release of the aortic clamp, when hemodynamic alterations are the most dramatic. Finally, the technique should not be used when the operator cannot access the patient's head to reposition the probe. In other words, surgical settings where the anesthesiologist is away from the head (e.g., neurosurgery; ear, nose, and throat; cervical spine surgery) are not suitable for the use of this monitor.

Hemodynamic Optimization in High-Risk Surgical Patients

Esophageal Doppler can be used to titrate fluids (i.e., to conduct "hemodynamic optimization") in patients. By giving small fluid challenges while measuring the response in terms of stroke volume, it is easy to maximize stroke volume without the risk of volume overload (Fig. 35.6). Failure to

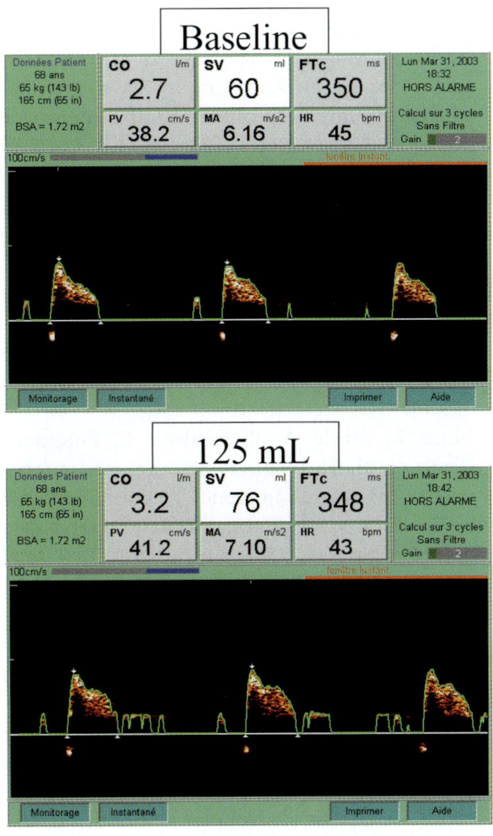

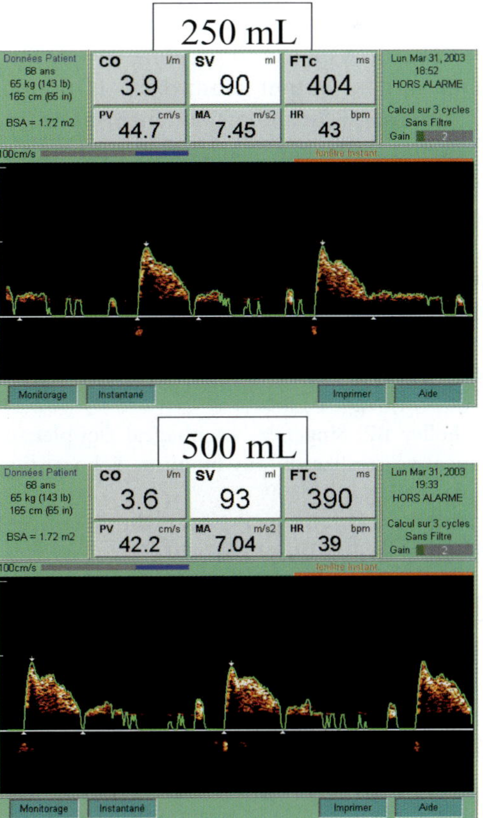

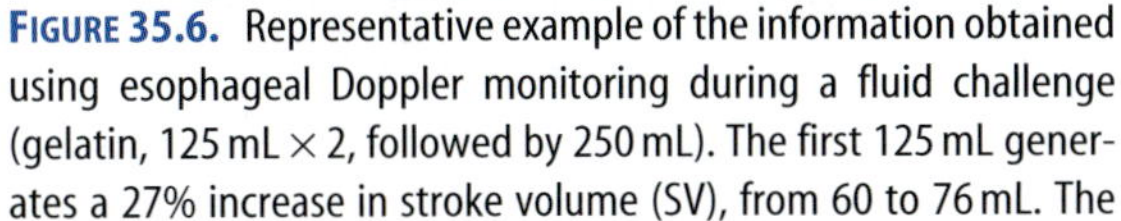

FIGURE 35.6. Representative example of the information obtained using esophageal Doppler monitoring during a fluid challenge (gelatin, 125 mL × 2, followed by 250 mL). The first 125 mL generates a 27% increase in stroke volume (SV), from 60 to 76 mL. The second 125 mL results in 18% increase (from 76 to 90 mL), while the last 250 mL does not produce any change in stroke volume (90 and 93 mL, respectively), indicating that the plateau of the cardiac function curve has been reached.

increase cardiac output after a fluid challenge indicates that the patient operates on the flat portion of the cardiac function curve and that further loading might result in venous congestion and not in perfusion improvement. This strategy has proven beneficial in several randomized studies involving limited numbers of high-risk surgical patients[13–17]. It is remarkable that a resuscitation strategy based on the use of a monitoring device leads to a reduction in postoperative morbidity and hospital length of stay. However, a large-scale, multicenter randomized trial remains desirable to confirm that esophageal Doppler-guided fluid resuscitation can effectively improve outcome in this setting. In ventilated intensive care unit patients, esophageal Doppler could be a useful help to conduct early goal-directed therapy and to monitor cardiovascular alterations. Indeed, since flow is less narrowly regulated than systemic arterial pressure, stroke volume will be affected prior to pressure, and therapeutic interventions elicited by flow reduction will certainly be earlier than those in response to pressure drops. Stroke volume/cardiac output monitoring is undoubtedly very useful for the management of critically ill patients, especially variations with patient's illness or resulting from therapeutic interventions. Esophageal Doppler offers the advantages of being poorly invasive in sedated patients, requiring minimal training to obtain data, and providing "beat-by-beat" monitoring.

References

1. Cholley BP, Singer M. Esophageal Doppler: noninvasive cardiac output monitor. Echocardiography 2003;20(8):763–9.
2. Farthing S, Peronneau P. Flow in the thoracic aorta. Cardiovasc Res 1979;13:607–20.
3. Dumans-Nizard V, Nizard J, Payen D, Cholley BP. Redistribution of cardiac output during hemorrhagic shock in sheep. Crit Care Med 2006;34(4):1147–51.
4. Singer M, Clarke J, Bennett ED. Continuous hemodynamic monitoring by esophageal Doppler. Crit Care Med 1989;17(5):447–52.
5. Gan TJ, Arrowsmith JE. The esophageal Doppler monitor: a safe means of monitoring the circulation. BMJ 1997;315:893–4.
6. Freund PR. Transesophageal Doppler scanning versus thermodilution during general anesthesia. An initial comparison of cardiac output techniques. Am J Surg 1987;153(5):490–4.
7. Lefrant JY, Bruelle P, Aya AG, et al. Training is required to improve the reliability of esophageal Doppler to measure cardiac output in critically ill patients. Intensive Care Med 1998;24:347–52.
8. Lavandier B, Cathignol D, Muchada R, Bui Xuan B, Motin J. Noninvasive aortic blood flow measurement using an intraesophageal probe. Ultrasound Med Biol 1985;11(3):451–60.
9. Mark JB, Steinbrook RA, Gugino LD, et al. Continuous noninvasive monitoring of cardiac output with esophageal Doppler ultrasound during cardiac surgery. Anesth Analg 1986;65:1013–20.
10. Valtier B, Cholley BP, Belot J-P, de la Coussaye J-E, Mateo J, Payen D. Noninvasive monitoring of cardiac output in critically ill patients using transesophageal Doppler. Am J Respir Crit Care Med 1998;158:77–83.
11. Cholley BP. Benefits, risks and alternatives of pulmonary artery catheterization. Curr Opin Anaesthesiol 1998;11:645–50.
12. Dark PM, Singer M. The validity of trans-esophageal Doppler ultrasonography as a measure of cardiac output in critically ill adults. Intensive Care Med 2004;30(11):2060–6.
13. Mythen MG, Webb AR. Perioperative plasma volume expansion reduces the incidence of gut mucosal hypoperfusion during cardiac surgery. Arch Surg 1995;130:423–9.
14. Sinclair S, James S, Singer M. Intraoperative intravascular volume optimisation and length of hospital stay after repair of proximal femoral fracture: randomized controlled trial. BMJ 1997; 315:909–12.
15. Venn R, Steele A, Richardson P, Poloniecki J, Grounds M, Newman P. Randomized controlled trial to investigate influence of the fluid challenge on duration of hospital stay and perioperative morbidity in patients with hip fractures. Br J Anaesth 2002;88:65–71.
16. Gan TJ, Soppitt A, Maroof M et al. Goal-directed intraoperative fluid administration reduces length of hospital stay after major surgery. Anesthesiology 2002;97(4):820–6.
17. Conway DH, Mayall R, Abdul-Latif MS, Gilligan S, Tackaberry C. Randomised controlled trial investigating the influence of intravenous fluid titration using oesophageal Doppler monitoring during bowel surgery. Anaesthesia 2002;57(9):845–9.

36 Minimally Invasive Cardiac Output Monitoring: Pulse Contour and Pulse Power Analysis

Andrew Tillyard and Andrew Rhodes

In every area of medicine, adequate perfusion is vital to organ function and life. Tissue oxygen perfusion is dependent on two factors: cardiac output (CO) and blood oxygen content. The oxygen content is easily measured with an arterial blood gas analyzer. Cardiac output, though, is less easily measured. We still lack a universally accepted, reproducible, 100% specific and sensitive means of CO measurement despite CO monitoring in the intensive therapy unit (ITU) being a routine element of critical care provision. The clinical importance of CO assessment was emphasized by Schoemaker (1), who noted that the cardiac index (CO proportional to body mass) and oxygen delivery index (DO_2I) of patients who survived the ITU were consistently higher than for nonsurvivors. This led to the therapeutic aim of achieving supranormal CO and DO_2I values in a variety of patient populations. By the early 1990s it was realized that this one-size-fits-all approach to CO manipulation did not produce consistently improved outcomes. We now realize that CO monitoring and manipulation need to be individualized for the patient.

Until very recently, if a patient's CO needed to be established, then a pulmonary artery catheter (PAC) was required, because the ability to estimate CO based on the clinical examination and institute appropriate therapy has been questioned. The PAC is the current gold standard of CO monitoring. However, with advances in medical technology, less invasive methods of CO assessment have been developed, in an attempt to reduce iatrogenic complications and improve the ease of CO monitoring. These include techniques based on pulse contour analysis and the pulse power analysis.

This chapter describes the impetus behind the development of these two newer modes of CO measurement and summarizes their efficacy. Perhaps more importantly, this chapter emphasizes the significance of establishing the adequacy of the measured CO for the individual patient. This last point introduces an essential concept: the CO can be measured in a number of ways, none of which may be 100% accurate. But clinicians must ask themselves, Is the measured CO adequate for the patient?

The Drive to Less Invasive Cardiac Output Assessment

Clinical Assessment of Cardiac Output

As the CO falls, autoregulatory mechanisms divert blood flow from the periphery to more vital organs, namely, the brain, heart, kidneys, and gastrointestinal tract. The peripheries become cool as they become poorly perfused. If the CO continues to fall, the perfusion of the vital organs is also reduced. These changes can occur in high CO states as well, such as sepsis where the CO may be normal or high, but autoregulatory mechanisms fail to maintain adequate vital organ perfusion. The effects of an inadequate CO for the body's demands can be reflected by cool peripheries, tachycardia, a variable blood pressure, oliguria, and impaired cerebration. Biochemically, a low CO can also be inferred from a rising lactate, creatinine, and urea, and a low central venous oxygen saturation.

However, the evidence to suggest that this information is sufficient to accurately estimate CO clinically and titrate vasoactive drugs is limited and contradictory. Clinical assessment is vital, though, to prompt the physician to more accurately determine the CO as soon as possible. The work of Rivers et al. (2) confirms that the earlier correction of hemodynamic variables leads to an improved outcome. For many years, the PAC has been the sole means of continuous CO assessment.

The Pulmonary Artery Catheter and Less Invasive Technologies

The PAC is the gold standard of clinical CO monitoring. Numerous authors argue, though, that there is no gold standard of CO assessment because of the many confounding factors that exist with the PAC. The best estimate of CO using the PAC requires three or four cold-dilution measurements, spread equally over the respiratory cycle (3). This is a highly operator dependent technique that has been shown to still have a variability of calculated CO of up to 13% (4).

Despite this, all the recent, less invasive modes of CO assessment have been compared to the PAC and are deemed accurate if they have good reproducibility and are within 10% of the PAC estimate of CO. This means there is the potential for the measured CO to over- or underestimate the true CO by up to 25% or more. It must also be remembered that not all of the newer CO monitors have been compared to the triplicate cold bolus CO method of assessment, which is accepted to be the true gold standard. This serves to highlight the importance of the following:

1. Treating the patient as a whole and not as an isolated number
2. Looking at the trend—the change in the measured CO over time
3. Assessing the change in CO in response to treatment

Because of various limitations with the PAC and a suggestion that the PAC may be associated with an increased mortality, there was an impetus to find less invasive ways to estimate CO without loss of accuracy. The term *noninvasive* in this context does not refer to purely extravascular devices. It refers to monitors that do not require pulmonary artery catheterization for their operation. Thus the devices still require an arterial line and often still require a central line and are perhaps more accurately referred to as minimally invasive devices.

Minimally Invasive Monitors

The three minimally invasive techniques discussed in this chapter are the LiDCO-Plus System (LiDCO, Cambridge, United Kingdom), the PiCCO-Plus monitor (Pulsion, Munich, Germany), and the Vigileo monitor (Edwards Lifesciences, Irvine, CA). The PiCCO-Plus uses pulse contour analysis, the LiDCO-Plus uses pulse power analysis, and the Vigileo analyzes the standard deviation of the mean arterial pressure (MAP) (Table 36.1).

Table 36.1. Characteristics of the three minimally invasive techniques

	LiDCO-Plus	PiCCO-Plus	Vigileo
Setup time	Moderate	Moderate	Minimal
Ease of setup	Moderate	Moderate	Simple
Manual calibration	Necessary	Necessary	Not required
Access	Arterial only	Arterial + venous	Arterial only
Clinical accuracy	Established	Established	Awaited
Clinical efficacy	Established	Established	Awaited
Data recorded	CO, SV, SVV, SVR, DO2I	CO, SV, SVV, CFI, EVLW, GEDV	CO, SVR, SvO2, SV, SVV

CFI, cardiac function index; CO, cardiac output; DO_2I; oxygen delivery; EVLW, extravascular lung water; GEDV, global end-diastolic volume; SV, stroke volume; SvO_2, mixed venous oxygen saturation; SVR, systemic vascular resistance; SVV, stroke volume variation.

All three systems analyze the arterial pressure waveform to establish a stroke volume. This is then multiplied by the heart rate to calculate CO. Akin to the strength of the pulse palpated during a cardiovascular examination, each system relies on the fact that the arterial waveform is dependent on the volume of blood ejected from the left ventricle. This pressure waveform can be converted to a volume waveform, which then enables the calculation of the stroke volume (SV) and CO.

The determination of the SV from the arterial waveform is based on the concept that beat-to-beat changes in pulse pressure (systolic pressure – diastolic pressure) around a mean value will be due to changes in the SV. A correction factor for the nonlinear compliance of the aorta is required so the pressure change in the arterial circulation can be linearly related to the ejected blood volume. This enables analysis and integration of a linear arterial pressure waveform to produce an SV. The main difference among the three systems is the method used to analyze the waveform to convert it into an SV and the mechanism of correcting for individual differences in aortic compliance. The compliance of the aorta is inversely and nonlinearly related to the MAP and reflected pressure waves from the periphery, both of which are further influenced by age, sex, height, and weight (5).

Each monitor has specific derived values of cardiac performance that are calculated and displayed. All monitors, however, provide continuous CO monitoring, SV and SV variation, heart rate, and systemic vascular resistance.

Pulse Contour Analysis

Arterial pulse contour analysis uses Wesseling et al.'s (6) Cz method of measuring the area under the systolic portion of the arterial pressure wave and dividing it by the aortic impedance to calculate the SV. However, the pulse pressure of an arterial trace is a complex summation of various factors. First, it is affected by the aortic impedance, which is nonlinearly related to the MAP, age, sex, height, and weight. Second, it is a combination of the pressure wave created by the ejected SV and the reflected pressure waves from the periphery. The two types of pressure waves are different in shape and timing. Pulse contour analysis is only interested in the pressure wave due to the SV. It analyzes the area under the systolic portion of the arterial waveform—the upstroke of the arterial waveform to the dicrotic notch (Fig. 36.1). It depends on the morphology of the waveform, so it needs to analyze a central arterial trace, because the precise detection of the dicrotic notch is essential and it is least affected centrally by changes due to reflected peripheral pressure waves. The PiCCO formula for CO calculation needs to take account of all these factors (7):

$$CO = \text{Cal} \times HR \times (P(t) + C_{(P)} \times \Delta P/\Delta t)\Delta t$$

where

$P(t)$ is the area under the systolic portion of the pressure wave (shaded blue in Fig. 36.1)
$C_{(P)}$ is the aortic compliance
$\Delta P/\Delta t$ is the shape of the arterial pressure curve
$HR \times (P(t) + C_{(P)} \times \Delta P/\Delta t)\ \Delta t$ is the pulse contour CO
$(P(t) + C_{(P)} \times \Delta P/\Delta t)\Delta t$ is the pulse contour SV or nominal SV, determined from the analysis of the arterial trace
Cal is the patient specific calibration factor determined by thermodilution, and is the ratio of the actual CO as determined by the thermodilution to the measured CO by the pulse contour

The latest software analyzes the shape of the diastolic portion of the pressure waveform, that is, that part of the waveform after the dicrotic notch, which is affected by the peripheral vascular resistance, so changes in arterial tone over time will be compensated for.

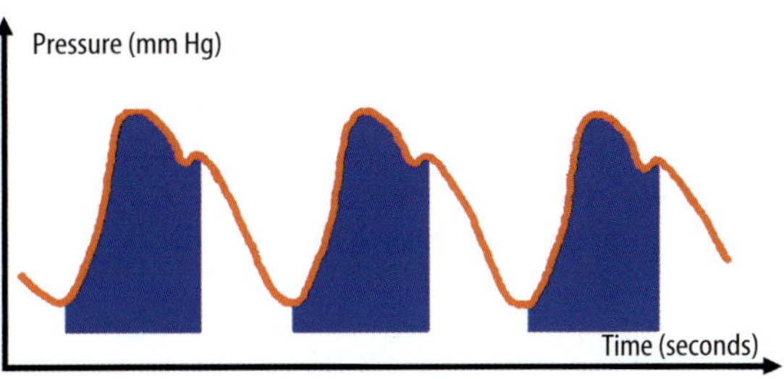

Figure 36.1. An arterial pressure trace with the systolic area under the curve analyzed by pulse contour analysis highlighted.

PiCCO-Plus: The Practical Method of Cardiac Output Calculation

A central venous injection of a known volume of ice-cold saline is injected into a central vein. This is detected by a thermistor in the product-specific arterial line that is placed in a central artery—preferably femoral or brachial. A transpulmonary thermodilution curve is created, using the modified Stewart-Hamilton equation, which calculates the area under the concentration-time curve. The area under the curve is inversely proportional to the CO. This establishes the actual CO and the actual SV.

The systolic portion of the arterial waveform is proportional to the volume of blood ejected from the left ventricle and is integrated to become the standardized or nominal SV. This is the SV that takes account of the nonlinear aortic compliance and the analysis and integration of the arterial pressure wave as described by the above formula. The calculation of the actual SV by the thermodilution allows a calibration factor to be derived by dividing the nominal SV by the calculated SV and adjusting for age, heart rate, and MAP. Each subsequent arterial waveform can then be integrated and multiplied by the calibration factor to achieve continuous CO measurement.

The transcardiopulmonary thermodilution method correlates well with the PAC thermodilution estimation for CO (8). It has also been shown to have excellent correlation reproducibility (9). Unlike the LiDCO-Plus, the PiCCO-Plus does require a central venous access and an arterial line that is specific for the PiCCO-Plus to be placed in a central artery.

Following acceptable calibration, the PiCCO-Plus provides continuous data regarding CO, arterial blood pressure, heart rate, SV, SV variation, and systemic vascular resistance. The transcardiopulmonary thermodilution allows several specific volumes to be estimated including intrathoracic blood volume, extravascular lung water, and cardiac function index. The last three parameters are unique to the PiCCO-Plus.

Intrathoracic Blood Volume

The thorax contains three fluid compartments: the intrathoracic blood volume, the intrathoracic gas volume, and extravascular lung water. The intrathoracic blood volume (ITBV) is composed of the pulmonary blood volume (20%), and the global end-diastolic volume (GEDV) of all four chambers of the heart (80%)(Fig. 36.2).

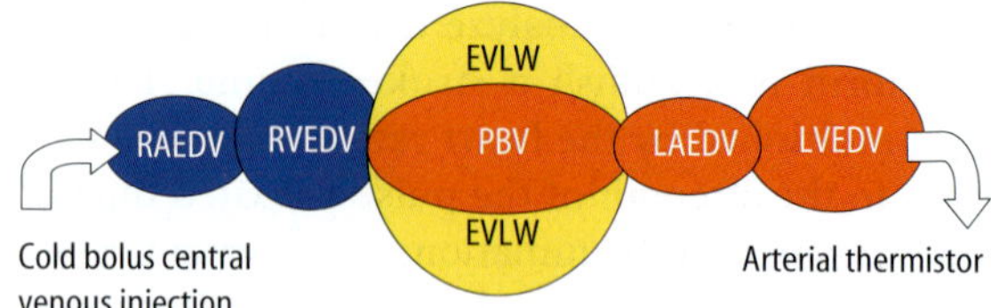

Figure 36.2. Intrathoracic volume compartments. Cold saline is injected centrally and the change in temperature is measured in the aorta by the arterial catheter after traversing the fluid compartments. RAEDV, right atrial end-diastolic volume; RVEDV, right ventricle end-diastolic volume; PBV, pulmonary blood volume; EVLW, extravascular lung water; LAEDV, left atrial end-diastolic volume; LVEDV, left ventricle end-diastolic volume.

Cold saline is injected via the central venous catheter. As it passes from the right atria to the aorta, the temperature is diluted by the surrounding fluid compartments that the saline passes through. The time taken to pass from the central vein to the aorta multiplied by the CO equates to the intrathoracic volume (ITV). The ITV consists of the extravascular lung water (EVLW) and the ITBV. The ITBV consists of the blood in the pulmonary vessels, the pulmonary blood volume (PBV), and the GEDV. There is a relatively constant relationship between the GEDV and the ITBV.

Global End-Diastolic Volume and Cardiac Function Index

The global end diastolic volume is equivalent to the preload of the four heart chambers: it is the sum of all the end-diastolic volumes of both atria and ventricles. It is determined by the PiCCO-Plus through the thermodilution technique as described above (10). Once this is calculated, the ejection fraction can be calculated by reference to the SV. This has been called the cardiac function index by the PiCCO-Plus.

A small CO with a large preload as determined by a high global end-diastolic volume may suggest volume overload or cardiomyopathy. Alternatively, a small CO with a small preload may indicate a restrictive myopathy or a hypovolemic patient. There is some evidence that the calculated cardiac function index correlates well with the transesophageal estimates of ejection fraction. If the cardiac function index is reduced, however, the PiCCO-Plus cannot determine if it is due to right or left ventricular impairment. But similar to the clinical suspicion of an inadequate CO prompting the clinician to use a CO monitor, a low cardiac function index should prompt the physician to consider investigating further with echocardiography.

Extravascular Lung Water

Extravascular lung water (EVLW) is the volume of fluid that is within the interstitium and alveoli. An approximate estimation of extravascular lung water can be made from the dilution of an indicator (such as the warming of a 20-mL cold saline bolus) between two points, which allows the calculation of the volume in between. As the cold saline traverses the pulmonary capillaries, heat energy is exchanged between the gaseous and liquid compartments. The extent of the heat exchange alters the slope of the temperature–time curve as measured at the arterial line. The area under the curve is inversely proportional to the CO as discussed. The shape and duration of the curve reflects the movement of thermal energy between the fluid compartments and has been validated as an accurate means of EVLW assessment (10).

In any acute lung injury, third spacing of fluid within the alveoli and pulmonary interstitium frequently occurs. This increase in extravascular lung water would be expected to be at the expense of the intrathoracic volume and gas exchange. The development of early pulmonary edema, with small changes in lung water, is often not detectable on a chest x-ray, or reflected in arterial blood gas analysis. Theoretically, the PiCCO-Plus may detect the development of pulmonary edema early as an increase from the initial EVLW measurement. There is some evidence to suggest that EVLW is more sensitive than chest x-rays or deterioration in oxygenation for detecting increasing pulmonary edema (11, 12). There is also some evidence that using EVLW to guide management improves morbidity and mortality (13). However, a patient with raised EVLW may still require fluid boluses rather than just diuretics due to the dynamic nature of fluid movement between the intra- and extravascular space in critically ill patients.

Sources of Error

The accuracy of the monitor is vitally dependent on the maintenance and correct use of the invasive arterial line and its transducer set. Arterial lines that are incorrectly zeroed or damped due to associated catheter site, transducer set, or pressure line problems can lead to incorrect CO values. The use of the PiCCO-Plus is contraindicated in patients who have restricted arterial access, either because of grafting of the femoral artery or an intraaortic balloon pump in situ. Patients who have intracardiac shunts, aortic aneurysms, aortic regurgitation, pneumonectomy, or who are receiving extracorporeal membrane oxygenation therapy would generate inaccurate thermodilution measurements.

The complications associated with the use of the PiCCO-Plus are related to those of cannulation of major arteries and veins. In the event of significant alterations in the patient's heart rate, arterial blood pressure, and vascular resistance, the pulse contour analysis has the potential to become unreliable. To overcome this problem, frequent recalibrations may be necessary to allow for changes in aortic impedance.

Pulse Power Analysis

Pulse power analysis addresses the entire area under the arterial waveform curve. Unlike the morphology-dependent algorithm utilized by pulse contour techniques, pulse power analysis is based on the physics of the conservation of mass and power. Each heartbeat produces a change in power (work done per unit time). This change is the balance between the input of mass (SV) minus the mass of blood lost to the periphery during the heartbeat. A linear relationship of net power change and flow can be created with a calibration factor, which takes into account the aortic compliance.

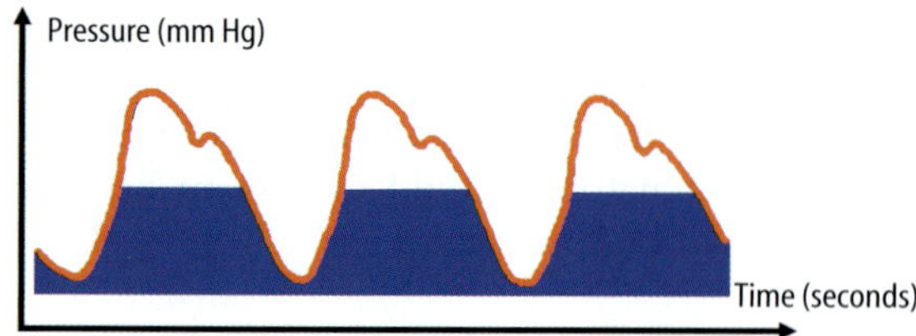

FIGURE 36.3. An arterial pressure trace with the area analyzed by pulse power analysis highlighted.

A benefit of pulse power analysis is that any arterial site can be used because it is not dependent on the dicrotic notch. The reflected peripheral waves are negated by analyzing the power of the entire waveform (Fig. 36.3).

LiDCO-Plus

The LiDCO-Plus uses a three-step transformation to convert the entire arterial pressure trace into a volume trace that can then be multiplied by the heart rate to calculate the CO. Using standardized tables to account for the nonlinear compliance variables of the arterial tree, the pressure waveform can be then be adjusted to a volume waveform to calculate the standardized or nominal SV.

The compliance algorithm that converts the arterial pressure waveform into a nominal SV one is as follows:

$$\Delta V/\Delta bp = \text{Calibration} \times 250 \times e^{-k \cdot bp}$$

where

$\Delta V/\Delta bp$ is the change in pressure divided by the change in volume
k is the curve coefficient
250 is the maximum distending volume of the aorta from diastolic volume

Autocorrelation of the nominal SV waveform derives the beat period (heart rate) and beat power, which is proportional to the nominal SV.

Converting this nominal SV into an actual SV requires the measurement of the actual CO by an indictor dilution technique. This scales the standardized or nominal SV to an actual SV by determining a calibration factor that accounts for the individual's arterial compliance in a similar way to the PiCCO-Plus. A venous bolus of lithium (0.002 to 0.004 mmol/kg) produces a lithium dilution curve that establishes the actual SV and CO. The lithium is analyzed by an ion-selective sensor (a lithium sensor) that is attached to a standard arterial line. The Nernst equation relates the voltage measured across the lithium sensor membrane to the plasma lithium over time, to produce a curve. The CO can be calculated using the modified Stewart-Hamilton equation. This is the LiDCO-Plus calibration. The nominal SV is adjusted by the calibration factor to derive the actual SV. All subsequent arterial waveforms can subsequently undergo the three-step calibration and then be adjusted according to the calibration factor to derive continuous CO assessment.

The LiDCO-Plus calibration (the initial calculation of CO) has been validated in adults and children (14, 15). It has been shown to have an excellent correlation and better reproducibility than the PAC estimation of CO (14). It has also been shown to work equally well if the lithium is injected peripherally as opposed to centrally (16). This has the added advantage of allowing CO assessment without the need for central access. However, as most vasoactive drugs necessitate delivery centrally, this benefit is in part self-limiting. Three studies in various patient groups have demonstrated that the pulse power analysis of the LiDCO-Plus when used as a continuous CO monitor has a good accuracy and precision over time (17).

The LiDCO-Plus also calculates SV, pulse pressure variation, systolic pressure variation, and SV variation. If the central venous pressure (CVP) is inputted manually, the LiDCO-Plus can calculate the systemic vascular resistance (SVR).

Sources of Error

As with the PiCCO-Plus, the accuracy of the monitor is dependent on the accuracy of the invasive arterial line and its transducer set. However, because the power of the waveform is unchanged by minor to moderate damping of the transducer system, its remains accurate (18). The LiDCO-Plus is like most hemodynamic monitoring regarding potential sources of inaccuracy; the presence of aortic valve regurgitation, left-to-right shunts, severe peripheral arterial vasoconstriction, irregular heart rates, hypothermia, or the use of intra aortic balloon pumps will affect accuracy. The LiDCO-Plus cannot be used in patients who are receiving therapeutic doses of lithium. Also, because of the interaction between the lithium ion-sensing electrode and muscle relaxants, especially vecuronium and atracurium, the accuracy of the LiDCO-Plus is reduced when these drugs are being administered.

Vigileo and Standard Deviation of the Pulse Pressure

The Vigileo, like the LiDCO-Plus, analyzes the entire arterial waveform and it does not necessarily require a central line. Unlike the LiDCO-Plus, the Vigileo does not require an initial calibration using an indicator, and it analyzes the standard deviation of the pulse pressure rather than purely the pulse power.

The mathematical algorithm analyzes the standard deviation of the pulse pressure. The pulse pressure is believed to more accurately reflect changes in left ventricular stroke work because it is less influenced by changes in the intrathoracic pressure due to respiration. "The pulse pressure is proportional to SV and is inversely related to aortic compliance" (19). Each waveform in every 20-second period is analyzed at a rate of 100 Hz. This means that over the 20 seconds, there are 2000 data points from which the Vigileo can reconstruct the pressure waveform into a volume waveform (Fig. 36.4). Then using the Langewouters principle, the calibration factor is determined that is used to adjust the volume waveform according to the patient's cardiovascular compliance to calculate the SV. The patient's arterial compliance variables are assumed on the basis of Langewouters ex-vivo research.

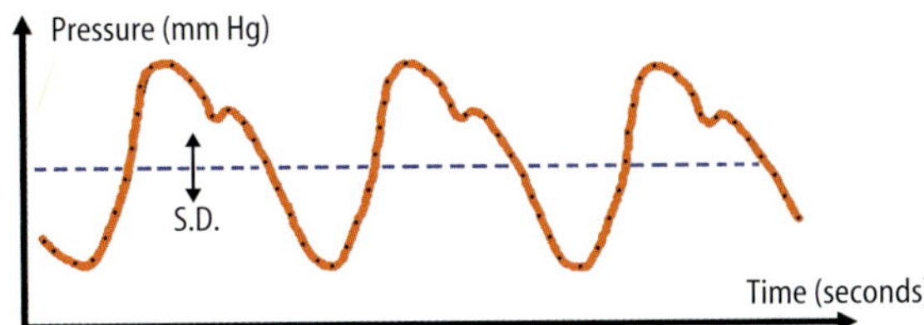

FIGURE 36.4. The Vigileo analysis of the arterial pressure trace with the standard deviation (S.D.) of the pulse pressure highlighted and the 2000 data points per 20 seconds marked.

Langewouters Principle

The Langewouters mathematical principle relates age, weight, height, gender, and MAP to aortic compliance on the basis of the shape of the waveform. The ejected volume of blood from the left ventricle is partially opposed by the elastic resistance of the arterial wall and the arterial tree impedance. These opposing forces are not constant and vary with the MAP: an increasing MAP leads to a reduction in the aortic compliance. Other factors that effect the aortic compliance include the distending pressure of the SV, the sympathetic tone, the volume status of the patient, and the patient's age, sex, height, and weight. The variations in aortic impedance and compliance are nonlinear in nature and were studied in vitro by Langewouters et al. (5). They developed mathematical equations based on population averages to create look-up tables that take account of the nonlinear compliance and impedance relationships proportional to the arterial pressure that is measured to allow integration and SV calculation from the systolic pressure waveform.

The Vigileo analyzes and then recalibrates the arterial waveform according to the look-up tables every 10 minutes. The shape of the waveform is assessed in terms of its skewness and kertosis to detect changes in arterial compliance. It therefore compensates for progressive changes in overall cardiovascular performance by recalibration every 10 minutes. The LiDCO-Plus and PiCCO-Plus update the SV for each arterial waveform. However, this updating is based on correcting each beat compared to the most recent calibration with either cold saline or lithium, which may have been as long as 12 hours ago. Therefore, this updating may potentially miss changes in the overall cardiac performance that have occurred in the intervening period leading to inaccurate CO estimation.

The Vigileo provides continuous information regarding the SV, CO, and systemic vascular resistance without requiring central access. It does not require a specific arterial line but does require its own transducer set. The Vigileo monitor can be used with its own specific central line, which provides continuous central venous saturation measurement. A benefit of this calculation is that it allows the clinician to directly and easily assess the adequacy of the CO by comparing it to a monitor of tissue oxygen performance.

The Vigielo is new to the CO market and has as yet very little data validating its accuracy clinically. Studies are ongoing.

Conclusion

The measurement of CO in critically ill patients remains an integral part of the patient's management. The clinical assessment can suggest that the CO may be inadequate but cannot be relied upon as a sole means of CO estimation and intervention. The clinical assessment should prompt the use of a minimally invasive monitor, which can easily and rapidly establish a reproducible and reliable CO. Although the measured CO may not be 100% accurate, it is reproducible over time and thus provides a useful trend that enables the clinician to quickly and easily assess the cardiovascular response to any therapeutic intervention.

The pulse contour and pulse power estimation of CO each have their specific benefits. They are most probably more accurate than clinical assessment alone and appear to be as accurate as the PAC at guiding therapy. They are undoubtedly less invasive than the PAC. They provide reproducible, continuous CO estimation relatively easily, and can be set up and maintained by nursing staff. They enable the clinician to concentrate on the data produced to formulate a therapeutic plan. As evidenced by the recent PAC-Man study, a monitor on its own will not improve patient outcome; it is how the information is used that proves vital (20).

References

1. Shoemaker WC. Cardiorespiratory patterns of surviving and nonsurviving postoperative patients. Surg Gynecol Obstet 1972;134:810–14.
2. Rivers E, Nguyen B, Havstad S, et al. Early goal-directed therapy in the treatment of severe sepsis and septic shock. N Engl J Med 2001;345:1368–77.
3. Jansen J, Verprille A. Improvement of cardiac output estimation by the thermodilution method during mechanical ventilation. Int. Care Med. 1985;12:71–9.
4. Stetz C, Miller R, Kelly G, et al. Reliability of the thermodilution method in the determination of cardiac output in clinical practice. Am. Rev. Respir. Dis. 1982;126:1001–4.
5. Langewouters G, Wesseling K, Goedhard W. The static elastic properties of 45 human thoracic and 20 abdominal aortas in vitro and the parameters of a new model. J. Biomech. 1984;17:425–35.
6. Wesseling K, Jansen J, Settels J, et al. Computation of aortic flow from pressure in humans in using nonlinear, three-element model. J. Appl. Physiol. 1993;74:2566–73.
7. Gödje O, Höeke K, Goetz A, et al. Reliability of a new algorithm for continuous cardiac determination by pulse-contour analysis during haemodynamic instability. Crit. Care Med. 2002;30:52–8.
8. Sakka S, Reinhart K, Meirer-Hellmann A. Comparison of pulmonary artery and arterial thermodilution cardiac output in critically ill patients. Int. Care Med. 1999;25:843–6.
9. Coedje O, Hoeke K, Lichtwarck-Aschoff M, et al. Continuous cardiac output by femoral arterial thermodilution calibrated pulse contour analysis: comparison with pulmonary arterial thermodilution. Crit. Care Med. 1999;27:2407–12.
10. Sakka S, Ruhl C, Pfeiffer U, et al. Assessment of cardiac preload and extravascular lung water by single transpulmonary thermodilution. Int. Care Med. 2000;26:180–7.
11. Halperin B, Feeley T, Mihm F, et al. Evaluation of the portable chest roentgenogram for quantitating extravascular lung water in critically ill adults. Chest 1985;88:649–52.
12. Baudendistel L, Shields J, Kaminski D. Comparison of double indicator thermodilution measurements of extravascular lung water (EVLW) with radiographic estimation of lung water in trauma patients. J. Trauma 1982;22:983–88.
13. Mitchell J, Schuller D, Calandrino F, et al. Improved outcome based on fluid management in critically ill patients requiring pulmonary artery catheterisation. Am. Rev. Respir. Dis. 1992;145:990–8.
14. Linton R, Band D, O'Brien T, et al. Lithium dilution cardiac output measurement: a comparison with thermodilution. Crit. Care Med. 1997;25:1796–1800.
15. Linton R, Young L, Marlin D, et al. Cardiac output measure by lithium dilution, thermodilution and transoesophageal Doppler echocardiography in anaesthetised horses. Am. J. Vet. Res. 2000;61:731–7.

16. Jonas M, Kelly F, Linton R, et al. A comparison of lithium dilution cardiac output measurement made using central line and antecubital venous injection of lithium chloride. J. Clin. Monitor 1999;15:525–8.
17. Jonas M, Hett D, Morgan J. Real-time, continuous monitoring of cardiac output and oxygen delivery. Internat. J. Int. Care 2002;9:33–42.
18. Pittman J, Bar-Yosef S, Sum-Ping J, et al. Continuous cardiac output monitoring by arterial pressure waveform analysis: a 24 hour comparison with the lithium dilution indicator technique. Crit. Care Med. 2005;33:2015–21.
19. Boulain T, Achard J-M, Teboul J-L, et al. Changes in BP Induced by Passive Leg Raising Predict Response to Fluid Loading in Critically Ill Patients. Chest. 2002;121:1245–52.
20. Harvey S, Harrison D, Singer M, et al. Assessment of the clinical effectiveness of pulmonary artery catheters in management of patients in intensive care (PAC-Man): a randomised controlled trial. Lancet 2005;366:472–7.

37
Oxygen Saturation Measurements in Acute Heart Failure Syndrome

Etienne Gayat, Alexandre Mebazaa, and Didier Payen de La Garanderie

The primary physiologic task of the cardiovascular system is to deliver enough oxygen (O_2) to meet the metabolic demands of the body. The monitoring of venous O_2 saturation measurements (venous oximetry) seems to be more sensible to hemodynamic changes than the simple monitoring of cardiac output in patients with acute heart failure. Indeed, a drop in mixed venous oxygen saturation is a marker not only of decreased cardiac output but also of decreased hemoglobin concentration, impaired arterial oxygenation, and increased tissue oxygen demand. Monitoring venous oxygen saturation is increasingly used as a clinical marker of systemic oxygen utilization in critically ill patients, particularly those with hemodynamic alteration (1,2).

Physiopathology of Venous Oximetry

Low values of SvO_2 (mixed oxygen saturation measured in pulmonary artery) or $ScvO_2$ (central venous oxygen saturation measured in the superior vena cava [SVC]) indicate a mismatch between O_2 delivery (i.e., O_2 delivered by the left ventricle) and global tissue O_2 requirement.

Considering O_2 dissolved in blood as negligible and based on the Fick equation, SvO_2 could be expressed as follows:

$$SvO\frac{Vo_2}{CO.Hb.OP}$$

where SaO_2 is the arterial oxygen saturation, VO_2 is the whole body oxygen consumption, CO is the cardiac output, Hb is the hemoglobin concentration, and OP is the oxyphoric power of hemoglobin (which is equal to 1.34 in physiologic status). Figure 37.1 shows several factors that can influence those five variables.

If the SaO_2, oxygen consumption and hemoglobin value remain stable, then SvO_2 is proportional to the cardiac output.

Normal Values

The physiologic values and the regional values of venous oximetry are shown in Figure 37.2.

How Can We Measure Venous Oximetry?

Mixed Venous or Central Venous Oxygen Saturation?

Pulmonary artery catheterization (PAC) facilitates measuring the oxygen saturation of the true mixed venous blood with an O_2 sensor at the tip of the PAC. It is the gold standard for measuring venous oxygen saturation. However, intensivists are increasingly performing measurements of $ScvO_2$ via a central venous catheter in the SVC.

Individual measurements of oxygen saturation from central venous and right atrial blood are slightly different from mixed venous blood values (around 10% differences versus mixed venous blood values). More importantly, a good correlation was found between the trend of $ScvO_2$ and SvO_2 values (2,3).

Figure 37.1. Main factors influencing mixed venous oxygen saturation. DPG, diphosphoglycerate; OP, oxyphoric power of hemoglobin.

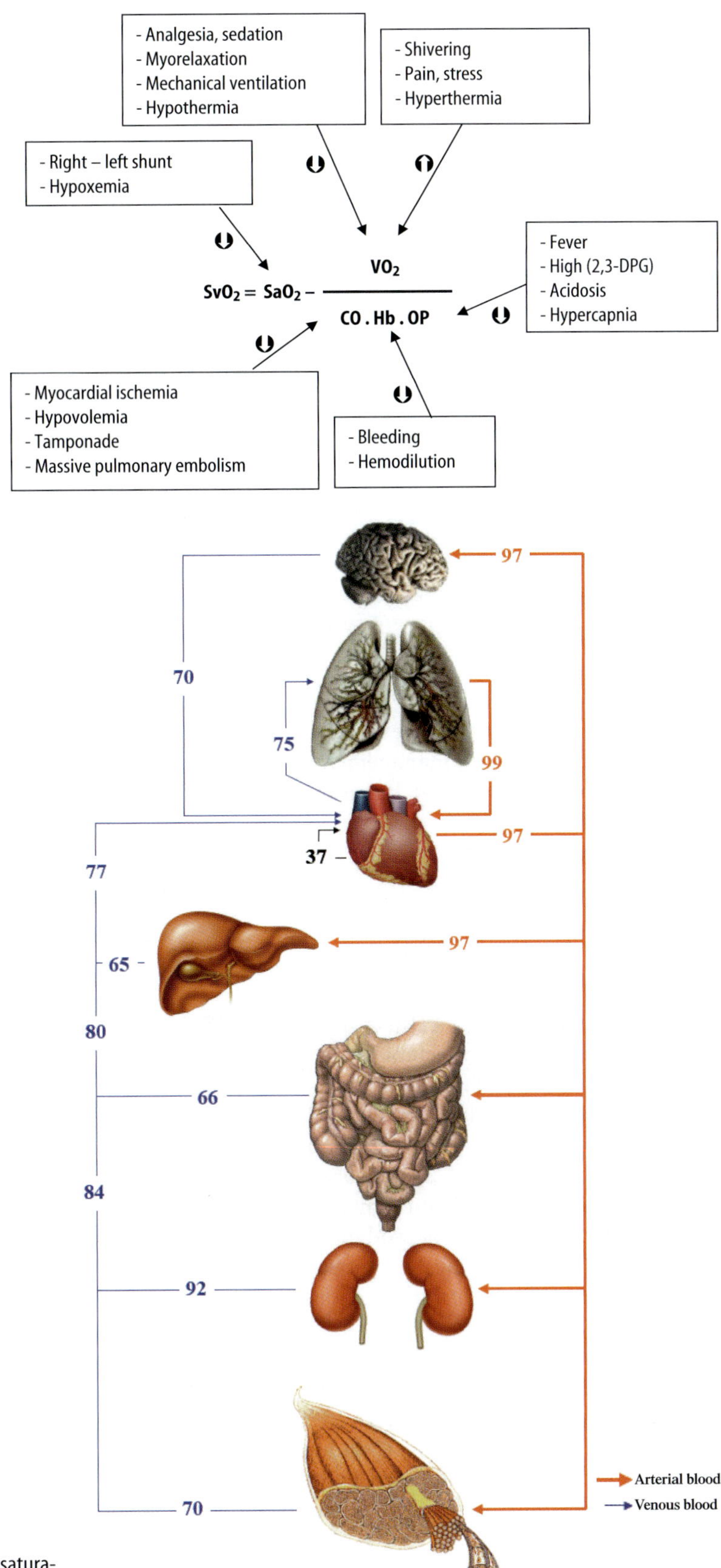

Figure 37.2. Physiologic values of oxygen saturation in both arterial and venous beds.

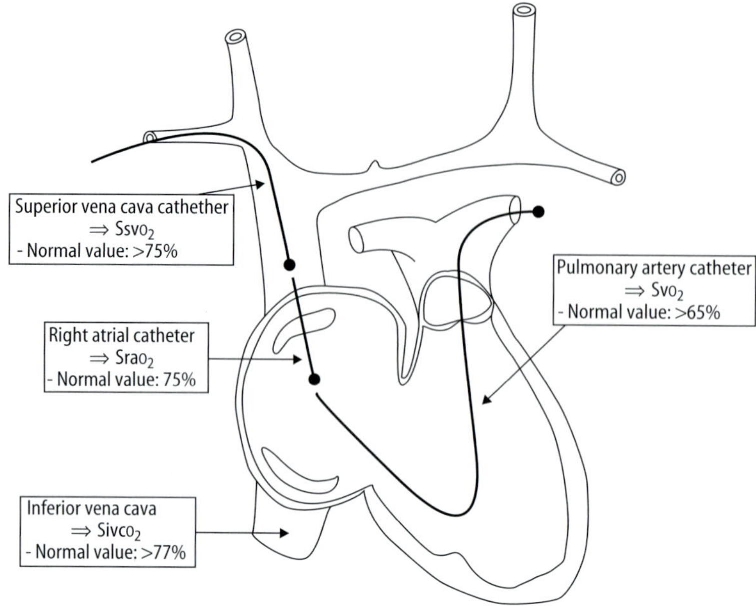

FIGURE 37.3. Measurement of venous oximetry.

Therefore, the clinical relevance of venous oximetry in heart failure management is not the absolute value but the trend in response to the therapeutic interventions.

The different ways for measuring venous oximetry are illustrated in Figure 37.3.

Continuous or Intermittent Monitoring?

Since the creation of a new catheter incorporating a fiberoptic photometric system in the beginning of the 1980s, continuous measurement of venous oximetry has been available to the physician. By providing continuous monitoring of venous oxygen saturation, this system permits the physician to identify hemodynamic changes much earlier, before any hemodynamic change occurs. This fiberoptic system now exists for both the PAC and he central venous catheter (CVC).

Intermittent monitoring can also be performed and even useful in those who have a CVC line, without a fiberoptic system. Intermittent venous blood withdrawn from the SVC should be performed before and after therapeutic intervention and every 4 to 6 hours together with arterial blood gas to assess pulmonary and cardiovascular diseases.

Use During Hemodynamic Instability

SvO_2 as a Continuous Marker of Cardiac Output

According to the Fick principle, SvO_2 follows the changes of cardiac output when SaO_2, VO_2, and hemoglobin values remain stable. This fact was illustrated in clinical work led by Gawlinski (4) in 1998, who studied 42 patients admitted to the cardiac care and observation unit of a university tertiary care center. Most patients had advanced heart failure due to dilated or ischemic cardiomyopathy. The mean left ventricular ejection fraction was 20%. The results indicated a significant relationship ($r = 0.54$, $p < .001$) between cardiac output and SvO_2 in patients with heart failure who had a low ejection fraction, even for those receiving vasoactive medications.

Management Algorithm of Low SvO_2

The etiologies of low SvO_2 are multiple. The physician has to consider all of them and proceed to

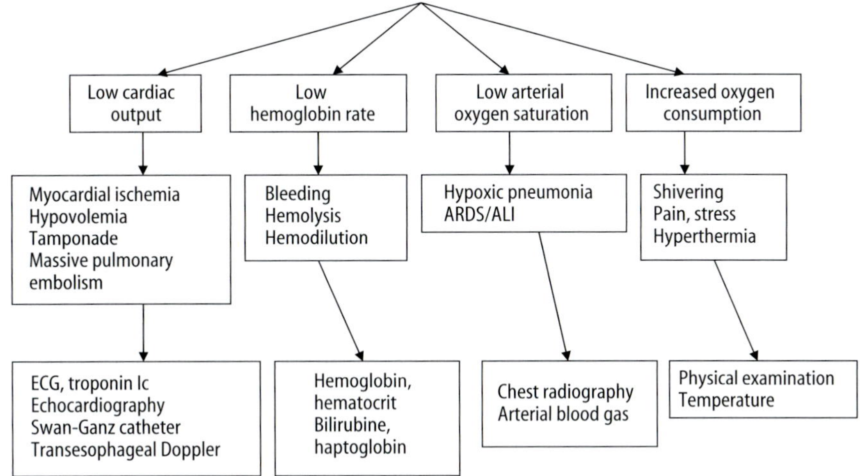

Figure 37.4. Physiopathology of low SvO_2. ARDS, acute respiratory distress syndrome; ALI, acute lung injury.

eliminate them one by one to define the correct diagnostic. We propose in the Figure 37.4 an algorithm that the physician can follow to determinate the etiology of low SvO_2 in the patient.

SvO_2 as a Marker of Prognosis

The relation of mixed venous oxygen saturation, the cardiac index, tissue oxygenation, and prognosis has been investigated by Sumimoto et al. (5) in 199 patients in the early phase of acute myocardial infarction. They found that a decreased mixed venous oxygen saturation in patients with acute myocardial infarction more reliably reflected the presence of lactic acidosis and predicted a fatal outcome than did the simultaneously measured cardiac index.

Discussion and Perspectives

As well as increasing cardiac output, maintaining adequate mixed venous oxygen saturation should also be a goal of the treatment of acute heart failure.

It may be interesting to design a trial similar to that led by Rivers et al. (1) regarding early goal-directed therapy in septic patients, but instead concerning goal-directed therapy for acute heart failure using venous oximetry optimization as one of the goals.

Case Report

A 65-year-old man is admitted to the emergency room for acute pulmonary edema. He presents a history of chronic anemia and chronic congestive heart failure related to ischemic cardiopathy treated with beta-blocker, angiotensin-conversion enzyme inhibitor, loop diuretics, and aspirin.

The blood pressure is 80/40 mm Hg, the heart rate is 96 bpm, and the respiratory rate is 27/min. A central venous catheter is placed through the jugular vein in the patient. The blood results show $ScvO_2$ at 58% with an SaO_2 at 91%. An echocardiography is performed and shows a left ventricular ejection fraction at 35%.

How can you explain this low $ScvO_2$ value? You initiate a treatment with dobutamine infusion. The latter increases $ScvO_2$ to 62% while SaO_2 remains at 99% under 6 L/min O_2 with a RR at 18/min. Hemoglobin value is 8.5 g/dL.

$ScvO_2$ is still below 75%. What is your analysis of the situation? What are you going to do? Following the algorithm reproduced in Figure 37.4, low $ScvO_2$ can be explained by a low cardiac output, anemia, or hypoxia. Hemoglobin value and arterial blood gas must be checked.

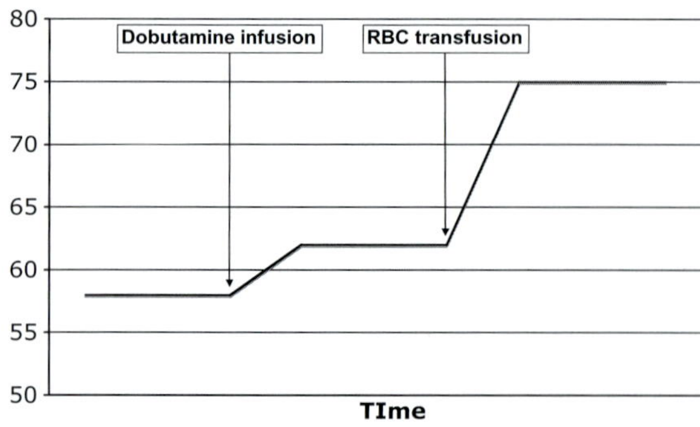

FIGURE 37.5. SvO_2 trend (see case report).

There persists an inadequacy between O_2 consumption and O_2 delivery. This is probably related to anemia. Red blood cell transfusion must be performed; diuretic, like furosemide, could be associated to the transfusion (Fig. 37.5).

Conclusion

Together with the use of PAC, venous oximetry remains a less invasive and useful tool that can be obtained with a simple CVC in patient with acute heart failure syndrome (AHFS).

We suggest, however, that venous oximetry should be combined with other cardiocirculatory parameters and indicators of organ perfusion such as serum lactate concentration and urine output (6) to assess the mechanism of AHFS and to follow effects of treatment.

References

1. Rivers E, Nguyen B, Havstad S, et al. Early goal-directed therapy in the treatment of severe sepsis and septic shock. N Engl J Med 2001;345:1368–77.
2. Reinhart K, Kuhn HJ, Hartog C, Bredle DL. Continuous central venous and pulmonary artery oxygen saturation monitoring in the critically ill. Intensive Care Med 2004;30:1572–8.
3. Dueck MH, Klimek M, Appenrodt S et al. Trends but not individual values of central venous oxygen saturation agree with mixed venous oxygen saturation during varying hemodynamic conditions. Anesthesiology 2005;103:249–57.
4. Gawlinski A. Can measurement of mixed venous oxygen saturation replace measurement of cardiac output in patients with advanced heart failure? Am J Crit Care 1998;7:374–80; quiz 81–2.
5. Sumimoto T, Takayama Y, Iwasaka T et al. Mixed venous oxygen saturation as a guide to tissue oxygenation and prognosis in patients with acute myocardial infarction. Am Heart J 1991;122:27–33.
6. Bloos F, Reinhart K. Venous oximetry. Intensive Care Med 2005;31:911–3.

38
Pulmonary Artery Catheter in the Intensive Care Unit

Xavier Monnet and Jean-Louise Teboul

After its initial description by Swan and Ganz more than 30 years ago (1), the pulmonary artery catheter (PAC) technique rapidly became more and more popular in the following years. To date, the PAC remains the monitoring tool that enables more extensive hemodynamic assessment of the critically ill. Furthermore, its use has stimulated the comprehension of physiologic concepts of hemodynamics and tissue oxygenation in various situations of acute circulatory failure. After years of debate about its adverse effects, recent large-scale studies clearly demonstrate that the use of the PAC does not alter the outcome of critically ill patients.

Practical Use of the Pulmonary Artery Catheter

Description

Among the commercially available models of PAC, the most commonly used is a water-filled catheter of 7 or 7.5 French (F) external diameter and 80 cm long that is connected to an electronic pressure transducer (Fig. 38.1). The distal lumen located at the tip of the catheter enables blood sampling and pressure measurement at the level of the pulmonary artery. A few millimeters before the catheter's termination, a latex balloon surrounds it. Balloon inflation by totally occluding the pulmonary artery branch (10 to 15 mm diameter), where the catheter has been placed, facilitates measuring the pulmonary artery occlusion pressure (PAOP). A proximal lumen that ends in the right atrium facilitates measuring the right atrial pressure. A thermistor placed at the distal segment of the catheter facilitates recording the changes in blood temperature induced by cold bolus infusion via the proximal lumen. This enables calculating the thermodilution cardiac output according to the Stewart-Hamilton principle.

On the basis of this minimal configuration (1), alternative PAC models can be equipped with:

- A right ventricular lumen for electrosystolic pacing
- A thermal filament for the continuous measurement of cardiac output (see below) (2, 3)
- A fiberoptic probe for reflectance photometry and continuous assessment of SvO_2 (see below) (4)
- An additional distal lumen for central venous injection

Insertion

The setting up of the PAC first requires the insertion of an introducer into a large vein using the Seldinger method. Any large vein can be used with the aim of inserting the PAC (5), but the subclavian and internal jugular veins are more commonly employed because the PAC insertion is easier by these routes. Once the introducer in place and fixed to the skin, the PAC is introduced into its lumen and moved through the venous network. The pressure recorded at the tip level of the PAC is simultaneously displayed and indicates the position of the catheter during its

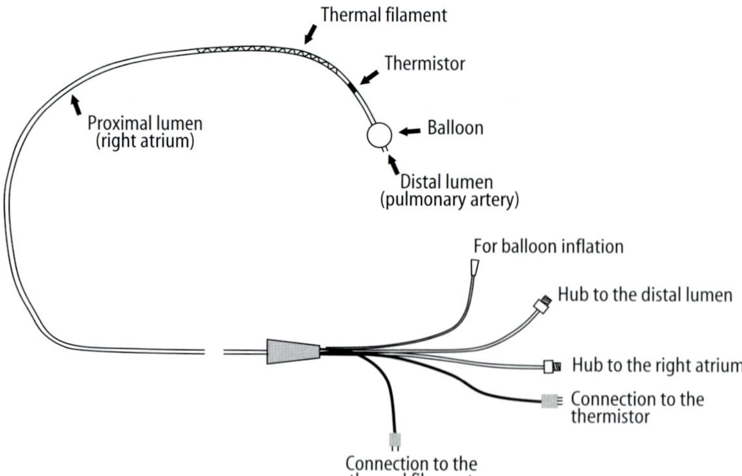

FIGURE 38.1. Schematic description of the pulmonary artery catheter.

course. The occurrence of a respiratory variation of the pressure waveform indicates that the PAC is located into the thorax. When a typical right atrial pressure waveform appears on the screen of the monitor, the distal balloon is inflated with 1.5 mL of air to allow the direction of the catheter by the bloodstream. The PAC crosses the tricuspid orifice and the pressure curve depicts a typical waveform of ventricular pressure. It crosses the pulmonary orifice and the pulmonary artery pressure curve is displayed. A further advance of the catheter while its balloon still inflated occludes a branch of the pulmonary artery, and a waveform of PAOP is finally obtained (Fig. 38.2). The deflation of the balloon relieves the occlusion, and the pressure trace comes back to the pulmonary artery pressure curve. The proximal side of the PAC is locked to the external orifice of the venous introducer by means of a clip that can be relieved for further PAC repositioning. The external tip of the PAC is covered by a sheath for allowing aseptic repositioning. The correct positioning of PAC and the absence of pneumothorax must be checked on a chest radiograph at the end of procedure. Note that the insertion of PAC by the classic subclavian or internal jugular routes does not require any radioscopic guidance.

The advance of the PAC toward the pulmonary artery can be difficult because of an anatomic

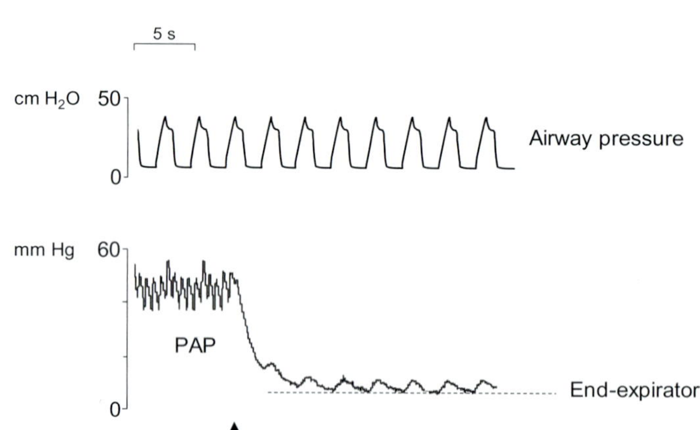

FIGURE 38.2. Waveform depicted by the pressure measured at the tip of the pulmonary artery catheter level before (pulmonary artery pressure, PAP) and after (pulmonary artery occlusion pressure, PAOP) balloon inflation. In this patient under mechanical ventilation, the PAOP must be measured at the end of expiration (see the airways pressure waveform).

abnormality (left-sided superior vena cava [6]), of a blockade of the catheter into the coronary sinus (7) or, more commonly, because a high pulmonary artery pressure with right cardiac cavities dilation impedes the advance of the catheter through the tricuspid or pulmonary valves.

Description and Clinical Use of the Pulmonary Artery Catheter–Derived Parameters

The PAC provides the physician with hemodynamic measures (cardiac output, right atrial, pulmonary artery and pulmonary artery occlusion pressures, and possibly right ventricular volumes) and also with tissue perfusion variables (oxygen venous saturation [SvO_2], oxygen consumption, oxygen delivery, oxygen extraction, and the venous carbon dioxide pressure).

Cardiac Output

The cardiac output is measured according to the thermodilution principle. Two methods of measurement are currently used. The intermittent thermodilution technique requires the injection of cold saline bolus through the atrial lumen of the catheter. The decrease of blood temperature is recorded downstream by the distal thermistor, and cardiac output is calculated from the Stewart-Hamilton equation by an external processor. At least three measurements must be averaged for a reliable estimation of cardiac output (8). One advantage of this technique is to provide the value of cardiac output at the time when it is measured.

The continuous thermodilution method is based on intermittent and automatic heating of blood by means of a proximal thermal filament and recording of the temperature changes by a distal thermistor (3). This measure has been demonstrated to agree with that provided by the intermittent technique (9–11), except for the high values of cardiac output that could be underestimated by the continuous method (10, 12). This technique presents the advantage of continuously displaying cardiac output and avoiding repeated manipulations of the lines and bolus injections. The major inconvenience is that it does not enable real-time monitoring of cardiac output since the average of successive cardiac output measurements is delayed as compared to the standard intermittent technique (13). This limitation may be important if one attempts to monitor rapid changes induced by a hemodynamic treatment. Nonetheless, the PAC remains the gold-standard tool for measuring cardiac output in the clinical setting.

Pulmonary Artery Occlusion Pressure

Technique of Measurement

The inflation of the distal balloon of the catheter with 1.5 mL of air occludes a branch of the pulmonary artery of around 13-mm diameter. This occlusion stops the blood flow distal to the balloon until it reaches a pulmonary vein of similar diameter. The PAOP is the pressure obtained after inflating the distal balloon (Fig. 38.2). Since a static column is created between the inflated balloon and the venous site where the blood flow resumes, PAOP is assumed to reflect the pressure in a large pulmonary vein and thus the left atrial pressure and eventually the left ventricular end-diastolic pressure (1) (Fig. 38.3).

Physiologic Relevance of Pulmonary Artery Occlusion Pressure

Since it reflects the left ventricular pressure at the end-diastole, PAOP is considered an estimate of

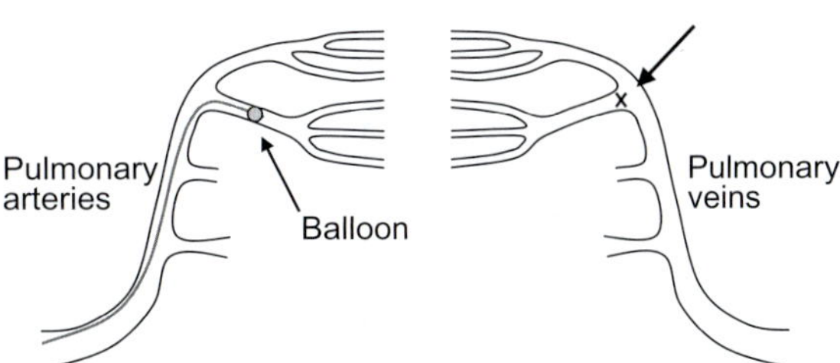

FIGURE 38.3. Significance of the pulmonary artery occlusion (PAOP). Since a static column is created between the inflated balloon (in a large artery) and the venous site where the blood flow resumes (cross), PAOP is assumed to reflect the pressure in a large pulmonary vein and thus the left atrial pressure and eventually the left ventricular end diastolic pressure.

the left ventricular filling pressure (14), and thus an index of left ventricular preload. On the other hand, the PAOP may also reflect the pulmonary filtration pressure and thus is often used to determine the mechanism of pulmonary edema.

Conditions for a Correct Pulmonary Artery Occlusion Pressure Measurement

The interpretation of PAOP is based on numerous assumptions which must be questioned (15).

Is the technique of pressure measurement suitable? The correct measurement of PAOP requires a cautious calibration of the zero of the pressure gauge with respect to the atmospheric pressure. The catheter tip must be placed at the midaxillary line. The fluid-filled catheter used for pressure measurement must be flushed for avoiding clotting.

Is PAOP influenced by the variations in the intrathoracic pressure? The intrathoracic pressure is transmitted to the pulmonary vasculature; PAOP is increased by inspiration during positive pressure ventilation and decreased during inspiration during spontaneous breathing. To minimize the influence of intrathoracic pressure on PAOP measurements, it is recommended to measure PAOP (as well as the other intravascular and intracardiac pressures) at the end of expiration, a time when intrathoracic pressure is close to atmospheric pressure (Fig. 38.4). However, positive end-expiratory pressure (PEEP) or auto-PEEP may lead to overestimation of PAOP at end-expiration (see below).

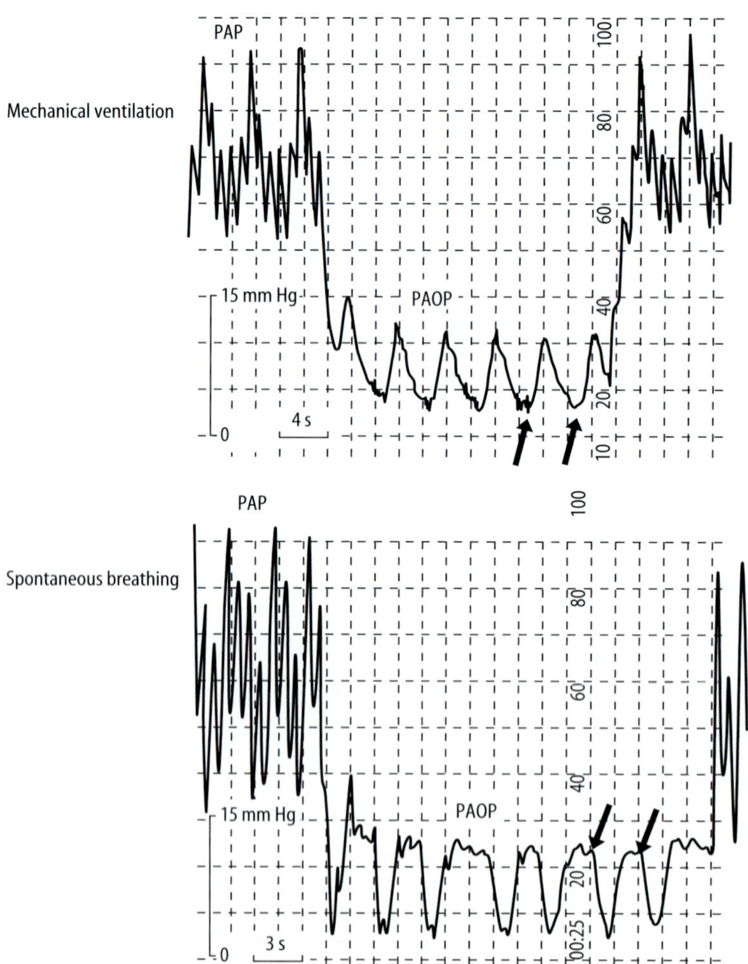

FIGURE 38.4. Measurement of the pulmonary artery occlusion (PAOP) depending on the ventilatory mode. To minimize the influence of intrathoracic pressure on PAOP measurements, it is recommended to measure PAOP at the end of expiration, a time when intrathoracic pressure is close to atmospheric pressure (arrows). During mechanical ventilation, the end-expiratory PAOP corresponds to the minimal pressure recorded during balloon inflation, while it corresponds to the maximal pressure recorded during balloon inflation in the case of spontaneous breathing.

Does PAOP always reflect the pressure in a large pulmonary vein? Considering that the PAOP senses the pressure in the pulmonary vein where the blood flow resumes, one must assume that the blood column immobilized by the balloon inflation is uninterrupted. This may not be the case in the presence of high PEEP (or auto-PEEP) or hypovolemia, conditions that may result in squeezing of alveolar microvessels downstream of the branch of the pulmonary artery where balloon inflation has occurred. This condition where PAOP may not reflect a pulmonary venous pressure but rather alveolar pressure can be easily identified by the observation of large changes of PAOP over the respiratory cycle in comparison with those of the pulmonary artery diastolic pressure, which are assumed to reflect the respiratory changes in intrathoracic pressure (16). If the ratio of the respiratory variation of PAOP over the respiratory variation of diastolic pulmonary artery pressure is close to 1, the PAOP is likely to actually reflect a pulmonary venous pressure. If the ratio is greater than 1.5, the PAOP is likely to reflect alveolar pressure and must not be interpreted as a pulmonary venous pressure (16). In fact, in the case of severe acute respiratory distress syndrome (ARDS), the low pulmonary and pulmonary vessels compliance can avoid the compression of pulmonary microvessels by the alveoli, even when PEEP as high as 15 or 20 mm Hg is applied.

Does the PAOP as a pulmonary venous pressure reflect the left ventricular end-diastolic pressure? Even if reflected by PAOP, the left atrial pressure may be different from the left ventricular end-diastolic pressure in some clinical situations. The PAOP overestimates the left ventricular end-diastolic pressure in the case of significant mitral stenosis or mitral insufficiency; it underestimates the left ventricular end-diastolic pressure in the case of severe aortic insufficiency or in case of reduced left ventricular compliance.

Does the left ventricular end-diastolic pressure reflect the left ventricular preload? The left ventricular preload is better related to the left ventricular transmural pressure (left ventricular end-diastolic pressure minus the intrathoracic pressure) than to the "intramural" left ventricular pressure. Accordingly, when high levels of PEEP are applied, the PAOP overestimates the left ventricular end-diastolic transmural pressure and hence the left ventricular preload, even at end-expiration.

Two simple methods have been proposed for correcting the overestimation and thus for calculating the true left ventricular filling pressure (17, 18). The first method consists of measuring the nadir PAOP after transiently (<3 seconds) disconnecting the patient from the ventilator during a PAOP recording (18). If the end-expiratory intrathoracic pressure influences the end-expiratory PAOP in a great extent, its fall during the disconnection is accompanied by an immediate fall in PAOP. After a few seconds, the PAOP value will rise again due to the increase in systemic venous return that follows the ventilatory support withdrawal with a short time delay. The lowest value of PAOP, called the nadir PAOP, has been demonstrated to reflect the on-PEEP left atrial pressure in patients receiving PEEP (18). Second, Teboul and coworkers (17) proposed evaluating the transmission of alveolar pressure to the intravascular system at end-expiration. This transmission index (I_t) can be estimated by the ratio of ΔPAOP (difference between the PAOP values at end-expiration and end-inspiration) over ΔPalv (difference between the plateau pressure and the total PEEP). Once this transmission index is calculated, the part of PAOP due to PEEP transmission can be estimated by the product of PEEP by I_t. This product must be subtracted to the end-expiratory PAOP and the corrected value of PAOP is obtained (Fig. 38.5) (17). Contrary to the nadir-PAOP measurement, this technique is also suitable in the case of intrinsic PEEP and pulmonary dynamic hyperinflation (18).

Finally, the question of whether the left ventricular preload is better assessed by left ventricular transmural end-diastolic pressure or volume is still a physiologic debate. Because left ventricular compliance is different from one patient to another, PAOP must not correlate with left ventricular end-diastolic volume when a vast population of patient is considered (19). Importantly, studies in healthy volunteers as well as in the critically ill reported that left ventricular end-diastolic dimensions were better correlated with stroke volume than was PAOP (20). In patients studied after myocardial infarction, higher than normal values of PAOP have been found associated with optimal left ventricular filling conditions. This

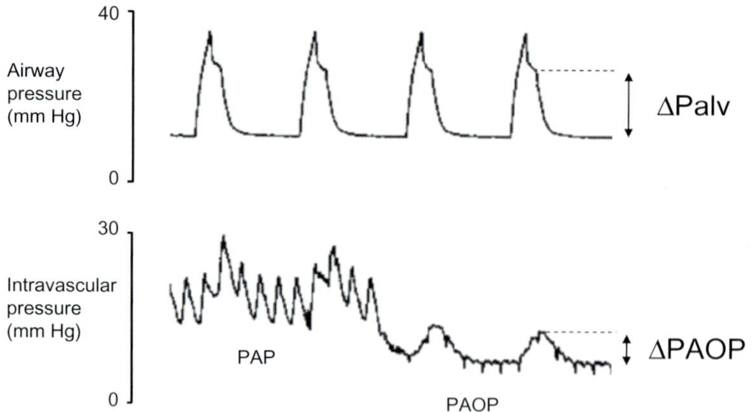

Figure 38.5. Transmural pulmonary artery occlusion pressure. The ΔPAOP/ΔPalv (I_t) reflects the percent transmission of airway pressure to intrathoracic vessels. A "transmural" PAOP value can be calculated by subtracting the product of PEEP by I_t. Palv, alveolar pressure; PAP, pulmonary artery pressure; PAOP, pulmonary artery occlusion pressure.

suggests that in the case of reduced left ventricular compliance, a PAOP in the normal range may reflect an abnormally reduced left ventricular preload (21).

Does PAOP adequately reflect the hydrostatic pulmonary filtration pressure? The main determinant of pulmonary edema formation is the hydrostatic pressure that exists in the capillary vessel (P_{cp}). Since the PAOP reflects the pressure in a large pulmonary vein, the P_{cp} is necessarily higher than the PAOP and the difference between these two pressures is proportional to the blood flow through the pulmonary venous bed and the resistance of the pulmonary venous bed. Thus, PAOP underestimates P_{cp}, particularly in the high blood flow states or in conditions where pulmonary venous resistance are elevated, such as during acute respiratory distress syndrome (ARDS) (22, 23).

In the clinical setting, P_{cp} can be estimated by observing the shape of the pulmonary artery pressure trace decay during the seconds following the inflation of the balloon. Schematically, the decreasing pressure profile is considered as biexponential: the initial fast decrease corresponds to the fast blood emptying through the low compliant arterial system; the ensuing slower decrease corresponds to the addition of the slower blood emptying through the capillary and venous beds (24). The pressure recorded at the intersection between the two parts of the curve can be assimilated to P_{cp} (24). However, this method is prone to numerous pitfalls in pathologic conditions (25) and requires rigorous conditions of measurement (e.g., mechanical ventilation with low respiratory rate and without any spontaneous breaths), which makes this method difficult to routinely apply. Moreover, this method provides a rough estimation of the P_{cp}, which would be better estimated by the extrapolation back toward time zero of the slow component. A computerized mathematical model would be mandatory for obtaining a valid P_{cp} measurement since the visual method weakly agrees with the mathematical method (22).

Another approach is to estimate the resistance of the venous pulmonary bed. For this purpose, the PAC can be advanced with deflated balloon until wedging against a small-diameter artery. The pressure measured at the distal tip of the PAC thus reflects the pressure into a small pulmonary vein of identical diameter at the opposite side of the pulmonary bed (23). The difference between the PAOP (reflecting the pressure into a large pulmonary vein) and the distal wedge pressure is high in the case of high pulmonary venous resistance (veno-occlusive disease [26], ARDS [22, 23], and α-agonist catecholamine therapy [27]).

For Which Clinical Purpose May the PAOP Be Used?

Using PAOP for Determining the Cause of Pulmonary Edema

The PAOP as a rough estimate of P_{cp} could be used to differentiate between hydrostatic and increased permeability-pulmonary edema. The value of 18 mm Hg is often considered a cutoff value.

However, hydrostatic pulmonary edema can still be present, although PAOP has already normalized (28), and increased permeability pulmonary edema can be associated with elevated PAOP (29).

Using PAOP for Assessing the Pulmonary Vasomotor Tone

The pulmonary vasomotor tone can be approached by dividing the pressure difference through the pulmonary vascular bed (estimated as mean pulmonary arterial pressure minus the PAOP) by the cardiac output. In the case of pulmonary hypertension, normal pulmonary vascular resistance (from 2 to 3 mm Hg/L/min or 150 to 200 dynes/s·cm^{-5}) indicates that pulmonary arterial hypertension results from a left cardiac disease while elevated pulmonary artery vascular tone indicates "precapillary" pulmonary hypertension (e.g., primary pulmonary arterial hypertension, chronic cor pulmonale). Nevertheless, this measurement is prone to pitfalls, particularly because the pulmonary vascular resistance may vary from a pulmonary region to another (25).

Using PAOP for Assessing Weaning-Induced Pulmonary Edema

One particular context of acute heart failure is the left ventricular dysfunction that occurs in some patients during weaning from mechanical ventilation. Several mechanisms may result in weaning-induced left ventricular dysfunction and hence in increased left ventricular filling pressure and in hydrostatic pulmonary edema, which may prevent successful weaning from positive pressure ventilation (30). So far, the measurement of PAOP remains the gold-standard for detecting pulmonary edema in this setting (31).

Using PAOP for Guiding Fluid Resuscitation/Fluid Restriction

As a reflection of the left ventricular filling pressure, the PAOP is considered a marker of left ventricular preload. Nonetheless, this static marker of cardiac preload has been demonstrated to be of little value for the guidance of fluid therapy in the critically ill or in the setting of the operating room since it is a poor predictor of volume responsiveness (32). This point can be explained in reference to the Frank-Starling principle (32). Indeed, the slope of the Frank-Starling curve (ventricular preload vs. stroke volume) also depends on systolic cardiac function. Thus, except for the lowest and the highest ranges of ventricular preload, a given value of ventricular preload can be associated with preload-dependency in the case of normal ventricular systolic function (steep part of the Frank-Starling curve) or with preload-independency in the case of decreased ventricular contractility (flat part of the Frank-Starling curve). As patients cared for in intensive care units often have been already resuscitated, ventricular preload is rarely low in contrast to what may happen in critically ill patients admitted in the emergency room. Therefore, a given value of a ventricular preload marker (and thus of PAOP) generally fails to predict the ability of the ventricle to positively respond to volume loading, except for very low values (32).

On the other hand, PAOP can be used to ensure that fluid administration has induced an effective increase in cardiac preload, independently of its effects on cardiac output. This is particularly important in the context of sepsis, where capillary leak can make fluid therapy ineffective for increasing central blood volume. Finally, PAOP is frequently used as a safety parameter during volume loading or fluid challenge (33). To prevent fluid-induced pulmonary edema, fluid administration could be discontinued when a predefined value of PAOP has been reached. The value of 18 mm Hg is often cited as the PAOP value above which pulmonary edema is at high risk to occur with fluid administration, although no study validated it.

Acute lung injury is a clinical situation where fluid management is a crucial issue. On the one hand, volume expansion may be required since this situation is frequently associated with sepsis and relative hypovolemia; on the other hand, volume infusion may enhance pulmonary edema formation since pulmonary vascular permeability is increased. Although there is some evidence of superiority of a conservative strategy over a liberal strategy in terms of fluid management in acute lung injury (34), PAOP-guided therapy was not found to perform better than central venous pressure–guided therapy (35).

Right Ventricular Volumes

The PAC equipped with a fast-response thermistor is able to measure the right ventricular ejection fraction by analyzing the changes in blood temperature induced by the right ventricular ejection on the thermodilution waveform. The end-systolic and end-diastolic right ventricular volumes are calculated from the right ejection fraction, the cardiac output, and the heart rate measured through electrodes fixed on the catheter (36).

This technique allows an estimation of the right ventricular volumes that is reliable as compared to the conventional ventriculographic method (37) but that is highly hampered if the tricuspid regurgitation is of significant importance (38). Furthermore, the clinical utility of such right ventricular volumes assessment has never been clearly defined, even in the context of right ventricular failure.

Mixed Venous Oxygen Saturation

The PAC enables measurement of oxygen saturation of the mixed venous blood (Svo_2). Since the mixed venous blood results from the mix of all venous territories of the body, measuring Svo_2 with the PAC enables assessment of global tissue oxygenation, which is not provided by peripheral blood samplings.

Techniques of Measurement of Svo_2

Two techniques are currently available. The first one requires a sampling of the pulmonary artery blood through the distal tip of PAC (with deflated balloon), with further classic blood gas analysis at the laboratory. The second technique uses commercially available PAC models, which enable a continuous in vivo monitoring of Svo_2 by means of fiberoptic spectrophotometry (4). This method is based on the principle that the amount of energy reflected by hemoglobin molecules during an infrared illumination is different if they carry an oxygen molecule or not. This method avoids cumbersome repeated blood samplings and provides a continuous monitoring of Svo_2.

Significance and Clinical Use of Svo_2

Svo_2 is related to arterial oxygen saturation (Sao_2), oxygen consumption, to cardiac output, and to hemoglobin concentration (Hb) according to the formula derived from the Fick equation applied to oxygen:

$$Svo_2 = Sao_2 - [\text{oxygen consumption}/(\text{cardiac output} \times Hb \times 13.4)]$$

Thus, Svo_2 is an integrative variable, which can be considered as a marker of the global balance between actual oxygen consumption and oxygen delivery, since cardiac output, Hb, and Sao_2 are the key determinants of oxygen delivery. The Svo_2 values range from 65% to 77% in healthy subjects.

In patients with acute heart failure, Svo_2 cannot be been taken as a surrogate of cardiac output (39, 40). A better approach is to consider Svo_2 as a marker of adequacy of cardiac output with actual metabolic conditions. In this regard, it has been proposed to use Svo_2 rather than cardiac output to adjust the dose of inotropic drugs, which have potential thermogenic effects (41, 42). For example, phosphodiesterase inhibitors as well as β-agonist agents can increase myocardial and global oxygen consumption and may result in unchanged Svo_2 despite increase in cardiac output (41, 42). Moreover, in patients with severe cardiac failure experiencing low cardiac output and potential tricuspid regurgitation, thermodilution cardiac output may be erroneous, and monitoring the cardiovascular treatment using Svo_2 could be a better approach (43).

The interpretation of Svo_2 and its changes is prone to some difficulties, which should be emphasized. First, a low value of Svo_2 can be the consequence of a decrease in Sao_2. In this condition, Svo_2 can no longer be considered a marker of the oxygen consumption/oxygen delivery balance. Second, a normal or high Svo_2 value can be observed in distributive shock states as septic shock. In these conditions and contrary to what occurs in cardiogenic or hypovolemic shock states, the decrease in oxygen consumption (relatively to oxygen demand) is not the consequence of a decrease in cardiac output but is related to impaired oxygen extraction capabilities. Therefore, in patients with septic shock where hemodynamic resuscitation has restored a normal or high cardiac output, values of Svo_2 >70% can be observed despite persistence of marked global tissue dysoxia and anaerobiosis. This emphasizes the fact that Svo_2 is a marker of the global balance between oxygen consumption and oxygen delivery but not between oxygen demand and oxygen delivery. Third, if oxygen consumption, Hb, and Sao_2 are constant, the relation between Svo_2 and cardiac output is not linear but rather hyperbolic. Under these conditions, while in low blood flow states changes in Svo_2 parallel changes in cardiac output, in hyperdynamic states marked changes in cardiac output will not significantly alter Svo_2. In this regard, when Svo_2 lies in its high or even normal range, any decrease in Svo_2 by at least 5% should be considered clinically significant since it indicates a dramatic fall in oxygen delivery or an increase in oxygen demand. This should prompt the checking of Hb, Sao_2, cardiac output, and potential causes of increased oxygen demand and lead to appropriate treatment. Fourth, in shock states characterized by oxygen supply/oxygen consumption dependency, changes in cardiac output result in changes in oxygen consumption in the same direction, such that Svo_2 does not change provided that oxygen delivery is less than its critical value. Fifth, Svo_2 is the flow-weighted average of the venous saturation values from all organs of the body. Organs with high blood flow and low oxygen extraction, such as the kidneys, have a greater influence on Svo_2 than organs with low blood flow and high O_2 extraction, such as the myocardium. In sepsis the interpretation of Svo_2 is further complicated by the fact that regional and local distribution of blood flow is disturbed.

In summary, in the shock states where oxygen consumption is lower that oxygen demand by essence, the interpretation of Svo_2 and its changes must be particularly cautious. However, in any shock state (even of septic origin), monitoring of Svo_2 can be helpful since a low value of Svo_2 (for example, <65%) would incite the clinician to attempt to increase oxygen delivery (mainly through an increase in cardiac output) in order to improve global tissue oxygenation. On the other hand, a high value of Svo_2 would suggest that attempts to increase further oxygen delivery have little chance to improve significantly tissue oxygenation and ultimately outcome (44).

Because of the above-mentioned difficulties in appropriately interpreting Svo_2 and its changes (or its absence of changes), it would be more judicious to monitor continuously both Svo_2 and cardiac output with special PAC models, rather than to monitor Svo_2 alone.

Venoarterial Carbon Dioxide Tension Difference

The venoarterial carbon dioxide tension (Pco_2) difference (ΔPco_2) is the difference between Pco_2 in mixed venous blood ($Pvco_2$) and the Pco_2 in arterial blood ($Paco_2$). Its normal value ranges from 2 to 5 mm Hg.

The Fick equation applied to carbon dioxide indicates that the carbon dioxide excretion (equivalent to carbon dioxide production in a steady state) equals the product of cardiac output by the difference between the carbon dioxide content in mixed venous blood ($Cvco_2$) and in arterial blood ($Caco_2$).

The normal relationship between CO_2 content and tension is almost linear over the usual physiologic range of the carbon dioxide contents. Thus, by substituting Pco_2 for dioxide content, $\Delta Pco_2 = k \times Vco_2/\text{cardiac output}$, where k is a constant. Accordingly, ΔPco_2 would be linearly related to carbon dioxide production and inversely related to cardiac output.

Clinical Interpretation of ΔPco_2

Contrary to what was initially thought, ΔPco_2, cannot serve as a reliable marker of tissue hypoxia. However, it could be considered as a marker of adequacy of venous blood flow (i.e., cardiac output) to remove the total carbon dioxide produced by the peripheral tissues.

The clinical implications of this concept can be summarized as follows: an increased ΔPco_2 suggests that the cardiac output is not high enough with respect to the global metabolic conditions; under suspected hypoxic conditions, a high ΔPco_2 could incite the clinician to increase cardiac output with the aim to reduce tissue hypoxia; under aerobic conditions, the presence of a high

ΔP_{CO_2} would mean that blood flow is not high enough, even if the cardiac output is in the normal range. This condition can be associated with an increased oxygen demand and hence increased carbon dioxide production. In patients with severe cardiac failure, ΔP_{CO_2} as well as S_{VO_2}, can serve to titrate inotropic drugs better than cardiac output can because of potential thermogenic effects of these agents (44, 45).

A normal ΔP_{CO_2}, by indicating that the cardiac output is high enough to washout the amount of the carbon dioxide produced from the peripheral tissues, suggests that increasing cardiac output has little chance to improve global oxygenation even in the case of prior hypoxic conditions.

Complications and Contraindications

The adverse effects related to the use of a PAC are relatively rare. They are undoubtedly related to the poor experience of the user and to the catheter length of stay.

Complications Related to Insertion

As with any venous puncture in the upper caval territory, the insertion of a PAC can lead to arterial puncture and bleeding, pneumothorax, the injury of the brachial plexus, and a gas embolism (46). The consequences of such complications are worsened since the diameter of the introducer needed for the PAC insertion is large. More specifically, the contact of the PAC with the atrioventricular node can induce transitory atrioventricular block, but this side effect is rare (47). The introduction of PAC through the tricuspid valve can induce ventricular extrasystoles and more rarely ventricular tachycardia (47–50). These rhythmic complications are related to the duration of the PAC insertion and to a preexisting risk for arrhythmias (47). They are spontaneously reversible in most cases (47, 49).

Infectious and Thrombotic Complications

The bacterial colonization of the PAC is relatively frequent, but infectious endocarditis is rare. This risk is related to the duration of the PAC use. Catheter infection is frequently associated with a venous thromboembolism. Heparin coating of the catheter could reduce such infectious and thromboembolic risks.

Complications Related to Inflation

If the position of the PAC in the pulmonary artery is too distal, the inflation of the balloon can induce a rupture of a pulmonary artery branch (51). This complication is rare but dramatic and can be treated by coil embolization (52). False aneurysm of the pulmonary artery related to the catheter is rare (53). Long-term inflation of the distal balloon in a pulmonary branch may rarely result in infarction in the corresponding pulmonary region.

Complications Related to Withdrawal

As well as its insertion, the withdrawal of PAC can induce transient ventricular arrhythmias (48). Knotting of the catheter is possible at any level (54), especially if its insertion has been long and difficult. Such a knot makes it difficult to extract the catheter. Although the percutaneous extraction of the catheter and the knot are usually still possible, it sometimes requires percutaneous untying (55) or surgical intervention (54).

To conclude, the adverse side effects related to the insertion or to the use of the PAC are relatively rare (56). They are clearly related either to the poor experience of the user or to the duration of the PAC insertion. Thus, the PAC should be carefully removed as soon as possible and it should not be used for longer than 3 or 4 days.

Contraindications

Contraindications for PAC insertion are the common contraindications for central venous catheterization, such as bleeding risk. More specifically, the risk of using a PAC should be considered in patients at high risk of arrhythmias, in patients at high risk of atrioventricular block, and in patients with a preexisting pacemaker.

Although various complications may occur during insertion and maintenance of the inserted PAC, these complications are most often minor. Serious complications occur in less than 0.5% of the patients (57–59). Furthermore, it must be emphasized that these complications are strongly reduced with the experience of the operator and if the PAC is not left indwelling for a long time.

Does the Use of Pulmonary Artery Catheter Alter the Outcome of Critically Ill Patients?

Considering advantages and disadvantages of the PAC, a debate has emerged concerning whether its use may cause harm or benefit in the critically ill. The debate was most seriously raised by the study by Connors et al. (60), showing an increase in the mortality rate, in the cost, and in the length of hospitalization related to PAC utilization. However, this study was observational and enrolled a very heterogeneous population of patients. A meta-analysis of 13 randomized studies showed that in critically ill patients, the use of the PAC neither increased mortality or hospital length of stay nor conferred benefit (59). These neutral results can be explained by three reasons. The first is the lack of management protocols triggered by PAC data in most of the studies included in the meta-analysis. However, in recent randomized studies, PAC-guided therapy did not perform better than clinical evaluation-guided therapy in congestive heart failure (61) or than central venous catheter-guided therapy in acute lung injury (34). The second reason is that the increased accuracy of diagnosis potentially provided by use of the PAC did not lead to improved survival since hemodynamic data triggered use of therapies, which do not affect or even worsen outcome. In this regard, the use of inotropic therapy in patients with decompensated heart failure may affect outcome negatively (62). The third reason for the neutral results of the meta-analysis is that inaccuracies in measurement and interpretation of PAC data may have resulted in inappropriate decisions. This emphasizes the need for physicians and nurses to undergo training in hemodynamic data interpretation to better use the PAC.

Conclusion

The PAC is a hemodynamic tool of considerable interest. It enables continuous monitoring of an extensive panel of hemodynamic variables including cardiac output and pressures in the pulmonary and systemic circulation. It is a unique tool for allowing extensive assessment of global tissue oxygenation. It still remains the gold-standard for the bedside measure of most of these variables. Furthermore, recent studies clearly demonstrate that, although invasive, the PAC does not worsen the outcome of critically ill patients.

References

1. Swan HJ, Ganz W, Forrester J, et al. Catheterization of the heart in man with use of a flow-directed balloon-tipped catheter. N Engl J Med 1970;283: 447–51.
2. Mihm FG, Gettinger A, Hanson CW, 3rd, et al. A multicenter evaluation of a new continuous cardiac output pulmonary artery catheter system. Crit Care Med 1998;26:1346–50.
3. Burchell SA, Yu M, Takiguchi SA, Ohta RM, et al. Evaluation of a continuous cardiac output and mixed venous oxygen saturation catheter in critically ill surgical patients. Crit Care Med 1997;25: 388–91.
4. Birman H, Haq A, Hew E, Aberman A. Continuous monitoring of mixed venous oxygen saturation in hemodynamically unstable patients. Chest 1984;86: 753–6.
5. Martin C, Auffray JP, Saux P, et al. The axillary vein: an alternative approach for percutaneous pulmonary artery catheterization. Chest 1986;90:694–7.
6. Leibowitz AB, Halpern NA, Lee MH, et al. Left-sided superior vena cava: a not-so-unusual vascular anomaly discovered during central venous and pulmonary artery catheterization. Crit Care Med 1992;20:1119–22.
7. Hanson EW, Hannan RL, Baum VC. Pulmonary artery catheter in the coronary sinus: implications of a persistent left superior vena cava for retrograde cardioplegia. J Cardiothorac Vasc Anesth 1998;12: 448–9.
8. Stetz CW, Miller RG, Kelly GE, et al. Reliability of the thermodilution method in the determination of cardiac output in clinical practice. Am Rev Respir Dis 1982;126:1001–4.
9. Boldt J, Menges T, Wollbruck M, et al. Is continuous cardiac output measurement using thermodilution reliable in the critically ill patient? Crit Care Med 1994;22:1913–8.
10. Jacquet L, Hanique G, Glorieux D, et al. Analysis of the accuracy of continuous thermodilution cardiac output measurement. Comparison with

intermittent thermodilution and Fick cardiac output measurement. Intensive Care Med 1996;22:1125–9.
11. Bottiger BW, Soder M, Rauch H, et al. Semi-continuous versus injectate cardiac output measurement in intensive care patients after cardiac surgery. Intensive Care Med 1996;22:312–8.
12. Dhingra VK, Fenwick JC, Walley KR, et al. Lack of agreement between thermodilution and Fick cardiac output in critically ill patients. Chest 2002; 122:990–7.
13. Poli de Figueiredo LF, Malbouisson LM, Varicoda EY, et al. Thermal filament continuous thermodilution cardiac output delayed response limits its value during acute hemodynamic instability. J Trauma 1999;47:288–93.
14. Teboul JL, Zapol WM, Brun-Buisson C, et al. A comparison of pulmonary artery occlusion pressure and left ventricular end-diastolic pressure during mechanical ventilation with PEEP in patients with severe ARDS. Anesthesiology 1989;70:261–6.
15. Pinsky MR. Pulmonary artery occlusion pressure. Intensive Care Med 2003;29:19–22.
16. Teboul JL, Andrivet P, Ansquer M, et al. A bedside index assessing the reliability of pulmonary occlusion pressure during mechanical ventilation with positive end-expiratory pressure. J Crit Care 1992; 7:22–9.
17. Teboul JL, Pinsky MR, Mercat A, et al. Estimating cardiac filling pressure in mechanically ventilated patients with hyperinflation. Crit Care Med 2000;28:3631–6.
18. Pinsky M, Vincent JL, De Smet JM. Estimating left ventricular filling pressure during positive end-expiratory pressure in humans. Am Rev Respir Dis 1991;143:25–31.
19. Raper R, Sibbald WJ. Misled by the wedge? The Swan-Ganz catheter and left ventricular preload. Chest 1986;89:427–34.
20. Kumar A, Anel R, Bunnell E, et al. Pulmonary artery occlusion pressure and central venous pressure fail to predict ventricular filling volume, cardiac performance, or the response to volume infusion in normal subjects. Crit Care Med 2004;32:691–9.
21. Crexells C, Chatterjee K, Forrester JS, et al. Optimal level of filling pressure in the left side of the heart in acute myocardial infarction. N Engl J Med 1973;289:1263–6.
22. Nunes S, Ruokonen E, Takala J. Pulmonary capillary pressures during the acute respiratory distress syndrome. Intensive Care Med 2003;29:2174–9.
23. Teboul JL, Andrivet P, Ansquer M, et al. Bedside evaluation of the resistance of large and medium pulmonary veins in various lung diseases. J Appl Physiol 1992;72:998–1003.
24. Cope DK, Allison RC, Parmentier JL, et al. Measurement of effective pulmonary capillary pressure using the pressure profile after pulmonary artery occlusion. Crit Care Med 1986;14:16–22.
25. Pinsky MR. Clinical significance of pulmonary artery occlusion pressure. Intensive Care Med 2003;29:175–8.
26. Wiedemann HP. Wedge pressure in pulmonary veno-occlusive disease. N Engl J Med 1986;315: 1233.
27. Teboul JL, Douguet D, Mercat A, et al. Effects of catecholamines on the pulmonary venous bed in sheep. Crit Care Med 1998;26:1569–75.
28. Bindels AJ, van der Hoeven JG, Meinders AE. Pulmonary artery wedge pressure and extravascular lung water in patients with acute cardiogenic pulmonary edema requiring mechanical ventilation. Am J Cardiol 1999;84:1158–63.
29. Ferguson ND, Meade MO, Hallett DC, et al. High values of the pulmonary artery wedge pressure in patients with acute lung injury and acute respiratory distress syndrome. Intensive Care Med 2002;28: 1073–7.
30. Lemaire F, Teboul JL, Cinotti L, et al. Acute left ventricular dysfunction during unsuccessful weaning from mechanical ventilation. Anesthesiology 1988;69:171–9.
31. Monnet X, Teboul JL. Invasive measures of left ventricular preload. Curr Opin Crit Care 2006;12:235–40.
32. Michard F, Teboul JL. Predicting fluid responsiveness in ICU patients: a critical analysis of the evidence. Chest 2002;121:2000–8.
33. Vincent JL, Weil MH. Fluid challenge revisited. Crit Care Med 2006;34:1333–7.
34. The National Heart, Lung, and Blood Institute Acute Respiratory Distress Syndrome (ARDS) Clinical Trials Network. Pulmonary-artery versus central venous catheter to guide treatment of acute lung injury. N Engl J Med 2006;354:2213–2224.
35. The National Heart, Lung, and Blood Institute Acute Respiratory Distress Syndrome (ARDS) Clinical Trials Network. Comparison of Two Fluid-Management Strategies in Acute Lung Injury. N Engl J Med 2006;354:2564–75.
36. Vincent JL, Thirion M, Brimioulle S, et al. Thermodilution measurement of right ventricular ejection fraction with a modified pulmonary artery catheter. Intensive Care Med 1986;12:33–8.
37. Spinale FG, Smith AC, Carabello BA, et al. Right ventricular function computed by thermodilution

and ventriculography. A comparison of methods. J Thorac Cardiovasc Surg 1990;99:141–52.
38. Spinale FG, Mukherjee R, Tanaka R, et al. The effects of valvular regurgitation on thermodilution ejection fraction measurements. Chest 1992;101: 723–31.
39. Hassan E, Roffman DS, Applefeld MM. The value of mixed venous oxygen saturation as a therapeutic indicator in the treatment of advanced congestive heart failure. Am Heart J 1987;113:743–9.
40. Richard C, Thuillez C, Pezzano M, et al. Relationship between mixed venous oxygen saturation and cardiac index in patients with chronic congestive heart failure. Chest 1989;95:1289–94.
41. Teboul JL, Annane D, Thuillez C, et al. Effects of cardiovascular drugs on oxygen consumption/ oxygen delivery relationship in patients with congestive heart failure. Chest 1992;101:1582–7.
42. Teboul JL, Graini L, Boujdaria R, et al. Cardiac index vs oxygen-derived parameters for rational use of dobutamine in patients with congestive heart failure. Chest 1993;103:81–5.
43. Nunez S, Maisel A. Comparison between mixed venous oxygen saturation and thermodilution cardiac output in monitoring patients with severe heart failure treated with milrinone and dobutamine. Am Heart J 1998;135:383–8.
44. Gattinoni L, Brazzi L, Pelosi P, et al. A trial of goal-oriented hemodynamic therapy in critically ill patients. SvO2 Collaborative Group. N Engl J Med 1995;333:1025–32.
45. Teboul JL, Mercat A, Lenique F, et al. Value of the venous-arterial PCO2 gradient to reflect the oxygen supply to demand in humans: effects of dobutamine. Crit Care Med 1998;26:1007–10.
46. Patel C, Laboy V, Venus B, et al. Acute complications of pulmonary artery catheter insertion in critically ill patients. Crit Care Med 1986;14: 195–7.
47. Sprung CL, Pozen RG, Rozanski JJ, et al. Advanced ventricular arrhythmias during bedside pulmonary artery catheterization. Am J Med 1982;72:203–8.
48. Damen J. Ventricular arrhythmias during insertion and removal of pulmonary artery catheters. Chest 1985;88:190–3.
49. Davies MJ, Cronin KD, Domaingue CM. Pulmonary artery catheterisation. An assessment of risks and benefits in 220 surgical patients. Anaesth Intensive Care 1982;10:9–14.
50. Iberti TJ, Benjamin E, Gruppi L, et al. Ventricular arrhythmias during pulmonary artery catheterization in the intensive care unit. Prospective study. Am J Med 1985;78:451–4.
51. Mullerworth MH, Angelopoulos P, Couyant MA, et al. Recognition and management of catheter-induced pulmonary artery rupture. Ann Thorac Surg 1998;66:1242–5.
52. Tayoro J, Dequin PF, Delhommais A, et al. Rupture of pulmonary artery induced by Swan-Ganz catheter: success of coil embolization. Intensive Care Med 1997;23:198–200.
53. Ferretti GR, Thony F, Link KM, et al. False aneurysm of the pulmonary artery induced by a Swan-Ganz catheter: clinical presentation and radiologic management. Am J Roentgenol 1996;167:941–5.
54. Koh KF, Chen FG. The irremovable swan: a complication of the pulmonary artery catheter. J Cardiothorac Vasc Anesth 1998;12:561–2.
55. Bhatti WA, Sinha S, Rowlands P. Percutaneous untying of a knot in a retained Swan-Ganz catheter. Cardiovasc Intervent Radiol 2000;23:224–5.
56. Boyd KD, Thomas SJ, Gold J, Boyd AD. A prospective study of complications of pulmonary artery catheterizations in 500 consecutive patients. Chest 1983;84:245–9.
57. Richard C, Warszawski J, Anguel N, et al. Early use of the pulmonary artery catheter and outcomes in patients with shock and acute respiratory distress syndrome: a randomized controlled trial. JAMA 2003;290:2713–20.
58. Ivanov R, Allen J, Calvin JE. The incidence of major morbidity in critically ill patients managed with pulmonary artery catheters: a meta-analysis. Crit Care Med 2000;28(3):615–9.
59. Shah KB, Rao TL, Laughlin S, et al. A review of pulmonary artery catheterization in 6,245 patients. Anesthesiology 1984;61:271–5.
60. Connors AF Jr, Speroff T, Dawson NV, et al. The effectiveness of right heart catheterization in the initial care of critically ill patients. SUPPORT Investigators. JAMA 1996;276:889–97.
61. Binanay C, Califf RM, Hasselblad V, et al; ESCAPE Investigators and ESCAPE Study Coordinators. Evaluation study of congestive heart failure and pulmonary artery catheterization effectiveness: the ESCAPE trial. JAMA 2005;294:1625–33.
62. Bayram M, De Luca L, Massie MB, et al. Reassessment of dobutamine, dopamine, and milrinone in the management of acute heart failure syndromes. Am J Cardiol 2005;96:47G–58G.

39 Assessment of Critically Ill Patients with Acute Heart Failure Syndromes Using Echocardiography Doppler

Philippe Vignon

Acute heart failure (AHF) is defined by the presence of symptoms of heart failure (at rest or during exercise) in conjunction with objective evidence of cardiac dysfunction (1). It may correspond to either a new-onset heart failure or a decompensation of chronic heart failure. Symptoms of AHF may predominantly reflect the decrease in cardiac output and associated peripheral hypoperfusion (e.g., fatigue, cardiogenic shock), the pulmonary congestion (e.g., breathlessness, pulmonary edema), or the peripheral congestion (e.g., hepatomegaly, peripheral edema, raised venous pressure) (Fig. 39.1). With the exception of mitral stenosis, pulmonary congestion usually develops secondary to a diastolic dysfunction of the left ventricle (LV) with elevated filling pressure, whereas peripheral hypoperfusion predominantly reflects LV systolic dysfunction. Other clinical presentations of AHF include hypertensive AHF, pulmonary edema, cardiogenic shock, high output failure, and right heart failure (1). The diagnosis of AHF relies on the clinical judgment based on patient history, physical signs, and appropriate investigations (1).

Recent guidelines recommend that objective documentation of cardiac dysfunction related to AHF should preferably be obtained by echocardiography (1). Echocardiography is currently the only diagnostic technique that provides real-time imaging of the heart at the bedside, allows a comprehensive hemodynamic assessment, and clearly identifies all clinical presentations of the AHF syndrome (Fig. 39.1). In the setting of patients presenting with AHF, echocardiography Doppler is an unparalleled diagnostic tool that yields crucial information on both the cardiac anatomy and function. Ease of use and instantaneous diagnostic capability allow accurate and expeditious quantitative assessment of cardiac pump function as well as the identification of both the mechanism and etiology of AHF. Accordingly, echocardiography became one of the most versatile imaging modalities for the assessment of patients with AHF in various clinical settings, including the intensive care unit (ICU), the emergency department, the operating theater, or the recovery room (2).

This chapter discusses the practical use of echocardiography Doppler as a first-line diagnostic technique, at the bedside, in patients presenting to the ICU with a AHF syndrome, in order to (1) document heart failure and quantify LV pump function at rest using simple and easy-to-obtain indices (ejection fraction, cardiac output); (2) identify the origin of AHF, according to predominantly left or right heart failure; and (3) guide initial management of AHF patients presenting with chest pain or cardiogenic shock. The use of echocardiography in AHF patients admitted to the ICU can be extrapolated to other clinical settings (e.g., emergency department, perioperative period). The long-term management of heart failure using ultrasound, the prognostic value of echocardiographic parameters in chronic heart failure patients, the use of stress echocardiography (3), and the potential clinical value of recently available hand-held echocardiography in ICU patients (4,5) are not discussed here.

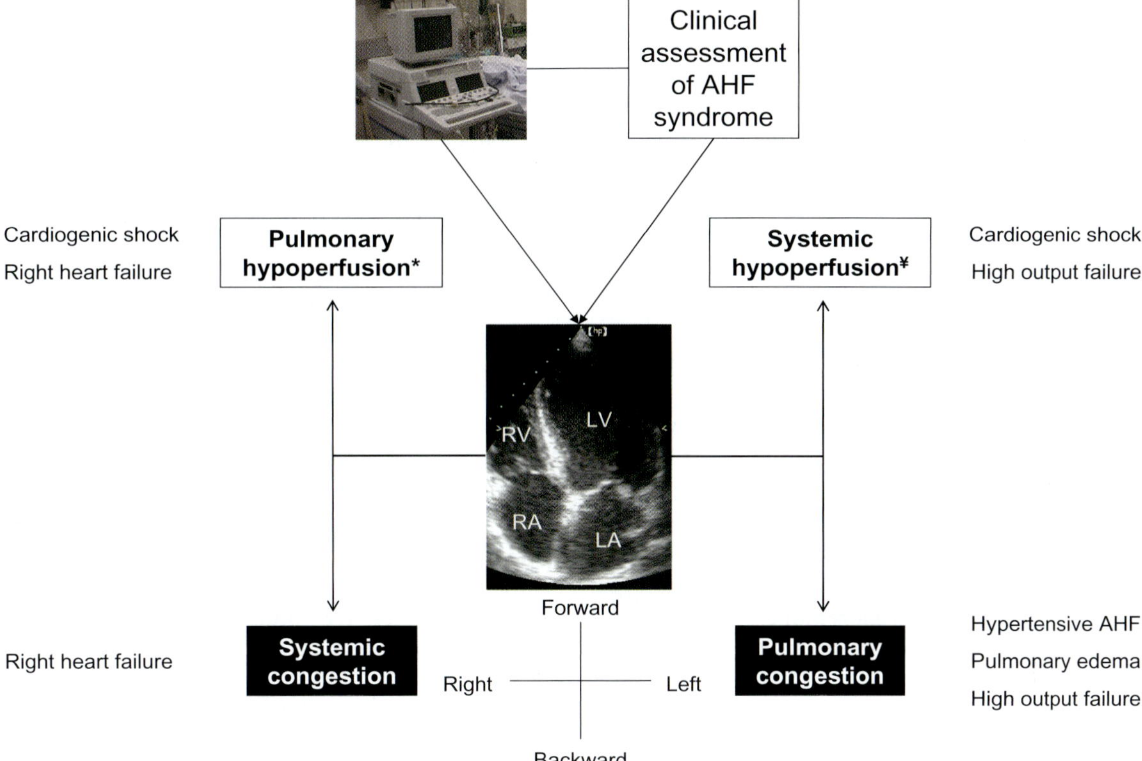

FIGURE 39.1. Summary of potential clinical presentations of acute heart failure (AHF) syndromes. Symptoms and physical signs may predominantly reflect venous congestion or hypoperfusion, and the left or the right heart may be principally involved. When guided by the clinical examination, echocardiography Doppler determines both the mechanism (e.g., systolic or diastolic dysfunction, left or right ventricular failure, high output failure) and etiology (e.g., cardiomyopathy, valvulopathy) of AHF (see text for details). *Decreased LV filling reserve. ¥May also be the result of a predominant RV systolic dysfunction. RV, right ventricle; RA, right atrium; LV, left ventricle; LA, left atrium.

Diagnosis of Left Heart Failure

Transthoracic echocardiography (TTE) is a widely available imaging modality that is currently the preferred method for the documentation of cardiac dysfunction at rest (1). Although transesophageal echocardiography (TEE) is not recommended in spontaneously breathing patients with suspected AHF (1), it is frequently required in ICU patients under ventilator who present with decompensated or new-onset heart failure or with cardiogenic shock. Transesophageal echocardiography is recommended in ventilated patients sustaining circulatory failure (6), especially in the perioperative period (7), and is frequently superior to TTE when a comprehensive hemodynamic assessment is required in complex clinical situations (2).

Regardless of the echocardiographic approach (TTE or TEE), the identification of left heart failure relies on the measurement of quantitative parameters of LV systolic function. Ejection fraction (EF) and cardiac output are the most frequently used echocardiographic indices of LV systolic function. Importantly, as all parameters of systolic function routinely used on clinical grounds, these indices are frequency and load-dependent. Accordingly, they should be considered as parameters of LV pump function rather than indices of myocardial contractility, and interpreted in light of LV loading conditions. Left ventricular ejection fraction (LVEF) and cardiac output reflect the complex interactions between heart rate, LV loading conditions (preload and afterload), and LV contractility (8). These indices facilitate the serial evaluation of LV systolic performance after acute therapeutic interventions (e.g., ventilator settings, administration of vasopressors, or inotropic support). Other echocardiographic parameters have been proposed to assess more precisely myocardial contractility, but their measurement is cumbersome and difficult to obtain routinely in clinical practice (9).

Ejection Fraction

Left ventricular ejection fraction is a frequently used parameter of pump function in AHF patients because it helps distinguish patients with LV systolic dysfunction from those with preserved systolic performance (e.g., diastolic heart failure, high output failure) (1). Since qualitative eyeball evaluation of LV pump function may be inaccurate (10), the measurement of LVEF remains advocated (11). Two-dimensional echocardiography facilitates the measurement of LV volumes and EF using different methods, the most widely recommended being the modified Simpson's rule applied in two orthogonal planes (0 degrees and ~90 degrees) (12). Although echocardiography usually underestimates true LV volumes when compared to reference imaging techniques (12), the evaluation of EF remains fairly accurate since both LV end-diastolic and LV end-systolic volumes are underestimated (12). Left ventricular ejection fraction is measured on two-dimensional still-frames and expressed as a percentage, as follows:

$$\text{LVEF (\%)} = (\text{LVEDV} - \text{LVESV})/\text{LVEDV} \quad (1)$$

where LVEDV denotes LV end-diastolic volume and LVESV denotes LV end-systolic volume, both expressed in milliliters.

This equation has several implications. First, LVEDV is physiologically the combined result of heart rate, LV compliance and preload, whereas LVESV is determined by both LV contractility and afterload (Fig. 39.2). Consequently, EF is conceptually a load-dependent parameter of cardiac function (8,9,13). This is particularly relevant in AHF patients since EF is maximally sensitive to changes in loading conditions when LV function is severely depressed (8). The LV volume overload (e.g., mitral insufficiency) may result in increased EF (proportionally to the regurgitated volume), whereas acute LV pressure overload (e.g., high systolic blood pressure) may decrease EF. Second, LV volumes are also influenced by the chronic remodeling of LV wall and cavity geometry (Fig. 39.2), with variable results on myocardial wall stress (9). The LV cavity tends to dilate in the presence of elevated end-diastolic pressure (e.g., severe LV systolic dysfunction, volume overload), while myocardial hypertrophy usually develops in the presence of chronic LV pressure overload (e.g., hypertension, aortic stenosis). Traditionally, EF tends to be underestimated in the presence of an enlarged LV cavity, whereas it tends to be overestimated in case of small LV cavity (e.g., concentric LV hypertrophy). Third, ventricular interactions may also influence LVEDV (Fig. 39.2) when the right ventricle (RV) acutely dilates in the stiff pericardium (i.e., acute cor pulmonale), or in the presence of increased pericardial pressure (i.e., tamponade). In these clinical circumstances, heart–lung interactions will also periodically alter LV volumes (abnormal ventricular septal motion).

All indices of LV systolic function based on the EF concept (i.e., fractional shortening, fractional area change) should be used with caution in patients with decompensated ischemic cardiomyopathy or in the presence of grossly distorted LV cavity anatomy (e.g., LV aneurysm). When located in the tomographic plane of LV cavity measurements, regional wall motion abnormalities (RWMAs) may lead to underestimate LV pump function. Conversely, LV systolic performance may be overestimated if an RWMA is present outside the tomographic plane in which LV cavity measurements are performed. In this specific setting, biplane LVEF measurement using the modified Simpson's rule is particularly recommended (12), and the measurement of cardiac output using spectral Doppler is a valuable alternative approach (see below). Conditions of validity of LVEF measurement are summarized in Table 39.1. Reference values of indices based on the EF concept are listed in Table 39.2 and their measurement is illustrated on Figure 39.3. In patients with a known cardiac disease, it is usually conceded that LVEF values in the range of 40% to 50% are of little clinical significance (9). In patients without cardiopathy, LVEF oscillates physiologically between 60% and 70% (8), and a reduction of LVEF below 45% usually indicates impaired myocardial function, regardless of loading conditions (13). Normal values of LV

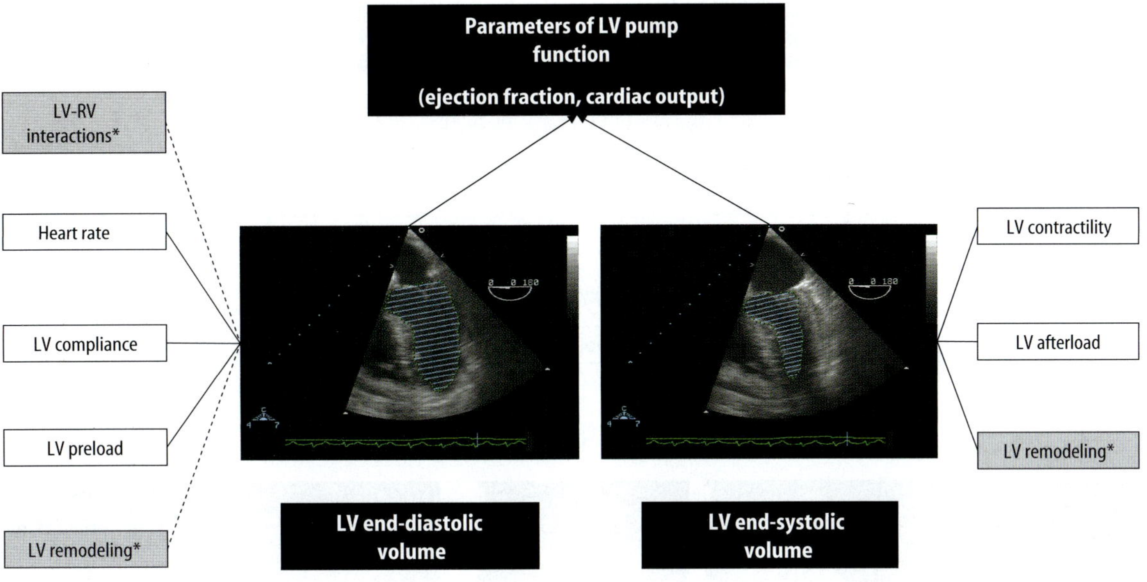

FIGURE 39.2. Factors influencing end-diastolic and end-systolic LV volumes, as well as LV ejection fraction and cardiac output. In this patient with a history of hypertension, LV volumes measured using the modified Simpson's rule were small, partly due to a mild concentric LV hypertrophy. The LV ejection fraction and cardiac output were within normal range (63% and 5.8 L/min, respectively). Note that cardiac output was mostly generated by elevated heart rate (131 bpm) since LV stroke volume was as low as 44 mL. *See text for details. LV, left ventricle; RV, right ventricle.

TABLE 39.1. Recommendations for the measurement of left ventricular (LV) ejection fraction

Step	Conditions for an accurate measurement of LV ejection fraction
1	Obtain a true apical transthoracic echocardiography (TTE) or transesophageal (TEE) four-chamber view of the heart that excludes the aortic valve
2	Position the transducer to clearly identify LV endocardial borders (especially the lateral wall) throughout the cardiac and ventilatory cycles
3	Avoid foreshortening the LV long axis, especially when using TEE
4	When using the modified Simpson's rule, incorporate mitral papillary muscles in the manual planimetry of LV cavity at both end-diastole and end-systole
5	In the presence of extended RWMA or grossly distorted LV anatomy, measure LV ejection fraction in two orthogonal planes (0 and 90 degrees) and consider using Doppler measurement of cardiac output
6	Perform several measurements at end-expiration, on nonconsecutive heart beats, check for consistency, and average values

RWMA, regional wall motion abnormality.

TABLE 39.2. Calculation and reference values of echocardiographic indices of LV pump function based on the ejection fraction concept

Parameter	Formula	Normal values*
Fractional shortening (parasternal long axis view, TTE)	(LVEDD—LVESD)/LVEDD (mm)	25–46%
Fractional area change (short-axis view, TTE or TEE)	(LVEDA—LVESA)/LVEDA (cm^2)	36–64%
Ejection fraction (four-chamber view, TTE or TEE)	(LVEDV—LVESV)/LVEDV (mL)	55–75% or male: 70% ± 7% female: 65% ± 10%

*Range or mean ± standard deviation (SD). TTE, transthoracic echocardiography; TEE, transesophageal echocardiography; LVEDD, left ventricular end-diastolic diameter; LVESD, left ventricular end-systolic diameter; LVEDA, left ventricular end-diastolic area; LVESA, left ventricular end-systolic area; LVEDV, left ventricular end-diastolic volume; LVESV, left ventricular end-systolic volume.

Source: Schiller et al. (12) and Caroll and Hess (13).

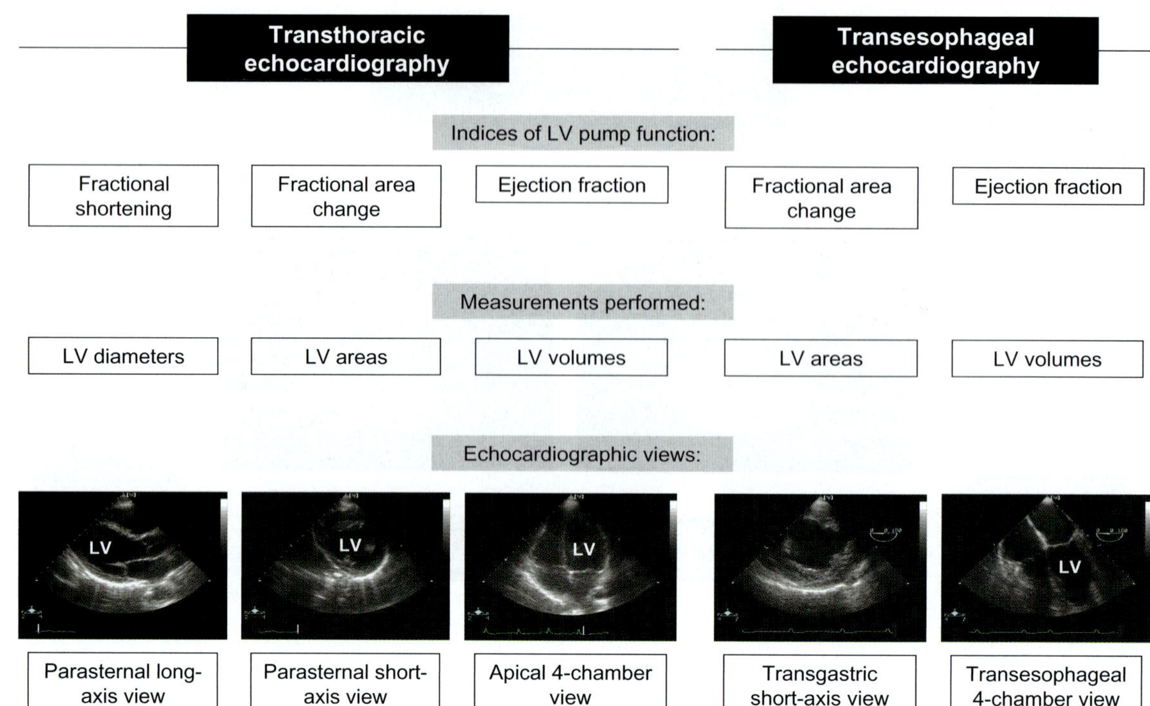

FIGURE 39.3. Two-dimensional end-diastolic still frames illustrating the measurement of indices based on the ejection fraction concept that are routinely used to quantitatively assess LV pump function, with transthoracic or transesophageal echocardiography. The same measurements are performed on end-systolic still frames in corresponding echocardiographic views, and the ejection fraction concept is applied to calculate indices of LV pump function [(end-diastolic measurement—end-systolic measurement)/end-diastolic measurement, expressed as a percentage] LV, left ventricle.

fractional shortening and LV fractional area change exceed 25% and 35%, respectively (Table 39.2).

Cardiac Output and Derived Indices

Combining the cross-sectional area (measured using two-dimensional imaging) and the stroke distance traveled by the column of blood at the same level (measured using spectral Doppler) enables the accurate determination of stroke volume—and hence cardiac output—at different anatomic sites of the heart (14). Most clinical trials support TEE as a reliable method for measuring cardiac output and tracking its changes after therapeutic interventions (15,16). In the absence of relevant aortic valvulopathy or subaortic obstruction, aortic annulus and LV outflow tract are the anatomical sites that appear to provide a lower failure rate and higher accuracy for the measurement of cardiac stroke volume when compared to the ascending aorta, the pulmonary artery, or other valvular orifices (14,17). Pulsed-wave Doppler is usually advocated since it enables matching the velocities measured with a corresponding cross-sectional area (14). In the absence of space resolution, continuous-wave Doppler measures maximal blood flow velocities, which are usually located at the aortic valve orifice. Accordingly, it may lead to an overestimate of cardiac output in the presence of a sclerotic aortic valve. In patients without aortic valvulopathy, continuous-wave Doppler has been shown to accurately determine cardiac output perioperatively when assuming a triangular shape for the measurement of aortic valve area (18). Finally, measurement of LV stroke volume appears more accurate when using the Doppler method rather than two-dimensional determination of LV volumes (19,20).

Conditions of validity of LV stroke volume measurement are summarized in Table 39.3. The LV stroke volume is usually measured at the level of LV outflow tract using the pulsed-wave Doppler method as follows (Fig. 39.4):

$$\text{LV stroke volume (mL)} = (\Pi \cdot d^2 / 4) \cdot VTI \quad (2)$$

where d is the diameter of LV outflow tract measured at the level of insertion of aortic cusps (cm) and VTI is the velocity-time integral of pulsed-wave Doppler pattern recorded at the same level (cm). The derived indices of cardiac function are then easily obtained using standard formulas:

$$\text{Cardiac output (L/min)} = \text{LV stroke volume} \cdot \text{heart rate} \quad (3)$$

$$\text{LV stroke index (mL/m}^2\text{)} = \text{LV stroke volume/Body surface area} \quad (4)$$

$$\text{Cardiac index (L/min/m}^2\text{)} = \text{Cardiac output/Body surface area} \quad (5)$$

In patients presenting with AHF, sinus tachycardia may represent a confounding factor by preserving cardiac output within a normal range despite a severely depressed LV systolic function. In this clinical setting, LV stroke volume is presumably a better index of LV pump function since it is less altered by heart rate. Similarly, LV stroke index may be used rather than the cardiac index to take into account the body size and allow between patient comparisons.

Indices of LV pump function have a fairly large normal range (21,22), according to proposed reference values in the literature (Table 39.4). Since the measurement of LV outflow tract diameter is squared for the calculation of LV stroke volume, any error will result in a substantial under- or overestimation. In addition, the reproducibility for measurement of velocity time integral is higher than that of aortic annulus diameter (mean percent error: 2.4% ± 1.5% and 6.0% ± 1.6%, respectively) (14), and a change in LV outflow tract diameter induced by acute care is unlikely to occur. Accordingly, it is usually preferable to use the same diameter value when serial determination of LV stroke volume is required, and to measure solely Doppler velocity time integral at each echocardiographic assessment.

Table 39.3. Recommendations for the measurement of cardiac output using the Doppler method at the level of LV outflow tract (see Fig. 39.4)

Step	Conditions for an accurate measurement of cardiac output
1	Exclude a relevant aortic valvulopathy or a subaortic obstruction using color Doppler mapping and continuous-wave Doppler
2	Obtain a parasternal long-axis view of the heart (TTE) or a transesophageal 120-degree view of the ascending aorta (TEE)
3	Magnify LV outflow tract when zooming on the aortic root and slightly rotate the transducer (TTE or multiplane TEE) as required to obtain a true longitudinal view of the aortic valve with symmetric Valsalva sinuses
4	Measure the maximal LV outflow tract diameter (*d*) during the cardiac cycle (select the corresponding still frame using the cine loop) at the precise level of aortic cusps insertion, from inner edge to inner edge
5	Repeat measurement on non consecutive heart beats, check for consistency and average three or more values
6	Calculate the cross-sectional area (CSA) of LV outflow tract as follows: CSA (cm^2) = ($\Pi \cdot d^2$)/4
7	When using TTE, obtain an apical five-chamber view of the heart with a clear visualization of the LV outflow tract and aortic valve; when using TEE, use the transgastric 120-degree view (16) or the deep transgastric transverse (0-degree) five-chamber view of the heart (15)
8	Place the pulsed-wave Doppler sample at the exact level where LV outflow tract diameter was measured (usually immediately proximal to the aortic annulus), while attempting to reduce the angle between the ultrasound beam and blood flow (<20 degrees)
9	Use a high recording speed (100 mm/s) Use ECG and respiratory tracings, especially in ventilated patients Set velocity filter as low as possible (200 to 600 Hz)
10	Trace manually the velocity time integral (VTI) of the (systolic) aortic Doppler pattern to obtain the stroke distance (in cm) of ejected blood flow Trace the external contour of the spectral display to improve reproducibility
11	Repeat measurement on nonconsecutive heart beats and respiratory cycles, check for consistency and average three or more values
12	Calculate LV stroke volume as follows: LV stroke volume (mL) = CSA (cm^2) · *VTI* (cm)*
13	Calculate cardiac output and cardiac index as follows: Cardiac output (L/min) = LV stroke volume (mL) · Heart rate (bpm) Cardiac index (L/min/m^2) = Cardiac output (L/min)/Body surface area (m^2)

*If one assumes the cosinus of the angle between the ultrasound beam and flow to be close to 1 (angle <20 degrees), the cross-sectional area of flow to be constant, the velocity profile to be flat (14). LV, left ventricle; TTE, transthoracic echocardiography; TEE, transesophageal echocardiography.

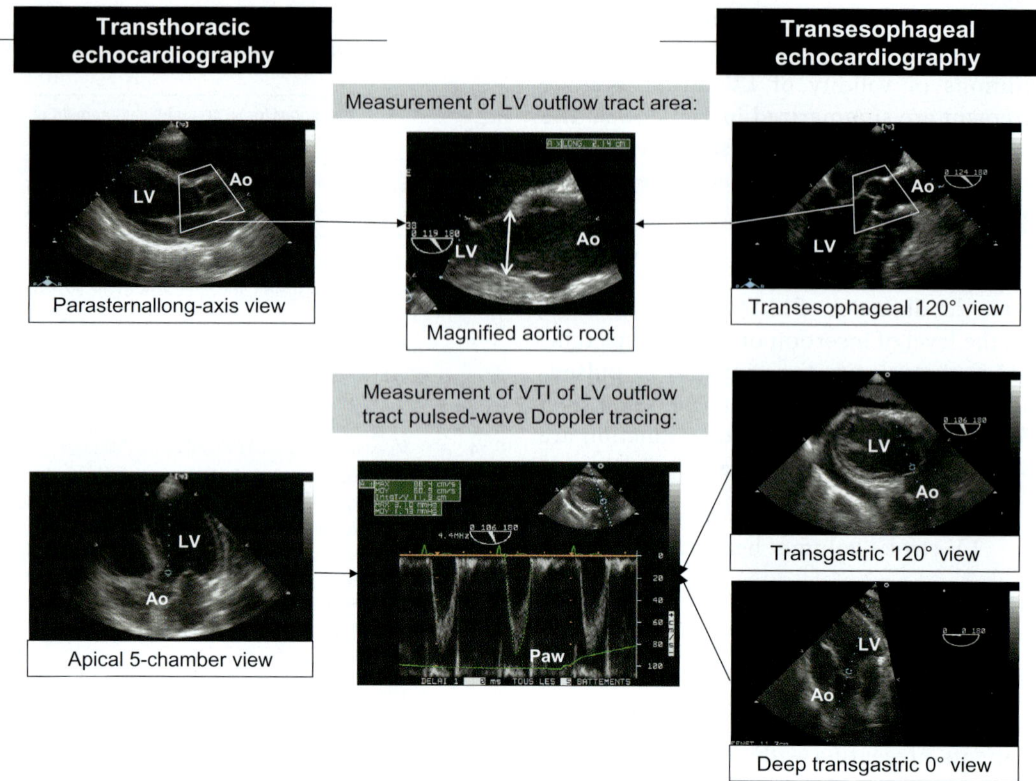

FIGURE 39.4. Measurement of LV stroke volume using the Doppler method applied to the LV outflow tract. Two-dimensional echocardiography is used to measure LV outflow tract diameter and calculate its surface. Pulsed-wave Doppler sample is applied at the same anatomic site (blue open circles overimposed on two-dimensional still frames) to record systolic blood flow velocities, and VTI is measured to obtain blood stroke distance. The LV stroke volume is then calculated as the product of LV outflow tract cross-sectional area and blood stroke distance (see text for details). In this ventilated patient (middle panel), LV outflow tract cross-sectional area was 3.59 cm^2 and VTI was 11.9 cm, resulting in a stroke volume of 43 mL. LV, left ventricle; Ao, ascending aorta; VTI, velocity time integral; Paw, airway pressure curve.

TABLE 39.4. Calculation and reference values of main indices of LV pump function measured using echocardiography Doppler (see text for details)

Parameter	Formula	Normal range
Stroke volume (mL)	$[(\Pi \cdot d^2)/4] \cdot VTI$	50–100*
Stroke index (mL/m^2)	Stroke volume/body surface area	30–65
Cardiac output (L/min)	Stroke volume · heart rate	–*
Cardiac index (L/min/m^2)	Cardiac output/body surface area	2.8–4.2

*Vary with body size. LV, left ventricle; *d*, diameter of LV outflow tract (cm); *VTI*, velocity-time integral of Doppler profile recorded at the level of the LV outflow tract (cm).
Source: Schlant and Sonnenblick (21) and Hall et al. (22).

Acute Heart Failure Syndrome with Pulmonary Venous Congestion

Pulmonary edema is the most severe clinical presentation of pulmonary venous congestion. The diagnosis of cardiogenic pulmonary edema relies on the documentation of (markedly) elevated pulmonary venous pressure, but not on the presence of a LV systolic dysfunction. High LV filling pressure enables the distinction between cardiogenic pulmonary edema and the acute respiratory distress syndrome (ARDS) (23). In contrast, LV systolic performance is not discriminative, since a preserved LV systolic function may be observed in the presence of a cardiogenic pulmonary edema (e.g., massive mitral regurgitation), whereas ARDS may be associated with a depressed LV pump function (e.g., septic shock). On clinical grounds, pulmonary artery occlusion pressure (PAOP) is used as a surrogate of pulmonary venous pressure and traditionally measured invasively. Although right heart catheterization remains the reference method for measuring PAOP, echocardiography Doppler appears to be an accurate and less invasive alternative diagnostic approach (2).

In the setting of cardiac patients presenting with AHF, several clinical studies have uniformly shown that Doppler indices could be valuable in assessing LV filling pressure using two distinct approaches: (1) the prediction of the absolute value of PAOP using complex equations that combine several Doppler parameters (quantitative approach); or (2) the prediction of different levels of PAOP using threshold values of a single Doppler parameter (semiquantitative approach). The latter diagnostic strategy appears adequately suited for the assessment of patients with suspected cardiogenic pulmonary edema, since the prediction of a pulmonary artery wedge pressure >18 mm Hg facilitates confidently ruling out an ARDS (23).

Estimation of Left Ventricular Filling Pressure with Doppler

Doppler velocities are generated by pressure gradients in the circulation. Accordingly, both the mitral and pulmonary vein pulsed-wave Doppler velocity profiles are markedly altered by variations in LV filling pressure. Importantly, these Doppler patterns are also influenced by numerous additional factors, such as age and LV diastolic properties (Fig. 39.5). Since cardiogenic pulmonary edema usually occurs in patients with a

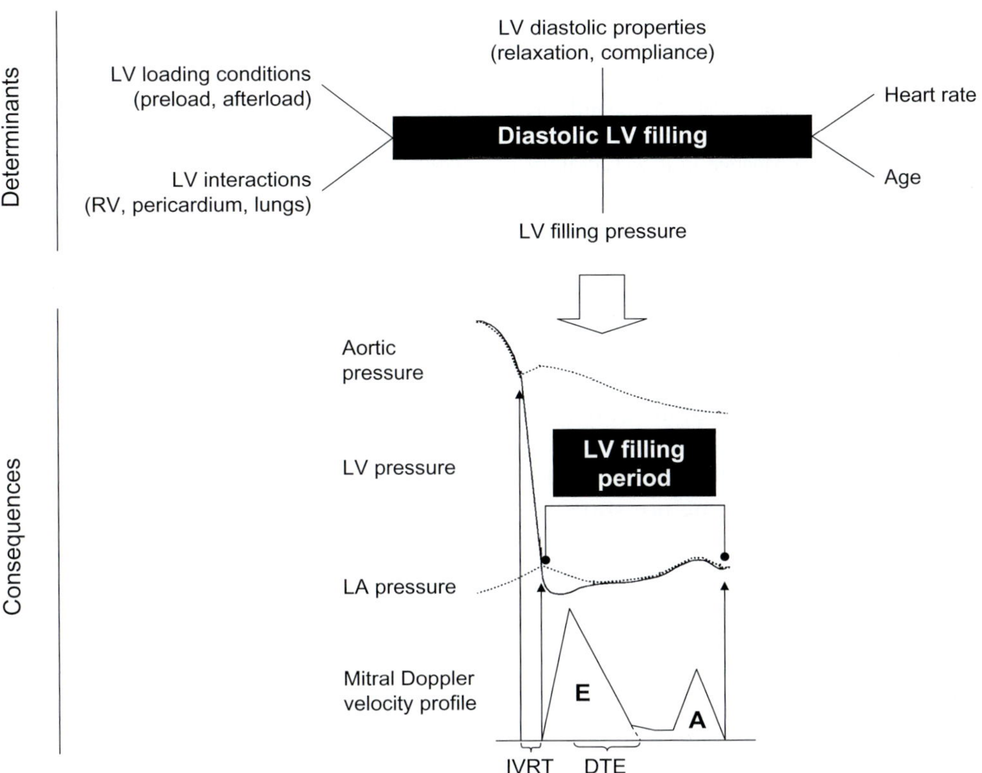

Figure 39.5. Determinants of LV diastolic filling and subsequent mitral Doppler velocity profile. Upper panel: Numerous factors, extrinsic or intrinsic to the heart, substantially alter LV filling during diastole. Lower panel: Mitral Doppler velocities reflect the variations of diastolic LA-LV pressure gradient throughout LV filling. LV, left ventricle; LA, left atrium; RV, right ventricle; IVRT, isovolemic relaxation time; DTE, deceleration time of early diastolic E wave.

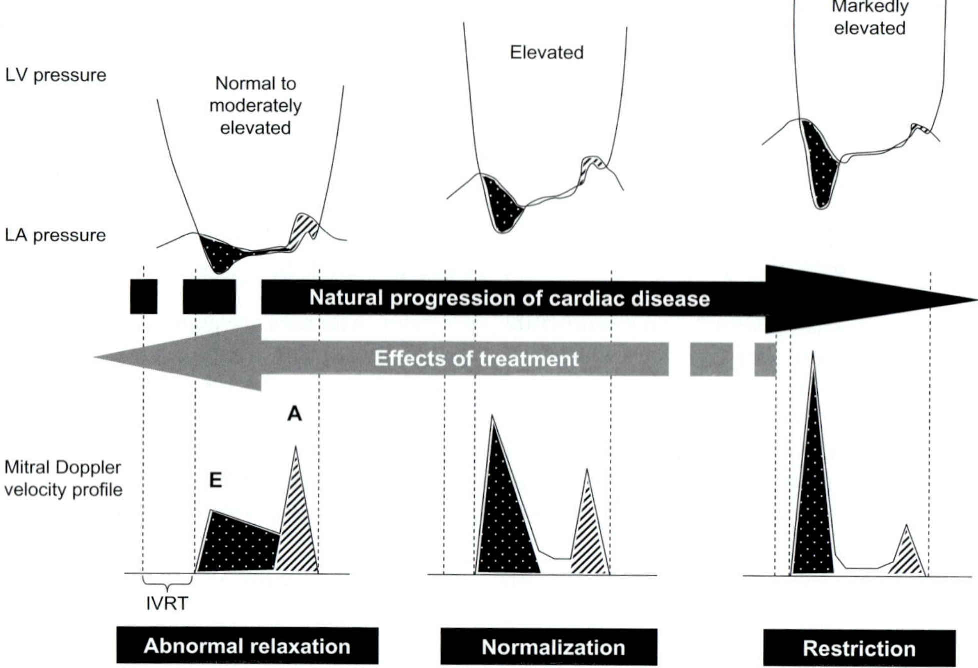

Figure 39.6. Schematic representation of the natural progression of LV filling pressures in the presence of a diastolic dysfunction (heart rate is assumed to be constant and within normal range). LA-LV pressure gradient determines instantaneous mitral Doppler velocities of early diastolic E wave (dotted areas) and late diastolic A wave (dashed areas). Note that the progressive elevation of left cardiac pressures results in a gradual reduction of the atrial contribution toward LV filling, as reflected by an increasingly prominent E wave on mitral Doppler velocity profiles. Note also that (acute) treatment may (abruptly) decrease LV filling pressures, and hence modify the mitral Doppler inflow pattern, with the exception of end-stage cardiac disease with severely restrictive LV filling. LV, left ventricle; LA, left atrium; IVRT, isovolemic relaxation time.

known cardiac disease, it should be emphasized that distinct mitral and pulmonary vein Doppler patterns have been described during the natural progression of LV diastolic dysfunction (24). Practically, the more prominent the early diastolic mitral E wave, when compared to the late diastolic A wave, the higher the LV filling pressures (Fig. 39.6). This holds true in the presence of a relevant mitral regurgitation (25). Thus, the documentation of either a normalized or a restrictive mitral Doppler pattern is consistent with elevated or markedly increased LV filling pressures (Fig. 39.6). Similarly, a prominent diastolic D wave, when compared to the systolic S wave, on the pulmonary vein Doppler pattern is usually consistent with elevated left atrial filling pressures (26). Figure 39.7 depicts how to obtain pulsed-wave Doppler tracings, and Figure 39.8 illustrates the

Figure 39.8. Schematic representation of main pulsed-wave Doppler indices that can be measured from mitral and pulmonary vein Doppler tracings. Left panels: Timing of mitral and pulmonary vein Doppler velocity profiles with respect to ECG tracing. Note that the S wave may be biphasic. Right panels: Pulsed-wave Doppler parameters routinely measured to assess LV filling pressure are maximal velocities and velocity time integrals of E, A, S, and D waves, the deceleration time of E and D waves, and the duration of Ar and A waves during atrial contraction. S, systolic pulmonary vein wave (with potentially two components S_1 and S_2); D, diastolic pulmonary vein wave; Ar, reversal pulmonary vein wave during atrial contraction; E, early diastolic mitral wave; A, late diastolic mitral wave (during atrial contraction); V_{max}, maximal velocity; VTI, velocity time integral; DT E, deceleration time of E wave; DT D, deceleration time of D wave.

Transthoracic echocardiography

Transesophageal echocardiography

Pulsed-wave Doppler velocity profiles

Pulsed-wave Doppler mitral inflow:

LV

LA

LA

RV

LV

TTE

TEE

Paw

Pulsed-wave Doppler pulmonary vein flow:

RV LV

RA LA

LA

RV

LV

TTE

Paw

TEE

Paw

FIGURE 39.7. Two-dimensional echocardiographic still frames illustrating the proper position of the pulsed-wave Doppler sample to record optimal tracings of mitral inflow and pulmonary vein flow, with both the transthoracic and transesophageal approaches (see Table 39.5 for details). Corresponding pulsed-wave Doppler velocity tracings are shown (right panel). TTE, transthoracic echocardiography; TEE, transesophageal echocardiography; LV, left ventricle; LA, left atrium; RV, right ventricle; RA, right atrium; Paw, airway pressure curve.

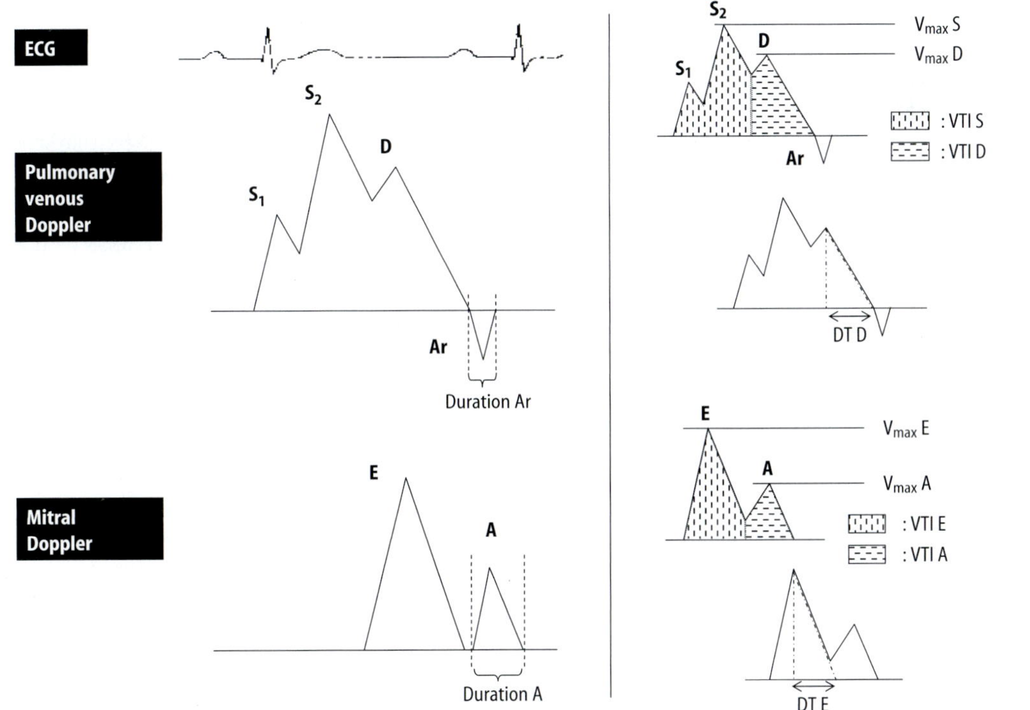

measurement of main indices used for a semiquantitative evaluation of LV filling pressure. Technical recommendations for optimal pulsed-wave Doppler velocity recordings have been described previously with TTE (27) and are summarized in Table 39.5. Since a physiologic progression of Doppler patterns has been described with aging (26), normal values of Doppler parameters depend on age (28).

Only a few studies have focused on the prediction of PAOP in ICU patients, especially when mechanically ventilated for acute respiratory failure (29–34). Currently proposed threshold values of easily obtained Doppler indices to predict elevated PAOP are summarized in Table 39.6. Of note, the prediction of PAOP using conventional pulsed-wave Doppler appears to be even more accurate in the presence of LV systolic dysfunction (35,36) and associated elevated filling pressure (37), a common scenario encountered in patients presenting with cardiogenic pulmonary edema.

Doppler tissue imaging (DTI) of mitral annulus motion and measurement of LV inflow propagation velocity during early diastole using color M-mode appear as promising additional tools in predicting PAOP in critically ill patients (32–34). Since these new Doppler indices are relatively load-independent, they are usually considered to be more reliable parameters of LV diastolic properties than conventional spectral Doppler measurements (38,39). Conse-

TABLE 39.5. Technical recommendations for obtaining optimal pulsed-wave Doppler flow velocity recordings of the mitral inflow and pulmonary venous flow during the assessment of LV filling pressure

Step	Conditions for optimal flow velocity recordings
1	Obtain a true apical (TTE) or TEE four-chamber view of the heart that excludes the aortic valve
2	Try to reduce the angle between the ultrasound beam and blood flow (visualized with color Doppler mapping) as much as possible (<20 degrees): • Mitral inflow: translate the transducer from the true apical four-chamber view to a slightly more lateral position (TTE) or adjust the depth of the probe into the esophagus or slightly rotate the esophageal probe (TEE) • Pulmonary venous flow: use a slight anterior angulation from the apical four-chamber view to visualize the right upper pulmonary vein (TTE) or slightly withdraw the esophageal probe and rotate the transducer (~20 to 40 degrees) to obtain a true long-axis view of the left upper pulmonary vein (TEE)
3	Use a small pulsed-wave Doppler sample volume: • Mitral inflow: 1 to 2 mm • Pulmonary venous flow: 2 to 3 mm
4	Place the sample volume adequately (Fig. 39.7): • Mitral inflow: between the tips of the mitral leaflets • Pulmonary venous flow: 1 to 2 cm into the pulmonary vein
5	Use a recording speed of 50 mm/s (appreciation of the influence of the respiratory cycle on Doppler velocities) or 100 mm/s (measurement of flow duration or deceleration time) Use ECG and respiratory tracings, especially in ventilated patients Set velocity filter as low as possible (200 to 600 Hz)
6	Perform all measurements at end-expiration (or during apnea) to limit the effects of heart–lung interactions on Doppler velocities (select appropriate Doppler velocity profiles with respiratory tracings)
7	Measure Doppler parameters as follows (Fig. 39.8): • Maximal velocities: determine the peak velocity of each Doppler wave (mitral E and A waves, pulmonary vein S and D waves) • Deceleration time: extend the deceleration slope from the peak wave velocity to the zero-velocity baseline (mitral E wave and pulmonary vein D wave) • Time velocity integral: trace manually the external contour of the spectral display to improve reproducibility (mitral E and A waves, pulmonary vein S and D waves) • Duration: perform measurement as close to the zero-velocity baseline as possible from the start of flow at the onset of atrial contraction to the end of flow at mitral valve closure (mitral A wave and pulmonary vein Ar wave)
8	Repeat measurements on nonconsecutive heart beats and respiratory cycles, check for consistency and average three or more values
9	Take into account patient's age to interpret obtained Doppler parameters (physiologic modification of LV diastolic properties with aging) (26,28)

TTE, transthoracic echocardiography; TEE, transesophageal echocardiography; LV, left ventricle.
Source: Adapted from Appleton et al. (27).

Table 39.6. Threshold values of simple mitral and pulmonary vein pulsed-wave Doppler indices currently proposed in critically ill patients to predict an elevated pulmonary artery occlusion pressure (PAOP)

Doppler parameter (reference)	Setting	Predicted PAOP	Threshold value	Sensitivity	Specificity
E/A ratio					
(35)	CCU	≥20 mm Hg	>2	43%	99%
(29)	ICU	>18 mm Hg[¥]	>2	–	–
(34)	ICU	>18 mm Hg[¥]	>1.4	85%	89%
DT E					
(35)	CCU	≥20 mm Hg	<120 ms	100%	99%
(34)	ICU	>18 mm Hg[¥]	<110 ms	77%	82%
S/D ratio					
(34)	ICU	>18 mm Hg[¥]	<0.65	85%	94%
Systolic fraction[¶]					
(30)	OR	>15 mm Hg[¥§]	<55%	91%	87%
(29)	ICU	>18 mm Hg[¥]	<40%	–	–
(31)	ICU	>18 mm Hg[¥]	<40%	100%	100%
(34)	ICU	>18 mm Hg[¥]	<44%	85%	88%

[¥] Ventilated patients.
[§] Perioperative assessment of left atrial pressure, rather than PAOP.
[¶] Systolic fraction corresponds to the ratio between the systolic pulmonary vein velocity time integral and the sum of the systolic and diastolic pulmonary vein velocity time integrals, expressed as a percentage (VTI S/VTI (S + D) · 100) (30).
E/A, ratio of maximal velocities of early diastolic mitral E wave and late diastolic mitral A wave; DT E, deceleration time of mitral Doppler E wave; S/D, ratio of maximal velocities of systolic pulmonary venous S wave and diastolic pulmonary venous D wave; CCU, coronary care unit; ICU, intensive care unit; OR, operating room.

quently, when combined with pulsed-wave Doppler indices that are the result of numerous factors, including LV diastolic properties and filling pressures (Fig. 39.5), DTI of the mitral annulus and color M-mode of LV diastolic inflow promise to help predict even more accurately PAOP (Table 39.7). Measurement of E′ maximal velocity is more reproducible than that of Vp (32,34). Accordingly, DTI measurement of mitral annulus motion, at its lateral aspect (36), should be preferably used by less experienced operators.

Table 39.7. Threshold values of combined Doppler indices (conventional pulsed-wave Doppler and DTI of mitral annulus motion or propagation velocity of LV early diastolic inflow measured by color M-mode) currently proposed in ventilated ICU patients to predict an elevated pulmonary artery occlusion pressure (PAOP)

Doppler parameter (reference)	Predicted PAOP	Threshold value	Sensitivity	Specificity
E/E′ lateral				
(32)	≥13 mm Hg	≥7	86%	92%
(33)	≥15 mm Hg	>7.5	86%	81%
(34)	>18 mm Hg	>9.5	100%	94%
E/E′ septal				
(33)	≥15 mm Hg	>9	76%	80%
E/Vp				
(32)	≥13 mm Hg	>2	55%	90%
(34)	>18 mm Hg	>2.6	100%	94%

DTI, Doppler tissue imaging; ICU, intensive care unit; E/E′, ratio of maximal velocities of mitral pulsed-wave Doppler E wave and DTI E′ wave of the mitral annulus at the level of the lateral or septal wall; Vp, propagation velocity of early diastolic LV inflow measured using color M mode.

In AHF patients with atrial fibrillation (AF), pulsed-wave Doppler atrial waves (A and Ar) are no longer observed and pulmonary vein Doppler S wave is usually reduced. In addition, beat-to-beat variation of the duration of ventricular diastole precludes reproducible measurements of Doppler indices. In this setting, measurements should be performed on three or more representative beats (duration of diastole within averaged values) (40). A deceleration time of mitral E wave ≤120 ms has been shown to predict a PAOP ≥20 mm Hg in AF patients with LV systolic dysfunction, with a sensitivity and a specificity of 100% and 96%, respectively (41). Conversely, a deceleration time of pulmonary vein D wave >220 ms enabled predicting a PAOP ≤12 mm Hg with a sensitivity and a specificity of 100% in AF patients (42). Finally, an E/E′ ratio ≥11 could predict elevated LV filling pressure (≥15 mm Hg) in AF patients, with a sensitivity of 75% and a specificity of 93% (43).

Diagnostic Algorithm: Pulmonary Edema

Although the prevalence of elevated LV filling pressure is high in patients with known systolic dysfunction, it is lower in dyspneic patients without cardiac history (44) and challenging to predict by the sole physical examination (45,46). In addition, patients with a known cardiopathy may present with a concomitant acute condition complicated by an ARDS that should be distinguished from AHF. In patients presenting with bilateral radiographic infiltrates and hypoxemia, a diagnostic algorithm based on a first-line echocardiographic assessment can be proposed (Fig. 39.9).

As previously mentioned, the diagnosis of cardiogenic pulmonary edema relies on the documentation of elevated LV filling pressure in a suggestive clinical setting. This finding is typically associated with LV systolic dysfunction (Fig. 39.9). In this case, echocardiography quantifies LV

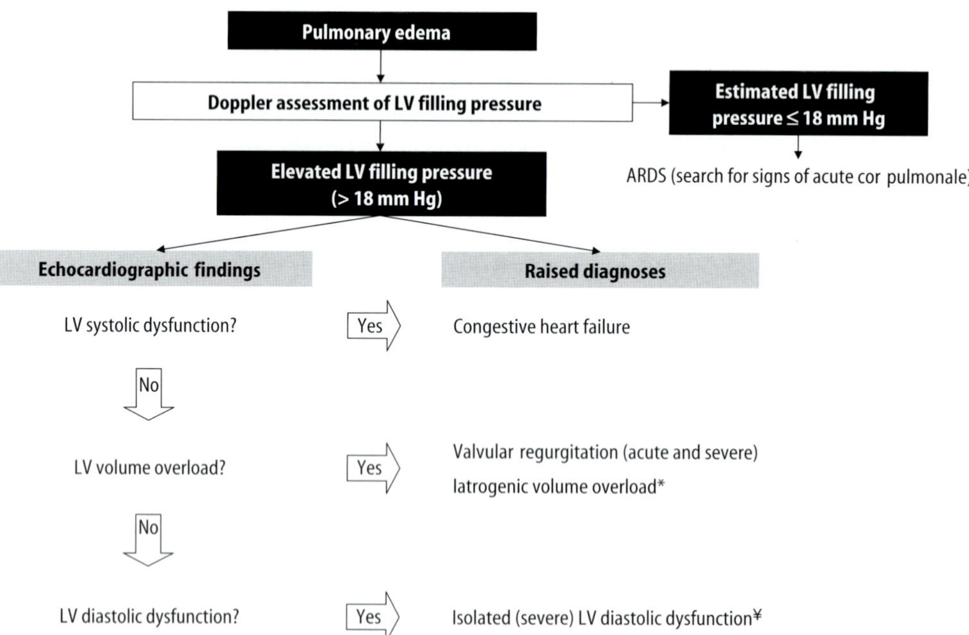

FIGURE 39.9. Proposed diagnostic algorithm using echocardiography Doppler to identify the mechanism and potential cause of pulmonary edema in hypoxemic AHF patients presenting with bilateral infiltrates on chest radiograph. *Usually associated with oliguria (renal failure). ¥Diagnostic criteria of diastolic dysfunction must be fulfilled (see text for details). LV, left ventricle; ARDS, acute respiratory distress syndrome.

pump function and identifies the underlying cardiomyopathy responsible for the congestive heart failure. Importantly, the clinical relevance of identified abnormalities should be addressed, as well as their imputability in the development of pulmonary edema. This task may be challenging, especially in the setting of chronic valvulopathy or combined cardiac abnormalities.

In the presence of a preserved LV systolic function—but still elevated LV filling pressure—a high output AHF should be ruled out (1) (Fig. 39.9). The absence of dilatation of left cardiac cavities is usually consistent with an acute volume overload (e.g., valvular regurgitation, iatrogenic volume overload). In contrast, markedly dilated left cardiac chambers reflect a progressive adaptation of the heart to a chronic volume overload. Associated LV hypertrophy is usually interpreted as a marker of associated LV pressure overload (e.g., aortic regurgitation). The level of pulmonary hypertension, which may accurately be assessed using continuous-wave Doppler interrogation of tricuspid or pulmonary regurgitation (47,48), may also help in distinguishing recent from rather chronic LV volume overload. Since a normal RV may barely generate a systolic pressure >60 mm Hg (49), higher values usually denote the presence of a subacute or chronic pulmonary hypertension rather than an acute increase of RV output impedance. Finally, echocardiography may clearly identify the cause of acute LV volume overload (e.g., endocarditis, ruptured papillary muscle, or mitral chordae) and confirms its severity.

When a congestive and a high output AHF have been confidently ruled out by echocardiography, the exclusion diagnosis of pure LV diastolic dysfunction can be raised (Fig. 39.9). This clinical scenario typically corresponds to hypertensive AHF and frequently involves elderly patients with a history of hypertension (1). Standardized diagnostic criteria of LV diastolic dysfunction have been proposed (50) and are summarized in Table 39.8. It has been recently shown that AHF patients who fulfilled these diagnostic criteria exhibited prolonged (active) LV relaxation and increased (passive) LV stiffness, thus supporting the clinical entity of diastolic heart failure (51). The main limitation of this classification approach (50) is the need for objective documentation of LV diastolic dysfunction with cardiac catheterization. In the setting of AHF patients presenting with pulmonary edema and preserved LV systolic function, echocardiography Doppler may represent a valuable alternative diagnostic method when depicting LV diastolic dysfunction, increased LV filling pressures (see above), and a cardiomyopathy known to be associated with LV filling impairment (e.g., LV hypertrophy). Diagnosis of LV diastolic dysfunction usually relies on the presence of decreased E′ maximal velocity (<8 cm/s) or decreased Vp (<45 cm/s) (52). Importantly, echocardiography must be performed as close as possible to the AHF event (i.e., when symptoms are still present), since LV filling pressure may rapidly change in response to treatment-induced variations of loading conditions (e.g., diuretics, nitrates, mechanical ventilation, sedation) (Fig. 39.10). In addition, precipitating events such as paroxysmal AF or small amount of intravenous fluid administration are suggestive of LV diastolic dysfunction (50), as illustrated in Figure 39.11. In hypertensive pulmonary edema, transient LV systolic dysfunction or mitral regurgitation is unlikely to occur (53). In AHF patients, the prevalence of primary LV diastolic dysfunction identified by echocardiography Doppler may reach 38% (54).

Table 39.8. Diagnostic criteria for diastolic heart failure*

Criteria	Objective evidence
1. Congestive heart failure	• Suggestive clinical presentation • Supporting tests (e.g., chest x-ray) • Positive response to diuretics • With or without the documentation of elevated LV filling pressure
2. Normal LV systolic function in proximity to the AHF event	LV ejection fraction ≥50% within 72 hours of AHF event
3. LV diastolic dysfunction	Abnormal LV relaxation, filling, distensibility indices on cardiac catheterization

*This classification approach is applicable to patients without congestive heart failure attributable to valvular heart disease, cor pulmonale, or a primary volume overload state. Diastolic heart failure is considered as *definite* when all three diagnostic criteria are fulfilled, *probable* when the first two criteria are present, and *possible* when a preserved ejection fraction has not been documented at the time of AHF event. LV, left ventricle; AHF, acute heart failure.

Source: Adapted from Vasan and Levy (50).

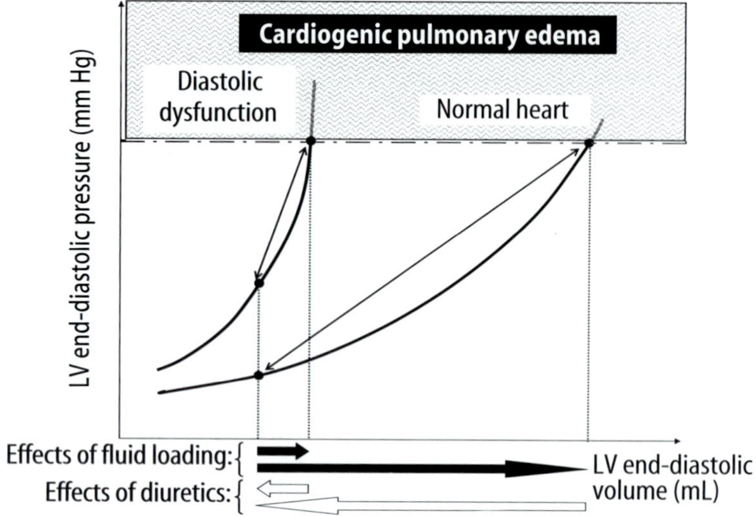

FIGURE 39.10. Examples of LV diastolic pressure-volume curves of a stiff heart with prolonged relaxation (e.g., LV hypertrophy) and of a normal heart for comparison. During diastole, the hypertrophied LV fills a smaller cavity (lower end-diastolic volume) with a higher pressure because its diastolic pressure-volume curve is shifter toward the left when compared to that of a normal heart. Accordingly, in patients with LV diastolic dysfunction, the administration of a small volume of fluid may rapidly decompensate diastolic heart failure or even lead to pulmonary edema (short solid single arrow). In contrast, a much larger volume of fluid loading would be necessary for a normal heart to reach LV filling pressure compatible with the development of pulmonary edema (long solid single arrow). Importantly, the steep curvilinear shape of diastolic pressure-volume curve of the hypertrophied LV accounts for the fact that decreasing preload by first-line therapy of AHF may rapidly and dramatically reduce LV filling pressures (short open single arrow). In this setting, the diagnosis of pulmonary edema secondary to diastolic heart failure is more challenging (see text for details). Double arrows indicate the therapeutic index of fluid loading according to the characteristics of LV diastolic pressure-volume curves. LV, left ventricle.

Acute Heart Failure Syndrome with Systemic Venous Congestion

Patients with right heart failure typically present with acute-onset dyspnea at rest, physical signs of peripheral congestion, and clear lung fields (1). The proposed diagnostic algorithm using echocardiography Doppler in patients presenting with right heart failure is summarized in Figure 39.12. Specific aspects of RV dysfunction in the ICU are discussed in Chapter 23.

In a patient presenting with systemic venous congestion but no RV dilatation, a tamponade

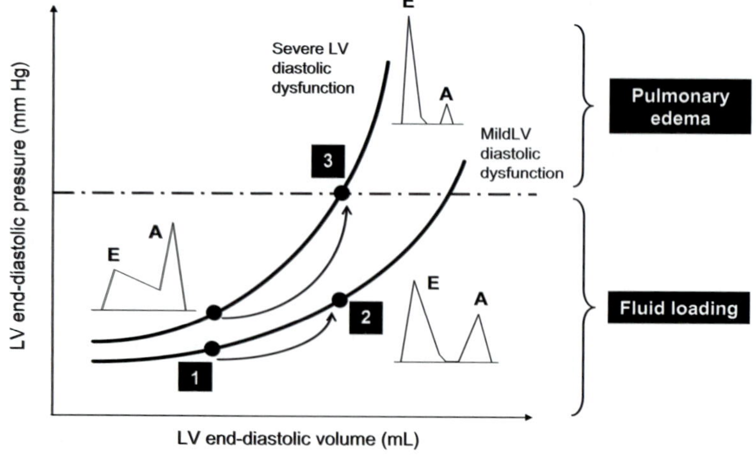

FIGURE 39.11. Illustration of the preload dependence of mitral Doppler pattern, according to LV diastolic properties. Fluid loading increases LV end-diastolic volume—referred to as cardiac preload—and alters mitral Doppler profiles. Since the LV diastolic pressure-volume curve is steeper in the presence of a severe diastolic dysfunction, the same fluid loading may precipitate the development of a pulmonary edema. A modification of mitral Doppler profile from an abnormal relaxation pattern (point 1) to a normalized pattern (point 2) should alert the physician. When a restrictive pattern is observed (point 3), the risk of pulmonary edema is high. LV, left ventricle.

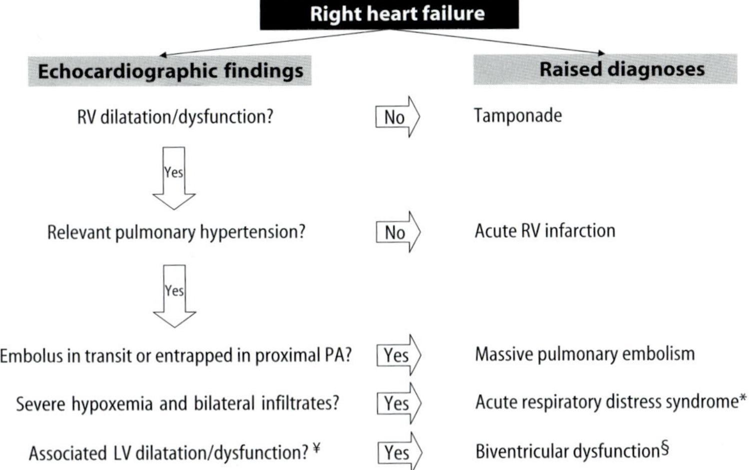

FIGURE 39.12. Proposed diagnostic algorithm in patients presenting with right heart failure when primarily assessed by echocardiography Doppler. *Acute cor pulmonale is present in only one fourth of patients with currently recommended ventilator settings. [¥]Usually denotes a chronic heart disease that can be readily identified by echocardiography. [§]Echocardiography may quantify cardiac pump function and allow serial comparisons with previous examinations. RV, right ventricle; LV, left ventricle; PA, pulmonary artery.

physiology should be sought for (Fig. 39.12). Echocardiographic diagnosis of cardiac tamponade is straightforward in the presence of a pericardial effusion with diastolic compression of right cardiac cavities. Increased and opposite respiratory variations of mitral and tricuspid Doppler velocities are also diagnostic of tamponade (55). Unfortunately, these hemodynamic findings are no longer applicable in mechanically ventilated patients (56). In this clinical setting, the diagnosis of tamponade remains challenging, especially when the volume of pericardial effusion is small or when impaired cardiac filling is secondary to a localized compressive hematoma (57).

A dilated RV with marked systolic dysfunction but no relevant pulmonary hypertension is frequently related to a RV infarction (Fig. 39.12). Right ventricular systolic pressure is not increased, as reflected by a low peak tricuspid regurgitation velocity, and associated RWMA of the LV inferior wall is frequently observed (58). In contrast, the association of RV dilatation and pump failure in the setting of a sudden increase of RV output impedance is suggestive of acute cor pulmonale (59). Right ventricular afterloading is usually reflected by pulmonary hypertension, provided that RV systolic function can still generate a substantial systolic pressure. In this clinical setting, the identification of an embolus-in-transit within right cardiac cavities or the documentation of an entrapped embolus in proximal pulmonary artery is pathognomonic of massive pulmonary embolism (Fig. 39.12). Importantly, acute cor pulmonale is consistent with, but not specific for, massive pulmonary embolism, since it may be observed in up to 25% of ARDS (60). Finally, the observation of a concomitant RV and LV systolic dysfunction associated with a biventricular dilatation is usually the marker of an underlying long-standing cardiomyopathy (Fig. 39.12). Regardless of the origin of right heart failure, echocardiography enables a comprehensive evaluation of both global and regional RV systolic function (61).

Acute Heart Failure and Chest Pain

Chest pain may be associated with AHF. In this setting, AHF may have various clinical presentations, such as pulmonary edema, right heart failure, or cardiogenic shock. Acute aortic syndrome (AAS) involving the ascending aorta should first be ruled out by echocardiography since it requires prompt surgical repair (Fig. 39.13). The clinical entity of AAS, proposed by Vilacosta and San Román (62), refers to patients presenting with

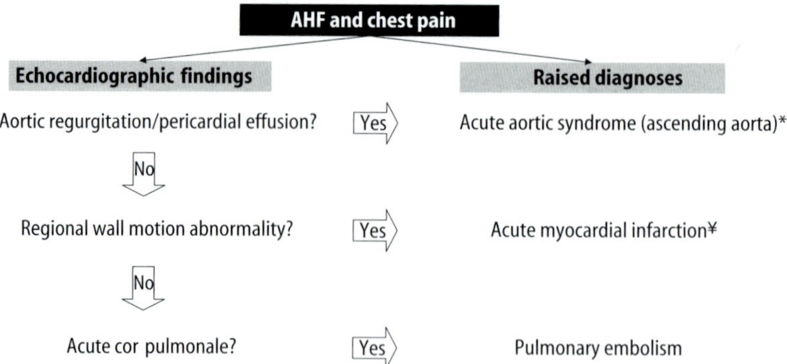

FIGURE 39.13. Proposed diagnostic algorithm in patients assessed using echocardiography for chest pain and AHF syndrome. *Acute aortic syndrome refers to a typical "aortic pain" in a patient with a history of hypertension (62) and may be secondary to acute aortic dissection, intramural aortic hematoma, or penetrating aortic ulcer (see text for details). ¥Echocardiography depicts the extension of regional wall motion abnormality, the presence of a mechanical complication (papillary muscle rupture, ventricular septal rupture, left ventricular free wall rupture), and the potential involvement of the right ventricle. AHF, acute heart failure.

an aortic pain (i.e., severely intense, acute, searing or tearing, throbbing, and migratory chest pain) and a coexisting history of hypertension. Acute aortic syndrome is usually symptomatic of a distended and stretched aorta (62), with associated risk of fissuration or rupture, and may be secondary to any acute aortic disease with increased aortic wall stress (e.g., acute aortic dissection, intramural aortic hematoma, penetrating aortic ulcer). Acute heart failure is usually a complication of AAS, which involves the aortic root rather than the descending aorta. Accordingly, TTE plays a key role in the evaluation of these patients since it is accurate for the diagnosis of acute condition of the ascending aorta and better tolerated than TEE in this specific clinical setting. Although there is no evidence for an intimal flap or an intramural hematoma based on TTE examination, the presence of a dilated ascending aorta and findings consistent with blood extravasation (i.e., hemopericardium) or aortic regurgitation is highly suggestive of AAS. Then TEE may be safely performed in the operating room, in a ventilated patient under general anesthesia in whom immediate pericardial decompression can be eventually performed. In this environment, TEE is superior to TTE to clearly identify the acute aortic disease responsible for AAS and to describe precisely its anatomic characteristics, thereby guiding ongoing surgical repair (6,63).

In the absence of acute disease of the ascending aorta, echocardiographic documentation of a new RWMA is indicative of acute myocardial infarction (Fig. 39.13). In the setting of patients presenting with AHF and chest pain, RWMA is usually extended to a large LV coronary artery territory, or may be associated with an ischemic-induced severe mitral regurgitation or with a mechanical complication. In patients presenting with chest pain, AHF may also be related to a RV infarction leading to right heart failure (Fig. 39.12). Finally, the documentation of an acute cor pulmonale with echocardiography is highly suggestive of pulmonary embolism in this scenario (Fig. 39.13).

Cardiogenic Shock

Cardiogenic shock is the most severe clinical presentation of peripheral hypoperfusion related to AHF syndrome (1). In contrast to obstructive shock in which hypotension results from impeded circulation (e.g., pulmonary embolism, tamponade), cardiogenic shock is attributable to a failing cardiac pump, regardless of the nature of the insult. In this setting, echocardiography has the unparalleled advantage of enabling (1) documenting and assessing the severity of cardiac pump failure, as previously described; (2) excluding any preload-dependency of the heart; (3) differentiat-

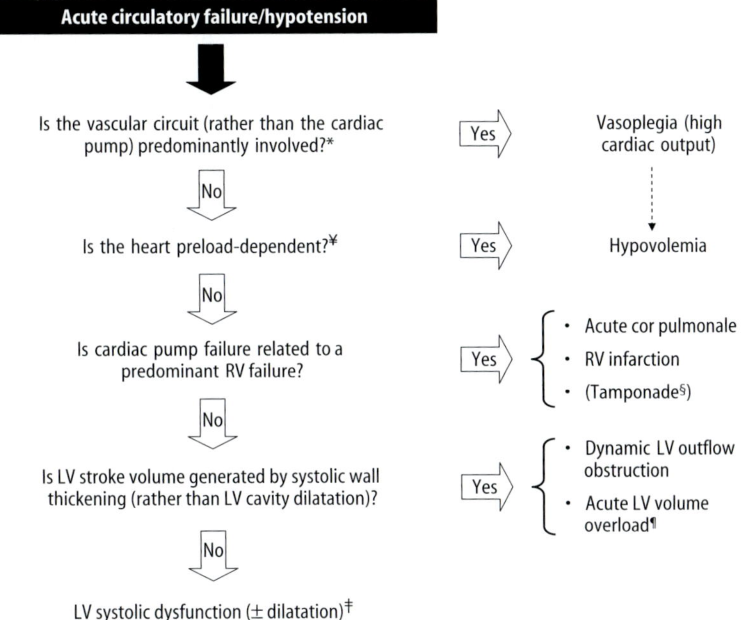

FIGURE 39.14. Pragmatic diagnostic approach to identify the leading mechanism of a circulatory failure using echocardiography Doppler. *In specific clinical settings such as postoperative (extracorporeal circulation) cardiogenic shock, the circulatory failure may result from a dysfunction of both the cardiac pump and vascular system. ¥A failing heart is rarely preload-dependent since it usually operates on the flat portion of the Frank-Starling curve. §Tamponade refers to an impeded RV filling rather than a true RV failure; left heart filling may be specifically impeded when the pericardial effusion is loculated or when a hematoma develops outside the pericardial space, at the vicinity of left cardiac cavities (e.g., after cardiac surgery or chest trauma). ¶See Figure 39.9 and corresponding text for details. ‡Echocardiography clearly depicts structural changes secondary to LV remodeling and potential consequences on pulmonary artery pressure and right heart function. LV, left ventricle; RV, right ventricle.

ing between a low cardiac output due to a failing LV and a right heart failure; and (4) determining if LV stroke volume is mostly generated by myocardial contractility rather than LV cavity dilatation (Fig. 39.14) (2). In patients with severe RV systolic dysfunction (e.g., ARDS, RV infarction), specific therapeutic interventions aimed at decreasing RV output impedance (e.g., inhalation of NO) may improve hemodynamics (64,65). Although reduced stroke volume may result from a dynamic LV outflow obstruction in the presence of a small (hypertrophied) hyperkinetic ventricle, low cardiac output is most frequently attributable to a (dilated) failing LV (Fig. 39.14). Thus, echocardiography allows the identification of the predominant mechanism of circulatory failure, but also documents the etiology of cardiogenic shock (e.g., extended or complicated myocardial infarction, severe endocarditis, acute dissection of the ascending aorta).

Case Presentation

A 17-year-old boy was hospitalized in the ICU for septic shock. This patient with no medical history complained of persistent headache and fever despite repeated administrations of paracetamol for 24 hours. Two hours before ICU admission, he had dizziness, fainted, and became slightly agitated, confused, and drowsy.

Upon admission, his level of consciousness deteriorated; he did not open his eyes in response to a loud voice or localized pain. A subtle meningismus was observed without cranial nerve palsies. Body temperature was 40°C. Rapidly extensive and necrotic petechiae were noted on the torso and extremities, all cutaneous lesions consistent with purpura fulminans. Ceftriaxone was immediately administered intravenously. Blood pressure rapidly fell to 75/55 mm Hg, despite a rapid blood volume expansion with 3 L of crystalloids and the introduction of norepinephrine. The patient became tachypneic and pulmonary auscultation noted diffused crackles in the lower lobes. Urine output remained low. Chest radiograph showed a diffuse bilateral infiltrate consistent with an acute respiratory distress syndrome (ARDS).

The white blood cell counts was 3.0×10^9/L and the platelet count was 127×10^9/L. Prothrombin time was 27 seconds (control: 12 seconds), fibrinogen was 1.2 g/L, and fibrin degradation products titer was 718 µg/L. Glucose was 12 mmol/L, creatinine was 250 µmol/L, and lactate was 9 mmol/L. Lumbar puncture withdrew clear cerebrospinal fluid (CSF) with the following characteristics: white cell count 75/mm^3 (95% of neutrophils), glucose concentration 0.70 g/L, and protein concentration 1.2 g/L. The CSF examination by Gram stain failed to identify any bacteria, and specific antigens were negative. Several blood cultures yielded *Neisseria meningitidis* susceptible to ampicillin. The patient was placed on a ventilator and received adjunctive therapy by intravenous hydrocortisone (300 mg/day) and recombinant human activated protein C.

A TEE was performed to assess patient hemodynamics. A short-axis transesophageal view depicted a moderate dilatation of the left ventricle, which had a severely depressed systolic function secondary to global hypokinesis. The transesophageal four-chamber view confirmed these findings and showed a right ventricle with a normal size and systolic function, excluding a cor pulmonale physiology secondary to ARDS. The transesophageal longitudinal view of the left ventricle depicted a severe hypokinesis of both anterior and inferior walls and enabled precise measurement of left ventricular outflow tract to calculate stroke volume and cardiac output. In the transgastric transverse view of the left ventricle, M-mode clearly depicted a severe hypokinesis of both its inferior and anterior walls, and a moderate enlargement of its cavity with a diastolic diameter of 57 mm. The left ventricular outflow tract diameter was 1.9 cm, corresponding to an orifice area of 2.83 cm^2. The velocity time integral of pulsed Doppler profile obtained at the level of the left ventricular outflow tract was less than 10 cm, resulting in a stroke volume of 28 mL. Both the transmitral and pulmonary venous Doppler velocity profiles indicated fairly low left ventricular filling pressures. This was confirmed by a normal early diastolic velocity recorded by tissue Doppler imaging at the lateral aspect of the mitral ring. The absence of elevated left ventricular filling pressures enabled confidently ruling out a cardiogenic pulmonary edema despite the presence of a severely depressed left ventricular systolic function. Finally, a nonsignificant acceleration of Doppler aortic velocities was observed during tidal volume insufflation, a finding consistent with the absence of preload dependence of the left ventricle.

Based on TEE evaluation, the patient received an inotropic support. He progressively recovered from this severe septic shock and another TEE study was performed on day 6. Transgastric transverse view of the left ventricle showed a total recovery with the presence of both a normal cavity size and systolic function of the left ventricle, after the cessation of vasopressor and inotropic agents. The transesophageal four-chamber view confirmed these findings. In the transgastric transverse view, M-mode clearly depicted the reduction of left ventricular cavity size and the recovery of left ventricular walls thickening during systole. The velocity time integral of the pulsed wave Doppler recorded at the level of left ventricular outflow tract was 21 cm, a normal value corresponding to a stroke volume of 60 mL. The patient was extubated on day 8 and the subsequent course was uneventful.

This clinical presentation illustrates the severe left ventricular systolic dysfunction that may promote circulatory failure at the early course of septic shock. It also illustrates the potential recovery of the severe yet reversible left ventricular pump dysfunction. Acute respiratory distress syndrome is frequently associated with severe septic shock, as in this representative example. In this case, left ventricular filling pressures remain fairly low despite the presence of a depressed systolic function. This enables excluding a cardiogenic origin of the pulmonary edema, although extravascular lung water may accumulate in perialveolar and alveolar spaces for relatively low pulmonary venous pressure in the setting of ARDS, due to diffuse damage of lung alveolar–capillary barrier integrity.

Conclusion

In the environment of critical care with unstable critically ill patients who present with AHF syndrome and may not tolerate lengthy and invasive diagnostic procedures, echocardiography Doppler is ideally suited for a prompt and comprehensive hemodynamic assessment. In allowing the quantification of cardiac pump function, the identification of both mechanism and cause of heart failure associated with pulmonary venous or systemic venous congestion, echocardiography Doppler constitutes a valuable first-line diagnostic technique for the acute assessment of AHF patients. In addition, this alternative approach enables the documentation of the etiology of chest pain in AHF patients and the identification of the mechanism of circulatory failure in patients with cardiogenic shock. As such, echocardiography Doppler has supplanted right heart catheterization and currently represents the cornerstone of acute modern assessment of AHF patients.

References

1. Swedberg K, Cleland J, Dargie H, et al. Guidelines for the diagnosis and treatment of chronic heart failure (update 2005). The task force for the diagnosis and treatment of CHF of the European Society of Cardiology. Eur Heart J 2005;26:1115–40.
2. Vignon P. Hemodynamic assessment of critically-ill patients using echocardiography Doppler. Curr Opin Crit Care 2005;11:227–34.
3. Armstrong WF, Zoghbi WA. Stress echocardiography. Current methodology and clinical applications. J Am Coll Cardiol 2005;45:1739–47.
4. Vignon P, Chastagner C, François B, et al. Diagnostic ability of hand-held echocardiography in ventilated critically-ill patients. Crit Care 2003;7:R84–91.
5. Vignon P, Frank MBJ, Lesage J, et al. Hand-held echocardiography with Doppler capability for the assessment of critically-ill patients: is it reliable? Intensive Care Med 2004;30:718–23.
6. ACC/AHA guidelines for the clinical application of echocardiography. A report from the American College of Cardiology/American Heart Association Task Force on Practice Guidelines (Committee on Clinical Application of Echocardiography). Circulation 1997;95:1686–744.
7. American Society of Anesthesiologists and the Society of Cardiovascular Anesthesiologists Task Force on Transesophageal Echocardiography. Practice guidelines for perioperative transesophageal echocardiography. Anesthesiology 1996;84:986–1006.
8. Robotham JL, Takata M, Berman M, et al. Ejection fraction revisited. Anesthesiology 1991;74:172–83.
9. Aurigemma GP, Douglas PS, Gaash WH. Quantitative evaluation of left ventricular structure, wall stress, and systolic function. In: Otto CM, ed. The Practice of Clinical Echocardiography, 2nd ed. Philadelphia: WB Saunders, 2002:65–87.
10. Schiller NB, Foster E. Analysis of left ventricular systolic function. Heart 1996;75 (suppl 2):17–26.
11. Schiller NB. Ejection fraction by echocardiography: the full Monty or just a peep show? (Editorial). Am Heart J 2003;146:380–2.
12. Schiller NB, Shah PM, Crawford M, et al. Recommendations for quantification of the left ventricle by two-dimensional echocardiography. American Society of Echocardiography Committee on Standards, Subcommittee on Quantification of Two-dimensional Echocardiograms. J Am Soc Echocardiogr 1989;2:358–67.
13. Caroll JD, Hess OM. Assessment of normal and abnormal cardiac function. In: Zipes DP, Libby P, Bonow RO, Braunwald E, eds. Heart Disease, 7th ed. Philadelphia: Elsevier Saunders, 2005:491–507.
14. Zoghbi WA, Quinones MA. Determination of cardiac output by Doppler echocardiography: a critical appraisal. Herz 1986;11:258–68.
15. Katz WE, Gasior TA, Quilan JJ, et al. Transgastric continuous-wave Doppler to determine cardiac output. Am J Cardiol 1993;71:853–7.
16. Perrino AC, Harris SN, Luther MA. Intraoperative determination of cardiac output using multiplane transesophageal echocardiography. A comparison to thermodilution. Anesthesiology 1998;89:350–7.
17. Poelaert J, Schmidt C, Van Aken H, et al. A comparison of transesophageal echocardiographic Doppler across the aortic valve and the thermodilution technique for estimating cardiac output. Anaesthesia 1999;54:128–36.
18. Darmon PL, Hillel Z, Mogtader A, et al. Cardiac output by transesophageal echocardiography using continuous-wave Doppler across the aortic valve. Anesthesiology 1994;80:796–805.
19. Darmon PL, Axler O. Mesure du débit cardiaque. In: Vignon P, Goarin JP, eds. Echocardiographie Doppler en Réanimation, Anesthésie et Médecine d'Urgence. Paris: Elsevier, 2002:172–92.

20. Axler O, Megarbane B, Lentschener C, et al. Comparison of cardiac output measured with echocardiographic volumes and aortic Doppler methods during mechanical ventilation. Intensive Care Med 2003;29:208–17.
21. Schlant RC, Sonnenblick EH. Normal physiology of the cardiovascular system. In: Hurst JW, Schlant RC, eds. The Heart, 7th ed. New York: McGraw-Hill, 1990:35–71.
22. Hall JB, Schmidt GA, Wood LDH. Principles of Critical Care. New York: McGraw Hill, 1992.
23. Bernard GR, Artigas A, Brigham KL, et al. The American-European Consensus Conference on ARDS. Definitions, mechanisms, relevant outcomes, and clinical trial coordination. Am J Respir Crit Care Med 1994;149:818–24.
24. Appleton CP, Hatle LK, Popp RL. Relation of transmitral flow velocity patterns to left ventricular diastolic function: new insights from a combined hemodynamic and Doppler echocardiographic study. J Am Coll Cardiol 1988;12:426–40.
25. Temporelli PL, Scapellato F, Corra U, et al. Chronic mitral regurgitation and Doppler estimation of left ventricular filling pressures in patients with heart failure. J Am Soc Echocardiogr 2001;14:1094–9.
26. Appleton CP, Hatle LK. The natural history of left ventricular filling abnormalities: assessment by two-dimensional and Doppler echocardiography. Echocardiography 1992;9:437–57.
27. Appleton CP, Jensen JL, Hatle LK, et al. Doppler evaluation of left and right ventricular diastolic function: a technical guide for obtaining optimal flow velocity recordings. J Am Soc Echocardiogr 1997;10:271–91.
28. Oh JK, Seward JB, Yajik AJ. Assessment of diastolic function. In: Oh JK, Seward JB, Yajik AJ, eds. The Echo Manual, 2nd ed. Philadelphia: Lippincott Williams & Wilkins, 1999:45–57.
29. Boussuges A, Blanc P, Molenat F, et al. Evaluation of left ventricular filling pressure by transthoracic Doppler echocardiography in the intensive care unit. Crit Care Med 2002;30:362–7.
30. Kuecherer HF, Muhiudeen IA, Kusumoto FM, et al. Estimation of left atrial pressure from transesophageal pulsed Doppler echocardiography of pulmonary venous flow. Circulation 1990;82:1127–39.
31. Vargas F, Gruson D, Valentino R, et al. Transesophageal pulsed Doppler echocardiography of pulmonary venous flow to assess left ventricular filling pressure in ventilated patients with acute respiratory distress syndrome. J Crit Care 2004;19:187–97.
32. Bouhemad B, Nicolas-Robin A, Benois A, et al. Echocardiographic Doppler assessment of pulmonary capillary wedge pressure in surgical patients with postoperative circulatory shock and acute lung injury. Anesthesiology 2003;98:1091–100.
33. Combes A, Arnoult F, Trouillet JL. Tissue Doppler imaging estimation of pulmonary artery occlusion pressure in ICU patients. Intensive Care Med 2004;30:75–81.
34. Vignon P, François B, Pichon N, et al. Evaluation non invasive de la PAPO par échocardiographie Doppler chez les patients ventilés: quelle est sa précision et quel est l'apport des nouvelles techniques? Réanimation 2006;15:S235(abstr).
35. Gianuzzi P, Imparato A, Temporelli PL, et al. Doppler-derived mitral deceleration time of early filling as a strong predictor of pulmonary capillary wedge pressure in postinfarction patients with left ventricular systolic dysfunction. J Am Coll Cardiol 1994;23:1630–7.
36. Rivas-Gotz C, Manolios M, Thohan V, et al. Impact of left ventricular ejection fraction on estimation of left ventricular filling pressures using tissue Doppler and flow propagation velocity. Am J Cardiol 2003; 91:780–4.
37. Vanoverschelde JL, Robert AR, Gerbaux A, et al. Noninvasive estimation of pulmonary arterial wedge pressure with Doppler transmitral flow velocity pattern in patients with known heart disease. Am J Cardiol 1995;75:383–9.
38. Nagueh SF, Middleton KJ, Kopelen HA, et al. Doppler tissue imaging: a noninvasive technique for evaluation of left ventricular relaxation and estimation of filling pressure. J Am Coll Cardiol 1997;30:1527–33.
39. Garcia MJ, Smedira NG, Greenberg NL, et al. Color M-Mode Doppler flow propagation velocity is a preload insensitive index of left ventricular relaxation: animal and human validation. J Am Coll Cardiol 2000;35:201–8.
40. Nagueh SF, Kopelen HA, Quinones MA. Assessment of left ventricular filling pressures by Doppler in the presence of atrial fibrillation. Circulation 1996;94;2138–45.
41. Temporelli PL, Scapellato F, Corrà U, et al. Estimation of pulmonary wedge pressure by transmitral Doppler in patients with chronic heart failure and atrial fibrillation. Am J Cardiol 1999;83: 724–7.
42. Chirillo F, Brunazzi MC, Barbiero M, et al. Estimating mean pulmonary wedge pressure in patients with chronic atrial fibrillation from transthoracic Doppler indexes of mitral and pulmonary venous flow velocity. J Am Coll Cardiol 1997;30:19–26.
43. Sohn DW, Song JM, Zo JH, et al. Mitral annulus velocity in the evaluation of left ventricular dia-

stolic function in atrial fibrillation. J Am Soc Echocardiogr 1999;12:927–31.
44. Badgett RG, Lucey CR, Mulrow CD. Can the clinical examination diagnose left-sided heart failure in adults. JAMA 1997;277:1712–9.
45. Connors AF, Mc Caffree DR, Gray BA. Evaluation of right-heart catheterization in the critically ill patient without acute myocardial infarction. N Engl J Med 1983;263–7.
46. Eisenberg PR, Jaffe AS, Schuster DP. Clinical evaluation compared to pulmonary artery catheterization in the hemodynamic assessment of critically-ill patients. Crit Care Med 1984;12:549–53.
47. Yock PG, Popp RL. Noninvasive estimation of right ventricular systolic pressure by Doppler ultrasound in patients with tricuspid regurgitation. Circulation 1984;70:657–62.
48. Masuyama T, Kodama K, Kitabatake A, et al. Continuous-wave Doppler echocardiographic detection of pulmonary regurgitation and its application to non-invasive estimation of pulmonary artery pressure. Circulation 1986;74:484–92.
49. Weber KT, Janicki JS, Shroff SG, et al. The right ventricle: physiologic and pathophysiologic considerations. Crit Care Med 1983;11:323–8.
50. Vasan RS, Levy D. Defining diastolic heart failure. A call for standardized diagnostic criteria. Circulation 2000, 101:2118–21.
51. Zile MR, Baicu CF, Gaasch WH. Diastolic heart failure—abnormalities in active relaxation and passive stiffness of the left ventricle. N Engl J Med 2004;350:1953–9.
52. Garcia MJ, Thomas JD, Klein AL. New Doppler echocardiographic applications for the study of diastolic function. J Am Coll Cardiol 1998;32:865–75.
53. Gandi SK, Powers JC, Nomeir A, et al. The pathogenesis of acute pulmonary edema associated with hypertension. N Engl J Med 2001;344;17–22.
54. Yamada H, Goh PP, Sun JP, et al. Prevalence of left ventricular diastolic function by Doppler echocardiography: clinical application of the Canadian consensus guidelines. J Am Soc Echocardiogr 2002;15:1238–44.
55. Appleton CP, Hatle LK, Popp RL. Cardiac tamponade and pericardial effusion: respiratory variation in transvalvular flow velocities studied by Doppler echocardiography. J Am Coll Cardiol 1988;11:1020–30.
56. Faehnrich JA, Noone RB, White WD, et al. Effects of positive-pressure ventilation, pericardial effusion, and cardiac tamponade on respiratory variation in transmitral flow velocities. J Cardiovas Vasc Anesth 2003;17:45–50.
57. Kochar GS, Jacobs LE, Kotler MN. Right atrial compression in postoperative cardiac patients: detection by transesophageal echocardiography. J Am Coll Cardiol 1990;16:511–6.
58. Kinch JW, Ryan TJ. Right ventricular infarction. N Engl J Med 1994;330:1211–7.
59. Vieillard-Baron A, Prin S, Chergui K, et al. Echo-Doppler demonstration of acute cor pulmonale at the bedside in the medical intensive care unit. Am J Respir Crit Care Med 2002;166:1310–9.
60. Vieillard-Baron A, Schmitt JM, Augarde R, et al. Acute cor pulmonale in ARDS submitted to protective ventilation: incidence, clinical implications and prognosis. Crit Care Med 2001;29:1551–5.
61. Vignon P, Weinert L, Mor-Avi V, et al. Quantitative assessment of regional right ventricular ventricular function with color kinesis. Am J Respir Crit Care Med 1999;159:1949–59.
62. Vilacosta I, San Román JA. Acute aortic syndrome (Editorial). Heart 2001;85:365–8.
63. Erbel R, Alfonso F, Boileau C, et al. Diagnosis and management of aortic dissection. Eur Heart J 2001;22:1642–81.
64. Bhorade S, Christenson J, O'Connor M, et al. Response to inhaled nitric oxide in patients with acute right heart syndrome. Am J Respir Crit Care Med 1999;159:571–9.
65. Inglessis I, Shin JT, Lepore JJ, et al. Hemodynamic effects of inhaled nitric oxide in right ventricular myocardial infarction and cardiogenic shock. J Am Coll Cardiol 2004;44:793–8.

40
Portable Echocardiography and Acute Heart Failure Syndromes in the Emergency Room

Gerasimos S. Filippatos, Ioannis A. Paraskevaidis, and Dimitrios Th. Kremastinos

Acute heart failure (AHF) is characterized by the presence of signs and symptoms of heart failure requiring urgent intervention (1). More than 70% of patients with AHF have decompensation of chronic heart failure and 30% have heart failure of new onset (2). In the emergency room most patients have signs and symptoms of pulmonary or peripheral congestion (e.g., breathlessness, pulmonary edema, hepatomegaly, peripheral edema, raised venous pressure), and only a minority of patients have symptoms and signs of hypoperfusion (e.g., fatigue, cardiogenic shock). Many patients present with congestion, elevated left ventricular filling pressures, and preserved ejection fraction. In most of these patients blood pressure is elevated (hypertensive AHF). Some patients also have isolated right heart failure or high-output heart failure secondary to a systemic disease (1).

For the differential diagnosis of AHF in the emergency room (ER), clinical history, clinical examination, chest x-ray, and appropriate blood tests are necessary (1). The electrocardiogram is necessary to identify early the patients with AHF and acute ischemia and especially those with ST elevation acute myocardial infarction who could benefit from immediate reperfusion (3). The recent European guidelines recommend objective documentation of cardiac anatomy and function by echocardiography in all patients with AHF (1). Chapter 40 presented the exact role of Doppler echocardiography in AHF. This chapter presents the role of echocardiography, especially of the portable hand-held devices, in the initial triage of patients with AHF in the ER.

Portable Echocardiography: Hand-Held Devices

In the emergency room, the evaluation of the ventricular contractility and of the morphology and function of the valves, and the examination of the pericardiac sac help in the differential diagnosis and the initiation of appropriate therapy in the AHF patient (Fig. 40.1). However, the cost and the size of the standard echocardiographic systems do not allow their routine use in the ER (4). Thus, echocardiography was usually performed in selected patients. Recently, it has been suggested that hand-held echocardiography could add to the clinical cardiologic assessment in patients presenting with dyspnea, chest pain, or hypertension (5, 6). Moreover, the final diagnostic conclusions of the hand-held device evaluation were comparable to those of the standard echocardiographic examination, reducing waiting list time and costs (5).

The first portable ultrasounds, presented in the 1970s, had limited capabilities, with only a two-dimensional (2D) mode on small screens, but the rapid development of computer technology changed the field of clinical echocardiography. After this first generation of portable ultrasounds, the continuous development of technology and the need of cardiologists for better resolution and more capabilities led to the new generation of portable ultrasound systems of light weight and small volume, while at the same time implementing new techniques (7). Today, new hand-held devices are available in the market, some

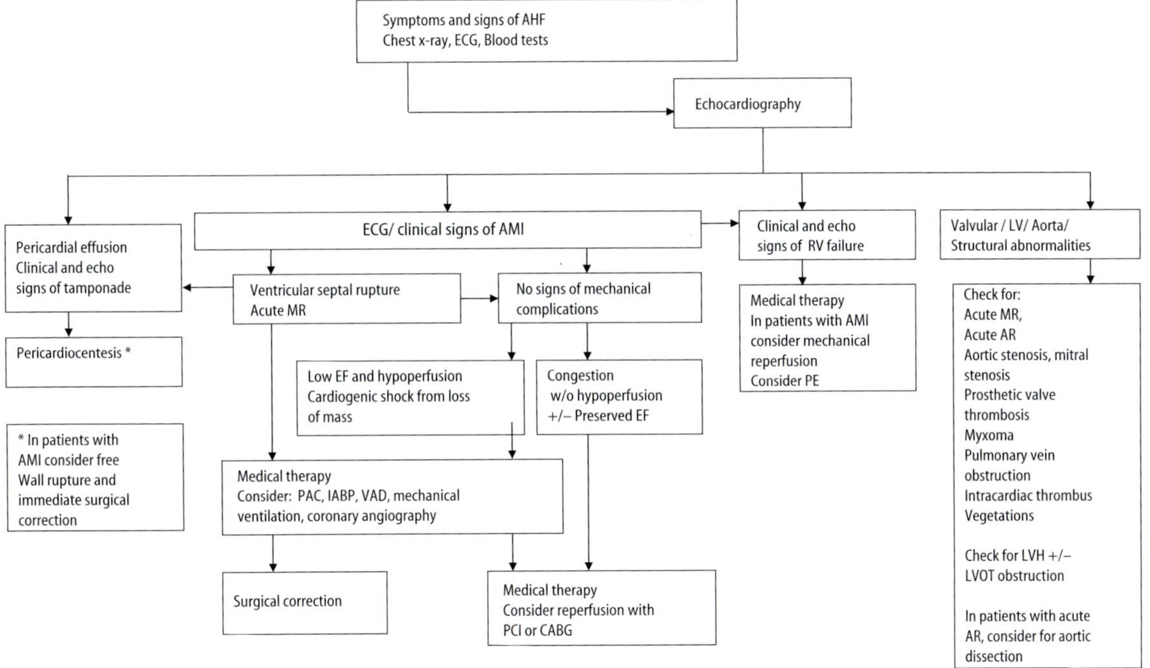

FIGURE 40.1. Diagnostic and treatment algorithm for the initial clinical and echocardiographic evaluation. AHF, acute heart failure; AMI, acute myocardial infarction; AR, aortic regurgitation; CABG, coronary artery bypass graft; EF, ejection fraction; IABP, intraaortic balloon pump; LVH, left ventricular hypertrophy; LVOT, left ventricular outflow tract; MR, mitral regurgitation; PAC, pulmonary artery catheter; PCI, percutaneous coronary intervention; VAD, ventricular assist device.

including complete instrumentations following the recommendations of the American Society of Echocardiography (8) and others with very low weight and cost but limited technologic capabilities. The top-level portable ultrasound systems have all the measurement and analysis software and the display techniques of the big systems, such as 2D, color Doppler, pulse-wave (PW) Doppler, continuous-wave (CW) Doppler, harmonics, tissue Doppler, and contrast agent–enhanced display modes, and they can accept transesophageal probes (7). Moreover, conventional and wireless imaging transfer systems are available in some of these devices (7). Thus, the field of application of a portable system is similar to the conventional big and heavy standard echocardiographic systems. Most of these systems have not been evaluated in the ER in patients with AHF. However, the new echo techniques are very useful for the diagnosis and treatment of patients with AHF. The use of these techniques in AHF are presented in details in Chapter 40.

Echocardiographic/Doppler Evaluation in the Emergency Room

In general, echocardiography is necessary for all patients presenting with AHF in the ER, especially if they present with signs and symptoms of acute ischemia and heart failure or if they do not respond to the initial treatment (9). Figure 40.1 is a diagnostic and treatment algorithm for the initial clinical and echocardiographic evaluation. Table 40.1 lists the echo/Doppler parameters that should be measured in patients with suspected valvular heart disease after the initial evaluation. It is possible to measure flow in stenosis, estimate insufficiencies and valve anatomy, and evaluate the function of prosthetic valves.

Other parameters that can be measured:

Mitral valve: With the 2D mode, the mitral valve area can be measured with an area caliper. With the color Doppler, the area of the mitral valve regurgitation, the mitral valve regurgitation

Table 40.1. Echo/Doppler parameters that should be measured when valvular heart disease is suspected after the initial echocardiographic evaluation

Valvular heart disease	Echo parameters
Acute decompensation of preexisting heart valve disease	2D echo: wall motion abnormalities
Prosthetic valve failure or thrombosis	Evaluate RV function, RV systolic pressure
Acute mitral regurgitation from:	Inferior vena cava
(a) Ischemic papillary muscle rupture	Pulsed and continuous Doppler for max and mean transvalvular pressure gradient
(b) Ischemic papillary muscle dysfunction	Color Doppler for valve regurgitation
(c) Myxomatous chordal rupture	(consider transesophageal echo)
(d) Endocarditis	CO measurement
Acute aortic regurgitation from:	Vegetations (?); consider TEE
Endocarditis	
Aortic dissection	

CO, cardiac output; RV, right ventricle; TEE, transesophageal echocardiography.

orifice area with the phase-invariant signature algorithm (PISA) method, and the flow propagation can be calculated. With the spectral Doppler mode (PW, CW) in mitral valve stenosis, it is possible to measure the pressure gradient, calculate the mitral valve area from the pressure half-time, and measure the acceleration time, maximum pulmonary gradient (PG), the mean and maximum velocities and pressures, and the E/A filling waves' ratio. In mitral valve regurgitation, measurement of pressure gradient, acceleration time, mean and maximum velocities, and severity calculation with PISA are possible.

Aortic valve: With the 2D mode, the measurement of the aorta with an area caliper and calculation of the left ventricular outflow tract (LVOT) are possible. With color Doppler the severity of the insufficiency can be assessed with the PISA method. With the spectral Doppler mode (PW, CW) in atrioventricular (AV) stenosis, measurement of the pressure gradient, mean and maximum pressures and velocities, and application of the continuity equation are possible. In AV regurgitation, measurement of the pressure gradient, mean and maximum pressures and velocities, and severity can be done with the PISA method.

Tricuspid valve: In tricuspid valve stenosis, measurement of the pressure gradient and mean and maximum pressures and velocities is possible. In tricuspid valve regurgitation, measurement of the pressure gradient, acceleration time, mean and maximum pressures and velocities for the estimation of pulmonary hypertension, and calculation of the severity can be done with the PISA method.

Pulmonary valve: With the 2D mode, it is possible to measure the diameter of the pulmonary valve for the calculation of Qp/Qs. With color Doppler

Table 40.2. Echo/Doppler parameters that should be measured when cardiac muscle disease is suspected after the initial echocardiographic evaluation

Cardiac muscle disease	Echo parameters
Cardiogenic shock after acute myocardial infarction	2D echo: Wall motion abnormalities,
Postinfarction free wall rupture	LVEF; LVEF > or <40%, consider diastolic dysfunction
Postinfarction ventricular septal defect	Evaluation of RV function, RV systolic pressure
Acute decompensation of chronic cardiomyopathy	Inferior vena cava
Dilated cardiomyopathy	2D echo: pericardial effusion
Septic cardiomyopathy	Color Doppler for valve incompetence and/or intracardiac shunts
Hypertrophic cardiomyopathy	Left ventricular outflow tract obstruction
Acute anterior myocardial infarction with akinetic apex and hyperdynamic basal IVS and LVOT obstruction	

IVS, intraventricular septum; LVEF, left ventricular ejection fraction; LVOT, left ventricular outflow tract.

Table 40.3. Echo/Doppler parameters that should be examined when extracardiac disease is suspected after the initial echocardiographic evaluation

Extracardiac	Echo parameters
Aortic aneurysm or aortic dissection rupture into the pericardial sac	2D echo: pericardial effusion—aortic valve regurgitation—intima flap
Trauma	(consider transesophageal echo)
Ruptured aneurysm of the sinus of Valsalva	2D echo: Wall motion abnormalities
Aortic dissection	
Closed chest trauma	

continuous flow motion (CFM) the area of the pulmonary valve regurgitation flow can be measured. With spectral Doppler (PW, CW) in pulmonary valve stenosis, the pressure gradient, acceleration time, mean and maximum pressure for the Qp/Qs calculation, and mean and maximum velocity can be estimated.

Table 40.2 lists the echo/Doppler parameters that should be measured when cardiac muscle disease is suspected after the initial evaluation. The introduction of the new technology of the portable ultrasound systems and the evolution of high-speed microprocessors enabled the rapid frame rate increase. The increase of the frame rate from 30 to above 150 enabled the study of each of the myocardial segments with greater accuracy. Using tissue Doppler, the velocities of the mitral valve ring, the interventricular septum, and the right ventricle can be compared. The evaluation of patients with right ventricular failure is presented in Chapter 23.

Table 40.3 lists the Echo/Doppler parameters that should be measured when extracardiac disease is suspected after the initial evaluation. With the display of the harmonics and the increase in the resolution in the new generation of hand-held devices, structures like myxoma, thrombus, vegetations, and pericardiac fluid can be easily seen. Through the use of harmonic imaging on contrast agents with pulse inversion techniques, the walls of the left ventricle can be evaluated in difficult cases and in mechanically ventilated patients in search of apical thrombi and intraventricular flow.

Transesophageal Echocardiography

The evaluation of the AHF patient with transesophageal echocardiography (TEE) in the emergency room is not common, but the new portable ultrasound systems with the ability to carry a TEE probe enables a fast evaluation of the aorta in cases of rupture from trauma or dissection, prosthetic valve thrombosis, and acute valvular catastrophes (10). Recent data suggest that portable echocardiography could be useful at the prehospital setting where it can be used by cardiologists or emergency physicians after formal training (11).

Conclusion

Echocardiography/Doppler is useful for the initial evaluation of patients presenting with AHF syndromes in the emergency room. It enables the identification of the etiology of heart failure, the hemodynamic evaluation, and the prompt assessment of the effects of treatment. With the portable hand-held devices, echocardiography can be used for AHF evaluation in the emergency rooms of most hospitals.

References

1. Nieminen MS, Bohm M, Cowie MR, et al.; ESC Committee for Practice Guideline (CPG). Executive summary of the guidelines on the diagnosis and treatment of acute heart failure: the Task Force on Acute Heart Failure of the European Society of Cardiology. Eur Heart J 2005;26:384–416.
2. Gheorghiade M, Zannad F, Sopko G, et al.; International Working Group on Acute Heart Failure Syndromes. Acute heart failure syndromes: current state and framework for future research. Circulation 2005;112:3958–68.
3. Bassand JP, Danchin N, Filippatos G, et al. Implementation of reperfusion therapy in acute myocardial infarction. A policy statement from the European Society of Cardiology. Eur Heart J 2005;26:2733–41.
4. Oh JK, Meloy TD, Seward JB. Echocardiography in the emergency room: is it feasible, beneficial, and cost-effective? Echocardiography 1995;12:163–70.
5. Giannotti G, Mondillo S, Galderisi M, et al. Hand-held echocardiography: added value in clinical cardiological assessment. Cardiovasc Ultrasound 2005;3:7.

6. Kobal SL, Atar S, Siegel RJ. Hand-carried ultrasound improves the bedside cardiovascular examination. Chest 2004;126:693–701.
7. Mondillo S, Giannotti G, Innelli P, Ballo PC, Galderisi M. Hand-held echocardiography: Which usefulness? Who user? Int J Cardiol 2005;111:1–5.
8. Seward JB, Douglas PS, Erbel R, et al. Hand-carried cardiac ultrasound (HCU) device: recommendations regarding new technology. A report from the Echocardiography Task Force on new technology of the nomenclature and Standard Committee of the American Society of Echocardiography. J Am Soc Echocardiogr 2002;15:369–73.
9. Vargas Barron J. Echocardiography at the emergency room. Arch Cardiol Mex 2004;74(suppl 1): S103–5.
10. Petkov MP, Napolitano CA, Tobler HG, Ferrer TJ, Palacios JM, Wangler MD. A rupture of both atrioventricular valves after blunt chest trauma: the usefulness of transesophageal echocardiography for a life-saving diagnosis. Anesth Analg 2005;100:1256–8.
11. Lapostolle F, Petrovic T, Lenoir G, et al. Usefulness of hand-held ultrasound devices in out-of-hospital diagnosis performed by emergency physicians. Am J Emerg Med 2006; 24: 237–242.

41
Coronary Angiography in Acute Heart Failure

Patrick Henry

The decision to perform a coronary angiography in acute heart failure must be well balanced. On the one hand, the decision to perform a coronary angiography supposes that an acute cause (mainly coronary) can be diagnosed by this exam and that a specific treatment (mainly revascularization) could help the patient. On the other hand, coronary angiography means that the patient must remain still in a prone position during the exam, unless intubated. This exam is also associated with the injection of a notable amount of contrast media, which increases the loading conditions and can impair renal function.

Is Coronary Angiography Mandatory When Coronary Disease Is Suspected?

There are several causes of coronary artery–related cardiogenic shock that can be diagnosed without coronary angiography, mainly using echocardiography; these causes include acute mitral regurgitation, and septal or free wall rupture. In these settings, coronary angiography can evaluate the severity of coronary artery disease before surgery. However, these pathologies are usually so critical that coronary angiography cannot be performed[1].

ST Elevation Acute Myocardial Infarction

The main reason to perform a coronary angiography during the acute phase of heart failure is ST elevation myocardial infarction (STEMI). Where there is doubt, portable echocardiography can clarify the diagnosis of STEMI, especially if the diagnosis is confounded by left bundle branch block or pacing. Bedside biomarkers can be helpful only if they are positive and if they do not delay the revascularization procedure[1].

ST Elevation Acute Myocardial Infarction and Cardiogenic Shock

Acute heart failure and particularly cardiogenic shock occur in 5% to 10% of patients who suffer a myocardial infarction[1]. Despite therapeutic advances in the management of acute myocardial infarction, prior reports, including those from large thrombolytic trials, suggest no change in the incidence or overall mortality (55% to 80%) of cardiogenic shock in this setting[3,4].

Two randomized clinical trials[4–6] by them have examined the role of emergency revascularization in STEMI complicated by cardiogenic shock. Both trials showed a clinically important (even if statistically insignificant) absolute 9% reduction in 30-day mortality. In the Should We Emergently Revascularize Occluded Coronaries in Cardiogenic Shock (SHOCK) trial, the survival curves continued to progressively diverge over time with a significant mortality reduction. In this trial, almost two thirds of hospital survivors with cardiogenic shock who were treated with early revascularization were alive 6 years later[5].

The prespecified subgroup analysis of patients less than 75 years old showed an absolute 15% reduction in 30-day mortality, whereas there was no apparent benefit for the small cohort of patients more than 75 years old. However, several registries[7,8] have demonstrated a marked survival benefit for elderly patients who are clinically selected for revascularization (approximately 20% of patients), so age alone should not disqualify a patient for early revascularization.

These data strongly support having patients younger than 75 years with STEMI complicated by cardiogenic shock undergo emergency revascularization associated with support measures, such as intraaortic balloon pump (IABP) and ventricular assist devices that can stabilize hemodynamics so that revascularization procedures can be performed easier. Post hoc analyses[8] have suggested that glycoprotein (GP) IIb/IIIa inhibitors may help to reduce mortality.

These data further underscore the need for direct admission or early transfer of patients in cardiogenic shock or who are at risk of cardiogenic shock[8].

Predictors of Cardiogenic Shock in a Patient with ST Elevation Myocardial Infarction

In several cases, heart failure appears progressively after STEMI. The main predictors of developing cardiogenic shock in patients with STEMI are as follows[3,9]:

- Killip class III
- Killip class II
- Anterior location
- Inferior location with extension to right ventricle
- Age
- Tachycardia
- Low systolic blood pressure
- Previous coronary artery bypass graft (CABG)
- Previous myocardial infarction (MI)
- Female gender

Angioplasty of Culprit Lesion or All Lesions, or Coronary Artery Bypass Graft?

Although percutaneous coronary intervention (PCI) in a noninfarct artery is not recommended in stable patients, it can be beneficial in hemodynamically compromised patients if the stenotic artery perfuses a large area of myocardium and the procedure can be performed efficiently. In patients with significant left main disease or severe three-vessel disease and without right ventricular infarction or major comorbidities such as renal insufficiency or severe pulmonary disease, CABG can also be considered as the revascularization strategy[8,10].

American College of Cardiology (ACC)/American Heart Association (AHA) Recommendation Concerning Percutaneous Coronary Intervention for Cardiogenic Shock (2005)[8] (Fig. 41.1)

Class I

Primary PCI is recommended for patients less than 75 years old with ST elevation or left bundle branch block who develop shock within 36 hours of MI and are suitable for revascularization that can be performed within 18 hours of shock, unless further support is futile because of the patient's wishes or contraindications/unsuitability for further invasive care (level of evidence: A).

Class IIa

Primary PCI is reasonable for selected patients 75 years of age or older with ST elevation or left

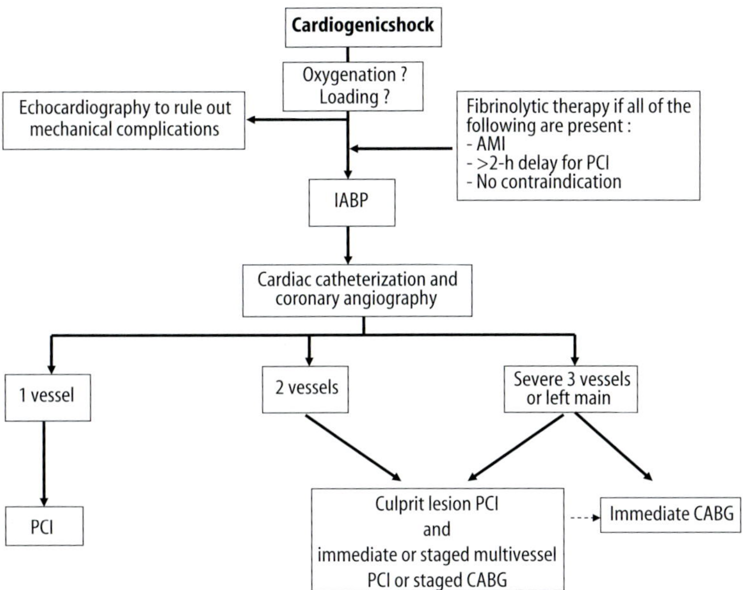

Figure 41.1. Recommendation concerning percutaneous coronary intervention for cardiogenic shock. AMI, acute myocardial infarction; CABG, coronary artery bypass graft; IABP, intraaortic balloon pump; PCI, percutaneous coronary intervention. (Adapted from Hochman.[11])

bundle branch block who develop shock within 36 hours of MI and are suitable for revascularization that can be performed within 18 hours of shock. Patients with good prior functional status who are suitable for revascularization and agree to invasive care may be selected for such an invasive strategy (level of evidence: B).

Coronary Angiography in Non–ST Elevation Myocardial Infarction

An early invasive treatment strategy defined as coronary angiography and revascularization within 12 to 48 hours after presentation is appropriate in patients with non–ST elevation myocardial infarction (NSTEMI) with a high-risk level[12].

The patients with a high-risk level are those with any of the following:

- Recurrent ischemia with associated heart failure (S_3 gallop, pulmonary edema, worsening rales, or new or worsening mitral regurgitation)
- Depressed systolic LV function (ejection fraction <0.40 on noninvasive study)
- Sustained ventricular tachycardia

Intraaortic balloon pump is probably underused in this setting.

References

1. Antman EM, Anbe DT, Armstrong PW, et al. ACC/AHA guidelines for the management of patients with ST-elevation myocardial infarction: A report of the American College of Cardiology/American Heart Association Task Force on Practice Guidelines (Committee to Revise the 1999 Guidelines for the Management of patients with acute myocardial infarction). J Am Coll Cardiol. 2004;44(3):E1–211.
2. Berger PB, Tuttle RH, Holmes DR Jr, et al. One-year survival among patients with acute myocardial infarction complicated by cardiogenic shock, and its relation to early revascularization: results from the GUSTO-I trial. Circulation. 1999;99(7):873–8.
3. Hasdai D, Califf RM, Thompson TD, et al. Predictors of cardiogenic shock after thrombolytic therapy for acute myocardial infarction. J Am Coll Cardiol. 2000;35(1):136–43.
4. Urban P, Stauffer JC, Bleed D, et al. A randomized evaluation of early revascularization to treat shock complicating acute myocardial infarction. The

(Swiss) Multicenter Trial of Angioplasty for Shock-(S)MASH. Eur Heart J. 1999;20(14):1030–8.
5. Hochman JS, Sleeper LA, Webb JG, et al. Early revascularization and long-term survival in cardiogenic shock complicating acute myocardial infarction. JAMA. 2006;295(21):2511–5.
6. Hochman JS, Sleeper LA, Webb JG, et al. Early revascularization in acute myocardial infarction complicated by cardiogenic shock. SHOCK Investigators. Should We Emergently Revascularize Occluded Coronaries for Cardiogenic Shock. N Engl J Med. 1999;341(9):625–34.
7. Dzavik V, Sleeper LA, Picard MH, et al. Outcome of patients aged > or = 75 years in the SHould we emergently revascularize Occluded Coronaries in cardiogenic shocK (SHOCK) trial: do elderly patients with acute myocardial infarction complicated by cardiogenic shock respond differently to emergent revascularization? Am Heart J. 2005;149(6):1128–34.
8. Smith SC Jr, Feldman TE, Hirshfeld JW Jr, et al. ACC/AHA/SCAI 2005 guideline update for percutaneous coronary intervention: a report of the American College of Cardiology/American Heart Association Task Force on Practice Guidelines (ACC/AHA/SCAI Writing Committee to Update 2001 Guidelines for Percutaneous Coronary Intervention). Circulation. 2006;113(7):e166–286.
9. Chase M, Robey JL, Zogby KE, et al. Prospective validation of the Thrombolysis in Myocardial Infarction Risk Score in the emergency department chest pain population. Ann Emerg Med. 2006;48(3):252–9.
10. Lee MS, Kapoor N, Jamal F, et al. Comparison of coronary artery bypass surgery with percutaneous coronary intervention with drug-eluting stents for unprotected left main coronary artery disease. J Am Coll Cardiol. 2006;47(4):864–70.
11. Hochman JS. Cardiogenic shock complicating acute myocardial infarction: expanding the paradigm. Circulation. 2003;107(24):2998–3002.
12. Gibler WB, Cannon CP, Blomkalns AL, et al. Practical implementation of the Guidelines for Unstable Angina/Non-ST-Segment Elevation Myocardial Infarction in the emergency department. Ann Emerg Med. 2005;46(2):185–97.

42
Arterial Blood Gas Analysis in Acute Heart Failure Syndrome

Martin J. Cook and Andrew Rhodes

Arterial blood gas analysis is a fundamental component of assessing critically ill patients. It allows rapid near-patient testing, giving vital information on oxygenation, ventilation, metabolic harmony, and an indication of tissue hypoxia.

Oxygen and carbon dioxide were first discovered in the 18th century, but the ability to measure both the partial pressure of these gases in solution and hydrogen ion concentration was not discovered until the middle of the 20th century. Subsequent analytical developments have progressed such that blood gas analyzers are no longer the preserve of laboratories, but are instead found in most critical care settings.

Blood gas analyzers measure the partial pressures of oxygen (PO_2), carbon dioxide (PCO_2) and pH. The percentage saturation of hemoglobin with oxygen (SpO_2) is either calculated using the oxygen dissociation curve (assuming the normal form of adult hemoglobin) or directly measured using a co-oximeter. The actual bicarbonate (HCO_3^-), standard HCO_3^-, base deficit/excess are not measured but are derived variables using the pH and PCO_2. Modern blood gas analyzers often measure a number of other variables: sodium, potassium, and chloride ion concentrations, and blood glucose and lactate.

Arterial Blood Gas Sampling and Measurement

Arterial blood can be obtained either through a single stab or from an indwelling arterial catheter. The most common sites are the radial artery and femoral artery. The risks from a single stab are small but include pain, paresthesia, hematoma, vasospasm, infection, arterial thrombosis, and aneurysm formation. Indwelling arterial catheters allow continuous accurate blood pressure monitoring along with easy access for repeated blood gas analysis. The complications of an indwelling arterial catheter are the same as for a simple stab, but clearly the risks of infection and arterial thrombosis are significantly higher.

The blood gas sample should be taken into a preheparinized syringe, and all air bubbles must be expelled. Excess heparin can interfere with the accuracy of the results obtained and should constitute less than 5% of the sample volume (1). The sample needs to be analyzed immediately (within 15 minutes); otherwise it should be cooled in an ice bath (to slow cellular respiration).

Normal Values

The normal range for arterial blood gases are listed in Table 42.1. Advancing age is associated with the development of ventilation/perfusion mismatches, which leads to an expected gradual decline in PaO_2. An approximate method for predicting the normal PaO_2 (breathing room air) corrected for age is as follows (1):

$$100\,\text{mm Hg} - 0.3 \times \text{Age (years)}$$

Temperature Correction

The solubility of a gas in a solution alters with temperature. With reducing temperature there is increased solubility of gases in liquids, which

Table 42.1. Normal arterial blood gas values breathing room air

pH	7.35–7.45
PCO_2	35–45 mm Hg
PO_2	86–100 mm Hg
HCO_3^-	22–26 mmol/L
Base excess/deficit	−2–+2 mmol/L
Arterial oxygen saturation SpO_2	94–100%

leads to a fall in the measured partial pressure of the gases in solution. Since blood gas analyzers actually measure the blood sample at 37°C, this may mean that the results obtained in vitro may not correlate with those actually found in vivo. Most blood gas analyzers can give temperature-corrected results (corrected to the patient's measured core temperature), as well as those measured at 37°C. Despite the theoretical advantages of temperature corrected results, there is little clinical evidence of any benefit (2).

Assessment of Gas Exchange

Oxygen

Oxygen is transported in blood principally bound to hemoglobin, with only a small fraction dissolved in the blood:

$$\text{Oxygen content (mL/dL)} = [\text{Hb (g/dL)} \times Sp\text{O}_2 \times 1.34] + [0.003 \times Pa\text{O}_2 \text{ (mm Hg)}]$$

where 1.34 is oxygen carrying capacity of 1 g of hemoglobin, and 0.003 is the solubility of oxygen in plasma at room temperature at 37°C.

The adequacy of oxygen delivery to the tissues is dependent on the cardiac output, hemoglobin, and oxygen saturation.

Hypoxemia is reduced arterial oxygen content, which may be caused by low inspired oxygen, hypoventilation, ventilation/perfusion mismatch, intrapulmonary shunts, and impaired diffusion across the alveoli. Hypoxia is a lack of oxygen at the cellular/mitochondrial level, which can be caused by hypoxemia, anemia, or an inadequate cardiac output.

As the vast majority of oxygen is carried by hemoglobin, noninvasive pulse oximeters are routinely used to assess oxygenation. Pulse oximeters are accurate with saturations above ~85%, but below this level they are poorly calibrated. Pulse oximeters may also become unreliable in a number of clinical settings that may be relevant to critically ill patients (Table 42.2). Although a normal arterial saturation is reassuring, it is not a marker of adequacy of ventilation; hypoxia often develops late in the setting of hypoventilation, especially if supplementary oxygen is supplied.

Arterial blood gas analyzers, via an electrochemical method, measure the partial pressure of oxygen in blood (Po_2). The percentage saturation of hemoglobin with oxygen is either estimated using the oxygen dissociation curve (assuming normal adult hemoglobin) or calculated using a co-oximeter.

Oxygen therapy should be taken into account when interpreting arterial blood gases. The ideal alveolus-to-arterial gradient (A-a gradient) is one way of assessing oxygenation as it takes into account oxygen therapy (3). The A-a gradient is the difference between the partial pressure of oxygen in the ideal alveolus (P_AO_2) and that found in arterial blood (Pao_2). This gradient can help differentiate hypoxemia caused by either hypoventilation or low inspired oxygen from that caused by impaired gas exchange. The P_AO_2 is calculated using the ideal alveolar gas equation:

$$\text{A-a Gradient} = P_AO_{22} - Pao_2$$

where Pao_2 is the measured arterial Po_2, P_AO_2 is the partial pressure of oxygen in the ideal alveolus:

$$P_AO_2 = Fio_2 \times (760 - 47) - (Paco_2/0.8)$$

where Fio_2 is the fractional inspired oxygen concentration, 760 is the atmospheric pressure (mm Hg), and 47 is the saturated water vapor pressure at 37°C (mm Hg).

Table 42.2. Causes of inaccurate pulse oximeter readings

Severe hypoxemia, SpO_2 <85%
Poor peripheral perfusion
Shivering
Strong ambient lighting
Severe tricuspid regurgitation
Abnormal hemoglobins (met- and carboxy-hemoglobin)
Intravenous dyes (e.g., methylene blue and indocyanine green)
Nail varnish

Due to the development of ventilation/perfusion mismatches, the A-a gradient changes with age. The normal A-a gradient (age corrected) is approximately

$$\text{A-a gradient} = (\text{Age}/4) + 4.$$

The A-a gradient also changes with oxygen therapy, increasing by 5 to 7 mm Hg for every 10% increase FiO_2.

In health, right-to-left shunts from both the bronchial veins and the thebesian veins draining the coronary circulation cause the A-a gradient. Hypoxemia associated with a normal A-a gradient implies hypoventilation, whereas an increased gradient indicates either lung pathology or a right-to-left shunt. The lung pathology may be due to ventilation/perfusion mismatch, shunt, or impaired alveolar diffusion.

Carbon Dioxide

Carbon dioxide (CO_2) is produced as a by-product of cellular respiration; it is then transported to and cleared by the lungs. The $PaCO_2$ is determined by the rate of production of CO_2 (VCO_2) and is inversely proportional to the minute ventilation of the lungs:

$$(PaCO_2 \propto VCO_2)/\text{Minute Ventilation}$$

CO_2 production (VCO_2) is usually constant, and so $PaCO_2$ is determined by minute ventilation, which in turn is controlled by central and peripheral chemoreceptors whose primary function is to maintain a steady $PaCO_2$ (35–45 mm Hg). $PaCO_2$ in association with pH is thus used to assess adequacy of ventilation.

The majority of carbon dioxide is carried in blood as HCO_3^-, and the rest is bound to proteins as carbamino compounds (most notably to deoxygenated hemoglobin) and a small amount is found dissolved in blood ($PaCO_2$). CO_2 slowly and reversibly combines with water H_2O to form carbonic acid (H_2CO_3), which then dissociates into bicarbonate (HCO_3^-) and hydrogen (H^+) ions:

$$CO_2 + H_2O \leftrightarrow H_2CO_3 \leftrightarrow HCO_3^- + H^+$$

Carbonic anhydrase is a catalyst to the above reaction and is found in red blood cells. CO_2 diffuses into red cells and there, under the influence of carbonic anhydrase, it combines with H_2O to form H^+ and HCO_3^-. The HCO_3^- exits into the plasma, and chloride ions (Cl^-) enter the red blood cell to maintain electroneutrality (chloride shift). In the lungs CO_2 is cleared. Increasing minute ventilation causes a fall in CO_2, which shifts the balance of the above equation to the left; this reduces H^+ levels and thereby increases the pH (respiratory alkalosis). Conversely, a fall in minute ventilation leads to an increased CO_2, which shifts the balance of the equation to the right, with an associated increased H^+ concentration and fall in pH (respiratory acidosis). The ability of the body to rapidly alter CO_2 clearance means that $PaCO_2$ acts as an intrinsic component of acid–base regulation.

Arterial blood gas analyzers measure the partial pressure of carbon dioxide in blood via electrochemical methods. In ventilated patients the arterial $PaCO_2$ may be estimated using capnometry, which measures end tidal expired CO_2.

Acid–Base Balance

pH is the negative logarithm of the hydrogen ion concentration. The hydrogen ion concentration in blood is solely dependent on the relative dissociation of water:

$$H_2O \leftrightarrow H^+ + OH^-$$

In blood the balance of the equation is such that the normal $[H^+]$ is 40 nmol/L or pH = 7.4 at 37°C. Any factor affecting the dissociation of water alters the pH of blood; the degree to which each factor affects pH is dependent on their ionic charge, quantity, and relative dissociation. Normally the pH of arterial blood is maintained between 7.35 and 7.45 by intracellular and extracellular buffers along with renal and respiratory regulatory systems. The central nervous system and respiratory systems regulate the $PaCO_2$. The renal system affects the pH by means of alterations in retention and excretion of acid and alkali (principally by regulation of Cl^- elimination).

The terms *acidosis* and *alkalosis* express the presence of excess acid and base in the blood, respectively; *acidemia* (pH < 7.35) and *alkalemia* (pH > 7.45) describe the net effect on blood pH. As the acid–base balance defines the pH, alterations in either acid or base can affect the pH, but alterations in both cause a mixed picture that may compound or cancel each other out. Thus a normal pH does not necessarily mean there is no acid–base disturbance.

There are two components of acid–base balance: respiratory and metabolic. Disturbance in either will cause an acid–base disturbance. Respiratory acid–base disorders are related to alterations in $Paco_2$. All other factors affecting pH are considered metabolic.

Assessing the respiratory component of acid–base balance is relatively simple, with high $Paco_2$ causing a respiratory acidosis and a low $Paco_2$ causing alkalosis. Interpretation of the metabolic component is more complex. There are now three differing methods of assessing the metabolic component; they focus on either bicarbonate, standard base deficit/excess or the physiochemical approach (4)

Bicarbonate Approach

The traditional approach interprets the pH in terms of the CO_2 and HCO_3^- according to the Henderson-Hasselbalch equation.

$$H_2O + CO_2 \leftrightarrow H_2CO_3 \leftrightarrow H^+ + HCO_3^-$$

$$pH = 6.1 + \log[HCO_3^-]/(Paco_2 \times 0.03)$$

As alterations in $Paco_2$ directly alter HCO_3^- levels, the calculated HCO_3^- needs to be corrected to a normal CO_2; the result obtained is known as the standard HCO_3^-. The standard HCO_3^- is the actual HCO_3^- concentration corrected to a $Paco_2$ of 40 mm Hg at 37°C, using the Siggard-Anderson nomogram (5). Increases in standard HCO_3^- above 26 mmol/L indicate a metabolic alkalosis, and a fall below 22 mmol/L indicate a metabolic acidosis. A criticism of this approach is that it does not does not reliably quantify the severity or the mechanism of the metabolic disturbance (6).

Standard Base Deficit/Excess

The base deficit or excess (BDE) quantifies the metabolic component of acid–base balance. By definition it is the quantity of strong acid (or strong base) that has to be added to 1 L of fully saturated whole blood at 37°C to bring its pH to 7.4 when the $Paco_2$ is 40 mm Hg. The BDE was originally measured on whole blood, which meant that alterations in hemoglobin affected the validity of the results. To resolve this, the standard BDE is now used, which is corrected to a hemoglobin concentration of 5 g/dL. The standard BDE is independent of the actual hemoglobin concentration. A BDE less than −2 mmol/L indicates the presence of a metabolic acidosis, and a BDE greater than +2 mmol/L indicates the presence of a metabolic alkalosis. Acute changes in $Paco_2$ will alter the pH but do not alter the BDE.

The BDE is calculated using the Van Slyke equation (7), which assumes normal total body water, normal plasma electrolyte concentrations, and normal plasma proteins (most notably albumin). Changes in any of these assumed normal variables can cause alterations in the calculated BDE.

Anion Gap

In conjunction with either the bicarbonate or base BDE approach, the anion gap is used to help elucidate the cause of a metabolic acidosis (8). Electroneutrality assumes that the net positive ions (cations) in a system must equal the net negative ions (anions). The anion gap is the difference between the sum of the measured cations (sodium and potassium) and anions (chloride and bicarbonate):

$$\text{Anion Gap} = (Na^+ + K^+) - (HCO_3^- + Cl^-)$$

The normal calculated anion gap is 8 to 16 mmol/L and is made up of unmeasured anions (mainly albumin, but also other proteins, phosphates, sulfates, and organic anions). An elevated anion gap indicates the presence of excess unmeasured anions. The causes of a raised anion-gap metabolic acidosis include lactic acidosis and ketoacidosis. A metabolic acidosis associated with a normal anion gap is due to an elevated Cl^- concentration relative to Na^+. The HCO_3^- concentration changes with pH and so does not independently affect acid–base balance.

As albumin is a significant component of the normal anion gap, alterations in albumin levels can directly affect the accuracy of the calculated anion gap. Hypoalbuminemia and hypophosphatemia, often present in critical illness, reduce the calculated anion gap and may mask the presence of other unmeasured anions. To address this, the corrected normal anion gap has been formulated, which calculates what the normal anion gap should be for any given albumin or phosphate level (6):

Corrected normal anion gap = 0.2 [Albumin (g/L)] + 1.5 [Phosphate (mmol/L)]

If the calculated anion gap is greater than the corrected normal anion gap, then unmeasured anions are present.

Physiochemical (Stewart) Approach

The physiochemical approach is a relatively new understanding of acid–base balance that uses modern quantitative methods of analysis. Stewart (9) first described this approach in 1983; it has been subsequently modified by Fencl and Leith (10).

At first glance it appears similar to the traditional approach, but in actuality it is fundamentally different. Whereas the traditional approaches, bicarbonate and BDE, have two independent variables (HCO_3^- and CO_2) affecting pH, the physiochemical approach recognizes that acid–base balance is determined by three independent factors: CO_2, strong ion difference (SID), and total weak acid concentration (A_{TOT}). Bicarbonate is viewed as a dependent variable and as such does not have any affect on acid–base balance; alterations in HCO_3^-, therefore, do not alter pH but instead just reflect changes in the other independent variables.

As with the traditional approach, carbon dioxide is an independent variable and represents the respiratory component of acid–base balance.

The SID is the difference between all the completely dissociated positively charged ions (strong cations) and negatively charged ions (strong anions) in plasma. The normal SID is 40 to 42 mmol/L. The SID independently affects water dissociation via electroneutrality (assuming all other factors are kept constant):

[Total positive charged ions] – [Total negatively charged ions] = 0

A reduced SID increases liberation of H^+ from water, causing an acidosis, and an increased SID reduces liberation of H^+, causing an alkalosis.

The SID is always positive and is balanced by an equal amount of negative charge from HCO_3^- (total CO_2), A_{TOT} (phosphate and albumin), and unmeasured anions, which is also known as the effective SID (eSID). For clinical practice the SID can be simplified to the apparent SID (aSID). The aSID is calculated using the routinely measured strong ions:

$$\text{Apparent SID} = (Na^+ + K^+ + Mg^{2+} + Ca^{2+}) - (Cl^-)$$

The difference between the effective and apparent strong ion difference is known as the strong ion gap (SIG):

$$\text{SIG} = \text{eSID} - \text{aSID}$$

The strong ion gap is composed of unmeasured ions. An elevated SIG is in essence similar to an elevated anion gap (Fig. 42.1), the main exception being that the anion gap is directly affected by changes in albumin and phosphate (A_{TOT}).

The third independent variable is the total charge derived from weak acids (A_{TOT}). Proteins (most notably albumin) and phosphates are the main constituents. The charge derived from weak acids is complex, as it depends on absolute

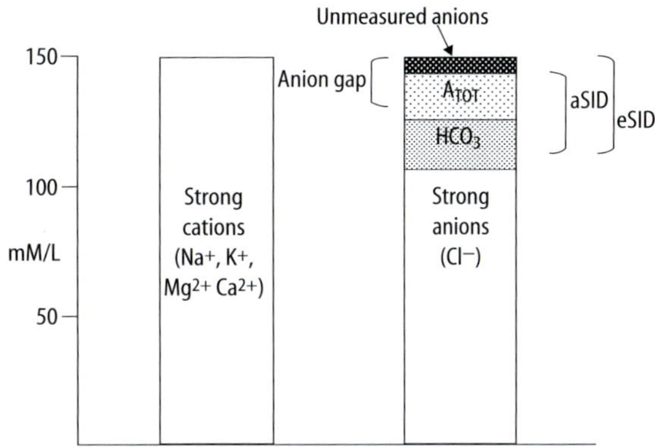

FIGURE 42.1. Diagrammatic representation of the strong ion gap (SIG) and the anion gap. The SIG is the difference between the effective SID and the apparent SID. It is composed of unmeasured anions such as lactate or ketones. The anion gap is calculated from the difference between measured cations and anions [anion gap = $(Na^+ + K^+) - (HCO_3^- + Cl^-)$]. The anion gap is composed of both unmeasured anions and A_{TOT}, alterations in either will affect the anion gap. The corrected anion gap corrects for alterations in A_{TOT}.

quantities and on factors affecting dissociation (pH) (11). In health, these compounds have little effect on acid–base balance. Critical illness can lead to alterations in A_{TOT} that can have a significant affect on acid–base balance. Hypoalbuminemia and hypophosphatemia both cause a reduction in total weak acid and so will cause a metabolic alkalosis. Hyperphosphatemia, as found in renal failure, increases total weak acid concentration and so causes a metabolic acidosis.

The benefit of the Stewart approach to interpreting acid–base balance is most apparent in the critically ill. These patients often have marked disturbances of their albumin, total body water, and sodium and chloride levels, all of which can have an impact on acid–base balance that would otherwise be missed by the traditional approaches. A criticism of this approach is its complexity, as it requires six simultaneous equations and fourth-power polynomials for resolution. Any error in measurement of any of the variables can have a significant effect on the accuracy of the final calculation.

In view of the relative complexity of the physiochemical approach, Storey et al. (12) have formulated two simple bedside calculations that adapt the base deficit/excess model so that it is compatible with the physiochemical approach (12). These calculations correct for acid–base disturbance caused by changes in sodium ions, chloride ions, free water, and albumin levels.

$$BDE_{NaCl} = (Na^+ - Cl^-) - 38$$

$$BDE_{Alb} = 0.25 \times [42 - \text{measured albumin concentration (g/L)}]$$

where BDE_{NaCl} is the base deficit/excess caused by alterations in sodium or chloride ions, and BDE_{Alb} is the base deficit/excess caused by alterations in albumin concentration.

The combination of the BDE_{NaCl} and BDE_{Alb} is known as the calculated BDE. The difference between the actual BDE obtained from the arterial blood gases and that contributed by albumin and Na^+ and Cl^- is known as the BDE gap and is made up of unmeasured ions. The BDE gap should normally be zero and is similar to the strong ion gap (SIG):

$$\text{BDE gap} = \text{Actual BDE} - (BDE_{NaCl} + BDE_{Alb}) = \text{Unmeasured ions}$$

Clinical Example

A 74-year-old man was admitted to the intensive care unit (ICU) 2 days previously with pneumonia and acute heart failure. An arterial blood gas is taken, with the following results:

pH	7.37
$Paco_2$	44 mm Hg
HCO_3^-	22 mmol/L
BDE	−2 mmol/L
Na^+	145 mmol/L
K^+	4 mmol/L
Cl^-	111 mmol/L
Fio_2	0.2
Pao_2	104 mmHg
Serum albumin	16 g/L

At first glance these arterial blood gas results appear unremarkable. Oxygenation is adequate. The pH is normal, as is the $Paco_2$, BDE, and $HCO3^-$. But then we assess the BDE using the Storey calculations:

$$BDE_{NaCl} = (Na^+ - Cl^-) - 38 = (145 - 111) - 38 = -4\ \text{mmol/L}$$

$$BDE_{Alb} = 0.25 \times (42 - \text{albumin}) = 0.25 \times (42 - 14) = +7\ \text{mmol/L}$$

From these calculations we can see that the hyperchloremia is causing a metabolic acidosis (BDE_{NaCl} = −4 mmol/L) and the hypoalbuminemia is causing a metabolic alkalosis (BDE_{Alb} = +7 mmol/L). If we combine the BDE due to NaCl and albumin we get a calculated BDE:

$$\text{Calculated BDE} = BDE_{NaCl} + BDE_{Alb} = -4 + 7 = 3\ \text{mmol/L}$$

As discussed above the difference between the actual and calculated BDE is known as the BDE gap. This is made up from unmeasured ions:

$$\text{BDE gap} = \text{Actual BDE} - \text{Calculated BDE} = -2 - 3 = -5\ \text{mmol/L}$$

The BDE gap should normally be zero; an elevated BDE gap indicates unmeasured anions are present. A lactate concentration was subsequently measured at 3.5 mmol/L (normal lactate <1 mmol/L).

This example shows that despite apparently normal arterial blood gas results, there may still be marked metabolic acid–base balance disorder. In this example there is a metabolic acidosis caused by both hyperchloremia (reduced SID) and lactic acidosis, but these are hidden by the metabolic alkalosis caused by hypoalbuminemia. All of these abnormalities are clinically relevant.

Types of Acid-Base Disturbance

Respiratory Alkalosis

Excess removal of CO_2 from the body leads to a respiratory alkalosis. In a primary respiratory alkalosis the $Pa{CO_2}$ is <35 mm Hg and the pH is >7.45. The main causes of a respiratory alkalosis are cerebral (e.g., pain, anxiety, raised intracranial pressure) and respiratory disturbance (e.g., acute asthma, pneumonia, and pulmonary emboli). A common cause of respiratory alkalosis in the critical care setting occurs when patients are overventilated with an excessive minute volume. In acute respiratory alkalosis the BDE should be normal. Chronic respiratory alkalosis is unusual, and metabolic compensation is slow, involving decreased urinary loss of Cl^-; this decreases the SID and thereby causes a compensatory metabolic acidosis. A formula to calculate the expected compensatory metabolic response for a chronic respiratory alkalosis is as follows (13):

$$\text{BDE (mmol/L)} = 0.4 \times [40 - Pa{CO_2}\ \text{(mmHg)}]$$

Respiratory Acidosis

This is a primary disturbance when the pH is <7.35 associated with a $Pa{CO_2}$ that is >45 mm Hg. An elevated $Pa{CO_2}$ may be caused by central nervous system (CNS) depression (e.g., drugs, trauma, infection), lung disease (e.g., obstructive airways disease and pulmonary fibrosis), musculoskeletal disease (e.g., exhaustion, myopathies, and neuropathies), or dramatically increased CO_2 production (e.g., malignant hyperthermia). Hypercapnea causes CNS depression and can lead to CO_2 narcosis, which in turn can lead to further CO_2 retention. In the setting of an acute disease such as asthma or acute heart failure, the development of a respiratory acidosis indicates severe fatigue and is an ominous sign. In acute uncomplicated respiratory acidosis the BDE is unchanged. Metabolic compensation for chronic respiratory acidosis is slow and limited. The kidneys eliminate more Cl^-; this increases the SID and thus causes a compensatory metabolic alkalosis. In chronic CO_2 retention, the metabolic compensation may be adequate to correct the pH disturbance, which will become inadequate in the face of a further deterioration. The expected metabolic response to a chronic respiratory failure is as follows (13):

$$\text{BDE (mmol/L)} = 0.4 \times [40 - Pa{CO_2}\ \text{(mmHg)}]$$

Metabolic Alkalosis (Table 42.3)

A primary metabolic alkalosis is associated with a pH >7.45, HCO_3^- >26 mmol/L, and BDE >+2 mmol/L. Metabolic alkalosis can be caused by an increased SID or reduced A_{TOT}. Examples include hypochloremia caused by severe vomiting and hypernatremia caused by excess diuresis (contraction alkalosis); both of these increase the SID and cause a metabolic alkalosis. Fluids with sodium coupled to weak ions (e.g., citrate in blood products, acetate in parenteral nutrition and bicarbonate) have a high SID; administration of large volumes of these fluids increases the SID and can cause a metabolic alkalosis. Hypoalbuminemia and hypophosphatemia both cause a metabolic alkalosis due to a reduced A_{TOT}.

Respiratory compensation for a metabolic alkalosis is rapid and involves relative hypoventilation, causing a respiratory acidosis. This compensatory response returns the pH toward normal. The expected respiratory response is for a metabolic alkalosis is as follows (13):

$$Pa{CO_2}\ \text{(mm Hg)} = 40 + (0.6 \times \text{BDE})$$

Table 42.3. Causes of a metabolic alkalosis

Increased SID
Chloride loss
• Severe vomiting
• Gastric drainage
• Chloride wasting diarrhea (villous adenoma)
• Mineralocorticoid excess
• Excess liquorice intake
• Diuretic use (contraction alkalosis)
Sodium load
• Administration sodium linked to weak ions (sodium acetate, sodium citrate, or sodium bicarbonate)
Reduced weak acid (decreased A_{TOT})
• Hypoalbuminemia
• Hypophosphatemia

Table 42.4. Causes of a metabolic acidosis

Normal anion gap acidosis
Reduced SID (increased Cl^- in relation to Na^+)
• Hyperchloremic acidosis–intravenous fluids with low SID (e.g., 0.9% saline based solutions and suspensions)
• Excess gastrointestinal Na^+ loss (diarrhea and high output fistulas)
• Renal mishandling of ions (renal tubular acidosis)
Increased weak acids (A_{TOT})
• Hyperphosphatemia (renal failure)
• Hyperproteinemia
Elevated anion gap acidosis
Increased unmeasured anions
• Lactic acidosis
• Ketoacidosis
• Renal failure (sulfates and other acids)
• Toxins (methanol, ethylene glycol, salicylates and paraldehyde)

Metabolic Acidosis (Table 42.4)

Metabolic acidosis is the most common acid–base disturbance in the critical care setting. In a simple metabolic acidosis the arterial blood gas shows a pH < 7.35 with the HCO_3^- <22 mmol/L and the BDE <–2 mmol/L.

Metabolic acidosis can be caused by either a fall in SID or an increased concentration of weak acids (A_{TOT}). A fall in the SID can be caused by the generation of strong organic anions (e.g., ketones and lactate), loss of cations (e.g., Na^+ loss from diarrhea), mishandling of ions (e.g., in renal tubular acidosis there is increase urinary Na^+ loss in comparison to Cl^-), or due to the addition of exogenous anions (e.g., iatrogenic acidosis and poisonings). The administration of large volumes of intravenous fluid with a low SID causes a dilutional acidosis (14). Dilutional acidosis occurs when there is an increase in Cl^- in relation to Na^+ (net Cl^- gain or Na^+ loss); this causes a reduction in SID. Normal (0.9%) saline has a SID of zero (Na^+ 154 and Cl^- 154); administration of large volumes of normal saline-based solutions increases extracellular Cl^-, which reduces the SID, thereby causing a hyperchloremic acidosis. Hyperphosphatemia (renal failure) and hyperproteinemia both increase A_{TOT} and also cause a metabolic acidosis.

Respiratory compensation for a metabolic acidosis involves hyperventilation, which causes a compensatory respiratory alkalosis. Respiratory compensation is rapid and usually effective in returning the pH toward normal. The expected $Pa{CO_2}$ from respiratory compensation in metabolic acidosis is as follows (13):

$$\text{Expected } Pa{CO_2} = 40 + \text{BDE (mm Hg)}$$

Lactic Acidosis (Table 42.5)

Lactate is normally produced from pyruvate as a by-product of anaerobic glycolysis (Embden-Meyerhof pathway). All tissues produce lactate under anaerobic conditions, but some tissues (skin, red blood cells, brain, muscle, and gut) routinely metabolize glucose to lactate; excess lactate then leaks into the bloodstream. The excess lactate is metabolized predominantly by the liver (60%) and kidneys (30%). The internal cycling with production by the tissues and transport to and metabolism by the liver and kidney is known as the Cori cycle. Half of the lactate is converted to glucose (gluconeogenesis) and half is further metabolized to CO_2 and water in the citric acid cycle. Other tissues can use lactate as a substrate

Table 42.5. Causes of lactic acidosis (Cohen and Woods classification)

Type A (hypoxia)
• Inadequate cardiac output (cardiogenic, hypovolemic, and septic shock)
• Regional hypoperfusion (peripheral or mesenteric ischemia)
• Acute severe hypoxemia
• Severe anemia
• Carbon monoxide poisoning
Type B (no tissue hypoxia)
Type B1–associated with underlying disorders
• Diabetes mellitus
• Renal failure
• Liver failure
• Leukemia/lymphoma
• Abnormal bowel flora
• Severe infections (e.g., cholera, malaria)
Type B2–drugs or toxins
• Metformin/phenformin
• Antiretroviral drugs
• Ethanol
• Methanol
• Ethylene glycol
• Isoniazid
Type B3–hereditary metabolic disorders

and oxidize it to CO_2 and water, but it is only the liver and kidney that have the enzymes that can convert lactate to glucose. Normally any lactate produced is rapidly metabolized. The balance between release into the bloodstream and hepatorenal uptake maintains plasma lactate at about 1 mmol/L.

At physiologic pH, lactate is 99% ionized and as such is considered a strong ion. Elevations in lactate reduce the SID and therefore can cause a metabolic acidosis. Lactic acidosis is a common cause of a raised anion gap acidosis.

The normal lactate concentration is <1 mmol/L; lactic acidosis is hyperlactatemia (>2 mmol/L), associated with a metabolic acidosis. Elevated lactate levels may be caused by either excess production (e.g., extreme exercise, convulsions, or sepsis) or when there is impaired lactate clearance (liver disease). In the critically ill, lactic acidosis is usually caused by a combination of both increased production (cellular hypoxia) and reduced clearance (liver dysfunction).

Lactic acidosis has been classified into two types: A and B (15). Type A results from inadequate oxygen delivery to the tissues (cellular hypoxia). Type B is thought to be due to impaired carbohydrate metabolism; it is not associated with inadequate oxygen delivery. Type A lactic acidosis is of greater clinical importance. Transient tissue hypoxia associated with lactic acidosis is not necessarily harmful; there is even evidence suggesting that elevated lactate levels are associated with improved endurance in athletes. Persistent tissue hypoxia is harmful and can lead to isolated organ dysfunction or even multiorgan failure. Treatment should be directed to the underlying cause, and attempts must be made to optimize global oxygen delivery (16–18). Improved oxygen delivery to the tissues requires accurate assessment and optimization of cardiac output, hemoglobin, and arterial oxygen content.

Prognostically, an isolated elevated lactate level is of limited use (very high levels may be seen following a convulsions, yet the mortality is low). Of greater importance is the trend of lactate levels with time (19, 20). The failure of improvement in lactic acidosis following appropriate treatment has been shown to be associated with a poor outcome.

A Practical Approach to Assessing Acid–Base Balance

Assess the pH

A pH > 7.45 indicates an alkalemia and a pH <7.35 indicates an acidemia; the direction of the pH change indicates the overriding primary acid–base disturbance. Although a normal pH (7.35 to 7.45) is likely to indicate that there is no acute major acid–base disturbance, a complex acid–base disturbance may still be occurring.

Assess the Respiratory Component ($Paco_2$)

A $Paco_2$ <35 mm Hg indicates a respiratory alkalosis and a $Paco_2$ >45 mm Hg indicates a respiratory acidosis. Acute respiratory acid–base disorders do not cause changes in the BDE. If the BDE is abnormal, a metabolic acid–base disturbance must also be present.

Assess the Metabolic Component

A BDE <–2 mmol/L or a HCO_3^- <22 mmol/L indicates the presence of a metabolic acidosis, and a BDE >+2 mmol/L or a HCO_3^- >26 mmol/L indicates a metabolic alkalosis. If the Na^+, Cl^-, albumin, or phosphate is abnormal, then further assessment of acid–base balance is required, which should be via the physiochemical approach or alternatively using the corrected BDE (see earlier).

If a Metabolic Acidosis Is Present, Calculate the Anion Gap

The normal calculated anion gap is 8 to 16 mmol/L. The corrected normal anion gap should be used if the albumin or phosphate concentration is abnormal (see earlier). An elevated the anion gap indicates the presence of unmeasured anions and should prompt the measurement of blood lactate levels, and urine should be analyzed for ketones. Consideration should be given to other causes of raised anion gap acidosis (Table 42.4).

TABLE 42.6. Expected compensatory responses in primary acid–base disorders

Disorder	Expected response
Acute respiratory acidosis	No change in BDE
Acute respiratory alkalosis	No change in BDE
Chronic respiratory acidosis	$BDE = 0.4 \times (PaCO_2 - 40)$
Chronic respiratory alkalosis	$BDE = 0.4 \times (PaCO_2 - 40)$
Acute metabolic acidosis	$PaCO_2 = 40 + BDE$
Acute metabolic alkalosis	$PaCO_2 = 40 + (0.6 \times BDE)$

BDE, base deficit or excess.

Elicit the Primary Disturbance

In simple acid–base disturbances, the primary disturbance is the process that causes the overriding pH change; the compensatory mechanisms, either renal or respiratory, attempt to return the pH toward the normal range. Typically a low pH and BDE <–2 mmol/L or HCO_3^- <22 mmol/L indicate a primary metabolic acidosis, and a high pH and an elevated BDE >+2 mmol/L or HCO_3^- >26 mmol/L indicate a primary metabolic alkalosis. A low pH with an elevated $Paco_2$ indicates a primary respiratory acidosis, and a high pH with a low $Paco_2$ a primary respiratory alkalosis.

Assess the Compensatory Response

The expected compensatory response to a simple acid–base disorder can be estimated using simple calculations (Table 42.6) (13). If the actual response does not correlate with the expected response, then a mixed respiratory and metabolic acid–base disorder is occurring.

Clinical Example

Mr. X., a 64-year-old man with known ischemic heart disease is admitted through the emergency department with chest pain and severe breathlessness. Clinical evaluation reveals a heart rate 120, blood pressure 190/100 mm Hg, jugular venous pressure 10 cm, and a third heart sound. He is dyspneic (respiration rate [RR] 32, Spo_2 98%, Fio_2 0.8), and has end expiratory crepitations throughout his chest. A chest radiograph is consistent with pulmonary edema, and an electrocardiograph demonstrates sinus rhythm with an old inferior myocardial infarct) and ST depression in leads V_3 to V_6. A diagnosis of acute pulmonary edema is made, with a possible underlying acute coronary syndrome.

Arterial blood gases on admission are as follows:

pH	7.25
$Paco_2$	33 mmHg
HCO_3^-	17 mmol/L
BDE	–8 mmol/L
Na^+	140 mmol/L
K^+	4 mmol/L
Cl^-	102 mmol/L
Fio_2	0.8
Pao_2	110 mmHg

Serum albumin and phosphate results are within normal range.

Assessment of Oxygenation

At first glance the patient has adequate oxygenation, but given the fact that the patient is on high flow oxygen therapy, one would expect the Pao_2 to be greater. To further assess oxygenation, we can use the A-a gradient (as discussed earlier). For Mr. X., the expected A-a gradient is as follows:

$$(\text{Age}/4) + 4 = (64/4) + 4 = 20$$

The actual A-a gradient is as follows:

$$\text{A-a gradient} = (P_AO_2) - (Pao_2)$$

where P_AO_2 is the ideal alveolar oxygen tension, and Pao_2 is the actual arterial oxygen tension.

$$\begin{aligned} PAO_2 &= Fio_2 \times (760 - 47) - Paco_2/0.8 \\ &= 0.8 \times (760 - 47) - 33/0.8 \\ &= 570 - 41 \\ &= 529\,\text{mm Hg} \end{aligned}$$

$$\begin{aligned} \text{A-a gradient} &= 529 - 110\,\text{mm Hg} \\ &= 419\,\text{mm Hg} \end{aligned}$$

The actual A-a gradient of 419 mm Hg is grossly elevated, indicating impaired gas exchange; this is consistent with impaired gas exchange such as in acute pulmonary edema.

Assessment of Acid–Base Balance

Assess the pH

The pH is less than 7.35; the overriding acid–base disturbance is causing an acidemia.

Assess the $Pa{CO_2}$

The $Pa{CO_2}$ is reduced at 33 mm Hg (normal 35 to 45 mm Hg). A respiratory alkalosis is present.

Assess the Metabolic Component

The BDE is −7 mmol/L and the HCO_3^- is 17 mmol/L. A metabolic acidosis is present.

In the Presence of a Metabolic Acidosis, Calculate the Anion Gap

$$\text{Anion Gap} = (Na^+ + K^+) - (HCO_3^- + Cl^-) = (140 + 4) - (17 + 102) = 25\,\text{mmol/L}$$

The normal anion gap is 8 to 16 mmol/L (there is no need to use the corrected normal anion gap, as albumin and phosphate levels are normal).

The anion gap is elevated at 25 mmol/L. A serum lactate level is subsequently measured at 4 mmol/L (normal <1 mmol/L); ketones are absent on urine analysis.

In view of the elevated lactate level and the metabolic acidosis, a lactic acidosis is present.

Elicit the Primary Disturbance

The arterial blood gas results are consistent with a primary metabolic acidosis and a secondary compensatory respiratory alkalosis.

Assess the Compensatory Response to the Underlying Acid–Base Disturbance

The expected $Pa{CO_2}$ in a metabolic acidosis is as follows:

$$\text{Expected } Pa{CO_2} = 40 + \text{BDE} = 40 - 7 = 33\,\text{mm Hg}$$

The actual $Pa{CO_2}$ is consistent with the expected $Pa{CO_2}$ for this degree of metabolic acidosis. Hence the compensatory respiratory alkalosis is appropriate.

The diagnosis is of a metabolic lactic acidosis with a compensatory respiratory alkalosis. The patient is treated with aspirin, a glyceryl trinitrate infusion, and low molecular weight heparin. He is also started on continuous positive airway pressure (CPAP) via a tight-fitting face mask. On this therapy his condition stabilizes. A repeat arterial blood gas shows improvement in oxygenation, and the lactic acidosis has also improved; the lactate is now 2 mmol/L. He is transferred to the coronary care unit.

Unfortunately, 2 hours later Mr. X. has a further deterioration. He is now very sweaty, agitated, and intolerant of the CPAP mask. He is tachycardic and hypotensive (the glyceryl trinitrate having being stopped earlier). He is put on high flow oxygen with a $Fi{O_2}$ of 1.0, but despite this a pulse oximeter measures the $Sp{O_2}$ at 84%. Further clinical examination is impossible due to severe patient agitation.

An arterial gas is performed, with the following results:

pH	7.05
$Pa{CO_2}$	45 mmHg
HCO_3^-	14 mmol/L
BDE	−12 mmol/L
Na^+	142 mmol/L
K^+	65 mmol/L
Cl^-	101 mmol/L
$Fi{O_2}$	1.0
$Pa{O_2}$	63 mmHg

Serum albumin and phosphate results are within normal range.

Assessment of Oxygenation

The patient is now significantly hypoxic despite the $Fi{O_2}$ of 1.0. As the A-a gradient is clearly increased, a formal calculation of the A-a gradient is unnecessary.

Assessment of Acid–Base Balance

Assess the pH

The pH is 7.05; a severe acidemia is present.

Assess the $Pa{CO_2}$

The $Pa{CO_2}$ is within the normal range at 45 mm Hg.

Assess the Metabolic Component

The BDE is −12 mmol/L and the HCO_3^- is 14 mmol/L. A metabolic acidosis is present.

In the Presence of a Metabolic Acidosis, Calculate the Anion Gap

$$\text{Anion gap} = (Na^+ + K^+) - (Cl^- + HCO_3^-) = (141 + 6) - (101 + 14) = 32\,\text{mmol/L}$$

There is a raised anion gap metabolic acidosis. A lactate level is measured at 9 mmol/L; a lactic acidosis is present.

Elicit the Primary Disturbance

A metabolic acidosis is the primary acid–base disturbance. The $Pa{CO_2}$ is within the normal range.

Assess the Compensatory Response to the Underlying Acid–Base Disturbance

The expected $Pa{CO_2}$ for this severe metabolic acidosis is as follows:

$$\text{Expected } Pa{CO_2} = 40 + \text{BDE} = 40 - 12 = 28\,\text{mm Hg}$$

There is a marked difference between the actual and expected $Pa{CO_2}$. The respiratory compensatory response is inadequate, and respiratory failure is now ensuing.

The patient is critically ill. He has a severe lactic acidosis along with respiratory failure. This is a mixed acid–base disorder.

Mr. X. continued to deteriorate; he required intubation and ventilation and was transferred to the intensive care unit. Invasive hemodynamic monitoring was established, and he was started on ionotropes to optimize his cardiac output. Once stabilized, he was transferred to the cardiac catheter room for further management.

Conclusion

Arterial blood gas measurement enables allows rapid near-patient testing that gives objective information about ventilation, oxygenation, and acid–base balance, all of which may be abnormal in acute heart failure. Accurate interpretation of the results obtained is vital, and this should be matched to the clinical assessment. The physiochemical approach to interpreting acid–base balance is preferable, as it quantifies and qualifies the cause of any disturbance. Despite this, the bicarbonate and BDE approaches remain clinically relevant, especially at the bedside, and usually result in similar interpretations.

References

1. Gross R, Dellinger R. Arterial blood gas interpretation. In: Fink M, Abraham E, Vincent JL, et al. Textbook of Critical Care Medicine. Philadelphia: Elsevier Saunders, 2005:463–70.
2. Shapiro BA. Temperature correction of blood gas values. Respir Care Clin North Am 1995;1:69–76.
3. Mellemgaud K. The alveolar-arterial oxygen difference. Its size and components in normal man. Acta Physiol Scand 1966;67:10–20.
4. Sirker AA, Rhodes A, Grounds RM et al. Acid base physiology: the "traditional" and the "modern" approaches. Anaesthesia 2002;57:348–56.
5. Siggard-Anderson O, Engel K. A new acid base nomogram. An improved method for calculation of the relevant blood acid-base data. Scand J Clin Lab Invest 1960;12:177–86.
6. Kellum JA. Determination of blood pH in health and disease. Crit Care 2000;4:6–14.
7. Siggard Anderson O. The Van Slyke equation. Scand J Clin Lab Invest Suppl 1977;37:15–20.
8. Narins RG, Emmett M. Simple and mixed acid-base disorders. A practical approach. Medicine 1980;59: 161–87.
9. Stewart P. Modern quantitative acid-base chemistry. Can J Physiol Pharmacol 1983;61:1444–61.
10. Fencl V, Leith DE. Stewart's quantitative acid-base chemistry applications in biology and medicine. Respir Physiol 1993;91:1–16.
11. Rossing TH, Maffeo N, Fencl V. Acid base effects of altering plasma protein concentration in human blood in vivo. J Appl Physiol 1986;61:2260–5.
12. Storey DA, Morimatsu H, Bellomo R. Strong ions, weak acids and base excess, a simplified Fencl-Stewart approach to clinical acid base disorders. Br J Anaesth 2004;92:54–60.
13. Schlichtig R, Grogono AW, Severinghaus JW. Human PaCO2 and standard base excess compensation for acid–base imbalance. Crit Care Med 1998;26:1173–9.
14. Waters JH, Miller LR, Clark S, et al. Cause of metabolic acidosis in prolonged surgery. Crit Care Med 1999;27:2142–6.
15. Cohen RD, Woods HF. Lactic acidosis revisited. Diabetes 1983;32:181–91.
16. Boyd O, Grounds RM, Bennett ED. A randomized clinical trial of the effect of deliberate perioperative increase of oxygen delivery on mortality in high-risk surgical patients. JAMA 1993;270:2699–707.

17. Shoemaker WC, Appel PL, Kram HB, Waxman K, Lee TS. Prospective trial of supranormal values of survivors as therapeutic goals in high-risk surgical patients. Chest 1988;94:1176–86.
18. Rivers E, Nguyen B, Havstad S. Early goal-directed therapy in the treatment of severe sepsis and septic shock. N Engl J Med 2001;345:1368–77.
19. Bakker J, Gris P, Coffernils M, et al. Serial blood lactate concentrations can predict the development of multiple organ failure following septic shock. Am J Surg 1996;171:221–6.
20. McNelis J, Marini CP, Jurkiewitz A, et al. Prolonged lactate clearance is associated with increased mortality in the surgical intensive care unit. Am J Surg 2001; 182:481–5.

43

B-Type Natriuretic Peptide Testing in the Emergency Room and Intensive Care Unit for the Patient with Acute Heart Failure

Damien Logeart and Alain Cohen Solal

The natriuretic peptide family includes two major peptides that are secreted by myocardial cells: A-type (ANP) and B-type natriuretic peptide (BNP). While ANP is stored in both atria and ventricles, the major source of BNP are the ventricles (1). Both are synthesized as precursors; BNP is synthesized as pro-BNP in ventricular myocytes, and pro-BNP cleavage leads to two secreted fragments: BNP (32 amino acids [aa]) and N-terminal pro-BNP (NT-pro-BNP) (76 aa). B-type natriuretic peptide is an active hormone with cyclic guanosine monophosphate (cGMP)-mediated vasodilator and natriuretic properties, as well as ANP, and is eliminated by the neutral endopeptidase. N-terminal pro-BNP is mainly eliminated through kidneys and biologically inactive. The half-life of BNP and NT-pro-BNP are 20 and 120 minutes, respectively. Natriuretic peptides blood levels reflect the severity of cardiac diseases and, further, the decompensated state of cardiac dysfunction. Indeed, the main stimulus of the constitutive pro-BNP synthesis is the mechanical strain within the ventricular wall, which depends on ventricular mass, geometry, and diastolic pressures. Close relations have been demonstrated between left ventricular end-diastolic pressures and BNP/NT-pro-BNP blood levels (2). In contrast, natriuretic peptide levels are poorly related to left ventricular ejection fraction. Others direct stimuli include catecholamines, angiotensin, cytokines, and hypoxemia. Because of such characteristics, BNP/NT-pro-BNP has been tested as cardiac biomarker for both diagnosis and prognosis of heart failure. Recent improvements in point-of-care assays have extended their use in the clinical practice.

B-type Natriuretic Peptide Testing and Diagnosis of Acute Heart Failure in the Emergency Room

The diagnostic value of natriuretic peptides blood levels in assessing acute heart failure (AHF) in the emergency room (ER) has been extensively studied (3–13). A number of studies examined how well BNP testing classifies patients with dyspnea, using simple protocols. The final diagnosis of dyspnea was assessed, after discharge, from all in-hospital data except the BNP level, which was blinded. The global diagnostic value, such as suggested by the area under the receiver operating characteristic (ROC) curve, was high in each study (Table 43.1). In the ER, such a bedside biomarker is particularly interesting because of the high rate of clinical misjudgments or uncertainties on admission and because of potentially dramatic consequences of such misdiagnoses. Dao et al. (5) showed that BNP measurements added significant, independent explanatory power to others clinical variables for predicting heart failure (HF). They also demonstrated that a number of clinical misdiagnoses could have been avoided by BNP testing. Among 250 patients, the use of BNP testing with a cutoff value of 80 pg/mL would have corrected 29 of 30 misdiagnosed cases in the ER. In the multicenter BNP study (7), which included 1586 patients with acute dyspnea, the diagnostic value of BNP testing (using a 100 pg/mL cutoff) was more accurate than National Health and Nutrition Examination Survey (NHANES) or Framingham criteria–based clinical

TABLE 43.1. Main studies with B-type natriuretic peptide (BNP) and N-terminal pro-BNP (NT-pro-BNP) for diagnosing AHF in the emergency room

	Sample	Area under ROC curve	Cutoff (pg/mL)	Sensitivity (%)	Specificity (%)	PPV (%)	NPV (%)	Accuracy (%)
BNP								
Davis et al. (4)	52		76	93	90	94	90	92
Dao et al. (5)	250	0.97	80	98	92	90	98	95
Morrison et al. (6)	321		94	86	98	98	83	91
			240	96	79	86	93	89
Maisel et al. (7)	1586	0.91	50	97	62	71	96	79
			100	90	76	79	89	83
			150	85	83	83	85	84
Logeart et al. (8)	163	0.93	80	97	27	76	93	78
			400	79	93	98	66	83
Lainchbury et al. (9)	205	0.89	208	70	94	61	96	78
Ray et al. (10)	202	0.91	250	73	91	86	81	83
Mueller et al. (11)	251	0.91	295	80	86	87	78	83
NT-pro-BNP								
Lainchburry et al. (9)	205	0.89	2875	87	80	76	89	85
Bayes-Genis et al. (12)	100	0.96	254	99	47	90	100	91
			973	91	93	99	70	92
Ray et al. (10)	202	0.80	1500	75	76	71	80	76
Januzzi et al. (13)	599	0.94	300	99	68	62	99	79
			900	90	85	78	94	87
Mueller et al. (11)	251	0.90	825	87	81	84	84	84

Cutoff values are optimal thresholds regarding ROC curves or accuracy.
NPV, negative predictive value; PPV, positive predictive value; ROC, receiver operating characteristics.

judgment (83%, 67%, and 73%, respectively). B-type natriuretic peptide testing strongly reduced the rate of clinical uncertainty from 43% to 11% using a 100 pg/mL cutoff. The BNP levels are not significantly different in both acute diastolic and systolic HF (8,18). In a randomised study, Mueller et al. (19) demonstrated that the use of BNP testing in the ER (single BNP cutoff of 100 pg/mL) improves the efficiency of treatment; the rate of admission to the intensive care unit (ICU), the duration of stay, as well as the cost of in-hospital stays were reduced when BNP testing was performed on admission (19).

How to Use Results of B-Type Natriuretic Peptide Testing for Diagnosis?

The ROC curves give optimal cutoff values which are the best compromise between sensitivity and specificity in a population. Such compromises are not necessarily the most relevant cutoff at the patient's bedside if it results in a significant risk of a false positive or false negative. From the "Breathing Not Properly" (BNP) Multinational Study's data, McCullough et al. (20) proposed a BNP-nomogram, which gives a final AHF probability from both the first clinical judgment and the BNP level. Such a nomogram is not easily usable at the bedside because it is difficult to translate clinical judgment to probability. We pointed out the importance of a "gray zone" including moderate increase in BNP levels; within this range, the diagnostic value of BNP levels is unrelevant regarding clinical practice (8). Consequently, a two-threshold–based three-arm algorithm can be preferred (8,21): the AHF diagnosis is ruled out under the low cutoff while the AHF diagnosis is highly probable above the second cutoff; between these two thresholds is the gray zone. Figure 43.1 shows a BNP-based algorithm using consensual cutoffs. The gray zone is due to a number of causes that can increase blood levels of natriuretic peptides, irrespective of left ventricular dysfunction.

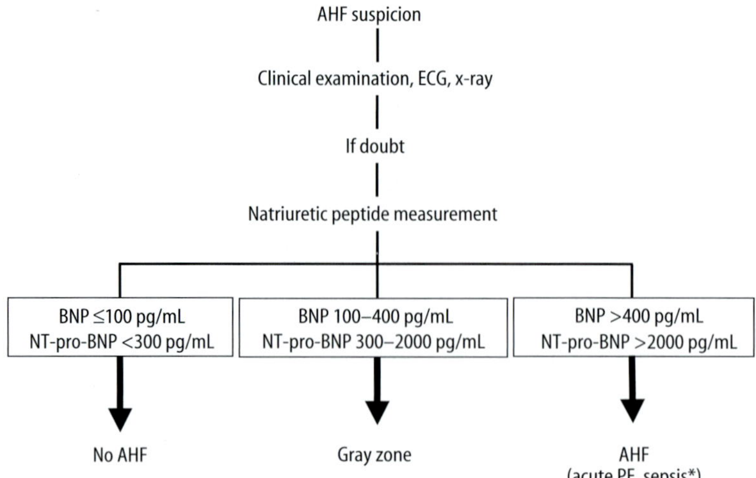

Figure 43.1. Algorithm for diagnostic use of BNP and NT-pro-BNP measurements in the emergency room. Within the gray zone, natriuretic peptides are poorly helpful (see text). *High BNP/NT-pro-BNP levels can also be due to acute pulmonary embolism (PE) as well as severe sepsis. AHF, acute heart failure.

Figure 43.2 illustrates the main factors leading to this gray zone.

Chronic renal failure induces volume overload and cardiovascular abnormalities that explain the increase in natriuretic peptides levels. The increase in natriuretic peptides with aging is explained by the presence in the elderly people of a number of comorbidities and possibly by some degree of asymptomatic diastolic left ventricular dysfunction, especially in women. Physicians have to discriminate AHF-related dyspnea from other causes including acute bronchitis, pneumonia, decompensated chronic obstructive pulmonary disease (COPD), and asthma, but each of these conditions can induce some degree of pulmonary hypertension or cor pulmonale with subsequent release of natriuretic peptides from the right ventricle. Such an increase in BNP/NT-pro-BNP levels is moderate except in some patients with primary pulmonary hypertension or severe acute pulmonary embolism as well as in patients with severe sepsis (14). Such a secretion of natriuretic peptides is easily explained in pulmonary hypertension because of the overloaded right ventricle, and it has been shown that the increase in BNP levels in acute pulmonary embolism was related to right ventricular (RV) dysfunction (15–17).

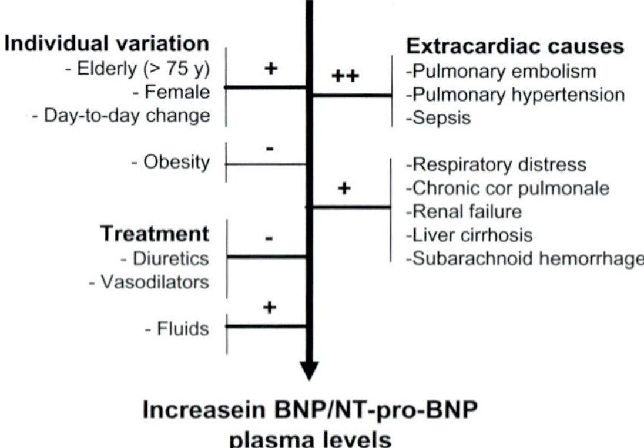

Figure 43.2. Cardiac dysfunction is the main determinant of natriuretic peptide levels, but many others parameters affect BNP/NT-pro-BNP levels.

In contrast, mechanisms of the sepsis-related increase in natriuretic peptides levels are more complex, including sepsis-mediated cardiac dysfunction, respiratory failure-mediated right ventricular dysfunction, the direct role of cytokines and hypoxemia, as well as renal failure (14). On the other hand, normal BNP levels have been observed in some patients with evidence of flash pulmonary edema (9). Natriuretic peptides levels decrease during treatment-related ventricular unload (diuretics, vasodilators), and thus BNP results have to be interpreted according to the time between the blood sample and the beginning of intensive treatment. Another important confounding factor is the chronic increase in natriuretic peptide levels in patients with severe chronic heart failure.

Finally, BNP/NT-pro-BNP testing should never been used as a stand-alone diagnostic test but must be interpreted within the clinical context; BNP testing is useful when the clinical diagnosis is uncertain and its best use is for ruling out a diagnosis of HF. This last point is underlined in the recently updated guidelines for acute as well as chronic HF (22,23). It should be emphasized that HF diagnosis requires the assessment of structural/functional cardiac abnormalities, which is obtained mainly from echographic examination. Low BNP levels can avoid useless echography, but an increase in BNP levels does not substitute for echography.

B-Type Natriuretic Peptide and N-Terminal Pro-BNP: Similar Usefulness But Different Cutoffs

Both BNP and NT-pro-BNP assays have relevant diagnostic values. By comparing them in the ER, different studies demonstrated similar areas under the ROC curve (9–11) and good correlation between BNP and NT-pro-BNP ($r = 0.54 - 0.90$) have been reported (9,11). Because of different biologic characteristics, such as molecular weights or half-life, for examples, NT-pro-BNP cutoffs are higher than BNP cutoffs, especially when they are expressed in units of picograms per milliliter.

Table 43.1 summarizes the mains results of diagnostic studies in the ER. According to ROC curves obtained from the largest multicenter population with dyspnea (7,24), optimal cutoffs are between 100 and 250 pg/mL for BNP (Biosite®) and 450 pg/mL for NT-pro-BNP (Roche Diagnostics). For ruling out the diagnosis of AHF, the BNP cutoff is about 100 pg/mL and the NT-pro-BNP cutoff is 300 pg/mL. Natriuretic peptides levels increase with age irrespective of HF (25). In patients older than 65 years, a better diagnostic value was shown with BNP compared to NT-pro-BNP (10). From an pooled analysis of four studies, the diagnostic value of NT-pro-BNP in acute dyspnea decreased across the increase in age (24), and the authors proposed different optimal cutoff points: 450 pg/mL in patients younger than 50 years, 900 pg/mL in patients 50 to 75 years of age, and 1800 pg/mL in patients older than 75 years. Such differences could be explained by the worsening of renal function with age. Indeed, NT-pro-BNP is only eliminated through the kidneys, and the NT-pro-BNP blood level has been shown to depend on renal function ($r = -0.55$) (26) more than do the BNP levels ($r = -0.20$) (27). A higher NT-pro-BNP cutoff, such as 1200 pg/mL, has been proposed for a glomerular filtration rate less than 60 mL/min/1.73 m^2. At last, different BNP assays using different BNP antibodies are commercialized available, but correlation between these assays are not always clearly established across the whole range of values. Physicians should be familiar with the assay that is used in their hospital and with respective cutoff values.

B-Type Natriuretic Peptide/ N-Terminal Pro-BNP Levels as Surrogate Hemodynamic End Points in the Intensive Care Unit

Natriuretic peptides levels are positively related to left ventricular (LV) end-diastolic pressure as well as pulmonary capillary wedge pressure (2,28), which explains their diagnostic value in patients with dyspnea. However, such a relation is relatively poor in patients admitted to the ICU. In a nonselected critically ill population requiring invasive hemodynamic monitoring, the BNP and NT-pro-BNP levels were weakly or not correlated with pulmonary capillary wedge pressure (PCWP) (29–31). Comparing BNP measurement and echography for the assessment of LV filling pressures in ICU, Dokainish et al. (32) also showed weak correlation between BNP and PCWP ($r = 0.32$); however, they demonstrated interesting diagnostic values of BNP levels for predicting a PCWP >15 mm Hg: an accuracy of 82% was obtained with BNP >250 pg/mL in patients without underlying cardiac disease and BNP >400 pg/mL in patients with cardiac diseases. In patients with

AHF and invasive hemodynamic monitoring, it has been shown that BNP changes correlate with change in PCWP (28,32). In the management of various diseases, in ICU, such a relation between change in BNP levels and PCWP is lacking (29,33), which can be easily explained by the number of "extracardiac" factors that can alter natriuretic peptide levels (Fig. 43.2), vigorous treatment of respiratory distress, sepsis, renal failure, as well as in day-to-day variations.

B-Type Natriuretic Peptide Testing and Prognosis

The prognostic relevance of natriuretic peptides levels have been well established in chronic heart failure for several years (34–36). In the ER, natriuretic peptides measurement also gives relevant prognostic information. In their pooled analysis, Januzzi et al. (24) showed that NT-pro-BNP >5180 pg/mL was strongly predictive of deaths (odds ratio [OR], 5.2; 95% confidence interval [CI], 2.2–8.1). In the Rapid Emergency Department Heart Failure Outpatient Trial (REDHOT) study, there was a mismatch between the perceived severity by physicians and severity as determined by BNP levels, which were more predictive of 90-day mortality than was the New York Heart Association (NYHA) functional class as well as initial clinical judgment (37). Such results suggest that BNP/NT-pro-BNP levels could help physicians in stratifying patients on admission and in deciding to admit or not. Among patients admitted with AHF, serial BNP measurements give additional prognostic information (38–40). When both the admission and the following BNP levels have prognostic value, early changes in BNP levels as well as predischarge BNP levels give the best information. Indeed, it has been shown than a decrease in BNP >10% on day 2 or a predischarge BNP level <300 to 350 pg/mL was strongly and independently related to the lowest rate of 6-month mortality or readmissions after discharge, while a predischarge BNP level >750 was associated with the poorest outcome (39,40). Similar results were demonstrated with NT-pro-BNP measurements (41).

The prognostic value of these biomarkers is of interest in other settings and is potentially relevant in the ER and in the ICU. In acute pulmonary embolism, the increase in BNP/NT-pro-BNP levels predicts right ventricular dysfunction and the risk of in-hospital death (42,43), which could be helpful information on admission for determining the early therapeutic strategy. Prognostic value has also been observed in sepsis (44,45) and cardiac surgery (46,47), but confirmatory studies are required. A number of studies have demonstrated that BNP levels displays a strong prognostic value in acute coronary syndromes, which is independent and additive to cardiac troponins (48–50). In acute coronary syndromes, natriuretic peptide release can be explained by the very early diastolic dysfunction of the ischemic LV wall. The BNP/NT-pro-BNP levels could correlate with the magnitude of insult of the LV wall when troponins relate to the severity/unstability of the culprit lesion.

Conclusion

Testing of BNP/NT-pro-BNP is a powerful biomarker for the diagnosis and prognosis of HF in both the cardiology setting and the emergency room. Low natriuretic peptide levels on admission rule out AHF and high-risk patients. Any increase in natriuretic peptide levels have to be interpreted from the clinical context and do not replace echocardiography for assessing cardiac abnormalities and dysfunction. BNP testing can be a part of the therapy monitoring. Its usefulness in the ICU is less obvious because of a number of confounding factors, including sepsis, renal failure, respiratory distress, and intensive treatment.

References

1. Levin ER, Gardner DG, Samson WK. Natriuretic peptides. N Engl J Med 1998;339:321–8.
2. Maeda K, Tsutamoto T, Wada A, et al. Plasma brain natriuretic peptide as a biochemical marker of high left ventricular end-diastolic pressure in patients with symptomatic left ventricular dysfunction. Am Heart J 1998;135:825–32.

3. Rodeheffer RJ. Measuring plasma B-type natriuretic peptide in heart failure. J Am Coll Cardiol 2004;44:740–9.
4. Davis M, Espiner E, Richards G. Plasma brain natriuretic peptide in assessment of acute dyspnea. Lancet 1994;343:440–4.
5. Dao Q, Krishnaswamy P, Kazanegra R, et al. Utility of B-type natriuretic peptide in the diagnosis of congestive heart failure in an urgent-care setting. J Am Coll Cardiol 2001;37;379–85.
6. Morrison LK, Harrison A, Krishnaswamy P, et al. Utility of a rapid B-natriuretic peptide assay in differentiating congestive heart failure from lung disease in patients. J Am Coll Cardiol 2002;39: 202–9.
7. Maisel AS, Krishnaswamy P, Nowak RM, et al, for the Breathing Not Properly Multinational Study Investigators. Rapid measurement of B-Type Natriuretic Peptide in the emergency diagnosis of heart failure. N Engl J Med 2002;347:161–7.
8. Logeart D, Saudubray C, Beyne P, et al. Comparative value of Doppler echocardiography and B-Type natriuretic peptide assay in the etiologic diagnosis of acute dyspnea. J Am Coll Cardiol 2002;40:1794–800.
9. Lainchburry JG, Campbell E, Frampton CM, et al. Brain natriuretic peptide and N-terminal brain natriuretic peptide in the diagnosis of heart failure in patients with acute shortness of breath. J Am Coll Cardiol 2003;42:728–35.
10. Ray P, Arthaud M, Birolleau M, et al. Comparison of brain natriuretic peptide and probrain natriuretic peptide in the diagnosis of cardiogenic pulmonary edema in patients aged 65 and older. J Am Geriatr Soc 2005;53:643–8.
11. Mueller T, Gegenhuber A, Poelz W, Haltmayer M. Diagnostic accuracy of B type natriuretic peptide and amino terminal proBNP in the emergency diagnosis of heart failure. Heart 2005;91:606–12.
12. Bayes-Genis A, Santalo-Bel M, Zapico-Muniz E, et al. N-terminal probrain natriuretic peptide (NT-proBNP) in the emergency diagnosis and in-hospital monitoring of patients with dyspnea and ventricular dysfunction. Eur J Heart Fail 2004;6: 301–8.
13. Januzzi JL, Camargo CA, Anwarudidin S, et al. The N-terminal pro-BNP investigation dyspnea in the emergency department (PRIDE) study. Am J Cardiol 2005;95:948–54.
14. Jason P, Keang LT, Hoe LK. B-type natriuretic peptide: issues for the intensivist and pulmonologist. Crit Care Med 2005;33:2094–103.
15. Kucher N, Printzen G, Goldhaber SZ. Prognostic role of brain natriuretic peptide in acute pulmonary embolism. Circulation 2003;107: 2545–7.
16. Kruger S, Graf J, Merx MW, et al. Brain natriuretic peptide predicts right heart failure in patients with acute pulmonary embolism. Am Heart J 2004;147: 60–5.
17. Pruszczyk P, Kostrubiec M, Bochowicz A, et al. N-terminal pro-brain natriuretic peptide in patients with acute pulmonary embolism. Eur Respir J 2003;22:649–53.
18. Maisel AS, McCord J, Nowak RM, et al. Bedside B-type natriuretic peptide in the emergency diagnosis of heart failure with reduced or preserved ejection fraction. J Am Coll Cardiol 2003;41:2010–7.
19. Mueller C, Scholer A, Laule-Kilian K, et al. Use of B-type natriuretic peptide in the evaluation and management of acute dyspnea. N Engl J Med 2004;350:647–54.
20. McCullough PA, Nowak RM, McCord J, et al. B-Type natriuretic peptide and clinical judgment in the emergency diagnosis of heart failure: an analysis from the Breathing Not Properly (BNP) Multinational Study. Circulation 2002;106:416–22.
21. Maisel AS. B-type natriuretic peptide measurements in diagnosing congestive heart failure in the dyspneic emergency department patient. Rev Cardiovasc Med 2002;3:S10–S17.
22. Task Force for the Diagnosis and Treatment of Chronic Heart Failure of the European Society of Cardiology. Guidelines for the diagnosis and treatment of chronic heart failure: executive summary (update 2005). Eur Heart J 2005;26:1115–40.
23. Guidelines on the diagnosis and treatment of acute heart failure. The task force on acute heart failure of the European society of cardiology. Eur Heart J 2005;26:1115–40.
24. Januzzi JL, van Kimmenade R, Lainchbury J, et al. NT-proBNP testing for diagnosing and short-term prognosis in acute destabilized heart failure: an international pooled analysis of 1256 patients. Eur Heart J 2006;27:330–7.
25. Redfield MR, Jacobsen S, et al. Plasma brain natriuretic peptide concentration: impact of age and gender. J Am Coll Cardiol 2002;40:976–82.
26. Anwaruddin S, Lloyd-Jones DM, Baggish A, et al. Renal function, congestive heart failure, and amino-terminal pro-brain natriuretic peptide measurement. J Am Coll Cardiol 2006;47:91–107.
27. McCullough PA, Omland T, Maisel AS. B-type natriuretic peptide: a diagnostic breakthrough for clinicians. Rev Cardiovasc Med 2003;4:72–80.
28. Kazanegra R, Cheng V, Garcia A, et al. A rapid test for B-type natriuretic peptide correlates with falling wedge pressures in patients treated for

decompensated heart failure: a pilot study. J Card Failure 2001;7:21–9.
29. Tung RH, Garcia C, Morss AM, et al. Utility of B-type natriuretic peptide for the evaluation of intensive care in unit shock. Crit Care Med 2004; 32:1643–7.
30. Forfia PR, Watkins SP, Rame JE, Stewart KJ, Shapiro EP. Relationship between B-type natriuretic peptides and pulmonary capillary wedge pressure in the intensive care unit. J Am Coll Cardiol 2005;45: 1667–71.
31. Jefic D, Lee JW, Jefic D, et al. Utility of B-type natriuretic peptide and N-terminal pro B-type natriuretic peptide in evaluation of respiratory failure in critically ill patients. Chest 2005;128: 288–95.
32. Dokainish H, Zoghbi WA, Lakkis NM, et al. Optimal non-invasive assessment of left ventricular filling pressures. Circulation 2004;109:2432–9.
33. McLean AS, Huang SJ. B-type natriuretic peptide to assess cardiac function in the critically ill. In: Vincent J-L, ed. Yearbook of Intensive Care and Emergency Medicine 2005. Heidelberg: Springer-Verlag, 2005:151–60.
34. Tsutamoto T, Wada A, Maeda K, et al. Attenuation of compensation of cardiac natriuretic peptide system in chronic heart failure: prognostic role of plasma brain natriuretic peptide concentration in patients with chronic symptomatic left ventricular dysfunction. Circulation 1997;96:509–16.
35. De Groote P, Dagorn J, Soudan B, et al. B-type natriuretic peptide and peak exercise oxygen consumption provide independent information for risk stratification in patients with stable congestive heart failure. J Am Coll Cardiol 2004;43:1584–9.
36. Doust JA, Pietrzak E, Dobson A, Glasziou PP. How well does B-type natriuretic peptide predicts death and cardiac events in patients with heart failure: systematic review. BMJ 2005;330:625–33.
37. Maisel A, Hollander JE, Guss D, et al. Preliminary results of the Rapid Emergency Department Heart Failure Outpatient Trial (REDHOT). J Am Coll Cardiol 2004;44:1328–33.
38. Cheng V, Kazanegra R, Garcia A, et al. A rapid bedside test for B-Type natriuretic peptide predicts treatment outcomes in patients admitted for decompensated heart failure: a pilot study. J Am Coll Cardiol 2001;37:386–91.
39. Logeart D, Thabut G, Jourdain P, et al. Predischarge B-type natriuretic peptide assay for identifying patients at high risk of readmission after decompensated heart failure. J Am Coll Cardiol 2004;43: 635–41.
40. Gackowski A, Isnard R, Golmard JL, et al. Comparison of echocardiography and plasma B-type natriuretic peptide for monitoring the response to treatment in acute heart failure. Eur Heart J 2004; 25:1788–96.
41. Bettencourt P, Azevedo A, Pimenta J, et al. N-terminal probrain natriuretic peptide predicts outcome after hospital discharge in heart failure patients. Circulation 2004;110:2168–74.
42. ten Wolde M, Tulevski II, Mulder JWM, et al. Brain natriuretic peptide as a predictor of adverse outcome in patients with pulmonary embolism. Circulation 2003;107:2082–4.
43. Binder L, Pieske B, Olschewski M, et al. N-terminal probrain natriuretic peptide or troponin testing followed by echocardiography for risk stratification of acute pulmonary embolism. Circulation 2005; 112:1573–9.
44. Charpentier J, Luyt CE, Fulla Y, et al. Brain natriuretic peptide: a marker of myocardial dysfunction and prognosis during severe sepsis. Crit Care Med 2004;32:660–5.
45. Roch A, Alardet-Servent J, Michelet P, et al. NH2 terminal pro-brain natriuretic peptide plasma levels as an early marker of prognosis and cardiac dysfunction in septic shock patients. Crit Care Med 2005;33:1001–7.
46. Chello M, Mastroroberto R, Perticone F, et al. Plasma levels of atrial and brain natriuretic peptide as indicators of recovery of left ventricular systolic function after coronary artery bypass. Eur J Cardiothorc Surg 2001;20:140–6.
47. Berendes E, Schmidt C, Van Aken H, et al. A-type and B-type natriuretic peptide in cardiac surgical procedure. Anesth Analg 2004;98:11–9.
48. De Lemos JA, Morrow DA, Bentley JH, et al. The prognostic value of B-type natriuretic peptide in patients with acute coronary syndromes. N Engl J Med 2001;345:1014–21.
49. Morrow DA, de Lemos JA, Sabatine MS, et al. Evaluation of B-type natriuretic peptide for risk assessment in unstable angina/non-ST-elevation myocardial infarction. J Am Coll Cardiol 2003;41: 1264–72.
50. Sabatine MS, Morrow DA, DeLemos JA, et al. Multimarker approach to risk stratification in non-ST elevation acute coronary syndromes. Simultaneous assessment of troponin I, C-reactive protein, and B-type natriuretic peptide. Circulation 2002;105: 1760–3.

2.2
Treatment of Acute Heart Failure Syndrome: Airway and Lung Management

44
Noninvasive Ventilation and Acute Heart Failure Syndrome

Laurent Ducros and Patrick I. Plaisance

Noninvasive ventilation (NIV) is a modality of ventilatory support without endotracheal intubation and sedation and is usually delivered through a face mask, sometimes through a helmet, and infrequently through a nasal mask. It is now recognized as a very simple and efficient treatment of acute pulmonary edema due to acute heart failure (AHF), and it is also nondeleterious and associated with a low cost/effectiveness ratio. The effect of positive airway pressure is rapid and sometimes spectacular, even in case of hypercapnia and severe acute pulmonary edema. Surprisingly, NIV is not yet widely used in the intensive care unit and emergency department for this indication, possibly because it is erroneously believed that NIV is a complicated technique requiring a specialist, such as for acute respiratory failure in chronic obstructive pulmonary disease (COPD). Nowadays, some techniques of NIV do not require more than 1 hour of training, and can be used by every physician and nurse in treating patients suffering from acute heart failure and pulmonary edema. This chapter reviews the positive physiologic effect of the NIV in acute pulmonary edema and demonstrates the simplicity of this technique.

Description

For treating acute pulmonary edema secondary to AHF, two techniques of NIV are effective: noninvasive pressure support ventilation (NIPSV) and continuous positive airway pressure (CPAP). Noninvasive pressure support ventilation is delivered by a mechanical ventilator that provides pressure support during the inspiratory phase and a positive end-expiratory pressure (PEEP). Noninvasive pressure support ventilation is sometimes called bi-level positive airway pressure (BiPAP) despite some differences in the way this latter mode provides the inspiratory support. Both modes deliver a pressure support that actively helps the patient during inspiration but requires the use of a mechanical ventilator with energy, air, and oxygen fluids. The patient needs to make an effort (very little effort with new ventilators) to trigger the inspiratory flow.

Continuous positive airway pressure is simpler, does not require a ventilator, and is widely considered to be another NIV technique. As compared to NIPSV, there is no active help in the inspiratory phase of respiration, that is, no real pressure support. Breathing is entirely spontaneous, and baseline pleural, alveolar, and airway pressures are simply shifted toward positive values. Continuous positive airway pressure requires a simple generator designed to provide a high air/oxygen flow to the face mask during inspiration. A flow higher than the patient's maximum instantaneous inspiratory flow allows maintenance of a constant positive airway pressure. Some ventilators provide a CPAP mode, but in this case the patient always needs to make an inspiratory effort in order to open a valve and receive the flow. Figure 44.1 describes the differences between NIPSV and CPAP. Figure 44.2 shows different CPAP flow generators and conditions required for maximal efficiency. Figure 44.3 shows the practical use of CPAP and explains the

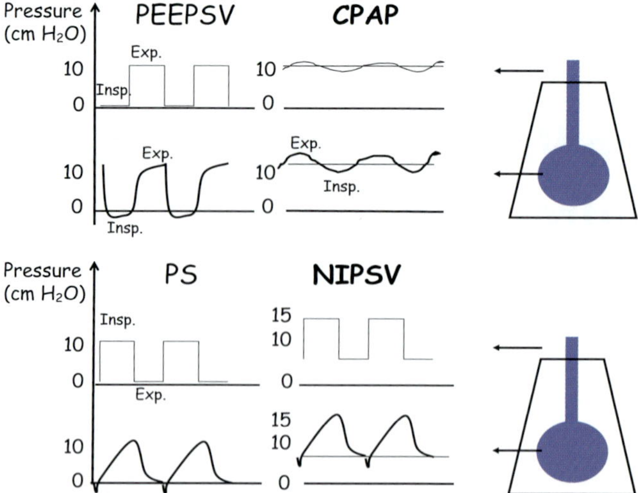

FIGURE 44.1. Differences between noninvasive pressure support ventilation (NIPSV) and continuous positive airway pressure (CPAP): airway pressure at the mouth level (top) and at the alveolar level (bottom), during four ventilation modes: spontaneous ventilation with PEEP valve (PEEPSV), CPAP, pressure support (PS), and noninvasive pressure ventilation that associates PS with PEEP (NIPSV). During PEEPSV, airway pressure is positive during expiration only, resulting in large variations of intrathoracic pressure from PEEP to negative values. Addition of high oxygen/air flow during inspiration with a CPAP generator stabilizes intrathoracic pressure at the PEEP level leading to the continuous positive airway pressure CPAP (see Fig. 44.2). Figure 44.2B explains the conditions for stabilization of the pressure, which is crucial to decrease both afterload and preload. PS is delivered during inspiration and only with the help of a ventilator. With NIPSV, a PEEP is added to the noninvasive pressure support.

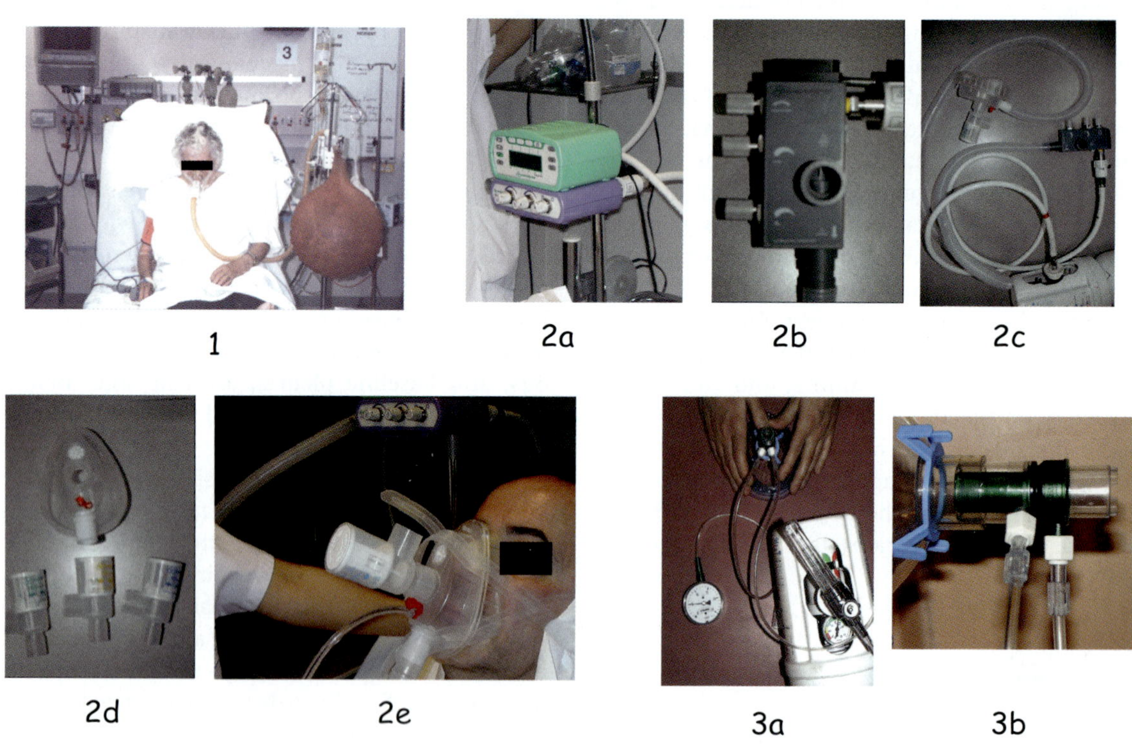

FIGURE 44.2. (A) Three CPAP devices: (1) With the older system the patient inspires in a latex balloon filled by an air/oxygen flow, which remains lower than the patient's maximal instantaneous inspiratory flow. The patient expires through a PEEP valve. (2) The high-flow CPAP is a device that uses the Venturi effect to deliver a 120 to 140 L/min flow from a pressurized oxygen supply (c) with (a) or without (b) FiO_2 and pressure monitor (here the Caradyne® Gamida model). FiO_2 can be varied from 33% to 60% without any decrease in flow. The patient inspires through a facial mask (d,e) and expires through a PEEP valve calibrated at 5, 7.5, or 10 cm H_2O (d,e). (3) The Boussignac CPAP is based on a different scientific principle and also gives a high oxygen/air flow to the patient (a) with a special device directly attached to the mask (b) but FiO_2 and PEEP values cannot be altered independently.

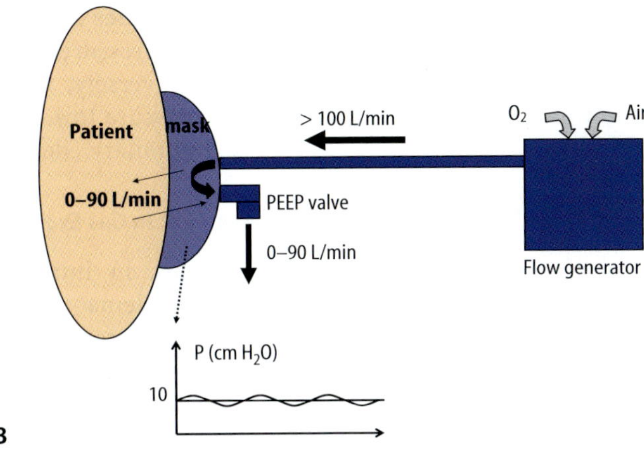

FIGURE 44.2. (B) Conditions required to create a high-flow CPAP. The generator must produce a flow superior to the maximal inspiratory flow of a patient, which can reach 90 L/min. High flow CPAP is able to produce flow of 120 to 140 L/min. Thus, there is always a flow passing through the PEEP valve and pressure is maintained in the mask and in the airways. Conversely, in case of flow reduction under 90 L/min, pressure cannot be maintained continuously throughout the respiratory cycle. In such a case, the mode should be called PEEPSV rather than CPAP.

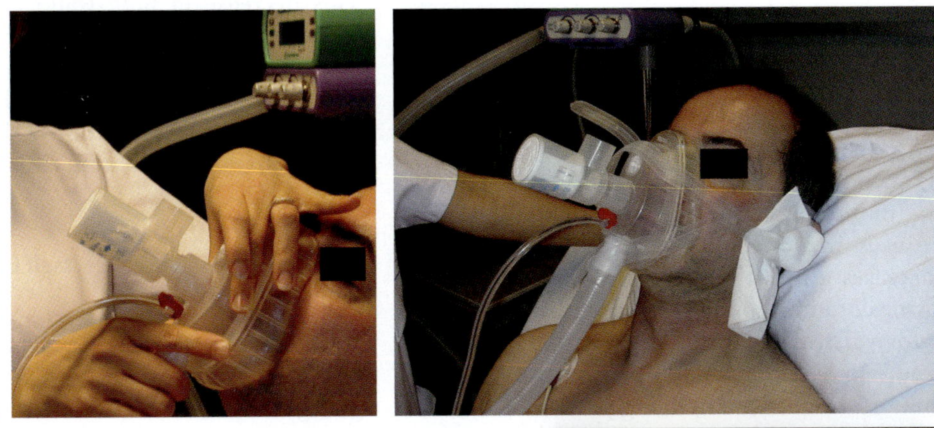

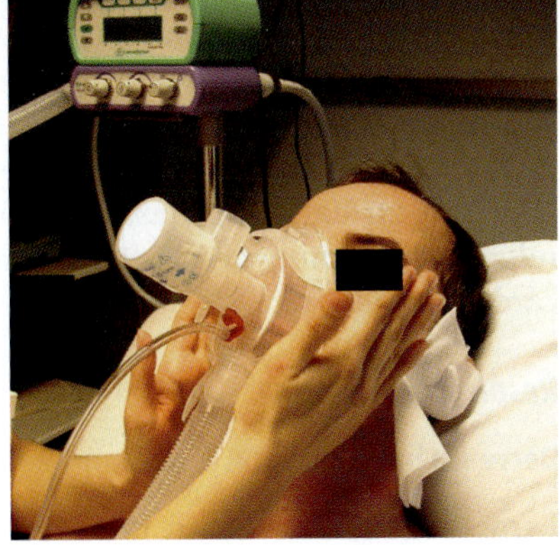

FIGURE 44.3. In practice, for a better immediate tolerance of the mask by the patient, three steps should be followed: (A) Apply the mask to the patient's face and inform the patient that a positive effect will occur in few minutes. (B) When the patient is becoming comfortable, the mask can be attached tightly but with the minimal stretch on the face with the four straps and with two precautions: avoid hurting the patient and (C) check for the absence of air leaks.

few precautions that must be taken for the patient's immediate tolerance. The choice between CPAP and NIPSV in treating acute pulmonary edema is discussed later in this chapter.

Mechanism of Improvement in Acute Heart Failure

Pathophysiology

The effects of NIV are mainly related to the intrathoracic positive pressure and are as follows.

Haemodynamic Effects

Reduction in Preload

This reduction, proportional to the level of the mean intrathoracic pressure, is due to a decrease in venous return to the right heart.[1,2] Positive pressure also increases afterload to the right heart and thus further reduces the preload to the left heart.

Reduction in Afterload

In the case of heart failure, myocardial function is much more sensitive to afterload than to preload.[3,4] It has been demonstrating in animals[5] and humans[6] that application of a positive pressure in the thorax decreases afterload to the left heart, reduces myocardial oxygen consumption, and increases cardiac output. Conversely, negative swings of intrathoracic pressure, that is, in respiratory distress, contribute to an increased afterload.[7] In clinical situations, increase in stroke volume[8] or decrease in filling pressures[9] has been demonstrated during application of a positive intrathoracic pressure in heart failure with pulmonary edema. Maximal venous oxygen consumption (MVO_2) is decreased together with heart rate, leading to an increase in coronary perfusion and endocardial flow; thus, myocardial function might also be improved without any increase in cardiac output.[6]

Respiratory Effects

Decrease in Lung Water

Large negative swings in intrathoracic pressure, such as those that occur in severe asthma, are known to produce lung edema due to the increase in filtration pressure through the alveolar membrane.[10] Conversely, the increase in airway and alveolar pressure toward positive values tends to reduce pulmonary edema.

Improvement in Gas Exchange

The increase in intrathoracic pressure during pulmonary edema induces an alveolar recruitment and a decrease in the pulmonary shunt with a proportional increase in blood arterial oxygen pressure.[11] Patient's oxygenation is rapidly improved in the first minutes with NIV as compared to conventional treatment.[12–15] These results have now been confirmed with both CPAP and NIPSV.[9,16–23]

Work of Breathing

Application of a positive intrathoracic pressure is followed by an improvement in pulmonary compliance because of the reduction in lung water. This decrease in lung water also reduces small airways congestion and therefore airway resistance.[24,25] These effects have been demonstrated in clinical situations.[9,26] Compared to CPAP, NIPSV provides a greater reduction in the work of breathing because of the addition of inspiratory pressure support.[26]

Hemodynamic Disturbance Itself Contributes to the Respiratory Distress

In the case of pulmonary edema, the proportion of the systemic blood flow devoted to the diaphragm and other respiratory muscles is increased from 4% to 20%.[27] However, since cardiac output is limited, this increase in metabolic demand is not satisfied, and respiratory muscle weakness is exacerbated along with development of lactic acidosis[28] and a resultant worsening in respiratory distress. Thus, acute pulmonary edema is the result of a progressive exacerbation of heart failure and respiratory distress. Pulmonary congestion increases resistance of breathing and decreases lung compliance in parallel with pulmonary congestion, shunt, and hypoxia. All these disorders result in a large increase in the work of breathing and respiratory distress. They are also responsible for a large negative swing of the intrathoracic

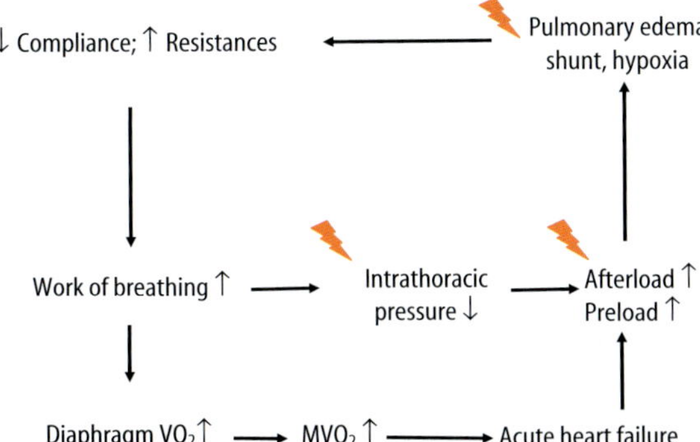

FIGURE 44.4. Acute pulmonary edema autoaggravation between respiratory and heart failure. The cycle is broken by CPAP due to positive airway pressure application and reduction of preload, afterload, and shunt.

pressure with a simultaneous increase in preload, afterload, and diaphragm oxygen consumption, which further worsen heart failure and pulmonary congestion. In summary, the positive airway pressure provided by NIV strongly contributes to stopping rapidly the negative feedback loop between heart failure and respiratory distress by acting at all the steps of this deleterious mechanism: reduction in preload and afterload, and pulmonary shunt (Fig. 44.4).

Evidence to Support the Use of Noninvasive Ventilation in the Initial Management of Acute Pulmonary Edema

Historically, NIPSV was developed in the 1980s and has demonstrated its benefit in both the reduction in endotracheal intubation rate and in-hospital mortality in respiratory failure of COPD patients.[29] Continuous positive airway pressure is a very old technique. The first description was published 70 years ago as a "pulmonary-plus machine," helpful in treating pulmonary edema.[30] During the last 20 years, several studies have reported the benefit of CPAP in acute heart failure syndrome (AHFS). The first recommendations from societies of critical care[31] were based on the more rapid improvement in vital parameters with CPAP and the significant reduction in endotracheal intubation rate and mechanical ventilation, compared to the conventional medical treatment with oxygen.[9,13–15,20] By 2001, none of the studies had proved a significant reduction in mortality with CPAP or NIPSV in acute pulmonary edema. In 1998, a meta-analysis reported only a trend toward reduction in mortality with CPAP.[32] More recently, a randomized trial in a population older than 75 years found a reduction in in-hospital mortality with CPAP compared to the conventional treatment.[33] A second meta-analysis from 15 randomized controlled studies found a significant reduction in mortality with NIV compared to conventional treatment (–46% with CPAP; –37% with NIPSV) as well as in endotracheal intubation rates (–60% with CPAP; –49% with NIPSV).[34] Despite a higher level of agreement with CPAP compared to NIPSV, the authors conclude that both techniques should be used as a first-line therapy in acute pulmonary edema. In the recent first international guidelines on acute heart failure,[35] both NIPSV and CPAP have been considered by the European Society of Cardiology as a full treatment for pulmonary edema (type IIa, level of evidence C). The previous guidelines of NIV in acute pulmonary edema were edited by the societies of critical care that approved the use of CPAP but did not recommend NIPSV due to a controversy regarding its potential to cause myocardial ischemia.[31] This was based on two studies in which NIPSV was associated with a higher mortality due to myocardial infarction.[20,23] This result has not been confirmed in further studies.[17,36,37] Moreover, in the last meta-analysis, myocardial infarction rate was found to be reduced with NIV when compared to the conventional treatment (–27% versus –22%, respectively), whatever the technique of NIV.

Indications of Noninvasive Ventilation in Acute Heart Failure Syndrome

Severe Acute Pulmonary Edema Only?

According to the recent European guidelines, since the use of NIV is associated with a significant reduction in endotracheal intubation and mechanical ventilation, NIV is recommended when the patient meets the criteria for endotracheal intubation, that is, in severe acute pulmonary edema. However, considering the immediate beneficial effect on oxygenation with NIV and the fact that a rapid improvement of oxygenation and hemodynamic parameters may limit myocardial damage and improve long-term survival, indications might be spread out to include all acute pulmonary edema as soon as the patient presents with signs of respiratory failure.

CPAP or NIPSV?

Although the level of evidence is higher for CPAP than for NIPSV, both techniques are recommended in the last guidelines; CPAP is less expensive and easier to use than NIPSV and can even be used at home by patients with obstructive sleep apnea syndromes. However, when COPD is associated with AHFS, NIPSV is preferable, as it provides inspiratory pressure support and a greater reduction in the work of breathing.[26]

Which Level of Positive End-Expiratory Pressure and Pressure Support?

With CPAP, most of the studies have been realized with a 10 cm H_2O PEEP without any side effect. With NIPSV, the mean PEEP and pressure support values were 5 and 15 cm H_2O, respectively.[35] In practice, pressure support level should be set in order to provide enough tidal volume for the patient.

Duration of Noninvasive Ventilation Therapy?

Regarding published studies, patients were treated with NIV for 1 to 6 hours, rarely 24 hours, and never continuously except in the first hours. In practice, NIV is stopped when the patient feels better or when respiratory distress has disappeared.

With or Without Medical Treatment?

There is no reason not to give diuretics or vasodilators to patients receiving NIV, except for the potential hazardous reduction in preload and cardiac output associated with both therapies. Noninvasive ventilation alone has been shown to be more effective than drugs in the first 15 minutes of treatment and, more interestingly, its benefit continues even after drugs have been added.[12]

Side Effects

Side effects are infrequent and reported only in a few patients in all studies. They include nausea and vomiting due to abdominal distention (especially when airway pressure is abnormally high), skin reactions, and claustrophobia. Barotrauma and arterial collapse due to positive intrathoracic pressure have never been observed. Thus, NIV is advantageous as it has the same positive effects of medical therapy by reducing both preload and afterload without the associated side effects.

Contraindications

It is recognized that NIV should not be used in the presence of the following contraindications: impaired level of consciousness, bradypnea and the need for immediate endotracheal intubation, vomiting, and systolic arterial pressure <80 mm Hg. As we previously noted, myocardial infarction associated with acute pulmonary edema is not a contraindication to NIV use. In several studies, severe mitral or aortic stenosis were considered exclusion criteria for NIV. However, the theoretical risk of excessive decrease in preload or afterload is probably less important with NIV than with any drug therapy that has a prolonged half-life; with the cessation of NIV, the potent side effects due to positive pressure are immediately removed. Also, in pulmonary edema, a decreased level of consciousness is probably a relative contraindication as the patient may respond favorably to NIV within a short period, thus avoiding the need for tracheal intubation. This response is due to the rapid decrease in hypercapnia and respiratory distress, and occasionally a spectacular reduction in encephalopathy may be observed.

Case Report

An 82-year-old man presents to the emergency room with acute dyspnea and severe respiratory distress. He does not complain of chest pain despite a long past medical history of coronary heart disease. On examination, he is unable to speak in full sentences and exhibits signs of hypercapnic encephalopathy. His skin feels clammy and he is cyanotic, with pulse oxymetry of 72% on air. The jugular venous pressure is not raised. His respiratory rate is 45 breaths per minute with excessive use of accessory muscles. On auscultation, crackles are heard throughout both lung fields. Immediate high-flow oxygen increases the SpO_2 to 82%. Arterial blood pressure is 102/67 mm Hg. Heart rate is 125 bpm. The electrocardiogram does not exhibit signs of acute myocardial ischemia.

Questions

The following questions are raised by this case:

1. What kind of treatment should be immediately discussed?
2. Are there any drug therapies indicated?
3. What is the best therapeutic solution?
4. When should treatment stop?

Answers

1. Because of severe respiratory distress with encephalopathy and persistence of hypoxia, tracheal intubation is theoretically the best solution. However, advanced age and potential difficulties in weaning the patient from the ventilator are associated with a high mortality rate, and thus any other alternative treatment would be preferred.

2. In the present case of heart failure without arterial hypertension and probably severe left ventricular systolic dysfunction, both vasodilators and diuretic drugs are hazardous, with an increased risk in arterial hypotension due to excessive arterial vasodilation or venous return reduction, more so with associated coronary disease. Dobutamine is not a good therapeutic alternative in the absence of shock and in the presence of coronary disease.

3. Application of a CPAP facial mask with 50% high-flow oxygen and a 10 cm H_2O pressure valve was followed by rapid reduction in respiratory frequency and distress. Arterial blood pressure was conserved and small doses of diuretics were prescribed.

4. The patient wanted to keep the mask for 3 hours continuously and fell asleep. He was weaned from CPAP 4 hours later. As we noticed above, the key point is to keep the pressure positive in the airway. Therefore, the care team must carefully check the absence of air leak between the face skin and the mask. To verify it, one can observe or listen to the flow of air passing through the expiratory valve during both expiration and inspiration (Fig. 44.2B).

References

1. Guyton AC, Jones CE, Coleman TG. Circulatory Physiology: Cardiac Output and Its Regulations. Philadelphia: Saunders, 1973.
2. Fessler HE, Brower RG, Wise RA, Permutt S. Effects of positive end-expiratory pressure on the gradient for venous return. Am Rev Respir Dis 1991;143: 19–24.
3. Cohn JN, Franciosa JA. Vasodilator therapy of cardiac failure: (first of two parts). N Engl J Med 1977;297:27–31.
4. Cohn JN, Franciosa JA. Vasodilator therapy of cardiac failure (second of two parts). N Engl J Med 1977;297:254–8.
5. Pinsky MR, Summer WR, Wise RA, Permutt S, Bromberger-Barnea B. Augmentation of cardiac function by elevation of intrathoracic pressure. J Appl Physiol 1983;54:950–5.
6. Naughton M, Rahman M, Hara K, Floras J, Bradley D. Effect of continuous positive airway pressure on intrathoracic and left ventricular transmural pressures in patients with congestive heart failure. Circulation 1995;91:1725–31.
7. Buda AJ, Pinsky MR, Ingels NB Jr, Daughters GT 2nd, Stinson EB, Alderman EL. Effect of intrathoracic pressure on left ventricular performance. N Engl J Med 1979;301:453–9.
8. Bradley TD, Holloway RM, McLaughlin PR, Ross BL, Walters J, Liu PP. Cardiac output response to continuous positive airway pressure in congestive heart failure. Am Rev Respir Dis 1992;145:377–82.
9. Lenique F, Habis M, Lofaso F, Dubois-Rande JL, Harf A, Brochard L. Ventilatory and hemodynamic effects of continuous positive airway pressure in

left heart failure. Am J Respir Crit Care Med 1997; 155:500–5.

10. Stalcup SA, Mellins RB. Mechanical forces producing pulmonary edema in acute asthma. N Engl J Med 1977;297:592–6.
11. Ashbaugh DG, Petty TL, Bigelow DB, Harris TM. Continuous positive-pressure breathing (CPPB) in adult respiratory distress syndrome. J Thorac Cardiovasc Surg 1969;57:31–41.
12. Plaisance P, Pirracchio R, Berton C, Payen D. Benefit of immediate continuous positive airway pressure (CPAP) in out-of-hospital management of cardiogenic pulmonary edema. Eur Heart J 2008, in press.
13. Bersten AD, Holt AW, Vedig AE, Skowronski GA, Baggoley CJ. Treatment of severe cardiogenic pulmonary edema with continuous positive airway pressure delivered by face mask. N Engl J Med 1991;325:1825–30.
14. Lin M, Yang YF, Chiang HT, Chang MS, Chiang BN, Cheitlin MD. Reappraisal of continuous positive airway pressure therapy in acute cardiogenic pulmonary edema. Short-term results and long-term follow-up. Chest 1995;107:1379–86.
15. Rasanen J, Heikkila J, Downs J, Nikki P, Vaisanen I, Viitanen A. Continuous positive airway pressure by face mask in acute cardiogenic pulmonary edema. Am J Cardiol 1985;55:296–300.
16. Crane SD, Elliott MW, Gilligan P, Richards K, Gray AJ. Randomised controlled comparison of continuous positive airways pressure, bilevel non-invasive ventilation, and standard treatment in emergency department patients with acute cardiogenic pulmonary oedema. Emerg Med J 2004;21:155–61.
17. Kelly CA, Newby DE, McDonagh TA, et al. Randomised controlled trial of continuous positive airway pressure and standard oxygen therapy in acute pulmonary oedema; effects on plasma brain natriuretic peptide concentrations. Eur Heart J 2002;23:1379–86.
18. L'Her E. Noninvasive mechanical ventilation in acute cardiogenic pulmonary edema. Curr Opin Crit Care 2003;9:67–71.
19. L'Her E, Deye N, Lellouche F, et al. Physiological effects of noninvasive ventilation during acute lung injury. Am J Respir Crit Care Med 2005;4:4.
20. Mehta S, Jay G, Woolard R, et al. Randomized, prospective trial of bilevel versus continuous positive airway pressure in acute pulmonary edema. Crit Care Med 1997;25:620–8.
21. Nava S, Carbone G, DiBattista N, et al. Noninvasive ventilation in cardiogenic pulmonary edema: a multicenter randomized trial. Am J Respir Crit Care Med 2003;168:1432–7. Epub 2003 Sep 4.
22. Park M, Sangean MC, Volpe Mde S, et al. Randomized, prospective trial of oxygen, continuous positive airway pressure, and bilevel positive airway pressure by face mask in acute cardiogenic pulmonary edema. Crit Care Med 2004;32:2407–15.
23. Rusterholtz T, Kempf J, Berton C, et al. Noninvasive pressure support ventilation (NIPSV) with face mask in patients with acute cardiogenic pulmonary edema (ACPE). Intensive Care Med 1999;25: 21–8.
24. Snashall PD, Chung KF. Airway obstruction and bronchial hyperresponsiveness in left ventricular failure and mitral stenosis. Am Rev Respir Dis 1991;144:945–56.
25. Sharp JT, Griffith GT, Bunnell IL, Greene DG. Ventilatory mechanics in pulmonary edema in man. J Clin Invest 1958;37:111–7.
26. Chadda K, Annane D, Hart N, Gajdos P, Raphael JC, Lofaso F. Cardiac and respiratory effects of continuous positive airway pressure and noninvasive ventilation in acute cardiac pulmonary edema. Crit Care Med 2002;30:2457–61.
27. Aubier M, Trippenbach T, Roussos C. Respiratory muscle fatigue during cardiogenic shock. J Appl Physiol 1981;51:499–508.
28. Aubier M, Viires N, Syllie G, Mozes R, Roussos C. Respiratory muscle contribution to lactic acidosis in low cardiac output. Am Rev Respir Dis 1982; 126:648–52.
29. Brochard L, Mancebo J, Wysocki M, et al. Noninvasive ventilation for acute exacerbations of chronic obstructive pulmonary disease. N Engl J Med 1995; 333:817–22.
30. Poulton P. Left-sided heart failure with pulmonary oedema: its treatment with the "pulmonary plus pressure machine". Lancet 1936;2:981–3.
31. International Consensus Conferences in Intensive Care Medicine: noninvasive positive pressure ventilation in acute Respiratory failure. Am J Respir Crit Care Med 2001;163:283–91.
32. Pang D, Keenan SP, Cook DJ, Sibbald WJ. The effect of positive pressure airway support on mortality and the need for intubation in cardiogenic pulmonary edema: a systematic review. Chest 1998;114: 1185–92.
33. L'Her E, Duquesne F, Girou E, et al. Noninvasive continuous positive airway pressure in elderly cardiogenic pulmonary edema patients. Intensive Care Med 2004;30:882–8. Epub 2004 Feb 28.
34. Masip J, Roque M, Sanchez B, Fernandez R, Subirana M, Exposito JA. Noninvasive ventilation in acute cardiogenic pulmonary edema: systematic review and meta-analysis. JAMA 2005;294:3124–30.

35. Nieminen MS, Bohm M, Cowie MR, et al. Executive summary of the guidelines on the diagnosis and treatment of acute heart failure: the Task Force on Acute Heart Failure of the European Society of Cardiology. Eur Heart J 2005;26:384–416. Epub 2005 Jan 28.
36. Masip J, Betbese AJ, Paez J, et al. Non-invasive pressure support ventilation versus conventional oxygen therapy in acute cardiogenic pulmonary oedema: a randomised trial. Lancet 2000;356:2126–32.
37. Bellone A, Monari A, Cortellaro F, Vettorello M, Arlati S, Coen D. Myocardial infarction rate in acute pulmonary edema: noninvasive pressure support ventilation versus continuous positive airway pressure. Crit Care Med 2004;32:1860–5.

45
Invasive Ventilation and Acute Heart Failure Syndrome

Jean-Damien Ricard and Damien Roux

Because utilization of noninvasive ventilatory techniques considerably reduces the need for endotracheal intubation and invasive mechanical ventilation during acute heart failure syndrome (AHFS) (1, 2), the recent guidelines issued by the European Society of Cardiology (3) recommend that invasive mechanical ventilation in the setting of acute heart failure (AHF) should be considered only after failure of noninvasive methods, such as continuous positive airway pressure (CPAP) and noninvasive positive pressure ventilation (NIPPV). Overall failure rate (i.e., need for intubation) of noninvasive ventilation is approximately 13% during AHF (2), but may affect up to 25% of patients in some studies (4). Because inadequate ventilatory settings may be harmful and may directly influence outcome in patients with (5) and in those at risk of (6, 7) acute lung injury, appropriate ventilatory management of such patients is crucial to avoid the deleterious effects of mechanical ventilation (8). The mortality rate of patients with AHF who require intubation can be high as 50% (9), but encouraging results have been published in elderly patients discharged after intubation and mechanical ventilation for cardiogenic pulmonary edema, with a 1-year survival rate of 69% (10). Taken together, these data suggest that intubation and mechanical ventilation should be undertaken in AHF patients failing noninvasive ventilation, provided mechanical ventilation can be conducted appropriately.

Quality assurance programs (7) in hospitals and intensive care units (ICUs) should ensure that mechanical ventilation is adequately and uniformly delivered, taking into account the pathophysiology of the disease. In the setting of AHF, the aim of mechanical ventilation is to relieve respiratory distress due to AHF-induced respiratory muscle fatigue, improve pulmonary gas exchange, and protect airways, without harming the injured lung. This may be achieved by reducing tidal volume (V_T) in order to avoid lung overdistention and by adding moderate levels of positive end-expiratory pressure (PEEP). Close monitoring of plateau pressure is mandatory, and patients should be regularly evaluated for weaning, so as to reduce the duration of mechanical ventilation.

Physiologic Effects of Mechanical Ventilation

Acute respiratory failure complicating acute heart failure and cardiogenic pulmonary edema is due to hypoxemia, increased work of breathing, augmented oxygen consumption, and ultimately muscle fatigue.

Contrary to other forms of acute respiratory failure in which mechanical ventilation usually worsens cardiac function, cardiogenic pulmonary edema is probably the situation in which mechanical ventilation will alleviate both pulmonary and cardiac dysfunction.

Effects of Mechanical Ventilation on Pulmonary Dysfunction

Intrapulmonary shunt is believed to be the primary cause of hypoxemia in cardiogenic pulmonary edema, due to the filling of alveolar by edema fluid. Hypoxemia may be further worsened by a decrease in PvO_2 caused by the drop in cardiac output encountered in AHF. Mechanical ventilation, by increasing intrathoracic pressure, will augment functional residual capacity (FRC), thereby decreasing intrapulmonary shunting. Pulmonary shunt will be further decreased by the application of PEEP, which will help recruit fluid-filled alveoli and further increase FRC. As a consequence, arterial oxygen content will rise, enabling greater oxygen transport. Cardiac consequences of severe hypoxemia (myocardial ischemia, arrhythmias) may thus be prevented.

Patients with AHF display restrictive respiratory deficiency with reduced vital capacity. Replacement of air in the lungs with blood and edema fluid reduces pulmonary compliance, and engorgement of blood vessels—by reducing the caliber of the peripheral airways—increases airway resistance. Thus the work of breathing is increased to compensate for the reduction in tidal volume, and respiratory muscle oxygen demand is in turn, considerably augmented. Unfortunately, this demand cannot be met because of low cardiac output, hypoxemia, and ensuing acidosis that all concur to reduce oxygen delivery to the respiratory muscles. In the absence of ventilatory support, hypercapnia and impaired consciousness occur as the consequence of respiratory exhaustion.

By placing respiratory muscles at rest, invasive mechanical ventilation greatly reduces their oxygen consumption, thereby improving global oxygen distribution in the organism. Restoration of adequate V_T provides appropriate alveolar ventilation, enabling correction of hypercapnia. It should be noted, however, that too rapid correction of hypercapnia may be responsible for coronary vasoconstriction, as suggested by a greater incidence of myocardial infarction in patients with AHF treated with noninvasive positive pressure support ventilation in comparison with CPAP (1).

Effects of Mechanical Ventilation on Cardiac Dysfunction

Heart–lung interactions during mechanical ventilation were described over 50 years ago (11), and have been extensively studied (12). There has been renewed interest with the study of arterial pulse variation (13, 14) combined with the contribution of echocardiographic techniques (15, 16).

Invasive mechanical ventilation increases intrathoracic pressure, which affects systemic venous return to the right ventricle and left ventricle ejection. Right atrial pressure is increased with increasing intrathoracic pressure, that, at the same time, decreases transmural left ventricle systolic pressure, both resulting in decreased intrathoracic blood volume. Therefore, in normal subjects, invasive mechanical ventilation, by reducing right ventricle preload through altered venous return, decreases cardiac output.

In the presence of AHF, however, an increase in right atrial pressure and a reduction in transmural left ventricle systolic pressure are highly beneficial. Consequently, improvement of cardiac output observed with rises in intrathoracic pressure during mechanical ventilation is suggestive of congestive heart failure. Mechanical ventilation not only affects right and left pressure gradients but also affects left ventricle function through changes in left ventricular afterload. As detailed above, during AHF, spontaneous breathing is associated with increased inspiratory efforts to overcome augmented airway resistance and reduced compliance. These efforts result in large negative swings in intrathoracic pressure that increase left ventricle transmural pressure and, thus, left ventricle afterload. This increase in ventricle afterload further decreases left ventricle ejection. Therefore, invasive mechanical ventilation improves left ventricle ejection and cardiac function during AHF not only by increasing intrathoracic pressure but also by simply withdrawing the negative swings in intrathoracic pressure. Finally, increasing intrathoracic pressure with mechanical ventilation, will reduce myocardial oxygen demand by reducing left ventricle end-diastolic volume and left ventricle ejection pressure.

Additional Effects of Positive End-Expiratory Pressure

In the presence of pulmonary edema, addition of PEEP during mechanical ventilation improves

PaO_2 by increasing alveolar recruitment, thereby increasing FRC and reducing intrapulmonary shunt.

Effects of PEEP on cardiac output have been comprehensively and exhaustively reviewed recently (17). In the setting of AHF, it seems that only very moderate levels of PEEP may be beneficial. Grace and Greenbaum (18) studied the effect of a stepwise increase in PEEP on cardiac function during mechanical ventilation of AHF. Cardiac output increased in four of six patients with a pulmonary artery occlusion pressure between 14 and 18 mm Hg and in 12 of 13 patients whose occlusion pressure exceeded 18 mm Hg, with a mean level of PEEP of 3.9 cm H_2O. In patients with lower occlusion pressures, application of PEEP decreased cardiac output. Schuster et al. (19) studied by transesophageal echocardiography the effect of increasing levels of PEEP in 11 patients with severe left ventricle failure. They found an almost linear decrease in cardiac output with increasing levels of PEEP. It should be noted, however, that patients were being treated for their cardiac dysfunction at the time of the measurements and that mean index cardiac was 3.5 ± 0.7 L/min/m^2. It therefore may well be that cardiac function was already improving and that left ventricle became more susceptible to the decrease in right ventricle filling induced by PEEP.

Finally, there is some experimental evidence suggesting that excessive PEEP reduces coronary blood flow (20, 21), which could be deleterious in the presence of ischemic heart disease.

Indications for Invasive Mechanical Ventilation

The recent guidelines issued by the European Society of Cardiology (3) recommend that invasive mechanical ventilation should be initiated only after failure of noninvasive methods (CPAP, NIPPV). However, intubation and invasive mechanical ventilation should be performed without delay in these situations: acute respiratory failure with respiratory exhaustion, hemodynamic instability, cardiogenic shock, impaired consciousness, and severe cardiac arrhythmias.

Adjusting the Ventilator (Tables 45.1–45.3)

Ventilatory Mode

Volume assist-control ventilation is a mode in which the ventilator delivers the same V_T during each inspiration, whether it be patient-triggered or machine initiated. This mode has been repeatedly shown as the most utilized ventilatory mode around the world (22, 23).

Inspired Fraction of Oxygen (FiO_2)

Following tracheal intubation, patients should be (at least transiently) ventilated under 100% O_2 ($FiO_2 = 1$) until arterial blood gases are performed (approximately 30 minutes later). The value of PaO_2 after FiO_2 increases to 1 will help assess the severity of gas exchange abnormalities (including shunt), guide therapy (addition of PEEP), and evaluate response to therapy. PaO_2 should be kept between 80 and 100 mm Hg. Occurrence of reabsorption atelectasis with the use of high FiO_2 is debated during acute lung injury, and in any case its importance is outweighed by potentially life-threatening hypoxemia. The same holds true for oxygen toxicity.

Table 45.1. Practical steps to mechanical ventilation initiation

1. Intubation	
2. Ensure adequate sedation: Continuous IV infusion: fentanyl 25–100 µg/h with midazolam: 2–10 mg/h (use neuromuscular blocking agents should be restricted to patients with sustained ventilator dyssynchrony despite high dose sedation)	
3. Initial ventilatory parameters:	VT: 6 to 8 mL/kg*
	Respiratory rate: 15 bpm
	FiO2: 100%
	PEEP: 5 cm H_2O
	I/E ratio: 1:1
	Inspiratory flow: 40–60 L/min
4. Perform chest x-ray to ensure appropriate positioning of the endotracheal tube (ETT) (possible selective intubation), absence of aspiration pneumonia, absence of barotraumas	
5. Measure plateau pressure with initial parameters and adjust if pressure >30 cm H_2O	
6. Perform arterial blood gas 30 minutes after intubation and adjust ventilatory parameters	

*V_T should be reduced to avoid not only ventilator-induced lung injury but also a too rapid correction of hypercapnia (if present) that could induce coronary vasoconstriction.

Table 45.2. Daily management of the intubated patient (at least once a day)

At the bed side:	Routine clinical examination
	Check for patient discomfort, evaluate for weaning
	Check ventilatory parameters (consistency with medical prescription) and adjust if necessary.
	Measure plateau pressure (several times a day) (inspiratory pause)
	Look for possible auto-PEEP (expiratory pause)
Daily chest x-ray:	Verify ETT position (avoid endobronchial intubation)
	Check central line and gastric tube position
	Look for barotrauma, new infiltrate infection
Daily arterial blood gas	

Tidal Volume

Choice of V_T is of great importance when initiating mechanical ventilation because of the potentially life-threatening effects of inappropriate settings (24). Too large V_T will lead to excessive end-inspiratory lung volume, the main culprit of barotrauma (extraalveolar air) and ventilator-induced lung injury (permeability-type pulmonary edema) (8). In noncardiogenic pulmonary edema (acute lung injury and acute respiratory distress syndrome [ARDS]), it has been clearly shown that patients ventilated with 12 mL/kg V_T had a 23% greater mortality than those ventilated with 6 mL/kg V_T (5). Although there is still a debate as to whether or not 6 mL/kg V_T should be applied to all patients ventilated for acute lung injury (25), there is a general agreement that end-inspiratory plateau pressure (which best approximates end-inspiratory lung volume at the bedside) should be kept below 30 cmH_2O. Rather than setting V_T according to predicted or ideal body weight (and not actual body weight!), it may be preferable to tailor V_T adjustment to the corresponding plateau pressure. This attitude offers the benefit of taking into account the added risk of both excessive V_T and PEEP. To resume, V_T greater than 10 mL/kg must be avoided and V_T should be best adjusted to keep plateau pressure below 30 cm H_2O.

Positive End-Expiratory Pressure

By recruiting atelectatic areas and by redistributing extravascular lung water form alveoli to peribronchial and perivascular spaces, PEEP is one of the cornerstones of pulmonary edema treatment. As discussed above, applying PEEP conveys both positive pulmonary effects and potentially negative cardiac and hemodynamic effects. In the setting of AHF, however, these hemodynamic effects of PEEP may prove beneficial. If there are sufficient data to support and promote the use of CPAP to achieve cardiopulmonary improvement and reduce intubation rate in spontaneously breathing patients with cardiogenic pulmonary edema (26), data are less abundant and conclusive on the additional benefits of PEEP once invasive mechanical ventilation has been instituted. Nevertheless, because alveolar flooding remains the main cause of hypoxemia in these patients, PEEP should be applied to hypoxemic patients ventilated for AHF. Obviously, application of PEEP

Table 45.3. Main causes of worsening hypoxemia during mechanical ventilation for acute heart failure

Inappropriate ventilator settings, ventilator malfunction	
Selective intubation:	Deflate the cuff of the endotracheal tube and pull slightly the tube so as to leave 3 to 4 cm between the tip of the tube and the carina
	Check correct position of the tube with a chest x-ray
	Check and secure external fixation of the tube
Airway obstruction, mucus plugging, retained secretions:	Perform endotracheal suctioning, check humidification device
Atelectasis:	Check for selective intubation in the controlateral lung
	Verify natremia, even moderate hypernatremia may enhance atelectasis
	Consider patient positioning, bronchoscopy,
Pneumothorax:	Consider chest tube insertion
Aspiration :	Check cuff inflation
Ventilator-associated pneumonia (see Chapter 75), sepsis, shock	
Pulmonary edema:	Either reoccurrence of AHF or occurrence of ARDS
Decompensation of concomitant lung disease (COPD, asthma)	
Pulmonary embolism	

should be delayed in patients with severe cardiogenic shock until a more stable hemodynamic condition is restored. Considering the possible worsening effect of PEEP on cardiac output in patients with AHF, adequate continuous monitoring is warranted. Moderate levels of PEEP (3 to 5 cm H_2O) should be applied initially and adjusted according to hemodynamic tolerance, effect on oxygenation, and plateau pressure. In some rare instances, much higher levels of PEEP (15 to 18 cm H_2O) may be used in case of massive and life-threatening alveolar flooding.

Respiratory Rate and I/E Ratio

In the absence of expiratory flow limitation, respiratory rate will be set between 15 and 20 cpm and further adjusted according to the patient's rate demand and $PaCO_2$. Inspiratory-to-expiratory time (I/E) ratio should be set in order to ensure optimal lung recruitment and oxygenation. This can be achieved by setting I/E = 1 : 1. The I/E ratio can be modulated by changing inspiratory flow or respiratory rate. In patients with coexisting chronic obstructive pulmonary disease (COPD), dynamic hyperinflation will be minimized by increasing expiratory time (I/E ratio of 1 : 2 or 1 : 3). This can be obtained by increasing inspiratory flow and reducing respiratory rate by about 12 to 15 cpm. Decreasing V_T should also be considered in patients with important expiratory flow limitation.

Weaning and Extubation

Discontinuation of mechanical ventilation should be considered as soon possible so as to avoid unnecessary prolonging of mechanical ventilation and minimize related complications. Partial or complete reversal of the underlying cause of respiratory failure is warranted before thinking of withdrawing mechanical ventilation. In that respect, FiO_2 should be less than 40% to 50%. Patients should also satisfy a number of criteria before extubation (27) is considered: absence of uncontrolled ongoing infection (temperature ≤38°C), hemodynamic stability without vasopressors (moderate levels of dobutamine can be maintained, and may even be helpful in patients with severe cardiac insufficiency), hemoglobin ≥8 g/dL), no sedation or sedative infusion, adequate cough, adequate neurologic status (answer to simple orders, no agitation or confusion).

For the majority of patients, weaning and successful extubation is uneventful. Some patients, however, may worsen their cardiopulmonary status during weaning. This situation has been described in COPD patients, in which cardiogenic pulmonary edema occurs when positive pressure mechanical ventilation is withdrawn (28). These patients warrant careful evaluation and monitoring during this process, and withdrawal of positive pressure should be particularly progressive to prevent occurrence of pulmonary edema.

There are two ways to wean patients: (1) daily 30-minute T-piece trials, in which the patient is disconnected from the ventilator and left to breathe spontaneously through the endotracheal tube, with oxygen added laterally at the upper extremity of the tube with an adaptor, hence the name T-piece or T-tube; (2) progressive decrease in the level of positive pressure support ventilation. Although there is still a debate as to whether or not one method is superior to the other, both have proved to be effective and are widely used. One can also combine these two methods (which is our preference): when sedation is decreased (or interrupted) and the patient is awakening, the assist-control ventilation mode is changed to pressure support ventilation; when the patient is comfortable with levels of about 12 to 14 cm H_2O, a T-piece trial is performed. The T-piece trial helps evaluate a patient's ability to sustain spontaneous breathing. The first successful T-piece trial should be followed by extubation. A successful T-piece trial is one at the end of which the patient has not developed respiratory distress. Conversely, patients who develop severe tachypnea, increased accessory muscle activity, diaphoresis, oxygen desaturation, tachycardia, hyper- or hypotension, and arrhythmias are considered to have failed their trial. In case of failure, another T-piece trial should be considered at least 24 hours later, in order to allow respiratory muscles to recover. Stopping enteral feeding at midnight preceding the T-piece trial should be considered, enabling immediate extubation if the trial is successful.

Clinical Case

A 59-year-old man is brought to the emergency room of a general hospital because of rapid increasing dyspnea. He has a history of ischemic cardiopathy and had undergone stenting of the anterior interventricular and circumflex arteries 5 years ago. At that time, left ventricular ejection fraction (LVEF) was 50% and electrocardiogram (ECG) showed a left bundle branch block. Other antecedents are a right carotid endarterectomy and an aortofemoral bypass. Cardiovascular risk factors are hypertension, tabagism, and dyslipidemia. His daily treatment includes aspirin 75 mg, diltiazem, rilmenidine, lisinopril, hydrochlorothiazide, and molsidomine.

Dyspnea started 2 days prior to admission without chest pain and worsened right until his arrival at the emergency room. On examination, the patient is confused with a Glasgow Coma Scale score of 13/15, arterial oxygen saturation is 72% while breathing high-concentration oxygen through a face mask, blood pressure 150/60 mm Hg, heart rate 115/minute, respiratory rate 35/minute, and temperature 37.6°C. A thoracoabdominal asynchrony with intercostal indrawing is observed. There are diffuse crackles throughout both lung fields. Cardiac examination reveals no sign of right-sided heart failure. No gallops or rubs are heard. No signs of deep vein thrombosis are noted. The electrocardiogram shows a regular rhythm with a left bundle branch block.

In view of the antecedents and clinical symptoms, a diagnosis of severe AHF seems the most probable. The patient is immediately treated with furosemide 80 mg IV and receives a bolus of isosorbide dinitrate 2 mg followed by 2 mg/h infusion.

How Should This Patient Be Immediately Managed?

Immediate ventilatory support is warranted. Because of the severity of the respiratory failure, the presence of confusion and somnolence, invasive mechanical ventilation with tracheal intubation should be preferred to noninvasive ventilation. Orotracheal intubation can be performed after rapid-sequence induction. However, the patient's lying down could worsen his cardiopulmonary status and precipitate cardiorespiratory arrest. One would therefore prefer to leave the patient in a sitting position and perform nasotracheal intubation after adequate local anesthesia.

Continuous intravenous sedation is initiated with midazolam and fentanyl. Initial ventilator parameters are as follows: assist control ventilation mode with $FiO_2 = 1$, tidal volume = 500 mL, respiratory rate = 15 bpm, and PEEP = 5 cm H_2O. With these settings, oxygen saturation remains low, around 85%. To optimize muscle relaxation and minimize ventilator dyssynchrony, the patient is paralyzed. Blood pressure remains stable (120/75 mm Hg), and thus PEEP is gradually increased to 10 and then to 15 cm H_2O. Under 15 cm H_2O PEEP, blood pressure is 110/73 mm Hg, and oxygen saturation has increased to 98%. Given the high levels of PEEP, it is vital to check the level of plateau pressure. This is done by performing an inspiratory pause on the ventilator and by reading the value of end-inspiratory pressure on the airway pressure curve. In the present case, plateau pressure is 35 cm H_2O. The high level of PEEP should be maintained because it enabled a significant improvement in oxygenation and is well tolerated. Hence, V_T must be decreased from 500 mL to 420 mL, to reduce plateau pressure. After this adjustment, plateau pressure is 29 cm H_2O.

Laboratory Exams

Chest X-ray: diffuse perihilar infiltrates and cardiac enlargement; endotracheal tube correctly positioned

Arterial blood gas: pH 7.25, PCO_2 60 mm Hg, PO_2 140 mm Hg, HCO_3^- 25 mM

Laboratory tests: Na 138 mM, K 3.6 mM, Cl 100 mM, CO_2 28 mM, creatinine 85 µM (9.5 mg/L), glucose 8.8 mM (160 mg/dL)

Complete blood count: hemoglobin 11 g/dL, white blood count 17,000/µL, platelets 406,000/µL

Troponin Ic 0.87 ng/mL (nL <0.15), creatine phosphokinase (CPK) 182 UI/L (nL <171)

Echocardiogram: visual estimation of LVEF 40%, septoapical hypokinesia, mild left ventricular hypertrophy (LVH), E/A ratio >2, nondilated right ventricle (RV), systolic pulmonary artery pessure 35 mm Hg (evaluated by trans-tricuspid gradient), inferior vena cava (IVC) dilated without respiratory variation, no valvulopathy

How Should This Patient's Management Proceed?

The slight increase in troponin Ic with apical hypokinesia on transthoracic echocardiogram suggests an acute coronary syndrome even if it could be due to hypoxemia only. Thus, anticoagulation therapy is started with clopidogrel. Coronary angiography should be performed as soon as possible to confirm or rule out acute coronary syndrome. In the present case, the coronarography is stable in comparison with previous exams.

During the next 24 hours, persistent improvement in oxygenation allows reduction of PEEP at 10 cm H_2O and FiO_2 at 70%. A slight degree of hypercapnia was tolerated when V_T was reduced in order to maintain plateau pressure below 30 cm H_2O (permissive hypercapnia). The present reduction of PEEP enables a moderate increase in V_T so as to augment minute ventilation and gradually correct hypercapnia and respiratory acidosis. With these ventilatory settings, arterial blood gas is pH 7.39, $PaCO_2$ 45 mm Hg, PO_2 164 mm Hg, and HCO_3^- 27 mM.

The patient's oxygen saturation drops to 90%. Peak inspiratory and plateau pressure increase. Clinical examination shows a decreased left thoracic expansion with diminished vesicular murmur in the left lung. Hemodynamic parameters are stable.

What Is the Diagnosis?

Because both peak and plateau pressure increase, one should suspect an sudden decrease in aerated lung volume, rather than an increase in airway resistance, that would have been responsible for an isolated increase peak inspiratory airway pressure. Thus, the two principal hypotheses are left side pneumothorax and selective intubation of the left mainstem bronchus.

A chest x-ray is immediately performed and reveals endobronchial intubation, with major atelectasis of the right lung. The endotracheal tube cuff is deflated and the tube is gently pulled out 2 to 3 cm. The cuff is inflated again and the tube is securely fixed. A chest x-ray confirms the adequate positioning of the tube. A couple of hours later, the patient has resumed his initial respiratory condition.

Conclusion

The recognition of ventilator-induced lung injury has prompted clinicians to pay attention to the way they ventilated their patients and to the potential harm they were doing to some of them because of inappropriate ventilator settings. This change in attitude has been comforted by the unambiguous demonstration that taking into account simple ventilatory parameters such as V_T improves outcome in acute lung injury and ARDS. The same may hold true for AHF, and clinicians should strive to deliver mechanical ventilation to all their patients according to sound physiologic reasoning and validated guidelines.

References

1. Peter JV, Moran JL, Phillips-Hughes J, et al. Effect of non-invasive positive pressure ventilation (NIPPV) on mortality in patients with acute cardiogenic pulmonary oedema: a meta-analysis. Lancet 2006;367:1155–63.
2. Masip J, Roque M, Sanchez B, et al. Noninvasive ventilation in acute cardiogenic pulmonary edema: systematic review and meta-analysis. JAMA 2005; 294:3124–30.
3. Nieminen MS, Bohm M, Cowie MR, et al. Executive summary of the guidelines on the diagnosis and treatment of acute heart failure: the Task Force on Acute Heart Failure of the European Society of Cardiology. Eur Heart J 2005;26:384–416.
4. Delclaux C, L'Her E, Alberti C, et al. Treatment of acute hypoxemic nonhypercapnic respiratory insufficiency with continuous positive airway pressure delivered by a face mask: a randomized controlled trial. JAMA 2000;284:2352–60.
5. The Acute Respiratory Distress Syndrome Network. Ventilation with lower tidal volumes as compared with traditional tidal volumes for acute lung injury and the acute respiratory distress syndrome. N Engl J Med 2000;342:1301–8.
6. Gajic O, Dara SI, Mendez JL, et al. Ventilator-associated lung injury in patients without acute lung injury at the onset of mechanical ventilation. Crit Care Med 2004;32:1817–24.
7. Dreyfuss D. Acute lung injury and mechanical ventilation: need for quality assurance. Crit Care Med 2004;32:1960–1.
8. Dreyfuss D, Saumon G. Ventilator-induced lung injury: lessons from experimental studies. Am J Respir Crit Care Med 1998;157:294–323.

9. Nava S, Carbone G, DiBattista N, et al. Noninvasive ventilation in cardiogenic pulmonary edema: a multicenter randomized trial. Am J Respir Crit Care Med 2003;168:1432–37.
10. Adnet F, Le Toumelin P, Leberre A, et al. In-hospital and long-term prognosis of elderly patients requiring endotracheal intubation for life-threatening presentation of cardiogenic pulmonary edema. Crit Care Med 2001;29:891–5.
11. Cournand A, Motley H, Werko L, et al. Physiologic studies of the effect of intermittent positive pressure breathing on cardiac output in man. Am J Physiol 1948;152:162–74.
12. Pinsky M. Effects of mechanical ventilation on heart-lung interactions. In: Hill NS, Levy M, eds. Ventilator Management Strategies for Critical Care. New York: Marcel Dekker, 2001:655–92.
13. Jardin F. Cyclic changes in arterial pressure during mechanical ventilation. Intensive Care Med 2004; 30:1047–50.
14. Perel A. The physiological basis of arterial pressure variation during positive pressure ventilation. Reanimation 2005;14:162–71.
15. Vieillard-Baron A, Chergui K, Augarde R, et al. Cyclic changes in arterial pulse during respiratory support revisited by Doppler echocardiography. Am J Respir Crit Care Med 2003;168:671–6.
16. Vieillard-Baron A, Prin S, Chergui K, Dubourg O, Jardin F. Hemodynamic instability in sepsis: bedside assessment by Doppler echocardiography. Am J Respir Crit Care Med 2003;168:1270–6.
17. Luecke T, Pelosi P. Clinical review: positive end-expiratory pressure and cardiac output. Crit Care 2005;9:607–21.
18. Grace MP, Greenbaum DM. Cardiac performance in response to PEEP in patients with cardiac dysfunction. Crit Care Med 1982;10:358–60.
19. Schuster S, Erbel R, Weilemann LS, et al. Hemodynamics during PEEP ventilation in patients with severe left ventricular failure studied by transesophageal echocardiography. Chest 1990;97:1181–9.
20. Tucker HJ, Murray JF. Effects of end-expiratory pressure on organ blood flow in normal and diseased dogs. J Appl Physiol 1973;34:573–7.
21. Beyer J, Conzen P, Schosser R, et al. The effect of PEEP ventilation on hemodynamics and regional blood flow with special regard to coronary blood flow. Thorac Cardiovasc Surg 1980;28:128–32.
22. Esteban A, Anzueto A, Alia I, et al. How is mechanical ventilation employed in the intensive care unit? An international utilization review. Am J Respir Crit Care Med 2000;161:1450–8.
23. Esteban A, Anzueto A, Frutos F, et al. Characteristics and outcomes in adult patients receiving mechanical ventilation: a 28-day international study. JAMA 2002;287:345–55.
24. Dreyfuss D, Saumon G, Hubmayer RD. Ventilator-induced lung injury. In: Lenfant C, ed. Lung Biology in Health and Disease. New York: Taylor & Francis, 2006.
25. Ricard J-D. Are we really reducing tidal volume—and should we? Am J Respir Crit Care Med 2003;167:1297–8.
26. Navalesi P, Maggiore S. Positive end-expiratory pressure. In: Tobin M, ed. Principles and Practice of Mechanical Ventilation. New York: McGraw-Hill, 2006:273–325.
27. MacIntyre NR, Cook DJ, Ely EW Jr, et al. Evidence-based guidelines for weaning and discontinuing ventilatory support: a collective task force facilitated by the American College of Chest Physicians; the American Association for Respiratory Care; and the American College of Critical Care Medicine. Chest 2001;120:375S–95S.
28. Lemaire F, Teboul JL, Cinotti L, et al. Acute left ventricular dysfunction during unsuccessful weaning from mechanical ventilation. Anesthesiology 1988;69:171–9.

46
Chest X-Ray in Acute Heart Failure

Laurence Monnier-Cholley

This chapter discusses the consequences of chest x-ray of acute left heart failure due to left ventricular failure or mitral valve disease. Valuable interpretation of a chest x-ray in such conditions requires knowledge of the normal appearance of a chest x-ray and the technical parameters that may change it to avoid misinterpretation. A better understanding of the images also requires some knowledge of the physiopathology of pulmonary edema.

Normal Chest Radiograph

Under normal conditions, there is a linear increase in pulmonary blood flow from the apex to the base of the lung due to gravity, when the chest radiograph is performed with the patient in the erect position. Pulmonary blood flow is equally distributed throughout the lung when the patient lies in the supine position. In consequences, one needs to know the patient position when looking at his chest radiograph. If the radiograph is taken with the patient supine or semierect, the position has to be documented. The presence of an air-fluid level in the stomach is the landmark of an erect position.

Cardiac size also depends on technical parameters. On a posteroanterior view of the chest, cardiac size is almost the real-life size, but if the radiograph is taken with the x-ray beam oriented in the anteroposterior direction, the size of the heart is artificially enlarged on the film and may be mistaken for a cardiomegaly. The degree of inspiration–expiration can dramatically change the appearance of the cardiothoracic (C/T) ratio, which corresponds to the ratio of the width of the heart to the width of the thoracic cavity (Fig. 46.1). Normal C/T is less than 50%. Cardiothoracic ratio has to be measured at end inspiration (more than six to seven anterior ribs above the diaphragm) to be of value (Fig. 46.1). On expiration, cardiomegaly can be erroneously diagnosed (Fig. 46.2). On the other hand, patients with emphysema often have cardiac enlargement, although heart size appears normal due to pulmonary distention.

Typical Aspect and Physiopathology of Acute Heart Failure

In acute left heart failure, there is a progressive increase in pulmonary venous pressure. The first stage of elevation of venous hypertension, when pulmonary capillary wedge pressure is between 10 and 15 mm Hg, is a uniformization of blood flow with equalization from bases to apices accomplished through capillary distention and recruitment.

For a capillary wedge pressure between 15 and 25 mm Hg, a vascular redistribution of blood flow to the apices is observed and vessels appear larger than basal vessels (Figs. 46.3 and 46.4). Modest elevations in pulmonary venous pressure are accommodated in this manner without the development of pulmonary edema.

At higher filling pressures, fluid begins to cross the microvascular barrier, and edema can develop. The interstitial compartment is first involved and

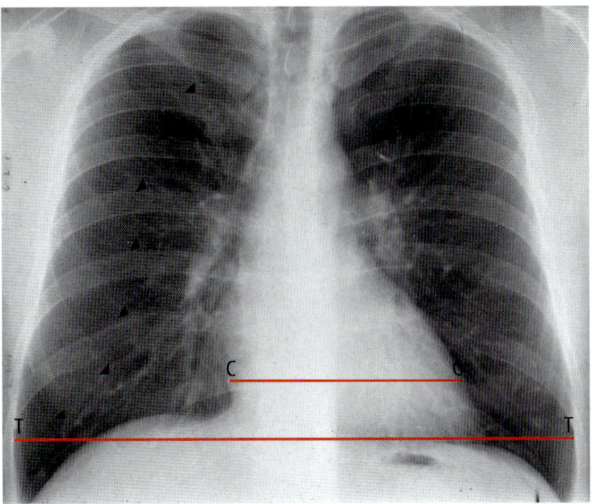

FIGURE 46.1. Posteroanterior chest radiograph taken in the upright position, at end inspiration. Seven anterior ribs are visualized above the diaphragm (black arrowheads). Cardiothoracic (C/T) ratio corresponds to the ratio of the width of the heart to the width of the thoracic cavity.

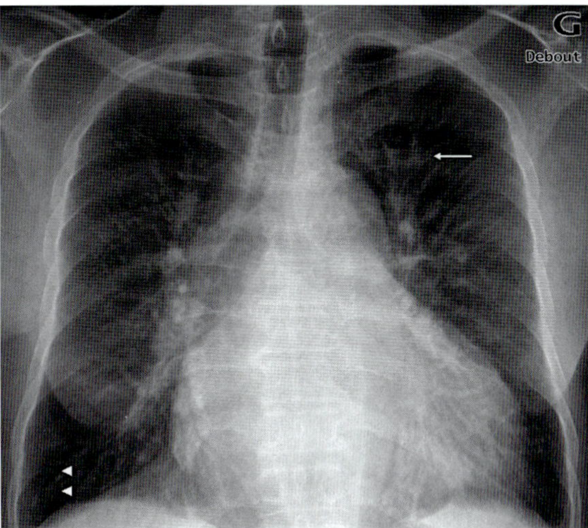

FIGURE 46.3. Posteroanterior chest radiograph taken in the upright position showing cardiomegaly, vascular redistribution (arrow) to the apices, and fairly discrete Kerley B lines (arrowheads).

fluid fills up successively in the interlobular septa and the peribronchovascular spaces, and reaches the hila. The radiologic signs are therefore Kerley lines corresponding to septal thickening (Figs. 46.4 and 46.5), and peribronchovascular and hilar haziness (Fig. 46.6). Kerley lines include Kerley A lines situated at the apices and Kerley B lines located at the bases.

If the pressure raises a value above 35 mm Hg, alveolar pulmonary edema can occur and produces a bilateral alveolar syndrome in a medullary distribution, with sparing of the periphery of the

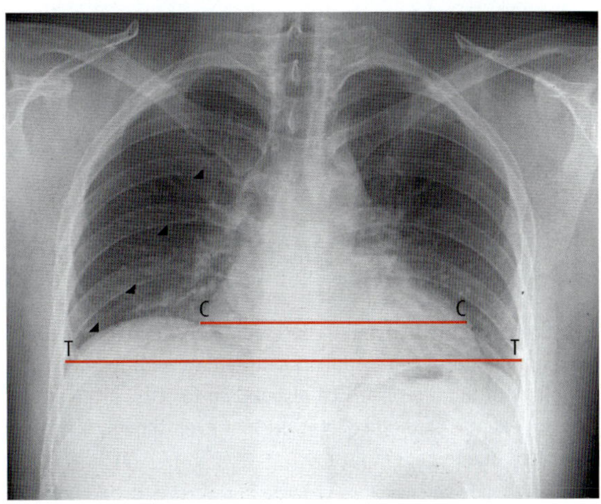

FIGURE 46.2. Same patient as in Figure 46.1 with chest radiograph taken at end expiration. Four anterior ribs are visualized above the diaphragm (black arrowheads). C/T should not be measured in such conditions because it is artificially increased and could erroneously lead to the diagnosis of cardiomegaly.

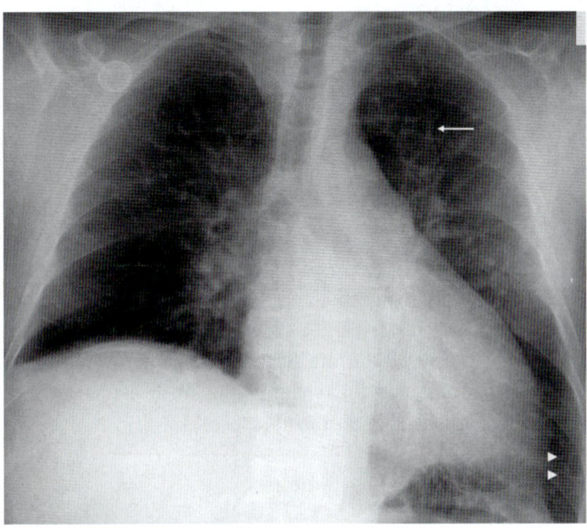

FIGURE 46.4. Posteroanterior chest radiograph in an upright position showing marked cardiomegaly, vascular redistribution (arrow), and Kerley B lines (arrowheads).

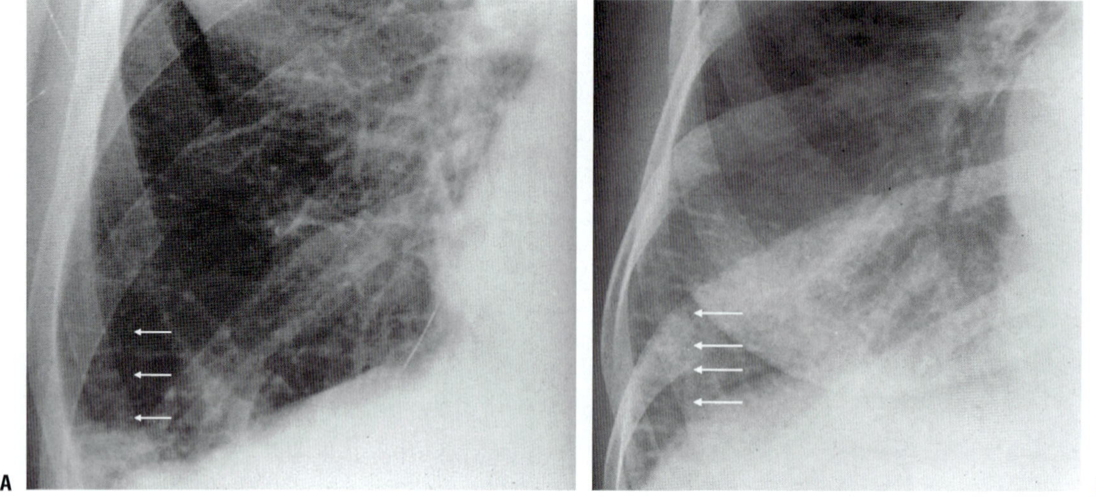

Figure 46.5. (A,B) Zoom on the right base showing marked Kerley B lines (arrows).

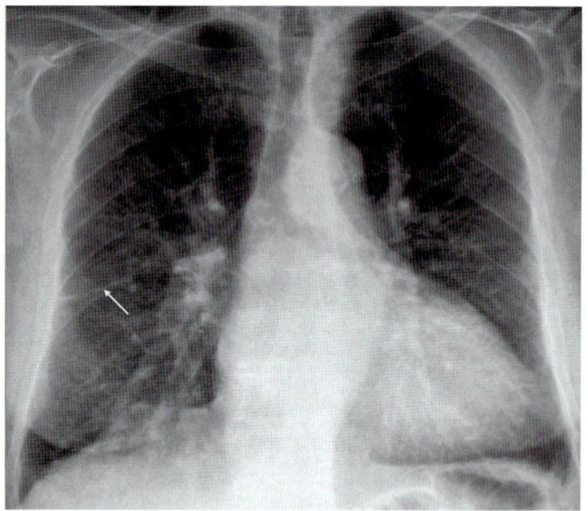

Figure 46.6. Anteroposterior chest radiograph taken in a semi-erect position. Heart size is artificially enlarged, but this patient has cardiomegaly. Kerley B lines are associated to peribronchovascular and hilar haziness and thickening of the small fissure (arrow), corresponding to fluid in the pleural space.

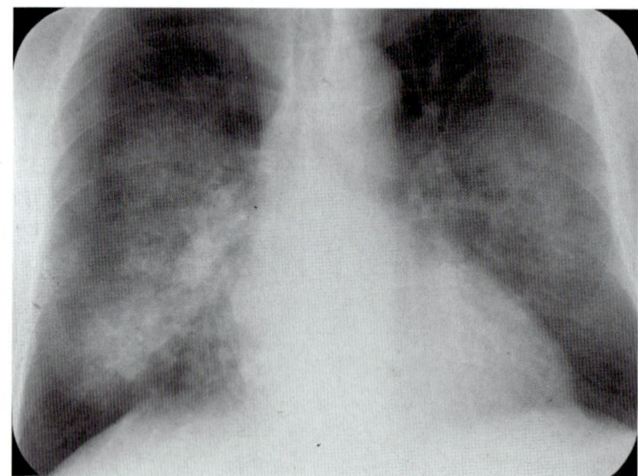

Figure 46.7. Anteroposterior chest radiographs showing bilateral air-space infiltrates in a medullary distribution, with sparing of the periphery of the lung fields corresponding to acute alveolar pulmonary edema. Cardiomegaly is present even though it is overestimated due to patient position.

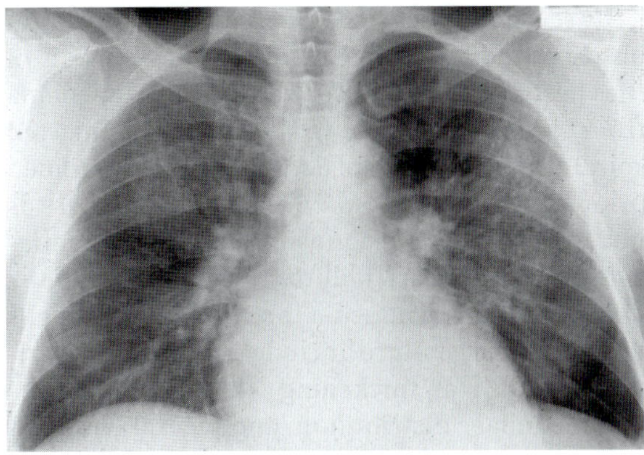

FIGURE 46.8. Same patient as in Figure 46.7. Also notice smoothing of the costophrenic angles due to accumulation of fluid in the pleural space.

lung fields known as "bat's wing" or "butterfly" pattern (Figs. 46.7 and 46.8).

Fluid also collects in the pleural space (Figs. 46.8 and 46.9). Lymphatic vessels that are present in the connective tissue of the interstitial compartment are recruited to increase the clearance of the lung. Diagnosis of left ventricular insufficiency is therefore made on the presence of a cardiomegaly associated with one of the previous signs described above.

Chest Radiograph Limitation

Chest radiography may show some limitations in the diagnosis of pulmonary edema when presentation is atypical.

Alveolar edema is not always uniformly distributed owing to gravity. Lower lobe predominance can be observed when the patient is upright, and posterior distribution is more likely if the patient is supine. When the patient lies on one side, edema favors the dependent side.

Coexisting lung disease may obscure pulmonary edema. For example, emphysema may modify aspects of alveolar pulmonary edema and present as an asymmetric alveolar syndrome (Figs. 46.9 and 46.10) or may be mistaken for an interstitial process (Fig. 46.11). Destruction of the vascular bed in the emphysematous areas of the lung results in the development of edema in more normal areas.

Pulmonary edema may also present differently depending on the course of the disease. Patients with long-standing elevations in pulmonary wedge pressure like severe mitral stenosis undergo remodeling of their alveolocapillary membranes, which protects the lung from pulmonary edema. Chest radiograph may show pleural effusion, but little evidence of pulmonary edema. On the other hand, a previously healthy patient with acute heart failure from acute myocardial infarction or massive volume overload may show dense

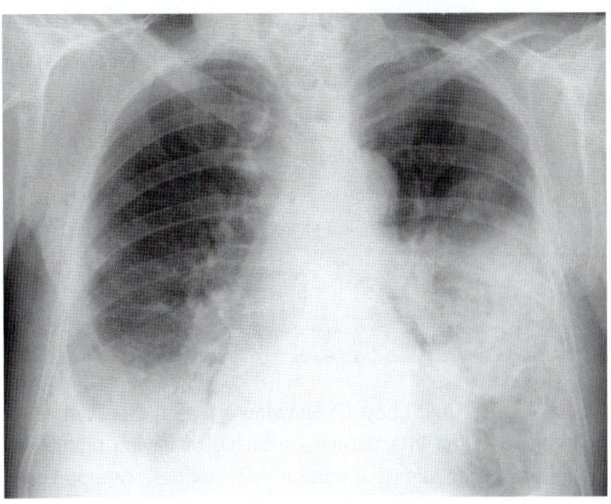

FIGURE 46.9. Chest radiograph showing an asymmetrical airspace infiltrate predominant in the left lung associated with bilateral pleural effusion.

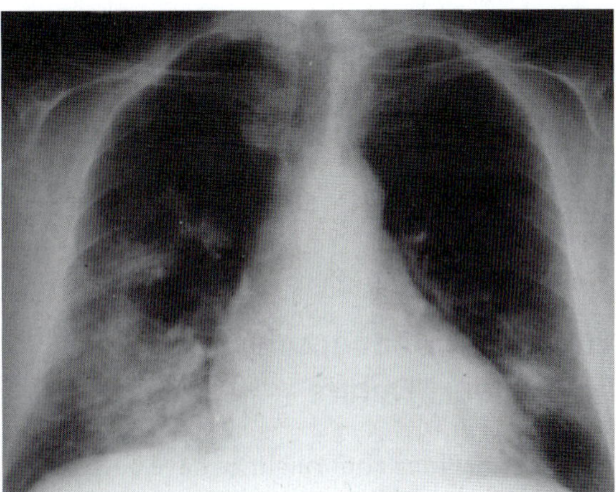

FIGURE 46.10. Chest radiograph showing an asymmetrical, patchy air-space infiltrate predominant on the right.

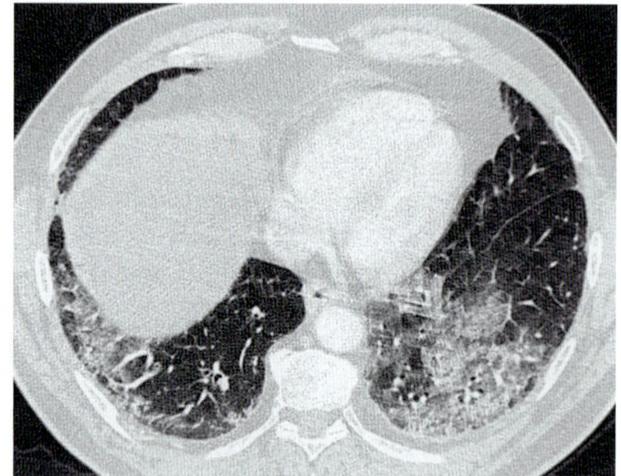

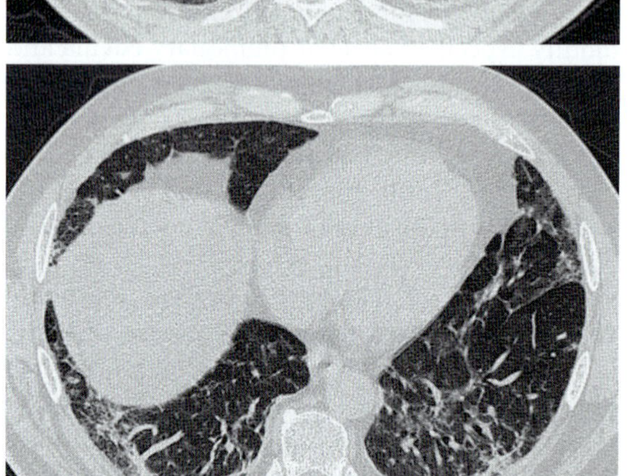

Figure 46.11. (A) Patient with acute alveolar pulmonary edema. (B) Chest computed tomography (CT) shows a fibrosing-like process after a few days of treatment.

alveolar perihilar infiltrates with little pleural effusion.

Cardiomegaly may be absent especially in diastolic heart failure with subnormal ejection fraction (>40%) or in iatrogenic pulmonary edema due to fluid overload. Acute myocardial infarction and acute cardiac arrhythmias can also result in pulmonary edema of cardiac origin with a normal-sized heart.

Computed Tomography in Acute Heart Failure

Parenchymal lung abnormalities have been found on chest computed tomography (CT) in patients with acute left heart failure syndrome.

In selected cases, when diagnosis is uncertain on chest radiograph, high-resolution CT scan of the chest may help differentiate pulmonary edema from parenchymal lung disease. Noninjected spiral CT of the lung fields can also be performed prior to a CT pulmonary angiogram if there is uncertainty about diagnosing pulmonary embolism or acute heart failure, to avoid potentially dangerous contrast media injection. The CT signs of acute heart failure include septal lines, peribronchovascular thickening, air space infiltrates in a medullary distribution, and pleural effusions (Fig. 46.12).

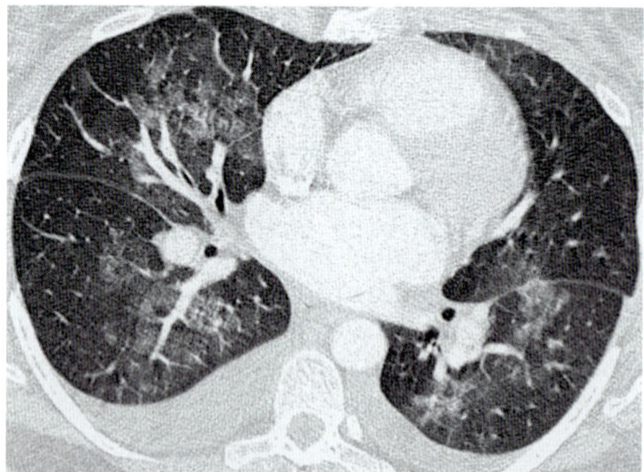

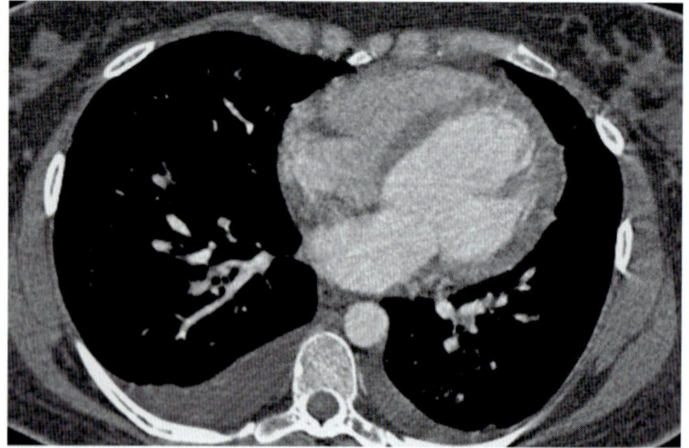

Figure 46.12. (A,B) Chest CT showing a typical aspect of acute pulmonary edema in a patient suspected of having pulmonary embolism. Septal lines, ground-glass opacities, cardiomegaly, and pleural effusions are present. Unfortunately, CT scan was performed with contrast injection, which is not recommended in acute heart failure.

Further Readings

Gehlbach BK, Geppert E. The pulmonary manifestations of left heart failure. Chest 2004, 125:669–682.

Müller ND, Fraser RS, Colman NC, Paré PD. Radiologic Diagnosis of Diseases of the Chest. Philadelphia: WB Saunders, 2001:432–451.

Reed JC. Chest Radiology. Plain Film Patterns and Differential Diagnoses, 4th ed. St. Louis: Mosby, 1996:229–234.

Vasile N, Monnier JP. Cœur et vaisseaux. In: Radiodiagnostic, 5th ed. JP Monnier, JM Tubiana, et al., eds. Paris: Masson, 1996:265–295.

2.3
Treatment of Acute Heart Failure Syndrome: Fluid Management

47 Management of Volume Overload in Acute Heart Failure: Diuretics and Ultrafiltration

Maria Rosa Costanzo

Loop Diuretics

Approximately 1 million hospitalizations, with an estimated cost of $28 billion, occur annually in the United States due to acutely decompensated heart failure[1]. Data from the Acute Decompensated Heart Failure National Registry (ADHERE) show that 90% of hospitalizations for acutely decompensated heart failure are due to fluid overload in patients who have failed treatment with oral diuretics[2]. The average length of stay for acutely decompensated heart failure is 4.3 days, and 42% of the patients are discharged without complete resolution of symptoms. With current treatment strategies, 50% of the patients lose ≤5 lbs from the admission weight and 20% gain weight during the hospitalization[2]. The failure to effectively resolve congestion and reduce weight may contribute to readmission rates, which may be as high as 50% at 6 months[3].

It is not surprising that pulmonary and systemic congestion precipitate heart failure decompensation. The abnormal systolic or diastolic function leads to increased left ventricular diastolic pressure and impaired volume regulation. These may be further aggravated by progressive activation of neurohormonal systems, such as the sympathetic nervous system (SNS), the renin-angiotensin-aldosterone system (RAAS), and vasopressin. The increased blood volume and increased left ventricular diastolic pressure, often aggravated by mitral regurgitation, increase pulmonary capillary wedge pressure, which, in turn, leads to increased pulmonary artery pressure, increased right ventricular and atrial pressures, and tricuspid regurgitation. In addition, depending on the hydrostatic pressure of the pulmonary capillaries, the plasma oncotic pressure, the permeability and integrity of the alveolar-capillary membrane, and the pulmonary lymphatic drainage of the lungs, the increased pulmonary capillary wedge pressure leads to redistribution of the excess fluid in the pulmonary vascular bed, interstitial edema, and alveolar edema. All these processes, together with abnormalities in lung and respiratory muscle function, contribute to the development of dyspnea in heart failure patients. The increased right ventricular and atrial pressures and the resulting tricuspid regurgitation lead to the development of the systemic signs of congestion, such as jugular venous distention, hepatomegaly, and leg edema[4].

Data from the ADHERE Registry shows that 88% of the patients hospitalized for acutely decompensated heart failure are treated with intravenous loop diuretics[2]. Although many patients with chronic heart failure can be successfully treated with orally administered loop diuretics, 25% to 30% of patients develop diuretic resistance, defined as reduced diuresis and natriuresis before resolution of congestion[5]. Causes include neurohormonally mediated sodium retention, functional renal failure, hyponatremia, altered diuretic pharmacokinetics, and increased distal tubular reabsorption of the sodium that escapes from the loop of Henle. In salt-restricted patients fractional excretion of sodium decreases with continued exposure to the loop diuretics, and intermittent diuretic administration causes postdiuretic sodium retention[5]. Therapies to ameliorate diuretic resistance, including fluid and sodium restriction, increase in angiotensin-converting enzyme inhibitors doses, use of diuretic combinations, and changes in the timing and route of diuretic administration, have limited success[5]. Finally, hospital stay may be inappropriately prolonged when aggressive use of intravenous diuretics leads to worsening renal function[6].

Renal insufficiency and diuretic resistance worsen the outcomes of heart failure patients[6,7]. In 1153 heart failure patients enrolled in the Prospective, Randomized Amlodipine Survival Evaluation (PRAISE), high diuretic doses independently increased mortality, sudden death, and pump failure, associating diuretic resistance with a poor prognosis in heart failure patients[7]. Recently, the safety of diuretics in heart failure patients with acutely decompensated heart failure has been questioned[6]. Intravenous diuretic use can decrease cardiac output, increase pulmonary capillary wedge pressure and total systemic vascular resistance, and reduce renal blood flow and glomerular filtration rate[8,9]. An increase of serum creatinine of >0.3 mg/dL, which occurs in nearly one third of acutely decompensated heart failure patients, is associated with poorer prognosis and longer hospitalization[6]. Mechanical fluid removal may be a promising alternative for the treatment of congestion. Ultrafiltration of isotonic plasma water from peripheral veins using a rate-controlled peristaltic pump and filter is an alternative treatment for decompensated heart failure and volume overload[10].

Loop Diuretics in Acutely Decompensated Heart Failure

Mechanism of Action

The entry of filtered sodium chloride (NaCl) into the cells of the thick ascending limb of the loop of Henle is mediated by a neutral Na-K-2Cl cotransporter in the apical (luminal) membrane; the energy for this process is provided by the favorable inward electromechanical gradient for Na (low cell Na concentration and electronegative cell interior). Reabsorbed Na is pumped out of the cell by the Na-K–adenosine triphosphatase (ATPase) pump in the basolateral (peritubular) membrane. Although K plays an important role in this process, the concentration of K in the filtrate and tubular fluid is much less than that of Na and Cl; thus K must recycle back to the lumen through K channels in the apical membrane to allow continued NaCl reabsorption. This movement of cationic K into the lumen plus the movement of reabsorbed Cl (via a Cl channel) out of the cell into the peritubular capillary generates a net positive current from the capillary to the lumen. The ensuing electropositivity creates an electrical gradient that promotes passive reabsorption of Na cations, and, to a lesser degree, calcium (Ca) and magnesium (Mg) via the paracellular pathway between the cells. The loop diuretics inhibit Na, K, and Cl (as well as Ca and Mg) reabsorption by competing for the Cl site on this transporter[11] (Fig. 47.1).

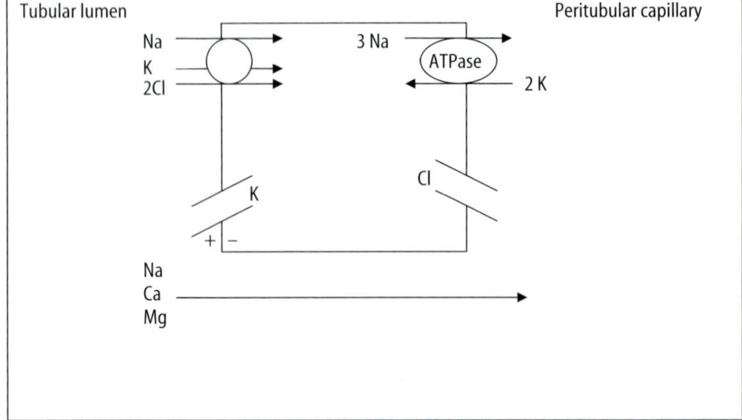

FIGURE 47.1. Ion transport in the loop of Henle. The loop diuretics inhibit Na, K, Cl, Ca, and Mg reabsorption by competing for the Cl site on the transporter. ATPase, adenosine triphosphatase.

Pharmacokinetics

All loop diuretics reach the luminal transport sites through the tubular fluid and are actively secreted into the urine by the cells of the proximal tubule. A high degree of binding to serum proteins (>95%) keeps the diuretic into the vascular space so that it can be delivered to the secretory sites of proximal tubular cells. Loop diuretics are secreted through the organic-acid pathway[12]. Approximately 50% of a furosemide dose is excreted unchanged into the urine, while the remaining 50% is conjugated to glucuronic acid in the kidneys[13]. In patients with renal insufficiency, the plasma half-life of furosemide is prolonged because both urinary excretion and renal conjugation are decreased[13]. In contrast, the half-lives of bumetanide and torsemide are not prolonged in patients with renal insufficiency because these two drugs are largely metabolized by the liver (50% and 80%, respectively); however with renal disease the delivery of bumetanide and torsemide to the tubular fluid is impaired[14,15] (Table 47.1). Ethacrynic acid is used only in patients allergic to other loop diuretics because of its greater ototoxicity[13].

Plasma half-life determines the frequency of intravenous administration of loop diuretics. Plasma half-life is shortest for bumetanide (≈1 hour), intermediate for furosemide (≈1.5 to 2 hours), and longest for torsemide (3 to 4 hours). Once a dose of a loop diuretic has been administered, its effect dissipates before the next dose is given. During this time, the nephron avidly reabsorbs sodium, resulting in rebound sodium retention, which may negate the prior natriuresis[16].

Pharmacodynamics

The pharmacodynamics of loop diuretics are determined by the relation between the arrival of the drug at its site of action, which depends on urinary excretion rate, and the natriuretic response[17] (Fig. 47.2). This relation is similar for all loop diuretics, although the curve may be shifted to the right or the left[17]. Thus in any given patient, the maximal response to each loop diuretic is the same. However, because a threshold quantity of drug must reach the site of action to elicit a response, the diuretic must be titrated in each patient to identify the effective dose. In addition, the lowest diuretic dose that elicits a maximal response should not be exceeded. In normal subjects, a 40-mg intravenous furosemide dose or an equivalent dose of other loop diuretics produces a maximal response, which is the excretion of 200 to 250 mmol of Na in 3 to 4 L of urine over a period of 3 to 4 hours.

Intravenous Loop Diuretics in Patients with Congestive Heart Failure and Normal Renal Function

Large doses of intravenous loop diuretics are unnecessary in patients without significant renal dysfunction because drug delivery to the tubular fluid is normal[18]. However, renal responsiveness to loop diuretics may be decreased[19]. As compared with normal subjects, patients with New York Heart Association (NYHA) class II or III heart failure have one fourth to one third the natriuretic response to maximally effective doses of loop diuretics, and the response is even smaller in patients with more severe heart failure[19]. Therefore, natriuresis is enhanced more by increasing the frequency rather than the amount of diuretic doses. Although sometimes helpful in improving diuresis and natriuresis, the addition of a thiazide diuretic may be associated with excessive volume and electrolyte depletion[17]. In addition, substantial kaliuresis usually occurs with sequential blockade of nephron sites at which potassium is normally reabsorbed. In some patients, the

Table 47.1. Pharmacokinetics of loop diuretics

		Elimination alf-life hours)		
Loop diuretic	Oral bioavailability (%)	Normal subjects	Patients with renal insufficiency	Patients with heart failure
Furosemide	10–100	1.5–2	2.8	2.7
Bumetanide	80–100	1	1.6	1.3
Torsemide	80–100	3–4	4–5	6

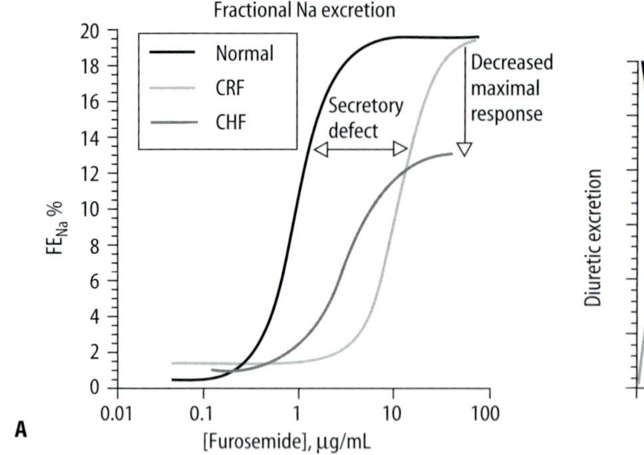

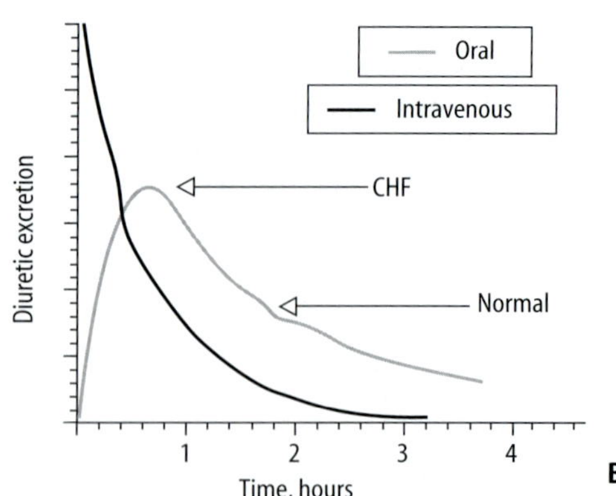

FIGURE 47.2. Dose-response curves for loop diuretics. (A) Fractional Na excretion (FE$_{Na}$) as a function of loop diuretics concentration. Compared with normal subjects, patients with chronic renal failure (CRF) show a rightward shift in the curve, due to impaired diuretic secretion. The maximal response is preserved when expressed as FE$_{Na}$ but not when expressed as absolute Na secretion. Patients with congestive heart failure (CHF) demonstrate a rightward and downward shift, even when the dose response is expressed as FE$_{Na}$, and thus are relatively diuretic resistant. (B) Comparison of the response to intravenous and oral doses of loop diuretics. In a normal individual, an oral dose may be as effective as an intravenous dose because the time above the natriuretic threshold (indicated by the "Normal" line) is approximately equal. If the natriuretic threshold increases (indicated by the "CHF" line), then the oral dose may not provide a high enough serum level to elicit natriuresis. (From Ellison [5], with permission.)

addition of a potassium-sparing diuretic that acts at distal nephron sites, may slightly increase sodium excretion. However, if urinary sodium and potassium concentrations are both low, a distal diuretic will be ineffective because an insufficient amount of sodium is delivered to the distal nephron. If the urinary sodium concentration is low and the urinary potassium concentration is high, sodium is being exchanged for potassium distally, and the addition of a diuretic that acts on distal tubules will increase natriuresis[17].

Intravenous Loop Diuretics in Patients with Congestive Heart Failure and Decreased Renal Function

The hemodynamic abnormalities and neurohormonal activation occurring in heart failure patients lead to progressive deterioration of renal function. Therefore, it is not surprising that in a significant proportion of patients heart failure and renal insufficiency coexist. The ADHERE Registry documents that 30% of patients hospitalized with acutely decompensated heart failure have significant renal dysfunction[2], defined as an admission serum creatinine ≥2 mg/dL. As renal function decreases, so does the secretion of a loop diuretic into the tubular fluid. In patients with a creatinine clearance of 15 mL/min, the amount of loop diuretic secreted into the tubular fluid is five to ten times smaller than in normal subjects[13]. Thus, a large dose must be given to attain an effective amount of diuretic in the tubular fluid.

The relation between the rate at which the diuretic is excreted and the response to it is similar in patients with and without renal insufficiency[20]. Because in patients with renal insufficiency the remaining nephrons retain diuretic responsiveness, the challenge is to deliver enough drug to the site of action to elicit a response. The maximal natriuretic response occurs with intravenous bolus doses of 160 to 200 mg of furosemide or the equivalent doses of bumetanide and torsemide, and no additional gain results from larger doses[20]. Some patients may require these large doses several times a day. The maximal achievable response is the excretion of about 20% of filtered Na. In a patient with a creatinine clearance of 15 mL/min, approximately 25 mmol of Na will be excreted. If the patient ingests 75 mmol of Na per

TABLE 47.2. Maximal intravenous doses of loop diuretics in patients with diminished responses to oral therapy

Maximal intravenous dose (mg)	Moderate renal insufficiency	Severe renal insufficiency	Heart failure
Furosemide	80–160	160–200	40–80
Bumetanide	4–8	8–10	1–2
Torsemide	20–50	50–100	10–20

day, then the single dose causing 25 mmol to be excreted must be administered three times per day, and Na will be retained if the intake is higher. The transient tinnitus occasionally caused by a single intravenous bolus dose of 160 to 200 mg of furosemide can be minimized by administering the dose over a period of 20 to 30 minutes[21].

Because the bioavailability of loop diuretics is the same in patients with and without renal insufficiency, the intravenous and oral doses of bumetanide and torsemide are similar[17]. For furosemide, the usual maximal intravenous dose is one half of the oral dose (80 to 160 mg in patients with moderate renal insufficiency and 160 to 200 mg in those with severe renal insufficiency) (Table 47.2).

In patients who have poor responses to intermittent doses of a loop diuretic, a continuous intravenous infusion can be tried. If an effective amount of the diuretic is maintained at the site of action over time, a small but clinically important increase in the response may occur[17]. Depending on the diuretic used, 6 to 20 hours are required to achieve a steady state with continuous infusion, so a loading dose of the loop diuretic is recommended before initiation of continuous infusion to achieve therapeutic drug concentrations sooner. The rate of the continuous infusion is guided by the patient's renal function. If after 1 hour the response is inadequate, the loading dose should be repeated before increasing the infusion rate (Table 47.3). The differential effects of loop diuretics given by bolus injections or continuous infusions are discussed in detail later in this chapter.

Cardiovascular Effects

Decreased pulmonary edema by intravenous diuretics can improve oxygenation. Reduction of pulmonary pressures decreases the sensation of dyspnea, the symptom that most commonly causes hospitalization of heart failure patients. Acute vasodilation mediated by prostaglandin E_2 (PGE_2) may explain the increase in venous capacitance observed within 5 minutes of intravenous furosemide administration[22]. The improvement in cardiac index and other load-dependent indices of cardiac performance occurring after diuresis may be due to decreased afterload, as suggested by the finding that increases in stroke volume following diuresis correlate with drops in systemic vascular resistance, but not with decreases in preload[23]. Diuretic-induced volume reduction may also increase cardiac output by reducing mitral regurgitation. Reduced wall stress resulting from reduced left ventricular size may be beneficial. Lower filling pressures may also reduce myocardial ischemia[23]. Cardiac output may also be enhanced by the inotropic effect of diuretic-induced neurohormonal activation. However, excessive reduction of left ventricular filling pressures by diuretics can excessively reduce cardiac output, particularly in patients with advanced heart failure[23].

Neurohormonal Effects

In patients with congestive heart failure, increased angiotensin II (AII) concentration and plasma rennin activity (PRA) often reflect the intensity of

TABLE 47.3. Doses for continuous intravenous infusion of loop diuretics

Diuretic	Intravenous loading dose (mg)	Infusion rate (mg/hour)		
		Creatinine clearance <25 mL/min	Creatinine clearance 25–75 mL/min	Creatinine clearance >75 mL/min
Furosemide	40	20, then 40	10, then 20	10
Bumetanide	1	1, then 2	0.5, then 1	0.5
Torsemide	20	10, then 20	5, then 10	5

diuretic treatment. Renin release may be caused by volume contraction and stimulation of baroreceptors and the macula densa. Indeed, many studies have documented increased PRA and plasma concentration of AII after administration of loop diuretics[8,24]. The effects of loop diuretics on aldosterone are highly variable. In one study, aldosterone concentrations decreased with initial diuretic treatment and symptomatic improvement but rose as weight and therefore sodium delivery to the renal tubule decreased[25]. It is difficult to determine the risk/benefit ratio of RAAS activation by diuretics. It is unknown whether preservation of renal function by RAAS stimulation outweighs the deleterious clinical and hemodynamics consequences of neurohormonal activation. In a porcine heart failure model, intravenous furosemide shortened time to left ventricular dysfunction and elevated serum aldosterone levels independent of cardiac preload[26]. In addition, aldosterone stimulates collagen production[27]. Diuretic-induced AII stimulation may be responsible for the increased concentration of antidiuretic hormone (ADH) observed after acute diuresis. To date clinically important effects of loop diuretics on the production of natriuretic peptides have not been documented.

The stimulation by loop diuretics of renal PGE_2 production may be responsible for the symptomatic improvement observed after administration of diuretics before any increase in urine output. In addition, renal prostaglandins may help maintain renal blood flow compromised by diuretic-induced neurohormonal activation[28].

In contrast to RAAS activation, catecholamine concentrations frequently decrease as symptoms improve with diuresis[24].

Metabolic Effects

Diuretic-induced volume contraction leads to avid Na and bicarbonate reabsorption and metabolic alkalosis. Gout can result from inhibition of renal uric acid excretion by loop diuretics. Excretion of K in the distal tubule, metabolic alkalosis, decreased Na intake, and neurohormonal activation all contribute to the hypokalemia that can occur with diuretic therapy[29]. Hypokalemia has known arrhythmogenic effects[30]. The rate of change in serum K may influence cardiac rhythm more than the degree of hypokalemia[31]. Therefore, the hypokalemia produced by intravenously administered diuresis may be more arrhythmogenic than that observed with chronic diuretic use. The mechanisms and rates of diuretic-induced hypomagnesemia are uncertain. However, hypomagnesemia may exacerbate the development of hypokalemia and indirectly cause arrhythmias. Magnesium administration should be considered in the settings of intractable ventricular arrhythmias or refractory hypokalemia coexisting with hypomagnesemia[32]. Although rare, acute hyponatremia can be dangerous. When secondary to overdiuresis, it is easily corrected with modification of the diuretic regimen and without administration of Na. A syndrome of inappropriate antidiuretic hormone (ADH) secretion should be considered when severe hyponatremia is refractory to modification of diuretic therapy[33].

Loop diuretics increase Ca excretion[33]. Because low serum Ca concentration may not adequately reflect ionized Ca or intracellular Ca concentration, it is difficult to determine the significance of altered Ca excretion. At present it is unclear if the effects of loop diuretics on Ca excretion alter myocardial function.

Renal Effects

Intravenous loop diuretics have both direct and indirect effects on renal function. If intravascular Na and volume depletion is sufficiently severe, the physiologic mechanisms aimed at maintaining blood pressure will cause decreased glomerular filtration rate and, at times, cause frank renal failure[8,9,24]. Neurohormonal activation is the most likely culprit of renal dysfunction caused by diuretic-induced volume contraction. On the other hand, plasma volume may actually increase when diuretics enhance venous capacitance, decrease capillary hydrostatic pressure, and augment colloid pressure[34]. Renal artery vasodilation due to increased PGE_2 may explain the acute increase in renal plasma flow and glomerular filtration observed after intravenous administration of furosemide and ethacrynic acid[35].

Clinical Implications of the Effects of Intravenous Loop Diuretics in Acutely Decompensated Heart Failure

In symptomatic heart failure patients there is little question about diuretics' efficacy in decreasing pulmonary congestion and dyspnea and in improving cardiovascular hemodynamics[36]. Intravenous loop diuretics reduce pulmonary capillary wedge pressure and increase venous capacitance within a few minutes, before any discernible increase in urinary output[22]. This rapid hemodynamic improvement is likely due to the release of vasodilatory prostaglandins, since it does not occur when the renal release of prostaglandins is suppressed or when the release of vasopressor hormones attenuates loop diuretic-mediated release of PGE_2[28]. The hypoxia, hypercapnia, and metabolic acidosis occurring with severe pulmonary edema can depress myocardial function[37]. By correcting these acid-base disorders, treatment with diuretics may improve not only pulmonary symptoms, but also cardiac function. On the other hand, the use of diuretics in some patients with acutely decompensated heart failure may lead to deterioration of renal function.

Thus, the question emerges whether these patients should be maintained in a volume overloaded state that, by maximizing cardiac index, will result in preserved renal function. In clinical practice, intravenous loop diuretics are often stopped before achievement of euvolemia in patients whose blood urea nitrogen and serum creatinine levels increase during treatment. Recent observations, however, suggest that hypervolemia per se contributes to the progression of cardiac and renal dysfunction[37]. In fact, in some patients with acutely decompensated heart failure presenting with increased blood urea nitrogen and serum creatinine levels, renal function improves after diuretic-induced weight loss. On the other hand, the use of large doses of loop diuretics may have deleterious effects on cardiac function because of diuretic-induced K and Mg losses[33].

When weighing the benefits and risks of diuretic therapy in patients with acutely decompensated heart failure, it is important to keep in mind that loop diuretics block NaCl transport at the macula densa and thus activate the RAAS, which plays a critical role in the progression of heart failure[38]. Perhaps the lowest level of neurohormonal activation is the best indicator of optimal volume status, since catecholamines and aldosterone concentration decrease as symptoms improve after the onset of diuresis, but increase as dry weight is approached. Assessment of total body fluid, as manifested by peripheral edema, ascites, and sacral edema, indicates the need for additional diuresis. Often hospitalized patients are discharged after elimination of pulmonary edema, but before resolution of total body fluid overload[2]. This inadequate diuresis may contribute to high rehospitalization rates[3].

Patients hospitalized with severe volume overload can typically lose 1 kg/day with only mild deterioration of renal function, which will normalize when weight stabilizes due to resolution of intravascular depletion. However, significant increases in serum creatinine concentrations and decreases in glomerular filtration rates can occur with diuretics and can have serious consequences. It is controversial whether decreased renal function in patients with acutely decompensated heart failure is a reflection of the rate or of the extent of diuresis. Among 382 patients hospitalized with decompensated heart failure, those who developed worsening renal function, defined as an increase in serum creatinine level >3 mg/dL, had received higher intravenous loop diuretic doses than those without significant renal function changes (199 ± 195 mg versus 143 ± 119 mg of loop diuretic; $p < .05$). Interestingly there were no differences in weight or fluid loss between patients with and without worsening renal function[6]. These findings suggest that the effects of intravenous loop diuretics on renal function in patients with acutely decompensated heart failure may be influenced by the degree of underlying renal dysfunction and diuretic resistance.

If significant increases in serum creatinine and decreases in glomerular filtration rates occur, the rate of diuresis should be slowed. To prevent renal failure complicating therapy with angiotensin-converting enzyme inhibitors or angiotensin receptor blockers in Na and volume-depleted patients, initiation or up-titration of these drugs should be delayed until euvolemia is achieved[39].

Hypokalemia can be prevented even during aggressive diuresis by frequent measurements of serum K concentration and appropriate K replacement.

Comparison of Continuous Infusion Versus Bolus Injection of Loop Diuretics in Acutely Decompensated Heart Failure

Loop diuretics, when given as intermittent bolus injections in patients with acutely decompensated heart failure, may be associated with fluctuations in intravascular volume, increased toxicity, and development of tolerance. Continuous intravenous infusion of loop diuretics may avoid these complications and result in greater diuresis, faster symptom resolution, and decreased morbidity and possibly mortality. The differential effects of these two treatment modalities were recently evaluated in a meta-analysis of eight randomized controlled trials comparing the efficacy of continuous intravenous infusion versus bolus intravenous administration of loop diuretics in a total of 254 patients with acutely decompensated heart failure[40]. In seven studies that reported urine output, fluid loss (measured in cc/24 hours) was greater in patients given continuous infusion, with a weighted mean difference (WMD) of 271 cc/24 hour (95% confidence interval [CI], 93.1 to 449; $p < .01$)[41–47]. Clinically relevant serum electrolyte disturbances (hypokalemia and hypomagnesemia), as reported in three studies, were not significantly different in the two treatment groups with a relative risk (RR) of 1.47 (95% CI, 0.52 to 4.15; $p = .5$)[45,47,48], although higher serum creatinine levels were noted in the bolus injection group, WMD −0.54 (95% CI, 0.57 to −0.51; $p < .01$)[43,46,48]. Less adverse effects (tinnitus and hearing loss) were noted when continuous infusion was used: RR 0.06 (95% CI, 0.01 to 0.44; $p = .005$)[43,46–48]. Based on a single study, the duration of hospital stay was shortened by 3.1 days with continuous infusion, WMD −3.1 (95% CI, −4.1 to −2; $p < .01$)[46]. All cause-mortality, evaluated in two studies, was significantly reduced in the infusion group with an RR of 0.52 (95% CI, 0.38 to 0.71; $p < .01$)[46,48]. Cardiac mortality, reported in a single study, was also significantly lower in the infusion group with an RR 0.47 (95% CI, 0.33 to 0.69; $p < .0001$)[46]. Thus based on small and relatively heterogeneous studies, the meta-analysis showed greater diuresis and a better safety profile when loop diuretics were given as continuous infusion. The authors of the meta-analysis conclude that existing data do not allow definitive recommendations for clinical practice, and larger studies should be done to more adequately settle this issue.

Ultrafiltration

The Process

The process of ultrafiltration consists of the production of plasma water from whole blood across a semipermeable membrane (hemofilter) in response to a transmembrane pressure gradient[10]. The pressure gradient across ultrafiltration membranes is generated by the classic Starling forces, which include the hydrostatic pressures in the blood and in the filtrate compartments, and the oncotic pressure generated by plasma proteins. Hydrostatic pressure is determined by the blood pressure in the filtering device, generated by either the patient's endogenous blood pressure or an extracorporeal pump plus the siphoning effect of suction occurring in the ultrafiltrate compartment[10]. With isolated ultrafiltration, the solute is passively removed by accompanying the solvent flow (convective transport)[49]. In convective transport, the sodium concentration in the ultrafiltrate is essentially equal to the solute concentration in the water component of the plasma on the blood side of the membrane[49]. The process of ultrafiltration is performed on blood extracted from the patient after cannulation of an artery or vein. The blood is then returned to the patient via separate access to the venous circulation[10]. Based on frequency and duration, ultrafiltration techniques can be classified as isolated, intermittent, or continuous. With appropriate ultrafiltration rates, the extracellular fluid gradually refills the intravascular space and blood volume is maintained. If the ultrafiltration rate is too high, blood volume may decrease, because intravascular volume depletion exceeds reabsorption of fluid from the interstitium into the vascular space. Therefore, the three key factors for the removal of an adequate amount of fluid without hemodynamic compromise are accurate determination of the amount of fluid to be removed, optimization of fluid removal rate, and maintenance of circulating blood volume[50].

To understand the differential effects of diuretics and ultrafiltration on hemodynamic and neurohormonal abnormalities occurring in heart failure, it is critical to recognize the distinctive characteristics of fluid removal with these therapies. The fluid removed with diuretics has a sodium concentration lower than that of the plasma. In contrast, the ultrafiltrate is essentially isoosmotic and isonatremic compared with plasma. Therefore, for any amount of fluid withdrawn, more sodium is removed with ultrafiltration than with diuretics[10].

With diuretics, intravascular volume contraction is prolonged, and inhibition of NaCl uptake in the macula densa enhances renal secretion of renin[10]. These effects augment neurohormonal activation, which in turn promotes sodium and water retention, ultimately reducing the diuretics' ability to relieve the signs and symptoms of circulatory congestion[4].

In contrast, ultrafiltration does not stimulate macula densa-mediated neurohormonal activation, nor does it produce prolonged intravascular volume contraction because ultrafiltration removes fluid from the blood at the same rate at which fluid is reabsorbed from the edematous interstitium[51]. Thus, the basis for maintenance of cardiovascular stability during ultrafiltration relates to many factors, including minimal osmolar shifts, appropriate neurohormonal sympathetic responses, and rapid redistribution of volume.

Rationale for the Use of Ultrafiltration in Heart Failure

Due to the characteristics described above, ultrafiltration techniques appear ideally suited to interrupt the vicious circle of volume overload, neurohormonal activation, and worsening renal dysfunction occurring in heart failure[52]. Ultrafiltration has been consistently shown to improve the symptoms of congestion, lower right atrial and pulmonary arterial wedge pressures, improve cardiac output, decrease neurohormone levels, correct hyponatremia, restore diuresis, and reduce diuretics requirements[53].

Sixteen heart failure patients were randomly allocated to receive either a single ultrafiltration treatment ($n = 8$) or intravenous furosemide ($n = 8$, mean furosemide dose = 248 mg) to remove approximately the same amount of fluid (↔ 0111600 mL)[54]. Soon after fluid withdrawal by either method, biventricular filling pressures and body weight were reduced, and plasma renin, norepinephrine, and aldosterone levels were increased. After furosemide, neurohormones levels remained elevated for the next 4 days, and during this period patients had positive water balance, recurrent elevation of filling pressures, and lung congestion without improvement of VO_{2max}. In contrast, after ultrafiltration, neurohormones levels fell below baseline within 48 hours, whereas water metabolism was equilibrated at a new set point (less fluid intake and diuresis without weight gain). Favorable circulatory and neurohormonal changes were correlated with lung water reabsorption, which was increased only in ultrafiltration-treated patients. Improvement was sustained at 3 months after ultrafiltration[54].

Thus while ultrafiltration and furosemide are equally effective in terms of acute volume of fluid removed and resolution of congestive symptoms, their long-term effects are significantly different. Specifically, the effects of ultrafiltration on pulmonary water metabolism and neurohormone levels are due to mechanisms not occurring with diuretics. The fluid removed by ultrafiltration has different sodium content compared to the fluid removed with diuretics. Indeed, ultrafiltration removes fluid with a sodium concentration similar to that of plasma, so that approximately 150 mmol of sodium are withdrawn with each liter of ultrafiltrate. In contrast, the urine of heart failure patients is hypotonic compared with plasma, and the 50 mmol of sodium usually present in 1 L of urine increases to only 100 mmol with furosemide administration[55]. It is possible that the different amounts of sodium removed with similar amounts of fluid account for the differential effects of ultrafiltration and diuretics on neurohormonal responses, which in turn result in different renal sodium and water reabsorption.

Among 32 NYHA class II to IV heart failure patients with varying degrees of hypervolemia, the baseline 24-hour diuresis and natriuresis were inversely correlated with neurohormones levels and renal perfusion pressure (mean aortic pressure—mean arterial pressure)[56]. The response to ultrafiltration ranged from neurohormonal activation and reduction of diuresis in patients with the mildest hypovolemia and urine output >1000 mL per 24 hours, to neurohormonal inhibition and potentiation of diuresis and natriuresis in those with the most severe volume overload and urine output <1000 mL per 24 hours[56]. In the majority of cases, the decrease in norepinephrine level was proportional to the potentiation of diuresis. This finding suggests that subtraction of total body water uncovers enough cardiac reserve to increase cardiac output and attenuate neurohormonal activation. These benefits are then maintained because the resulting enhancement of diuresis leads to improved norepinephrine clearance from the circulation[57]. The earliest effect of ultrafiltration may be the reduction of the extravascular pulmonary fluid, with a subsequent decrease in pulmonary extravascular resistance, improvement of ventilation and gas exchange, and a decrease in hypoxia-induced vasoconstriction.

Ultrafiltration itself via baroreceptor-mediated reflexes may reset neurohormonal activation, which in turn may explain the intermediate- and long-term benefits observed after ultrafiltration[57].

The removal of myocardial depressant factors has also been invoked as an explanation for the clinical benefits associated with ultrafiltration[58]. In 36 patients with acutely decompensated heart failure, ultrafiltration was associated with an increased cardiac index and oxygenation status, decreased pulmonary artery pressure and vascular resistance, as well as reduced requirement for inotropic support[59]. It is not known if the clinical benefits of ultrafiltration translate into improved survival.

In the setting of decompensated heart failure ultrafiltration has been used predominantly after diuretics have failed or in the presence of acute renal failure. Earlier utilization of ultrafiltration can expedite and maintain compensation of acute heart failure by simultaneously reducing volume overload without causing intravascular volume depletion and reestablishing acid–base and electrolyte balance.

However, overly aggressive ultrafiltration in patients with decompensated heart failure can convert nonoliguric renal dysfunction into oliguric renal failure by increasing neurohormonal activation and decreasing renal perfusion pressure, with minimal opportunity of recovery of renal function.

Continuous Ultrafiltration Techniques

The continuous ultrafiltration techniques include continuous hemofiltration in the arteriovenous (CAVH) or venovenous mode (CVVH) and slow continuous ultrafiltration (SCUF) in arteriovenous or venovenous modes[60].

Using a large-bore catheter inserted into the femoral artery and the patients' own blood pressure, arterial blood is delivered to a hemofilter. Systemic blood pressure provides the driving force to achieve sufficient blood flow. When hydrostatic pressure exceeds oncotic pressure, ultrafiltrate is generated. Ultrafiltrate drains by gravity through tubing into a collection bag, creating mild negative pressure in the blood chamber of the filter, favoring further ultrafiltration[61].

With SCUF, replacement volumes are much lower than with CAVH. The most recent advance in this area has been the reintroduction of extracorporeal blood pumps[62,63].

Because the blood flow provided by the pump eliminates the need for an arteriovenous pressure gradient, the technique does not require arterial cannulation and can be performed with venovenous vascular access (CVVH). Until the introduction of simplified intermittent *peripheral* venovenous ultrafiltration techniques, CVVH and SCUF were the recommended therapies for the more critically ill, hypotensive patients with congestive heart failure[62,63].

Because CVVH requires an extracorporeal blood pump, air embolism and blood loss can occur. In contrast with SCUF, air embolism is uncommon and blood loss is self-limited. On the other hand, extracorporeal blood pumps, by producing a constant blood flow, can provide ultrafiltration rates not achievable with SCUF.

All continuous therapies require anticoagulation. Volume depletion can be avoided by careful clinical management. Published reports suggest that complication rates are acceptable[64–66].

With SCUF, ultrafiltration rate can vary from 0 to 20 mL per minute with a practical goal of about 5 mL per minute. The clinical urgency will dictate the ultrafiltration rate, which can be easily adjusted. For CVVH, an ultrafiltration rate of 40 mL per minute can be achieved. In the absence of an extracorporeal blood pump, the vascular access must guarantee an adequate arteriovenous gradient. Thus, catheters must transmit the arterial pressure to the filter with minimal pressure loss due to the resistance within the access itself. The placement of large-bore percutaneous catheters requires specific technical skills. In CVVH, the extracorporeal blood pump produces flow rates of 100 to 150 mL per minute. The venovenous double-lumen catheters can be placed in the internal jugular, subclavian, or femoral veins. The extracorporeal blood pump system includes a roller pump, arterial pressure sensor, air detector, and venous pressure alarms. Use of this equipment requires trained hemodialysis personnel. The ultrafiltration rate can be controlled directly by a pump on the ultrafiltration line or indirectly by altering blood flow. Alternatively, venous pressure can be raised by placing a screw clamp on the venous bloodline, or negative pressure can be applied by suction to the ultrafiltrate compartment.

Intermittent Isolated Ultrafiltration with Central Venovenous Access

With intermittent isolated ultrafiltration the blood is pumped through a filter by an extracorporeal blood pump aided either by suction applied to the ultrafiltrate compartment (negative pressure) or from resistance induced in the venous line (positive pressure). Because of the extracorporeal blood pump, a dual lumen venovenous catheter will generate a blood flow of 500 to 1000 mL per hour. Hemodynamic tolerance is the limiting factor of ultrafiltration rate[67].

Slower ultrafiltration rates over longer periods of time improve hemodynamic tolerance. Intermittent isolated ultrafiltration is effective in removing salt and water in overhydrated patients with moderate and severe congestive heart failure[67].

Many patients regain responsiveness to diuretics after one or more ultrafiltration treatments, suggesting that untapped cardiac functional reserve is recruited by ultrafiltration[67]. In addition, ascites, peripheral edema, and respiratory compromise may dramatically improve. Serum sodium concentration normalizes without worsening of renal function. As expected, plasma volume falls and plasma oncotic pressure rises[65]. Ultrafiltration increases the colloid osmotic pressure of plasma and the transcapillary gradient[68]. The increase in plasma oncotic pressure is maximal in the first 60 minutes of ultrafiltration and then levels off as refilling occurs. After ultrafiltration, the decreased venous pressure further enhances the net transcapillary pressure gradient change, favoring interstitial fluid reabsorption.

Most reports note that heart rate does not change and that blood pressure or systemic vascular resistance does not fall if the ultrafiltration rate is limited to 500 to 1000 mL per hour for only a few hours[52,53,69]. Cardiac output either rises or is stable. Pulmonary capillary wedge pressure is unchanged or decreased. Right atrial pressure and pulmonary vascular resistance fall. An improved ejection fraction and a decrease radiographic cardiothoracic ratio have also been described[52,53].

Advantages of intermittent isolated ultrafiltration include the avoidance of an arterial puncture and the short exposure to systemic anticoagulation. Disadvantages include the need for specialized dialysis equipment and personnel, which may limit the feasibility of the procedure, and the removal of large amounts of fluid in one limited session per day. Thus, the extracellular fluid space may be filling and emptying in a nonphysiologic manner. Slower, more protracted ultrafiltration minimizes these problems. Hemorrhage from anticoagulation and extracorporeal blood pump complications, such as air embolism, can occur.

Intermittent isolated ultrafiltration has been described in more than 100 NYHA class IV heart failure patients who have failed aggressive vasodilator, diuretic, and inotropic therapy[70]. Of 52 such patients treated with slow isolated ultrafiltration, 13 died less than 1 month into treatment (nonresponders), 24 had both cardiac and renal improvement (responders) for either <3 months ($n = 6$) or for >3 months ($n = 18$), and 15 (partial responders) had hemodynamic improvement but worsening renal function requiring either long-term weekly ultrafiltration ($n = 8$), continuous ambulatory peritoneal dialysis ($n = 1$), or intermittent renal replacement therapy ($n = 6$). Adequate diuresis was restored in 1 month in 24 of the 39 responders and partial responders. Four of the 15 partial responders had sufficient recovery of renal function to undergo heart transplantation 3 to 9 months after isolated ultrafiltration. Thus, intermittent ultrafiltration can be used as a non-pharmacologic approach for the treatment of congestive heart failure refractory to maximally tolerated medical therapy. Restoration of diuresis and natriuresis after intermittent ultrafiltration identified patients with recoverable cardiac functional reserve. Intermittent isolated ultrafiltration is valuable in partial responders because it improves quality of life and may be used as a bridge to heart transplantation. The high short-term mortality in this and in another study, in which 23 of 86 patients (27%) died within 2 months after ultrafiltration, is consistent with the poor prognosis associated with advanced heart failure.

Simplified Intermittent Isolated Ultrafiltration with Peripheral Venovenous Access

All ultrafiltration techniques described above require cannulation of a central vein for fluid withdrawal, blood return, or both. Recently, a new device (Aquadex System 100, CHF-Solutions, Minneapolis, MN) has become clinically available that permits both withdrawal of fluid and blood return through peripheral veins (Fig. 47.1).

However, central venous access remains an option with this device. Fluid removal can range from 10 to 500 mL per hour, blood flow can be set at 10 to 40 mL per minute, and total extracorporeal blood volume is only 33 mL. The device consists of a console, an extracorporeal blood pump, and venous catheters. The console controls the rate at which blood is removed from the patient and extracts ultrafiltrate at a user-set maximum rate. The device is designed to monitor the extracorporeal blood circuit and to alert the user to abnormal conditions. The device has one user setting that determines the rate of ultrafiltrate removal. Liquid removed during treatment drains into an ultrafiltrate bag. Blood is withdrawn from a vein through the withdrawal catheter. Tubing connects the withdrawal catheter to the blood pump. Blood passes through the withdrawal pressure sensor just before it enters the blood pump tubing loop. During operation, the pump loop is compressed by rotating rollers that propel the blood through the tubing. After exiting the blood pump, blood passes through the air detector and enters the hemofilter. The hemofilter is bonded to a clip-on cartridge that mounts onto the ultrafiltrate pump raceway on the side of the console. Blood enters the filter through a port on the bottom, exits through the port at the top of the filter, and passes through the infusion pressure sensor before returning to the patient. Inside the hemofilter, there is a bundle of hollow fibers. The ultrafiltrate passes through the fiber walls, fills the space between the fibers inside the filter case, and exits the filter through a port near the top of the filter case. After exiting the filter, ultrafiltrate passes through a blood leak detector. Ultrafiltrate sequentially passes through the ultrafiltrate pressure sensor, the ultrafiltrate pump, and the collecting bag that is suspended from the weight scale. Treatment can be performed by any nurse trained in the use of the device and does not require specialized dialysis personnel.

To date, three clinical trials of intermittent peripheral venovenous ultrafiltration have been published. In the first study, 21 fluid-overloaded patients, removal of an average of 2611 ± 1002 mL (range 325 to 3725 mL) over 6.43 ± 1.47 hours reduced weight from 91.9 ± 17.5 kg to 89.3 ± 17.3 kg ($p < .0001$), and also reduced signs and symptoms of pulmonary and peripheral congestion without associated changes in heart rate, blood pressure, electrolytes, or hematocrit[71].

The aim of the second study was to determine if ultrafiltration with this same Aquadex System 100 before intravenous diuretics in patients with decompensated heart failure and diuretic resistance results in euvolemia and hospital discharge in 3 days, without hypotension or worsening renal function (Fig. 47.3). Ultrafiltration was initiated within 4.7 ± 3.5 hours of hospitalization and before intravenous diuretics in 20 heart failure patients with volume overload and diuretic resistance (age

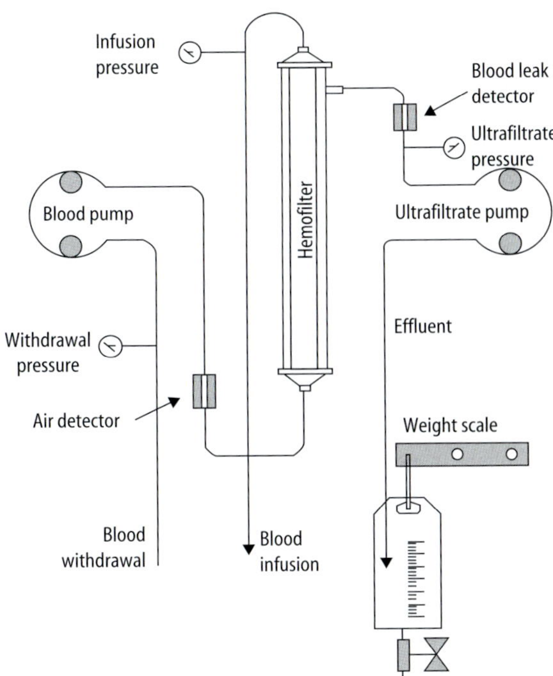

Figure 47.3. The Aquadex System 100 peripheral venovenous system (CHF Solutions, Minneapolis, MN).

74.5 ± 8.2 years; 75% ischemic disease; ejection fraction 3%±15%), and continued until euvolemia. Patients were evaluated at each hospital day, at 30 days, and at 90 days. An average of 8654±4205 mL was removed with 2.6 ± 1.2 eight-hour ultrafiltration courses. Twelve patients (60%) were discharged in 3 days. One patient was readmitted in 30 days and two patients in 90 days. Weight (p = .006), Minnesota Living with Heart Failure scores (p = .003), and Global Assessment (p = .00003) were improved after ultrafiltration, at 30 and 90 days. B-type natriuretic peptide levels were decreased after ultrafiltration (from 1236±747 pg/mL to 988 ± 847 pg/mL) and at 30 days (8l6 ± 494 pg/mL; p = .03. Blood pressure, renal function, and medications were unchanged. The results of this study suggest that in heart failure patients with volume overload and diuretic resistance, early ultrafiltration before intravenous diuretics effectively and safely decreases length of stay and readmissions. Clinical benefits persisted at 3 months after treatment[72].

The aim of the third study was to compare the safety and efficacy of ultrafiltration with the Aquadex System 100 device versus those of intravenous diuretics in patients with decompensated heart failure. Compared to the 20 patients randomly assigned to intravenous diuretics, the 20 patients randomized to a single 8-hour ultrafiltration session had greater median fluid removal (2838 mL versus 4650 mL; p = .001) and median weight loss (1.86 kg versus 2.5 kg; p = .24). Ultrafiltration was well tolerated and not associated with adverse hemodynamic renal effects. The results of this study show that an initial treatment decision to administer ultrafiltration in patients with decompensated congestive heart failure results in greater fluid removal and improvement of signs and symptoms of congestion than those achieved with traditional diuretic therapies[73].

Conclusion

In symptomatic heart failure patients, loop diuretics play a positive role in treating symptoms and signs of congestion. On the other hand, the use of diuretics in some heart failure patients may lead to deterioration of renal function. If diminished renal function and volume overload contribute to progression of heart failure, the use of loop diuretics poses a therapeutic dilemma. Fluid removal by ultrafiltration may be helpful when the use of loop diuretics is associated with deterioration of renal function. Fluid removal by ultrafiltration in patients with advanced heart failure may be preferable to loop diuretics. Relative or absolute diuretic resistance is common in patients with advanced heart failure. In these patients the use of large doses of loop diuretics may have deleterious effects on cardiac function due to diuretic-induced electrolyte abnormalities and neurohormonal activation. In addition, the fluid removed by ultrafiltration is isotonic with plasma, whereas urine produced in response to loop diuretics is hypotonic. Thus, for the same volume of fluid removal, ultrafiltration removes more sodium than loop diuretics. Because sodium and its anion are the major determinants of extracellular fluid volume, ultrafiltration decreases edema more than a comparable fluid loss induced by loop diuretics. Fluid removal by ultrafiltration may have sustained benefits in patients with acutely decompensated heart failure and volume overload.

References

1. Thom T, Haase N, Rosamond W, et al. Heart Disease and Stroke Statistics—2006 Update. A Report from the American Heart Association Statistics Committee and the Stroke Statistics Subcommittee. Circulation 2006;113:e85–151.
2. Adams KF, Fonarow GC, Emerman CL, et al. Characteristics and outcomes of patients hospitalized for heart failure in the United States: rationale, design, and preliminary observations from the first 100,000 cases in the Acute Decompensated Heart Failure National Registry (ADHERE). Am Heart J 2005;149:209–16.
3. Aghababian RV. Acutely decompensated heart failure: opportunities to improve care and outcomes in the emergency department. Rev Cardiovasc Med 2002;3(suppl 4):S3–9.
4. Schrier RW, Abraham WT. Hormones and hemodynamics in heart failure. N Engl J Med 1999; 341:577–85.
5. Ellison DH. Diuretic therapy and resistance in congestive heart failure. Cardiology 2001;96:132–43.
6. Butler J, Forman DE, Abraham WT, et al. Relationship between heart failure treatment and development of worsening renal function among hospitalized patients. Am Heart J 2004;147:331–8.
7. Neuberg GW, Miller AB, O'Connor CM, et al. for the PRAISE Investigators. Prospective Randomized Amlodipine Survival Evaluation. Diuretic resistance predicts mortality in patients with advanced heart failure. Am Heart J 2002;144:31–8.
8. Francis GS, Benedict C, Johnstone DE, et al. Comparison of neuroendocrine activation in patients with left ventricular dysfunction with and without congestive heart failure. A substudy of the Studies Of Left ventricular Dysfunction (SOLVD). Circulation 1990;82:1724–9.
9. Gottlieb SS, Brater DC, Thomas I, et al. BG9719 (CVT-124), an A1 adenosine receptor antagonist, protects against the decline in renal function observed with diuretic therapy. Circulation 2002; 105:1348–53.
10. Ronco C, Ricci Z, Bellomo R, Bedogni F. Extracorporeal ultrafiltration for the treatment of overhydration and congestive heart failure. Cardiology 2001;96:155–68.
11. Rose BD. Diuretics. Kidney Int 1991;39:336.
12. Odlind B, Beermann B Renal tubular secretion and effects of furosemide. Clin Pharmacol Ther 1980; 27:784–90.
13. Brater DC. Diuretics pharmacokinetics and pharmacodynamics. In: van Boxtel CJ, Holford NHG, Danhof M, eds. In Vivo Study of Drug Action: Principles and Applications of Kinetic-Dynamic Modeling. Amsterdam: Elsevier Science, 1992: 253–75.
14. Davies DL, Lant AF, Millard NR, Smith AJ, Ward JW, Wilson GM. Renal action, therapeutic use, and pharmacokinetics of the diuretic bumetanide. Clin Pharmacol Ther 1974;15:141–55.
15. Schwartz S, Brater DC, Pound D, Greene PK, Kramer WG, Rudy D. Bioavailability, pharmacokinetics, and pharmacodynamics of torsemide in patients with cirrhosis. Clin Pharmacol Ther 1993;54:90–7.
16. Ferguson JA, Sundblad KJ, Becker PK, Gorski JC, Rudy DW, Brater DC. Role of duration of diuretic effect in preventing sodium retention. Clin Pharmacol Ther 1997;62:203–8.
17. Brater DC. Diuretic therapy. N Engl J Med 1998;339:387–95.
18. Greither A, Goldman S, Edelen JS, Benet LZ, Cohn K. Pharmacokinetics of furosemide in patients with congestive heart failure. Pharmacology 1979;19: 121–31.
19. Brater DC, Chennavasin P, Seiwell R. Furosemide in patients with heart failure: shift in dose-response curves. Clin Pharmacol Ther 1980;28:182–6.
20. Voelker JR, Cartwright-Brown D, Anderson S, et al. Comparison of loop diuretics in patients with chronic renal insufficiency. Kidney Int 1987;32: 572–8.
21. Gerlag PGG, van Meijel JJM. High-dose furosemide in the treatment of refractory congestive heart failure. Arch Intern Med 1988;148:286–91.
22. Dikshit K, Vyden JK, Forrester JS, Chatterjee K, Prakash R, Swan HJC. Renal and extrarenal hemodynamic effects of furosemide in congestive heart failure after acute myocardial infarction. N Engl J Med 1973;288:1087–90.
23. Wilson JR, Reicheck N, Dunkman WB, Goldberg S. Effect of diuresis on the performance of the left ventricle in man. Am J Med 1981;70:234–9.
24. Bayliss J, Norell M, Canepa-Anson R, Sutton G, Poole-Wilson P. Untreated heart failure: clinical and neuroendocrine effects of increasing diuretics. Br Heart J 1987;57:17–22.
25. Knight RK, Miall PA, Hawkins LA, Dacombe J, Edwards CRW, Hamer J. Relation of plasma aldosterone concentration to diuretic treatment in patients with severe heart disease. Br Heart J 1979;42:316–25.
26. McCurley JM, Hanlon SU, Wei S, et al. Furosemide and the progression of left ventricular dysfunction in experimental heart failure. J Am Coll Cardiol 2004;44:1301–27.

27. Weber KT, Barilla CG. Pathological hypertrophy and cardiac interstitium: fibrosis and renin-angiotensin-aldosterone system. Circulation 1991; 83:1849–65.
28. Johnston GD, Hiatt WR, Nies AS, Payne A, Murphy RC, Gerber JG. Factors modifying the early non-diuretic vascular effects of furosemide in man. Circ Res 1983;53:630–5.
29. Morgan DB, Davidson C. Hypokalemia and diuretics: an analysis of publications. Br Med J 1980; 280:905–8.
30. Dyckner T, Helmers C, Lundman T, Wester PO. Initial serum potassium level in relation to early complications and prognosis in patients with acute myocardial infarction. Acta Med Scand 1975; 197;201–10.
31. Pelleg A, Mitamura H, Price R, Kaplinski E, Menduke H, Dreifus LS, Michelson EL. Extracellular potassium ion dynamics and ventricular arrhythmias in the canine heart. J Am Coll Cardiol 1989;13:941–50.
32. Gottlieb SS. Importance of magnesium in congestive heart failure. Am J Cardiol 1989;63:39G–42G.
33. White MG, van Gelder J, Estes G. The effect of loop diuretics on the excretion of Na^+, Ca^{2+}, Mg^{2+} and Cl^-. J Clin Pharmacol 1981;21:610–14.
34. Schuster CJ, Weil MH, Besso J, Carpio M, Henning RJ. Blood volume following diuresis induced by furosemide. Am J Med 1984;76:585–92.
35. Scherer B, Weber PC. Time-dependent changes in prostaglandin excretion in response to furosemide in man. Clin Sci 1979;56:77–81.
36. Kramer BK, Schweda F, Riegger GAJ. Diuretic treatment and diuretic resistance in heart failure. Am J Med 1999;106:90–6.
37. Schrier RW, Abdallah J, Weinberger H, Abraham WT. Therapy of heart failure. Kidney Int 2000; 57:1.
38. He XR, Greenberg S, Briggs J, Schnerman J. Effects of furosemide and verapamil on the NaCl dependency of macula densa-mediated secretion. Hypertension 1995;26:137–9.
39. Hrich DE. Captopril-induced renal insufficiency and the role of sodium balance. Ann Intern Med 1985;103:222–3.
40. Salvador DRK, Rey NR, Ramos GC, Punzalan FER. Continuous infusion versus bolus injection of loop diuretics in congestive heart failure. Cochrane Database Syst Rev 2005;3:CD003178.
41. Aaser E, Gullestad L, Tollofsrud S, et al. Effect of bolus injection versus continuous infusion of furosemide on diuresis and neurohormonal activation in patients with severe congestive heart failure. Scand J Lab Invest 1997;57:361–8.
42. Bagatin J, Sardelic S, Gancevic I, et al. Diuretic efficiency of furosemide in continuous intravenous infusion vs. bolus injection in congestive heart failure: results of a pilot study. Pharmaca 1993; 31:279–86.
43. Dormans TPJ, van Meyel JJM, Gerlag PGG, et al. Diuretic efficacy of high dose furosemide in severe heart failure: bolus injection versus continuous infusion. J Am Coll Cardiol 1996;28:376–82.
44. Kramer WG, Smith WB, Ferguson J, et al. Pharmacodynamics of torsemide administered as intravenous injection and as a continuous infusion to patients with congestive heart failure. J Clin Pharmacol 1996;36:265–70.
45. Lahav M, Regev A, Ra'anani P, Theodor E. Intermittent administration of furosemide vs. continuous infusion preceded by a loading dose for congestive heart failure. Chest 1992;102:725–31.
46. Licata G, Di Pasquale P, Parrinello G, et al. Effects of high-dose furosemide and small volume hypertonic saline solution infusion in comparison with a high dose of furosemide as a bolus, in refractory congestive heart failure. Am Heart J 2003; 145:459–66.
47. Pivac N, Rumboldt D, Sardelic S, et al. Diuretic effects of furosemide infusion versus bolus injection in congestive heart failure. Int J Clin Pharmacol Res 1998;18:121–8.
48. Schuller D, Lynch J, Fine D. Protocol-guided diuretic management: comparison of furosemide by continuous infusion and intermittent bolus. Crit Care Med 1997;25:1969–75.
49. Paganini EP, Flague J, Whiman G, et al. Amino acid balance in patients with oliguric renal failure undergoing slow continuous ultrafiltration (SCUF). Trans Am Soc Artif Int Org 1982;28:615–20.
50. Metha RL. Fluid management in CRRT. Contrib Nephrol 2001;132:335–48.
51. Marenzi GC, Lauri G, Grazi M, et al. Circulatory response to fluid overload removal by extracorporeal ultrafiltration in refractory congestive heart failure. J Am Coll Cardiol 2001;38:963–8.
52. Rimondini A, Cipolla CM, Della Bella P, et al. Hemofiltration as short-term treatment for refractory congestive heart failure. Am J Med 1987;83: 43–8.
53. Marenzi G, Grazi S, Lauri G, et al. Interrelation of humoral factors, hemodynamics and fluid and salt metabolism in congestive heart failure: effects of extracorporeal ultrafiltration. Am J Med 1993; 94:49–56.
54. Agostoni PG, Marenzi GC, Lauri G, et al. Sustained improvement in functional capacity after removal of body fluid with isolated ultrafiltration in chronic

cardiac insufficiency: failure of furosemide to provide the same result. Am J Med 1994;96:191–9.

55. Canaud B, Leray-Moragues H, Garred, et al. Slow isolated ultrafiltration for the treatment of congestive heart failure. Am Kidney Dis 1996;28(suppl): S67–73.
56. Cipolla CM, Grazi S, Rimondini A, et al. Changes in circulating norepinephrine with hemofiltration in advanced congestive heart failure. Am J Cardiol 1990;66:987–94.
57. Bergerone S, Golzio PG, Pacitti A. Atrial natriuretic factor and concomitant hormonal, hemodynamic and renal function changes after slow continuous ultrafiltration. Int J Cardiol 1992;36:305–7.
58. Blake P, Hasewaga Y, Khosla MC, et al. Isolation of "myocardial depressant factor(s)" from the ultrafiltrate of heart failure patients with acute renal failure. ASAIO J 1996;42:M911–5.
59. Coraim FI, Wolner E. Continuous hemofiltration for the failing heart. New Horiz 1995;3:725–31.
60. Burchardi H. History and development of continuous renal replacement techniques. Kidney Int 1998;66(suppl):S120–4.
61. Kramer P, Wigger W, Rieger J, et al. Arteriovenous haemofiltration: a new and simple method for treatment of overhydrated patients resistant to diuretics. Klin Wochenschr 1977;55:1121–2.
62. Canaud B, Cristol JP, Klouche K, et al. Slow continuous ultrafiltration: a means of unmasking myocardial functional reserve in end stage cardiac disease. Contrib Nephrol 1991;93:79–85.
63. Lepape A, Bene B, Pedrix JP, et al. Double pump driven continuous haemofiltration (CVVH). In: Siebert HG, Mann H, eds. Continuous Arteriovenous Haemofiltration. Basel: S Karger, 1985: 53–8.
64. Kramer P, Buhler J, Kehr A, et al. Intensive care potential of continuous arteriovenous hemofiltration. Trans Am Soc Artif Intern Org 1982;28: 28–32.
65. Grone HJ, Kramer P. Puncture and long term cannulation of the femoral artery and vein in adults. In: Kramer P, ed. Arteriovenous Hemofiltration. Berlin: Springer-Verlag, 1985:35–47.
66. Olbricht CJ, Schurek HJ, Stolte H, et al. The influence of vascular access mode on the efficiency of CAVH. In: Sieberth HG, Mann H, eds. Continuous Arteriovenous Hemofiltration. Basel: S Karger, 1985:14–24.
67. Dileo M, Pacitti A, Bergerone S, et al. Ultrafiltration in the treatment of refractory heart failure. Clin Cardiol 1988;11:449–59.
68. Kishore K, Yagi N, Paganini E. Renal replacement therapy in congestive heart failure. Semin Dialysis 1997;10:259–66.
69. Guazzi M, Agostoni P, Perego B. Apparent paradox of neurohumoral axis inhibition after body fluid volume depletion in patients with congestive heart failure and water retention. Br Heart J 1994; 72:534–9.
70. Silverstein ME, Ford CA, Lysaght MJ, et al. Treatment of severe volume overload by ultrafiltration. N Engl J Med. 1974;291:747–51.
71. Jaski BE, Ha J, Denys BG, et al. Peripherally inserted veno-venous ultrafiltration for rapid treatment of volume overloaded patients. J Card Fail 2003;9: 227–31.
72. Costanzo MR, Saltzberg MT, O'Sullivan JE, et al. Early ultrafiltration in patients with decompensated heart failure and diuretic resistance. J Am Coll Cardiol 2005;46:2043–51.
73. Bart BA, Boyle A, Bank AJ, et al. Randomized controlled trial of ultrafiltration versus usual care for hospitalized patients with heart failure: relief for acutely fluid overloaded patients with decompensated congestive heart failure. J Am Coll Cardiol 2005;46:2043–6.

48
Role of Anemia in Acute and Chronic Heart Failure and the Role of Erythropoietin in Its Correction

Donald S. Silverberg, Dov Wexler, Adrian Iaina, and Doron Schwartz

The World Health Organization considers anemia in adults to be present when the hemoglobin (Hb) of men is <13 g/dL and of women is <12 g/dL (1). The average lower limit of a normal Hb for men and women together, therefore, is about 12.5 g/dL, and anything less than this would be considered to be anemia. In a study of 32,229 consecutive patients admitted to 263 United States hospitals with a primary diagnosis of congestive heart failure (CHF) (the Acute Decompensated Heart Failure National Registry [ADHERE] study), the mean Hb was 12.4 g/dL and the mean serum creatinine was 1.8 mg/dL (2) (roughly equivalent to a calculated creatinine clearance of about 40 mL/min/1.73 m^2). Clearly, then, about half the patients admitted to hospital with a primary diagnosis of CHF in the U.S. have anemia and, since a creatinine clearance of <60 mL/min/1.73 m^2 is considered to be chronic kidney insufficiency (CKI), the great majority also have CKI.

Is this anemia important? How does the anemia affect the CHF and the CKI? What are the causes of this anemia? Is it worth treating, and with what?

In the last 5 years there has been an enormous upsurge in interest in the role of anemia in CHF. In the U.S. guidelines on diagnosis and treatment of CHF in 1999 (3), anemia was not even mentioned, but since then the number of papers published on this subject has increased dramatically. These include reanalysis of several key CHF studies including the CHARM, COMET, COPERNICUS, ELITE II, IN-CHF, OPTIME, PRAISE, RENAISSANCE, SOLVD, and VAL-HEFT studies. There have also been analyses of the prevalence and significance of anemia of hospitalized and clinic CHF patients throughout the world by several large medical centers, as recently summarized by us and others (4–8). As summarized in these reviews, the vast majority of epidemiological studies have shown the following:

1. Anemia is common in CHF, with a prevalence of anywhere from 10% to 60%, with the average prevalence being around 40% (4–8). Examination of these CHF studies shows that the differences in prevalence were dependent on many factors. The anemia was generally more common in the elderly, in diabetics, in those with more severe renal damage, and in those with more severe CHF. It was also more common in those who were hospitalized than in those treated in the community, and more common in those in whom the anemia was defined as an Hb level of <12 to 13.5 g/dL as compared to <11 g/dL. In many of the larger controlled intervention studies of angiotensin-converting enzyme inhibitors (ACEIs), angiotensin receptor blockers (ARBs), and beta-blockers in CHF, patients with CKI or severe anemia were specifically excluded, which could partially explain the low prevalence of anemia in these studies. In some studies anemia was not present when first seen but developed over the period of follow-up. Some of the CHF studies defined anemia as merely a physician's recorded diagnosis of anemia in the medical discharge chart without actual values of Hb being given. The problem with this is that some doctors may recognize the presence of anemia only if it is very severe.

2. Compared to CHF patients without anemia, the presence of anemia in CHF patients has been associated with many more cardiovascular abnormalities (4–8) (Table 48.1). On average, in these many studies, the mortality and hospitalization rate in CHF increased by about 15% to 20% for every fall in the Hb level of 1 g/dL (4–8). Thus a fall in Hb from 15 to 10 g/dL would be associated with about double the mortality rate and double the rate of hospitalization. This is similar to the odds ratio of mortality and hospitalization seen in CHF with four other common risk factors: smoking, diabetes, hypertension, and hypercholesterolemia. For this reason anemia could be called the fifth cardiovascular risk factor.

Brain natriuretic peptide (BNP) is now used commonly for both the diagnosis of CHF and for assessing its prognosis. It reflects the volume, stretch, and pressure in the ventricles. Studies in CHF have found that the BNP levels in cardiac patients both with and without CHF were related inversely and independently to Hb levels: the lower the Hb, the higher the BNP (4–8). Even in studies in the general population, the level of BNP is inversely related to the level of Hb. In some studies anemia was found to be an even better

Table 48.1. Characteristics of congestive heart failure (CHF) patients who are anemic compared with those who are not anemic

Clinical findings	*Abnormal laboratory findings*
Older age	Higher serum creatinine
Higher percentage with diabetes	Lower glomerular filtration rate (GFR)
It is more likely that the patient is hospitalized than in an outpatient CHF clinic	Higher brain natriuretic peptide (BNP)
Higher mortality	Higher C-reactive protein (CRP)
Lower left ventricular ejection fraction (LVEF)	More rapid rate of decrease of GFR
More likely to be on an angiotensin-converting enzyme (ACE) inhibitor	Higher blood levels of the bone marrow suppressor *N*-acetyl-seryl-aspartyl-lysyl proline (Ac-SDKP)
More severe systolic CHF with higher New York Heart Association (NYHA)	Hyponatremia
More severe diastolic CHF with higher NYHA	Lymphopenia
More hospitalizations	Hyperuricemia
Longer hospitalization stays	Signs of malnutrition and inflammation:
Higher hospital costs	Lower caloric intake
Lower cognitive function	Reduced body mass index
More severe renal failure	Reduced serum albumin
More rapid progression of renal failure	Reduced total serum protein
More likely to require dialysis	Reduced serum cholesterol
More resistant to medical therapy	Evidence of iron deficiency
Lower quality of life	Higher serum tumor necrosis factor-alpha (TNF-α)
Higher percentage requiring intravenous diuretics	Higher serum interleukin-6 (IL-6)
Higher dose of oral diuretics required	Increased blood cortisol/decreased blood androgens (i.e., signs of catabolism)
Higher percentage requiring digoxin	Blunted serum erythropoietin (EPO) response to anemia
Reduced body mass index	Abnormal blood and body water changes
More serious cardiovascular abnormalities	Lower red cell mass
Higher right and left ventricular pressures	Higher plasma volume
Higher pulmonary artery pressure	Higher interstitial volume
Increased pulmonary capillary wedge pressure	Higher total water volume
Greater left ventricular hypertrophy and left ventricular mass index	
Larger LV end systolic and end diastolic volumes	
Greater atrial dimensions	
Lower oxygen utilization (MVO_2) during maximal exercise	
Poorer peripheral perfusion	
Lower blood pressure	
Higher heart rate	
Lower exercise tolerance on exercise testing	

predictor of long-term survival in CHF than the BNP level. All this suggests that part of the elevated BNP seen in CHF may simply be due to the associated anemia (4–8)!

Approximately 5% of CHF patients have hyponatremia, and these patients have a poorer prognosis than those with a normal serum sodium concentration. Anemia is not included among the causes of hyponatremia in CHF. In a study we have just completed (unpublished data) in 200 patients with severe CHF and anemia (Hb < 12 g/dL), 40 (20%) were found to be hyponatremic with a serum Na of less than 136 mEq/L. Correction of the anemia with subcutaneous (SC) erythropoietin (EPO) and intravenous (IV) iron increased the mean Hb from 10.6 ± 0.9 to 13.7 ± 1.1 g/dL over 3 months, and this was associated with an increase of the mean serum Na from 133.9 ± 2.7 to 138.3 ± 2.9 mEq/L. Thus anemia may be a treatable cause of hyponatremia. This is perhaps not so surprising since anemia is known to increase antidiuretic hormone (ADH) levels (9).

3. The Hb levels alter with time. A fall in Hb over a period of time in CHF patients has been associated with an increase in mortality, an increase in hospitalization, an increase in left ventricular mass index, and a fall in cognitive function (4–8).

How Does Anemia Cause or Worsen CHF?

It has been known for years that anemia, if severe enough, can cause heart failure even in normal individuals (9) (Fig. 48.1). The tissue hypoxia and peripheral vasodilation present in anemia causes a lowering of blood pressure, leading to an increased sympathetic response, which leads to tachycardia, increased stroke volume, renal vasoconstriction, reduced renal blood flow, and salt and water retention (Fig. 48.1). This leads to an increase in extracellular fluid (ECF), including an increase in plasma volume (9). The reduced renal blood flow also causes an increased secretion of renin, angiotensin, aldosterone, and ADH, further augmenting the renal vasoconstriction and salt and water retention, and further increasing the ECF and plasma volume (9). In addition, norepinephrine, renin, angiotensin, and aldosterone are all toxic to renal, cardiac, endothelial, and other cells (4–9). The tachycardia and increased stroke

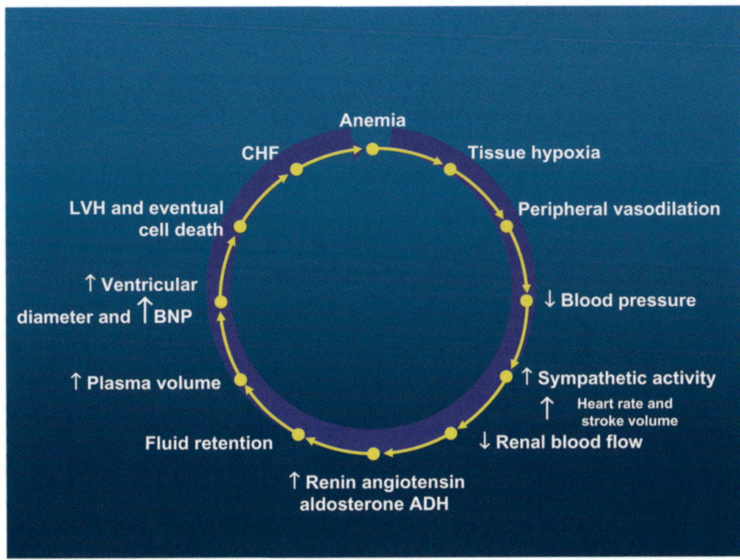

FIGURE 48.1. The mechanism for fluid retention and heart failure in anemia (9). ADH, antidiuretic hormone; BNP, brain natriuretic peptide; CHF, congestive heart failure; LVH, left ventricular hypertrophy.

volume can eventually lead to ventricular dilation and hypertrophy, and to myocardial cell death, cardiac fibrosis, and CHF (4–9).

Is Anemia Actually Causing Worsening of the CHF? Results of Correcting the Anemia (Table 48.2)

Does anemia actually contribute to the worsening of the CHF or is it just an innocent bystander, merely a marker of more severe CHF? One way of finding out is to actually treat the anemia and see if this improves the CHF. In both uncontrolled and controlled studies (10–13), we showed that when anemia was corrected to an Hb of 12.0 to 13.5 g/dL by SC EPO and IV iron (ferric sucrose; Venofer, Vifor Int St Gallen, Switzerland), the CHF improved, as evidenced by improvement of the New York Heart Association (NYHA) functional class, increased left ventricular ejection fraction (LVEF), reduced number and days of hospitalization, reduced doses of oral and IV furosemide required, and improved self-assessed shortness of breath and fatigue. In the uncontrolled studies (10,12,13) we also found that the creatinine clearance (CCr), which had been falling at a rate of about 1 mL/min/month before the anemia, was corrected, and stabilized after its correction. All these patients had been under a cardiologist's care before we intervened to treat the anemia, and had been on maximally tolerated doses of all the recommended CHF medications but were still resistant to therapy and were highly symptomatic. In the controlled study (11), the group in which anemia was treated (16 patients) had an improvement in NYHA class, LVEF, days in hospital, dose of oral and IV furosemide, and no change in mean serum creatinine, whereas in the untreated group (also 16 patients) all the above parameters worsened and the mean serum creatinine levels increased significantly (11). In addition, one quarter of the patients in the controlled group died, all due to severe progressive CHF, whereas none died in the treatment group in which the anemia had been corrected.

TABLE 48.2. Causes of anemia in congestive heart failure (CHF)

1. Renal failure with reduced EPO production in the kidney
2. Increased secretion of the inflammatory cytokines TNF-α and IL-6 which causes:
   a. Reduced EPO production in the kidney
   b. Resistance to EPO in the bone marrow
   c. Reduced release of iron from iron stores in the reticuloendothelial system
   d. Increased hepcidin causing reduced release of iron from iron stores in the reticuloendothelial system
3. Diabetes with low EPO production caused by damage to the EPO-producing cells in the kidney
4. Increased gastrointestinal blood loss from aspirin and uremia
5. Loss of iron, transferrin, and EPO in the urine in those CHF patients with proteinuria
6. Malabsorption of iron from the gut due to bowel edema
7. Hemodilution
8. Decreased food intake from anorexia
9. ACE inhibition by ACE inhibitors, which causes anemia by
   a. Increasing Ac-SDKP in the blood and thus causing bone marrow suppression and
   b. Reducing angiotensin II production which thus reduces bone marrow stimulation
10. Angiotensin receptor blockers (ARBs), which cause anemia probably by interfering with the angiotensin II stimulating effects in the bone marrow
11. Beta-blockers may also cause anemia

In a randomized, placebo-controlled, single-blind study of 22 patients with anemia and severe CHF, Mancini et al. (14) evaluated the use of SC EPO 15,000 to 30,000 IU weekly and oral iron over a 3-month period. Exercise duration, 6-minute walking distance, peak oxygen utilization during maximal exercise (MVO_2), oxygen utilization at the anaerobic threshold, and the quality of life all improved in the treated group (whose mean Hb increased from 11.0 to 14.3 g/dL) and did not change significantly in the placebo group. The degree of improvement in MVO_2 was proportional to the degree of change in the Hb. This is important, since MVO_2 is an important prognostic predictor of survival in CHF (14). In another study by the same group the anemia was found to be associated with a reduced red cell mass in the majority of cases and with an increased plasma volume (PV) in the rest (15). Correction of the anemia reduced the PV to normal and increased the red cell mass (14). In a recent 1-year controlled study of 38 patients with CHF and anemia, and treatment with EPO and oral iron compared to oral iron alone (16), the NYHA class, endurance time, distance walked in exercise testing, MVO_2, BNP, and renal function all improved with correction of the anemia but remained the same in the control group.

In a randomized double-blind multicenter study, the effect on exercise tolerance of darbopoietin-α, a long- lasting erythropoietin preparation, was compared to placebo in patients with CHF (17); 19 patients were randomized to darbopoietin given SC every 2 weeks for 26 weeks. The remaining 22 received placebo. Exercise duration was increased by 109 seconds in the treated group (p = .075). The Patient Global Assessment of change showed a benefit in favor of darbopoietin (79% vs. 49%, p = .014).

In an uncontrolled study of 16 patients with anemia and CHF, IV iron alone was associated with an improvement in NYHA, quality of life, and distance walked in 6 minutes (18).

All these studies suggest that correction of anemia with either erythropoietin or darbopoietin as well as with oral or IV iron, or oral iron alone, may have a positive effect of CHF, but larger studies clearly are needed to confirm these findings.

The Effect of Erythropoietin in Patients with Renal Failure

Another piece of evidence suggesting that control of anemia is important is the large literature on the use of EPO in renal failure (Table 48.3). A recent meta-analysis of CKI patients not on dialysis showed that correction of the anemia with EPO was associated with a decrease in the number of patients requiring transfusion, an improvement in quality of life and exercise capacity, no statistical difference in rate of progression in renal disease, and no increase in adverse effects (19). A meta-analysis on the effect of EPO on ventricular structure and function in patients with CKI or patients on dialysis showed that EPO caused significant reductions in left ventricular mass and left ventricular mass index, an increase in left ventricular ejection fraction, and a reduction in left ventricular end diastolic volume and end systolic volume (20). Since severity of left ventricular hypertrophy (LVH) is closely related to mortality (20), these data suggest that EPO might reduce mortality in patients with renal failure and LVH, although long-term controlled studies on this subject are not available. Uncertainty about the level to which to correct the anemia in renal failure is partly due to a randomized double-blind trial in hemodialysis patients with known heart disease, evaluating the impact on outcomes of normalization of hematocrit (Hct) to 42% versus a lower Hct (30%) (21). The trial was stopped early because of failure to demonstrate a survival benefit for patients in the higher Hct group and an increase in vascular access thrombosis in the higher Hct group. In a recent meta-analysis of treatment of anemia in CKI, it was concluded that there was a 17% greater cardiovascular risk if the Hb is increased beyond 12 g/dL (22). Whether this is true for the anemia of CHF will require large controlled studies, and indeed these are now being performed.

TABLE 48.3. Summary of effects of treatment of the anemia in CHF with EPO and oral or IV iron seen in uncontrolled, controlled single blind and controlled double-blind studies

Improved NYHA class
Reduced number of hospitalizations
Reduced number of hospital days
Stabilized renal function or slower rate of deterioration of renal function
Improved quality of life
Increased exercise duration
Improved exercise tolerance
Improved MVO_2
Improved systolic function
Improved diastolic function
Reduced BNP
Reduced need for oral and IV diuretics
Reduced number of attacks of pulmonary edema

The Additive Effects of Anemia on CHD, CHF, CKI, Diabetes, and Other Conditions (4–8)

As seen in Table 48.4, anemia is associated with an increased risk of the development or worsening of cardiovascular complications in many conditions. The question as to whether correction of the anemia with EPO will reduce the incidence of these cardiovascular complications will only be answered by randomized, controlled, double-blind studies.

All three conditions, CHF, CKI and anemia (4–8), are associated with an increase in four mechanisms that can damage the tissues: sympathetic activity, the activity of the renin-angiotensin-aldosterone system (RAAS), oxidative stress, and inflammation. Even more worrisome is the fact that all four of these mechanisms, if present in increased levels, not only can destroy body cells but also can activate each other (4–8)! This suggests that the only way to improve CHF and CKI is by a broad-based treatment that controls all four of the mechanisms, something that we do when we use ACEI/ARBs, beta-blockers, and spironolactone in addition to controlling the anemia.

Anemia can cause or worsen CHF and CKI, CKI can cause or worsen CHF and anemia, and CHF can cause or worsen CKI and anemia. So what we frequently see in our hospital wards and clinics is this unholy trio, each causing and worsening each other. We have called this vicious circle the cardiorenal anemia syndrome (4–8,10–13) (Fig. 48.2).

The sensitivity of the damaged heart to anemia has been shown in many animal studies; CHF develops at much milder degrees of anemia in those animals with damaged hearts than in those with normal hearts (4–8). This is consistent with our findings in CHF and those of others (4–14).

Table 48.4. Anemia: an independent risk factor for increasing or worsening cardiovascular events such as sudden death, CHF, myocardial infarction (MI), acute coronary syndromes (ACS), and stroke

In normal middle aged and elderly people
In diabetics
In patients with diabetes and CKI
In patients on dialysis
In patients with asymptomatic left ventricular dysfunction
In patients with systolic CHF
In patients with diastolic CHF
In patients with pulmonary hypertension
In patients with LVH
In renal transplant patients
In heart transplant patients
In acute coronary syndromes
In patients with percutaneous coronary intervention (PCI)-proven coronary artery disease
It also increases the risk of developing contrast media-induced acute renal failure

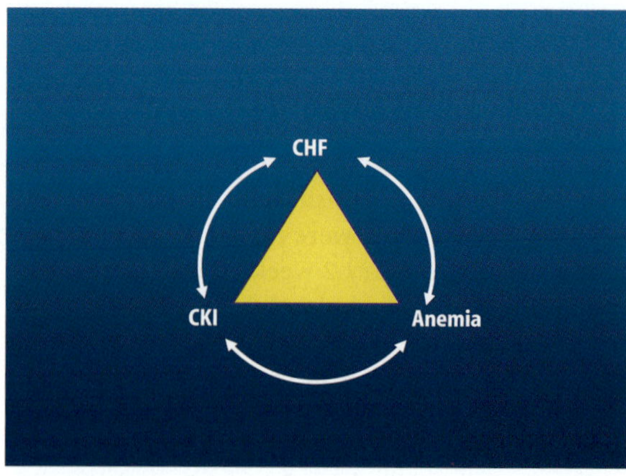

Figure 48.2. The vicious circle of congestive heart failure (CHF), chronic kidney insufficiency (CKI), and anemia: the cardiorenal anemia syndrome.

The etiology of the anemia in CHF is listed in Table 48.2 (4–8).

Nonhematopoietic Actions of Erythropoietin

Erythropoietin modulates a broad array of cellular processes outside of the hematopoietic system including increasing both the number and the activity of endothelial progenitor stem cells and improving neoangiogenesis (23,24). It also inhibits the apoptotic mechanisms of injury of the endothelial and myocardial cells and inhibits inflammatory damage. It may offer similar protection in other areas as well, such as the central and peripheral nervous system, the eyes, the kidney, and the blood vessels (23,24). Not only does EPO administration at the time of an induced myocardial infarction in animals reduce the size of the infarct, but it also maintains its cardiac function (23,24). How much of the improvement in CHF with EPO administration is due to the increase in Hb and how much due to the direct effects of EPO on tissues is still not determined.

Antioxidant Effects of Erythropoietin

The improvement in the cardiac and renal function that we see when the anemia is corrected with EPO may not be related only to the increased oxygen carrying capacity of the blood and the delivery of more oxygen to the tissues. The erythrocyte has many antioxidants that can neutralize the oxidative stress produced by radical oxygen species (ROS) that are produced in excessive amounts in CHF and CKI and can damage all the cells of the body by causing increased collagen synthesis and fibrosis, lipid peroxidation, the release of inflammatory cytokines, and apoptosis of endothelial cells and smooth muscle cells. (25). The neutralization of ROS by the red cell is partly caused by the glutathione system in the erythrocyte as well as by enzymes such as superoxide dismutase and catalase, which react with the ROS and limit their effect on surrounding tissues. Thus simply increasing the number of erythrocytes can cause a major improvement in oxidative stress. In addition, EPO itself may also have other antioxidant effects that are unrelated to anemia correction. It may, for example, directly reduce ROS production in polymorphonuclear cells (26).

Attitude of Cardiologists and Internists to Anemia in Congestive Heart Failure

In a preliminary report from the Cleveland Clinic (27), 2011 consecutive ambulatory patients with chronic CHF seen in tertiary care cardiology or internal medicine clinics were studied. Anemia was defined as an Hb ≤ 12 g/dL in men and ≤11 g/dL in women; 29% of these CHF patients had or developed anemia. Yet anemia was recognized as a diagnosis in only 11.1% of those cases by the internists and in only 4.4% of those cases seen by cardiologists! Diagnostic evaluation was performed in only 6% of these anemic patients, and only 10% received medical therapy for the anemia! The conclusion of the investigators was that anemia in ambulatory patients with CHF was underrecognized, underdiagnosed, and undertreated by cardiologists and internists.

Treatment of the Anemia of Congestive Heart Failure (4–7,10–13)

Clearly secondary causes of anemia such as gastrointestinal bleeding must be diagnosed and treated. We attempt to achieve a final target Hb of 12 g/dL. If the initial Hb is less than 9 g/dL and the patient is still symptomatic after standard acute treatment of pulmonary edema, administer packed cells carefully so as to reach an Hb of 9 g/dL and then begin standard therapy of anemia, as follows:

1. Erythropoietin (EPO) alpha or beta or Darbopoietin can be given subcutaneously or IV. We start with subcutaneous EPO alpha or beta in a dose of 10,000 IU once weekly or Darbopoietin in a dose of 50 μg once weekly.
2. If the percent of transferrin saturation (%TSat) is below 20% and serum ferritin less than 800 μg/L we also start IV iron. We use the IV iron preparation Venofer (ferric sucrose) since it has an excellent safety record. We give it weekly in a dose of 200 mg (2 ampules) in 150 mL normal saline over 45 minutes. (On the first visit we administer a test dose of 25 mg over 30 minutes in 150 mL normal saline, and if this is well tolerated we then give the other 175 mg in another 150 mL). We then administer 200 mg once weekly in a similar manner over 45 minutes until either the %TSat has reached 20%, the Hb has reached our target of 12 g/dL, or the serum ferritin reaches 800 μg/L, at which point we stop the IV iron.

When the target Hb is attained, we maintain the same dose of the erythropoietin preparation weekly for another 2 weeks. If the Hb is stable at around 12 g/dL, we begin to reduce the frequency or doses of the EPO preparations as needed. Other investigators use only oral iron preparations (not IV) to achieve and maintain the %TSat of at least 20%. Only if they fail to reach or maintain this level do they switch to the IV iron preparation

Conclusion

The final evidence about the effect of correction of the anemia of CHF with EPO and iron is not yet in. The epidemiologic studies overwhelmingly attest to the strong association between anemia and increased mortality, increased hospitalizations, increased severity of CHF, and reduced quality of life in those who are anemic. The present clinical evidence on the correction of the anemia in CHF suggests that this may improve many aspects of CHF including cardiac function, renal function, hospitalizations, exercise capacity, and quality of life. However, large randomized, controlled, double-blind studies, which are really needed to answer this question, are only now being completed.

In CHF patients who are being maximally treated with all the recommended CHF medications in the recommended doses but who are still not doing well and who have Hb levels below 11.5 to 12 g/dL, physicians should at least be aware that this form of therapy is available, appears to be safe, and in the studies available appears highly effective in improving CHF.

Clearly cooperation must exist between cardiologists and nephrologists in treating these anemic CHF patients since the vast majority will also have moderate to severe renal insufficiency.

The value of anemia correction using these agents in other types of cardiac disease with anemia—from acute coronary syndromes to chronic coronary heart disease (CHD), to asymptomatic ventricular dysfunction and LVH, etc.—are fascinating questions for future investigation as well, especially since EPO may also have many positive nonhematologic effects on endothelial, myocardial, renal, brain, and other cells.

References

1. World Health Organization. Nutritional anemias: report of a WHO Scientific Group. WHO Tech Rep Series 1968;405:5–37.
2. Fonarow GC, Adams KF Jr, Abraham WT, et al. Risk stratification for in hospital mortality in acutely decompensated heart failure. JAMA 2005; 293;572–580.
3. Packer M, Cohn JN, et al. Consensus recommendations for the management of chronic heart failure. Am J Cardiol 1999;83:1A–38A.
4. Silverberg DS, Wexler D, Iaina A, Schwartz D. The interaction between heart failure and other heart disease and anemia. Semin Nephrol 2006;26: 296–306.
5. Silverberg DS, Wexler, Iaina A. The role of anemia in the progression of congestive heart failure. Is there a place for erythropoietin and intravenous iron? J Nephrology 2004;17:749–761.
6. Mitchell JE. Emerging role of anemia in heart failure. Am J Cardiol 2007;99(6B):15D–20D.
7. Tang YD, Katz SD. Anemia in chronic heart failure: prevalence, etiology, clinical correlates, and treatment options. Circulation 2006;113:2454–2461.
8. Lindenfeld JA. Prevalence of anemia and the effects on mortality in patients with heart failure. Am Heart J 2005;149:391–340.
9. Anand IS, Chandrashekhar Y, Ferrari R, Poole-Wilson PA, Harris PC. Pathogenesis of edema in chronic anemia: Studies of body water and sodium, renal function, haemodynamics and plasma hormones. Br Heartt J 1993;70:357–362.
10. Silverberg DS, Wexler D, Blum M, et al. The use of subcutaneous erythropoietin and intravenous iron for the treatment of the anemia of severe, resistant congestive heart failure improves cardiac and renal function, functional cardiac class, and markedly reduces hospitalizations. J Am Coll Cardiol 2000; 35:1737–1744.
11. Silverberg DS, Wexler, Sheps D et al. The effect of correction of mild anemia in severe, resistant congestive heart failure using subcutaneous erythropoietin and intravenous iron: a randomized controlled study. J Am Coll Cardiol 2001;37: 1775–1780.
12. Silverberg DS, Wexler D, Blum M et al. The effect of correction of anemia in diabetic and non diabetics with severe resistant congestive heart failure and chronic renal failure by subcutaneous erythropoietin and intravenous iron. Nephrol Dial Transplant 2003;18:141–146.
13. Silverberg DS, Wexler D, Blum M, et al. Effects of treatment with EPO beta on outcomes in patients with anaemia and chronic renal failure. Kidney Blood Pressure Res 2005;28:41–47.
14. Mancini DM, Katz SD, Lang C, et al. Effect of erythropoietin on exercise capacity in patients with moderate to severe chronic heart failure. Circulation 2003;107:294–299.
15. Androne AS, Katz SD, Lund L, et al. Hemodilution is common in patients with advanced heart failure. Circulation 2003;107:226–229.
16. Palazzuoli A, Silverberg DS, Iovine F, et al. Erythropoietin improves anemia, exercise tolerance, and renal function and reduces B-type natriuretic peptide and hospitalization in patients with heart failure and anemia. Am Heart J 2006;152: e9–15.
17. Ponikowski P, Anker SD, Szachniewicz J, et al. Effect of darbepoetin alpha on exercise tolerance in anemic patients with symptomatic chronic heart failure. J Am Coll Cardiol 2007;49:753–762.
18. Bolger AP, Bartlett FP, Penston HS, et al. Intravenous iron alone for the treatment of anemia in patients with chronic heart failure. J Am Coll Cardiol 2006;48:1225–1227.
19. Cody J, Daly C, Campbell M, et al. Recombinant human erythropoietin for chronic renal failure

anaemia in pre-dialysis patients. Cochrane Database Syst Rev 2005 July 20;(3):CD003266.

20. Jones M, Schenkel B, Just J. Epoetin alpha's effect on left ventricular hypertrophy and subsequent mortality. Int J Cardiol 2005;100:253–265.
21. Besarab A, Bolton WK, Browne JK, et al. The effects of normal as compared with low hematocrit values in patients with cardiac disease who are receiving hemodialysis and epoetin. N Engl J Med 1998; 339:584–590.
22. Phrommintikul A, Haas SJ, Elsik M, Krum H. Mortality and target hemoglobin concentrations in anaemic patients with chronic kidney disease treated with erythropoietin: a meta-analysis. Lancet 2007;369:381–388.
23. van der meer P, Voors AA, Lipsic E, van Gilst WH, van Veldhuisen DJ. Erythropoietin in cardiovascular diseases. Eur Heart J 2004;13:285–291.
24. Maiese K, Li F, Chong ZZ. New avenues of exploration for erythropoietin. JAMA 2005;293:90–95.
25. Grune T, Sommerburg O, Siems WG. Oxidative stress in anemia. Clin Nephrology 2000;53(suppl 1): S18–S22.
26. Kristal B, Shurtz-Swirski R, Sasha SM, et al. Interaction between erythropoietin and peripheral polymorphonuclear leucocytes in hemodialysis patients. Nephron 1999;81:406–413.
27. Tang WHW, Miller H, Partin M, et al. Anemia in ambulatory patients with chronic heart failure: A single-center clinical experience derived from electronic medical records. J Am Coll Cardiol 2003;41(suppl A):157A.

2.4
Treatment of Acute Heart Failure Syndrome: Cardiovascular Management

2.4.1
Vasodilators

49
Management of Chronic Heart Failure Therapy in the Setting of Acute Heart Failure

Luigi Tavazzi, Aldo Pietro Maggioni, and Donata Lucci

Clinical research on the treatment of chronic heart failure (CHF) has developed significantly over the last 20 years, leading to substantial changes in therapeutic practices and notable improvements in patients' outcome. Research on the treatment of acute heart failure (AHF) has not developed in parallel, and only in the last few years have researchers turned their interest toward this important public health problem. This shift in interest has been predominantly caused by the development of new drugs for use in cardiology and the consequent resources made available by the pharmaceutical industry. However, the two areas of interest remain distinct. Neither research nor the medical literature has so far dealt with the link between ongoing treatments in patients with CHF and acute clinical destabilization or with the therapeutic changes induced by the event in survivors. In reality, patients with CHF typically fluctuate between periods of clinical stability and other periods of instability, and the diagnostic-therapeutic strategy in these patients is continuously reshaped by the occurrence of acute events. Therefore, it is useful to reconstruct the dynamics of the therapeutic approach in order to evaluate its rationality and to establish appropriate lines of conduct.

Trends and Current Treatments in Patients with Chronic Heart Failure

Many factors can gradually or suddenly upset the cardiocirculatory balance in a patient with CHF. It is important to identify the factors precipitating such destabilizations because they may provide a key to how to prevent further episodes of AHF. Table 49.1 reports the precipitating factors observed in a recent Italian survey of 2807 patients with AHF (1). Although it is not always possible to identify the cause of a destabilization, ischemic events, arrhythmias (in particular new-onset atrial fibrillation), and hypertensive crises seem to be the most frequent triggers (1–10). A lack of compliance with drug therapy, dietary rules, or lifestyle changes is also an important destabilizing factors, although its frequency as a precipitating factors varies greatly in the different series. In fact, the variability of the precipitating factors precludes certain prediction of acute episodes only with standard heart failure management rules. Long-term pharmacologic treatment is important in stabilizing the clinical status, as shown by the reduced incidence of hospital admissions observed in all trials investigating currently recommended treatments. Furthermore, long-term treatment is the pharmacologic context in which the doctor deciding the therapeutic strategy for a patient with AHF must act.

The changes that have taken place in the treatment of CHF over the last decade emerge clearly from an analysis of the database of heart failure outpatients enrolled in the Italian Network on Congestive Heart Failure (IN-CHF) Registry. This registry was set up in 1995 and contains data on about 25,000 patients enrolled through 130 Italian cardiology centers over a period of 10 years. Figure 49.1 illustrate the frequencies of prescriptions of drugs affecting the adrenergic systems, the renin-angiotensin-aldosterone system (RAAS),

Table 49.1. Italian Survey on acute heart failure (AHF): precipitating factors recorded in 2807 patients hospitalized with acute heart failure (de novo, $n = 1347$; acute-on-chronic, $n = 1460$)

Factor	Percent
Acute myocardial infarction	20.3
Arrhythmia	15.0
Uncontrolled hypertension	13.4
Infections	6.1
Poor treatment compliance	5.4
Treatment reduction	5.3
Excessive sodium/fluid ingestion	4.6
Valvular disease	4.4
Renal failure	3.2
Noncardiovascular factors	2.6
High output	2.2
New dosages/change of dosages	0.6
Alcohol	0.2
Other factors	2.9
Not identified	13.8

and digitalis in the last decade. The use of RAAS modulators, angiotensin-converting enzyme inhibitors (ACEIs), and angiotensin-receptor blockers (ARBs), which was already high in 1995, increased moderately (from 82% to 87%), mainly due to the increase in prescriptions of ARBs (from 0% in 1995 to 15% in 2005). The doses of ACEI are frequently inadequate; only about half of the patients receive the recommended doses of these drugs. Prescriptions of beta-blockers rose gradually from 7% in 1995 to 58% in 2003, partly as a result of two observational studies carried out in Italy in 2000 (BRING-UP) (11) and in 2002 (BRING-UP 2) (12) that were explicitly designed to increase the use of beta-blockers in CHF, and then settled around 50%. Thus, the use of beta-blockers in everyday clinical practice is still far below that observed in recent trials (70% to 80%). Furthermore, the prescribed doses of beta-blockers are, on average, much lower than those recommended. For example, in the IN-CHF Registry, the average daily dose of carvedilol, used in 80% of the patients prescribed a beta-blocker, was no more than 20 mg and tended to decrease rather than increase in recent years. The prescriptions of digitalis decreased from 70% to about 27%.

The overall profile of pharmacologic treatment being received at the moment patients with CHF had an acute destabilization was analyzed in the previously mentioned Italian survey (1) (Table 49.2). In general, the main treatments recommended in CHF were largely underprescribed: ACEI/ARBs 72%, beta-blockers 32%, aldosterone antagonists 34%. ACEI/ARBs were being taken by 53% of patients and beta-blockers by 48% in the Acute Decompensated Heart Failure National Registry (ADHERE) Registry (8) and by 60% and 50%, respectively, in the initiation management pre-discharge assessment of carvedilol heart failure (IMPACT-HF) Registry (4). Data reported in these United States registries and the Italian survey are not comparable because the U.S. observational studies include both de novo and worsening HF. However, it is conceivable that greater care and continuity in the choice of long-term therapy could increase efficacy in preventing acute events.

A comparison of the therapy being received at the time of admission to hospital because of an acute event and that prescribed at discharge in 1460 survivors of acute-on-chronic heart failure demonstrates that the therapeutic management was reconsidered by doctors (Table 49.2): the frequencies of prescriptions increased for ACEI/ARBs from 73% to 84%, for beta-blockers from 32% to 45%, and for aldosterone antagonists from 34% to 66%. The prescription of diuretics increased from 81% to 94%. In the ADHERE Registry, the frequencies of discharge prescriptions following an acute destabilization were 69% for ACEI/ARBs and 59% for beta-blockers (13). According to data collected in the Euroheart Survey I, ACEI/ARBs were administered at discharge to 86% of patients, beta-blockers to 64%, and aldosterone antagonists to 47% (2,14). The IMPACT–HF Registry documented that the use of ACEI/ARBs increased from 60% at admission to 71% at discharge, while the use of beta-blockers rose from 50% to 61% (4) and the medication rates remained similar in a control 2 months after discharge. The discharge doses of drugs were considered appropriate in 58% of cases for ACEIs and in only 25% of cases for beta-blockers (4). However, it should be considered that the recommended dose in patients with stable CHF can be different from the effective dose in patients with a recent destabilization or those with advanced CHF. In such patients even low doses, for example 6.25 mg of carvedilol twice daily, have been

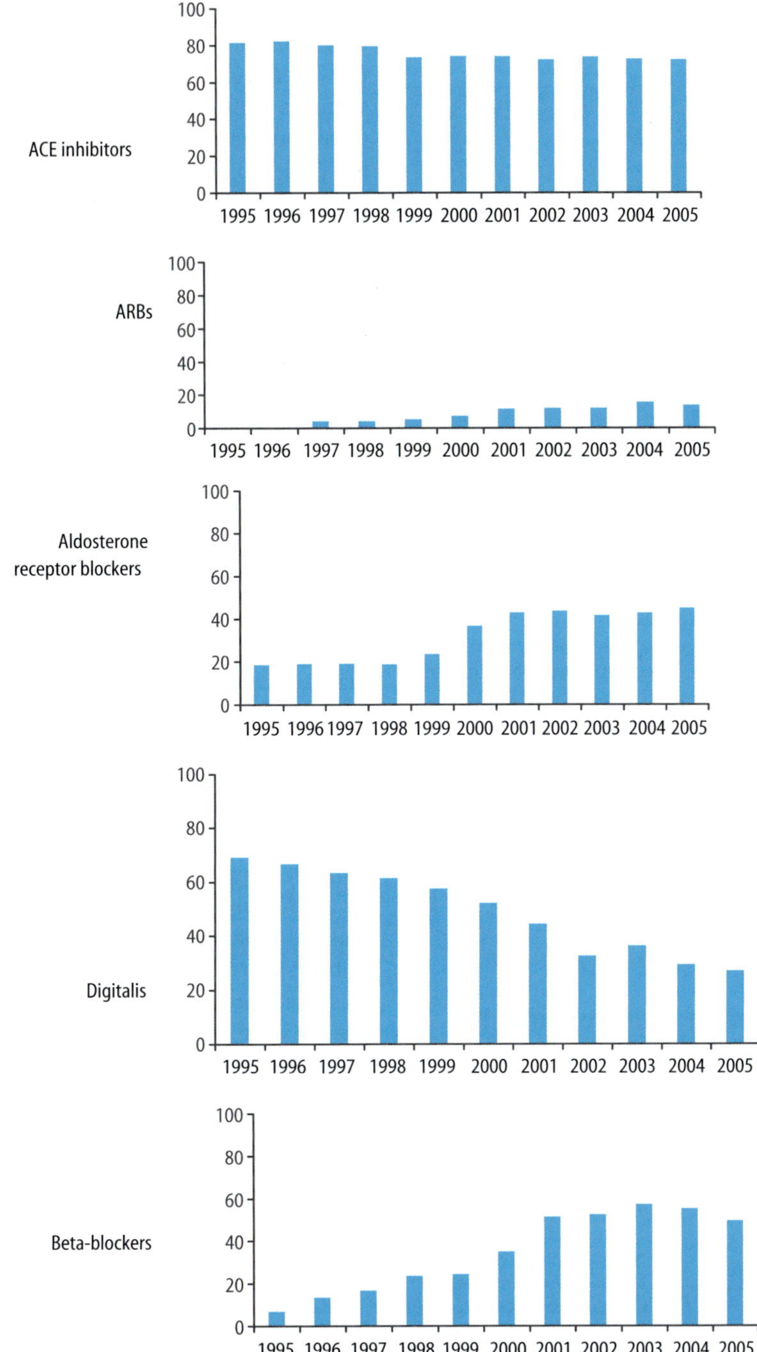

FIGURE 49.1. IN-CHF database: drug prescription by year in the last decade. ACE, angiotensin-converting enzyme; ARB, angiotensin-receptor blocker.

Table 49.2. Italian survey on AHF: pharmacologic treatments in patients discharged alive after an admission for acute-on-chronic heart failure ($n = 1460$)

Pharmacologic treatment	Before hospitalization n (%)	At discharge n (%)
ACEIs	920 (63.0)	1070 (73.3)
ARBs	173 (11.9)	200 (13.7)
ACEI/ARBs	1067 (73.1)	1229 (84.2)
Aldosterone blockers	503 (34.5)	968 (66.3)
Diuretics	1181 (80.9)	1375 (94.2)
Beta-blockers	476 (32.6)	658 (45.1)
Digitalis	549 (37.6)	601 (41.2)
Amiodarone	276 (18.9)	363 (24.9)
Nitrates	481 (33.0)	575 (39.4)
Calcium channel blockers	206 (14.1)	189 (13.0)
Statins	360 (24.7)	450 (30.8)
Oral anticolagulants	428 (29.3)	480 (32.9)
Antiplatelets	634 (43.4)	752 (51.5)

ACEI, angiotensin-converting enzyme inhibitor; ARB, angiotensin-receptor blocker.
All (except for Ca-channel blockers) $p < 0.05$.

reported to be effective, also on hard end points (15,16). Anticoagulants or antiplatelet agents are frequently prescribed despite the paucity of published data supporting their systematic use; they were being taken by 73% of patients admitted to hospital because of acute-on-chronic heart failure, by 84% of patients at discharge in the Italian survey (1), and by 75% of the patients in the ADHERE Registry (8).

Therapeutic Patterns According to Clinical Profiles

The guidelines recently released by the European Society of Cardiology (ESC) distinguish various different clinical profiles of AHF; the most relevant of them are reported in Table 49.3 (17). One other fundamental distinction is the differentiation between de novo AHF and worsening in patients with CHF. Although the clinical presentation may be similar, the biologic background of the patients can be very different in the two cases. In the largest multicenter registries (1,8), the frequencies of de novo AHF and worsening heart failure are approximately equal. In this chapter we consider the patients with acute-on-chronic heart failure, focusing only on their pharmacologic therapy. It should be appreciated that the hemodynamic and clinical pictures of AHF patients with previous CHF can also vary considerably from patient to patient with important therapeutic and prognostic implications. However, the frequencies of the different clinical profiles are hard to determine from the data available in registries of AHF patients. For example, in the IMPACT-HF Registry (4), progressive volume overload without acute pulmonary edema was recorded as the primary cause of AHF in 48% of the patients, pulmonary edema accounted for 8% of admissions, and low-output heart failure was reported as the cause of admission in only 1% of the cases. The remaining patients were classified according to the factor precipitating the acute episode: a pulmonary process in 10%, atrial fibrillation in 8%, an acute coronary syndrome in 12%, and uncontrolled hypertension in 3%. In a survey carried out in two referral centers, the cases of AHF were classified as cardiogenic shock, acute pulmonary edema and congestive HF (exclusive of cardiogenic shock and pulmonary edema), accounting for approximately 5%, 13%, and 82% of the cases, respectively (5). The Italian survey on AHF (1) retrospectively used the clinical classification suggested by the ESC guidelines (17) (Table 49.3). A

Table 49.3. Clinical profiles of AHF according to guidelines on AHF of the European Society of Cardiology (17)

- *Acute decompensated heart failure*: with signs and symptoms of acute heart failure, which are mild and do not fulfill criteria for cardiogenic shock, pulmonary edema, or hypertensive crisis
- *Hypertensive AHF*: signs and symptoms of heart failure are accompanied by high blood pressure and relatively preserved left ventricular function with a chest radiograph compatible with acute pulmonary edema
- *Pulmonary edema* (verified by chest x-ray): accompanied by severe respiratory distress, with crackles over the lung and orthopnea, with O_2 saturation <90% on room air prior to treatment
- *Cardiogenic shock*: evidence of tissue hypoperfusion induced by heart failure after correction of preload; is usually characterized by reduced blood pressure (systolic BP < 90 mm Hg or a drop of mean arterial pressure >30 mm Hg) or low urine output (<0.5 mL/kg/h), with a pulse rate >60 bpm with or without evidence of organ congestion

TABLE 49.4. Italian Survey on AHF: pharmacologic therapy on board 1 week before hospital admittance and prescribed at discharge, according to clinical profiles in patients with acute-on-chronic HF

	Hypertensive HF ($n = 131$)		Acute pulmonary edema ($n = 590$)		Acute HF ($n = 656$)		Cardiogenic shock ($n = 83$)	
Drug	Before %	Discharge %	Before %	Discharge %	Before %	Discharge %	Before %	Discharge %
Diuretics	67*	96	80	95	85	94	80*	89
ACEI-ARBs	76*	84*	77	88	70	81	66*	77*
Beta-blockers	29	43	33	47	32	44	36	42
Aldosterone blockers	20*	47*	33	66	40	71	30*	63*
Digitalis	22*	31*	33	38	46	48	29	28
Oral nitrates	39*	55*	37	47	26	29	45	42*
Anticoagulants	16*	22*	23	27	40	43	14*	16*
Antiplatelets	44*	60*	52	60	34	40	55*	70*
Amiodarone	13	19	20	26	19	25	19	26
Ca-antagonists	25*	38*	16	12	10	9	13*	11*
Statins	31*	37*	28	38	21	23	24	36*

*Indicate the drugs whose prescription rates were significantly different among groups, either before admission or at discharge. $p < 0.05$.

systolic blood pressure of 160 mm Hg was taken as the cutoff to define hypertensive heart failure (the guidelines do not provide a cutoff). A clinical profile of acute decompensated heart failure was identified in 45% of patients, pulmonary edema in 40%, hypertensive heart failure in 9%, and cardiogenic shock in 7% of the patients with acute-on-chronic heart failure.

The drugs being taken before the acute event and those prescribed at discharge to the survivors are reported in Table 49.4. There are some trends in common to all the clinical pictures. There were increases in the prescriptions of diuretics, already chronically administered to about 80% of the patients, ACEI/ARBs and beta-blockers. Aldosterone antagonists, being taken by only about one third of patients at admission, were prescribed to approximately two thirds at discharge. The pattern for antiplatelets was similar. Although the increased prescription of beta-blockers can be noted in all the groups, the use of these drugs nevertheless remained relatively modest, being prescribed to well below 50% of discharged patients. It is possible that cardiologists still have concerns about starting beta-blocker therapy immediately after an acute decompensation despite the reassuring results, in particular concerning the safety of this strategy, observed in the carvedilol prospective randomized cumulative survival (COPERNICUS) (15), IMPACT-HF (4) and BRING-UP 2 (12) studies. On the other hand, a general practitioner rarely takes the initiative to start a recently discharged patient on a beta-blocker that was not prescribed by a cardiologist. For patients admitted with hypertensive AHF, there appears not to be a particular tendency to prescribe blood pressure–lowering drugs from among those recommended for use in heart failure. This is particularly noteworthy for the lack of increase in the use of beta-blockers (43% of prescriptions at discharge). Calcium antagonists, not recommended in heart failure, are used more frequently in hypertensive patients than in AHF patients who are not hypertensive. Oral nitrates, whose long-term benefit/risk profile, at least in Caucasian patients with CHF and in the absence of hydralazine, has yet to be demonstrated, are prescribed to more than half the patients with acute-on-chronic heart failure and hypertension, whereas they are prescribed to only one third of nonhypertensive AHF patients. Furthermore, it seems that aldosterone antagonists are used less frequently in the hypertensive patients.

Overall, it does not appear that the different clinical profiles defined in the ESC guidelines are treated with substantially different maintenance therapies. In other words, the specific clinical presentations characterizing acute clinical patterns do not seem to prompt cardiologists to use different maintenance therapies.

TABLE 49.5. Italian Survey on AHF: pharmacologic therapy on board 1 week before hospital admittance and prescribed at discharge in patients with acute-on-chronic HF according to age

Age (No.)	<65 (298)		65–80 (858)		>80 (304)	
Drugs	Before %	Discharge %	Before %	Discharge %	Before %	Discharge %
Diuretics	79	92*	81	95	82	93
ACEI-ARBs	71	84	73	85	74	81
Beta-blockers	39*	54*	32	46	28*	34*
Aldosterone blockers	42*	70*	34	67	27	59*
Digitalis	38	45*	38	42	36	35
Oral nitrates	23*	29*	33	39	43*	51*
Anticoagulants	36*	36*	31	36	17*	20*
Antiplatelets	36*	48*	43	50	51*	60*
Amiodarone	19	23	19	26	18	24
Ca-antagonists	7*	7*	15	13	18*	17*

*Indicate the drugs whose prescription rates were significantly different among groups, either before admission or at discharge. $p < 0.05$.

Therapeutic Patterns According to Age, Etiology of the Underlying Disease, and Comorbidities

Age

The treatments received prior to admission and at discharge from the hospital in relation to the patients' age are reported in Table 49.5. In general, a trend toward a decrease in the frequency of prescription of all drugs recommended in CHF can be noted with increasing age, whereas the prescription of oral nitrates and CA antagonists increases. Antithrombotic drugs are prescribed to over 80% of patients in all age ranges, but in the elderly the preference for antiplatelets rather than anticoagulants is more marked. Overall, the lower rate of drug prescriptions in the elderly is confirmed, while it seems that any change of therapeutic strategies following an acute event is not influenced by the patients' age.

Etiology

The underlying disease in the patients with acute-on-chronic heart failure enrolled in the Italian survey was ischemic in 669, nonischemic in 742, and could not be determined in 49 (Table 49.6). The most marked differences in therapeutic prescriptions at discharge between patients with an ischemic or a nonischemic etiology concerned nitrates, which were prescribed to 53% and 29%

TABLE 49.6. Italian Survey on AHF: pharmacologic therapy on board 1 week before hospital admittance and prescribed at discharge in patients with acute-on-chronic HF according to etiology

Etiology (No.)	Ischemic (669)		Nonischemic (742)		Not determined (49)	
Drug	Before %	Discharge %	Before %	Discharge %	Before %	Discharge %
Diuretics	80*	94	83	94	63	98
ACEI-ARBs	76	85	71	83	67	92
Beta-blockers	40*	49*	27	42	18*	39*
Aldosterone blockers	38*	69	32	65	26	59*
Digitalis	30*	33*	44	48	45	53
Oral nitrates	46*	53*	22	29	18*	18*
Anticoagulants	21*	23*	37	42	22	31
Antiplatelets	56*	68*	32	37	35*	49*
Amiodarone	21	27	18	24	12	16
Ca-antagonists	14*	11*	13	14	29*	27*
Statins	37*	44*	15	20	12*	12*

*Indicate the drugs whose prescription rates were significantly different among groups, either before admission or at discharge. $p < 0.05$.

Table 49.7. Italian Survey on AHF: pharmacologic therapy on board 1 week before hospital admittance and prescribed at discharge in patients with acute-on-chronic HF according to history of arterial hypertension

	Hypertension (971)		No hypertension (489)	
Drug	Before %	Discharge %	Before %	Discharge %
Diuretics	80	95	82	93
ACEI-ARBs	78*	87*	64	79
Beta-blockers	32	46	33	44
Aldosterone blockers	33	64*	38	72
Digitalis	32*	37*	48	49
Oral nitrates	36*	45*	26	29
Anticoagulants	25*	29*	39	41
Antiplatelets	47*	56*	37	42
Amiodarone	20	24	17	26
Ca-antagonists	18*	17*	6	4
Statins	28*	35*	19	23

*Indicate the drugs whose prescription rates were significantly different between groups, either before admission or at discharge. $p < 0.05$.

of these patients, respectively, and antiplatelets (68% and 37%). Beta-blockers, taken by 40% of the ischemic patients and by 27% of the nonischemic ones prior to admission, were prescribed to 49% and 42% of the patients, respectively, at discharge. Statins, as expected, were also administered more frequently to ischemic patients than to nonischemic ones, the respective prescription rates at discharge being 44% and 20%.

Comorbidities

Hypertension

Most of the patients with acute-on-chronic heart failure (67%) had a history of systemic hypertension (Table 49.7). As already noted for hypertensive AHF in relation to other forms of AHF, substantial differences were not seen in changes of prescription rates before admission and at discharge between patients with and without underlying hypertension. Prior to the admission for AHF, hypertensive patients were taking all the recommended drugs more frequently than were their nonhypertensive counterparts, with the exception of beta-blockers (32% vs. 33%), and the frequency of prescriptions increased for all, hypertensives and nonhypertensives, at discharge. This increase in prescriptions also involved beta-blockers, whose prescription rates rose to 46% among hypertensives and to 44% among the nonhypertensives. The prescription rates for calcium antagonists were low before the acute event (6% in nonhypertensives and 18% in hypertensives) and remained so at discharge (4% vs. 17%).

Renal Dysfunction

Of the 1460 patients with acute-on-chronic heart failure, 443 had a history of renal disease, but only 218 had a serum creatinine above 2 mg/dL on admission to hospital (Table 49.8). The most important observations regarding treatment prior to the acute event in these patients compared with

Table 49.8. Italian Survey on AHF: pharmacologic therapy on board 1 week before hospital admittance and prescribed at discharge in patients with acute-on-chronic HF according to the presence of renal dysfunction (creatinemia >2 mg%) at admittance

	≤2 mg% (1197)		>2 mg% (218)	
Creatinine (No.) Drug	Before %	Discharge %	Before %	Discharge %
Diuretics	80	94	84	94
ACEI-ARBs	75*	87*	63	66
Beta-blockers	32	47*	34	35
Aldosterone blockers	35	70*	30	48
Digitalis	38	42	37	36
Oral nitrates	32	38*	41	45
Anticoagulants	29	34	26	28
Antiplatelets	44	51	43	53
Amiodarone	18	23*	23	33

Data available in 1415 patients.
*Indicate the drugs whose prescription rates were significantly different between groups, either before admission or at discharge. $p < 0.05$.

patients with a serum creatinine ≤2 mg/dL was a lesser use of ACEI/ARBs (63% vs. 75%). At discharge the prescription of ACEI/ARBs remained unchanged in patients with serum creatinine >2 mg/dL on admission (63% vs 66%), whereas these prescriptions increased further in patients with serum creatinine ≤2 mg/dL (from 75% to 87%). Prescriptions of aldosterone antagonists, increased in both, much more in patients with serum creatinine ≤2 mg%.

Diabetes

Before admission to hospital, there were not marked differences in therapy between diabetic ($n = 611$) and nondiabetic ($n = 849$) patients: only nitrates, antiplatelets, calcium-antagonists, and statins appeared to be prescribed slightly (but significantly, $p < .05$) more frequently to diabetic patients. At discharge these differences were confirmed together with a lack of substantial changes for the other drugs except beta-blockers, whose use increased from 32% to 43% among the nondiabetics and from 34% to 48% among the diabetics.

Anemia

Thirty-five percent of the patients enrolled in the Italian survey had a hemoglobin concentration <12 g/dL at entry into hospital and can be classified as anemic (Table 49.9). The treatments being administered prior to admission to these patients were similar to those in the patients who were not anemic; only aldosterone antagonists and diuretics were being used slightly more frequently by anemic patients than by nonanemic ones. At discharge the general trend in an increase in prescriptions of recommended drugs was noted in the anemic patients, but to a significantly lesser extent than in the nonanemic patients, for ACEI/ARBs, beta-blockers, and aldosterone antagonists. It should be noted that the administration of anticoagulants and antiplatelets increased similarly in the anemic and nonanemic patients.

TABLE 49.9. Italian Survey on AHF: pharmacologic therapy on board 1 week before hospital admittance and prescribed at discharge in patients with acute-on-chronic HF according to the presence of anemia (Hb <2 g%)

Drug	Anemia (498)		No anemia (911)	
	Before %	Discharge %	Before %	Discharge %
Diuretics	86*	94	78	94
ACEI-ARBs	73	78*	73	88
Beta-blockers	34	39*	32	48
Aldosterone blockers	39*	61*	31	69
Digitalis	39	39	37	42
Oral nitrates	34	41	32	39
Anticoagulants	31	31	28	34
Antiplatelets	44	50	44	52
Amiodarone	21	25	18	24
Ca-antagonists	14	15	14	12
Statins	25	30	25	32

Data available in 1409 patients.

*Indicate the drugs whose prescription rates were significantly different between groups, either before admission or at discharge. $p < 0.05$.

Symptoms, Signs, and Biomarkers as Guides to Long-Term Therapy

To implement chronic therapy after an acute event, the patient must achieve a stable state, which is not always easy to evaluate. About 66% of patients improve substantially with the therapy used in the acute phase, and more than 80% improve in about 3 days (18). In the ADHERE registry, 52% of the patients stated that they were asymptomatic at discharge and 37% reported an improvement in symptoms (13). However, since congestion is the dominant clinical feature during AHF, it is worth noting that about half the patients had no weight change or lost less than 2 kg during their hospital admission (and 16% had a weight gain), despite therapy, presumably indicating that the congestion was incompletely relieved notwithstanding the remission of symptoms (13). In patients with CHF the threshold for symptoms can be increased because of physiologic or perceptive adaptation. This means that a level of congestion that could constitute a permanent signal of neurohormonal activation, although not generating symptoms, is not picked up. Thus, while symptoms may be a useful guide to the initial treatment of patients with AHF, they may not be a suitable guide to maintenance therapy. In a prospective analysis of patients admitted to hospital with New York Heart Association (NYHA) class IV CHF, signs of congestion were recorded 4 to 6 weeks after discharge, and the patients were followed up for 2 years. It was found that the 2-year survival rate among patients without congestion at about 1 month after discharge was 87% compared with 67% among patients with one or two criteria of congestion, and 41% among those who had three to five signs of congestion (19). In the ACTIVE study, the association with tolvaptan, a drug blocking V2 vasopressin receptors, led to better resolution of the congestion prior to discharge from hospital (20).

Many patients with systolic heart failure can have pulmonary congestion without crepitations because of increased lymph drainage and perivascular remodeling (18). The presence of a third heart sound and an altered response to the Valsalva maneuver are more sensitive indicators of raised left ventricular filling pressure than are lung crepitations (21). The clinical signs of raised right ventricular filling pressure, such as jugular swelling, are also reliable indicators of raised left ventricular filling pressure (22). Judging from the results of the evaluation study of congestive heart failure and pulmonary artery catheter effectiveness (ESCAPE) trial, the clinical evaluation of low output states is more difficult (18). However, clinical stability can reasonably be assumed to have been achieved when symptoms have disappeared, edema has resolved, the jugular venous pressure is <8 cm, and the patient has an acceptable systolic arterial pressure, no postural symptoms during ambulation, a steady fluid balance, and a not overtly disturbed renal function (18). A consistent reduction (>100%) of B-type natriuretic protein (BNP) is another element suggestive of stabilization (18).

Two biomarkers, troponin and BNP, reflect the degree of myocyte damage and ventricular dysfunction during an episode of AHF. Troponin is raised in almost all episodes of AHF related to myocardial ischemia and in many episodes that occur in patients in whom an ischemic etiology of the heart disease has not been demonstrated (1,11,23). While troponin is a sensitive indicator of the severity of myocardial distress, BNP is an expression of ventricular overload and wall stress, and BNP levels reflect ventricular functional and hemodynamic compromise during the acute episode. Although individual values of BNP can vary considerably, there is a relatively strong relationship between serial changes in BNP and pulmonary wedge pressure (PWP) (18). Plasma BNP levels can continue to decrease even after the PWP has stabilized and the value of BNP at discharge from hospital is a reliable predictor of midterm outcome (18,24,25). For this reason, both troponin and, even more, BNP can act as guides to the type and intensity of treatment for AHF during and after the period in hospital.

The literature on pharmacologic treatment of AHF is completely focused on the immediate management, in particular infusion therapy. There is very limited clinical information, and consequently a lack of guidelines, on how to manage the chronic, ongoing therapy during an acute event and on how to adapt the subsequent therapy. Furthermore, the randomized studies carried out so far to study the effects of new therapeutic approaches to AHF have not taken into consideration the specific clinical profiles of the patients enrolled and therefore the background therapies, corresponding to the various clinical pictures, being used in the patients. There is a considerable body of data on the use of ACE inhibitors during acute or postacute myocardial infarction associated with left ventricular dysfunction or heart failure. In general, these drugs, unquestionably useful in the long-term management of heart failure, have given only moderately positive results in the short term (26). They should be used with care: the doses can be reduced or the drugs temporarily withdrawn in patients with marked hypotension or worsening renal failure during the acute event (14,27). Euvolemia is important for their efficacy: fluid retention can blunt the therapeutic effects of ACEIs, and fluid depletion can potentiate their adverse effects (27).

Similar recommendations have been made for the use of beta-blockers in AHF, a conceptually critical problem considering both the short-term negative inotropic effects of these drugs and the abrupt hemodynamic and biohumoral changes that an acute destabilization involves. It is generally recommended that the doses of beta-blockers are reduced during AHF, without suspending the drugs (14,17,27), but no study has been carried out to investigate this specifically. The positive results of COPERNICUS, in which carvedilol treatment was cautiously started in euvolemic patients with NYHA class IV and a left ventricular ejection fraction <25%, encourage maintaining the use of beta-blockers even in patients with signs and symptoms of severe heart failure (15). It has also been demonstrated, in patients who were not receiving treatment with ACEIs and beta-blockers and who did not have contraindications to their use, that starting treatment during a hospital admission for worsening heart failure is safe and can improve the use of drugs and the compliance with treatment, thus favoring their greatest possible efficacy through appropriate use (3,28). Indeed, the IMPACT-HF trial showed the safety and good compliance of beta-blocker therapy started early before discharge with midterm increase in prescriptions, a strategy that had raised the greatest doubts concerning feasibility and safety (4). Aldosterone antagonists have been demonstrated to be effective when started in patients with advanced CHF (29) and in patients with left ventricular dysfunction and clinical signs of heart failure after acute myocardial infarction (30). It is therefore considered appropriate to maintain or start treatment with these drugs if renal function is not greatly compromised (creatinemia >2.5 mg/dL) and serum potassium is not elevated (>5.5 mEq/L).

Conclusion

Acute heart failure is a very high risk event. In the Italian Survey, from which some of the data reported here were drawn, 7.2% of the patients died during their hospital admission and the 6-month mortality rate was nearly 22% (1). While the in-hospital mortality varies between about 4% and 8% in the different registries and trials, mainly in relation to the time spent in hospital (which, in its turn, varies from an average of 4 to 11 days) (1–7), the mortality at 2 to 3 months is very similar on different continents and in different health care contexts, being about 12% to 13% (1,2,8). The acute event in those patients who do survive is one further step toward progressively worsening heart failure. In this setting, a few considerations can be made from the observation of the background therapy prior to the decompensation and the maintenance therapy at discharge.

First, as repeatedly noted in the past, the frequency of prescriptions and the doses of recommended drugs are well below those advised. It is difficult to determine whether this is related to inadequate assimilation of the guidelines or to an objective difficulty in implementing the recommendations in real patients, who are notoriously different from those enrolled in the trials that generated the results on which the therapeutic recommendations are based and then generalized to populations in which they have not always been exhaustively documented. This is of particular relevance for age: patients enrolled in surveys and registries are, on average, much older than patients enrolled in trials. However, it seems reasonable to consider that since this underprescribing has been recorded in patients who shortly afterward were to have a destabilization, more intense and careful treatment would be advisable in order to provide greater protection against possible decompensations.

Second, comorbid conditions are often considered an important factor limiting the use of drugs, as well as factors worsening prognosis. These considerations are partly confirmed by the data presented but without their entity being exaggerated. Drug prescriptions are not markedly different in subgroups divided by comorbidity. The impact of a comorbid condition is probably more due to its role in the progression of heart failure than to the therapeutic differences that it may induce. However, it should be noted that comorbidities have been analyzed here in isolation, whereas they are actually often associated and this could have a greater impact on the therapeutic patterns.

Third, the therapeutic modifications decided by doctors after an acute event are substantial. There is a clear effort to review the maintenance treatment. Nevertheless, there seems to be unbridgeable gaps. The lack of use of beta-blockers in more than half of the patients, even in the face of evidence that the previous therapy was not able to prevent an acute decompensation, remains difficult to understand. On the other hand, given the limited therapeutic adjustments, once these have been undermined by the imperfect adherence of general practitioners to hospital prescriptions and by the notorious decrease in the compliance of patients over time, one may wonder how much treatment can really change the evolution of CHF. Although the beneficial impact of recommended therapies is beyond discussion, much remains to be done to improve the immediate therapeutic approach to acute decompensation of heart failure and the maintenance therapy that is intended to halt the progressive evolution of the heart failure and prevent destabilizations and the factors precipitating them.

References

1. Tavazzi L, Maggioni AP, Lucci D, on behalf of Italian Survey on Acute Heart Failure Investigators. A nationwide survey on acute heart failure. Eur Heart J 2006;27:1207–15.
2. Cleland JG, Swedberg K, Follath F, et al. The Euroheart Failure Survey Programme: a survey on the quality of care among patients with heart failure in Europe. Part 1: patients characteristics and diagnosis. Eur Heart J 2003;24:442–63.
3. Fonarow GC, Abraham WT, Albert NM, et al. Initial hospital, patient, and performance measure characteristics of the organized program to initiate lifesaving treatment in hospitalized patients with heart failure (OPTIMIZE-HF) program. J Cardiac Fail 2004;10(suppl):S112.
4. O'Connor C, Gattis Stough W, Gallup D, et al. Demographics, clinical characteristics and outcomes of patients hospitalized for decompensated heart failure: observations from the IMPACT-HF Registry. J Cardiac Fail 2005;11:200–205.
5. Rudiger A, Harjola VP, Muller A, et al. Acute heart failure: clinical presentation, one-year mortality and prognostic factors. Eur J Heart Fail 2005;7:662–70.
6. Lee DS, Austin P, Rouleau JL. Predicting mortality among patients hospitalized for heart failure. JAMA 2003;290:2581–7.
7. Goldberg R, Spencer FA, Farmer C, et al. Incidence and hospital death rates associated with heart failure: a community-wide perspective. Am J Med 2005;118:728–34.
8. Adams KF Jr, Fonarow GC, Emermann CL, et al. Rationale, design and preliminary observations from the first 100,000 cases in the Acute Decompensated Heart Failure National registry (ADHERE). Am Heart J 2005;149:209–16.
9. Opasich C, Rapezzi C, Lucci D, et al. Precipitating factors and decision-making processes or short term worsening heart failure treatment (from the IN-CHF Registry). Am J Cardiol 2001;88:382–7.
10. Ghali JK, Kadakis S, Cooper E, et al. Precipitating factors leading to decompensation of heart failure. Arch Intern Med 1988;148:2013–16.
11. Maggioni AP, Sinagra G, Opasich C, et al. Treatment of chronic heart failure with beta-adrenergic blockade beyond controlled clinical trials: the BRING-UP experience. Heart 2003;89:299–305.
12. Opasich C, Boccanelli A, Cafiero M, et al. Programme to improve the use of beta-blockers for heart failure in the elderly and in those with severe symptoms: results of the BRING-UP 2 Study. Eur J Heart Fail 2006;8:649–57.
13. Gheorghiade M, Filippatos G. Reassessing treatment of acute heart failure syndromes: the ADHERE Registry. Eur Heart J Suppl 2005;7:B13–B19.
14. The Task Force for the Diagnosis and Treatment of Chronic Heart Failure of the European Society of Cardiology. Guidelines for the diagnosis and treatment of chronic heart failure: HF. Eur Heart J 2005;26:1115–40.
15. Krum H, Roecker EB, Mohacsi P, et al. Effects of initiating carvedilol in patients with severe chronic heart failure. JAMA 2003;289:712–18.
16. Bristow M, Gilbert EM, Abraham WT, et al. Carvedilol procedures dose-related improvements in left ventricular function and survival in subjects with chronic heart failure. Circulation 1996;94:2807–16.
17. The task force on acute heart failure of the European Society of Cardiology. Executive summary of the guidelines on the diagnosis and treatment of acute heart failure. Eur Heart J 2005;26:384–416.
18. Nohria A, Mileniczuk LM, Warner Stevenson L. Evaluation and monitoring of patients with acute heart failure syndromes. Am J Cardiol 2005;96:32G–40G.
19. Lucas C, Johnson W, Hamilton MA, et al. Freedom from congestion predicts good survival despite previous class IV symptoms of heart failure. Am Heart J 2000;140:840–7.
20. Gheorghiade M, Gattis WA, O'Connor CM, et al. Effects of tolvaptan, a vasopressin antagonist, in patients hospitalized with worsening heart failure. JAMA 2004;291:1963–71.
21. Schmidt DE, Shah PK. Accurate detection of elevated left ventricular filling pressure by a simplified bedside application of the Valsalva maneuver. Am J Cardiol 1993;71:462–5.
22. Chakko S, Wodska D, Martinez H, et al. Clinical, radiographic and hemodynamic correlations in chronic congestive heart failure: conflicting results may lead to inappropriate care. Am J Med 1991;90:353–9.
23. Horwich TB, Patel J, MacLellan WR, et al. Cardiac troponin I is associated with impaired hemodynamics, progressive left ventricular dysfunction, and increased mortality rates in advanced heart failure. Circulation 2003;108:833–38.
24. Gackowski A, Isnard R, Golmard JL, et al. Comparison of echocardiography and plasma B-type natriuretic peptide for monitoring the response to treatment in acute heart failure Eur Heart J 2004;25:1788–96.

25. Metra M, Nodari S, Brentana L, et al. Time course and prognostic value of NT-proBNP plasma levels in the patients with acute heart failure. J Am Coll Cardiol 2005;45(suppl A):139A.
26. Teo KK, Yusuf S, Pfeffer M, et al. Effects of long-term treatment with angiotensin-converting enzyme inhibitors in the presence or absence of aspirin: a systematic review. Lancet 2002;360:1037–43.
27. ACC/AHA 2005 Guideline Update for the diagnosis and management of chronic heart failure in the adult. J Am Coll Cardiol 2005;46:1116–43.
28. Tarantini L, Cioffi G, Opasich C, et al. Pre-discharge initiation of beta-blockers therapy in elderly hospitalized for acute decompensation of chronic heart failure: an effective strategy for the implementation of beta-blockade in heart failure. Ital Heart J 2004;5:441–9.
29. Pitt B, Zannad F, Remme WJ, et al., for the randomized Aldactone evaluation study investigators: the effect of spironolactone on morbidity and mortality in patients with severe heart failure. N Engl J Med 1990;341:709–17.
30. Pitt B, William G, Remme W, et al. The EPHESUS trial: eplerenone in patients with heart failure due to systolic dysfunction complicating acute myocardial infarction: eplerenone postAMI heart failure efficacy and survival study. Cardiovascular Drugs Ther 2001;15:79–87.

50
Nitrates in Acute Decompensated Heart Failure

Jean-Michel Tartière and Alain Cohen Solal

Acute decompensated heart failure (ADHF) is associated with ventriculoarterial mismatch. In this case, the left ventricular afterload is usually increased, leading to modifications of ventricular performance (iniotropy and lusitropy). According to myocardial properties and the initial left-ventricular ejection fraction (LVEF) defining systolic or diastolic heart failure, the left-ventricular output impedance could be defined by three components (Fig. 50.1): the steady component or systemic vascular resistance, the pulsatile component or characteristic impedance, and the wave component corresponding to a reflected pulse wave returning to the heart. All of these components are increased in patients with heart failure[1–6]. This ventriculoarterial mismatch is associated with decreasing cardiac output[7]. Moreover, the lower the contractility, the more load dependent the cardiac output[8], which implies that from diastolic to systolic heart failure, the heart changes from a flow source whatever the pressure to a pressure source whatever the flow. Impaired relaxation and increased left-ventricular filling pressure are common in patients with heart failure whatever the LVEF. This increasing left-ventricular filling pressure is directly related to symptoms and pulmonary edema. Moreover, heart failure is associated with a load dependence of relaxation[9], especially in patients with a low LVEF[10].

Because oxygen consumption of the heart depends on afterload, heart rate, and contractility, ADHF is unbalanced in terms of myocardial oxygen consumption and cardiac output, the final result of myocardial work. In this setting, vasodilators are logical for the treatment of ADHF by improving ventriculoarterial coupling without deleterious effect (increase of myocardial oxygen consumption and cytosolic calcium concentration). Vasodilators such as nitric oxide (NO) donors (sodium nitroprusside or organic nitrates) improve ventriculoarterial coupling by decreasing all the components of left-ventricular output impedance and left-ventricular filling pressure and by decreasing forward cardiac flow (described in Figs. 50.1 and 50.2). These hemodynamic effects are associated with improved symptoms and an optimal effect on the energetic balance.

Treatment of ADHF is based on the initial hemodynamic assessment by clinical examination, bedside echocardiography, or, more rarely, use of a Swan-Ganz catheter.

Nitrates

Glyceride trinitrate (or nitroglycerin), isosorbide mononitrate, and isosorbide dinitrate are frequently used in the management of ADHF. Therapeutic effects are based on the degradation of organic nitrates in the presence of sulfhydryl groups with liberation of nitric oxide (NO) molecules.

Hemodynamic Effects

Nitrates, by liberating NO molecules, induce relaxation of smooth muscle cells of arteries and veins. Whatever the dosage, nitrates are associated with a constant venodilatation, but arterial vasodilatation increases progressively

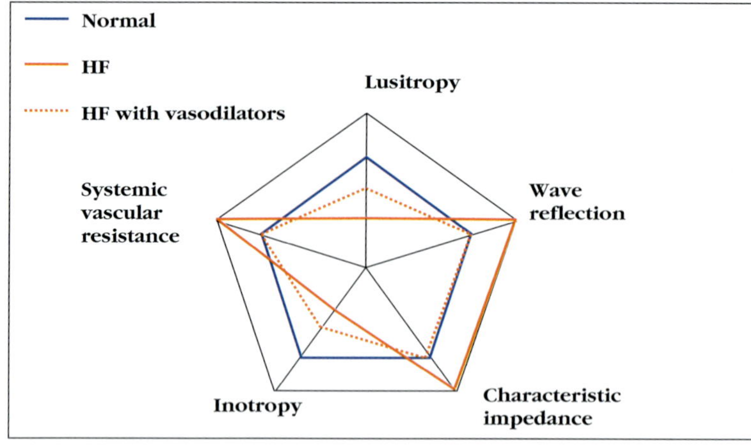

Figure 50.1. Pentagonal representation of ventriculoarterial coupling.

with increased plasma nitrate concentration[11]. This vasodilatation is associated with decreased preload and afterload and coronary vasodilatation. The final consequences of these hemodynamic modifications are decreased blood pressure and left-ventricular filling pressure[11,12]. As the blood pressure decreases, characteristic impedance decreases and reflected waves decrease in amplitude and are delayed after the aortic valve closure, which improves blood flow in the coronary arteries. The effect of nitrates on cardiac output is therefore the result of their combined effect on arterial and venous beds and dependent on left-ventricular performance. With left-ventricular systolic dysfunction and biventricular dilatation, the net effect on stroke volume, at least at moderate doses, is an increase secondary to decreased afterload and, in cases of biventricular dilatation, by improving afterload and interventricular dependence. On the contrary, in cases of a nonenlarged left ventricle with preserved LVEF, the reduction in venous return and preload may predominate and result in reduced stroke volume. The decreased aortic blood pressure is generally underestimated by use of brachial or radial, invasive or noninvasive blood pressure assessment because of the pulse amplification from the aorta to the peripheral arteries.

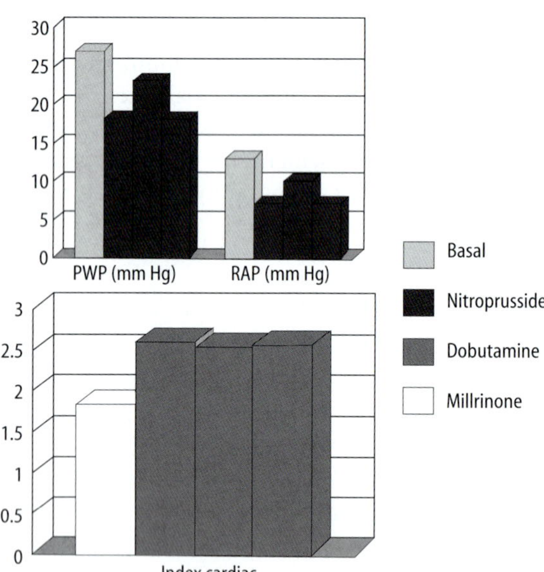

Figure 50.2. Comparison of sodium nitroprusside, dobutamine and milrinone in cardiac output after acute decompensated heart failure (ADHF). For the same modification of cardiac output, nitroprusside offers more important improvement in terms of pulmonary wedge pressure and right atrial pressure than dobutamine and milrinone.[13] PWP, pulmonary wedge pressure; RAP, right atrial pressure.

Clinical Trials

Cotter et al.[13] compared the efficacy and safety of high-dose isosorbide dinitrate plus low-dose furosemide versus high-dose furosemide plus low-dose isosorbide dinitrate in 110 patients with severe pulmonary edema. In the isosorbide dinitrate arm, after receiving intravenous furosemide (40 mg) and morphine (3 mg bolus), patients received a 3-mg bolus of nitrate every 5 minutes until oxygen saturation was greater than 96% or mean arterial blood pressure had decreased by 30% or was below 90 mm Hg. This regimen was associated with a reduced need for mechanical ventilation and a lower rate of myocardial infarction.

In the Vasodilatation in the Management of Acute Congestive Heart Failure (VMAC) study,[12] 489 patients with dyspnea at rest due to decompensated heart failure were randomly assigned to receive nesiritide infusion, nitroglycerin, or placebo, and were compared in the first 24 hours. Relatively low doses of nitroglycerin were associated with significant hemodynamic effects but lesser than that for nesiritide. Symptoms were similar after both therapies. Moreover, the 6-month death rate was comparable between the groups receiving nesiritide (25.1%) and nitroglycerin (20.8%).

Unfortunately, no trial results comparing nitrates with placebo in ADHF are available. However, short-term studies of ADHF show major hemodynamic and clinical benefits and safe use, and long-term use of vasodilators (fixed dose of hydralazine and isosorbide dinitrate) during chronic HF has been shown to increase survival among black patients under standard therapy for advanced heart failure[14].

Doses

Isosorbide dinitrate is clearly recommended during acute pulmonary edema. Moreover, nitrates can be given by sublingual pulverization, especially in an emergency, before venous catheterization, or by intravenous administration (bolus or continuous infusion). Continuous infusion doses must be adapted according to the drug. During congestive heart failure, recommended doses are usually 1 to 8 mg/h for nitroglycerin and 2 to 15 mg/h for isosorbide dinitrate, with a ratio of approximately 1 mg of nitroglycerin for 2.5 mg of isosorbide dinitrate.

Adverse Effects

Because degradation of nitrates needs the presence of sulfhydryl groups in an organism, exhaustion of these groups, especially after a long exposure to nitrates, leads to a loss of therapeutic activity. Tachyphylaxis can occur during the first 24 hours after treatment. Adverse effects of nitrates are usually dose dependent and consist of headache, flush, tachycardia and palpitations, and hypotension. These effects are reversed by withdrawal of the drug, but because of the half-life (1 to 5 hours), hemodynamic recovery can be delayed. A rare and serious adverse effect is the occurrence of methemoglobinemia. This complication is treated by use of methylene blue, restoring the normal function of hemoglobin.

Nitrates are indicated in ADHF, especially in cases of high blood pressure and left-ventricular filling pressure, or with myocardial ischemia without right-ventricular myocardial infarction. Because these drugs are easily obtainable, efficient and have different modes of administration (sublingual, intravenous bolus, or continuous infusion), they are helpful in emergencies or in intensive care units.

Sodium Nitroprusside

Sodium nitroprusside is metabolized in erythrocytes and degraded with NO and cyanide. The NO molecule is responsible for the drug's effects, and cyanide, a toxic molecule, is rapidly converted in the liver to thiocyanate.

Hemodynamic Effects

Sodium nitroprusside, by liberation of NO molecules such as nitrates, induces relaxation of smooth muscle cells in arteries and veins. This vasodilatation is also associated with decreased systemic vascular resistance, characteristic decrease in impedance, and wave reflection phenomenon. In patients with left ventriculoarterial mismatch and low cardiac output, compared with dobutamine or phosphodiesterase inhibitors, sodium nitroprusside is associated with a major increase in stroke volume and cardiac output[15–17] (Fig. 50.3) without increasing myocardial oxygen consumption. Hemodynamic improvement is associated with increasing diuresis and

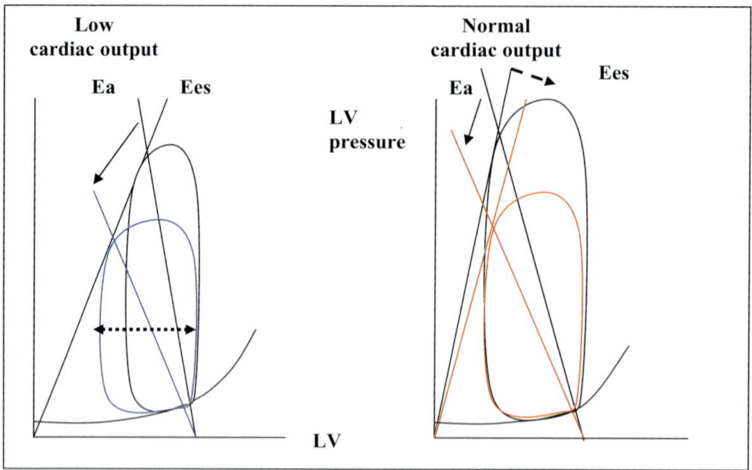

FIGURE 50.3. Two types of vasodilator effect on the pressure-volume loop in ADHF according to initial cardiac output. Subjects without ADHF show balanced ventriculoarterial coupling. Heart failure (HF) is associated with impaired inotropy and lusitropy and increasing afterload (systemic vascular resistance, characteristic impedance, and wave reflection). In HF, nitrate vasodilators improve ventriculoarterial coupling by decreasing all the components of afterload, with an indirect effect on myocardial function. In patients with low cardiac output and high arterial elastance (Ea; left), arterial vasodilatation (VD) (blue line) is associated with decreasing arterial elastance and an indirect improvement of stroke volume and cardiac output. In patients with normal cardiac output but high Ea (right), arterial vasodilatation (red line) is associated with decreasing Ea and end systolic elastance (Ees), without modification of stroke volume or cardiac output.

natriuresis[17] and improved renal function[16]. However, sodium nitroprusside exacerbates myocardial ischemia in coronary occlusion[18]. In acute myocardial infarction with heart failure, nitroprusside is associated with worsening prognosis when the dosage begins in the first 9 hours after heart attack[19]. However, the use of nitroprusside during stable coronary disease has never been associated with worsening myocardial ischemia, and myocardial effects are comparable with those of nitrate in patients with coronary stenosis[20]. Moreover, in severe pulmonary insufficiency, the ventilation-perfusion mismatch could be adversely altered. When the decrease in systemic vascular resistance is not balanced by the increased cardiac output, or when cardiac output is initially normal, blood pressure could therefore quickly fall, with severe hypotension.

Clinical Trials

Khot et al.[16] showed that nitroprusside rapidly and safely improved cardiac index, stroke volume, and pulmonary wedge pressure in patients with ADHF due to severe left-ventricular systolic dysfunction and severe aortic stenosis. However, although the authors showed that sodium nitroprusside is usable even in severe situations, it is not recommended for this indication; as well, the absence of controls in this study is a major issue. Further studies are therefore necessary in this setting.

Other studies have shown a rapid decrease in neurohormonal activation (A- and B-type natriuretic peptides, endothelin) after short-term use of nitroprusside during class IV heart failure[21].

Dosage

The recommended dosage of sodium nitroprusside is usually 0.5 to 10 μg/kg/min. Hemodynamic features must be strictly monitored during infusion, especially during dosage changes. The starting dose should be low, about 0.25 μg/kg/min. The maximal dose is generally obtained after a prespecified target is reached: cardiac output, systemic vascular resistance, mean blood pressure, or alleviated symptoms. The therapeutic dosage is usually well below 10 μg/kg/min.

Adverse Effects

Cyanide toxic effects are a major issue in nitroprusside use. The effects can be precipitated by severe liver or renal insufficiency. Hydroxycobalamin is an antidote for cyanide poisoning, but its use requires high doses. However, this serious adverse effect is rare with the dosage and infusion duration usually used for ADHF, and thiocyanate level can be assessed regularly during infusion if necessary.

Methemoglobinemia is also a rare adverse effect and is treated by methylene blue infusion. Finally, sodium nitroprusside is a light-sensitive molecule requiring special light protection during infusion.

Other adverse effects of nitroprusside, including headache, nausea, vomiting, anorexia, pain, and hypotension, are usually dose dependent. These effects are rapidly reversed by withdrawal of the drug, because of the short half-life (2 minutes).

Sodium nitroprusside is indicated in ADHF, especially in cases of high blood pressure and high left ventricular filling pressure associated with low cardiac output, to improve ventriculoarterial coupling and to increase cardiac output. Cardiogenic shock is an indication for nitroprusside, but the hemodynamic profile of the patient must be clearly defined, by low cardiac output and high systemic vascular resistance corresponding to normal or subnormal mean blood pressure.

References

1. Pepine CJ, Nichols WW, Conti CR. Aortic input impedance in heart failure. Circulation. 1978;58: 460–5.
2. Merillon JP, Fontenier G, Lerallut JF, et al. Aortic input impedance in heart failure: comparison with normal subjects and its changes during vasodilator therapy. Eur Heart J. 1984;5:447–55.
3. Laskey WK, Kussmaul WG. Arterial wave reflection in heart failure. Circulation. 1987;75:711–22.
4. Hundley WG, Kitzman DW, Morgan TM, et al. Cardiac cycle-dependent changes in aortic area and distensibility are reduced in older patients with isolated diastolic heart failure and correlate with exercise intolerance. J Am Coll Cardiol. 2001;38:796–802.
5. Mitchell GF, Tardif JC, Arnold JM, et al. Pulsatile hemodynamics in congestive heart failure. Hypertension. 2001;38:1433–9.
6. Kawaguchi M, Hay I, Fetics B, Kass DA. Combined ventricular systolic and arterial stiffening in patients with heart failure and preserved ejection fraction. Implications for systolic and diastolic reserve limitations. Circulation. 2003;107:714–20.
7. Maruyama Y, Nishioka O, Nozaki E, et al. Effects of arterial distensibility on left ventricular ejection in the depressed contractile state. Cardiovasc Res. 1993;27:182–7.
8. Westerhof N, O'Rourke MF. Haemodynamic basis for the development of left ventricular failure in systolic hypertension and for its logical therapy. J Hypertens. 1995;13:943–52.
9. Leite-Moreira AF, Correia-Pinto J, Gillebert TC. Afterload induced changes in myocardial relaxation: a mechanism for diastolic dysfunction. Cardiovasc Res. 1999;43:344–53.
10. Eichhorn EJ, Willard JE, Alvarez L, et al. Are contraction and relaxation coupled in patients with and without congestive heart failure? Circulation. 1992;85:2132–9.
11. Imhof PR, Ott B, Frankhauser P, Chu LC, Hodler J. Difference in nitroglycerin dose-response in the venous and arterial beds. Eur J Clin Pharmacol. 1980;18:455–60.
12. Intravenous nesiritide vs nitroglycerin for treatment of decompensated congestive heart failure: a randomized controlled trial. JAMA. 2002;287: 1531–40.
13. Cotter G, Metzkor E, Kaluski E, et al. Randomised trial of high-dose isosorbide dinitrate plus low-dose furosemide versus high-dose furosemide plus low-dose isosorbide dinitrate in severe pulmonary oedema. Lancet. 1998;351:389–93.
14. Taylor AL, Ziesche S, Yancy C, et al. Combination of isosorbide dinitrate and hydralazine in blacks with heart failure. N Engl J Med. 2004;351:2049–57.
15. Monrad ES, Baim DS, Smith HS, Lanoue AS. Milrinone, dobutamine, and nitroprusside: comparative effects on hemodynamics and myocardial energetics in patients with severe congestive heart failure. Circulation. 1986;73:III168–74.
16. Khot UN, Novaro GM, Popovic ZB, et al. Nitroprusside in critically ill patients with left ventricular dysfunction and aortic stenosis. N Engl J Med. 2003;348:1756–63.
17. Guiha NH, Cohn JN, Mikulic E, Franciosa JA, Limas CJ. Treatment of refractory heart failure with infusion of nitroprusside. N Engl J Med. 1974;291: 587–92.

18. Pearlman AS, Engler RL, Goldstein RA, Kent KM, Epstein SE. Relative effects of nitroglycerin and nitroprusside during experimental acute myocardial ischemia. Eur J Cardiol. 1980;11:295–313.
19. Cohn JN, Franciosa JA, Francis GS, et al. Effect of short-term infusion of sodium nitroprusside on mortality rate in acute myocardial infarction complicated by left ventricular failure: results of a Veterans Administration cooperative study. N Engl J Med. 1982;306:1129–35.
20. Ramanathan KB, Yamazaki H, Bodenheimer MM, Banka VS, Helfant RH. Regional coronary flow and contraction after partial coronary obstruction. Comparative effects of nitroglycerin and nitroprusside. Chest. 1981;80:481–6.
21. Johnson W, Omland T, Hall C, et al. Neurohormonal activation rapidly decreases after intravenous therapy with diuretics and vasodilators for class IV heart failure. J Am Coll Cardiol. 2002; 39:1623–9.

51
Use of Nesiritide in the Management Algorithm of Acute Decompensated Heart Failure

Clyde W. Yancy

Acute decompensated heart failure (ADHF) is an emerging component of heart failure that is incompletely understood, lacks clear pathophysiologic mechanisms, is associated with worrisome outcomes, and is confounded by only minimally effective treatment options. Currently, treatment is targeted toward abnormal hemodynamics and includes diuretics, vasodilators, and inotropes. Nesiritide (B-type natriuretic peptide), represents a novel therapeutic option for ADHF that lowers elevated filling pressures and improves dyspnea. However, the risk/benefit ratio represents an unresolved issue, as important questions persist regarding drug-related morbidity and mortality. More research is needed to address safety, identify the ideal clinical scenario, and to resolve the absence or presence of drug associated risks.

Acute decompensated heart failure has become a major clinical challenge in the field of heart failure. Whether defined as new-onset heart failure or an exacerbation of chronic heart failure, it is apparent that ADHF must be considered an important disease entity. The most recent estimates demonstrate that heart failure as a primary discharge diagnosis accounts for over 1 million hospital discharges and over 6.5 million hospital days. (1) This represents a financial burden that is largely borne by public health resources (e.g., Medicare, and Medicaid). Coincident with the financial considerations are the prognostic implications of a hospitalization for acute decompensated heart failure. The subsequent 6-month readmission rate is 50%, the short-term mortality rate (i.e., at 60 to 90 days) is ~10%, and the 1-year mortality risk is ~30%. (2,3) Thus, when compared to evidence-based standard therapy of chronic heart failure, the 1-year mortality risk after an episode of acute decompensated heart failure is tripled. Whereas an impressive portfolio of effective evidence-based strategies exists as therapy for chronic heart failure, such is not the case for acute heart failure. Guideline-based therapy adjudicated by oversight committees ensures that best practices in the management of heart failure are acknowledged and appropriately encouraged, but efforts to generate guidelines for ADHF have been thwarted by a dearth of clinical trial data addressing this disease entity. Nevertheless, there have been recent guideline iterations that address acute decompensated heart failure (Table 51.1). (2,4) It should be noted that no medical treatment strategy for ADHF has yet been proven to favorably impact the natural history of the disease.

The challenge to identify best treatment practices for ADHF is complicated by an incomplete understanding of the pathophysiology of ADHF. It might be inferred from the abrupt change in the natural history that follows an episode of ADHF that any of several circumstances may be operative: a change in the ventricular substrate, that is, ventricular injury; an act of commission as in a treatment option that results in deleterious outcomes; an act of omission, that is, failure to address a critical risk factor or failure to introduce the correct therapies; or faulty disease management after an episode of ADHF. It may also be probable that the standard of care for chronic heart failure with improved outcomes has actually shifted the morbidity/mortality risk profile of

Table 51.1. Heart Failure Society of America heart failure practice guidelines: acute decompensated heart failure (ADHF)

Evaluation and management of patients with ADHF: overall recommendations:
- Patients admitted with ADHF and evidence of fluid overload should be treated initially with loop diuretics
- When congestion fails to improve in response to diuretic therapy, the following options should be considered:
  —Sodium and fluid restriction
  —Increased doses of loop diuretics
  —Continuous infusion of a loop diuretic
  —Addition of a second type of diuretic
  —Ultrafiltration
- In the absence of symptomatic hypotension, IV NTG, NTP, or nesiritide may be considered as an addition to diuretic therapy for rapid improvement of congestive symptoms in patients with ADHF

Evaluation and management of patients with acute decompensated heart failure: specific recommendations
- 12.15: In the absence of hypotension, IV NTG, sodium nitroprusside or nesiritide may be considered as an addition to diuretic therapy for rapid improvement of congestive symptoms in patients admitted with ADHF (strength of evidence: B)
- 12.16: IV vasodilators (IV NTG or NTP) and diuretics are recommended for rapid relief in patients with acute pulmonary edema or severe hypertension
- 12.17: Intravenous vasodilators (nitroprusside, nitroglycerin, or nesiritide) may be considered in patients with ADHF and advanced HF who have persistent severe HF despite aggressive treatment with diuretics and standard oral therapies (strength of evidence: C)
- IV inotropes (milrinone or dobutamine) may be considered to relieve symptoms and improve end-organ function in patients with advanced HF

HF, heart failure; IV NTG, intravenous nitroglycerin; NTP, nitroprusside.
Modified from Adams et al. (4).

those who are hospitalized for heart failure toward a higher risk cohort, thus adverse outcomes may not be unexpected.

Irrespective of the uncertain issues related to the pathophysiology of ADHF, it is clear that hemodynamic alterations are responsible for the presenting signs and symptoms of ADHF. As such, our current approach to therapy is driven by hemodynamic targets. It is important to recognize that targeting hemodynamics may not be targeting the actual pathophysiology of ADHF, and thus improvements in the natural history of heart failure after an episode of ADHF may unfortunately need to await further elucidation of operative mechanisms in this disease process.

Current treatment approaches focus on relieving congestion, improving cardiac output, and elevating or stabilizing systemic blood pressure. Data acquired in the Acute Decompensated Heart Failure National Registry (ADHERE) database clearly demonstrate congestion to be the predominant clinical scenario associated with an episode of ADHF. (5) The Evaluation Study of Congestive Heart Failure and Pulmonary Artery Catheterization Effectiveness (ESCAPE) trial was completed at a select group of tertiary care medical centers with investigators highly experienced in the management of advanced heart failure. In the patient population studied, both congestion and low output states were associated with acute decompensation. (6)

Current Therapies

Diuretics, mechanical volume removal, inotropes, and vasodilators represent the currently available treatment options for ADHF. Background therapy should be consistent with evidence-based guidelines for chronic heart failure. Each of these approaches has been addressed elsewhere in this text. In brief, diuretic therapy represents the most conventional approach in the management of ADHF, but no prospectively acquired data exist to demonstrate a favorable effect of diuretic therapy on the natural history of ADHF. Registry data from ADHERE in fact raise a concern that diuretic therapy for ADHF is not without risk. In an evaluation of >50,000 hospital admissions from ADHERE, use of intravenous diuretics increased the risk of in-hospital mortality (odds ratio [OR], 1.29; 95% confidence interval [CI], 1.04–1.59) after adjusting for baseline covariates and treatment propensity. (7) It is also well known that acute parenteral administration of loop diuretics results in an elevation in pulmonary artery pressures, an increase in systemic vascular resistance, and a reduction in glomerular filtration rate. (8,9) Additionally, there is a well-described increase in neurohormonal activation associated with loop diuretic therapy, and the associated electrolyte disturbances are likewise well known. (10) Similarly, diuretic therapy given for chronic heart failure raises similar concerns (11,12), and animal data would suggest that morphological changes in the renal tubule do occur in the setting of chronic administration of high-dose loop diuretics. (13) Despite these questions, diuretic therapy is effective, appropriate, and inexpensive and remains at the core of conventional therapy for ADHF.

Recent data testing the benefit of ultrafiltration are promising. The Ultrafiltration vs. IV Diuretics for Patients Hospitalized for Acute Decompensated Congestive Heart Failure (UNLOAD) trial, demonstrated that patients randomized to ultrafiltration instead of diuretic therapy for ADHF experienced a greater weight loss and volume removal, a similar improvement in the symptom of dyspnea (primary end points), and a provocative signal of a reduction in near-term rehospitalization (secondary end point). These findings are promising, but the correct incorporation of mechanical volume removal with conventional therapy for ADHF remains an unresolved issue. (14)

Inotropic Therapy

Inotropic therapy has been consistently demonstrated to be problematic in the treatment of ADHF. When inodilator therapy, that is, milrinone, was compared to placebo in the Outcomes of a Prospective Trial of Intravenous Milrinone for Exacerbations of Chronic Heart Failure (OPTIME) trial, more adverse clinical events occurred on active therapy than with placebo. (15) In the aforementioned ESCAPE trial, the use of inotropic agents was associated with an increased risk of death (hazard ratio [HR], 1.75; 95% CI, 1.05–2.92) and death or rehospitalization (HR, 2.12; 95% CI, 1.52–2.97) after adjustment for blood pressure and renal function. (6)

A new class of inotropes, calcium sensitizers, has recently been investigated. The Survival of Patients with Acute Heart Failure in Need of Intravenous Inotropic Support (SURVIVE) trial assessed the benefit of levosimendan. This trial found no significant differences between patients randomized to levosimendan vs. dobutamine in the primary end point of all-cause mortality at 180 days (HR, 0.91; 95% CI, 0.74–1.13) or the secondary end points of all-cause mortality at 5 days (HR, 0.72; 95% CI, 0.44–1.16) or 31 days (HR, 0.85; 95% CI, 0.63–1.15). (16) In the Randomized Evaluations of Levosimendan (REVIVE–II) trial, the secondary end point of 90-day mortality revealed a nonstatistically significant increase in patients randomized to levosimendan (15.1%) vs. placebo (11.6%). (17) These investigations revealed a worrisome mortality concern, and additional development of levosimendan is uncertain. Despite these concerns, available inotropic therapy remains indicated in the setting of ADHF but should be reserved only for those patients with overt hypotension or abject evidence of compromised organ perfusion.

Vasodilator Therapy

Vasodilator therapy represents yet another treatment option for ADHF, given that filling pressures are lowered, cardiac output is improved without increasing myocardial oxygen consumption, and blood pressure can be preserved. Again, there are no data to suggest a survival advantage or a benefit on rehospitalization after an episode of ADHF, but sufficient data do exist to suggest that outcomes are better on vasodilator therapy than on inotropic therapy for ADHF. (18) The available vasodilators include nitroglycerin, nitroprusside, and B-type natriuretic peptide, that is, nesiritide. Nitroglycerin is a venodilator that also increases coronary artery blood flow and has an acute hemodynamic effect that is favorable. Intravenous nitroglycerin administered for ADHF is associated with acute symptom relief without a signal of apparent increase in risk. Nitrate tolerance, however, is well described and may occur early if the dose administered is elevated. Headache may make the therapy difficult to administer or titrate. No clinical trials to date have demonstrated a survival advantage associated with the use of nitroglycerin, but similarly there has been no evidence of risk due to parenteral therapy with nitroglycerin.

Nitroprusside is a balanced vasodilator that promotes both arterial and venous vasodilation. For those hemodynamic profiles in ADHF that are characterized by a low cardiac output and increased systemic vascular resistance, the administration of nitroprusside can lead to dramatic clinical improvement with marked increases in cardiac output and subsequent hemodynamic stability. These benefits are not long-lasting, as thiocyanide toxicity does occur and can be quite problematic requiring acute intervention. The risk for thiocyanide toxicity is increased in the older patient, in the setting of chronic liver disease, and with chronic renal disease. Reflex tachycardia, profound hypotension, and activation of neurohormonal systems may also be associated with both nitroglycerin and nitroprusside therapy. (19)

Nesiritide: a Therapeutic Application of B-Type Natriuretic Peptides

Nesiritide is an available formulation of human B-type natriuretic peptide. It is synthesized using recombinant technology from *Escherichia coli* and is structurally identical to the endogenous hormone. (20) It has a ligand-receptor interaction with natriuretic peptide receptor A, which results in activation of guanylate cyclase and yields a subsequent intracellular increase in the second messenger, cyclic guanosine monophosphate (cGMP). Among the properties exerted by the production of cGMP is a direct relaxant effect on human vascular tissue. (20,21) In both healthy volunteers and individuals with heart failure, this effect of nesiritide produces vasodilation, and significantly reduces mean arterial pressure, pulmonary capillary wedge pressure (PCWP), and right atrial pressure. (22) In an evaluation of 19 patients with severe heart failure, nesiritide produced a 48% reduction in mean PCWP and a 56% reduction in mean right atrial pressure (both $p < .01$ vs. placebo). (23) In another evaluation of 16 patients with ADHF, nesiritide produced a 17% reduction in mean arterial pressure ($p < .001$), a 41% reduction in PCWP ($p < .001$), and a 31% reduction in right atrial pressure ($p < .001$) versus placebo. Both cardiac index and coronary blood flow were increased. (22) In an evaluation of 10 patients undergoing heart catheterization, nesiritide increased coronary artery diameter by 15% ($p = .007$), coronary velocity by 14% ($p = .015$), coronary blood flow by 35% ($p = .007$), and reduced coronary resistance by 23% ($p = .036$) versus placebo. (24) These changes occurred without a significant increase in heart rate, that is, a crude marker of myocardial oxygen consumption.

Nesiritide differs from other parenterally administered compounds in that it has at least a neutral neurohormonal profile. (25–27) Nesiritide inhibits sympathetic stimulation, both centrally and in the periphery. Circulating levels of norepinephrine are diminished after administration of nesiritide. (25) In a randomized, multicenter evaluation, nesiritide at a dose of 0.015 μg/kg/min improved several markers of heart rate variability—another marker of sympathetic activation. These data included standard deviation of the R-R intervals over 24 hours, $p = .001$; standard deviation of all 5-minute mean R-R intervals, $p = .02$; and the square root of mean squared differences of successive R-R intervals, $p = .01$ in patients with severely depressed heart rate variability at baseline. (28) This observation is consistent with sympathetic nervous system inhibition and at least a partial correction of the sympathetic-parasympathetic balance.

Data also demonstrate the potential of nesiritide to inhibit the renin-angiotensin-aldosterone system. (25, 27) It is intriguing to acknowledge that aldosterone has emerged as an important marker of left ventricular remodeling, with its greatest effect on left ventricular fibrosis. Major clinical trial data, from both the Randomized Aldactone Evaluation Study (RALES) (29) and the Eplerenone Post-Acute Myocardial Infarction Heart Failure Efficacy and Survival Study (EPHESUS) (30), have confirmed the significant advantages of aldosterone antagonism in the setting of chronic heart failure or post–myocardial infarction (MI) left ventricular dysfunction. Both in the setting of acute heart failure and chronic decompensated heart failure, nesiritide has been demonstrated to lower aldosterone levels. (25,27,31) Additional data demonstrate that nesiritide inhibits the endothelin system. (32) Endothelin-1 is a potent vasoconstrictor and growth promoter, and it also generates cytokine activation, especially via its effects on transforming growth factor-β_1. In patients with decompensated heart failure, nesiritide (0.015 μg/kg/min) has been shown to lower endothelin-1 levels by 20% ($p < .001$) (32). It is important to acknowledge that these observations of neurohormonal modulation with nesiritide have not yet been demonstrated to be clinically important, and this property of nesiritide, although intriguing, should not be used as a rationale to initiate therapy with natriuretic peptides in heart failure.

In healthy volunteers, nesiritide increases glomerular filtration rate and produces both a diuresis and natriuresis in a dose-dependent fashion. (33–35) In the kidney, it inhibits sodium resorp-

Table 51.2. Randomized, controlled trials of nesiritide in ADHF

Study	Control	Patients: Nesiritide	Patients: Control	Nesiritide dose (μg/kg/min)	Median (IQR) duration of infusion (hours)
Mills et al.	Placebo	74	29	0.015, 0.03, or 0.06	24.0 (24.0–24.1)
Efficacy trial	Placebo	85	42	0.015 or 0.03	24.2 (7.8–47.7)
Comparative trial	Standard care	203	102	0.015 or 0.03	30.4 (23.0–65.1)
PRECEDENT	Dobutamine	163	83	0.015 or 0.03	24.1 (24.0–46.5)
VMAC	Nitroglycerin or standard care	273	216	0.01	24.3 (24.0–44.2)
PROACTION	Standard care	120	117	0.01	16.9 (12.2–21.9)

ADHF, acute decompensated heart failure; IQR, interquartile range; PRECEDENT, Prospective Randomized Evaluation of Cardiac Ectopy with Dobutamine or Natrecor Therapy trial; VMAC, Vasodilation in the Management of Acute Congestive Heart Failure trial; PROACTION, Prospective Randomized Outcomes Study of Acutely Decompensated Congestive Heart Failure Treated Initially as Outpatients with Nesiritide trial.
See references 25, 39, 40, 41, and 43.

tion in both the proximal and distal nephron, with its major effect occurring in the distal nephron. (34) Nesiritide also inhibits the tubuloglomerular feedback response that would typically occur in response to increased salt delivery in the distal tubule, preserving this natriuretic effect. (36) In patients with heart failure, the renal effects of nesiritide are less well established and may indeed be deleterious for as of yet undetermined reasons.

A very small study of hospitalized patients with stable left ventricular dysfunction randomized patients to nesiritide vs. placebo. There was no incremental increase in natriuresis in those patients treated with nesiritide. (37) Several factors may be operative, including intravascular volume status, concomitant medications, especially diuretics, and the underlying degree of comorbid renal insufficiency. Multiple small studies have shown nesiritide to have variable effects on renal blood flow, glomerular filtration rate, urinary sodium excretion, and water excretion. (37,38) It is clear that no definitive statement can be made that nesiritide is renoprotective as it is currently administered, and concerns remain (addressed below) that nesiritide is associated with treatment-induced renal insufficiency.

Nesiritide as a Therapeutic Option for Acute Decompensated Heart Failure

As a therapeutic strategy for patients with ADHF, nesiritide has been evaluated in six randomized, controlled clinical trials involving more than 1500 subjects (Table 51.2).

Mills et al. (39) performed a multicenter, double-blind, placebo-controlled evaluation of nesiritide therapy in 103 subjects with symptomatic heart failure (New York Heart Association [NYHA] class II, III, or IV) and left ventricular systolic dysfunction (left ventricular ejection fraction [LVEF] <0.35). Subjects were randomized to one of three regimens of nesiritide therapy: 24-hour infusion therapy with nesiritide 0.015 μg/kg/min, 0.03 μg/kg/min, or 0.06 μg/kg/min vs. placebo, with the study drug infusion initiated at least 2 hours after insertion of a pulmonary artery catheter. The primary end point was the change from pre- to postinfusion of study drug on cardiac hemodynamics. Compared with placebo, nesiritide produced significant reductions in PCWP, mean right atrial pressure, and systemic vascular resistance, and significant increases in stroke volume index and cardiac output with no effect on heart rate. These beneficial effects were evident at 1 hour and were sustained throughout the 24-hour infusions. Worsening heart failure necessitating termination of study drug occurred in 1% of nesiritide vs. 17% of control subjects ($p = .014$). (39)

The Efficacy trial was a multicenter, double-blind, placebo-controlled evaluation of nesiritide therapy in 127 subjects with acute decompensated heart failure (94% NYHA class III or IV. This study was likewise guided by measurement of cardiac hemodynamics, and all subjects were required to have a systolic blood pressure ≥90 mm Hg, a PCWP ≥18 mm Hg, and a cardiac index ≤2.7 L/min/m^2. Treatment arms consisted of nesiritide 0.015 μg/kg/min or 0.03 μg/kg/min or placebo for at least 6 hours. All other parenteral vasoactive agents were withheld during this initial 6-hour period. The primary outcome parameter was the change in PCWP from baseline to 6 hours. Secondary outcomes were global clinical status, clinical symptoms, and other hemodynamic parameters. In this trial, nesiritide produced a dose-dependent decrement in PCWP, right atrial pressure, systemic vascular resistance, and systolic blood pressure, and a moderate increase in cardiac index but no substantial change in heart rate. Global clinical status, as judged by the patient, was statistically better for the patients on nesiritide, both 0.015 μg/kg/min and 0.03 μg/kg/min vs. placebo groups ($p < .001$ for both nesiritide vs. placebo comparisons). Physician assessments of global status paralleled those of the patients. Dyspnea was improved and fatigue was reduced in the nesiritide subjects vs. placebo subjects ($p < .001$ for both comparisons). (25)

The Comparative trial was a multicenter, open-label evaluation of nesiritide versus usual therapy in 305 subjects with acute decompensated heart failure (92% NYHA class III or IV). Subjects were randomized to nesiritide 0.015 μg/kg/min or 0.03 μg/kg/min or other therapy consisting of a single parenteral vasoactive agent, either inotropes or other vasodilators, used for the short-term management of ADHF. In all subjects, intravenous diuretics and oral medications could be added at any time. The prespecified primary outcomes were global clinical status and clinical symptoms. In the standard therapy group, 57% of subjects received dobutamine, 19% received milrinone, 18% received nitroglycerin, 6% received dopamine and 1% received amrinone. Global clinical status, dyspnea, and fatigue improved in all three treatment groups, with no significant differences between treatment groups at 6 hours, 24 hours, and the end of therapy. Weight loss was similar in the three treatment groups. However, intravenous diuretics were required in fewer nesiritide than standard therapy subjects ($p < .001$). (25)

The Prospective Randomized Evaluation of Cardiac Ectopy with Dobutamine or Natrecor Therapy (PRECEDENT) study was a multicenter, open-label, active-controlled evaluation of nesiritide therapy in 255 subjects with ADHF (100% NYHA class III or IV) in which single-agent intravenous therapy with nesiritide or dobutamine, with or without diuretics, was administered. Subjects were stratified based on the presence or absence of a known history of ventricular tachycardia and were randomized to nesiritide 0.015 μg/kg/min or 0.03 μg/kg/min or dobutamine ≥5 μg/kg/min. The minimum infusion duration was 24 hours. All patients had three-channel, 24-hour Holter monitor recordings for the 24 hours immediately before (baseline) and after initiation of study drug. The primary outcome parameters were the changes from baseline in mean heart rate, mean hourly premature ventricular beats, and mean hourly repetitive beats. Secondary outcomes included the frequency of complex ventricular rhythm disturbances. Proarrhythmia was assessed using two established criteria, Velebit and Cardiac Arrhythmia Pilot Study (CAPS). (40) At baseline, all three treatment groups had similar heart rates and rates of ventricular ectopy. During treatment, heart rate and ventricular ectopy were increased significantly from baseline in dobutamine but not in nesiritide subjects. Velebit proarrhythmia criteria were met by 23% of dobutamine vs. 2% of nesiritide subjects ($p < .001$), and CAPS proarrhythmia criteria were met by 10% of dobutamine versus 0% of nesiritide subjects ($p = .001$). (40)

The Vasodilation in the Management of Acute Congestive Heart Failure (VMAC) trial was a multicenter, double-blind, placebo- and active-controlled evaluation of nesiritide therapy in 489 subjects with ADHF and dyspnea at rest or with minimal activity. Subjects were stratified based on the investigator's decision to measure cardiac hemodynamics with a right heart catheter as part of the management regimen. Patients were then randomized to nesiritide 0.01 μg/kg/min fixed dose in the noninstrumented patient; fixed- or adjustable-dose nesiritide in the instrumented group, with nitroglycerin (adjustable dose) or placebo for the initial 3 hours; after this, placebo subjects were randomly crossed over to nesiritide (fixed dose) or nitroglycerin therapy. The minimum infusion duration was 24 hours. Primary outcome parameters were the absolute change in

PCWP (when applicable) and relief of dyspnea at 3 hours. Secondary outcome parameters included the change in PCWP, relief of dyspnea, and global clinical status at 24 hours. At 3 hours, the mean change in PCWP was −2 mm Hg on placebo therapy, −3.8 mm Hg on nitroglycerin therapy ($p = .09$ vs. placebo), and −5.8 mm Hg on nesiritide therapy ($p < .001$ vs. placebo; $p = .03$ vs. nitroglycerin). In addition, at 3 hours, nesiritide produced a decrease in dyspnea compared with placebo ($p = .03$) but not nitroglycerin ($p = .56$). At 24 hours, patients on nesiritide had significantly greater reduction in PCWP (−8.2 mm Hg) than those on nitroglycerin (−6.3 mm Hg; $p = .04$), with no significant difference in dyspnea ($p = .13$) (Fig. 51.1). (41)

The Prospective Randomized Outcomes Study of Acutely Decompensated Congestive Heart Failure Treated Initially as Outpatients with Nesiritide (PROACTION) trial was a multicenter, double-blind, placebo-controlled study of nesiritide therapy in 237 emergency department/observation unit patients with ADHF and dyspnea at rest or with minimal activity (walking <20 feet). Patients were randomized to usual care plus nesiritide 0.01 μg/kg/min versus usual care plus placebo, with study medication initiated within 3 hours of presentation in the emergency department and continued for a minimum of 12 hours. Standard care was at the investigator's discretion and could include diuretics, oxygen, and one or more medications to reduce systemic vascular resistance and improve cardiac contractility. The primary outcome parameters were the safety profile and clinical effects of nesiritide when added to standard care in the emergency department/observation unit setting. Compared with placebo, subjects who received nesiritide had small, statistically insignificant reductions in the requirement for inpatient admission (49% vs. 55%; $p = .44$) and mean total hospital length of stay if admitted (5.1 days vs. 5.5 days; $p = .62$). Of

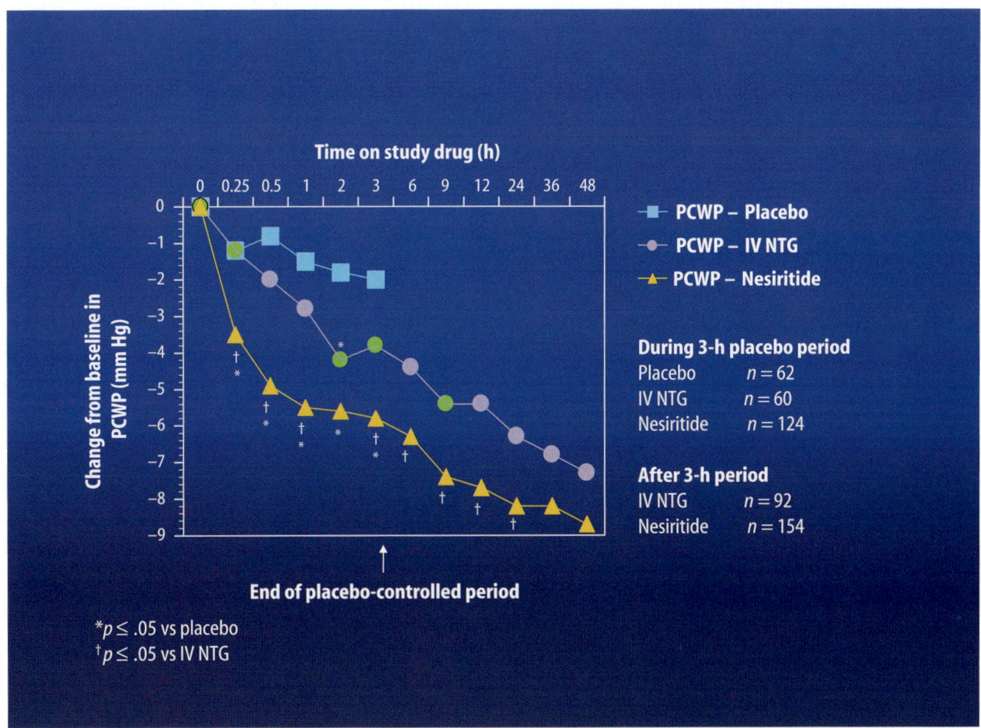

FIGURE 51.1. Hemodynamic effects of nesiritide versus placebo versus intravenous nitroglycerin (IV NTG). (From Publication Committee for the VMAC Investigators [41].)

the subjects admitted, those who received nesiritide had fewer readmissions (10% vs. 23%; $p = .06$) and a significantly shorter mean total duration of hospitalization through study day 30. (42) Eight patients enrolled in the PROACTION trial died from all causes, mostly noncardiac, within 30 days after treatment, seven (5.9%) in the nesiritide group and one (0.9%) in the placebo group (HR, 7.03; 95% CI, 0.87–57.15; $p = .066$). A narrowing of the difference in all-cause mortality between the nesiritide and placebo treatment groups was observed at the 180-day time point—24 (20.6%) patients receiving nesiritide and 20 (17.5%) patients receiving placebo died (HR, 1.24; 95% CI, 0.68–2.24; $p = .479$). (42,43)

The Risk-Benefit Profile of Nesiritide

The safety of nesiritide remains an issue of great concern. Similar to other vasodilators, nesiritide produces dose-related hypotension, which may occur even at currently recommended doses (0.01 μg/kg/min). The clinician should remain aware of this risk whenever nesiritide is initiated. Since early evaluations of nesiritide used higher than the currently approved starting dose (0.01 μg/kg/min), the frequency and potential complications of hypotension are difficult to assess but it is apparent that with higher doses, the incidence of hypotension does increase. In the study by Mills et al. (39), symptomatic hypotension developed in 15% of the patients receiving 0.06 μg/kg/min of nesiritide and 5% of those receiving 0.015 μg/kg/min. In the Efficacy trial, 2% and 5% of subjects randomized to nesiritide 0.015 μg/kg/min and 0.03 μg/kg/min, respectively, developed symptomatic hypotension, versus no patients randomized to placebo ($p = .55$). (25) In the Comparative trial, the incidence of symptomatic hypotension was higher occurring in 11% and 17% of patients randomized to nesiritide 0.015 μg/kg/min and 0.03 μg/kg/min, respectively. (25) Finally, in the PRECEDENT study, symptomatic hypotension developed in 17% and 24% of subjects randomized to nesiritide 0.015 μg/kg/min and 0.03 μg/kg/min, respectively, compared with 2% of subjects randomized to dobutamine ($p < .001$). (40)

In the VMAC trial, with nesiritide being given at a dose of 0.01 μg/kg/min, symptomatic hypotension developed in 4% of subjects randomized to nesiritide. This compares to an incidence of symptomatic hypotension of 5% in patients randomized to nitroglycerin ($p > .99$). (41) The hypotension noted in the VMAC trial with nesiritide was more troublesome than the hypotension noted with nitroglycerin due to the longer half-life of nesiritide, 18 minutes vs. 3 minutes. Similarly, in the PROACTION trial with nesiritide being given at a dose of 0.01 μg/kg/min, the frequency of symptomatic hypotension was not significantly different between nesiritide (2%) and standard care (1%) subjects ($p > .99$). (43) The degree of blood pressure reduction in subjects receiving nesiritide was related directly to the baseline blood pressure; the greatest reduction in blood pressure occurred in those subjects with the greatest degree of baseline hypertension. Overall, the mean reduction in systolic blood pressure with nesiritide was 1.2 mm Hg, 12.3 mm Hg, and 28.7 mm Hg in subjects with baseline systolic blood pressures <101 mm Hg, 101 to 140 mm Hg, and >140 mm Hg, respectively. (42)

Nesiritide is associated with an increased risk of acute serum creatinine elevation. (44) This acute increase in serum creatinine may be a hemodynamic consequence of blood pressure reduction in patients who are volume depleted or have underlying kidney dysfunction with loss of renal blood flow autoregulatory capability. (45,46) An analysis of five nesiritide trials demonstrated that the risk of an acute increase in serum creatinine is directly related to the prevalence of symptomatic hypotension. (47) An additional observation from the VMAC trial is that nesiritide was not associated with an increased risk of acute serum creatinine elevation in subjects who were receiving low-to-moderate-dose diuretics but was seen in those subjects who were receiving high-dose diuretics, defined as a maximum daily dose of furosemide >160 mg, bumetanide >4 mg, torsemide >80 mg, metolazone >10 mg, chlorothiazide >1000 mg, hydrochlorothiazide >50 mg or concurrent treatment with two or more of these diuretics regardless of dose. (48)

The risk of acute serum creatinine elevation in patients receiving nesiritide is also dose related, and consequently this effect was seen more often in early trials than in later studies. (47) In the VMAC trial, the frequency, onset, and persistence of acute serum creatinine elevations in patients on nesiritide was similar to those in patients on nitroglycerin, and nearly all episodes (~90%)

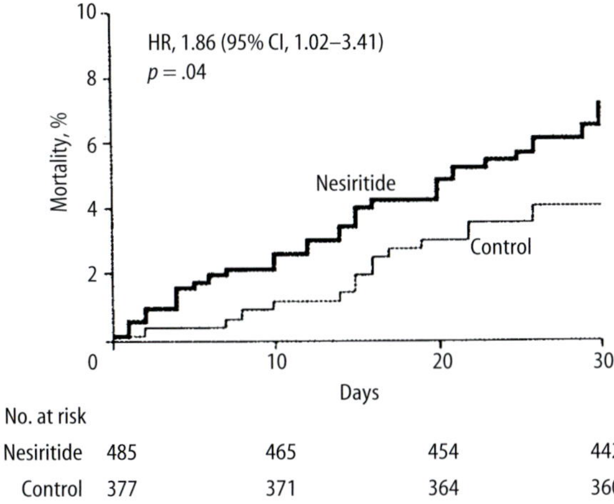

FIGURE 51.2. Kaplan-Meier curves of 30-day mortality associated with control and nesiritide therapies based on NSGET, VMAX, and PROACTION studies. NSGET, Nesiritide Study Group Efficacy Trial; VMAC, Vasodilation in the Management of Acute Congestive Heart Failure; PROACTION, Prospective Randomized Outcomes Study of Acutely Decompensated Congestive Heart Failure Treated Initially in Outpatients with Natrecor; CI, confidence interval; HR, hazard ratio. (From Sackner-Bernstein, et al. [49].)

resolved within 30 days of instituting either nesiritide or nitroglycerin therapy. (41)

The effect of nesiritide on mortality risk is the most troublesome issue and may be one that is difficult to definitively determine, given the short duration of nesiritide therapy, numerous potential confounding factors, and low background mortality rates. A pooled analysis of data from three nesiritide trials involving 862 subjects reported that nesiritide may be associated with an increased 30-day mortality risk compared with other non–inotrope-based control therapies. In this analysis, the 30-day mortality hazard ratio for nesiritide therapy after adjusting for study was 1.80 (95% CI, 0.98–3.31; $p = .06$; unadjusted $p = .04$) (Fig. 51.2). (49) The trials included in this analysis were not designed or powered to assess mortality. Consequently, there are substantial differences both between studies and between treatment groups within these studies in mortality risk factors, including heart failure severity, prevalence of acute coronary syndromes, and concomitant therapies. In the VMAC trial, which accounts for >50% of the subjects in this pooled analysis, there was significantly greater concomitant use of dobutamine in subjects randomized to nesiritide compared to nitroglycerin (50), and overall in the three trials used in this 862-patient meta-analysis, inotrope use was greater in subjects randomized to nesiritide compared with controls both before and during study drug infusion. (51)

In yet another meta-analysis, the effect on 30-day mortality from acute exposure to nesiritide therapy yielded a hazard ratio of 1.34 (95% CI, 0.84–2.15; $p = .22$) and a 6-month hazard ratio of 1.05 (95% CI, 0.81–1.36; $p = .73$). These are pooled data from all 1507 subjects who have participated in randomized, controlled clinical trials evaluating nesiritide infusion therapy in patients with ADHF (Table 51.3). (52) Neither of these pooled analyses is sufficiently robust to resolve the

TABLE 51.3. Kaplan-Meier estimates of mortality in randomized, controlled HF trials of nesiritide

		30-day mortality		180-day mortality	
Study	Control	Nesiritide	Control	Nesiritide	Control
Mills et al.	Placebo	2.7%	7.5%	n/a	n/a
Efficacy trial	Placebo	5.9%	4.8%	23.1%	19.3%
Comparative trial	Standard care	6.9%	4.9%	20.8%	23.5%
PRECEDENT	Dobutamine	3.7%	6.1%	16.3%	22.2%
VMAC	Nitroglycerin/standard care	8.1%	5.1%	25.1%	20.8%
PROACTION	Standard care	4.2%	0.9%	n/a	n/a
FUSION	Standard care	1.4%	2.9%	9.4%	13.5%
Pooled (6 studies)[a]		5.9%	4.4%	n/a	n/a
Pooled (7 studies)		5.3%	4.3%	n/a	n/a
Pooled (4 studies)[a]		n/a	n/a	21.7%	21.5%

[a]Excludes FUSION.

HF, heart failure; PRECEDENT, Prospective Randomized Evaluation of Cardiac Ectopy with Dobutamine or Natrecor Therapy trial; VMAC, Vasodilation in the Management of Acute Congestive Heart Failure trial; PROACTION, Prospective Randomized Outcomes Study of Acutely Decompensated Congestive Heart Failure Treated Initially as Outpatients with Nesiritide trial; FUSION, Follow-Up Serial Infusion of Nesiritide; n/a, not applicable.

Source: Adapted from Abraham (52).

Table 51.4. In-hospital mortality odds ratios for vasoactive therapies in the Acute Decompensated Heart Failure National Registry (ADHERE)

Comparison	Odds ratio[a]	95% confidence interval
Nesiritide vs.		
Nitroglycerin	0.94	0.77–1.16
Dobutamine	0.47	0.39–0.56
Milrinone	0.59	0.48–0.73
Nitroglycerin vs.		
Dobutamine	0.46	0.37–0.57
Milrinone	0.69	0.53–0.89
Dobutamine vs.		
Milrinone	1.24	1.03–1.55

[a]Adjusted for covariates and propensity score.
Source: Adapted from Abraham et al. (18).

question, and neither was fully adjusted for baseline differences that may have influenced mortality. However, both analyses appropriately raise the question of risk but in the absence of prospectively acquired data in a well-designed mortality trial, the question remains unresolved.

An analysis of data from the ADHERE Registry involving >15,000 patient episodes of ADHF requiring intravenous vasoactive therapy with nesiritide ($n = 5220$), nitroglycerin ($n = 6549$), dobutamine ($n = 4226$), or milrinone ($n = 2021$), demonstrated that vasodilatory therapy with nesiritide or nitroglycerin was associated with significant reductions in risk-adjusted in-hospital mortality compared with inotropic therapy with dobutamine or milrinone. There was no significant difference in risk-adjusted mortality between nesiritide and nitroglycerin therapy (Table 51.4). (18) Similarly, nesiritide significantly reduced in-hospital mortality risk compared with milrinone (adjusted OR, 0.24; $p < .001$) or dobutamine (adjusted OR, 0.29; $p < .001$) in a retrospective cohort analysis of data from 2130 patients with ADHF treated with nesiritide ($n = 386$), milrinone ($n = 433$), or dobutamine ($n = 1311$) at 32 academic health centers. (53)

Conclusions and Recommendations for Therapy

The problem of acute decompensated heart failure represents a major challenge in the continuum of care for patients with symptomatic left ventricular dysfunction. Clearly more insight into the pathophysiological mechanisms affecting both exacerbations of chronic heart failure and symptomatic new-onset heart failure is required. The current therapeutic options remain those focused on hemodynamic perturbations responsible for the signs and symptoms of decompensated heart failure. These treatments are applied in the context of sparse data regarding any interventions that may favorably influence this disease.

The ideal approach is to address the specific hemodynamic malady that is present: thus, the use of diuretics is appropriate for patients with volume overload; vasodilators for patients with volume overload and relative hypoperfusion who are not frankly hypotensive; and inotropes only for those patients with impending or frank cardiogenic shock. Although it is beyond the scope of this chapter, aggressive use of evidence-based therapies for chronic heart failure and referral to effective disease management programs should be strongly considered as appropriate treatment strategies for ADHF.

When the choice of treatment is vasodilator therapy, nesiritide represents one of several options. Nesiritide is a synthetic natriuretic peptide with a protean physiologic profile that includes natriuresis, balanced vasodilation, a decrement in filling pressures, an indirect increase in cardiac output, and modulation of neurohormonal activation. Nesiritide remains a Food and Drug Administration (FDA)-approved treatment option for ADHF. The available data demonstrate a significant effect on elevated filling pressures and at least a moderate effect on the symptom of dyspnea. Concern should be given to avoid the use of nesiritide in patients with blood pressure <90 mm Hg, to administer the drug only at the 0.01 μg/kg/min dose, and additional concern might be expressed if the patient is concomitantly receiving high doses of diuretic therapy. There is an associated risk of drug-induced renal insufficiency that may be enhanced when the drug is given concomitantly with higher dose loop diuretics. Mortality issues remain unresolved. However, there is clear evidence of neither harm nor benefit, and if symptom relief is felt to require vasodilator therapy, the use of nesiritide is a therapeutic option. It is hoped that a soon to be commenced 7000 patient mortality trial will resolve the issue of mortality risk.

Table 51.5. Recommendations of the nesiritide review panel, June 2005

Nesiritide is approved for inpatient management of acute heart failure (HF)
• Use of nesiritide should be limited to patients presenting to the hospital with acute HF who have dyspnea at rest
• Physicians considering the use of nesiritide should consider
—Its efficacy in reducing dyspnea
—Possible risks of the drug
—Availability of alternate therapies to relieve HF symptoms
Nesiritide is not recommended
• for intermittent outpatient infusion
• for scheduled, repetitive use
• to improve renal function
• to enhance diuresis

See reference 54.

Table 51.1 includes the new Heart Failure Society of America guidelines for management of ADHF, and Table 51.5 restates the opinions of the nesiritide review panel regarding the best profile for the use of nesiritide in clinical practice. (54)

References

1. Kozak LJ, Owings MF, Hall MJ. National Hospital Discharge Survey: 2002 annual summary with detailed diagnosis and procedure data. Vital Health Stat 13 2005;(158):1–199.
2. Nieminen MS, Böhm M, Cowie MR, et al. Executive summary of the guidelines on the diagnosis and treatment of acute heart failure: the Task Force on Acute Heart Failure of the European Society of Cardiology. Eur Heart J 2005;26;(4):384–416.
3. Jong P, Vowinckel E, Liu PP, Gong Y, Tu JV. Prognosis and determinants of survival in patients newly hospitalized for heart failure: a population-based study. Arch Intern Med 2002;162:1689–94.
4. Adams KF, et al. Heart Failure Society of America Guideline Writing Committee. Executive Summary: HFSA 2006 Comprehensive Heart Failure Practice Guideline. J Card Fail 2006;12:10–38.
5. Fonarow GC, for the ADHERE Scientific Advisory Committee. The Acute Decompensated Heart Failure National Registry (ADHERE): opportunities to improve care of patients hospitalized with acute decompensated heart failure. Rev Cardiovasc Med 2003;4(suppl 7):S21–30.
6. The ESCAPE Investigators and ESCAPE Study Coordinators. Evaluation study of congestive heart failure and pulmonary artery catheterization effectiveness: the ESCAPE trial. JAMA 2005;294: 1625–33.
7. Emerman CL, DeMarco T, Costanzo MR, Peacock WF, for the ADHERE® Scientific Advisory Committee. Impact of intravenous diuretics on the outcomes of patients hospitalized with acute decompensated heart failure: insights from the ADHERE® Registry (abstract 368). J Card Fail 2004;10(suppl 4):S116.
8. Ikram H, Chan W, Espiner EA, et al. Haemodynamic and hormone responses to acute and chronic furosemide therapy in congestive heart failure. Clin Sci 1980;59(6):443–9.
9. Gottlieb SS, Brater DC, Thomas I, et al. BG9719 (CVT-124), an A_1 adenosine receptor antagonist, protects against the decline in renal function observed with diuretic therapy. Circulation 2002; 105(11):1348–53.
10. Francis GS, Siegel RM, Goldsmith SR, et al. Acute vasoconstrictor response to intravenous furosemide in patients with chronic congestive heart failure. Activation of the neurohumoral axis. Ann Intern Med 1985;103(1):1–6.
11. Domanski M, Norman J, Pitt B, et al. Diuretic use, progressive heart failure, and death in patients in the studies of left ventricular dysfunction (SOLVD). J Am Coll Cardiol 2003;42(4):705–8.
12. Cooper HA, Dries DL, Davis CE, et al. Diuretics and risk of arrhythmic death in patients with left ventricular dysfunction. Circulation 1999;100(12): 1311–5.
13. Ellison, DH. Diuretic drugs and the treatment of edema from clinic to bench and back again. Am J Kidney Dis 1994;23(5):623–43.
14. Costanzo MR, for UNLOAD: Ultrafiltration vs. IV Diuretics for Patients Hospitalized for Acute Decompensated Congestive Heart Failure. Late Breaking Clinical Trials. ACC Scientific Meeting March 14, 2006, Atlanta, Georgia.
15. Cuffe, MS, Califf RM, Adams KF, et al., OPTIME-CHF. Outcomes of a prospective trial of intravenous milrinone for exacerbations of chronic heart failure). Short-term intravenous milrinone for acute exacerbation of chronic heart failure. A randomized controlled trial. JAMA 2002;287:1541–7.
16. Stiles S. SURVIVE: no levosimendan survival benefit over dobutamine in acute HF. http://www.theheart.org.
17. Stiles S. REVIVE-2: levosimendan improves five-day clinical status in acute HF. http://www.theheart.org.
18. Abraham WT, Adams KF, Fonarow GC, et al., the ADHERE Scientific Advisory Committee and

Investigators and the ADHERE Study Group. In-hospital mortality in patients with acute decompensated heart failure treated with intravenous vasoactive medications: an analysis from the Acute Decompensated Heart Failure National Registry (ADHERE). J Am Coll Cardiol 2005;46(1):57–64.
19. Ferreira A, Bettencourt P, Dias P, et al. Neurohormonal activation, the renal dopaminergic system and sodium handling in patients with severe heart failure under vasodilator therapy. Clin Sci 2001;100(5):557–66.
20. Keating GM, Goa KL. Nesiritide: a review of its use in acute decompensated heart failure. Drugs 2003; 63(1):47–70.
21. Boerrigter G, Burnett JC Jr. Recent advances in natriuretic peptides in congestive heart failure. Expert Opin Invest Drugs 2004;13(6):643–52.
22. Abraham WT, Lowes BD, Ferguson DA, et al. Systemic hemodynamic, neurohormonal, and renal effects of a steady-state infusion of human brain natriuretic peptide in patients with hemodynamically decompensated heart failure. J Card Fail 1998;4(1):37–44.
23. Marcus LS, Hart D, Packer M, et al. Hemodynamic and renal excretory effects of human brain natriuretic peptide infusion in patients with congestive heart failure. A double-blind, placebo-controlled, randomized crossover trial. Circulation 1996;94(12): 3184–9.
24. Michaels AD, Klein A, Madden JA, et al. Effects of intravenous nesiritide on human coronary vasomotor regulation and myocardial oxygen uptake. Circulation 2003;107(21):2697–701.
25. Colucci WS, Elkayam U, Horton DP, et al., for the Nesiritide Study Group. Intravenous nesiritide, a natriuretic peptide, in the treatment of decompensated congestive heart failure. N Engl J Med 2000; 343(4):246–53.
26. Brunner-La Rocca HP, Kaye DM, Woods RL, et al. Effects of intravenous brain natriuretic peptide on regional sympathetic activity in patients with chronic heart failure as compared with healthy control subjects. J Am Coll Cardiol 2001;37(5):1221–7.
27. Cataliotti A, Boerrigter G, Costello-Boerrigter LC, et al. Brain natriuretic peptide enhances renal actions of furosemide and suppresses furosemide-induced aldosterone activation in experimental heart failure. Circulation 2004;109(13):1680–5.
28. Aronson D, Burger AJ. Effect of nesiritide (human b-type natriuretic peptide) and dobutamine on heart rate variability in decompensated heart failure. Am Heart J 2004;148(5):920–6.
29. Pitt B, Zannad F, Remme WJ, et al. The effect of spironolactone on morbidity and mortality in patients with severe heart failure. N Engl J Med 1999;341:709–17.
30. Pitt B, Remme WJ, Zannad F, et al. Eplerenone, a selective aldosterone blocker, in patients with left ventricular dysfunction after myocardial infarction. N Engl J Med 2003;348:1309–21.
31. Yancy CW. Treatment with B-type natriuretic peptide for chronic decompensated heart failure: insights learned from the follow up serial infusion of nesiritide (FUSION) trial. Heart Fail Rev 2004; 9(3, special issue):209–16.
32. Aronson D, Burger AJ. Intravenous nesiritide (human B-type natriuretic peptide) reduces plasma endothelin-1 levels in patients with decompensated congestive heart failure. Am J Cardiol 2002;90(4): 435–8.
33. Holmes SJ, Espiner EA, Richards AM, et al. Renal, endocrine, and hemodynamic effects of human brain natriuretic peptide in normal man. J Clin Endocrinol Metab 1993;76(1):91–6.
34. Jensen KT, Carstens J, Pedersen EB. Effect of BNP on renal hemodynamics, tubular function and vasoactive hormones in humans. Am J Physiol 1998;274(1 pt 2):F63–72.
35. Jensen KT, Eiskjaer H, Carstens J, et al. Renal effects of brain natriuretic peptide in patients with congestive heart failure. Clin Sci (Lond) 1999;96(1):5–15.
36. Akabane S, Matsushima Y, Matsuo H, et al. Effects of brain natriuretic peptide on renin secretion in normal and hypertonic saline-infused kidney. Eur J Pharmacol 1991;198(2–3):143–8.
37. Wang DJ, Dowling TC, Meadows D, et al. Nesiritide does not improve renal function in patients with chronic heart failure and worsening serum creatinine. Circulation 2004;110(12):1620–5.
38. Elkayam U, Singh H, Akhter MW, et al. Effects of intravenous nesiritide on renal hemodynamics in patients with congestive heart failure (abstr 256). J Card Fail 2004;10(suppl 4):S88.
39. Mills RM, LeJemtel TH, Horton DP, et al., on behalf of the Natrecor Study Group. Sustained hemodynamic effects of an infusion of nesiritide (human b-type natriuretic peptide) in heart failure: a randomized, double-blind, placebo-controlled clinical trial. J Am Coll Cardiol 1999;34(1):155–62.
40. Burger AJ, Horton DP, LeJemtel T, et al. Effect of nesiritide (B-type natriuretic peptide) and dobutamine on ventricular arrhythmias in the treatment of patients with acutely decompensated congestive heart failure: The PRECEDENT Study. Am Heart J 2002;144(6):1102–8.

41. Publication Committee for the VMAC Investigators. Intravenous nesiritide vs. nitroglycerin for treatment of decompensated congestive heart failure: a randomized controlled trial. JAMA 2002; 287(12):1531–40.
42. Peacock WF IV, Emerman CL, Silver MA, et al. Nesiritide added to standard care favorably reduces systolic blood pressure compared with standard care alone in patients with acute decompensated heart failure. Am J Emerg Med 2005;23(3):327–31.
43. Peacock WF, Holland R, Gyarmathy R, et al. Observation unit treatment of heart failure with nesiritide: results from the PROACTION trial. J Emerg Med 2005;29(3):243–52.
44. Sackner-Bernstein JD, Skopicki HA, Aaronson KD. Risk of worsening renal function with nesiritide in patients with acutely decompensated heart failure. Circulation 2005;111(12):1487–91.
45. Epstein BJ. Elevations in serum creatinine concentration: concerning or reassuring? Pharmacotherapy 2004;24(5):697–702.
46. Butler J, Forman DE, Abraham WT, et al. Relationship between heart failure treatment and development of worsening renal function among hospitalized patients. Am Heart J 2004;147(2):331–8.
47. Abraham WT. Serum creatinine elevations in patients receiving nesiritide are related to starting dose (abstr 2789). Circulation 2005;112(17, suppl II):589.
48. Heywood JT. Combining nesiritide with high-dose diuretics may increase the risk of increased serum creatinine (abstr 240). J Card Fail 2005;11(6, suppl): S154.
49. Sackner-Bernstein JD, Kowalski M, Fox M, et al. Short-term risk of death after treatment with nesiritide for decompensated heart failure: a pooled analysis of randomized controlled trials. JAMA 2005;293(15):1900–5.
50. Gortney JS, Porter KB. Risk of death with nesiritide. JAMA 2005;294(8):897–8.
51. Burger AJ. Risk of death with nesiritide. JAMA 2005;294(8):897.
52. Abraham WT. Nesiritide does not increase 30-day or 6-month mortality risk. Circulation 2005;112 (17, suppl II):676.
53. Arnold LM, Carroll NV, Oinonen M, Crouch MA. Mortality and length of hospital stay in patients receiving dobutamine, milrinone, or nesiritide for acute decompensated heart failure. J Card Fail 2004;10(suppl 4):S103.
53. http://www.sciosinc.com/scios/pr_1118721302.

2.4.2
Positive Inotropes and Vasopressors

52 Dobutamine in the Management of Acute Heart Failure Syndrome

Rohit Mehta and Carl V. Leier

Case Study

A 56-year-old businessman was awakened at 2:15 a.m. by a "heavy feeling" across his chest, followed by generalized weakness; he reports, "I just couldn't get a deep breath." His wife called emergency services, and within 15 minutes he was in the emergency room of the local hospital.

He had been treated over the previous 4 to 5 years for systemic hypertension and hyperlipidemia with the medications valsartan and simvastatin. He stopped smoking about 10 years ago. His father died suddenly at age 62 and a brother required coronary artery bypass surgery at age 49 years.

Upon arrival in the emergency room, he was noted to be anxious and diaphoretic with a respiratory rate of 22 to 26 breaths/minute, blood pressure of 76/60 mm Hg, and a sinus tachycardia of 108 beats/minute. Peripheral pulses were rapid and diminished in amplitude, and his hands and feet were cool and moist ("clammy"). Finger and ear pulse oxygen saturation was 90% on room air and 94% on 2 L/min via nasal cannula. His jugular venous pressure was elevated at 11 to 12 cm H_2O. A summation gallop was noted over the precordium. Crepitant rales were heard over the posterobasal regions of both lungs.

The electrocardiogram showed a Q wave in V_1 and 3 to 5 mm ST segment elevation in V_1 to V_4. Aspirin and clopidogrel were administered and heparin was ordered. In the meantime, the cardiology catheterization-intervention service was called. Because this service can get the patient on the catheterization table within 30 minutes for placement of intraaortic balloon counterpulsation and diagnostic-interventional catheterization, thrombolytic therapy was held.

For hemodynamic and clinical stabilization and augmentation of systemic and coronary-myocardial perfusion until, and perhaps during, cardiac catheterization, dobutamine was started at 2.0 μg/kg/min.

Mechanism of Action and Metabolism

Dobutamine, a member of the catechol-catecholamine family of adrenergic agents, was systematically formulated to augment ventricular systolic function (↑ contractility) with a paucity of adverse effects.[1] Because dobutamine best achieved this objective, it was selected out of over a dozen molecules generated in this quest. The molecular structure is shown in Figure 52.1.

Dobutamine acts principally through stimulation of β_1-adrenergic receptors with lesser stimulation of β_2- and α-adrenergic receptors.[1–4] Therefore, dobutamine enhances ventricular contraction with little net direct effect on peripheral vasculature.[1,2] In normal animal models and in normal humans, dose incrementation increases heart rate. In the setting of human heart failure, the cardiac β_1-adrenergic receptors are generally downregulated from chronic stimulation (elevated circulating catecholamines) or blocked by β_1-selective adrenergic blockers; most of dobutamine's hemodynamic effects are then most likely rendered through β_2-adrenergic stimulation.

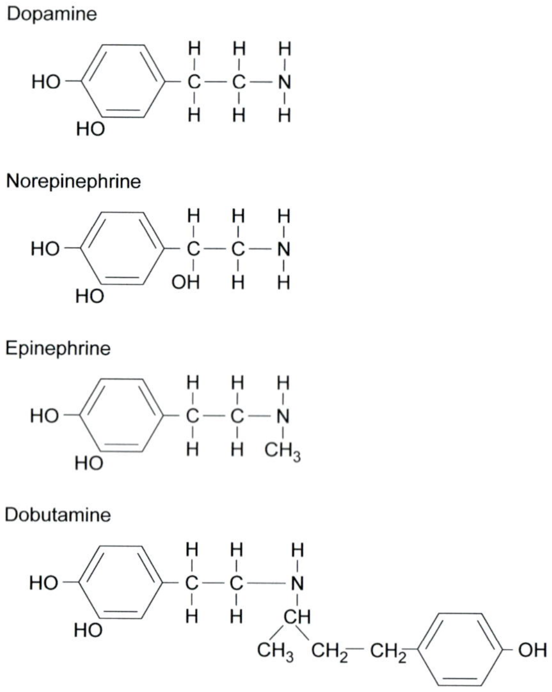

Dopamine

Norepinephrine

Epinephrine

Dobutamine

FIGURE 52.1. The molecular structures of the most commonly used catechols in critical cardiovascular medicine.

In states of ventricular systolic dysfunction, dobutamine increases contractility, stroke volume, and cardiac output. In the laboratory or clinical setting where ventricular systolic dysfunction has resulted in high ventricular filling pressures, reduced stroke volume and cardiac output, and systemic and organ hypoperfusion, dobutamine increases stroke volume, cardiac output, systemic pressure (through an increase in pulse pressure), and systemic and organ perfusion, and reduces ventricular filling pressures and systemic and pulmonic vascular resistances.[5–9] Proper dose selection and incrementation achieve these favorable responses without significantly increasing heart rate or provoking other adverse effects.[5–9] This relatively wide separation of positive inotropic and chronotropic effects is an ideal pharmacologic property of an agent intended for short-term therapy of systolic cardiac failure, but this wide separation cannot be maintained for dobutamine if the initial dose is too high, the dose is advanced too rapidly, or the patient's hemodynamic status is not appropriate (e.g., low ventricular filling pressures). The sinus tachycardia and dysrhythmias noted during dobutamine administration in more recently conducted pharmaceutical-funded trials (for which dobutamine served as a positive control) are generally a consequence of improper dosing and patient selection. Dobutamine also appears to have a favorable effect on ventricular diastolic properties, and on ventricular-vascular coupling by reducing aortic impedance.[10–13]

As a positive inotropic agent, dobutamine increases myocardial oxygen consumption. In the presence of nonobstructed coronary arteries and at dosing levels that do not provoke an increase in heart rate, the rise in oxygen consumption is matched by an adequate and proportional rise in coronary blood flow and myocardial oxygen delivery.[14–18] This balance can be disturbed, resulting in myocardial hypoperfusion and ischemia, in the presence of occlusive coronary artery disease or excessive dosing; this clinical scenario is intentionally created during high-dose dobutamine-stress imaging studies directed at detecting problematic occlusive coronary artery disease.

In human low-output cardiac failure, the patient substrate for dobutamine use, this agent increases enterohepatic, renal, and limb blood flow proportional to the augmentation in cardiac output.[19]

Because dobutamine is rapidly metabolized by gastrointestinal, hepatic, and circulating enzymes, it must be administered intravenously to provide adequate bioavailability. In human heart failure, its half-life is 2.37 ± 0.70 minutes, plasma clearance is 2.33 L/min/m^2, and volume of distribution is 20% of body weight.[20] The short half-life, attributable to metabolism by circulating catechol-o-methyltransferase and rapid redistribution, is a distinctly favorable property in critical care medicine in that its desired hemodynamic effects are attainable within 10 to 15 minutes of dose initiation or incrementation, and most adverse effects dissipate within 10 to 15 minutes of stopping the infusion or reducing the infusion rate. Dobutamine blood levels correlate well with both its infusion rate (dose) and its hemodynamic effects, yet another favorable property (i.e., a predictable dose response) of an agent used for acute inotropic support in the critical care setting[21] (Fig. 52.2). Bolus infusion is never necessary, and generally is not a safe or rational mode of administration for most positive inotropic drugs.

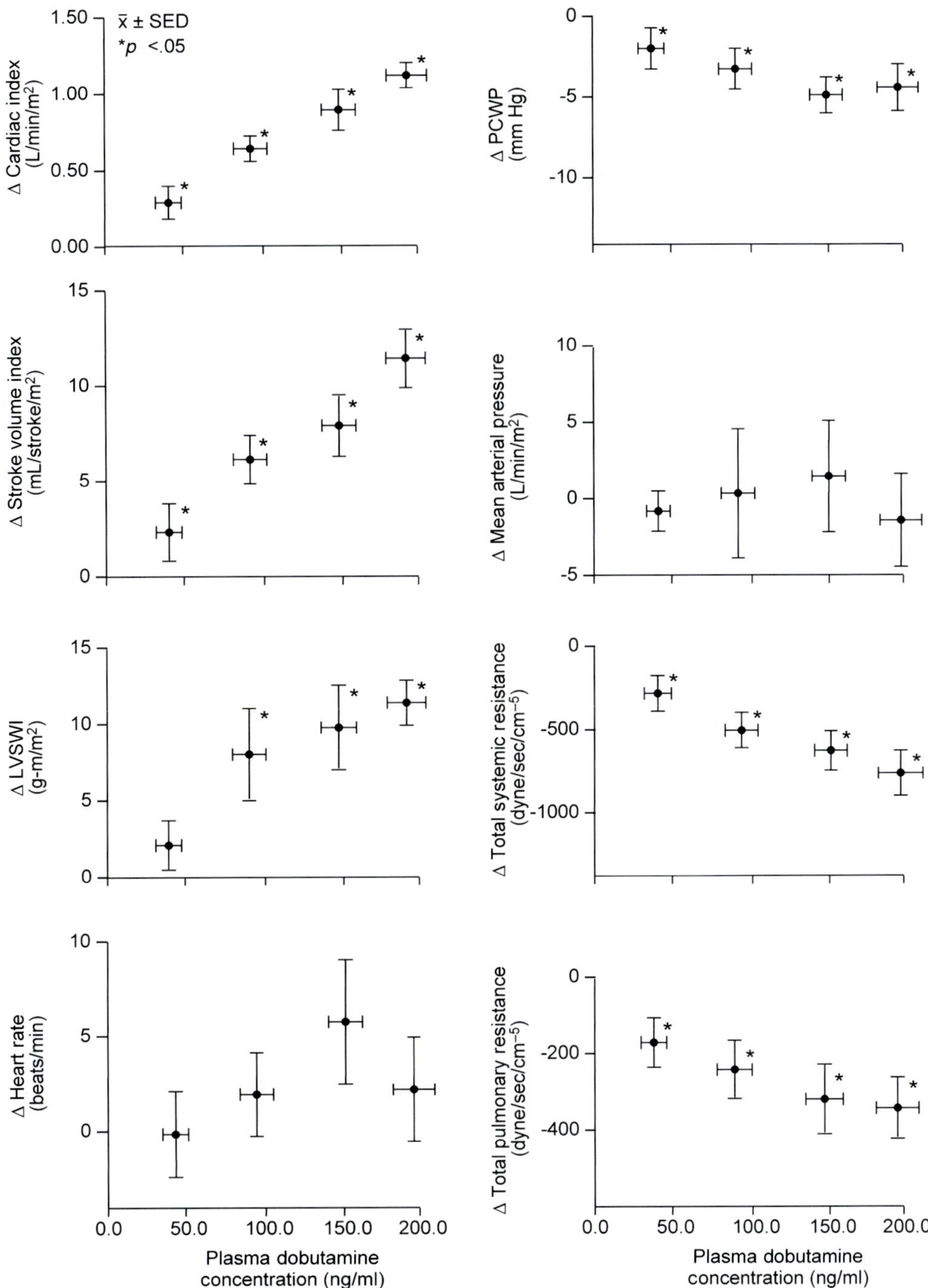

FIGURE 52.2. Graphs showing the relationships among dobutamine dosing, plasma concentrations, and hemodynamic responses in patients with decompensated heart failure. The data points from left to right represent dosing at 2.5, 5.0, 10.0, and 15 μg/kg/min. The data points and brackets represent mean ± 1 standard error. Δ, change from baseline; LVSWI, left ventricular stroke work index; PCWP, pulmonary capillary wedge pressure. (From Leier et al.,[21] with permission.)

Clinical Investigations and Trials

Dobutamine was approved to provide short-term hemodynamic support for patients with decompensated heart failure. The clinical situations for which dobutamine is a therapeutic option, often the initial drug of choice, are acute heart failure syndrome (AHFS) and acute or subacute decompensation of chronic heart failure. In concert with the subject of this book, this chapter discusses dobutamine in the setting of AHFS. Additional clinical applications for dobutamine include hemodynamic support for patients with severe chronic heart failure undergoing major diagnostic or surgical procedures and as a "pharmacologic bridge" to a more definitive intervention (e.g., placement of a ventricular assist device, cardiac transplantation).

Acute Heart Failure Syndrome

There are no double-blind, placebo-controlled trials to support the use of dobutamine in AHFS, but then the same is true for virtually all other agents used in this clinical setting. The profound difficulties in properly conducting such a trial are obvious. Much of the information on the application of drugs in AHFS is inferred from studies on patients with decompensated chronic heart failure.

As depicted in the introductory case study, above, dobutamine is indicated for short-term hemodynamic stabilization and support of the patient with systemic hypotension and hypoperfusion secondary to loss of cardiac systolic function, reduced stroke volume and cardiac output, and adequate or high left ventricle filling pressures (>15 mm Hg).

The choice of dobutamine in this clinical setting follows a rational algorithm. If the hypotensive-hypoperfused patient shows any evidence of low ventricular diastolic filling pressures, fluid volume is administered first to augment stroke volume, cardiac output, systemic pressure and perfusion. Once adequate or high ventricular filling pressures are established and the patient remains hypoperfused, the choice is then largely guided by the level of systemic blood pressure. At systolic pressures over 90 to 100 mm Hg, vasodilators (with or without a diuretic) represent first-line intervention; these include nitroglycerin (sublingual, then intravenous administration), nesiritide, and nitroprusside. The inodilator milrinone may in some instances also be appropriate for this patient profile. At the other end of the spectrum, namely cardiogenic shock or systolic pressures <70 mm Hg, vasopressor therapy with dopamine in vasoconstricting doses (>4 μg/kg/min) is initiated with dose incrementation as needed to raise systemic blood pressure to levels required for adequate coronary artery and systemic perfusion; other vasopressor options include phenylephrine, norepinephrine, and vasopressin. Dobutamine is initiated for patients who fall between these extremes, namely the hypoperfused AHFS patient with a systemic systolic pressure of 70 to 100 mm Hg; this profile represents a sizable portion of patients who present with AHFS.

In this very clinical setting, dobutamine can be expected to increase stroke volume, cardiac output, pulse pressure, systemic blood pressure, and systemic and organ perfusion, while reducing pulmonary and systemic resistances and ventricular filling pressures. The symptoms of dyspnea, weakness, and malaise, and the physical signs of peripheral and organ hypoperfusion should improve during the course of the dobutamine infusion. Proper dosing, beginning at 1 to 2 μg/kg/min with incrementation as needed, achieves these responses without increasing heart rate, the principal determinant of myocardial oxygen consumption.

Dobutamine is frequently used in acute or intensive care in combination with other agents or interventions to augment cardiac performance and systemic perfusion. Examples include dopamine-dobutamine for cardiogenic shock, and dobutamine-nitroglycerin, -nitroprusside, or -nesiritide for near-normotensive severe low output conditions. Dobutamine can augment right and left heart systolic function and cardiac output, if needed, and improve overall hemodynamics and clinical status in patients instrumented with intraaortic balloon counterpulsation or a ventricular assist device.

For AHFS caused by conditions other than coronary artery disease (e.g., myocarditis, decompensated nonischemic dilated cardiomyopathy), properly dosed dobutamine improves hemodynamics with favorable myocardial metabolism.[14,15,17,18] As a positive inotropic drug, dobutamine increases myocardial oxygen consumption. However, studies in human heart failure have shown that coronary blood flow and oxygen supply increase with dobutamine to meet the metabolic demands of enhanced contractility.[14,15,17,18] In addition, a number of dobutamine's favorable hemodynamic effects in the setting of ventricular systolic failure also lessen the metabolic burden of increased contractility by reducing myocardial work and increasing coronary blood flow and oxygen delivery. Right and left ventricular wall stress in both systole and diastole is reduced by dobutamine-induced decrease in vascular resistances, aortic impedance, ventricular filling pressures, and ventricular systolic and diastolic volumes. Coronary blood flow, myocardial perfusion, and myocardial oxygen delivery are augmented by dobutamine through an increase in diastolic coronary perfusion pressure (fall in ventricular diastolic pressure with unchanged or increased aortic diastolic pressure), by an increase in diastolic coronary perfusion time, and by direct vasodilatation of coronary arteries.[18,22–29] In the absence of occlusive coronary disease, patients with low output ventricular failure generally experience enhanced subendocardial perfusion and a drop in the coronary arterial-venous oxygen difference during properly administered dobutamine.[18,24] The critical factors regarding safe, metabolically friendly, and effective administration are proper patient selection, proper dosing, and avoiding an increase in heart rate beyond 10% over baseline.

The same concepts apply to AHFS patients with occlusive coronary artery disease; however, restricted coronary blood flow and flow reserve in these patients place them at a disadvantage from the standpoint of regional myocardial oxygen balance and metabolism. Because dobutamine's coronary vasodilating effects will not likely dilate a fixed high-grade lesion, the chances of evoking ischemia in areas of compromised flow or reserve are far greater in this patient population, particularly if the heart response or enhanced contractility exceed the augmentation of coronary blood flow and the other favorable hemodynamic effects noted above.[29–31]

Nevertheless, dobutamine is still indicated for short-term clinical and hemodynamic stabilization of the patient who presents with problematic coronary disease (e.g., acute coronary syndromes, decompensated ischemic cardiomyopathy), failing ventricle, elevated ventricular filling pressures, and reduced stroke volume, cardiac output and systemic perfusion, and a systemic systolic pressure of 70 to 100 mm Hg[32–39]—short term until the patient undergoes placement of intraaortic counterpulsation or ventricular assist device, a definitive intervention (e.g., angioplasty-stent deployment, coronary artery bypass surgery), or recovers clinically and hemodynamically. Parenthetically, dobutamine infusion may be beneficial in reversing myocardial hibernation and stunning,[40] not uncommon conditions in AHFS patients with underlying problematic occlusive coronary artery disease or following cardiac arrest.

Comparative Treatment Trials in Acute Heart Failure Syndrome

A study and report by Goldstein and colleagues[33] presented the relative safety and hemodynamic efficacy of dobutamine in AHFS after acute myocardial infarction, and demonstrated a limited to negligible role of intravenously administered digoxin (parallel control) in this clinical setting.

Several studies comparing dobutamine and dopamine in decompensated heart failure or cardiogenic shock have shown that, in general, dopamine (at doses of >4 μg/kg/minute) primarily evokes vasoconstriction and mild positive inotropy, while dobutamine greatly enhances contractility with a mild net vasodilatory effect.[19,36,41] Therefore, dopamine is more effective at raising blood pressure and dobutamine at raising cardiac output. At vasopressor doses, dopamine either does not alter or increases ventricular filling pressures, while dobutamine generally lowers them. It is, therefore, reasonable that these agents are often administered together in AHFS patients with low output and hypotension, with or without cardiogenic shock.[41]

Dobutamine and the phosphodiesterase inhibitor milrinone have similar hemodynamic effects, except that milrinone is a more powerful vasodilator.[42–45] Therefore, for the same rise in stroke volume and cardiac output, milrinone will evoke a greater reduction in ventricular filling pressures and pulmonary artery pressures. The vasodilating properties of milrinone may give this agent a more favorable myocardial metabolic profile. Unfortunately, milrinone generally lowers systemic blood pressure considerably more than dobutamine, such that milrinone is not recommended for patients with lower systemic blood pressure. In short, dobutamine is a positive inotropic agent with mild vasodilating properties, and milrinone is a vasodilating agent with mild inotropic effects. It is perhaps only in the AHFS patient with systemic systolic pressures residing somewhere between 90 and 100 mm Hg should there even be a quandary as to which agent to choose for initial intervention. As positive inotropic agents, dobutamine and milrinone are much more complementary than competitive in their clinical and hemodynamic profiles.

The most recent trials on dobutamine in AHFS involved its role as a parallel positive control for infusions of the hormonal vasodilator, nesiritide.[46–48] Unfortunately, these trials do not provide meaningful information on dobutamine because patient, drug, and dose selection were generally inappropriate for this agent. Entry criteria required that the patients not be hypotensive, and the starting, incremental, and maintenance doses for dobutamine were too high. Inappropriate drug and dosing in an inappropriate patient group offers no meaningful or useful information, other than providing a misleading platform or background to make another drug appear better than an agent already approved for use and applied differently in another clinical setting. Therefore, it is not surprising that the positive inotrope with mild vasodilating effects, dobutamine, was found to have more adverse effects and poorer outcomes than the vasodilator, nesiritide. More appropriate positive controls for these trials are other vasodilating agents such as nitroglycerin, nitroprusside, or even milrinone. Nesiritide has not yet been used as a parallel control infusion at inappropriately high doses in hypotensive AHFS patients for comparison with appropriately dosed dobutamine in this population.

Except for the AHFS patient with a systemic systolic pressure of 90 to 100 mm Hg, it is unusual that dobutamine and nesiritide should ever compete as the first best choice in any other AHFS patient. Dobutamine and nesiritide, when properly used, are also complementary and rarely competitive in day-to-day clinical application. In fact, in good clinical practice, it is not uncommon to arrive at simultaneous infusions of these two agents to optimize the clinical and hemodynamic condition of a markedly compromised AHFS patient.

For the same reasons noted above, comparative data on dobutamine versus nesiritide obtained from the pharmaceutical-sponsored Acute Decompensated Heart Failure National Registry (ADHERE) registry also add little meaningful information with two exceptions.[49] First, dobutamine is more likely to be used in hypotensive patients rather than normo- or hypertensive patients, and thus dobutamine is selectively administered to those who begin with a more compromised clinical status and an inherently worse outcome. Second, the findings in ADHERE reinforce the general impression that the selection of cardiovascular support drugs in decompensated cardiac failure is not uniformly appropriate or optimal in general cardiovascular practice (academic and private settings).

Parenthetically, virtually all studies of dobutamine in AHFS were performed on patients with decompensated chronic heart failure. Patients with first-time AHFS, such as that which occurs with acute myocardial infarction, acute myocarditis, and acute valvular regurgitation, have not been investigated in a controlled trial with dobutamine (or any other agent, for that matter).

Practical Application and Considerations

While the dose is often started at >2.0 µg/kg/min, clinical experience has taught us that many patients have a favorable clinical response at initial doses as low as 1.0 µg/kg/min. The lower starting dose is especially recommended for patients who appear to be particularly susceptible to problematic dysrhythmias; frequent premature atrial or ventricular ectopic beats predosing, atrial fibrillation or flutter with rapid ventricular response, hypokalemia, hypomagnesemia, or digitalis toxicity often identify these patients. Lower initial doses should also be considered in those with an elevated resting heart rate and those prone to angina pectoris. Starting doses of 3 to 5 μg/kg/min, commonly employed in trials using dobutamine as parallel control therapy, should rarely be used clinically. Similar caution is recommended in patients with acute coronary syndromes.

Steady-state blood levels are usually attained within 10 to 15 minutes.[20,21] However, unless a patient remains unstable hemodynamically and clinically, there is rarely a need to advance dosing in such a short time interval. A more gradual dosing schedule (dose increase every 30 to 120 minutes) at 1 to 2 μg/kg/min increments averts the most common undesirable effects, increase in heart rate, or dysrhythmias. Dosing is advanced until the desired clinical or hemodynamic effects are attained. It is rare that maintenance doses ever have to exceed 15 μg/kg/min, and such a dose likely portends a poor outcome in most patients with AHFS.

As already noted, patient selection is pivotal in attaining an acceptable benefit-to-risk ratio for dobutamine in AHFS. The prototypical patient is one whose ventricular systolic dysfunction has resulted in elevated ventricular diastolic filling pressures (≥18 mm Hg), reduced stroke volume and cardiac output, mild to moderate systolic hypotension (systemic systolic pressures of 70 to 100 mm Hg), and decreased systemic and organ perfusion. The goal of selecting the proper dosing of dobutamine in this setting is to improve and stabilize the patient's tenuous clinical and hemodynamic condition over the short term until more effective and definitive interventions are instituted (e.g., intraaortic counterpulsation, revascularization procedure) or the patient recovers. In general, dobutamine should not be considered an end-point therapy in AHFS.

The clinical and hemodynamic objectives of dobutamine administration include bringing systemic blood pressure into an acceptable range (which is somewhat dependent on a patient's pre-AHFS blood pressure levels, but generally a systolic of ≥90, diastolic of ≥60, and mean of ≥70 mm Hg), augmenting systemic and organ perfusion and organ function and thus, reducing the symptoms and signs of low-output heart failure (e.g., disturbed mentation, dyspnea, malaise, weakness, cool-moist hands and feet, renal insufficiency). In most patients, it is possible to achieve these end points with properly administered dobutamine without evoking dysrhythmias or a rise in heart rate >10% above baseline. In fact, an elevated predosing heart rate often decreases as hemodynamics improve during dobutamine administration.

As noted above, other agents are often added to assist dobutamine in achieving the clinical-hemodynamic objectives; dopamine or other vasopressor agents are used to raise systemic blood pressure, and vasodilating agents to further reduce ventricular filling pressures and augment systemic and organ perfusion, typically when systemic systolic pressure reaches ≥90 mm Hg.

Dobutamine can also be used for patients on β-adrenergic blocking drugs, but may require slightly higher dosing to reverse the competitive blockade at the β-adrenergic receptor.[39,50,51] For β_1-selective blocking agents, dobutamine acts through β_2-receptors, and β_1-receptors if available, and when adequate competitive dosing is attained. Responses could be influenced by β-receptor polymorphisms, but this question remains to be studied for dobutamine in human heart failure and AHFS.

Most adverse effects can be avoided with proper patient and dose selection, particularly the most frequently encountered, namely a rise in heart rate and cardiac dysrhythmias. Dobutamine enhances atrioventricular (AV) node conduction, and thus can accelerate ventricular response in patients with atrial fibrillation or flutter. An unexpectedly high rise in systemic systolic blood pressure can occur in patients with a history of systemic hypertension or with peripheral vascular disease. Pharmacodynamic tolerance can occur to some degree during infusions lasting >72 hours, and can be overcome with careful dose escalation, but this is generally not a problem during the recommended short-term administration.[52] An increase in cardiac enzymes can be seen in patients with occlusive coronary disease,[46] particularly in the setting of higher-than-needed dosing, which typically evokes an elevation of heart rate >10% above baseline. Prolonged administration can elicit hypokalemia.[53]

Subcutaneous infiltration of highly concentrated dobutamine often causes local erythema, pruritus, and pain, and less commonly, dermal necrosis. Infrequent reactions to dobutamine infusions include generalized erythema-flushing and eosinophilia,[54] both likely secondary to the bisulfite adjuvant.

Case Study Follow-Up

Dobutamine at 3.0 μg/kg/min brought the patient's systemic pressure to 94/70 mm Hg with a heart rate of 102 beats/minute. In the catheterization laboratory, an intraaortic balloon counterpulsation device was introduced, which achieved further augmentation of his systemic pressure to 118/60 mm Hg, and heart rate to 96 beats/min. A high-grade occlusive (85% to 90% obstructive) lesion with recent thrombus formation was found along the proximal left anterior descending coronary artery. Several nonocclusive atherosclerotic lesions (all <30% obstructive) were scattered along the proximal right and left circumflex coronary arteries. The occlusive lesion was dilated and a stent was successfully deployed with little residual stenosis of the culprit lesion and reasonably recovered distal angiographic flow. His angiographic ejection fraction was depressed at 25% to 30% secondary to extensive anterior hypokinesis and apical akinesis. Mild mitral regurgitation was noted.

Dobutamine was gradually weaned over a 3-hour period about 12 hours later, and the counterpulsation was discontinued and removed 36 hours following insertion.

He was discharged 5 days after admission on the usual postinfarction medication plan (beta-blocker, angiotensin-converting enzyme inhibitor, statin, low-dose aspirin, and clopidogrel). He underwent 12 weeks of cardiac rehabilitation, attained a New York Heart Association (NYHA) functional class I status, and returned to his business. Three months following the infarction, an echocardiogram showed mild distal anteroseptal hypokinesis and an overall ejection fraction of 50% to 55%.

References

1. Tuttle RR, Mills J. Dobutamine: development of a new catecholamine to selectively increase cardiac contractility. Circ Res 1975;36:185–96.
2. Robie NW, Nutter DO, Moody C, McNay JL. In vivo analysis of adrenergic receptor activity of dobutamine. Circ Res 1974;67:663–71.
3. Williams RS, Bishop T. Selectivity of dobutamine for adrenergic receptor subtypes: in vitro analysis by radioligand binding. J Clin Invest 1981;67:1703–11.
4. Ruffolo RR. The pharmacology of dobutamine. Am J Med Sci 1987;294:244–8.
5. Jewitt D, Birkhead J, Mitchell A, Doller C. Clinical cardiovascular pharmacology of dobutamine, a selective inotropic catecholamine. Lancet 1974;2:363–7.
6. Beregovich J, Bianchi C, D'Angelo R, et al. Haemodynamic effects of a new inotropic agent (dobutamine) in chronic heart failure. Br Heart J 1975;37:629–34.
7. Aktar N, Mikulic E, Cohn J, Chaudry M. Hemodynamic effects of dobutamine in patients with severe heart failure. Am J Cardiol 1975;36:202–5.
8. Leier CV, Webel J, Bush CA. The cardiovascular effects of the continuous infusion of dobutamine in patients with severe heart failure. Circulation 1977; 56:468–72.
9. Andy JJ, Curry CL, Ali N, Mehrotra PO. Cardiovascular effects of dobutamine in severe congestive heart failure. Am Heart J 1977;94:175–82.
10. Little WC, Rassi A, Freeman GL. Comparison of effects of dobutamine and ouabain on left ventricular contraction and relaxation in closed-chest dogs. J Clin Invest 1987;80:613–20.
11. Carroll JD, Lang RM, Neumann AL, at al. The differential effects of positive inotropic and vasodilator therapy on diastolic properties in patients with congestive cardiomyopathy. Circulation 1986;74: 815–25.
12. Parker JD, Landzberg JS, Bittl JA, et al. Effects of beta-adrenergic stimulation with dobutamine on isovolumic relaxation in normal and failing human left ventricle. Circulation 1991;84:1040–8.
13. Binkley PF, VanFossen DB, Nunziata E, et al. Influence of positive inotropic therapy on pulsatile hydraulic load and ventricular-vascular coupling in congestive heart failure. J Am Coll Cardiol 1990;15: 1127–35.
14. Bendersky R, Chatterjee K, Parmley WW, et al. Dobutamine in chronic ischemic heart failure: alterations in left ventricular function and coronary hemodynamics. Am J Cardiol 1981;48: 554–8.
15. Pozen RG, DiBianco R, Katz RJ, et al. Myocardial metabolic and hemodynamic effects of dobutamine in heart failure complicating coronary artery disease. Circulation 1981;63:1279–185.

16. Meyer SL, Curry GC, Donsky MS, et al. Influence of dobutamine on hemodynamics and coronary blood flow in patients with and without coronary artery disease. Am J Cardiol 1976;38:103–8
17. Beanlands RS, Bach DS, Raylman R, et al. Acute effects of dobutamine on myocardial oxygen consumption and cardiac efficiency measured using carbon-11 acetate kinetics in patients with dilated cardiomyopathy. J Am Coll Cardiol 1993;22:1389–98.
18. Magorien RD, Unverferth DV, Brown GP, Leier CV. Dobutamine and hydralazine: comparative influences of positive inotropy and vasodilation on coronary blood flow and myocardial energetics in nonischemic congestive heart failure. J Am Coll Cardiol 1983;1:499–505.
19. Leier CV, Heban P, Huss P, et al. Comparative systemic and regional hemodynamic effects of dopamine and dobutamine in patients with cardiomyopathic heart failure. Circulation 1978;58:466–75.
20. Kates RE, Leier CV. Dobutamine pharmacokinetics in severe heart failure. Clin Pharmacol Ther 1978;24:537–41.
21. Leier CV, Unverferth DV, Kates RE. The relationship between plasma dobutamine concentrations and cardiovascular responses in cardiac failure. Am J Med 1979;66:238–42.
22. Boudoulas H, Rittgers SE, Lewis RP, et al. Changes in diastolic time with various pharmacologic agents: Implications for myocardial perfusion. Circulation 1979;60:164–9.
23. Barbato E, Bartunek J, Wyffels E, et al. Effects of intravenous dobutamine on coronary vasomotion in humans. J Am Coll Cardiol 2003;42:1596–601.
24. Unverferth DV, Magorien RD, Lewis RP, Leier CV. The role of subendocardial ischemia in perpetuating myocardial failure in patients with nonischemic congestive cardiomyopathy. Am Heart J 1983; 105:176–9.
25. Vatner SF, McRitchie RJ, Braunwald E. Effects of dobutamine on left ventricular performance, coronary dynamics, and distribution of cardiac output in conscious dogs. J Clin Invest 1974;53:1265–73.
26. Liang CS, Hood WB. Dobutamine infusion in conscious dogs with and without autonomic nervous system inhibition: Effects on systemic hemodynamics, regional flows and cardiac metabolism. J Pharmacol Exp Ther 1979;211:698–705.
27. Liang CS, Yi JM, Sherman LG, et al. Dobutamine infusion in conscious dogs with and without acute myocardial infarction. Circ Res 1981;49:170–80.
28. Tuttle RR, Pollock GD, Todd G, et al. The effect of dobutamine on cardiac oxygen balance, regional blood flow, and infarction severity after coronary artery narrowing in dogs. Circ Res 1977;41:357–64.
29. Vatner SF, Baig H. Importance of heart rate in determining the effects of sympathomimetic amines on regional myocardial function and blood flow in conscious dogs with acute myocardial ischemia. Circ Res 19779;45:793–803.
30. Willerson JT, Hutton I, Watson JT, et al. Influence of dobutamine on regional myocardial blood flow and ventricular performance during acute and chronic myocardial ischemia in dogs. Circulation 1976;53:828–33.
31. Rude RE, Izuierdo C, Buja LM, Willerson JT. Effects of inotropic and chronotropic stimuli on acute myocardial ischemia injury. Circulation 1982;65: 1321–8.
32. Gillespie TA, Ambos HD, Sobel BE, Roberts R. Effects of dobutamine in patients with acute myocardial infarction. Am J Cardiol 1977;39:588–94.
33. Goldstein RA, Passamani ER, Roberts R. A comparison of digoxin and dobutamine in patients with acute infarction and cardiac failure. N Engl J Med 1980;303:846–50.
34. Renard M, Bernard R. Clinical and hemodynamic effects of dobutamine in acute myocardial infarction with left heart failure. J Cardiovasc Pharmacol 1980;2:543–52.
35. Keung ECH, Siskind SJ, Sonnenblick EH, et al. Dobutamine therapy in acute myocardial infarction. JAMA 1981;245:144–6
36. Francis GS, Sharma B, Hodges M. Comparative hemodynamic effects of dopamine and dobutamine in patients with acute cardiogenic circulatory collapse. Am Heart J 1982;103:995–1000.
37. Iqbal MZ, Liebson PR. Counterpulsation and dobutamine: their use in the treatment of cardiogenic shock due to right ventricular infarct. Arch Intern Med 1981;141:247–9.
38. Dell'Italia LJ, Starling MR, Blumhart R, et al. Comparative effects of volume loading, dobutamine, and nitroprusside in patients with predominant right ventricular infarction. Circulation 1985;72: 1327–55.
39. Waagstein F, Malek I, Hjalmarson AC. The use of dobutamine in myocardial infarction for reversal of the cardiodepressive effect of metoprolol. Br J Clin Pharmacol 1978;5:515–21.
40. Rahimtoola SH. Hibernating myocardium has reduced blood flow at rest that increases with low-dose dobutamine. Circulation 1996;94:3146–54.

41. Richard C, Ricome JL, Rimailho A, et al. Combined hemodynamic effects of dopamine and dobutamine in cardiogenic shock. Circulation 1983;67: 620–6.
42. Biddle TL, Benotti JR, Creager MA, et al. Comparison of intravenous milrinone and dobutamine for congestive heart failure secondary to ischemic or dilated cardiomyopathy. Am J Cardiol 1987;59:1345–50.
43. Grose R, Strain J, Greenberg M, LeJemtel TH. Systemic and coronary effects of intravenous milrinone and dobutamine in congestive heart failure. J Am Coll Cardiol 1986;7:1107–13.
44. Karlsberg RP, DeWood MA, DeMaria AN, et al. Comparative efficacy of short-term intravenous infusions of milrinone and dobutamine in acute congestive heart failure following acute myocardial infarction. Clin Cardiol 1996;19:21–30.
45. Yamani MH, Haji SA, Starling RC, et al. Comparison of dobutamine-based and milrinone-based therapy for advanced decompensated congestive heart failure: hemodynamic efficacy, clinical outcome, and economic impact. Am Heart J 2001; 142:998–1002.
46. Silver MA, Horton DP, Ghali JK, Elkayam U. Effect of nesiritide versus dobutamine on short-term outcomes in the treatment of acutely decompensated heart failure. J Am Coll Cardiol 2002;39:798–803.
47. Gheorghiade M, Gattis Stough W, Adams K, et al. The pilot randomized study of nesiritide versus dobutamine in heart failure (PRESERVD-HF). Am J Cardiol 2005;96(6A):18–25.
48. Burger AJ, Horton DP, LeJemtel TH, et al. Effect of nesiritide (B-type natriuretic peptide) and dobutamine on ventricular arrhythmias in the treatment of patients with acutely decompensated congestive heart failure: the PRECEDENT study. Am Heart J 2002;144:1102–8.
49. Abraham WT, Adams KF, Fonarow GC, et al. In hospital mortality in patients with acute decompensated heart failure requiring intravenous vasoactive medications: an analysis from the acute decompensated heart failure national registry (ADHERE). J Am Coll Cardiol 2005;46:57–64.
50. Metra M, Nodari S, D'Aloia A, et al. Beta-blocker therapy influences the hemodynamic response to inotropic agents in patients with heart failure. J Am Coll Cardiol 2002;40:1248–58.
51. Bollano E, Tang MS, Hjalmarson A, et al. Different responses to dobutamine in the presence of carvedilol or metoprolol in patients with chronic heart failure. Heart 2003;89:621–4.
52. Unverferth DV, Blanford DM, Kates RE, Leier CV. Tolerance to dobutamine after a 72 hour infusion. Am J Med 1980;69:262–6.
53. Goldenberg IF, Olivari MT, Levine TB, Cohn J. Effect of dobutamine on plasma potassium in congestive heart failure secondary to idiopathic or ischemic cardiomyopathy. Am J Cardiol 1989;63: 843–6.
54. El-Sayed OM, Abdelfattah RR, Barcelona R, Leier CV. Dobutamine-induced eosinophilia. Am J Cardiol 2004;93:1078–9.

53
Therapeutic Role of Dopamine in Acute Heart Failure Syndrome

Vijay Karajala, Murugan Raghavan, Ramesh Venkataraman, and John A. Kellum

Acute heart failure syndromes (AHFSs) resulting in hospitalization remain a major cause of morbidity and mortality in the United States (1). Despite optimal medical therapy, many patients have refractory heart failure and remain symptomatic. Dopamine is widely used in the therapy of AHFS. However, the use of dopamine in the therapy of such patients is highly variable and remains controversial. This chapter summarizes the physiologic and pharmacologic effects of dopamine as well as its clinical rationale in the therapy of AHFS.

Brief Pharmacology of Dopamine

Dopamine was first described by British pharmacologists, Barger and Henry Dale in 1910 (2). The ability of dopamine to augment cardiac output, improve renal blood flow, and induce natriuresis was first described by Mcdonald and Goldberg et al. in the early 1960s (2,3), and has resulted in the widespread use of dopamine in heart failure management. However in recent years, the use of dopamine has fallen out of favor in the management of AHFS due to the advent of superior inotropes with better pharmacodynamics (4). Dopamine, however, is still predominantly used as a vasopressor agent in critically ill patients with vasodilatory shock (5).

Endogenous dopamine (3,4-dihydroxyphenylethylamine) is an immediate metabolic precursor of norepinephrine and epinephrine, and exhibits both central and peripheral autonomic effects (6). However, when administered exogenously, intravenous dopamine does not cross the blood–brain barrier and hence has no central effects. Dopamine's onset of action occurs within 5 minutes of intravenous administration, and its plasma half-life is about 2 minutes, with the total duration of action less than 10 minutes, once the infusion is stopped. Maximal concentrations in kidney occur within 2 minutes after intravenous infusion (7). Dopamine is generally dosed according to lean body weight, and no dose adjustments are required in renal or hepatic insufficiency. About 80% of the drug is excreted in the urine within 24 hours, primarily as homovanillic acid, its sulfate and glucuronide conjugates, and as 3,4-dihydroxyphenylacetic acid. Approximately 25% of the dose is also taken up into specialized neurosecretory vesicles, where it is hydroxylated to form norepinephrine.

Dopamine exerts its effects through five genetically distinct receptors (D_1 to D_5). These receptors, in turn, are classified into two main superfamilies: D_1-like receptors (includes D_1 and D_5) and D_2-like receptors (includes D_2, D_3, D_4), which are located post- and prejunctionally respectively. D_1 and D_5 receptor subtypes act by increasing the cyclic adenosine monophosphate (cAMP), while D_2, D_3, and D_4 receptor subtypes act by decreasing cAMP (8,9). The location of these receptors and their functions are described in the Table 53.1.

The pharmacodynamic effects of dopamine are dose-dependent. At doses of $\leq 2\,\mu g/kg/min$, based on estimated lean body weight, dopamine causes vasodilation by direct stimulation of dopamine postsynaptic type 1 and presynaptic type 2

Table 53.1. Peripheral effects of dopamine on human physiology

Structure	Effect	Receptor
Whole kidney	Increased blood flow; increased glomerular filtration; natriuresis; diuresis	D_1 like and α_1 adrenoreceptors
Juxtaglomerular apparatus and glomerular hemodynamics	Afferent arteriolar vasodilation; variant effect on efferent arteriole; inhibition of renin release	D_1 like
Proximal tubule	Inhibition of Na^+/K^+-ATPase; inhibition of Na^+-H^+ exchange; inhibition of Na^+-PO_4 cotransport; antagonism of angiotensin II	D_1 like and D_2 like
Thick ascending loop of Henle	Inhibition of Na^+/K^+-ATPase	D_1 like and D_2 like
Collecting duct	Inhibition of Na^+/K^+-ATPase; antagonism of ADH action; PGE_2 production	D_4
Sympathetic presynaptic nerve endings	Renal vasodilatation via inhibition of noradrenaline release	D_2 like
Systemic vasculature	Increased BP; decreased BP (direct D1 action)	α-adrenoreceptor D_1 like and D_2 like
Heart	Reduced heart rate; increased heart rate; increased contractility	D_2 like, β_1 adrenoreceptor
Hypothalamus	Facilitation of vasopressin release	D_2
Lungs, basolateral membrane of alveolar type 2	Activation of Na^+/K^+-ATPase; increased lung edema clearance	D_1 like and D_2 like
Human peripheral blood lymphocytes	Neuroimmune interactions	D_3, D_4, and D_5 receptors

ADH, antidiuretic hormone; ATPase, adenosine triphosphatase; BP, blood pressure; PGE_2, prostaglandin E_2.
Source: Adapted from Holmes and Walley (2), with permission.

receptors in the splanchnic and renal arterial beds. Dopamine also has direct effects on renal tubular epithelial cells, resulting in increased natriuresis. Intermediate infusion rates of 2 to 5 μg/kg/min cause direct stimulation of β-adrenergic receptors in the heart and induce norepinephrine release from vascular sympathetic neurons. This results in increased heart rate and cardiac output. Infusion rates of 5 to 15 μg/kg/min generally stimulate β- and α-adrenergic receptors, leading to an increased heart rate and peripheral vasoconstriction (6).

Dopamine Modulates Chemoreflex Sensitivity and Ventilation

The peripheral chemoreceptors (carotid bodies and aortic bodies) are essential for the immediate ventilatory and arterial pressure increases during acute hypoxic, hypercapnic and acute disturbances of acid–base balance (10). Normally, upon exposure to hypoxia, there is an abrupt increase in ventilation, mediated by peripheral chemoreceptors located in carotid bodies. Patients with advanced heart failure generally are hypoxic due to low cardiac output, and chronic lung edema. Hence, these patients generally have increased chemoreflex sensitivity. Dopamine suppresses the carotid body response to hypercapnia as well as to hypoxemia (11). A randomized, double-blind, and placebo-controlled trial was done by Van de Borne et al. (12), which showed that dopamine depresses minute ventilation and oxygen saturation and prolongs apnea in heart failure patients. Low-dose dopamine also has been implicated in impaired gas exchange by blunting the local pulmonary vasoconstrictive response to hypoxia impairing ventilation/perfusion (V/Q) matching in lung (13).

The blunting of chemoreceptor, and V/Q mismatch in the lungs can be very deleterious to heart failure patients. First, these patients may have associated sleep disorders and could lose normal compensatory ventilatory mechanisms to both hypoxia and hypercapnia; second, dopamine may prolong apneic episodes, which could potentiate fatal arrhythmias induced by hypoxemia (7). In heart failure patients, especially those with tenuous respiratory status, dopamine infusion could pose problems in ventilator weaning (2,7). These patients may paradoxically appear comfortable despite significant hypoxia because of attenuated carotid response. If not cautious, a clinician may prematurely extubate these patients, thereby precipitating acute respiratory failure (13). Finally, some recent animal studies (14,15) have shown that dopamine produced by alveolar epithelial cells increase lung fluid clearance, partly through activation of Na^+/K^+–adenosine triphosphatase (ATPase), suggesting a possible role for dopamine in AHFS management (14). However, some other animal experiments have shown that augmentation of cardiac output with dopamine did not significantly affect the extravascular lung water (16).

Cardiovascular Effects of Dopamine

No randomized trial has evaluated the short-term or intermittent use of dopamine infusions in patients with AHFS. While lower doses are used in heart failure management, higher doses are required in vasodilatory shock. Studies have compared dopamine to dobutamine and amrinone and have found that, although dopamine increased maximal cardiac index to a similar extent, dopamine did not significantly decrease pulmonary capillary wedge pressure (PCWP), but caused greater tachycardia (17). Hence, while dopamine may be useful in selected patients with AHFS (i.e., bradycardia with mild heart failure), its isolated role in advanced heart failure is debatable.

A major side effect of dopamine is tachycardia and arrhythmias, which tends to be more pronounced at higher doses (6). In addition, tachycardia may provoke ischemia in patients with coronary artery disease. In the acute setting, inappropriate dosing of dopamine is relatively common for several reasons. First, dopamine dose is based on lean body weight, which in turn can be difficult to estimate (1,6). Second, plasma concentrations of dopamine in individuals receiving the same dose of dopamine differ very widely. Third, there is a markedly huge variation of inter- and intraindividual distribution and metabolism of dopamine, leading to altered tissue and plasma levels (18,19). Fourth, the sensitivity of dopamine receptors shows inter- and intraindividual variation with time. Hence, unexplained tachyarrhythmias in patients on low-dose dopamine should warn the clinician about inappropriate dosing (1).

Decreased heart rate is considered a compensatory mechanism to decrease oxygen requirements in a failing heart, and although augmentation of contractility and heart rate by dopamine may produce temporary improvement in cardiac performance, it may also increase oxygen consumption and aggravate the already injured and hibernating (1,20) myocardium in ischemic heart disease (1,21). In recent years, studies have demonstrated a cardioprotective phenomenon called ischemic preconditioning, which is an adaptive response to a brief ischemic insult that results in slowing cell death to the subsequent prolonged ischemia (22). This has triggered the possibility of using pharmacologic mimetics for ischemic preconditioning (23,24). While dopamine has been shown to promote ischemic preconditioning through its alpha effects (25), these effects have not been confirmed in human studies.

Renal Actions of Dopamine

"Renal dose" or low-dose dopamine (a dose at which dopaminergic and β-adrenergic effects predominate over its alpha effects), generally considered to be $<5\,\mu g/kg/min$ (2), is effective in increasing the renal blood flow and results in increased urine output through various mechanisms (26). These include an increase in cardiac output, vasodilation through direct D_1 and D_2 receptor stimulation, natriuresis by acting directly on the tubules, and reduced sodium reabsorption in the collecting duct, which may be mediated both by decreased secretion of aldosterone and by diminished activity of the Na-K-ATPase pump in the renal tubular cells (19).

Clinicians use renal-dose dopamine in the hopes that such a maneuver might attenuate renal injury and improve survival. In addition, some clinicians often interpret an increase in urinary output as proof that these two assumptions are valid (26). However, there is no evidence that the favorable effects of dopamine on renal hemodynamics are beneficial in patients with, or at risk for, renal dysfunction. Several large trials (27,28) and one comprehensive meta-analyses (26) clearly argue against the routine use of renal-dose dopamine (Table 53.2).

TABLE 53.2. Comparing effects of catecholamines on hemodynamics and gas exchange

		Dopamine		
	Norepinephine	Low dose (<5 µg/kg/min)	High-dose (≥5 µg/kg/min)	Dobutamine
Cardiac output	↔	↔	↑	↑↑
Systemic blood pressure	↑↑	↔	↑	↔
Heart rate	↓	↔	↑	↑
Systemic vascular resistance	↑↑	↔	↓	↓↓
Renal blood flow	↓	↑↑	↑	↔
Glomerular filtration rate	↔	↑	↑	↔
Chemoreceptor function	↔	↓	↓	↔
A-aPO_2	↔	↑	↑↑	↔
O_2 transport	↔	↓	↑	↑↑

A-aPO_2, alveolar-arterial O_2 tension difference; ↔, no change; ↑, increase; ↓, decrease; ↑↑, more profound increase; ↓↓, more profound decrease.
Source: Johnson (13), with permission.

Currently there is overwhelming evidence against the use of low-dose dopamine for renal protection in critically ill patients. Dopamine's effects on the kidney are transient, with maximal effect during the first 8 hours but disappearing after 48 hours (19). It has been suggested that downregulation or desensitization occurs, and tolerance to dopamine develops after 2 to 48 hours (2). The addition of dopamine to furosemide was found to have no effect on urinary sodium excretion rates in patients with New York Heart Association class II or III congestive heart failure (29). Most patients in heart failure, because of neurohormonal activation, have higher levels of renin (30). Hence in these patients, the dopamine's diuretic action is dampened by the high circulating levels of renin (31). In addition, natriuresis produced by dopamine increases solute overload to the distal tubular cells that might increase medullary oxygen consumption, thereby increasing the risk of medullary ischemia. This could potentially explain why agents that increase renal blood flow have generally not been beneficial in the setting of ischemic acute tubular necrosis (ATN). Dopamine has also been shown to worsen renal injury secondary to radiocontrast and in postcardiac surgery patients despite an increase in renal blood flow (26). Even at low doses, dopamine may cause increased systemic resistance and has been reported to be associated with tissue necrosis and digital gangrene (26).

Apart from adverse cardiovascular, renal, and ventilatory effects, low-dose dopamine has several other adverse effects (2). Dopamine worsens sick thyroid syndrome, decreases pulsatile growth hormone secretion, and causes hypopituitarism, immune dysfunction, and early-onset gut ischemia in critically ill patients (26).

New dopamine agonists such as ibopamine have been shown to have favorable symptomatic and hemodynamic effects in early clinical studies. However, the enthusiasm for these drugs diminished significantly when phase 2 trials failed to demonstrate a consistent improvement in symptoms and exercise tolerance, and phase 3 trials were stopped early due to excess mortality. In addition, concomitant use of other antiarrhythmic drugs such as amiodarone led to excess mortality in ibopamine-treated patients with AHFS (32).

Bayram et al. (1) have demonstrated that inodilator therapy is inappropriately used in patients with higher ejection fraction and in patients with normal or higher blood pressures. Short-term, intermittent, or continuous inodilator therapy has been shown to be associated with higher post-discharge mortality (1). Therefore, dopamine, dobutamine, or milrinone should be used only in patients with hypotension secondary to low cardiac output who are not responsive to other modalities. Inodilator therapy may also be a reasonable choice (intermittent and continuous) for symptomatic relief in end-stage heart failure patients who are not suitable for transplantation.

Conclusion

On the basis of the existing evidence, the routine use of dopamine for inotropy, natriuresis, or diuresis, or to improve renal function cannot be recommended in patients with AHFS. Dopamine use should be restricted to modestly hypotensive patients with elevated cardiac filling pressures. Combined norepinephrine with or without dobutamine therapy may be a better option for patients requiring combination of inotrope and vasopressor therapy.

References

1. Bayram M, De Luca L, Massie MB, Gheorghiade M. Reassessment of dobutamine, dopamine, and milrinone in the management of acute heart failure syndromes. Am J Cardiol 2005;96(6A):47G–58G.
2. Holmes CL, Walley KR. Bad medicine: low-dose dopamine in the ICU. Chest 2003;123(4):1266–75.
3. Goldberg LI, McDonald RH Jr, Zimmerman AM. Sodium diuresis produced by dopamine in patients with congestive heart failure. N Engl J Med 1963;269:1060–4.
4. Varriale P. Role of dopamine in congestive heart failure: a contemporary appraisal. Congest Heart Fail 1999;5(3):120–4.
5. Holmes CL. Vasoactive drugs in the intensive care unit. Curr Opin Crit Care 2005;11(5):413–7.
6. Brunton LL, Lazo JS, Parker KL, et al. Pharmacological treatment of heart failure. In: Goodman and Gilman's The Pharmacological Basis of Therapeutics. New York: McGraw-Hill, 2005.
7. Van De BP, Somers VK. Dopamine and congestive heart failure: pharmacology, clinical use, and precautions. Congest Heart Fail 1999;5(5):216–21.
8. Amenta F, Ricci A, Tayebati SK, Zaccheo D. The peripheral dopaminergic system: morphological analysis, functional and clinical applications. Ital J Anat Embryol 2002;107(3):145–67.
9. Katzung BG. Basic and Clinical Pharmacology. New York: McGraw-Hill Medical, 2003.
10. O'Regan RG, Majcherczyk S. Role of peripheral chemoreceptors and central chemosensitivity in the regulation of respiration and circulation. J Exp Biol 1982;100:23–40.
11. Huckauf H, Ramdohr B, Schroder R. Dopamine induced hypoxemia in patients with left heart failure. Int J Clin Pharmacol Biopharm 1976;14(3):217–24.
12. Van de Borne P, Oren R, Somers VK. Dopamine depresses minute ventilation in patients with heart failure. Circulation 1998;98(2):126–31.
13. Johnson RL Jr. Low-dose dopamine and oxygen transport by the lung. Circulation 1998;98(2):97–9.
14. Bertorello AM, Sznajder JI. The dopamine paradox in lung and kidney epithelia: sharing the same target but operating different signaling networks. Am J Respir Cell Mol Biol 2005;33(5):432–7.
15. Helms MN, Chen XJ, Ramosevac S, Eaton DC, Jain L. Dopamine Regulation of Amiloride-Sensitive Sodium Channels in Lung Cells. Am J Physiol Lung Cell Mol Physiol 2006:290(4):L710–22.
16. Garcia-Delgado M, Colmenero-Ruiz M, Fernandez-Sacristan MA, Rus-Mansilla C, Fernandez-Mondejar E. Effect of a catecholamine-induced increase in cardiac output on extravascular lung water. Crit Care Med 2001;29(5):931–5.
17. Van Veldhuisen DJ, Crijns HJ, Girbes AR, Tobe TJ, Wiesfeld AC, Lie KI. Electrophysiologic profile of ibopamine in patients with congestive heart failure and ventricular tachycardia and relation to its effects on hemodynamics and plasma catecholamines. Am J Cardiol 1991;68(11):1194–202.
18. MacGregor DA, Smith TE, Prielipp RC, Butterworth JF, James RL, Scuderi PE. Pharmacokinetics of dopamine in healthy male subjects. Anesthesiology 2000;92(2):338–46.
19. Ichai C, Passeron C, Carles M, Bouregba M, Grimaud D. Prolonged low-dose dopamine infusion induces a transient improvement in renal function in hemodynamically stable, critically ill patients: a single-blind, prospective, controlled study. Crit Care Med 2000;28(5):1329–35.
20. Packer M, Medina N, Yushak M. Hemodynamic and clinical limitations of long-term inotropic therapy with amrinone in patients with severe chronic heart failure. Circulation 1984;70(6):1038–47.
21. Jain P, Massie BM, Gattis WA, Klein L, Gheorghiade M. Current medical treatment for the exacerbation of chronic heart failure resulting in hospitalization. Am Heart J 2003;145(2 suppl):S3–17.
22. Robinet A, Hoizey G, Millart H. PI 3-kinase, protein kinase C, and protein kinase A are involved in the trigger phase of beta1-adrenergic preconditioning. Cardiovasc Res 2005;66(3):530–42.
23. Kloner RA, Jennings RB. Consequences of brief ischemia: stunning, preconditioning, and their clinical implications: part 1. Circulation 2001;104(24):2981–9.
24. O'Leary M, Davis M, Bihari D. Myocardial protection in the intensive care unit. Curr Opin Crit Care 1999;5(S):400–7.

25. Lazou A, Markou T, Zioga M, Vasara E, Efstathiou A, Gaitanaki C. Dopamine mimics the cardioprotective effect of ischemic preconditioning via activation of β1-adrenoceptors in the isolated rat heart. Physiol Res 2005.
26. Kellum JA, Decker M. Use of dopamine in acute renal failure: a meta-analysis. Crit Care Med 2001; 29(8):1526–31.
27. Bellomo R, Chapman M, Finfer S, Hickling K, Myburgh J. Low-dose dopamine in patients with early renal dysfunction: a placebo-controlled randomised trial. Australian and New Zealand Intensive Care Society (ANZICS) Clinical Trials Group. Lancet 2000;356(9248):2139–43.
28. Marik PE, Iglesias J. Low-dose dopamine does not prevent acute renal failure in patients with septic shock and oliguria. NORASEPT II Study Investigators. Am J Med 1999;107(4):387–90.
29. Vargo DL, Brater DC, Rudy DW, Swan SK. Dopamine does not enhance furosemide-induced natriuresis in patients with congestive heart failure. J Am Soc Nephrol 1996;7(7):1032–7.
30. Lim PO, MacFadyen RJ, Struthers AD. Is there a role for renin profiling in selecting chronic heart failure patients for ACE inhibitor treatment? Heart 2000;83(3):257–61.
31. Marik PE. Low-dose dopamine in critically ill oliguric patients: the influence of the renin-angiotensin system. Heart Lung 1993;22(2):171–5.
32. Smit AJ, Girbes AR. Dopamine agonists in heart failure: an untimely death. Neth J Med 1997;51(5):151–3.

54
Vasopressors in Acute Severe Heart Failure

John H. Boyd and Keith R. Walley

The management of heart failure has traditionally rested on a paradigm centering on reducing cardiac work load, and more recently on the antagonism of endogenous chronic pathogenic (over)stimulation with stress hormones such as angiotensin, catecholamines, and aldosterone. Depending on the individual patient, cardiac work load is decreased through a combination of modulating the heart rate, contractility, and perhaps most importantly afterload. As the pressure against which the left ventricle must eject is a main determinant of energy expended, afterload reduction has been a foundation of modern therapy. It is thus counterintuitive that in severe heart failure there is a role for agents whose main effect is to increase afterload. There are, however, clinical situations in which acute heart failure coexists with shock states requiring the use of pressor agents. This chapter discusses the pharmacology of the vasopressor agents approved for use and the clinical situations in which they are useful, and offers general recommendations for their use in acute severe heart failure.

Clinical Diagnosis

Clinical Picture

Patients with severe acute heart failure exhibit signs of heart failure plus evidence of end-organ hypoperfusion including tachycardia, tachypnea, low mean blood pressure, low pulse pressure, diaphoresis, cold mottled extremities, altered mental status, and decreased urine output. In those patients who receive a central venous or pulmonary arterial catheter, global hypoperfusion is reflected by a low mixed venous oxygen saturation and low cardiac output. Urgent echocardiographic assessment can reveal the cause by demonstrating regional myocardial dysfunction (myocardial infarction), a dilated left ventricle having poor global function (acute on chronic heart failure), a thick hypertrophic ventricle (diastolic dysfunction), valvular dysfunction, evidence of tamponade, combinations of the above, and other valuable findings that may help establish the underlying etiology.

Treatment is in a general sense aimed at improving tissue oxygen delivery. When the cause of acute severe heart failure is evident, reversing the cause is a priority, for example, thrombolytic therapy or percutaneous coronary angioplasty for acute myocardial infarction or pericardiocentesis for tamponade. General resuscitation is achieved through judicious use of fluids, normalization of cardiac rate and rhythm, and the use of inotropic agents. Occasionally these first two steps (reversing the cause and general resuscitation) fail to restore adequate blood pressure and end-organ perfusion so that vasopressor agents are required. When this happens several important issues should be considered.

Increased Afterload Is Also Detrimental

Decreased left ventricular systolic contractility is characterized by decreased slope of the end-systolic pressure-volume relationship (Fig. 54.1). In this setting, stroke volume is very sensitive to changes in afterload (Fig. 54.2). Accordingly, afterload reduction therapy is highly beneficial in increasing stroke volume and cardiac output in patients with decreased left ventricular contractility. Therefore, it is important to recognize that when vasopressor agents are required to treat excessive hypotension and end-organ hypoperfusion in acute severe heart failure, vasopressor agents have the potential to substantially decrease stroke volume and cardiac output from their initially inadequate values. This is a difficult problem and generally requires the concomitant use of an inotropic agent (having its own adverse effect of increased myocardial oxygen demand) to increase left ventricular contractility (the slope of the end-systolic pressure-volume relationship) or the use of intraaortic balloon counterpulsation or a ventricular assist device to aid ventricular ejection (Fig. 54.2).

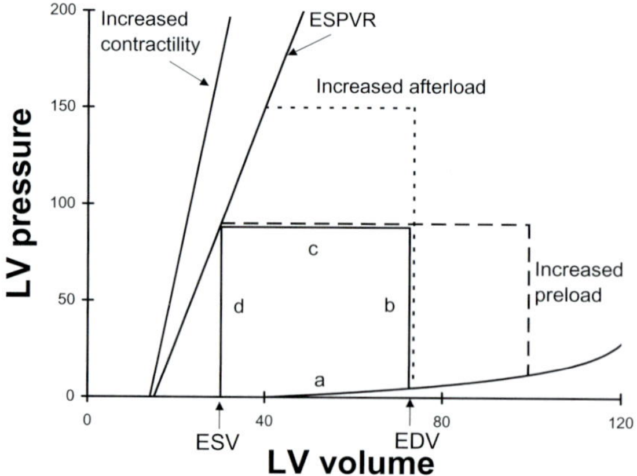

FIGURE 54.1. Ventricular pressure-volume relationships. During diastole the heart fills at quite low pressures along the normally compliant diastolic pressure-volume relationship of the ventricle (a). With the onset of isovolumic systole, the ventricle contracts raising intraventricular pressure at constant volume (in the absence of valvular heart disease) (b). When ventricular pressure exceeds aortic pressure, the aortic valve opens and ejection occurs (c) and continues to an end-systolic pressure-volume point. Intraventricular pressure decreases during the isovolumic relaxation phase (d), and the cardiac cycle starts again. It is not surprising that at high afterload (the blood pressure along segment c) the ventricle is not able to eject far, whereas at lower afterload the ventricle is able to eject further. End-systolic points for differently loaded ejections all fall along an approximately linear end-systolic pressure-volume relationship (ESPVR). The slope, E_{max}, of the end-systolic pressure-volume relationship is an excellent measure of ventricular contractility. That is, if E_{max} increases, it can be seen that the ventricle is able to eject further (to a smaller end-systolic volume [ESV]) at the same afterload. EDV, end-diastolic volume.

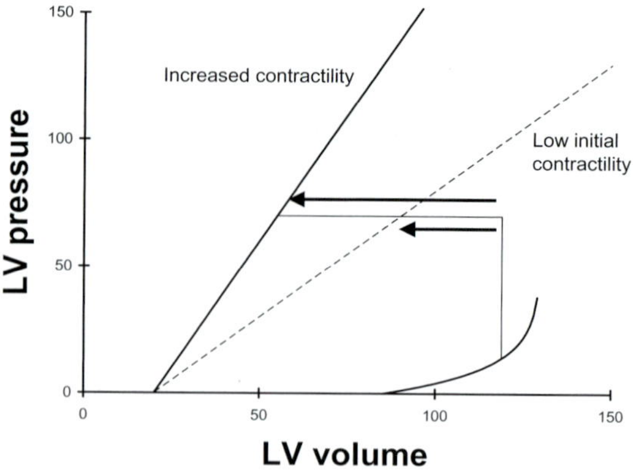

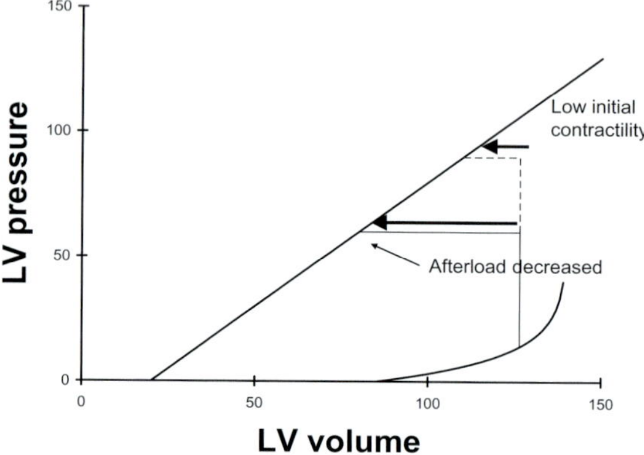

FIGURE 54.2. The left ventricular pressure-volume relationships in the setting of decreased ventricular systolic contractility. Stroke volume is determined by both contractility and afterload. Compared to Figure 54.1, the slope, E_{max}, of the end-systolic pressure-volume relationship is greatly decreased. The top panel demonstrates that stroke volume (horizontal arrows) can be greatly increased in this setting by using inotropic agents that increase the slope, E_{max}. The bottom panel illustrates that stroke volume (horizontal arrows) can be greatly increased by decreasing afterload. The corollary of this observation is that use of vasopressor agents to increase blood pressure afterload will have the undesired effect of decreasing stroke volume. To counteract this effect, concomitant use of an inotropic agent or support of stroke volume using, for example, an intraaortic balloon pump is often required.

Pure Cardiogenic Shock Versus a Component of Distributive Shock

Most textbooks characterize cardiogenic shock as having low cardiac output and high systemic vascular resistance. However, a subset of patients will present with mixed cardiogenic and vasodilatory shock. Patients presenting with a component of vasodilatory shock are reasonably common, particularly in view of current thrombolytic, angioplasty, surgical, and ventricular assist device therapy, which can all initiate a systemic inflammatory response syndrome characterized by increased concentrations of circulating inflammatory cytokines and other inflammatory mediators. While the underlying pathophysiology may differ, the hemodynamic profile and goals of therapy for these patients overlap with patients having severe sepsis combined with ventricular dysfunction. Vasopressor therapy is often required in this subset of patients.

Treatment

General Issues

Patients for whom the clinician considers vasopressor therapy are generally hemodynamically unstable. Thus some general recommendations can be made with respect to the location of treatment and the types of monitoring necessary in this group. Treatment should be given in a high acuity cardiac care unit or critical care unit where one-to-one nursing care and the capability to perform invasive hemodynamic monitoring are readily available. Given the concerns regarding end-organ perfusion and subsequent adequacy of resuscitation, the minimum monitoring includes continuous monitoring of urine output by bladder catheterization, continuous pulse oximetry for oxygen saturation levels, and continuous electrocardiographic monitoring to quickly identify disturbances of rate and rhythm. Noninvasive blood pressure monitoring in patients with shock is not accurate at low arterial pressures, and continuous pressure monitoring via arterial catheterization is the preferred method of monitoring. This also allows rapid assessment of the efficacy of any new therapy. Metabolic and hematologic monitoring upon admission are necessary, with frequent serum electrolytes, complete blood counts, lactate, and arterial blood gases guiding therapy and alerting the clinician to new problems.

Many vasopressors can cause serious local tissue necrosis due to profound vasoconstriction if peripheral intravenous infusions leak into surrounding tissues. For this reason, as well as to allow access to central venous pressure measurement, central venous catheterization is recommended in all patients. Of the two locations most often used to access the central circulation and right heart pressures, subclavian vein access has the fewest infectious complications and is generally less intrusive to the patient. For clinicians less experienced in central venous access techniques, however, there is a slightly increased risk of pneumothorax compared to the internal jugular route. The decision whether to place a pulmonary artery catheter via central vein access will be at the discretion of the treating physician, and depend in part on the ready availability of alternative measures of cardiac function such as echocardiography. This extensive monitoring enables the physician to pursue an aggressive integrated treatment plan with good measures of efficacy, an approach that in patients presenting with vasodilatory septic shock is one of the few treatments resulting in improved survival (1).

Specific Issues

Blood Pressure

Perhaps the most challenging aspect to the care of the patient with advanced heart failure is to decide at which level of arterial blood pressure therapeutic chronic lowering of afterload becomes pathologic and thus detrimental to the patient's physiology. It is not unusual (in fact it is the standard of care) to have patients with New York Heart Association (NYHA) class III/IV heart failure treated with afterload reduction using angiotensin-converting enzyme (ACE) inhibitors or AT2 blockers, combined with diuretics and beta-blockade. With these potent medications a systolic blood pressure of 80 to 90 mm Hg may be the therapeutic target, but it is the role of the clinician to determine when hypotension is negatively impacting global perfusion. Easily determined clinical variables rather than an absolute level of arterial pressure are key in making this diagnosis. Alteration in mental status, decreased urine output, hypoperfused extremities, along with an elevated blood lactate in the context of a drop in blood pressure from the usual should alert the treating physician that there is significant hypoperfusion with end-organ dysfunction. Although, as stated above, there is no absolute cutoff for blood pressure, a mean arterial pressure under 65 mm Hg or a drop in systolic pressure of more than 40 mm Hg is usually seen in this context.

Central Venous or Mixed Venous Oxygen Saturation

The use of pulmonary artery catheterization is becoming less common due to the increasing use and utility of echocardiographic examination and due to relatively recent reports suggesting that, depending on the experience of the center, pulmonary artery catheterization may result in increased morbidity and mortality (2–4). Measurement of oxygen saturation using co-oximetry principles or by sampling blood from the distal port of a thoracic central venous catheter provides useful information that may help guide management when a pulmonary artery catheter is not used. Central venous oxygen saturation slightly overestimates traditional mixed venous oxygen saturation measured using a pulmonary artery catheter, but central venous oxygen saturation changes closely correlate with simultaneous mixed venous oxygen saturation changes. Given these caveats, central venous oxygen saturation can be used with the Fick equation to estimate cardiac output and to primarily assess the adequacy of tissue oxygenation. In a randomized trial of early resuscitation of septic shock, early goal-directed therapy, which includes a central venous oxygen saturation goal exceeding 70%, dramatically improved patient outcome (1). The basic principles of early goal-directed therapy, including achieving a target central venous oxygen saturation, can be applied to resuscitation of acute severe heart failure. In view of the underlying pathophysiology, fluid resuscitation should be approached with care, and a target central venous oxygen saturation of 70% is very optimistic, but a slightly lower modified target is often achievable.

Initial Stabilization and Establishment of Treatment Goals

Once a patient is deemed to be in shock, with evidence of end-organ hypoperfusion, and careful fluid resuscitation has resulted in no clinical improvement, admission to a high acuity unit should not be delayed. Monitoring as outlined above should be instituted and goals of therapy established and communicated to all treating medical personnel. The clinical variables used to determine compromise, namely altered mental status, decreased urine output, cool peripheral skin, and elevated blood lactate are all excellent targets of resuscitation. Additionally, targeting a central venous mixed venous oxygen saturation of >65% to 70% should be added, where feasible, assuring adequate oxygen delivery. A target blood pressure should be set for the individual. Mean arterial pressure should be targeted to a level where signs of hypoperfusion are absent, or if this is unknown, choosing 65 mm Hg as the initial goal. Based on available data (1), fluids should be given, including blood products, to maintain a central venous pressure of 8 to 12 mm Hg and a hematocrit of >30%. If no improvement is observed with fluid resuscitation, then additional pharmacologic therapy must be instituted without delay.

Pharmacologic Therapy

If cardiac output is profoundly depressed, hypotension may be a result of isolated cardiogenic shock. In this case the increase in cardiac output with inotropic therapy such as intravenous dobutamine or milrinone may outweigh the peripheral vasodilation these agents tend to produce (Table 54.1). However, in a clinical setting where blood pressure is markedly reduced and one fears any further potential vasodilation might result in imminent cardiac arrest, it is prudent to begin therapy with a combination of inotropic agent (e.g., dobutamine) plus a vasopressor agent (e.g., noradrenaline) (Table 54.1). The peripheral β_1-adrenergic–mediated vasodilation caused by dobutamine is counteracted by the potent vasopressor activity of noradrenaline. While monotherapy with noradrenaline may often be advocated for vasodilatory shock states, when cardiac function is severely impaired one needs to temper the augmented afterload with more powerful inotropy than noradrenaline alone is able to provide. Both agents are started together, ensuring that neither blood pressure nor cardiac output is augmented at the expense of the other.

An alternative approach is to use monotherapy with an inotropic agent that also has vasopressor

TABLE 54.1. Cardiovascular effects of vasopressor agents

Vasopressor	Dose	Inotropy	Vasoconstriction
Dopamine	2.5–20 μg/kg/min	++	+
Noradrenaline	0.03–5 μg/kg/min	+	+++
Vasopressin	0.01–0.04 U/min	+ (low dose) – (high dose)	++
Phenylephrine	0.5–10 μg/kg/min	–	+

properties. Practically, first-line monotherapy is often dopamine, providing good inotropic effect with moderate pressor activity. At doses in the 5 to 10 μg/kg/min range, the hemodynamic effect is very similar to that of dobutamine, predominantly acting via β_1-adrenergic receptors to increase inotropy and reduce afterload. Should this dose range worsen the hypotension, dopamine can quickly be titrated over 10 μg/kg/min, thus taking advantage of its vasopressor properties at this dose. Tachycardia and tachyarrhythmias are frequent side effects of higher dose dopamine and may limit the doses tolerated by an individual. In some cases of intense vasodilatation such as in severe sepsis, dopamine alone may not suffice, and in this case therapy should be changed to a combination of dobutamine plus the more potent vasopressor noradrenaline, or the combined α- and β-agonist adrenaline alone. If hypotension persists despite maximal doses of noradrenaline, then low-dose vasopressin may be added at doses of 0.01 to 0.04 U/min. Given that vasopressin not only has vasoconstrictor properties via its own V1 receptors but potentiates catecholamine vasopressor activity, we generally recommend adding vasopressin to established therapy rather than substituting it for noradrenaline.

Specific Vasopressor Agents: Pharmacology and Hemodynamic Effects

Dopamine

Dopamine is synthesized from its precursor phenylalanine, converted in vivo first to noradrenaline by dopamine-β-hydroxylase, and then on to adrenaline by phenylalanine-*N*-methyltransferase. Due to its pharmacology, there are distinct effects depending on the dosage used. At doses of less than 5 μg/kg/min, dopaminergic receptors DA1 and DA2 are predominantly stimulated and result in vasodilation of the renal and mesenteric circulations, increasing urine output in healthy subjects (5). However, in patients with shock and early renal dysfunction, a large randomized control study showed no benefit in low-dose dopamine (2 μg/kg/min) with respect to improvement in creatinine, urine output or the need for renal replacement therapy (6). At doses between 5 and 10 μg/kg/min, β_1-adrenergic effects are strongest, leading to an increase in heart rate and contractility, while at doses in excess of 10 μg/kg/min, α_1-adrenergic receptor stimulation results in systemic vasoconstriction and increased arterial pressure.

In patients with hypotension, dopamine increases the mean arterial pressure mainly via an increased cardiac index with preservation or slight increase in vascular resistance (7–14). In those patients remaining hypotensive despite adequate fluid resuscitation, dopamine is able to increase the mean arterial pressure by nearly 25% at a median dose of 15 μg/kg/min. At doses under 20 μg/kg/min, an increase in stroke volume leading to improved cardiac index is the main hemodynamic effect, while as the dose is increased to over 20 μg/kg/min, tachycardia and increased pulmonary vascular resistance become more evident. While the increased cardiac output results in an increased oxygen delivery, there appears to be a decrease in the oxygen extraction ratio (15–17), implying a microcirculatory defect with no resultant gain in tissue oxygenation. Overall dopamine is a moderately effective agent in restoring arterial pressure, and given that its major effect is increased, the cardiac index may be well suited to those patients who have a cardiac component to their hypotension. Side effects are often dose limiting and include a propensity to induce tachyarrhythmias not seen as frequently with other vasopressor agents. At doses over 10 μg/kg/min, the increase in pulmonary artery occlusion pressure seen with dopamine may worsen hypoxia through increased lung water. Finally, there have been reports that dopamine infusion in the critically ill may the influence the endocrine system, with an inhibition in the secretion of prolactin observed in one study (14).

Noradrenaline

Noradrenaline stimulates both α- and β-adrenergic receptors, although α-adrenergic effects predominate. This profile results in an increase in mean arterial pressure via systemic vasoconstriction and increased systemic vascular resistance. The effect on cardiac output is much more modest, with reported increases in both stroke volume and cardiac index in the range of 10% to 15%, while some studies report no increase in cardiac output at all (18–20). Given the increase in mean arterial pressure seen with noradrenaline usage, when combined with a relatively static cardiac output, there is a resultant increase in ventricular stroke work index. Unlike dopamine there have been no reports of an increase in pulmonary artery occlusion pressures, and either no effect or a minimal increase in mean pulmonary artery pressure is produced by noradrenaline. Dosage of this drug is variable, possibly reflecting α-adrenergic downregulation in shock states (21). Published studies have doses ranging from 0.01 to a high of 5 μg/kg/min (22,23). When compared with dopamine in patients with shock unresponsive to fluids, noradrenaline has a favorable profile. In a randomized control study 32 patients with hyperdynamic shock states unresponsive to fluid resuscitation were treated to maintain a normal hemodynamic and oxygenation profile (7). Dopamine from 10 to 25 μg/kg/min achieved the goal in only 31% of the patients, while noradrenaline at a mean dose of 1.5 μg/kg/min was successful in 93% of those studied. Of the 11 patients who did not achieve the target physiology with dopamine, 10 normalized when noradrenaline was introduced. Although the studies were not designed to assess mortality, in this group of septic patients the survival also differed, with 59% surviving with noradrenaline while only 17% survived with dopamine.

Concerns have been raised regarding the vasoconstriction induced by noradrenaline, particularly with respect to renal and mesenteric blood flow. This effect is pronounced in those patients who are hypovolemic at the initiation of therapy (24–26), and has been found to induce renal ischemia. Even in the setting of normal physiology, infusion of noradrenaline has been found to reduce renal blood flow (27). However, unlike in normals or in shock states where the intravascular volume is depleted, the physiologic effect of noradrenaline in hypotensive but volume replete patients is more favorable. When used in hyperdynamic shock states, noradrenaline has been found in numerous studies to improve both urine output and creatinine clearance (13,27–29). This is felt to be due to an alteration in relative vasoconstriction between afferent and efferent arterioles. With respect to mesenteric blood flow and tissue oxygenation, in hypotensive patients treated with noradrenaline the results to date are inconclusive.

In summary, noradrenaline is an extremely efficacious drug to normalize blood pressure when used in patients who are volume replete. The adverse profile associated with noradrenaline usage in regard to organ ischemia are due to the powerful vasoconstrictive effects and are generally not seen in patients who are volume repleted prior to commencing therapy. Caution must be exercised, though, in patients who are kept chronically volume depleted to compensate for high left heart filling pressures. These patients are theoretically at high risk for renal dysfunction and possibly mesenteric ischemia.

Vasopressin

Vasopressin is a peptide endogenously produced in humans by the hypothalamus. Its effects are mediated via the tissue-specific receptors V1R, V2R, V3R, OTR, and P2R (30,31). Of the receptors thought to be mainly responsible for increased vascular tone, V1Rs mediate vasoconstriction and are found mainly on vascular smooth muscle, cardiac myocytes, and the kidney, and V2Rs are found in the renal collecting duct and are responsible for the antidiuretic effect associated with this hormone. Oxytocin receptors (OTRs) are found diffusely throughout the body and are likely responsible for tissue-specific vasodilation, interestingly allowing the same hormone to cause both vasoconstriction and vasodilation depending on the tissue-specific distribution of V1R vs OTR.

Vasopressin acts on vascular smooth muscle via a number of mechanisms in addition to stimulation of the V1R. Vasopressin is able to close potassium channels in the smooth muscle cells (32), which results in an enhanced depolarization and contraction of the vessels. Nitric oxide is a well-known vasodilator that acts through cyclic guanosine monophosphate (cGMP), and vasopressin both reduces the activity of inducible nitric oxide synthase (iNOS) and decreases the activity of cGMP (33,34). Finally, vasopressin is able via unknown mechanisms to enhance the effect of vasoconstrictor agents such as noradrenaline (35).

While its effect on vascular tone is relatively well understood, vasopressin has multiple effects on cardiac contractility and coronary arterial tone, many of which are dose dependent. Current understanding based on laboratory studies suggests that at low doses vasopressin counteracts coronary smooth muscle V1R-mediated vasoconstriction with P2R-mediated vascular endothelial vasodilation. With coronary flow unimpaired, there appears to be a mild but positive inotropic effect. At higher doses the relative effect of coronary arterial vasoconstriction outweigh any inotropic effects and results in a decrease in cardiac output. A variety of clinical data are available to support this. In patients with vasodilatory shock, it was observed that vasopressin increased systemic vascular resistance twofold, while only diminishing cardiac output by 14% (36). Further, in a study of 41 hypotensive postcardiotomy patients resistant to the effects of catecholamine infusions, the addition of low-dose (0.04 U/min) vasopressin resulted in a significant increase in left ventricular work index and a decrease in vasopressor use, inotrope use, and heart rate (37). When given to patients with advanced heart failure to counteract the vasodilatory effects of the phosphodiesterase inhibitor milrinone, vasopressin resulted in increased vascular tone and blood pressure with no resultant drop in cardiac output (38).

Clinically it is interesting to note that the hemodynamic effects of vasopressin are potentiated by the shock state. In normal subjects vasoconstriction only occurs at high doses, while in patients suffering from hypotension refractory to fluids, powerful vasopressor effects are seen at low doses. It is thought that this is due to a depletion of circulating vasopressin with subsequent hypersensitivity to its effects (13). Overall, vasopressin is a drug that, because of its many receptors, has very different effects depending on the dose used. At low (0.01 to 0.04 U/min) infusion rates, the predominant effects in those with vasodilatory shock are a potent increase in systemic vascular resistance and a milder positive effect on cardiac output, resulting in maintenance of forward flow despite an increased afterload.

Terlipressin

Terlipressin is a prodrug of vasopressin and has an extended half-life of 6 hours versus 24 minutes for vasopressin. It is available clinically in Europe and is undergoing safety and efficacy trials in North America. Terlipressin 1 to 2 mg given intravenously (IV) has significant hemodynamic effects in hypotensive patients for over 5 hours (39). The bulk of clinical experience has come with its use for control of portal pressures during variceal hemorrhage, a clinical situation for which it has found some utility.

Phenylephrine

Phenylephrine is an α-adrenergic agonist and as such increases systemic vascular resistance with no augmentation of cardiac output. Doses range from 0.5 μg/kg/min to 10 μg/kg/min as an intravenous infusion. Although widely used as a short-term pressor particularly well suited to counteract the vasodilatory effects of anesthesia, there are few studies looking at longer term infusions (40–42). When directly compared to noradrenaline infusion in patients with septic shock, phenylephrine infusion resulted in decreased oxygen delivery and splanchnic blood flow (42). Overall, concerns regarding using a powerful vasoconstrictor with no positive inotropic effects in critically ill patients who often exhibit cardiac dysfunction have precluded widespread use.

Case Study

A 55-year-old woman with idiopathic dilated cardiomyopathy is followed at the heart failure clinic and has been stably maintained on furosemide, an angiotensin-converting enzyme inhibitor (ACEI), beta-blocker, digoxin, and spironolactone. She has been ambulatory, although she gets short of breath with light exertion. She is brought to the emergency department by her husband, who reported she had become confused overnight and appeared to be more short of breath. There had been no recent change in medication, and the last clinic note 1 month ago noted no new issues. She is observed by the triage nurse to appear quite ill and is brought quickly to the acute care area of the emergency room (ER). On admission her vitals are noted as follows: temperature 38.6°C, oxygen saturation 88% on room air, heart rate (HR) 70 and regular, and systolic blood pressure (BP) 75 mmHg.

The patient is placed on a cardiac monitor and oxygen at FiO_2 50% is delivered by mask. An intravenous line is placed and a Foley catheter is inserted. A chest x-ray is taken and shows cardiomegaly with mild interstitial pulmonary edema, and arterial blood gas (ABG) taken on 50% O_2 is as follows: pH 7.25, pO_2 75, pCO_2 30, HCO_3 15. The lactate provided on the ABG is elevated at 4.6. A complete blood count (CBC) shows a white blood count (WBC) of 14.0 with 90% polymorphonuclear cells (PMNs), and hemoglobin (Hb) is 110. Electrolytes with creatinine, urea, and glucose show Na 141, K 4.0, Cl 111, HCO_3 15, BUN 10, Cr 190, and glucose 8 mmol/L. Urine dipstick reveals leukocytes and bacteria.

As the investigations return, the physician notes that the patient's blood pressure has not risen despite two 250-mL infusions of normal saline. After the second bolus her SaO_2 dropped from 95% to 89%. There has been only 5 mL of urine into the catheter system. Focused physical examination reveals systolic BP 70 mmHg and HR 70. Extremities are cold and mottled. The patient is alert but not oriented to place or time, which her husband says is new.

Cardiac exam reveals an elevated jugular veinous pressure (JVP), a II/VI pansystolic murmur at the left sternal border previously noted in the chart, and some moderate peripheral edema. There are bilateral crackles and occasional wheezes bilaterally. Abdominal exam reveals no pain or tenderness and the remainder of the medical exam is within normal limits.

Diagnosis

The diagnosis is severe urosepsis in a patient with impaired cardiac function. The patient is exhibiting signs of shock and end-organ dysfunction, including hypoperfused extremities, oliguria, and altered mental status. She has not responded to fluids, and given her tenuous cardiorespiratory status, the physician is reluctant to give further fluids at this time.

Treatment Plan

Urine and blood cultures are sent to the laboratory, 1 g intravenous cefotaxime is administered, and the patient is transferred to the intensive care unit (ICU). On arrival her blood pressure is obtained by palpation only, and she is now noted to be drowsy. A decision is made to intubate, and this is performed with 30 mg IV etomidate; the patient is sedated and placed on a ventilator. An arterial line and right subclavian line is placed, and IV dopamine is begun at 5 µg/kg/min and rapidly increased to 20 µg/kg/min with little blood pressure response. Central venous pressure (CVP) as measured by a central line is noted to be 15 mm Hg. Her infusions are changed from dopamine to dobutamine at 5 µg/kg/min and noradrenaline beginning at 1 µg/kg/min. There is some response to noradrenaline, but at a dose of 5 µg/kg/min the mean arterial pressure (MAP) remains quite low at 50 mm Hg compared to her normal BP of 120/70. IV vasopressin is added at a dose of 0.01 U/min and the MAP rises to 70 mm Hg. A central venous oxygen saturation that was sent to the lab when the central line was placed comes back at 40%.

The physician tells the patient's nurse that he wants to maintain her MAP at least 65 mm Hg and CVP at 8 to 12 mm Hg. To begin with, there will be glucose, electrolytes, lactate, and arterial and central venous blood gases drawn every 2 to 3 hours, and the dobutamine dose will be adjusted to arrive at a mixed venous saturation of over 70%. Should there be no urine output over the next 1 to 2 hours, the physician will be increasing the level of target MAP to 70 to 75 mm Hg in the hopes of better end-organ perfusion. As adjuncts to therapy, blood glucose will be kept between 4 and 8 mmol/L, and if there is a deterioration in her clinical picture, the physician will consider giving activated protein C.

Clinical Course

The patient required inotropic and vasopressor support for 24 hours, with a resultant increase in urine output to >45 cc per hour and an increase in central venous oxygen saturation to 70% within 2 hours. Normalization of lactate took 12 hours. *Escherichia coli* was identified as the causative organism from blood and urine cultures, and a 2-week course of intravenous antibiotics was instituted. Weaning off of vasopressors took place 1 day following admission, while the patient required inotropic support for a further 72 hours. She was extubated on day 3 of her ICU stay.

Discussion

This case highlights the often refractory nature of hypotension seen with cases of mixed cardiogenic and vasodilatory shock. It stresses the importance of a rapid diagnosis and institution of therapy to regain perfusion of vital organs, and shows that not infrequently multiple inotropes and vasopressors will be required for a given patient.

Conclusion

Patients with severe acute heart failure may present with shock due to a mixture of cardiogenic and distributive causes. In these cases, although inotropic support is important to maintain ventricular contractility and stroke volume, it is equally important to maintain perfusion of vital organs through maintenance of an adequate blood pressure. This is achieved through careful fluid resuscitation in conjunction with vasopressor agents. Noradrenaline combined with dobutamine is preferred for dual therapy, and dopamine may be considered as an agent for monotherapy. In most cases the toxicity associated with vasopressor use can be mitigated by avoiding volume depletion and targeting a central venous pressure of 8 to 12 mm Hg.

Acknowledgments. Support was provided by the Canadian Institutes of Health Research. Keith R. Walley is a Michael Smith Foundation for Health Research Distinguished Scholar. John H. Boyd is a Michael Smith Foundation for Health Research Postdoctoral Fellow.

References

1. Rivers E, et al. Early goal-directed therapy in the treatment of severe sepsis and septic shock. N Engl J Med, 2001;345(19):1368–77.
2. Binanay C, et al. Evaluation study of congestive heart failure and pulmonary artery catheterization effectiveness: the ESCAPE trial. JAMA, 2005;294(13): 1625–33.
3. Shah MR, et al. Impact of the pulmonary artery catheter in critically ill patients: meta-analysis of randomized clinical trials. JAMA, 2005;294(13): 1664–70.
4. Harvey S, et al. Assessment of the clinical effectiveness of pulmonary artery catheters in management of patients in intensive care (PAC-Man): a randomised controlled trial. Lancet, 2005;366(9484): 472–7.
5. McDonald RH, Jr, et al. Effect of dopamine in man: augmentation of sodium excretion, glomerular filtration rate, and renal plasma flow. J Clin Invest, 1964;43:1116–24.
6. Bellomo R, et al. Low-dose dopamine in patients with early renal dysfunction: a placebo-controlled randomised trial. Australian and New Zealand Intensive Care Society (ANZICS) Clinical Trials Group. Lancet, 2000;356(9248):2139–43.
7. Martin C, et al. Norepinephrine or dopamine for the treatment of hyperdynamic septic shock? Chest, 1993;103(6):1826–31.
8. Regnier B, et al. [Comparative study of the effects of dobutamine and dopamine in septic shock.] Ann Anesthesiol Fr, 1978;19(10):859–62.
9. Jardin F, et al. Effect of dopamine on intrapulmonary shunt fraction and oxygen transport in severe sepsis with circulatory and respiratory failure. Crit Care Med, 1979;7(6):273–7.
10. Samii K, et al. Hemodynamic effects of dopamine in septic shock with and without acute renal failure. Arch Surg, 1978;113(12):1414–6.
11. Drueck C, Welch GW, Pruitt BA, Jr. Hemodynamic analysis of septic shock in thermal injury: treatment with dopamine. Am Surg, 1978;44(7):424–7.
12. Wilson RF, Sibbald WJ, Jaanimagi JL, Hemodynamic effects of dopamine in critically ill septic patients. J Surg Res, 1976;20(3):163–72.

13. Winslow EJ, et al. Hemodynamic studies and results of therapy in 50 patients with bacteremic shock. Am J Med, 1973;54(4):421–32.
14. Van den Berghe G. de Zegher F, Anterior pituitary function during critical illness and dopamine treatment. Crit Care Med, 1996;24(9):1580–90.
15. Meier-Hellmann A, et al. The effects of low-dose dopamine on splanchnic blood flow and oxygen uptake in patients with septic shock. Intensive Care Med, 1997;23(1):31–7.
16. Marik PE, Mohedin M. The contrasting effects of dopamine and norepinephrine on systemic and splanchnic oxygen utilization in hyperdynamic sepsis. JAMA, 1994;272(17):1354–7.
17. Hannemann L, et al. Comparison of dopamine to dobutamine and norepinephrine for oxygen delivery and uptake in septic shock. Crit Care Med, 1995;23(12):1962–70.
18. Hesselvik JF, Brodin B. Low dose norepinephrine in patients with septic shock and oliguria: effects on afterload, urine flow, and oxygen transport. Crit Care Med, 1989;17(2):179–80.
19. Desjars P, et al. A reappraisal of norepinephrine therapy in human septic shock. Crit Care Med, 1987;15(2):134–7.
20. Desjars P, et al. Norepinephrine therapy has no deleterious renal effects in human septic shock. Crit Care Med, 1989;17(5):426–9.
21. Chernow B, Roth BL. Pharmacologic manipulation of the peripheral vasculature in shock: clinical and experimental approaches. Circ Shock, 1986;18(2):141–55.
22. Martin C, et al. Effect of norepinephrine on the outcome of septic shock. Crit Care Med, 2000;28(8):2758–65.
23. Martin C, et al. Septic shock: a goal-directed therapy using volume loading, dobutamine and/or norepinephrine. Acta Anaesthesiol Scand, 1990;34(5):413–7.
24. Murakawa K, Kobayashi A. Effects of vasopressors on renal tissue gas tensions during hemorrhagic shock in dogs. Crit Care Med, 1988;16(8):789–92.
25. Conger JD, Robinette JB, Guggenheim SJ. Effect of acetylcholine on the early phase of reversible norepinephrine-induced acute renal failure. Kidney Int, 1981;19(3):399–409.
26. Schaer GL, Fink MP, Parrillo JE. Norepinephrine alone versus norepinephrine plus low-dose dopamine: enhanced renal blood flow with combination pressor therapy. Crit Care Med, 1985;13(6):492–6.
27. Bellomo R, et al. Effects of norepinephrine on the renal vasculature in normal and endotoxemic dogs. Am J Respir Crit Care Med, 1999;159(4 pt 1):1186–92.
28. Fukuoka T, et al. Effects of norepinephrine on renal function in septic patients with normal and elevated serum lactate levels. Crit Care Med, 1989;17(11):1104–7.
29. Marin C, et al. Renal effects of norepinephrine used to treat septic shock patients. Crit Care Med, 1990;18(3):282–5.
30. Holmes CL, Landry DW, Granton J.T. Science review: vasopressin and the cardiovascular system part 2—clinical physiology. Crit Care, 2004;8(1):15–23.
31. Holmes CL, Landry DW, Granton J.T. Science review: Vasopressin and the cardiovascular system part 1—receptor physiology. Crit Care, 2003;7(6):427–34.
32. Wakatsuki T, Nakaya Y, Inoue I. Vasopressin modulates K(+)-channel activities of cultured smooth muscle cells from porcine coronary artery. Am J Physiol, 1992;263(2 pt 2):H491–6.
33. Kusano E, et al. Arginine vasopressin inhibits interleukin-1 beta-stimulated nitric oxide and cyclic guanosine monophosphate production via the V1 receptor in cultured rat vascular smooth muscle cells. J Hypertens, 1997;15(6):627–32.
34. Yamamoto K, et al. Arginine vasopressin inhibits nitric oxide synthesis in cytokine-stimulated vascular smooth muscle cells. Hypertens Res, 1997;20(3):209–16.
35. Noguera I, et al. Potentiation by vasopressin of adrenergic vasoconstriction in the rat isolated mesenteric artery. Br J Pharmacol, 1997;122(3):431–8.
36. Landry DW, et al. Vasopressin deficiency contributes to the vasodilation of septic shock. Circulation, 1997;95(5):1122–5.
37. Dunser MW, et al. Cardiac performance during vasopressin infusion in postcardiotomy shock. Intensive Care Med, 2002;28(6):746–51.
38. Gold J, et al. Vasopressin in the treatment of milrinone-induced hypotension in severe heart failure. Am J Cardiol, 2000;85(4):506–8, A11.
39. O'Brien A, Clapp L, Singer M. Terlipressin for norepinephrine-resistant septic shock. Lancet, 2002;359(9313):1209–10.
40. Gregory JS, et al. Experience with phenylephrine as a component of the pharmacologic support of septic shock. Crit Care Med, 1991;19(11):1395–400.
41. Flancbaum L, et al. A dose-response study of phenylephrine in critically ill, septic surgical patients. Eur J Clin Pharmacol, 1997;51(6):461–5.
42. Reinelt H, et al. Impact of exogenous beta-adrenergic receptor stimulation on hepatosplanchnic oxygen kinetics and metabolic activity in septic shock. Crit Care Med, 1999;27(2):325–31.

2.4.3
Novel Cardiovascular Therapy for Acute Heart Failure Syndrome

55
Calcium Sensitizer Levosimendan and Its Use in Acute Heart Failure and Related Conditions

Alexandre Mebazaa, John R. Teerlink, and Piero Pollesello

Mechanisms of Action of Levosimendan

The principal actions of levosimendan at therapeutic concentrations are as follows:

- Calcium sensitization of myocytes
- Arterial and venous dilatation mediated via the opening of adenosine triphosphate (ATP)-sensitive potassium channels in vascular smooth muscle.

This combination of actions endows levosimendan with the properties of both an energy-efficient inotrope and a balanced vasodilator. In addition, levosimendan exerts antiischemic and cardioprotective effects via potassium channels in cardiomyoctes.

Levosimendan as a Calcium Sensitizer

The essence of calcium sensitization with levosimendan is a qualitative alteration in the interactions between the contractile proteins actin and myosin. In brief, the formation of cross-bridges and the generation of contractile force are dependent on the binding of free ionic calcium to the troponin–tropomyosin complex associated with actin filaments. Saturation of troponin C with calcium induces conformational changes that expose binding sites on myosin that permit cross-bridge formation. Levosimendan facilitates this interaction by occupying a hydrophobic pocket formed near the N-terminal end of troponin C in response to initial calcium binding.[1,2] Binding of the drug molecule at this site maintains troponin C in the conformation that permits cross-bridge formation for longer than would otherwise be the case.[3] In the presence of levosimendan, therefore, more cross-bridges are created for any given concentration of calcium, and contractile force is augmented. An important aspect of this process is that it is calcium-dependent; the levosimendan–troponin C complex dissociates as calcium levels decline during diastole. Hence, systolic contractility is augmented without compromising diastolic function.[4,5]

Calcium sensitization is the mechanism through which levosimendan enhances cardiac contractility at therapeutically relevant concentrations.[6,7] Although levosimendan inhibits the phosphodiesterase (PDE) III isoenzyme in vitro, this inhibition is insufficient to exert any pharmacologic effects in vivo, because no elevation in cyclic adenosine monophosphate (cAMP) occurs without simultaneous inhibition of both PDE III and PDE IV. Unlike enoximone and milrinone, levosimendan in fact does not inhibit PDE IV at therapeutic concentrations and therefore does not elevate the intracellular calcium level via PDE inhibition.[8,9]

It is certainly the case, however, that levosimendan has other effects that are relevant to its clinical applications, including well-defined vasodilator, cardioprotective/antiischemic, and antistunning actions.

Effects on Potassium–Adenosine Triphosphate Channels

The ATP-dependent potassium (K-ATP) channels are inward rectifying channels inhibited by physiologic levels of intracellular ATP. The clinical opportunities presented by these channels have been the subject of a recent review.[10] In particular, the discovery of a link between the operation of mitochondrial K-ATP channels and cardiac preconditioning identified these channels as possible therapeutic targets in myocardial ischemia and in organ protection.[11]

Potassium–Adenosine Triphosphate Channels in Vascular Smooth Muscle

Levosimendan activates K-ATP channels in vascular smooth muscle cells, leading to hyperpolarization of the cells, reduction in intracellular calcium levels, relaxation, and vasodilatation.[12] A vasodilator action of levosimendan has been demonstrated in vitro in arteries, including coronary arteries, and veins.[12,13] Vasodilatation in the systemic vasculature may be expected to reduce ventricular loading; enhanced coronary perfusion secondary to vasodilatation may help to preserve ischemic tissue and improve cardiac function. Reduction in infarct size following coronary artery occlusion and reperfusion has been achieved in anesthetized dogs[14] and was blocked by glibenclamide, identifying the opening of K-ATP channels as the basis of this cardioprotective action. Inotropy was unaffected by glibenclamide, indicating that the cardioprotective action of levosimendan was not due to its calcium-sensitizing properties. Antiischemic and antiarrhythmic effects and attendant improvements in survival have been demonstrated in various other experimental models.[15,16]

Theoretical concerns that activation of K-ATP channels may exacerbate renal tubular injury in endotoxic acute renal failure have been at least partly allayed by recent experimental observations in a murine model by Zager and colleagues.[17] Preliminary experiences with levosimendan in critical care medicine are considered later in this commentary.

Potassium–Adenosine Triphosphate Channels in Mitochondria

Levosimendan activates mitochondrial K-ATP channels in rat hepatocyte and cardiac mitochondria.[18,19] The significance of these observations lies in the fact that mitochondrial K-ATP channels are implicated in potassium homeostasis within the mitochondrion. Agents that stimulate potassium flux through mitochondrial K-ATP channels represent a unique device for preserving cellular energy balance and protecting mitochondria from oxidative injury. Such effects are considered central to the phenomenon of ischemic preconditioning that protects myocardium and other tissues from ischemia–reperfusion injury.

Anti-Stunning Effect on Myocardium

Anti-stunning, the last of the ancillary properties of levosimendan, may in fact be a consequence of the primary action of levosimendan to enhance calcium sensitivity. Loss of sensitivity to calcium is considered a likely contributor to the compromise of contractile performance that characterizes myocardial stunning, the reversible state of contractile dysfunction that follows an episode or episodes of myocardial ischemia. Acidosis secondary to ischemia or heightened catecholaminergic levels may be contributory factors to this situation. Stunning may also be encountered after coronary artery surgery. Energy-neutral enhancement of calcium sensitivity might be expected to help in the resolution of episodes of stunning. Observations in experimental models,[20] including reperfusion after cardioplegic arrest,[21] support this expectation.

Pharmacokinetics of Levosimendan

Plasma concentrations of levosimendan increase linearly with dose across the therapeutic range after intravenous administration. The drug is distributed rapidly, reaches steady-state levels in plasma after about 2 hours when the drug is administered as a loading dose and subsequent infusion, and has a steady-state volume of distribution of about 0.2 L/kg in patients with mild or moderate heart failure.[22] The elimination half-life of the parent drug is about 1 hour, and almost all the drug is recovered from urine (~55% of total dose) or feces (~45% of total dose) as inactive cysteinyl or cysteinylglycine conjugates. About 5% of an administered dose is converted by acetylation to two active metabolites, of which one, designated OR-1896, has an elimination half-life of approximately 77 hours.

Clinical Trials of Levosimendan

Levosimendan has been the subject of an intensive clinical trials program in severe and acute heart failure and other critical care situations in the past decade. In acute heart failure, levosimendan has been subjected to clinical trials evaluation in more patients than any other agent currently in routine use for inotropic support.

Studies in Acute Heart Failure

A summary of studies of levosimendan in patients with acute or decompensated heart failure appears in Table 55.1.

Dose Ranging of Levosimendan

Nieminen et al.[23] identified the therapeutic range of intravenous levosimendan in heart failure as a 6 to 24 μg/kg loading dose followed by a 24-hour infusion at rates of 0.05 to 0.2 μg/kg/min. This conclusion was based on data from a randomized, double-blind, placebo- and active-controlled study in 151 patients with stable congestive heart failure of ischemic origin (New York Heart Association [NYHA] classes II to IV, but

Table 55.1. Summary of clinical studies using intravenous levosimendan in patients with acute or decompensated heart failure

Study	No. of patients; clinical status	Levosimendan dosage	Comparator	Results/observations
Nieminen et al. (2000)	151; NYHA II–IV HF	3–36 μg/kg + 0.05–0.6 μg/kg/min	Dobutamine 6 μg/kg/min or placebo	Dose-dependent favorable hemodynamic responses
Slawsky et al. (2000)	146; Advanced HF	6 μg/kg + 0.1–0.4 μg/kg/min	Placebo	Favorable hemodynamic effects and relief of symptoms
Kivikko et al. (2003)	146; Decompensated HF	6 μg/kg + 0.1–0.4 μg/kg/min	Placebo	Hemodynamic effects were maintained for at least 24 hours after discontinuation of a 24-hour infusion
Nanas et al. (2004)	18; HF refractory to dobutamine and furosemide	6 μg/kg + 0.2 μg/kg/min as adjunctive therapy	Dobutamine 10 μg/kg/min	Combined treatment improved hemodynamics and symptoms for 24 hours
Parissis et al. (2004)	27; Decompensated advanced HF	6 μg/kg + 0.1–0.4 μg/kg/min	Placebo	Levosimendan reduced the levels of IL-6, soluble Fas and Fas ligand; correlations between marker level change and ventricular wall stress
LIDO (2002)	203; Severe HF	24 μg/kg + 0.1 μg/kg/min	Dobutamine 5 μg/kg/min	Levosimendan improved: • Acute hemodynamics • Survival at 180 days
REVIVE-I & II (2005)	100 & 600; HF with symptoms at rest	6–12 μg/kg + 0.1–0.2 μg/kg/min	Placebo	Significantly larger proportion of patients regarded as improved according to clinical composite end point compared with placebo; dyspnea, global assessment, and BNP markedly improved in levosimendan-treated group
CASINO (2004)	227; Decompensated low-output HF	16 μg/kg + 0.2 μg/kg/min	Dobutamine 10 μg/kg/min or placebo	Study terminated early due to clear survival benefit from levosimendan
SURVIVE (2005)	1350; Decompensated HF requiring inotropes	12 μg/kg + 0.1–0.2 μg/kg/min	Dobutamine 5–40 μg/kg/min	Trend in favor of levosimendan vs. dobutamine for 180-day mortality; early and marked decrease in plasma BNP vs. dobutamine

CABG, coronary artery bypass graft; HF, heart failure; BNP, B-type natriuretic peptide; NYHA, New York Heart Association.

predominantly class III). Participants were randomized to one of five dose schedules of levosimendan, or to dobutamine (6 μg/kg/min), placebo, or an ethanol-containing vehicle. Levosimendan was initiated as a loading dose administered over 10 minutes, followed by continuous infusion for 24 hours.

Response rates* among levosimendan-treated patients ranged from 50% at the lowest dose to 88% at the highest dose. These rates were statistically better than those for placebo (14% response rate; $p = .038$) and statistically equivalent to those for dobutamine (70% response rate). The cardiovascular effects of levosimendan tended to be augmented with time, whereas response to dobutamine waned with continuing infusion. Headache (9%), nausea (5%), and hypotension (5%) were reported at higher dosages of levosimendan.

In other research, investigators in Finland and the United States[24,25] examined the hemodynamic effects of levosimendan in a dose-escalation/withdrawal study in a cohort of 146 patients with decompensated heart failure (NYHA functional class III [~66%] or IV [~34%]). Levosimendan was administered as an initial bolus of 6 μg/kg followed by an infusion of 0.1 μg/kg/min. Infusion rates were escalated over 4 hours to a maximum infusion rate of 0.4 μg/kg/min or to the maximum tolerated dose if lower than 0.4 μg/kg/min. The highest attained dose was then continued for another 2 hours. At 6 hours, the placebo was terminated and the dose of levosimendan was halved and continued, open label, for a further 18 hours. At 24 hours, the remaining patients ($n = 85$) were re-randomized, again double-blind, to levosimendan or placebo.

The primary efficacy end point of a 25% reduction in PCWP or a 25% increase in stroke volume at 6 hours was achieved in 80% of levosimendan-treated patients compared with 17% of placebo-treated controls ($p < .01$ by Cochran-Mantel-Haenszel test). Dose-related changes in mean cardiac index and PCWP were recorded (Fig. 55.1). These objective response criteria were supplemented by patient and investigator assessments of the signs and symptoms of heart failure. Adverse events were recorded in 17% of patients assigned to levosimendan and 19% of those given placebo during the first phase of the study.

Results from the succeeding phases of the study confirmed that the initial favorable hemodynamic effects of levosimendan were sustained during continuous infusion and persisted for 24 hours after discontinuation of infusion, an effect attributed to the persistence in plasma of the levosimendan active metabolite OR-1896.

*Patients were classified as responders to treatment if they fulfilled at least one of the following criteria during the period of the infusion: (1) stroke volume increase of ≥15% during the last hour of treatment; (2) pulmonary capillary wedge pressure (PCWP) reduction of ≥25% from baseline (and minimum absolute reduction ≥4 mm Hg) during the last hour of treatment; and (3) need for dose reduction at any time during the 24-hour period due to ≥50% reduction in PCWP or ≥40% increase in cardiac output, with a change in heart rate of <20%.

Levosimendan Infusion Versus Dobutamine Study

The Levosimendan Infusion Versus Dobutamine (LIDO) study[26] examined the effect of intravenous levosimendan on hemodynamic efficacy in heart failure. The 203 participating patients were predominantly (87%) men with an average age of just under 60 years and with low-output heart failure arising from a variety of causes including (but not limited to) deterioration of severe chronic heart failure despite maximum conventional oral therapy, heart failure subsequent to cardiac surgery, or acute heart failure arising from cardiac or noncardiac disorders of recent onset. Patients were also required to have left ventricular ejection fraction (LVEF) <35% and PCWP >15 mm Hg.

Treatment consisted of either levosimendan (24 μg/kg over 10 minutes followed by 0.1 μg/kg/min) or dobutamine (5 μg/kg/min). These doses could be doubled after 2 hours if cardiac index had not increased by ≥30% from baseline. Infusions were thereafter continued for up to 24 hours.

A significantly greater proportion of patients fulfilled the primary efficacy criterion* in the levosimendan group than with dobutamine (intention-to-treat analysis 28% vs. 15%; $p = .022$;

*A ≥ 30% increase in cardiac output and ≥25% reduction in PCWP, with a minimum absolute decline of 4 mm Hg.

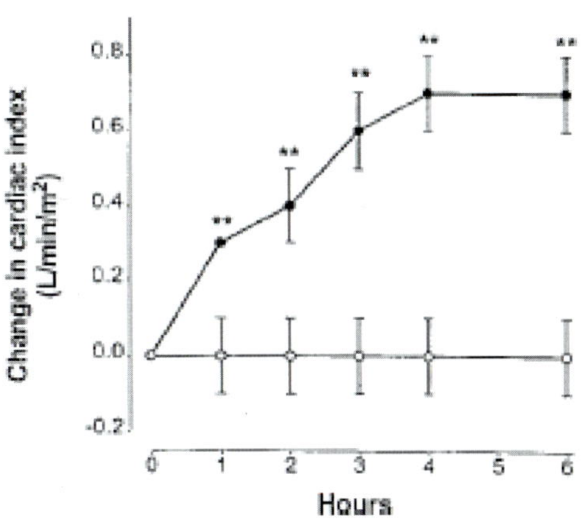

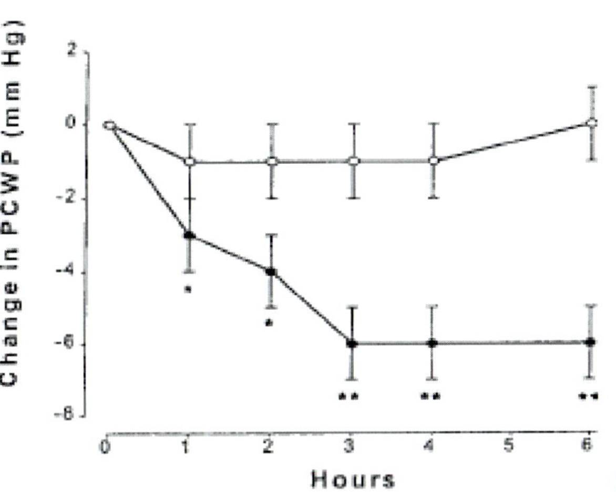

FIGURE 55.1. Effect of intravenous levosimendan and placebo on (A) cardiac index and (B) pulmonary capillary wedge pressure (PCWP). Absolute changes from baseline are shown over the course of a 6-hour infusion. $*p = .02$; $**p < .001$. (From Slawsky et al.,[24] with permission.)

per-protocol analysis 31% vs. 15%; $p = .021$). Levosimendan was quantitatively more effective than dobutamine for relief of dyspnea (68% improved vs. 59% improved) and fatigue (63% improved vs. 47% improved), but these differences were not statistically significant.

A marked interaction with beta-blocker use was revealed during LIDO, with attenuation of the effects of dobutamine on cardiac output and PCWP, but no comparable effect on levosimendan (Fig. 55.2). This effect did not significantly influence the primary end point ($p = .46$ in a post-hoc test for interaction). Thirty-seven percent of patients were being prescribed beta-blockers at baseline.

All-cause mortality at 31 days was recorded as a prespecified safety end point, and all-cause mortality at 180 days was monitored at the request of regulatory authorities. Fewer patients died at 31 and 180 days in the levosimendan group than with dobutamine, and these differences were statistically significant ($p = .049$ at 31 days, .029 at 180 days) (Fig. 55.3). The median number of days alive and out of hospital was also greater among patients randomized to levosimendan than to dobutamine (157 [range 101–173] vs. 133 [43.5–169]; $p = .027$).

The total number of adverse events was similar with both drugs (levosimendan, 48 episodes; dobutamine, 42 episodes), with headache the preponderant event recorded with levosimendan (14 vs. 5 events; $p = .052$).

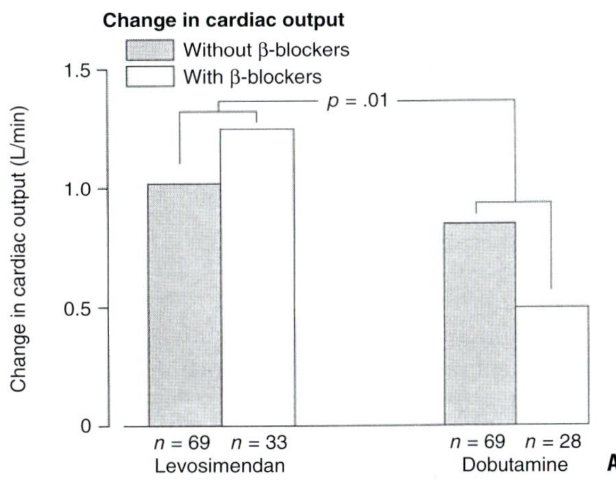

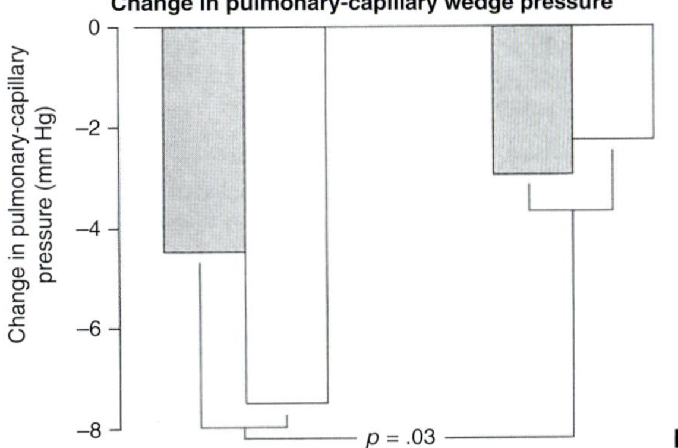

FIGURE 55.2. Effect of concomitant beta-blockade on (A) cardiac output and (B) PCWP in patients taking levosimendan or dobutamine in the Levosimendan Infusion Versus Dobutamine (LIDO) study. (From Follath et al.,[26] with permission.)

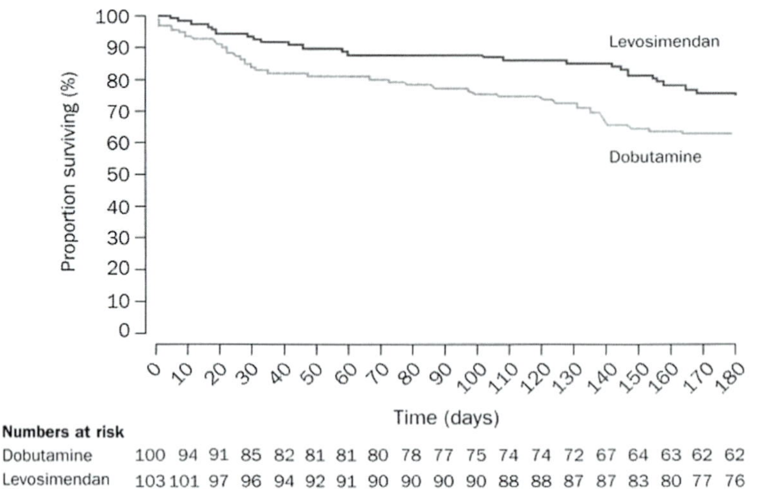

FIGURE 55.3. Kaplan–Meier estimates (analysis of time to first event) of risk of death during first 180 days after randomization (based on intention-to-treat analysis). (From Follath et al.,[26] with permission.)

The Randomized Evaluations of Levosimendan Studies

The Randomized Evaluations of Levosimendan (REVIVE) program was designed to assess the efficacy of levosimendan in improving clinical outcomes in patients with acute decompensated heart failure. REVIVE-I was a 100-patient pilot study that assessed the performance of a new, rigorous composite end point in acute decompensated heart failure trials and demonstrated an encouraging trend toward benefit with levosimendan.

The REVIVE-II study built on the experience gained in REVIVE-I and enrolled patients with a diagnosis of heart failure and LVEF <35% who remained symptomatic despite the use of intravenous diuretics and vasodilators. Six hundred patients were assigned in a randomized, double-blind manner to levosimendan 12 μg/kg followed by an infusion of 0.2 μg/kg/min for 24 hours or to matching placebo. Enrollment of patients within 48 hours of admission was encouraged but not mandatory.

The primary end point of REVIVE-II was a composite of patient-assessed changes in symptomatic status, worsening of heart failure, or death during the period of infusion and the ensuing 4 days. To be considered to have improved, patients had to report moderate or marked improvement at each time point (6 hours, 24 hours, and 5 days after study drug initiation), and report no worsening or require any additional medical interventions for heart failure during those 5 days. At the completion of follow-up, the distribution of patients who considered themselves improved, unchanged, or worse than at baseline was favorably influenced by levosimendan therapy ($p = .015$ vs. placebo), with approximately 30% more patients having improved and 30% fewer having worsened compared with patients treated with standard care.[27] This noteworthy treatment benefit was supported by significant improvements in patient global assessments and assessments of dyspnea, as well as rapid and sustained reductions in B-type natriuretic peptide (BNP).[28] Duration of hospitalization was reduced by about 2 days with levosimendan ($p = .001$ vs. placebo) and the proportion of patients requiring intravenous rescue therapy was lower with levosimendan than with standard care (15% vs. 26%). Ninety-day mortality, a secondary end point of the study, was 15.1% with levosimendan and 11.6% with placebo (difference not significant). Hypotension (49.2% vs. 35.5%), headache (29.4% vs. 14.6%), and ventricular tachycardia (24.1% vs. 16.9%), recorded as adverse events, occurred more often with levosimendan than placebo. REVIVE II is the first trial in patients with acute decompensated heart failure (ADHF) to demonstrate a beneficial clinical outcome.

Calcium Sensitizer or Inotrope or None in Low-Output Heart Failure (CASINO) Study and Survival of Patients with Acute Heart Failure in Need of Intravenous Inotropic Support (SURVIVE) Study

Two recently completed clinical end point trials—CASINO, and SURVIVE and REVIVE—have expanded the experience gained with levosimendan in LIDO and REVIVE-II. The first of these studies to be completed, CASINO, compared levosimendan with dobutamine and placebo. Subsequently, the SURVIVE (levosimendan versus dobutamine) and REVIVE-II (levosimendan versus placebo) studies examined the impact of levosimendan in patients with acute decompensated heart failure.

The Calcium Sensitizer or Inotrope or None in Low-Output Heart Failure (CASINO) study compared levosimendan (16-µg bolus over 10 minutes followed by 0.2 µg/kg/min for 24 hours), dobutamine (10 µg/kg/min), or placebo in patients with severe (NYHA class IV) heart failure. The study's primary end point was death from any cause or hospitalization for deterioration of heart failure during the ensuing year.[29] The study was halted after the recruitment of 299 of the planned 600 patients because of evidence of a substantial survival benefit with levosimendan (18.0% mortality at 6 months) compared with either dobutamine (42.0% mortality; $p = .0001$) or placebo (28.3% mortality; $p = .03$).[30]

The Survival of Patients with Acute Heart Failure in Need of Intravenous Inotropic Support (SURVIVE) study[31] is to date the largest randomized controlled trial of levosimendan in any indication and the largest mortality study of intravenous inodilator therapy yet undertaken in acute decompensated heart failure. The study, undertaken in nine European countries, enrolled 1327 patients who had LVEF ≤30% (mean 24%), persisting breathlessness despite intravenous diuretics and vasodilators, and other signs of a low-output state, including systolic blood pressure in the range of 80 to 130 mm Hg (mean 116 mm Hg), and considerably elevated plasma levels of BNP. Parallels with some of the enrollment criteria for REVIVE-II, reported above, will be evident. Patients were ineligible if they had serum creatinine >450 µmol/L.

Participating patients were randomized to receive either levosimendan 12 µg/kg followed by 0.1 to 0.2 µg/kg/min for 24 hours or dobutamine at doses of not less than 5 µg/kg for a minimum of 2 hours. The primary end point of the study was all-cause mortality at 180 days. All-cause mortality at 31 days was a prespecified secondary end point, and an analysis of deaths during the first 5 days was introduced retrospectively.

Death rates in this conspicuously at-risk population were high, with more than a quarter of patients in both treatment groups dead at the conclusion of follow-up. A trend for improved survival with levosimendan versus dobutamine was discernible after 5 days (hazard ratio, 0.72; 95% confidence interval [CI], 0.44–1.16). This effect was not statistically significant and became attenuated as duration of follow-up increased (180-day hazard ratio, 0.91; 95% CI, 0.74–1.13).[32]

Other outcomes of note from SURVIVE were as follows:

1. A marked trend for better outcomes at 5 days in patients with established (vs. new-onset) heart failure (hazard ratio 0.58; 95% CI, 0.33–1.01])
2. Significantly lower risk of worsening heart failure with levosimendan than with dobutamine (12.3% vs. 17%; $p < .02$)
3. A prompt, sustained, and large (~50%) reduction in plasma BNP levels soon after the start of levosimendan infusion ($p < .0001$ vs. dobutamine)
4. Indications of a treatment center interaction (the practical relevance of this observation has not been established)

No analysis of outcomes according to beta-blocker status (cf. LIDO, above) has yet been published for SURVIVE.

Other Studies in Acute Heart Failure

Combined use of levosimendan with dobutamine in patients with decompensated NYHA class IV

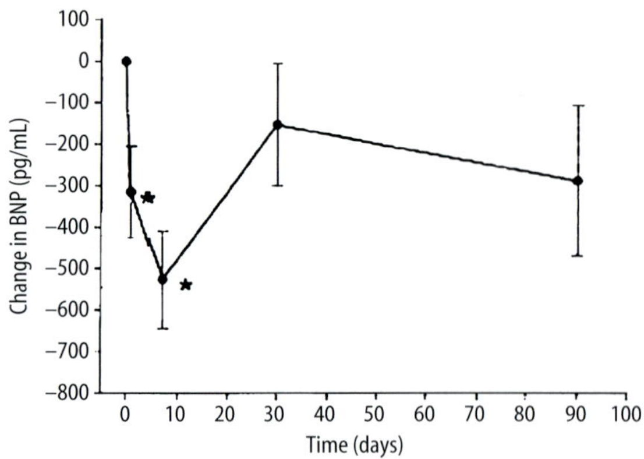

FIGURE 55.4. Change in BNP concentration from baseline (day 0). Levosimendan infusion started on day 0 and finished on day 1. *$p < .05$ vs. baseline. (From McLean et al.,[35] with permission.)

heart failure has been examined in a preliminary study by Nanas et al.[33] Supplementation of intravenous dobutamine (10 μg/kg/min) and intravenous furosemide (10 mg/h) with a 24-hour course of levosimendan (6 μg/kg/min bolus followed by 0.2 μg/kg/min infusion) led to attainment of the study primary end point of a ≥40% increase in cardiac index and a ≥25% reduction in PCWP in seven patients, compared with one patient in the control group ($p = .008$). Potentially favorable effects on cytokine mediators have been documented by Parissis et al.,[34] and pronounced reductions in BNP have been demonstrated by McLean et al.[35] in heart failure patients treated with levosimendan 12 μg/kg and then 0.1 μg/kg/min for 24 hours (Fig. 55.4). As noted previously, Teerlink and colleagues[28] have also documented pronounced reductions on BNP in heart failure patients treated with levosimendan.

Cardiac Surgery

Levosimendan has been evaluated as an intravenous inotropic support for patients emerging from cardiac surgery in five clinical trials (Table 55.2). Two of these studies examined the use of a bolus injection, two studied a combination of bolus plus infusion, and one evaluated infusion-only therapy.

Bolus Injection Studies

The first of the studies to evaluate levosimendan bolus therapy was a randomized, placebo-controlled trial in 23 patients who had undergone coronary artery bypass grafting (CABG).[36] These patients (17 men, six women) were a low-risk cohort with relatively good ventricular function and stable hemodynamics. Treatment consisted of levosimendan 8 or 24 μg/kg, initiated 30 to 60 minutes after restoration of coronary perfusion and administered over 5 minutes, or matching placebo. Responses to therapy were monitored for up to 1 hour.

Levosimendan augmented stroke volume and heart rate and reduced mean arterial pressure and PCWP modestly. Cardiac output was significantly enhanced by the higher dose, whereas systemic vascular resistance (SVR) was reduced ($p < .05$ for both parameters). Coronary vascular resis-

TABLE 55.2. Summary of experience with levosimendan in patients undergoing cardiac surgery

Study	No. of patients; clinical status	Levosimendan dosage	Comparator	Results/observations
Lilleberg et al. (1998)	23; post-CABG	8 or 24 μg/kg (B)	Placebo	Improved systemic and coronary blood flow with no increase in myocardial oxygen consumption or change in substrate utilization
Labriola et al. (2004)	11; severe LV dysfunction after CS	12 μg/kg + 0.1 μg/kg/min	None	Cardiac index was increased by >30% and PCWP reduced to <18 mm Hg within 3 hours ($n = 8$)
Nijhawan et al. (1999)	18; post-CABG	0.2–0.3 μg/kg/min (I)	Placebo	Increased cardiac output and reduced SVR
Barisin et al. (2004)	31; post-CABG	12–24 μg/kg (B)	Placebo	Increases in cardiac output and ejection fraction and decrease in SVR
Plöchl and Rajek (2004)	10; post-CABG	0.1–0.2 μg/kg/min (I) as adjunctive therapy	None	Increases in cardiac output and stroke volume and reduction in SVR

CABG, coronary artery bypass graft; CS, cardiac surgery; LV, left ventricular; (B), bolus only; (I), infusion only; PCWP: pulmonary capillary wedge pressure; SVR: systemic vascular resistance.

tance and perfusion pressure were reduced significantly ($p < .05$ vs. placebo) but the increment in coronary blood flow (~33% vs. placebo) was not statistically significant. There was no evidence of alterations in the profile of myocardial substrate utilization or myocardial oxygen consumption, and no electrocardiograph (ECG) evidence of an increased propensity to myocardial ischemia.

This demonstration of favorable acute effects of a levosimendan bolus on hemodynamic indices and cardiac function, with no untoward effect on cardiac energy consumption, was repeated in a study of 31 patients assigned randomly to single intravenous bolus doses of levosimendan (12 or 24 µg/kg delivered over 10 minutes) or to placebo in the course of off-pump CABG.[37]

Bolus-Plus-Infusion Studies

Prompt and sustained increases in cardiac output and stroke volume, and a reduction in SVR, were seen in 18 hemodynamically stable patients undergoing elective CABG, who were randomized to low-dose (18 µg/kg bolus and then 0.2 µg/kg/min infusion) or high-dose (36 µg/kg bolus and then 0.3 µg/kg/min infusion) levosimendan for 6.25 hours in a placebo-controlled study by Nijhawan et al.[38] Heart rate increased during the first 2 hours of treatment, with evidence of a dose effect and statistical differences between the higher dose of levosimendan and placebo during the first hour ($p < .05$).

Labriola et al.[39] examined the effects of a 12-µg/kg bolus of levosimendan (delivered over 10 minutes) followed by an infusion of 0.1 µg/kg/min for 12 hours in 11 patients with low-output syndrome after cardiac surgery and found that the overall effect of levosimendan was to reduce pre- and afterload, and increase cardiac output.

Infusion-Only Study

Hemodynamic data from an observational study of patients requiring inotropic support after surgery for cardiac ($n = 9$), cardiopulmonary ($n = 2$), or other ($n = 1$) causes documented progressive improvements in cardiac output and stroke volume and a reduction in SVR during the course of a 24-hour infusion of levosimendan at rates of 0.1 or 0.2 µg/kg/min. The drug was administered as an adjunct to other therapies, including catecholamines ($n = 10$).[40]

Ischemic Heart Disease

Experience with levosimendan in patients with left ventricular failure secondary to acute myocardial infarction (MI) is derived preeminently from the RUSSLAN study, with contributions from later exploratory studies. Appraisal of safety and efficacy data from this study identified bolus doses of 6 to 12 µg/kg with infusion rates of 0.1 to 0.2 µg/kg/min as the optimal schedule for levosimendan in this indication.

The RUSSLAN study was a placebo-controlled, double-blind trial that randomly assigned 504 patients to one of four schedules of levosimendan bolus plus infusion or to placebo for 6 hours.[41] Patients were eligible for the study if they had experienced an acute MI within the previous 5 days, had x-ray evidence of left ventricular failure (i.e., pulmonary edema or venous congestion), and were considered to have a clinical need for inotropic support. Exclusion criteria included low systemic blood pressure (<90 mm Hg), evidence of rhythm abnormalities, history of moderate-to-severe renal failure, and a diagnosis of septic shock. The primary study end point was hypotension or clinically significant myocardial ischemia, with a range of efficacy outcomes as secondary end points.

Evidence of improved survival and prognosis with levosimendan emerged during the first 24 hours of RUSSLAN and remained apparent for up to 180 days (22.6% vs. 31.4%; $p = .053$). Use of rescue medication was significantly lower in the levosimendan group ($p = .003$ vs. placebo). Rank analyses and patient self-assessments indicated that levosimendan reduced the proportion of patients experiencing a worsening of dyspnea ($p < .05$ vs. placebo) but there were no between-group differences for other clinical indices. There were no significant differences between groups in the incidence rates of reported adverse events except for myocardial rupture, which occurred more often in the placebo group ($p = .027$).

Several recent studies have supplemented the clinical data from RUSSLAN with insights into specific aspects of cardiac function in patients

Table 55.3. Results of studies of intravenous levosimendan in patients with ischemic heart disease

Study	No. of patients; clinical status	Levosimendan dosage	Comparator	Results/observations
Sonntag et al. (2004)	24; acute coronary syndromes	24 μg/kg (B)	Placebo	Improved function of stunned myocardium
De Luca et al. (2005)	26; acute MI	12 μg/kg (B)	Placebo	Improved hemodynamics and coronary flow reserve
Michaels et al. (2005)	10; coronary artery disease	24 μg/kg (B)	None	Reduction in myocardial oxygen extraction (attributed to vasodilator effects on coronary conductance and resistance arteries)
RUSSLAN (2002)	504; LV failure complicating acute MI	0.1–0.4 μg/kg/min (I)	Placebo	Improved survival at 14 and 180 days; incidence of ischemia and/or hypotension similar to placebo

with coronary vascular disease or acute MI treated with levosimendan. These include examination of changes in coronary artery diameter and blood flow,[42,43] use of Doppler echocardiography to demonstrate improvement in several indices of diastolic function, including isovolumetric relaxation time ($p = .001$),[44] and a significant ($p = .016$) reduction in the number of hypokinetic myocardial segments in 24 patients with stunned myocardium after percutaneous coronary angioplasty ($p = .016$ for levosimendan 24 μg/kg vs. placebo).[45]

The results of these studies of levosimendan in patients with ischemic heart disease are summarized in Table 55.3.

Critical Care

Levosimendan has been used to generally good effect in several small series of patients with cardiogenic or septic shock, although the participating investigators have emphasized that these data require confirmation in controlled trials among much larger patient populations.[46] These investigations are summarized in Table 55.4.

Representative findings from some of these studies include the report of Delle Karth et al.,[47] who added a 24-hour infusion of levosimendan 0.1 μg/kg/min to standard catecholamine therapy in 10 patients with cardiogenic shock and observed enhancement of mean cardiac index (2.4 ± 0.6 L/min/m^2 from 1.8 ± 0.4 L/min/m^2; $p = .023$) and reduction of mean SVR (1109 ± 202 dyn/sec/cm^{-5} from 1559 ± 430 dyn/sec/cm^{-5}; $p = .001$) at the conclusion of the infusion.

In patients with septic shock and associated dobutamine-refractory depression of left ventricular function, introduction of levosimendan as a 0.2 μg/kg/min infusion, maintained for 24 hours, was associated with increases in LVEF and cardiac index and reductions in end-diastolic ventricular volume and pulmonary artery pressure. Gastric mucosal flow and urine output were enhanced, and plasma lactate concentration was reduced.[48]

The successful use of adjunctive levosimendan in pediatric or infant patients with severe cardiac diseases requiring surgical intervention has also been documented by Braun and colleagues[49,50] in Berlin.

Table 55.4. Clinical series evaluating intravenous levosimendan in critically ill patients in critical care (cardiogenic or septic shock)

Study	Patients	Levosimendan dosage	Comparator	Results/observations
Delle Karth et al. (2003)	10; cardiogenic shock	0.1 μg/kg/min (I)	None	Significant increase in cardiac output together with a decrease in SVR
Lehmann et al. (2004)	10; cardiogenic shock	6 μg/kg + 0.2 μg/kg/min	None	8 patients survived without any multiorgan failure
Morelli et al. (2005)	28; septic shock	0.2 μg/kg/min (I)	Dobutamine 5 μg/kg/min	Levosimendan improved systemic hemodynamics and regional perfusion

References

1. Pollesello P, Ovaska M, Kaivola J, et al. Binding of a new Ca^{2+} sensitizer, levosimendan, to recombinant human cardiac troponin C. A molecular modeling, fluorescent probe, and proton nuclear magnetic resonance study. J Biol Chem 1994; 269:28584–90.
2. Levijoki J, Pollesello P, Kaviola J, et al. Further evidence for the cardiac troponin C mediated calcium sensitization by levosimendan: structure-response and binding analysis with analogs of levosimendan. J Mol Cell Cardiol 2000;32:479–91.
3. Sorsa T, Pollesello, Solaro RJ. The contractile apparatus as a target for drugs against heart failure: interaction of levosimendan, a calcium sensitiser, with cardiac troponin C. Mol Cell Biochem 2004; 266:87–107.
4. Haikala H, Nissinen E, Etemadzadeh E, et al. Troponin C-mediated calcium sensitization induced by levosimendan does not impair relaxation. J Cardiovasc Pharmacol 1995;25:794–801.
5. Janssen PM, Datz N, Zeitz O, et al. Levosimendan improves diastolic and systolic function in failing human myocardium. Eur J Pharmacol 2000;404: 191–9.
6. Pagel PS, Haikala H, Pentikainen PJ, et al. Pharmacology of levosimendan: a new myofilament calcium sensitizer. Cardiovasc Drug Rev 1996;14:286–316.
7. Haikala H, Kaheinen P, Levijoki J, et al. The role of cAMP- and cGMP-dependent protein kinases in the cardiac actions of the new calcium sensitizer, levosimendan. Cardiovasc Res 1997;34:536–46.
8. Szilagyi S, Pollesello P, Levijoki J, et al. The effects of levosimendan and OR-1896 on isolated hearts, myocyte-sized preparations and phosphodiesterase enzymes of the guinea pig. Eur J Pharmacol 2004;486:67–74.
9. Szilagyi S, Pollesello P, Levijoki J, et al. Two inotropes with different mechanisms of action: contractile, PDE-inhibitory and direct myofibrillar effects of levosimendan and enoximone. J Cardiovasc Pharmacol 2005;46:369–76.
10. Pollesello P, Mebazaa A. ATP-dependent potassium channels as a key target for the treatment of myocardial and vascular dysfunction. Curr Opin Crit Care 2004;10:436–4.
11. Yokoshiki H, Katsube Y, Sunagawa M, et al. The novel calcium sensitizer levosimendan activates the ATP-sensitive K^+ channel in rat ventricular cells. J Pharmacol Exp Ther 1997;283:373–83.
12. Pataricza J, Krassoi I, Hohn J, et al. Functional role of potassium channels in the vasodilating mechanism of levosimendan in porcine isolated coronary artery. Cardiovasc Drugs Ther 2003;17:111–3.
13. Pataricza J, Hohn J, Petri A, et al. Comparison of the vasorelaxing effect of cromakalim and the inodilator, levosimendan, in human isolated portal vein. J Pharm Pharmacol 2000;52:213–7.
14. Kersten JR, Montgomery MW, Pagel PS, et al. Levosimendan, a new positive inotropic drug, decreases myocardial infarct size via activation of K_{ATP} channels. Anesth Analg 2000;90:5–13.
15. Levijoki J, Pollesello P, Kaheinen P, et al. Improved survival with simendan after experimental myocardial infarction in rats. Eur J Pharmacol 2001; 419:243–8.
16. Leprán I, Papp JG. Effect of long-term oral pretreatment with levosimendan on cardiac arrhythmias during coronary artery occlusions in conscious rats. Eur J Pharmacol 2003;464:171–6.
17. Zager RA, Johnson AC, Lund S, et al. Levosimendan protects against experimental endotoxemic acute renal failure. Am J Physiol Renal Physiol 2006;290:F1453–62.
18. Kopustinskiene DM, Pollesello P, Saris NE. Levosimendan is a mitochondrial K(ATP) channel opener. Eur J Pharmacol 2001;428:311–4.
19. Kopustinskiene D, Pollesello P, Saris NE. Potassium-specific effects of levosimendan on heart mitochondria. Biochem Pharmacol 2004;68:807–12.
20. Jamali IN, Kersten JR, Pagel PS, et al. Intracoronary levosimendan enhances contractile function of stunned myocardium. Anesth Analg 1997;85: 23–9.
21. Lochner A, Colesky F, Genade S. Effect of a calcium-sensitizing agent, levosimendan, on the postcardioplegic inotropic response of the myocardium. Cardiovasc Drugs Ther 2000;14:271–81.
22. Kivikko M, Antilä S, Eha J, et al. Pharmacokinetics of levosimendan and its metabolites during and after a 24-hour continuous infusion in patients with severe heart failure. Int J Clin Pharmacol Ther 2002;40:465–71.
23. Nieminen MS, Akkila J, Hasenfuss G, et al. Hemodynamic and neurohumoral effects of continuous infusion of levosimendan in patients with congestive heart failure. J Am Coll Cardiol 2000;36:1903–12.
24. Slawsky MT, Colucci WS, Gottlieb SS, et al. Acute hemodynamic and clinical effects of levosimendan in patients with severe heart failure. Circulation 2000;102:2222–7.
25. Kivikko M, Lehtonen L, Colucci WS, et al. Sustained haemodynamic effects of intravenous levosimendan. Circulation 2003;107:81–6.

26. Follath F, Cleland JGF, Just H, et al. Efficacy and safety of intravenous levosimendan compared with dobutamine in severe low-output heart failure (the LIDO study): a randomised double-blind trial. Lancet 2002;360:196–202.
27. Styles S. REVIVE-2: levosimendan improves five-day clinical status in acute HF. www.theheart.org.
28. Teerlink JR, Massie BM, Colucci WS, et al. On behalf of the REVIVE II Investigators. Rapid and sustained reductions of plasma B-type natriuretic peptide concentrations in patients with acutely decompensated heart failure treated with levosimendan. J Am Coll Cardiol 2006;47(Suppl 1):343A (abstr).
29. Zairis MN, Apostolatos C, Anastasiadis P, et al. The effect of a calcium sensitizer or an inotrope or none in chronic low output decompensated heart failure: results from the calcium sensitizer or inotrope or none in low output heart failure study (CASINO). J Am Coll Cardiol 2004;43(suppl 1):206A–7A(abstr).
30. Coletta AP, Cleland JG, Freemantle N, et al. Clinical trials update from the European Society of Cardiology Heart Failure meeting: SHAPE, BRING-UP 2 VAS, COLA II, FOSIDIAL, BETACAR, CASINO and meta-analysis of cardiac resynchronisation therapy. Eur J Heart Fail 2004;6:673–6.
31. Mebazaa A, Cohen-Solal A, Kleber F, et al. Study design of a mortality trial with intravenous levosimendan (the SURVIVE study) in patients with acutely decompensated heart failure. Critical Care 2004;8(suppl 1):P87(abstr).
32. Styles S. SURVIVE: no levosimendan survival benefit over dobutamine in acute HF. www.theheart.org.
33. Nanas JN, Papazoglou PP, Terrovitis JV, et al. Haemodynamic effects of levosimendan added to dobutamine in patients with decompensated advanced heart failure refractory to dobutamine alone. Am J Cardiol 2004;94:1329–32.
34. Parissis JT, Adamopoulos S, Antoniades C, et al. Effects of levosimendan on circulating pro-inflammatory cytokines and soluble apoptosis mediators in patients with decompensated advanced heart failure. Am J Cardiol 2004;93:1309–12.
35. McLean AS, Huang SJ, Nalos M, Ting I. Duration of the beneficial effects of levosimendan in decompensated heart failure as measured by echocardiographic indices and B-type natriuretic peptide. J Cardiovasc Pharmacol 2005;46:830–5.
36. Lilleberg J, Nieminem MS, Akkila J, et al. Effects of a new calcium sensitizer, levosimendan, on hemodynamics, coronary blood flow and myocardial substrate utilization early after coronary artery bypass grafting. Eur Heart J 1998;19:660–8.
37. Barisin S, Husedzinovic I, Sonicki Z, et al. Levosimendan in off-pump coronary artery bypass: a four-times masked controlled study. J Cardiovasc Pharmacol 2004;44:703–8.
38. Nijhawan N, Nicolosi A, Montgomery MW, et al. Levosimendan enhances cardiac performance after cardiopulmonary bypass: a prospective, randomized placebo-controlled trial. J Cardiovasc Pharmacol 1999;34:219–28.
39. Labriola C, Siro-Brigiani M, Carrata F, et al. Haemodynamic effects of levosimendan in patients with low-output heart failure after cardiac surgery. Int J Clin Pharmacol Ther 2004;42:204–11.
40. Plöchl W, Rajek A. The use of the novel calcium sensitizer levosimendan in critically ill patients. Anaesth Intensive Care 2004;32:471–5.
41. Moiseyev VS, Poder P, Andrejevs. N, et al. Safety and efficacy of a novel calcium sensitizer, levosimendan, in patients with left ventricular failure due to an acute myocardial infarction. A randomized, placebo-controlled, double-blind study (RUSSLAN). Eur Heart J 2002;23:1422–32.
42. Michaels AD, McKeown B, Kostal M, et al. Effects of intravenous levosimendan on human coronary vasomotor regulation, left ventricular wall stress, and myocardial oxygen uptake. Circulation 2005;111:1504–9.
43. De Luca L, Proietti P, Celotto A, et al. Levosimendan improves hemodynamics and coronary flow reserve after percutaneous coronary intervention in patients with acute myocardial infarction and left ventricular dysfunction. Am Heart J 2005;150: 63–8.
44. De Luca L, Sardella G, Proietti P, et al. Effects of levosimendan on left ventricular diastolic function after primary angioplasty for acute anterior myocardial infarction: a Doppler echocardiographic study. J Am Soc Echocardiogr 2006;19: 172–7.
45. Sonntag S, Sundberg S, Lehtonen LA, et al. The calcium sensitizer levosimendan improves the function of stunned myocardium after percutaneous transluminal coronary angioplasty in acute myocardial ischemia. J Am Coll Cardiol 2004; 43:2177–82.
46. Lehmann A, Lang J, Boldt J, et al. Levosimendan in patients with cardiogenic shock undergoing surgical revascularization: a case series. Med Sci Monit 2004;10:89–93.
47. Delle Karth G, Buberl A, Geppert A, et al. Haemodynamic effects of a continuous infusion of levosimendan in critically ill patients with cardiogenic shock requiring catecholamines. Acta Anaesthesiol Scand 2003;47:1251–6.

48. Morelli A, De Castro S, Teboul JL, et al. Effects of levosimendan on systemic and regional hemodynamics in septic myocardial depression. Intensive Care Med 2005;31:638–44.
49. Braun JP, Schnieder M, Dohmen P, Dopfiner U. Successful treatment of dilative cardiomyopathy in a 12-year-old girl using the calcium sensitizer levosimendan after weaning from mechanical biventricular assist support. J Cardiothorac Vasc Anesth 2004a;18:772–4.
50. Braun JP, Schnieder M, Kastrup M, Liu J. Treatment of acute heart failure in an infant after cardiac surgery using levosimendan. Eur J Cardiothorac Surg 2004b;26:228–30.

56 Natriuretic Peptides

Markus Meyer, Hartmut Lüss, Veselin Mitrovic, and Alexandre Mebazaa

Peptide hormones belonging to the natriuretic peptide (NP) family play an important role in maintaining cardiac and renal function by regulating fluid volume, pressure, and sodium concentration. The principal members of this family are atrial natriuretic peptide (ANP); urodilatin (URO); brain natriuretic peptide (BNP); and C-type natriuretic peptide (CNP). The physiologic effects of these molecules generally lead to vasodilation, natriuresis, and diuresis, and regulate sodium and water homeostasis, rendering them promising candidates for potential therapeutic use in cardiovascular and renal dysfunction. This chapter reviews the biochemistry, physiology, and pharmacologic potential of the major natriuretic peptides, with particular emphasis on their clinical importance in the treatment of acute heart failure syndrome (AHFS).

Biochemistry

Structure and Synthesis

The natriuretic peptides are characterized by a highly conserved 17-amino-acid ring structure that varies little even among different species. Whereas the amino- and carboxy-terminal amino acid sequences vary markedly, the ring structure differs in only five positions between ANP/URO, BNP, and CNP (Fig. 56.1). The biologically active forms of these molecules are processed from precursor proteins encoded by two genes on chromosome 1 (ANP/URO and BNP) and a third gene on chromosome 2 (CNP). Atrial natriuretic peptide and URO share the same amino acid sequence from position 99 to 126 of the ANP-prohormone; however, URO has an additional N-terminal extension of 4 amino acids.

Atrial Natriuretic Peptide

Human ANP is a 28-amino-acid peptide synthesized in the myoendocrine cells of the heart atria, derived from a 151-amino-acid preprohormone through a series of proteolytic processing steps. An N-terminal, 126-amino-acid precursor, pro-ANP (ANP_{1-126}), is first derived from the preprohormone and stored in atrial myocyte granules. Pro-ANP is then cleaved into a 98-amino-acid N-terminal fragment and the biologically active, 28-amino-acid C-terminal atrial natriuretic peptide (ANP_{99-126}); both are released by exocytosis into the circulation.[1,2] Under normal conditions, ANP gene expression in the ventricles is seen only at very low levels (about 7% that in the atria), but increased ANP messenger RNA (mRNA) production may occur in pathologic conditions such as heart failure and left ventricular (LV) hypertrophy.[3] Atrial natriuretic peptide release is induced by elevations in cardiac-wall tension,[4] which may be due to physical exercise, neurohumoral stimuli, and other physiologic factors.[1]

Urodilatin

Urodilatin (URO/ANP_{95-126}) is a 32-amino-acid peptide that is produced by differential processing of the pro-ANP precursor peptide in distal renal tubule cells; therefore, it is identical to ANP except for the presence of four additional N-terminal amino acids. Urodilatin is found in urine

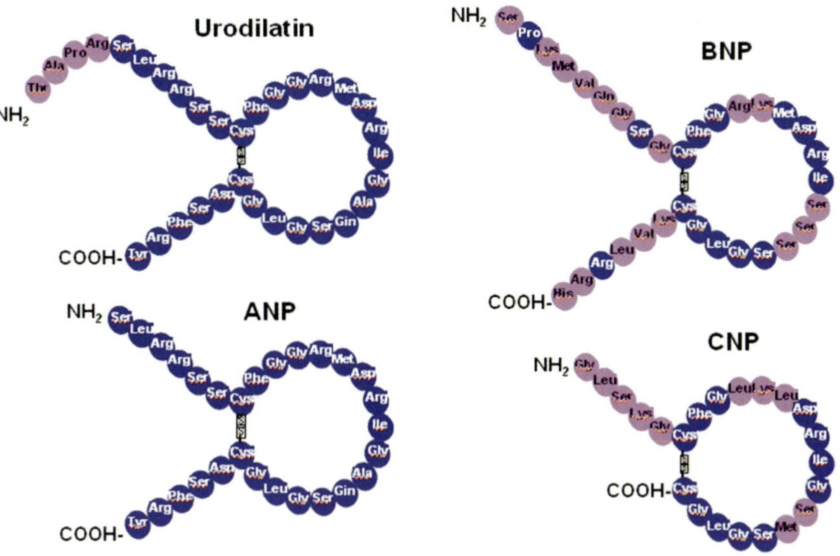

FIGURE 56.1. Structure of the natriuretic peptides ANP$_{99-126}$, urodilatin/ANP$_{95-126}$, BNP$_{77-108}$, and CNP$_{105-126}$ showing the conserved 17-amino-acid ring configuration. Nonconserved residues are indicated in pink.

and has not been detected and isolated from plasma. It is secreted into the tubular lumen and acts as a paracrine hormone, binding further downstream to receptors in the inner medullary collecting duct and inhibiting sodium reabsorption.[5,6] Urodilatin release occurs in response to acute volume load and selective increases in sodium concentration and dietary sodium intake,[7,8] and is closely correlated with the circadian rhythm of urinary sodium excretion.[9] In congestive heart failure (CHF), urinary urodilatin excretion was found to be increased, apparently to counteract antinatriuresis and fluid retention.[10]

Brain Natriuretic Peptide

Brain natriuretic peptide was originally isolated from porcine brain extracts and later identified from human cardiac tissue. It consists of 32 amino acids (BNP$_{77-108}$) derived from a 108-amino-acid pro-BNP precursor that is found, in humans, predominantly in the ventricles of the heart and in much smaller amounts in the atria, brain, and amniotic tissue.[11,12] N-terminal pro-BNP and mature BNP molecules are released from ventricular myocytes at a 1:1 molar ratio and circulate in plasma. Unlike ANP, which is stored in the form of the 126-amino-acid precursor pro-ANP, BNP is stored mainly as the mature peptide.[4,13] Whereas there is a threefold greater concentration of BNP mRNA in the ventricles than in the atria, the ventricles have only 1% of the amount of mature BNP that is in the atria.[14] Brain natriuretic peptide mRNA is transcribed in response to stretching of ventricle and atrial walls from increased blood pressure or elevated venous volume.[12,15–17]

C-Type Natriuretic Peptide

Processing of CNP starts with the removal of a 23-amino-acid signal peptide from the 126-amino acid preprohormone (prepro-CNP), converting it into pro-CNP (CNP$_{24-126}$). Pro-CNP is then cleaved to produce a 53-amino-acid intermediate peptide, CNP-53 (CNP$_{74-126}$); further cleavage of CNP-53 produces biologically active CNP-22 (CNP$_{105-126}$).[18] CNP-22 is produced in brain and endothelial cells and acts primarily as an autocrine or paracrine hormone that regulates vascular tone and blood pressure.[4,19] It is found in much lower concentrations than either ANP or BNP in the heart or in plasma. Like ANP, CNP is stored mainly in the 104-amino-acid propeptide (pro-CNP) form.[18]

Atrial natriuretic peptide and BNP secretion is regulated mainly by the degree of atrial and ventricular wall stress that results from volume or pressure overload and by several endogenous hormones, neurotransmitters, proinflammatory cytokines, and vasoactive factors. Both CNP production and secretion in vitro are stimulated by ANP, 20-fold more potently by BNP, and by several cytokines and growth factors, including transforming growth factor-β (TGF-β), tumor necrosis factor-α (TNF-α), interleukin-1 (IL-1), and lipopolysaccharide (LPS), although no relation has been established between CNP and any pathologic effects caused by these cytokines.[2]

Natriuretic Peptide Receptors and Metabolism

The three types of natriuretic peptide receptors (NPRs) are NPR-A, NPR-B, and NPR-C. NPR-A and NPR-B are expressed at high levels in the atria, ventricles, aorta, peripheral blood vessels, platelets, lungs, skin, tubules, smooth muscles of the kidney, and presynaptic sympathetic nerve fibers. Both are highly homologous transmembrane proteins composed of an extracellular binding domain (~440 amino acids), a transmembrane domain (37 amino acids), and intracellular domains with kinase (~280 amino acids) and guanylyl cyclase (~250 amino acids) activity. The guanylyl cyclase domain catalyzes the generation of cyclic guanosine monophosphate (cGMP), which mediates most of the physiologic effects of natriuretic peptides.[4] Atrial natriuretic peptide, BNP, and urodilatin all bind predominantly to NPR-A; ANP is the natural ligand for NPR-A and binds to it with a 10-fold higher affinity than BNP. C-type natriuretic peptide binds most strongly to NPR-B.[2,14]

Natriuretic peptide receptor C is expressed in cells of the kidney, adrenal gland, brain, lungs, and blood vessel walls. It is more abundantly expressed than any other NP receptor type, constituting 90% of all NP receptors in target tissues.[4] It has an extracellular binding domain that is approximately 30% homologous to its NPR-A and NPR-B counterparts and a short, noncatalytic 37-amino-acid intracellular domain that shares no homology with the corresponding domains of the other two receptor types. Natriuretic peptide receptor C is considered a "clearance" receptor whose action is geared toward internalization of receptor-ligand complexes and subsequent lysosomal degradation of the ligand.[20,21] One function of NPR-C may be the removal of excess natriuretic peptides in the circulation, although it may achieve other effects through signaling pathways involving other second messengers such as cyclic adenosine monophosphate (cAMP) or by coupling with G proteins. All natriuretic peptides bind avidly to NPR-C, although ANP and CNP bind with a somewhat higher affinity than BNP.[4,22,23]

Natriuretic peptide binding to NP receptors stimulates cGMP production and elevation of intracellular cGMP levels. Cellular responses depend on downstream cGMP signal transduction, mediated by cGMP-dependent protein kinases (PKGs) that catalyze phosphorylation of target proteins (reviewed by D'Souza et al.[4]). Two protein kinases, PKG-I and PKG-II, appear to be involved in this signaling pathway. PKG-I is a soluble cytoplasmic enzyme that modulates intracellular calcium levels and is present in cardiac myocytes, vasculature, lung, cerebellum, kidney, adrenal glands, and uterus. PKG-II regulates fluid homeostasis at the cell membrane and is found in brain, intestine, lung, kidney, and bone but is absent from the heart and vascular tissue. Cyclic GMP may also activate cAMP-dependent protein kinase A (PKA) or cGMP-regulated phosphodiesterases (PDEs) in certain tissues such as the heart, lung, liver, adrenals, brain, platelets, and smooth muscle.

Natriuretic peptides are cleared from the circulation by NPR-C uptake and the enzymatic action of neutral endopeptidase (NEP), a zinc metallopeptidase enzyme present in high concentrations in the brush border of renal proximal tubular cells and also in the vascular endothelium. Neutral endopeptidase digests other vasodilators such as bradykinin, substance P, and adrenomedullin, and vasoconstrictors such as angiotensin II and endothelin 1 (ET-1) (reviewed in Schmitt et al.[14]).

Physiology and Pharmacology

Atrial Natriuretic Peptide and Brain Natriuretic Peptide

Atrial natriuretic peptide and lower levels of BNP are produced in the atria and ventricles in response to changes in transmural atrial pressure or stretch as a consequence of pressure or volume expansion. Neurohumoral stimuli such as vasopressin, angiotensin II, endothelin (ET), enkephalin, morphine, and TNF-α also induce ANP release.[24–28]

The effects of ANP and BNP on the cardiovascular and renal systems are well documented.[17,29–36] Under physiologic conditions, ANP and BNP have similar physiologic effects, including vasodilation; suppression of the renin-angiotensin-aldosterone system (RAAS), endothelin, and sympathicoadrenergic systems; reduced blood pressure and peripheral vascular resistance; and enhanced diuresis, natriuresis, and kaliuresis.[29,30,36] In canine models and isolated arterial strips, ANP relaxes coronary arteries[37] and appears to be more selective for the renal arteries when compared to others (vertebral, femoral, and common carotid).[38] In humans, however, results of studies on the effects of BNP on coronary arteries and coronary flow rate have been equivocal.[39,40]

As natural antagonists of the RAAS, ANP and BNP inhibit Na^+ reabsorption in the inner medullary collecting duct and also modify the renal hemodynamics by increasing preglomerular vasodilation and postglomerular vasoconstriction, thereby increasing the glomerular filtration rate (GFR). All these actions have the end effect of enhancing natriuresis and diuresis. The pro-ANP fragment ANP_{31-67} also stimulates the release of prostaglandins, which induce natriuresis indirectly by blocking adenosine triphosphatase (ATPase)-dependent sodium exchange in the inner medullary collecting duct of the kidney.

Atrial natriuretic peptide or BNP infusions in healthy subjects increase urinary flow rate and Na^+ excretion in a dose-dependent manner and inhibit plasma renin secretion.[34,41] Brain natriuretic peptide also has predominantly central hemodynamic effects, such as decreased stroke volume and mean arterial pressure and increased heart rate, but it does not seem to affect the peripheral microcirculation in the skin and conjunctiva, capillary density, or skin oxygen capacity.[36]

Atrial natriuretic peptide also appears to play an important role in organogenesis and embryogenesis by regulating the differentiation and regulation of multiple organ systems, including the skeletal system, immune response, natural killer cell activation, histamine release, reproductive system, and central nervous system (reviewed in Schmitt et al.[14]). Additionally, other studies emphasize the potential role of ANP and BNP as important factors in cardiovascular remodeling as a result of their antiproliferative activity.[4] The mechanism by which these NPs modulate proliferation, cell growth, and apoptosis in cardiac myocytes, smooth muscle cells, and fibroblasts, as well as extracellular matrix production, is currently the subject of intensive research.

The biological half-life of ANP is approximately 3.5 minutes, whereas that of BNP is nearly seven times longer at 22.6 minutes as a result of its slower degradation by NEP and lower affinity for the NPR-C.[2]

Urodilatin

Because they are highly homologous to each other and are derived from the same precursor, the biologic actions of urodilatin and ANP are similar; however, the effects of urodilatin on renal sodium excretion are more critical than those of ANP. Urodilatin infusion in animal models results in a much stronger natriuretic and diuretic effect than that produced by an equimolar ANP infusion.[42,43] This is most likely due to the lesser susceptibility of urodilatin to degradation by the neutral endopeptidase as it passes the proximal tubules in the kidney.[44]

Urodilatin causes dilation of preglomerular and constriction of postglomerular vessels[45] and also increases GFR in animal models of acute renal failure.[46] In healthy human volunteers, urinary excretion of urodilatin is directly correlated to increased sodium intake and renal sodium excretion.[7] After prolonged diets with varying sodium doses, infused urodilatin at 20 ng/kg/min for 60 minutes increased diuresis and natriuresis in proportion to the amount of sodium in the diet, further suggesting an important role for endogenous urodilatin in sodium homeostasis.[35] The renal response to urodilatin appears to be exerted at the collecting duct where sodium reabsorption is inhibited. Even lower doses (5 and 10 ng/kg/min) of intravenously administered urodilatin to healthy subjects with normal LV function have significant systemic effects on the cardiovascular, endocrine, and renal systems. In contrast to the response in heart failure patients, in healthy volunteers these low doses led to a reduction in the cardiac output by 7% and 16%; in stroke volume by 10% and 20%, respectively, most likely due to venodilation; and in renal blood flow (hippurate clearance) by 13% to 37%, with no changes in arterial pressure or GFR.[47]

In addition to its effects on the kidney, in healthy volunteers, urodilatin at ≤20 ng/kg/min inhibits the neurohumoral axis, resulting in decreased secretion of renin, angiotensin II, aldosterone, vasopressin, and BNP into the plasma. At higher dosages, plasma renin, angiotensin II, aldosterone, and vasopressin levels actually increase in a compensatory fashion because of the decrease in blood pressure.[5,47,48]

In a randomized, placebo-controlled phase II study of subjects with bronchial asthma, urodilatin at various doses, alone or in combination with albuterol, improved bronchodilation parameters, including forced expiratory volume (FEV), maximum expiratory flow (MEF), and peak expiratory flow (PEF), and showed potential as an adjunct to β_2-adrenergic agonists for asthma management.[49]

Unlike ANP, urodilatin is more resistant to NEP degradation, probably because of the four additional amino acids at its N-terminal tail, and it seems to be cleared from circulation also by binding to NPR-C.[50] Infused urodilatin has a plasma half-life of approximately 5 to 24 minutes; with bolus injections, however, the half-life is shortened to 2 to 3 minutes.[48]

C-Type Natriuretic Peptide

C-type natriuretic peptide is produced in endothelial cells, acts in a paracrine/autocrine manner, and is rapidly inactivated so that plasma measurements do not always reflect changes in CNP levels. C-type natriuretic peptide has been shown to regulate vascular tone and induce arterial vasodilation and relaxation. Its potency varies with the size of the blood vessel and the type of NP receptor expressed on the vessel. It is more potent than ANP in relaxing smooth muscle and likely plays a more important role in dilating blood vessel walls than in inducing diuresis or natriuresis.[19]

Infused CNP has been shown to lower blood pressure in animal models as well as in healthy human volunteers.[18] C-type natriuretic peptide knockout mice, however, appear to compensate with increased ANP production so that they are not hypertensive as expected; rather, they are mildly hypotensive. C-type natriuretic peptide also suppresses adrenocorticotropic hormone (ACTH), vasopressin, and aldosterone synthesis.

C-type natriuretic peptide plays an important role in modulating vascular inflammation and in other vascular protective mechanisms (reviewed in Scotland et al.[18]). C-type natriuretic peptide production is stimulated by inflammatory cytokines such as IL-1 and TNF and by LPS; septic shock patients actually have significantly higher levels of circulating CNP. The antiinflammatory effect of CNP includes suppression of proinflammatory prostaglandin E_2 (PGE_2) production in isolated cells, reduced expression of vascular adhesion molecules, and inhibition of leukocyte migration, or "rolling." Vascular protection by CNP may also involve its beneficial effects on the vascular endothelium and smooth muscle and inhibition of coagulation and thrombus formation.

Clinical Significance

Studies of NPs have significantly expanded our understanding of homeostatic mechanisms underlying fluid volume and pressure regulation. Alterations in circulating levels of the cardiac NPs have been used as diagnostic and prognostic markers in various cardiovascular conditions, such as CHF, hypertension, LV dysfunction, acute coronary syndromes, and aortic valve diseases[2,51–53] (reviewed in D'Souza et al.[4]).

Natriuretic Peptides as Disease Indicators

Congestive Heart Failure

Increased mechanical strain in the atria and ventricles is a major stimulus for the synthesis and release of both ANP and BNP, resulting in a marked increase in ANP and BNP levels in circulation during the development of heart failure. Plasma ANP and BNP are negatively correlated with left ventricular ejection fraction (LVEF). Several studies have shown that plasma BNP, as well as the N-terminal pro-BNP fragment (NT-pro-BNP), may be a more powerful prognostic indicator of development of LV systolic or diastolic dysfunction and LV hypertrophy than is ANP.[2,17,51,52,54]

Rapid (15-minute) BNP immunofluorescence assays (Biosite Diagnostics, San Diego, CA, and Bayer Diagnostics, Tarrytown, NY) are currently approved as a tool for the diagnosis and prognosis of patients with acute coronary syndromes, including acute decompensated heart failure. There is also an 18-minute electrochemiluminescence assay for NT-pro-BNP (Roche Diagnostics, GmbH, Basel, Switzerland). Although BNP testing does not replace echocardiography and a full cardiologic assessment and should be used only within the clinical context, heart failure appears more likely with plasma BNP concentrations above 100 pg/mL.[51,52] At or above this level (100 pg/mL), BNP was more accurate than the National Health and Nutrition Examination Survey (NHANES) and Framingham criteria in diagnosing heart failure.[54] The ratio of plasma ANP to plasma BNP is significantly higher in patients with obstructive airway disease than in those who have heart failure, perhaps because of increased right atrial pressures secondary to severe primary lung disease.[4,55]

Serum BNP levels are useful guides for risk stratification for predicting mortality and for designing heart failure treatment regimens by titrating doses of standard medications to a desired BNP level.[56] The BNP levels rise in direct proportion to the severity of symptoms and cardiac damage, and BNP is an independent predictor of mortality in CHF patients. A pilot study of patients with decompensated heart failure has suggested that BNP concentration measured before discharge may help determine the risk of readmission within the month following discharge.[57]

Because BNP concentration is a good indicator of elevated end-diastolic pressure and LV wall tension, which in turn closely correlates with dyspnea, it also correlates well with the New York Heart Association (NYHA) classification scheme. However, tests are currently in progress to evaluate the prognostic and diagnostic value of NT-pro-BNP, which may be a better indicator of abnormal cardiac function than BNP itself in NYHA class I and II patients. In NYHA class III and IV patients, sensitivity and specificity are comparable. The NT-pro-BNP levels may also be more tightly linked to renal function, and negative predictive values for NT-pro-BNP are >95%.[54] The diagnostic value of NT-pro-BNP, however, depends on the patient's age, because NT-pro-BNP levels change with age and declining GFR (the cutoff for detecting CHF rises sharply from 125 pg/mL to 450 pg/mL after age 75), and there is a gray period coinciding with the peak incidence of CHF between 65 and 85 years of age when NT-pro-BNP is of little use to the clinician. Clearly, further research is required to determine how NT-pro-BNP measurements can be best applied in cardiovascular and cardiorenal management.

Acute Myocardial Infarction

Acute myocardial infarction is associated with compensatory activation of the RAAS and sympathetic nervous system, a low to moderate rise in ANP, and a 100-fold increase in plasma BNP via rapid synthesis in infarcted and periinfarcted areas. The ANP and BNP levels correlate with pulmonary capillary wedge pressure (PCWP), but BNP levels at 72 hours correlate inversely with the cardiac index (CI) and LVEF at day 5 and month 3 post-MI.[4] Although BNP gene expression and de novo synthesis occur rapidly in both ventricles, ANP is secreted from storage in the atrium, further indicating distinct pathologic roles for ANP and BNP in AMI.

Myocardial Ischemia and Coronary Artery Disease

In vivo models of experimental ischemia have shown that even brief periods of hypoxia generated by coronary artery occlusion trigger the rapid release of both ANP and BNP without any correlation to myocardial wall stress. In patients undergoing percutaneous transluminal coronary angioplasty (PTCA), inflation of the PTCA balloon induces transient myocardial ischemia, followed immediately by a rapid and transient increase in plasma BNP levels. However, no correlation was found between the magnitude of increase in BNP levels and the duration of myocardial ischemia from this procedure. The ANP levels also increased slightly after balloon inflation. Plasma BNP and pro-BNP levels are also elevated in patients with chronic coronary artery disease CAD without LV dysfunction.[58]

Natriuretic Peptides as Therapeutic Agents in Acute Heart Failure Syndrome

Acute heart failure syndrome (AHFS) comprises a set of severe, life-threatening symptoms resulting from congestion or fluid retention in the lungs and inadequate perfusion of tissues and organs.[59] Specific signs and symptoms of AHFS include dyspnea or orthopnea, fatigue, pulmonary congestion, rales, coughing, cachexia, peripheral edema, hypoperfusion, and jugular vein distention. Patients with AHFS may not have any previously known cardiac dysfunction but may suffer from symptoms following an acute coronary event such as a myocardial infarction (new-onset AHFS), or they may experience acute decompensation of chronic heart failure.[60]

Current Therapy of Acute Heart Failure Syndrome

The goals of AHFS therapy are (1) to improve clinical symptoms and hemodynamics without increasing the risk of short- and long-term mortality, (2) to preserve or improve renal function, and (3) to minimize myocardial damage. Current treatment strategies focus on rapidly improving hemodynamics and relieving congestion by reducing fluid volume with diuretics; increasing contractility and cardiac output with digoxin and inodilators such as dobutamine, dopamine, and milrinone; and enhancing pulmonary and peripheral circulation with vasodilators such as nitroglycerin and angiotensin-converting enzyme (ACE) inhibitors such as lisinopril and enalapril.

Current therapies have limitations, however. Controlled clinical trials have shown that hemodynamic improvements observed with AHFS interventions do not translate into long-term patient benefit, with most resulting in minimal or no benefit, some deleterious effects, or high mortality rates. For instance, vasodilators generally used when hypoperfusion is accompanied by congestion, normal or high blood pressure, and insufficient response to diuretics alone can also cause hypotension and induce tolerance with prolonged use. High-dose diuretics are associated with increased risk of renal deterioration and neurohormonal activation of the angiotensin-aldosterone and sympathetic nervous systems, perhaps affecting long-term outcomes such as mortality.[61] Some inodilators such as dobutamine and milrinone may increase the risk of ventricular arrhythmias, postdischarge morbidity, and mortality.[61,62] Digoxin increases cardiac contractility and improves symptoms with possible a reduction in the number of hospitalizations, but its long-term clinical outcomes are neutral at best.[63] Therefore, new therapeutic approaches that improve short-term outcomes without negatively affecting renal and cardiac function and long-term survival are desired.

Newer therapies include levosimendan, an inotropic, Ca^{2+}-sensitizing, K^+ channel opener with antiischemic and anti-stunning effects that increases myocardial contraction without increasing myocardial oxygen consumption, and tolvaptan, a vasopressin V2-receptor antagonist that increases urine volume and serum sodium with little or no sodium loss (reviewed in Gheorghiade et al.[64]). Levosimendan is well tolerated. Most common adverse effects include headache, hypotension, nausea, and dizziness believed to be secondary to its vasodilatory effects and slight reductions in red blood cell count, hemoglobin, and serum potassium, but no proarrhythmic effects.[65,66] However, a multicenter randomized trial (Survival of Patients with Acute Heart Failure in Need of Intravenous Inotropic Support [SURVIVE]) evaluating its efficacy in improving survival in AHFS patients showed no significant reduction in mortality when compared with dobutamine.[67]

Natriuretic Peptide Therapy for Acute Heart Failure Syndrome

Three natriuretic peptide agents are currently approved or undergoing development for the management of acute heart failure (Table 56.1). Carperitide and ularitide are synthetic analogues of ANP and urodilatin, respectively, and nesiritide is a recombinant form of human BNP. All three

Table 56.1. Characteristics of therapeutic natriuretic peptides

	Carperitide	Nesiritide	Ularitide
Peptide analogue	ANP_{99-126}	BNP_{77-108}	Urodilatin (ANP_{95-126})
Source	Synthetic	Recombinant	Synthetic
Development phase	Approved in Japan for acute heart failure	Approved in the U.S. for ADHF	Phase II–III
Secreted by	Atrial and ventricular myocytes	Ventricular myocytes	Renal tubular cells
Stimulus for secretion	↑ Blood pressure, venous volume; atrial wall stretching	↑ Blood pressure, venous volume; ventricular wall stretching	↑ Plasma Na^+; ↑ blood pressure
Receptor	NPR-A, NPR-C	NPR-A, NPR-C	NPR-A, NPR-C
Plasma half-life	2–5 min	18–23 min	2–24 min
Sensitivity to NEP	Yes	Yes	Yes, but less than ANP
Physiologic targets	Vascular wall endothelium and smooth muscle	Vascular-wall endothelium and smooth muscle	Collecting ducts
Pharmacologic effects: mechanism of action	↓ Na^+ reabsorption, ↓ renal perfusion rate; ↑ GFR; ↓ RAAS; predominantly venous vasodilation; bronchodilation	↓ Na^+ reabsorption, ↓ renal perfusion rate; ↑ GFR; ↓ RAAS; vasodilation; bronchodilation	↓ Na^+ reabsorption, ↓ renal perfusion rate; ↑ GFR; ↓ RAAS; vasodilation; bronchodilation
Clinical effects in ADHF patients	↓ PCWP, LVFP; ↑ CI	↓ PCWP and systemic arterial pressure; relief from dyspnea	↓ PCWP, PAP, and SVR; ↑ CI; ↑ relief from dyspnea
Adverse effects	Hypotension; renal dysfunction	Hypotension; renal dysfunction (azotemia, ↑ serum creatinine); potential ↑ mortality	Sweating; hypotension; nausea; dizziness; bradycardia

ADHF, acute decompensated heart failure; ANP, atrial natriuretic peptide; BNP, brain natriuretic peptide; LVFP, left ventricular filling pressure; NPR-A and NPR-C, natriuretic peptide receptor-A and -C; CI, cardiac index; RAAS, renin-angiotensin-aldosterone system; GFR, glomerular filtration rate; NEP, neutral endopeptidase; PAP, pulmonary arterial pressure; PCWP, pulmonary capillary wedge pressure; SVR, systemic vascular resistance.

restore hemodynamic balance and improve cardiac or renal function in patients experiencing AHFS.

Carperitide (Synthetic Atrial Natriuretic Peptide)

Carperitide is a synthetic form of human ANP that was approved for use in Japan in 1995 for the management of acute heart failure (AHF). In a 6-year open-label study of 3777 patients with AHF treated with 0.085 μg/kg/min carperitide for 65 hours, 82% of patients experienced clinical improvement in terms of severity of Killip classification and renal dysfunction.[68] A much smaller, earlier study in patients who had severe heart failure with AMI also demonstrated a decrease in PCWP by almost 50% (21 to 11 mm Hg) and plasma aldosterone from 148 to 56 pg/mL after carperitide infusion (0.05 to 1.0 μg/kg/min) without altering heart rate and systemic blood pressure.[69]

Studies on the effect of ANP infusion in CHF patients vary widely in design, patient population, and type of ANP analogue used, making interpretation difficult.[14] They all show an invariable reduction in cardiac filling pressure, however, that occurs too early to be due to a fluid shift or changes in diuresis and pulmonary or peripheral vascular resistance and has been attributed to ANP-induced venous vasodilation. This reinforces the concept of ANP as a vasodilator on veins rather than arteries in patients with high PCWP and plasma noradrenaline.[70]

Nesiritide (Recombinant Brain Natriuretic Peptide)

Nesiritide (Natrecor®) is a recombinant human B-type natriuretic peptide (hBNP) that was approved in the United States in 2001 for the treatment of AHFS patients with dyspnea at rest or minimal activity. The recommended dose is an intravenous bolus of 2 μg/kg followed by a continuous infusion of 0.01 μg/kg/min. Nesiritide improves short-term dyspnea and produces dose-dependent reductions in PCWP and systemic arterial pressure in patients with heart failure.[71] In clinical trials, the decrease in PCWP was observed within 15 minutes of the start of administration, and most of the effect was achieved at 60 minutes of the infusion.

Unlike dobutamine, nesiritide did not cause ventricular or supraventricular arrhythmias in patients with decompensated heart failure, and it actually reduced ventricular ectopy or had a neutral effect (Prospective Randomized Evaluation of Cardiac Ectopy with Dobutamine or Natrecor Therapy [PRECEDENT] study).[72] Urine output (mean change in volume status) during the first 24 hours of nesiritide infusion did not differ from that obtained with nitroglycerin treatment. Nesiritide may also cause hypotension (Vasodilation in the Management of Acute Congestive Heart Failure [VMAC] study).[73] The VMAC study also showed that relief from dyspnea was indeed reduced by nesiritide treatment but at levels not significantly different from the reduction caused by the relatively low dose of nitroglycerin used for comparison.

Controversy remains, however, as to whether nesiritide is associated with a significantly increased risk of worsening renal function and death after treatment.[74,75] This finding was based on meta-analyses of all available randomized clinical trials evaluating nesiritide in acute decompensated heart failure. Its use has not translated into long-term improvement in clinical outcome.[73]

Ularitide

Ularitide is a synthetic version of urodilatin that is currently under clinical development for the treatment of AHFS. Ularitide has the same ANP_{95-126} amino acid sequence as urodilatin. Like urodilatin, the synthetic version ularitide also binds to NPR-A receptors. Maximum concentration is reached 1.5 to 2 hours after the start of infusion. Various studies have reported a half-life range of 2 to 24 minutes.[48,76,77]

The primary pharmacodynamic effects of ularitide are preload and afterload reduction due to vasodilation of peripheral veins and arteries and increased diuresis and natriuresis at higher doses, lowering blood pressure. These effects result from its direct action on vascular smooth-muscle cells, causing dilation of renal, pulmonary, and coronary arterial vessels, and from inhibition of sodium reabsorption in the renal tubules. Ularitide activity is largely mediated by binding to NPR-A receptors, leading to increased intracellular cGMP levels. Consistent with this mode of action, dose-dependent ularitide-induced increases in plasma cGMP levels have been observed in both healthy subjects and subjects with AHFS.[78]

Ularitide restores fluid hemostasis by inducing diuresis and natriuresis, and vasodilation. In healthy volunteers, ularitide increased the renal filtration fraction by increasing GFR and reducing the effective renal plasma flow, and it increased the fractional excretion of sodium and the rate of urinary sodium excretion.[48] Additionally, administration of ularitide in healthy subjects at dosages up to 20 ng/kg/min leads to a decrease in plasma concentrations of renin, aldosterone, and angiotensin II, suggesting that ularitide may also have a downregulating effect on the RAAS that inhibits aldosterone secretion from the adrenal cortex.[47,48] Ularitide infusion into healthy volunteers also led to reduced cardiac preload, pulmonary arterial pressure (PAP) and PCWP, increased CI, and reduced systemic vascular resistance (SVR).[79] These mechanisms suggest that ularitide may provide a potential benefit to patients with AHF characterized by elevated left and right ventricular filling pressures and neuroendocrine activation.

The clinical efficacy of ularitide in patients with ADHF was evaluated in SIRIUS II, a parallel-dose, placebo-controlled, double-blinded study in 221 patients randomized to placebo or one of three ularitide dosing arms. Ularitide was administered by 24-hour intravenous infusions at 7.5, 15, or 30 ng/kg/min. Compared with placebo for change from baseline to +6 hours, all three ularitide doses were associated with significantly greater reductions in the co-primary efficacy end point of mean PCWP. Dyspnea at 6 hours (the second of two co-primary end points) was rated moderately or markedly improved by a greater percentage of subjects in each ularitide dose group than in the placebo group.[80]

Adverse effects of ularitide include increased sweating, nausea, dizziness, and hypotension (decreased blood pressure) with infusions of 5 ng/kg/min or greater. In the studies where these were observed, all side effects resolved without vasoconstrictor treatment. No apparent worsening of renal function was observed through 72 hours in the SIRIUS II study.

Conclusion

Natriuretic peptides are a family of peptide hormones with distinct biomolecular properties and clinical effects that have been well studied as a treatment modality for AHFS. Structurally, each has a 17-amino-acid loop differing in up to five positions among the different natriuretic peptides.

The vasodilators nesiritide and carperitide have been approved in the United States and Japan, respectively, for acute heart failure. The natural analogues of carperitide and nesiritide (ANP and BNP) are both produced by the atria and ventricles of the heart in response to increased blood pressure and stretching of the cardiac wall and generally cause vasodilation, RAAS inhibition, and reduction in blood pressure without affecting fluid volume. Plasma BNP has also been used as a diagnostic or prognostic marker for acute and chronic cardiac syndromes.

Ularitide, a synthetic form of the renal NP urodilatin, is currently undergoing clinical development. In contrast to the other peptides, urodilatin (ularitide), is produced in the kidney and acts in a paracrine fashion on collecting ducts, resulting in reduced Na^+ reabsorption and thereby increased natriuresis and diuresis. Intravenously applied ularitide also causes vasodilation, reduction in blood pressure, and bronchodilation.

Because of the capacity of the natriuretic peptides to restore hemodynamic balance and fluid homeostasis, they hold promise in the management of cardiopulmonary and renal symptoms of AHFS, although further studies are required to understand more completely their impacts on short- and long-term morbidity and mortality in AHFS patients.

References

1. Silver MA. The natriuretic peptide system: kidney and cardiovascular effects. Curr. Opin. Nephrol. Hypertens. 2006;15:14–21.
2. Stoupakis G, Klapholz M. Natriuretic peptides: biochemistry, physiology, and therapeutic role in heart failure. Heart Dis. 2003;5:215–23.
3. Saito Y, Nakao K, Arai H, et al. Augmented expression of atrial natriuretic polypeptide gene in ventricle of human failing heart. J. Clin. Invest. 1989; 83:298–305.
4. D'Souza SP, Davis M, Baxter GF. Autocrine and paracrine actions of natriuretic peptides in the heart. Pharmacol. Ther. 2004;101:113–29.
5. Carstens J, Jensen KT, Pedersen EB. Effect of urodilatin infusion on renal haemodynamics, tubular function and vasoactive hormones. Clin. Sci. (Lond.) 1997;92:397–407.
6. Forssmann W, Meyer M, Forssmann K. The renal urodilatin system: clinical implications. Cardiovasc. Res. 2001;51:450–62.
7. Heer M, Drummer C, Baisch F, Gerzer R. Long-term elevations of dietary sodium produce parallel increases in the renal excretion of urodilatin and sodium. Pflugers Arch. 1993;425:390–94.
8. Meyer M, Richter R, Brunkhorst R, Wrenger E, et al. Urodilatin is involved in sodium homeostasis and exerts sodium-state-dependent natriuretic and diuretic effects. Am. J. Physiol. 1996;271(3 Pt 2): F489–97.
9. Drummer C, Fiedler F, Konig A, Gerzer R. Urodilatin, a kidney-derived natriuretic factor, is excreted with a circadian rhythm and is stimulated by saline infusion in man. J. Am. Soc. Nephrol. 1991;1:1109–13.
10. Drummer C, Kentsch M, Otter W, Heer M, Herten M, Gerzer R. Increased renal natriuretic peptide (urodilatin) excretion in heart failure patients. Eur. J. Med. Res. 1997;2:347–54.
11. Nakamura S, Naruse M, Naruse K, et al. Atrial natriuretic peptide and brain natriuretic peptide coexist in the secretory granules of human cardiac myocytes. Am. J. Hypertens. 1991;4:909–12.
12. Ogawa Y, Nakao K, Mukoyama M, et al. Natriuretic peptides as cardiac hormones in normotensive and spontaneously hypertensive rats. The ventricle is a major site of synthesis and secretion of brain natriuretic peptide. Circ. Res. 1991;69:491–500.
13. Hino J, Tateyama H, Minamino N, Kangawa K, atsuo H. Isolation and identification of human brain natriuretic peptides in cardiac atrium. Biochem. Biophys. Res. Commun. 1990;167:693–700.
14. Schmitt M, Cockcroft JR, Frenneaux MP. Modulation of the natriuretic peptide system in heart failure: from bench to bedside? Clin. Sci. (Lond.) 2003;105:141–60.
15. Hama N, Itoh H, Shirakami G, et al. Rapid ventricular induction of brain natriuretic peptide gene expression in experimental acute myocardial infarction. Circulation 1995;92:1558–64.
16. Nakagawa O, Ogawa Y, Itoh H, et al. Rapid transcriptional activation and early mRNA turnover of brain natriuretic peptide in cardiocyte

hypertrophy. Evidence for brain natriuretic peptide as an "emergency" cardiac hormone against ventricular overload. J. Clin. Invest. 1995;96:1280–87.
17. Boomsma F, van den Meiracker AH. Plasma A- and B-type natriuretic peptides: physiology, methodology and clinical use. Cardiovasc. Res. 2001;51: 442–49.
18. Scotland RS, Ahluwalia A, Hobbs AJ. C-type natriuretic peptide in vascular physiology and disease. Pharmacol. Ther. 2005;105:85–93.
19. Sudoh T, Minamino N, Kangawa K, Matsuo H. C-type natriuretic peptide (CNP): a new member of natriuretic peptide family identified in porcine brain. Biochem. Biophys. Res. Commun. 1990; 168:863–70.
20. Porter JG, Arfsten A, Fuller F, Miller JA, Gregory LC, Lewicki JA. Isolation and functional expression of the human atrial natriuretic peptide clearance receptor cDNA. Biochem. Biophys. Res. Commun. 1990;171:796–803.
21. Shima M, Seino Y, Torikai S, Imai M. Intrarenal localization of degradation of atrial natriuretic peptide in isolated glomeruli and cortical nephron segments. Life. Sci. 1988;43:357–63.
22. Bennett BD, Bennett GL, Vitangcol RV, et al. Extracellular domain-IgG fusion proteins for three human natriuretic peptide receptors. Hormone pharmacology and application to solid phase screening of synthetic peptide antisera. J Biol. Chem. 1991;266:23060–7.
23. Mukoyama M, Nakao K, Hosoda K, et al. Brain natriuretic peptide as a novel cardiac hormone in humans. Evidence for an exquisite dual natriuretic peptide system, atrial natriuretic peptide and brain natriuretic peptide. J. Clin. Invest. 1991;87: 1402–12.
24. Ferrari R, Agnoletti G. Atrial natriuretic peptide: its mechanism of release from the atrium. Int. J. Cardiol. 1989;24:137–49.
25. Gardner DG, Newman ED, Nakamura KK, Nguyen KP. Endothelin increases the synthesis and secretion of atrial natriuretic peptide in neonatal rat cardiocytes. Am. J. Physiol. 1991;261:E177–82.
26. de Bold AJ, Bruneau BG, Kuroski de Bold ML. Mechanical and neuroendocrine regulation of the endocrine heart. Cardiovasc. Res. 1996;31:7–18.
27. Bruneau BG, de Bold AJ. Selective changes in natriuretic peptide and early response gene expression in isolated rat atria following stimulation by stretch or endothelin-1. Cardiovasc. Res. 1994;28: 1519–25.
28. Ruskoaho H, Vakkuri O, Arjamaa O, Vuolteenaho O, Leppaluoto J. Pressor hormones regulate atrial-stretch-induced release of atrial natriuretic peptide in the pithed rat. Circ. Res. 1989;64:482–92.
29. Atlas SA, Maack T. Effects of atrial natriuretic factor on the kidney and the renin-angiotensin-aldosterone system. Endocrinol. Metab. Clin. North Am. 1987;16:107–43.
30. Cody RJ, Atlas SA, Laragh JH, et al. Atrial natriuretic factor in normal subjects and heart failure patients. Plasma levels and renal, hormonal, and hemodynamic responses to peptide infusion. J. Clin. Invest. 1986;78:1362–74.
31. de ZD, Janssen WM, de Jong PE. Atrial natriuretic factor: its (patho)physiological significance in humans. Kidney. Int. 1992;41:1115–33.
32. Hobbs RE, Miller LW, Bott-Silverman C, James KB, Rincon G, Grossbard EB. Hemodynamic effects of a single intravenous injection of synthetic human brain natriuretic peptide in patients with heart failure secondary to ischemic or idiopathic dilated cardiomyopathy. Am. J. Cardiol. 1996;78:896–901.
33. Janssen WM, de Zeeuw D, van der Hem GK, de Jong PE. Antihypertensive effect of a 5-day infusion of atrial natriuretic factor in humans. Hypertension 1989;13:640–6.
34. Jensen KT, Carstens J, Pedersen EB. Effect of BNP on renal hemodynamics, tubular function and vasoactive hormones in humans. Am. J. Physiol. 1998;274:F63–72.
35. Meyer M, Richter R, Brunkhorst R, et al. Urodilatin is involved in sodium homeostasis and exerts sodium-state-dependent natriuretic and diuretic effects. Am. J. Physiol. 1996;271:F489–97.
36. van der Zander K, Houben AJ, Hofstra L, Kroon AA, de Leeuw PW. Hemodynamic and renal effects of low-dose brain natriuretic peptide infusion in humans: a randomized, placebo-controlled crossover study. Am. J. Physiol. Heart. Circ. Physiol. 2003;285:H1206–12.
37. Adachi H, Tomoike H, Nishijima H, Egashira S, Nakamura M. Sustained dilatation of large coronary artery by alpha-human atrial natriuretic peptide in conscious dogs: a comparison with nitroglycerin. Eur. J. Pharmacol. 1989;161:189–96.
38. Ishihara T, Aisaka K, Hattori K, et al. Vasodilatory and diuretic actions of alpha-human atrial natriuretic polypeptide alpha-hANP;Life. Sci. 1985;36:1205–15.
39. D'Souza SP, Yellon DM, Martin C, et al. B-type natriuretic peptide limits infarct size in rat isolated hearts via KATP channel opening. Am. J. Physiol. Heart Circ. Physiol. 2003;284:H1592–600.
40. Okumura K, Yasue H, Fujii H, et al. Effects of brain (B-type) natriuretic peptide on coronary artery

diameter and coronary hemodynamic variables in humans: comparison with effects on systemic hemodynamic variables. J. Am. Coll. Cardiol. 1995;25:342–8.
41. Levin ER, Gardner DG, Samson WK. Natriuretic peptides. N, Engl. J, Med 1998;339:321–8.
42. Riegger G, Elsner D, Forssmann WG, Kromer EP. Effects of ANP-(95–126) in dogs before and after induction of heart failure. Am. J, Physiol. 1990;259: H1643–8.
43. Schulz-Knappe P, Honrath U, Forssmann WG, Sonnenberg H. Endogenous natriuretic peptides: effect on collecting duct function in rat kidney. Am. J. Physiol. 1990;259:F415–8.
44. Gagelmann M, Hock D, Forssmann WG. Urodilatin (CDD/ANP-95–126) is not biologically inactivated by a peptidase from dog kidney cortex membranes in contrast to atrial natriuretic peptide/cardiodilatin (alpha-hANP/CDD-99–126). FEBS Lett. 1988;233: 249–54.
45. Endlich K, Steinhausen M. Natriuretic peptide receptors mediate different responses in rat renal microvessels. Kidney Int. 1997;52:202–7.
46. Schramm L, Heidbreder E, Lukes M, et al. Endotoxin-induced acute renal failure in the rat: effects of urodilatin and diltiazem on renal function. Clin. Nephrol. 1996;46:117–24.
47. Bestle MH, Olsen NV, Christensen P, Jensen BV, Bie P. Cardiovascular, endocrine, and renal effects of urodilatin in normal humans. Am. J, Physiol. 1999;276:R684–95.
48. Carstens J, Jensen KT, Pedersen EB. Metabolism and action of urodilatin infusion in healthy volunteers. Clin. Pharmacol. Ther. 1998;64:73–86.
49. Fluge T, Forssmann WG, Kunkel G, et al. Bronchodilation using combined urodilatin-albuterol administration in asthma: a randomized, double-blind, placebo-controlled trial. Eur. J, Med. Res. 1999;4:411–5.
50. Abassi ZA, Tate J, Hunsberger S, Klein H, Trachewsky D, Keiser HR. Pharmacokinetics of ANF and urodilatin during cANF receptor blockade and neutral endopeptidase inhibition. Am. J, Physiol. 1992;263:E870–6.
51. Cowie MR, Jourdain P, Maisel A, et al. Clinical applications of B-type natriuretic peptide (BNP) testing. Eur. Heart J, 2003;24:1710–8.
52. McCullough PA, Omland T, Maisel AS. B-type natriuretic peptides: a diagnostic breakthrough for clinicians. Rev. Cardiovasc. Med. 2003;4:72–80.
53. Suttner SW, Boldt J. Natriuretic peptide system: physiology and clinical utility. Curr. Opin. Crit Care 2004;10:336–41.
54. Maisel AS, Krishnaswamy P, Nowak RM, et al. Rapid measurement of B-type natriuretic peptide in the emergency diagnosis of heart failure. N. Engl. J Med. 2002;347:161–7.
55. Davis M, Espiner E, Richards G, et al. Plasma brain natriuretic peptide in assessment of acute dyspnoea. Lancet 1994;343:440–4.
56. Yu CM, Sanderson JE. Plasma brain natriuretic peptide–an independent predictor of cardiovascular mortality in acute heart failure. Eur. J. Heart Fail. 1999;1:59–65.
57. Cheng V, Kazanagra R, Garcia A, et al. A rapid bedside test for B-type peptide predicts treatment outcomes in patients admitted for decompensated heart failure: a pilot study. J. Am. Coll. Cardiol. 2001;37:386–91.
58. Goetze JP, Christoffersen C, Perko M, et al. Increased cardiac BNP expression associated with myocardial ischemia. FASEB J. 2003;17:1105–7.
59. Hunt SA, Abraham WT, Chin MH, et al. ACC/AHA 2005 Guideline Update for the Diagnosis and Management of Chronic Heart Failure in the Adult. Circulation. 2005 20;112(12):e154–235.
60. Gheorghiade M, Mebazaa A. Introduction to acute heart failure syndromes. Am. J, Cardiol. 2005a;96:1G–4G.
61. Gheorghiade M, Mebazaa A. The challenge of acute heart failure syndromes. Am. J, Cardiol. 2005b;96: 86G–9G.
62. Bayram M, De LL, Massie MB, Gheorghiade M. Reassessment of dobutamine, dopamine, and milrinone in the management of acute heart failure syndromes. Am. J. Cardiol. 2005;96:47G–58G.
63. Stough WG, O'Connor CM, Gheorghiade M. Overview of current noninodilator therapies for acute heart failure syndromes. Am. J, Cardiol. 2005; 96:41G–6G.
64. Gheorghiade M, Teerlink JR, Mebazaa A. Pharmacology of new agents for acute heart failure syndromes. Am. J, Cardiol. 2005;96:68G–73G.
65. Follath F, Franco F, Cardoso JS. European experience on the practical use of levosimendan in patients with acute heart failure syndromes. Am J, Cardiol. 2005;96:80G–5G.
66. Mebazaa A, Barraud D, Welschbillig S. Randomized clinical trials with levosimendan. Am. J, Cardiol. 2005;96:74G–9G.
67. Mebazaa A, Nieminen MS, Packer M, Cohen-Solal A, Kleber FX, Pocock SJ, Thakkar R, Padley RJ, Põder P, Kivikko M; SURVIVE Investigators. Levosimendan vs dobutamine for patients with acute decompensated heart failure: the SURVIVE Randomized Trial. JAMA. 2007;297(17):1883–91.

68. Suwa M, Seino Y, Nomachi Y, Matsuki S, Funahashi K. Multicenter prospective investigation on efficacy and safety of carperitide for acute heart failure in the "real world" of therapy. Circ. 2005; J. 69:283–90.
69. Kikuchi M, Nakamura M, Suzuki T, Sato M, Takino T, Hiramori K. Usefulness of carperitide for the treatment of refractory heart failure due to severe acute myocardial infarction. Jpn. Heart. 2001;J 42:271–80.
70. Schmitt M, Gunaruwan P, Payne N, et al. Effects of exogenous and endogenous natriuretic peptides on forearm vascular function in chronic heart failure. Arterioscler. Thromb. Vasc. Biol. 2004;24:911–7.
71. Scios, Inc. Nesiritide prescribing information. April 2005.
72. Burger AJ, Horton DP, LeJemtel T, et al. Effect of nesiritide (B-type natriuretic peptide) and dobutamine on ventricular arrhythmias in the treatment of patients with acutely decompensated congestive heart failure: the PRECEDENT study. Am. Heart J. 2002;144:1102–8.
73. Publication Committee for the VMAC Investigators Intravenous nesiritide vs nitroglycerin for treatment of decompensated congestive heart failure: a randomized controlled trial. JAMA. 2002;287:1531–40.
74. Sackner-Bernstein JD, Skopicki HA, Aaronson KD. Risk of worsening renal function with nesiritide in patients with acutely decompensated heart failure. Circulation 2005b;111:1487–91.
75. Sackner-Bernstein JD, Kowalski M, Fox M, Aaronson K. Short-term risk of death after treatment with nesiritide for decompensated heart failure: a pooled analysis of randomized controlled trials. JAMA. 2005a;293:1900–5.
76. Elsner D, Muders F, Muntze A, Kromer EP, Forssmann WG, Riegger GA. Efficacy of prolonged infusion of urodilatin [ANP-(95–126)] in patients with congestive heart failure. Am. Heart J. 1995; 129:766–73.
77. Kentsch M, Ludwig D, Drummer C, Gerzer R, Muller-Esch G. Haemodynamic and renal effects of urodilatin bolus injections in patients with congestive heart failure. Eur. J. Clin. Invest 1992a; 22:662–9.
78. Mitrovic V, Luss H, Nitsche K, et al. Effects of the renal natriuretic peptide urodilatin (ularitide) in patients with decompensated chronic heart failure: a double-blind, placebo-controlled, ascending-dose trial. Am. Heart J. 2005a;150:1239.
79. Kentsch M, Ludwig D, Drummer C, Gerzer R, Muller-Esch G. Haemodynamic and renal effects of urodilatin in healthy volunteers. Eur. J. Clin. Invest. 1992b;22:319–25.
80. Mitrovic V, Seferovic P, Simeunovic, D, et al. A randomized, double-blind, placebo-controlled phase II study of ularitide in patients with decompensated congestive heart failure. J. Card. Fail. 2005b;11:S151.

57
Vasopressin Antagonists in Acute Heart Failure Syndromes

Cesare Orlandi, Filippo Brandimarte, and Mihai Gheorghiade

The contribution of neurohormonal abnormalities in the pathophysiology of chronic heart failure (CHF) is well established. Attenuation of the excessive and continuous activation of angiotensin II and β-adrenergic receptors in patients with CHF with angiotensin-converting enzyme (ACE) inhibitors and beta-blockers, respectively, has resulted in substantial reductions in morbidity and mortality. However, it is not clear whether intervention with other neuroendocrine modulators (e.g., tumor necrosis factor [TNF] or endothelin) could result in similar benefits.

Data from the Studies of Left Ventricular Dysfunction (SOLVD) study have shown that arginine vasopressin levels are elevated in asymptomatic CHF patients prior to demonstrable elevations of plasma renin activity.[1] However, the assessment of the potential benefit associated with vasopressin receptor blockade in CHF has been hampered until recently by the lack of orally active, effective, and well-tolerated nonpeptide agents. Newly developed compounds targeting the V1 (vascular) and V2 (renal) vasopressin receptors are currently being studied in CHF patients and may represent the next generation of neuroendocrine modulators to show a beneficial impact in heart failure.

Arginine Vasopressin

Vasopressin, also known as vasopressin or antidiuretic hormone (ADH), is a neuropeptide produced in the supraoptic and paraventricular nuclei of the hypothalamus that is transported to the pituitary gland and released into the bloodstream. Secretion of this hormone from hypothalamic neurons is regulated by baroreceptors and osmoreceptors and is affected by such factors as malignancies, drugs, cardiopulmonary disease, central nervous system disorders, and endocrinopathies. Reduced blood pressure and increases in plasma osmolality lead to marked increases in vasopressin blood levels.

Vasopressin interacts with two receptors, V1 and V2. The V1 receptors increases intracellular calcium through the inositol-1,4,5-triphosphate (IP_3) pathway leading to vasoconstriction of smooth muscle and positive inotropic effects in cardiac muscle. Prolonged V1a stimulation leads to synthesis of proteins that promote cellular hypertrophy. The V1 receptor is localized in the vasculature, the uterus, and the brain. The V2 receptor primarily is localized in the collecting duct of the renal nephron, where it mediates changes in water permeability.

Vasopressin causes vasoconstriction via cyclic adenosine monophosphate (cAMP)-independent vascular V1a receptors and promotes water reabsorption in the kidneys via cAMP-dependent V2 receptors, thereby having an antidiuretic effect.[2] The absence of vasopressin, or its blockade by antagonists, leads to the excretion of large volumes of dilute urine and to an increase in plasma sodium concentration if water intake is unchanged.

Vasopressin in Congestive Heart Failure

Increased vasopressin levels have been demonstrated in patients with heart failure since the early 1980s.[1,3] These changes are similar to those observed for plasma renin and norepinephrine, with values that become higher as the severity of the disease increases. Vasopressin may contribute to the genesis and maintenance of congestive heart failure through a number of mechanisms mediated by activation of the V1a and V2 receptors. The activation of the V1a vascular receptor produces vasoconstriction, resulting in increased peripheral vascular resistance and afterload. Activation of the V2 renal tubular receptor produces water retention with consequent increased intra- and extracellular volumes and fluid overload. Vasopressin has also been shown to stimulate cell growth and contribute to the genesis of cardiac hypertrophy. Protein synthesis as well as the protein/DNA ratio are increased in cultured neonatal myocytes,[4] and enhanced DNA synthesis has also been observed in fibroblasts.

Interestingly, a large number of the potentially negative effects of vasopressin in heart failure are similar to those described for angiotensin II, and include vasoconstriction, cardiac hypertrophy, vascular smooth muscle cell remodeling and growth, central nervous system effects, and fluid retention. However, whether blockade of the vasopressin receptors will have a positive impact on clinical outcomes remains to be determined.

In a multivariate analysis from the SAVE study, Rouleau et al.[5] have also demonstrated that circulating vasopressin concentrations correlated independently with the occurrence of severe congestive heart failure, recurrent myocardial infarction (MI), and combined mortality, heart failure, and recurrent MI. Although these data are interesting, large well-controlled outcome studies with vasopressin receptor blockers are necessary to fully establish their potential role.

Hemodynamic Effects

The hemodynamic effects of conivaptan, a dual V1 and V2 vasopressin receptor antagonist, were studied by Udelson et al.[6] in patients with symptomatic heart failure. Compared with placebo, conivaptan reduced pulmonary capillary wedge pressure (PCWP) and right atrial pressure (RAP) without changing cardiac index (CI), systemic vascular resistance (SVR), pulmonary vascular resistance (PVR), blood pressure (BP), or heart rate (HR). There was a significant increase of urinary output in a dose-dependent manner. The trial was not designed to evaluate long-term hemodynamic effects. Similar results have also been recently reported for the selective V2 receptor antagonist, tolvaptan.[7]

Effects in Heart Failure

Gheorghiade et al.[8] studied the effects of tolvaptan, a new oral nonpeptide V2 antagonist, in patients with CHF who were not fluid restricted. Tolvaptan resulted in a significant reduction of body weight, reduced edema, and increased urine volume. Those beneficial effects were noted without changes in HR, serum potassium, or renal function.

Vasopressin and Serum Sodium in Congestive Heart Failure

Several reports have highlighted the common association between congestive heart failure and both sodium and water retention.[9–12] Increased vasopressin release is one of the postulated mechanisms for this imbalance.[13] In heart failure, the decrease in "effective" blood volume and arterial filling are sensed by the aortic and carotid sinus baroreceptors, resulting in stimulation of vasopressin release.[14,15] The importance of this mechanism is stressed in experimental models of heart failure, where abnormal dilution is also observed. Indeed, correction of the observed water excretory defect by a vasopressin receptor antagonist has been reported in rats with CHF induced by inferior vena cava constriction.[16]

Of particular interest is also the role played by vasopressin in the genesis and maintenance of hyponatremia in heart failure. Studies have demonstrated that patients with heart failure and hyponatremia have inappropriately elevated vasopressin levels, indicating that, in this condition, the normal osmotic control of vasopressin release is dysfunctional.[17,18] In these circumstances, the dominant pathways of vasopressin activation are likely to be the nonosmotic pathways (e.g., aortic and carotid baroreceptors). The inappropriately elevated vasopressin levels contribute to the development and maintenance of the hyponatremic and volume overloaded state due to ongoing stimulation of V2 renal receptors mediating water retention. The problem becomes greater and more evident in patients with worsening of chronic heart failure. In these patients, the concomitant presence of fluid overload and hyponatremia represents a particular challenge. Current treatment strategies for patients with decompensated heart failure and hyponatremia consist of additional loop diuretics to remove excess fluid and free-water restriction to correct the sodium imbalance. This approach is often inadequate. The effect of fluid restriction is limited and, additionally, diuretic therapy produces further stimulation of vasopressin secretion, and may result in maintenance or worsening of hyponatremia.[19] Indeed, loop diuretics produce reductions in plasma osmolality due to the excretion of isosmolar urine. The resulting elevated vasopressin levels provide a continuing stimulus to renal water retention, maintaining or even worsening the state of hyponatremia, even with restriction of water intake.

Thus, rather than just resulting in an improvement of a marker of the clinical state (i.e., correction of hyponatremia), treatment of this syndrome with a V2 receptor antagonist has the potential to directly address an important component of the pathophysiologic state that is driving the clinical signs of both hyponatremia and volume overload.

Vasopressin Receptor Antagonists in Development

Several orally active nonpeptide vasopressin antagonists are currently in clinical development and include selective V2- and mixed V1a/V2-receptor blockers. Limited published data are available from three compounds: VPA-985, conivaptan, and tolvaptan. Clinical data have shown the ability of all of these agents to mobilize fluid and increase serum sodium levels in heart failure patients.

In chronic heart failure patients with signs of mild fluid overload and on stable standard therapy including diuretics, chronic oral administration of tolvaptan showed an increase in urine volume accompanied by an acute, statistically significant reduction in body weight that was maintained for 25 days.[8] In the same study, a differential effect on serum sodium was observed in patients with normo- and hyponatremia at baseline. In normonatremic patients, an acute and nonsustained elevation in sodium levels was observed at day 1. However, patients with hyponatremia demonstrated statistically significant and sustained increases in serum sodium often leading to normalization.

Administration of a V1a receptor blocker is expected to produce vasodilation. However, results have been conflicting. Acute intravenous administration of conivaptan reduces pulmonary capillary wedge pressure; however, this effect did not appear to be related to a V1a receptor-mediated mechanism, but to the V2 receptor-mediated reduction in blood volume.[6] Indeed, while no changes in systemic vascular resistance were seen, large and dose-dependent increases in urine volume have been reported.

Tolvaptan has also been tested in patients who were hospitalized for heart failure with low left ventricular ejection fraction and systemic congestion that was resistant to standard therapy.[20] Treatment with tolvaptan was associated with significantly decreased body weight beginning at 1 day of treatment and lasting until the end of the trial.[20] Patients receiving tolvaptan also experienced reduced hyponatremia.[20] Although the incidence of worsening heart failure was not affected by tolvaptan, post-hoc analyses revealed that tolvaptan tended to reduce mortality in patients with renal dysfunction, and significantly reduced mortality in patients with severe systemic congestion.[20] The results of The Efficacy of Vasopressin Antagonism in Heart Failure Outcome Study With Tolvaptan (EVEREST) trials have recently been published.[21,22] These were 2 identical randomized, double-blind, placebo controlled, programs that evaluated the short term effects of tolvaptan when added to standard therapy (diuretics, ACE inhibitors, angiotensine receptor blockers [ARB] and β-blockers) as well as the long term (10-months) outcomes of post discharge mortality and hospitalization in more than 4,000 patients hospitalized for worsening heart failure. The addition of tolvaptan to standard therapy produced a significant and sustained reduction in body weight associated with a improvement in signs and symptoms of heart failure during hospitalization without significantly changing HR. BP or renal function. In addition, patients with hyponatremia (representing however only 8% of the overall population) achieved a significant improvement or normalization of their serum sodium concentration. There were no differences in post discharge outcomes (mortality and rehospitalization) between the Tolvaptan and the placebo groups.

Conclusion

It appears that acutely vasopressin antagonists decrease left ventricular filling pressure in patients with heart failure. They also have a potent "aquaretic" effect resulting in a significant decrease in body weight that is sustained during long-term therapy. The most common side effect was thirst and polyuria. The addition of oral Tolvaptan to standard therapy that included ACE inhibitors, ARB, B-blockers in patients admitted with heart failure and reduced ejection fraction resulted in significant improvement in signs and symptoms of heart failure without adversely affecting BP, HR, renal function and electrolytes. The sustained reduction in body weight and improvement/normalization of serum sodium in patients with hyponatremia in response to Tolvaptan that occurred after discharge was not associated with a decrease in mortality or rehospitalization.

References

1. Francis GS, Benedict C, Johnstone DE, et al. Comparison of neuroendocrine activation in patients with left ventricular dysfunction with and without congestive heart failure. A substudy of the Studies of Left Ventricular Dysfunction (SOLVD). Circulation. 1990;82:1724–29.
2. Michell RH, Kirk CJ, Billah MM. Hormonal stimulation of phosphatidylinositol breakdown with particular reference to the hepatic effects of vasopressin. Biochem Soc Trans. 1979;7:861–5.
3. Goldsmith SR, Francis GS, Cowley AW Jr, Levine TB, Cohn JN. Increased plasma arginine vasopressin levels in patients with congestive heart failure. J Am Coll Cardiol. 1983;1:1385–90.
4. Nakamura Y, Haneda T, Osaki J, Miyata S, Kikuchi K. Hypertrophic growth of cultured neonatal rat heart cells mediated by vasopressin V(1A) receptor. Eur J Pharmacol. 2000;391:39–48.
5. Rouleau JL, Packer M, Moye L, et al. Prognostic value of neurohumoral activation in patients with an acute myocardial infarction: effect of captopril. J Am Coll Cardiol. 1994;24:583–91.
6. Udelson JE, Smith WB, Hendrix GH, et al. Acute hemodynamic effects of conivaptan, a dual V(1A) and V(2) vasopressin receptor antagonist, in patients with advanced heart failure. Circulation. 2001;104:2417–23.
7. Udelson JE, Orlandi C, Ouyang J, et al. Acute hemodynamic effects of tolvaptan, a vasopressin V_2 receptor blocker, in patients with symptomatic heart failure and reduced LVEF: an international, multi-center, randomized, placebo-controlled trial. HFSA Annual Meeting, Washington, DC. J Card Fail. 2007.
8. Gheorghiade M, Niazi I, Ouyang J, et al. Vasopressin V2-receptor blockade with tolvaptan in patients with chronic heart failure: results from a double-blind, randomized trial. Circulation. 2003;107: 2690–6.
9. Dzau VJ, Colucci WS, Williams GH, Curfman G, Meggs L, Hollenberg NK. Sustained effectiveness of converting-enzyme inhibition in patients with severe congestive heart failure. N Engl J Med. 1980;302:1373–9.
10. Nitter-Hauge S, Brodwall EK, Rootwelt K. Renal function studies in hyponatremic cardiac patients with edema (dilution syndrome). Am Heart J. 1974;87:33–40.
11. Paller MS, Schrier RW. Pathogenesis of sodium and water retention in edematous disorders. Am J Kidney Dis. 1982;2:241–54.
12. Dzau VJ, Packer M, Lilly LS, Swartz SL, Hollenberg NK, Williams GH. Prostaglandins in severe congestive heart failure. Relation to activation of the renin–angiotensin system and hyponatremia. N Engl J Med. 1984;310:347–52.
13. Anderson RJ, Cadnapaphornchai P, Harbottle JA, McDonald KM, Schrier RW. Mechanism of effect of thoracic inferior vena cava constriction on renal water excretion. J Clin Invest. 1974;54:1473–9.
14. Schrier RW. Pathogenesis of sodium and water retention in high-output and low-output cardiac failure, nephrotic syndrome, cirrhosis, and pregnancy. N Engl J Med. 1988;319:1065–72.
15. Schrier RW, Humphreys MH, Ufferman RC. Role of cardiac output and the autonomic nervous system in the antinatriuretic response to acute constriction of the thoracic superior vena cava. Circ Res. 1971;29:490–8.

16. Ishikawa S, Saito T, Okada K, Tsutsui K, Kuzuya T. Effect of vasopressin antagonist on water excretion in inferior vena cava constriction. Kidney Int. 1986;30:49–55.
17. Riegger GA, Liebau G, Kochsiek K. Antidiuretic hormone in congestive heart failure. Am J Med. 1982;72:49–52.
18. Szatalowicz VL, Arnold PE, Chaimovitz C, Bichet D, Berl T, Schrier RW. Radioimmunoassay of plasma arginine vasopressin in hyponatremic patients with congestive heart failure. N Engl J Med. 1981;305:263–6.
19. Ikram H, Chan W, Espiner EA, Nicholls MG. Haemodynamic and hormone responses to acute and chronic frusemide therapy in congestive heart failure. Clin Sci (Lond). 1980;59:443–9.
20. Gheorghiade M, Gattis WA, O'Connor CM, et al. Effects of tolvaptan, a vasopressin antagonist, in patients hospitalized with worsening heart failure: a randomized controlled trial. JAMA. 2004;291:1963–71.
21. Konstam MA, Gheorghiade M, Burnett JC Jr, et al. Efficacy of Vasopressin Antagonism in Heart Failure Outcome Study With Tolvaptan (EVEREST) Investigators. Effects of oral Tolvaptan in patients hospitalized for worsening heart failure: the EVEREST Outcome Trial. JAMA. 2007;297:1319–31.
22. Gheorghiade M, Konstam MA, Burnett JC Jr, et al. Efficacy of Vasopressin Antagonism in Heart Failure Outcome Study With Tolvaptan (EVEREST) Investigators. Short-term clinical effects of tolvaptan, an oral vasopressin antagonist, in patients hospitalized for heart failure: the EVEREST Clinical Status Trials. JAMA. 2007;28;297:1332–43.

58
Endothelin Receptor Antagonists and Acute Heart Failure Syndromes

John R. Teerlink

As noted in the preceding chapters, the acute heart failure syndrome (AHFS) has been largely ignored until recently, despite its role as the primary hospital discharge diagnosis in 1million patients per year and accounting for over $14 billion in hospital costs in the United States alone.[1] The therapeutic approach to these patients has remained essentially unchanged for decades, despite, or perhaps due to, the relative absence of clinical trial evidence. Recent surveys have demonstrated that with current therapy, patients admitted for AHFS have a 45% chance of readmission[2] and a 20% to 40% risk of death in the following 6 months. Given these poor outcomes, the medical community is reevaluating the current therapeutic approach and searching for new therapies to treat patients with AHFS. One result of this reassessment of acute heart failure (AHF) has been the recognition of AHF as a vascular disorder and the need to develop therapies that can provide vascular protection. Endothelin receptor antagonists provide a potential novel approach to the treatment of AHF by addressing the underlying pathophysiologic abnormalities in this syndrome.

The Acute Heart Failure Syndrome as a Vascular Disorder

As described in earlier chapters, *acute heart failure* is a term of questionable value in describing the pathophysiology of the patients who present to hospitals afflicted with AHFS.

First, the development of the symptoms comprising the syndrome is not typically acute, but rather it usually results from a gradual increase in peripheral or pulmonary edema and the vascular responses to this fluid accumulation. In cases where there is an acute presentation, another type of vascular abnormality is often to blame, such as an acute coronary syndrome.

Second, the heart itself is often not the central organ in the pathophysiology of the syndrome. In approximately half of the patients, there is preserved left ventricular systolic function, and while an underlying abnormality of left ventricular diastolic or systolic dysfunction may instigate the syndrome, most of the symptoms, signs, and even therapies are directed to the vasculature. Pathologic vasoconstriction can be viewed as the central abnormality in acute heart failure (Fig. 58.1). Peripheral venoconstriction redistributes blood centrally, increasing pulmonary venous congestion and edema, resulting in the symptoms of dyspnea and fatigue. Peripheral arterial vasoconstriction results in increased afterload on the heart, elevation of left ventricular filling pressures, and increased postcapillary pulmonary venous pressures, resulting in worsening of pulmonary edema and dyspnea. This increased afterload results in elevation of ventricular wall stress and increased myocardial ischemia and cardiac arrhythmias. In addition, systemic vasoconstriction contributes to poor organ perfusion, such as the kidney, brain, and gut, contributing to renal failure and symptoms of fatigue, confusion, anorexia, and abdominal discomfort. Elevations in peripheral venous pressures and pathologic

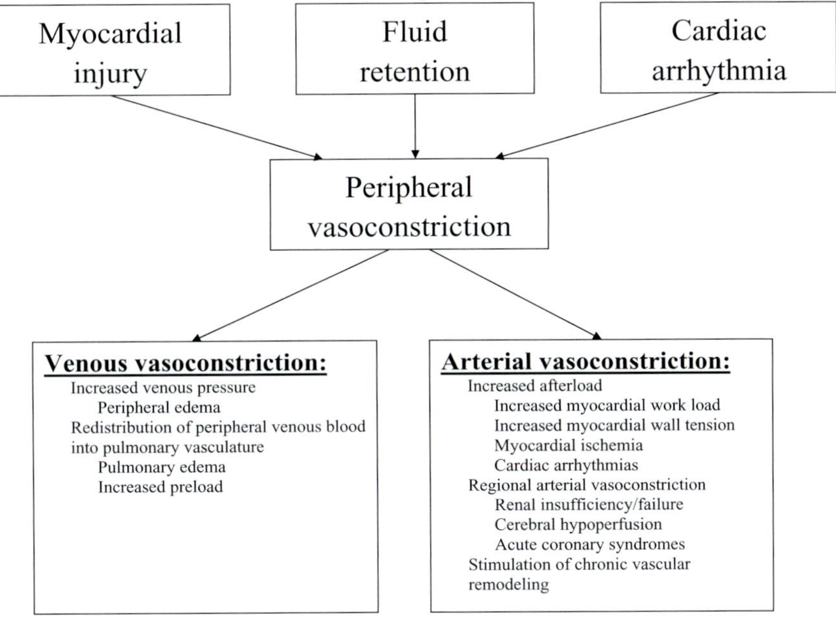

FIGURE 58.1. The central role of the vasculature in the pathogenesis of acute heart failure.

"leakiness" of the vessels result in the peripheral edema that often represents the most obvious sign of acute heart failure.

Third, therapies that are effective in the treatment of AHFS are often not directed at the heart, but rather influence the vasculature. Diuretics, such as furosemide, are the most commonly used therapies for these patients. The main effect of these agents is to reduce central venous pressures through diuresis and possibly via direct vasodilating properties,[3] not via any direct effect on the heart. The other commonly used agents, vasodilators, achieve symptom relief through their actions on the vasculature, rather than direct myocardial effects. Positive inotropes are used in a minority of acute heart failure patients, about 8% of the patients in the Acute Decompensated Heart Failure National Registry (ADHERE) registry,[4] but even the positive inotropes in common use, such as dobutamine and milrinone, have significant vasodilating effects. Thus, the main therapeutic target of the current therapies has been the vasculature via nonspecific vasodilation.

Viewing AHFS as a vascular syndrome has important implications for the clinical development of new therapies. For acute symptom resolution, the new therapy must be an effective vasodilator, relieving the elevated venous pressures that lead to congestion and dyspnea and reducing the abnormally high afterload that results in organ hypoperfusion and increased cardiac wall stress with the attendant increases in ischemia and arrhythmias. Yet, the new therapy must also target the underlying mediators of these vascular abnormalities to prevent acute and chronic damage. The neurohormonal hypothesis has been well established in chronic heart failure, where agents antagonizing the deleterious effects of neurohormones, such as angiotensin and adrenergic hormones, have improved clinical outcomes. Acute heart failure syndrome is accompanied by stimulation of these same neurohormones, as well as other toxic agents, such as endothelin. New therapies for acute heart failure need to improve clinical outcomes, and a vasodilator agent that can antagonize vascular and end-organ damage has the potential to have both short- and long-term benefits for patients. Almost 20 years of basic science and clinical research suggest that the endothelin receptor antagonists have this potential.

Theoretical and Scientific Basis for Endothelin Receptor Antagonism in Acute Heart Failure Syndrome

Endothelin-1 (ET-1)[5] is a 21-amino-acid peptide, homologous to the extraordinarily potent vascular toxins, known as sarafotoxins, isolated from the venom of *Atractaspis engadensis* or the Israeli burrowing asp. Although the brain and kidney also produce significant amounts of this peptide, ET-1 is synthesized predominantly by cardiovascular tissues in response to cardiovascular stressors, including vascular damage, other neurohormones (angiotensinII, epinephrine/norepinephrine), cytokines (interleukin-1 [IL-1], transforming growth factor-β [TGF-β]), and other stimuli (acidosis, thrombin, hypoxia. and shear stress). Endothelin-1 signals via two main types of receptors, known as ET_A and ET_B on the basis of their relative affinities for the endothelin isopeptides (Table 58.1). The ET receptors are members of the family of seven-transmembrane spanning G-protein–coupled receptors.

Endothelin is present in abnormally high concentrations in acute heart failure. Plasma ET-1 levels were first shown to be increased in patients with AHFS due to cardiogenic shock,[6] but subsequent studies have found increases in acute and chronic heart failure, pulmonary hypertension, systemic hypertension, and all forms of acute coronary syndromes, as well as many other conditions. Animal models demonstrated increased ET-1 in chronic heart failure,[7,8] and in patients with AHFS, elevated plasma endothelin levels have been shown to be very strong predictors of severe ventricular arrhythmias[9] and even long-term survival.[10] More importantly, there is substantial evidence demonstrating that these alterations have important effects on the vasculature, as well as the myocardium.

Table 58.1. Characteristics of endothelin (ET) receptors

	Relative affinities	Cardiovascular distribution	Selected effects of receptor stimulation
ET_A	ET-1 = ET-2 >> ET-3	Vascular smooth muscle cells Heart (myocytes > fibroblasts) Vascular fibroblasts	Vasoconstriction, hyperplasia "Pathologic" hypertrophy and fibrosis Fibrosis
ET_B	ET-1 = ET-2 = ET-3	Vascular endothelium Heart (fibroblast > myocytes) Vascular fibroblasts Vascular smooth muscle cell	Vasorelaxation, ET clearance Fibrosis, ? apoptosis, hypertrophy Fibrosis Vasoconstriction

The most apparent effect of endothelin is potent arterial and venous vasoconstriction,[11] mediated predominantly by the vascular smooth muscle cell ET_A receptors, as well as the vascular smooth muscle cell ET_B receptors.[12,13] The increased afterload caused by ET-1 is significant and at least additive to that caused by other neurohormones, such as angiotensin,[8,14] presenting a major specific target for afterload reduction therapy in the AHFS patient. However, ET-1 can induce marked regional vasoconstriction, which seems to be more specific for the renal, cerebral, and coronary vascular beds,[15] and plays an important role in end-organ damage.

Endothelin-1 exacerbates edema not only through changes in capillary hemodynamics, but also by promoting increased vascular permeability. Endothelin-1 increases capillary pressure and decreases precapillary/postcapillary resistance ratio resulting in net transcapillary fluid filtration with increased interstitial edema.[16,17] In addition to these hemodynamic effects, a part of this increased vascular permeability is thought to be due to local recruitment of inflammatory factors. In one study,[18] administration of endothelin to guinea pigs resulted in a two- to fourfold increase in pulmonary albumin extravasation, which appeared to be both ET_A and ET_B receptor-dependent. In addition, ET-1 has multiple other important vascular effects, including acting as a potent mitogen, an agent resulting in direct kidney injury,[19–21] which require only a brief exposure to produce sustained pathologic remodeling.[22] Thus, in the absence of antagonism, the transient marked elevations in ET-1 during acute heart failure could instigate deleterious long-term vascular remodeling.

Endothelin-1 has other deleterious effects that may be important in AHFS. Endothelin concentrations correlate with measures of ventricular remodeling in both the rat coronary artery ligation model of heat failure[23] and in patients.[24] It also stimulates the secretion of neurohormones known to be important in AHFS, such as norepinephrine, angiotensin II, vasopressin,[25] and aldosterone,[26] and conversely, vasopressin,[27] angiotensinII and norepinephrine also stimulate endothelin production. In addition, endothelin potentiates[28] and mediates[29] the effects of these neurohormones.

The effects of endothelin on myocardial contractility are complicated, since its primary hemodynamic effect is as a vasoconstrictor. In some studies of normal hearts, ET-1 acts as a mild positive inotrope, while in others there was no effect. In an elegant study in humans,[30] intracoronary infusion of the ET_A receptor antagonist BQ-123 increased contractility in heart failure patients while it decreased contractility in patients with normal ejection fraction. These studies suggest that ET-1 supports myocardial contractility in healthy subjects, but acts as a myocardial depressant in heart failure patients. The importance of these findings is unclear for patients with acute heart failure, but it suggests that endothelin receptor antagonism would have minimal effect on patients with preserved left ventricular (LV) function and, if anything, would improve contractility in patients with decreased function.

Endothelin-1 has proarrhythmic effects[31] on both ventricular[32] and atrial[33] tissue. Arrhythmias are a frequent and important complication of AHFS, and in a recent study of 83 patients hospitalized for AHF, there was a very significant positive relationship between plasma endothelin concentrations and multiple measures of ventricular ectopy, including the total of premature ventricular complexes, the frequency of ventricular pairs, and the number of ventricular tachycardia episodes.[9]

Endothelin-1 is also known to have profound adverse effects on renal function. In healthy human subjects, ET-1 infusion resulted in decreased renal blood flow, glomerular filtration rate, and urinary sodium excretion, and marked increases in sodium retention and renal vasoconstriction.[34,35] A significant interaction between renal failure and heart failure is increasingly apparent,[36] and renal function is one of the most important prognostic variables in patients with heart failure.[37]

Endothelin Antagonism in Preclinical Studies

A number of endothelin receptor antagonists (ERAs) have been developed and are broadly categorized as ET_A selective and dual (ET_A and ET_B) receptor antagonists. The ERAs reduce systemic[8] and pulmonary[38] vasoconstriction, as well as decrease left ventricular filling pressures[39] in rats with heart failure. Administration of ERA has also been shown to decrease vascular permeability[16,40] and pulmonary edema,[39] as well as inflammation and release of adhesion molecules.[41,42] The ERAs have also been shown to be protective against vascular-induced end-organ damage, such as progressive renal dysfunction[43] and cerebral injury[44,45] in animal models. The ERAs have had beneficial effects on renal function in a variety of models of intrinsic renal disease and in experimental models of heart failure,[46–49] as well as in healthy human volunteers.[50] Thus, there is ample preclinical evidence that ERA can provide vascular protection in multiple pathophysiologic disorders.

Most preclinical studies of ERA in heart failure have used chronic models. In these chronic heart failure models, a number of ET_A-selective antagonists have been shown to be effective in reducing myocardial infarct size,[51–53] ventricular remodeling,[54–56] as well as survival.[53] However, other studies have shown some adverse effects or no benefit from these agents.[57–59] The dual ET_A/ET_B receptor antagonists have also been shown to be effective in chronic heart failure animal models. Bosentan[60] is an oral nonpeptide, dual ERA, currently approved for the treatment of pulmonary arterial hypertension. Administration of bosentan to rats with congestive heart failure (CHF) resulted in significant reductions in blood pressure, which were at least additive, and possibly potentiating, to that caused by administration of maximal doses of the angiotensin-converting enzyme (ACE) inhibitor cilazapril.[8] Chronic administration of bosentan has also been shown to reduce adverse ventricular remodeling[61–65] and to increase survival[61] in animal models of chronic heart failure.

Tezosentan is structurally related to bosentan and is also a dual (ET_A/ET_B) ERA, designed specifically for intravenous use in hospitalized patients.[66] Acute administration of tezosentan to rats with heart failure effectively reduced systemic and left ventricular filling pressures with no effect on contractility, and these effects were additive to acute enalapril treatment.[67] In addition, acute tezosentan administration decreased renal vascular resistance and increased renal plasma flow, glomerular filtration rate, urine flow rate, and sodium excretion in rats with heart failure.[48] In rats with acute myocardial infarction,[39] two doses of tezosentan at 1 and 24 hours after coronary artery ligation resulted in attenuation of the increase in left ventricular end-diastolic pressure (LVEDP) and in marked decrease in pulmonary edema at 48 hours after ligation. Consistent with the hypothesis that short-term therapy for acute heart failure can provide long-term benefit, rats receiving these two doses of tezosentan during the first 24-hours had significantly reduced LV hypertrophy and improved survival 5 months later. These preclinical studies provided strong support for using the vascular protective therapies of endothelin receptor antagonists in patients with AHFS.

Clinical Studies of Acute Effects of Endothelin Antagonism in Chronic Heart Failure

The recognition of endothelin as an important target in the pathogenesis of AHFS and the beneficial effects of endothelin antagonists in experimental models encouraged the rapid clinical investigation of these agents, initially in patients with more stable, chronic heart failure. As noted above, endothelin antagonists have been shown to reduce vasoconstriction, and in general, systemically administered agents have decreased peripheral and pulmonary vascular resistance, pulmonary arterial pressures, and pulmonary capillary wedge pressure, while increasing cardiac output in patients with CHF. However, there are relatively few published studies with these agents and some differences among endothelin antagonists have emerged (for a summary of these results, see Tables 58.2 and 58.3).[68]

Bosentan was the first endothelin receptor antagonist to be tested in heart failure patients. In a study[69] of 24 patients with stable symptomatic chronic heart failure, left ventricular ejection fraction (LVEF) ≤30%, pulmonary capillary wedge pressure (PCWP) ≥15 mm Hg and a cardiac index ≤2.5L/min/m^2, bosentan infusion resulted in significant reductions in systemic, pulmonary right- and left-sided filling pressures, as well as systemic (SVR) and pulmonary (PVR) vascular resistances (Table 58.2). Cardiac index increased significantly with no change in heart rate (HR). Plasma endothelin concentrations increased with bosentan infusion, presumably due to receptor displacement or decreased clearance by the ET_B receptors. Another study[70] administered oral bosentan 1 g b.i.d. (24 patients) or placebo (12 patients) to

Table 58.2. Acute hemodynamic effects of dual (ET_A/ET_B) endothelin receptor antagonists in heart failure patients from selected studies

	Study				
% Change from baseline	Bosentan (i.v.)[69,a]	Bosentan (p.o)[70,b]	Tezosentan (i.v.)[73,c]	Tezosentan (i.v.)[74,d]	Tezosentan (i.v.)[75,e]
HR	0	−1	+3	+2	+1
MAP	−8†	−14†	−7	−10*	N/A
RAP	−18†	−20*	−11	N/A	−15†
MPAP	−14†	−13*	−10	−18*	N/A
PCWP	−9*	−14*	−10	−13*	−17†
CI	+14*	+15†	+27†	+50v	+19*
SVR	−16†	−24†	−25†	−34†	N/A
PVR	−33*	−20*	−39†	51†	N/A

HR, heart rate; MAP, mean arterial pressure; RAP, right atrial pressure' MPAP, mean pulmonary arterial pressure; PCWP, pulmonary capillary wedge pressure; CI, cardiac index; SVR, systemic vascular resistance; PVR, pulmonary vascular resistance.

*$p < .05$ versus baseline within study; †$p < .01$ versus baseline within study, otherwise p = not significant; N/A, data not available; NS, no statistically significant difference compared to placebo; [a]100-mg dose, then 200 mg 60 minutes later, 2-hour measurement; [b]1-g dose, 3-hour measurement; [c]5–100 mg/h ascending dose, 4-hour measurement, placebo-corrected; [d]5–100 mg/h parallel dose, 100 mg/h dose, 6-hour measurement, placebo-corrected; [e]20 and 50 mg/h groups combined, 48-hour hemodynamic measurement by Doppler echocardiography.

Source: Modified from Seed et al.[68]

Table 58.3. Acute hemodynamic effects of ETA-selective endothelin receptor antagonists in heart failure patients from selected studies

% Change from baseline	Study					
	BQ-123[76,a]	Darusentan (LU135252)[77,b]	Darusentan (LU135252)[78,c]	Sitaxsentan (TBC11251)[79,d]	BMS 193884[81,e]	ABT-627[82,f]
HR	+1	0	NS	−1	N/A	N/A
MAP	−8†	−10†	NS	−7	N/A	N/A
RAP	−14	−19†	NS	−15*	N/A	N/A
MPAP	−14†	−20†	NS	−12*	N/A	N/A
PCWP	−18	−25†	NS	−7	−33*	−33*
CI	+5*	+22†	+13%	+11	+28*	+28*
SVR	−12†	−27†	NS	−3	−26*	−26*
PVR	−14	−26†	NS	−20*	N/A	N/A

*$p < .05$ versus baseline within study; †$p < .01$ versus baseline within study, otherwise p = not significant; N/A, data not available; NS, no statistically significant difference compared to placebo; [a]100/200-nmol/min dose, 60-minute measurement; [b]300-mg dose, 2-hour measurement; [c]300-mg dose, 2-hour measurement; [d]6-mg/kg dose, 2-hour measurement; [e]100-mg dose, 4-hour measurement; [f]7–30 mg dose, time of measurement not given.

Source: Modified from Seed et al.[68]

heart failure patients with similar hemodynamic effects as noted above, with no change in heart rate (Table 58.2). The beneficial effects not only on both systemic and pulmonary vascular beds, but also on left ventricular filling pressures and cardiac output confirmed the promise of these agents for acute heart failure.

As noted above, tezosentan is also a dual ERA, designed as an intravenous formulation for acute use.[66] Initial pharmacokinetic and pharmacodynamic studies in healthy patients suggested that doses from 5 to 100 mg/h would be appropriate for further study[71] and that there were no clinically relevant adverse effects or need for dose adjustments with this tezosentan dose range in patients with markedly reduced renal function.[72] In 38 patients with chronic stable heart failure (Table 58.2),[73] reduced ejection fraction and cardiac index, and mildly elevated PCWP, tezosentan was administered in an ascending dose protocol (5, 20, 50, and 100 mg over 1 hour each) and invasive hemodynamic measurements demonstrated significant increases in cardiac index, and decreases in pulmonary and systemic vascular resistances. Dose-dependent increases in plasma endothelin and epinephrine were noted, without evidence of rebound or significant adverse events.

In another study of 61 patients with New York Heart Association (NYHA) class III or IV heart failure, LVEF <35%, PCWP >18 mm Hg, and cardiac index <2.5 L/min/m^2, the hemodynamic effects of 6-hour infusions of tezosentan in a placebo-controlled, parallel group design with doses of 5, 20, 50, and 100 mg/h were evaluated (Table 58.2).[74] Tezosentan caused up to a 50% dose-dependent increase in cardiac index, as well as significant decreases in PCWP. However, although only mildly elevated with the 5 mg/h dose, plasma endothelin levels were quite markedly increased in the 50 to 100 mg/h groups. There were no significant adverse events. Another study of 14 patients[75] assessed the safety of a 48-hour infusion of 20 and 50 mg/h tezosentan compared to dobutamine (Table 58.2), demonstrating no episodes of hypotension requiring discontinuation, although headache was quite common. There was no evidence of tachyphylaxis during, or rebound after, the infusion. Despite the significant increases in cardiac index and decreases in left-sided filling pressures, as well as systemic and pulmonary vascular resistances, there were no significant increases in heart rate in any of these trials. While these studies demonstrated that tezosentan effectively improved hemodynamics, larger studies would be performed to evaluate clinical efficacy.

The endothelin antagonists that are selective for the ET_A receptor were the first to be developed, and BQ-123 was the prototypical agent of this class. In 10 patients with stable CHF,[76] BQ-123 infusion resulted in significant decreases in mean arterial pressure (MAP), pulmonary arterial pressure (PAP), and SVR, with increased cardiac index. There was a trend toward decreased PVR, as well, and no comment is made in the publication of effects on right atrial or ventricular filling pressures (Table 58.3). Although this study was uncontrolled, the marked hemodynamic effects of BQ-123 were supportive of a beneficial response in these patients.

Darusentan (LU135252) is an orally available highly selective ET_A receptor antagonist that has been investigated in a number of studies (Table 58.3). In one study,[77] 95 NYHA class II to III heart failure patients with an LVEF ≤35% and PCWP ≥14 mm Hg or cardiac index ≤2.8 L/min/m^2 were randomized to one of five oral doses of darusentan (1, 10, 30, 100, or 300 mg). The 30- to 300-mg doses of darusentan produced significant reductions in all pertinent hemodynamic measures and increased cardiac index with minimal adverse effects. Plasma endothelin concentrations also increased in a dose-dependent fashion, supporting a mechanism of receptor displacement. In the Heart Failure ET_A Blockade Trial,[78] 157 NYHA class III patients with LVEF ≤35%, PCWP ≥12 mm Hg and cardiac index ≤2.6 L/min/m^2 were randomized to either placebo or one of three doses of darusentan (30, 100, or 300 mg p.o. once daily). These patients all took their regular medications on the morning of the study, and although definite trends were evident, there were no significant changes in any of the hemodynamics measured at 4 hours after oral administration of darusentan.

Sitaxsentan (TBC 11251) is also a nonpeptide, highly selective ET_A receptor antagonist that appeared to have preferential effects on the pulmonary vasculature in preclinical studies. In a multicenter, double-blind, placebo-controlled study of 48 NYHA class III to IV heart failure patients with LVEF ≤35%, PCWP ≥15 mm Hg, and cardiac index ≤2.5 L/min/m^2, three doses of a 15-minute sitaxsentan infusion (1.5, 3.0, and 6.0 mg/kg) were compared to placebo.[79] The infusion of sitaxsentan resulted in significant decreases in right atrial pressure (RAP) and mean PAP, as well as in PVR, but no significant effects on HR, MAP, PCWP, SVR, or cardiac index (Table 58.3). A smaller study confirmed the acute pulmonary vasodilating effects of sitaxsentan in eight heart failure patients, while there was no effect in four controls with normal LV systolic function.[80] Two other ET_A-selective antagonists (BMS-193884[81] and ABT-627[82]) have been used in studies reported only as abstracts to date (Table 58.3).

These studies and others on endothelin antagonists in patients with stable chronic heart failure have demonstrated favorable acute hemodynamic effects. However, few of these studies were placebo-controlled and few investigated the full-dose response of these agents or the time course of their effects. In addition, most drug development programs proceeded under the assumption that beneficial hemodynamic effects would translate into clinical benefit, an assumption that has proven wrong with other drug classes (e.g., phosphodiesterase inhibitors). Nonetheless, the findings from these acute studies encouraged some development programs to proceed to phase III clinical trials.

Clinical Trials of Endothelin Antagonists in Acute Heart Failure Syndromes

As noted above, the hemodynamic effects of tezosentan have been investigated in a number of trials, enrolling over 100 patients with advanced chronic heart failure using doses ranging from 5 to 100 mg/h as infusions for up to 48 hours.[73–75,83] These studies confirmed the predicted beneficial hemodynamic effects of tezosentan, which acutely reduced pulmonary artery pressures, left ventricular filling pressures and afterload, while increasing cardiac index with no change in heart rate. These studies were the basis for the design of the Randomized Intravenous TeZosentan (RITZ) trials.[84] This program was designed with two pivotal trials: RITZ-1, assessing symptom improvement without confounding from invasive hemodynamic monitoring, and RITZ-2, investigating the effect of tezosentan on invasive hemodynamics. Two other trials evaluated the safety of tezosentan in two specific high-risk groups: acute heart failure in patients with acute coronary syndromes (RITZ-4) and acute heart failure associated with fulminant pulmonary edema (RITZ-5).

The RITZ-2 trial[85] randomized 184 patients hospitalized for decompensated heart failure (NYHA class III/IV, cardiac index <2.5 L/min/m^2, PCWP>15 mm Hg) to 24-hour infusions of placebo or tezosentan (increased from 25 mg/h to either 50 mg/h or 100 mg/h). Both doses of tezosentan decreased PCWP by about 4 mm Hg (placebo-corrected; p <.0001) and increased cardiac index by about 0.4 L/min/m^2 (placebo-corrected; p <.0001), and there was a significant improvement in patient's dyspnea at 24 hours (p = .048). There was also a strong trend toward improving the time to worsening of heart failure or death at 30 days in the tezosentan-treated patients (p = .06). The most frequent side effects were related to vasodilation and included hypotension and headache, all of which were much more frequent in the high-dose group. Interestingly, most of the hemodynamic benefit in this trial was achieved by the initial 25-mg/h dose within the first hour of treatment, suggesting that lower doses could have fewer side effects and potentially equivalent hemodynamic effects.

The RITZ-1 trial randomized 669 patients with acute decompensated heart failure to at least 24 hours of tezosentan (50 mg/h IV) or placebo on top of standard therapy.[86,87] Due to concerns in previous trials with the potential confounding effects of invasive hemodynamic monitoring on symptom assessment, patients with pulmonary artery (PA) catheter monitoring were excluded. The primary end point, the change in dyspnea from baseline at 24 hours, was not statistically different between the two treatment groups, nor was there any difference in the main secondary end point of time to worsening of heart failure or death. However, adverse events related to excessive vasodilation, such as hypotension, nausea, headache, dizziness, and renal impairment were significantly more frequent in tezosentan-treated patients. These results were surprising in view of the findings from RITZ-2, and are probably explained by the RITZ-1 patient population being less acutely ill than the RITZ-2 groups (therefore less likely to show benefit), the absence of invasive monitoring, and the dose of tezosentan still being too high.

The RITZ-4 study investigated the effects of tezosentan in patients with acute decompensated heart failure and acute coronary syndrome,[88] randomizing 193 patients to placebo or tezosentan (50 mg/h). The composite primary end point (death, worsening of heart failure, recurrent ischemia, and recurrent or new myocardial infarction within 72 hours) was not significantly different between the two groups, an anticipated result given the marginal power of this safety study. Although symptomatic hypotension was greater in the tezosentan-treated patients, there was no evidence for proischemic effects. Other adverse events related to vasodilation, such as headache, dizziness, nausea, and renal failure/impairment, were more common in the tezosentan-treated patients. This study reassured the investigators that tezosentan was relatively safe in patients with acute coronary syndromes, and reinforced the impression from the other trials that the dose used in these trials was probably too high.

RITZ-5[89] studied the effect of tezosentan on changes in oxygen saturation in patients with acute heart failure and fulminant pulmonary edema. This study randomized 84 patients to either placebo or tezosentan, and tezosentan could be up-titrated from 50 to 100 mg/h at the investigator's discretion. The primary end point was the change from baseline to 60 minutes after study drug administration in oxygen saturation as measured by pulse oximetry. There was no difference between the placebo and tezosentan groups with regard to the primary end point, but in a post-hoc analysis, patients receiving tezosentan 50 mg/h had better outcomes, as assessed by time to death, cardiac failure, pulmonary edema, or cardiogenic shock, than those on placebo. Patients in the tezosentan 100 mg/h group had a high incidence of hypotension episodes and worse outcomes. Once again, RITZ-5 suggested that the tezosentan dose was too high, yet despite significant hypotension, there was no evidence of proischemic or proarrhythmic effects.

The evidence from the RITZ studies revealed a number of important lessons for clinical development programs for new acute heart failure therapies. First, tezosentan clearly produces favorable hemodynamic effects in patients with AHF. Second, demonstrating improved clinical outcomes can be very difficult in this patient population. Third, despite significant hypotension and related adverse effects, tezosentan was relatively safe and well tolerated. Fourth, the dose of tezosentan used in the RITZ program did not have a favorable risk/benefit profile, given the excess symptomatic hypotension and related renal failure observed in the studies. To address this issue, a recent dose-ranging study demonstrated that tezosentan doses of 1 to 5 mg/h (compared to 50 and 100 mg/h in the RITZ studies) improved cardiac index and pulmonary capillary wedge pressure with no hypotension or renal insufficiency/failure in patients with acute heart failure.[90] This low-dose, dose-ranging study strongly suggested that a lower dose of tezosentan would have a better risk/benefit profile.

The potential for providing improvement in clinical outcomes by administering a vascular protective agent such as tezosentan has led to a large, international, multicenter, randomized, placebo-controlled investigation of low-dose tezosentan (Value of Endothelin Receptor Inhibition with Tezosentan in Acute Heart Failure Study [VERITAS]).[91] The goal of VERITAS was to demonstrate the efficacy and safety of endothelin receptor antagonism in acute decompensated heart failure. The VERITAS program consisted of two identical, double-blind, randomized, placebo-controlled trials. The two trials (VERITAS-1 and VERITAS-2) were designed to enroll approximately 1760 patients total within 24 hours of admission to a hospital with dyspnea at rest due to heart failure and a respiratory rate of over 24 breaths per minute in need of intravenous therapy. In addition, the patient also had to have objective signs of pulmonary congestion or heart failure. Patients were randomized to 24 to 72 hours of tezosentan (5 mg/h IV for 30 minutes followed by 1 mg/h) or placebo and stratified based on the presence or absence of a pulmonary artery catheter. After a planned interim analysis, the VERITAS Data and Safety Monitoring Board (DSMB) recommended discontinuation of the trial, due to futility of reaching either of the primary end points, and the steering committee elected to terminate VERITAS in November 2004, with 1435 patients enrolled.[92] The primary end points were (1) incidence of death or worsening heart failure at 7 days in the combined trials and (2) area under the curve of the change from baseline in dyspnea assessment (measured using a visual analogue scale) from baseline over the first 24 hours of treatment in each trial. There were no significant differences in any of the secondary end points including time-to-event analysis for death or worsening HF, hospitalizations, and mortality, as well as other safety end points. Interestingly, in the small number of patients with invasive pulmonary artery catheter hemodynamic monitoring ($n = 83$), significant improvements in hemodynamics were once again noted. Although it was designed as a definitive study, VERITAS raised many questions about the future role of endothelin receptor antagonists in patients with AHFS. The apparent disconnect between improving hemodynamics and the failure to benefit symptoms will require further analysis.

Conclusion

Endothelin is one of the most potent vasoconstrictors known and clearly plays an important role in the pathogenesis of acute heart failure syndromes. Preclinical studies supported the potential of endothelin receptor antagonists for favorably improving clinical outcomes in patients with AHFS, by demonstrating the ability of these agents to acutely improve hemodynamics, pulmonary edema, and renal function in animal models of acute heart failure. In the early clinical studies, endothelin receptor antagonists consistently improved hemodynamics, reducing preload and afterload without increasing heart rate, while usually increasing cardiac output. However, larger clinical trials confirmed these beneficial hemodynamic effects, but were unable to demonstrate any improvement in symptoms (e.g., dyspnea[93]) or other clinical outcomes. The failure of these clinical trials in AHFS patients, as well as the negative trials in patients with chronic heart failure, have raised serious challenges for future development programs of endothelin receptor antagonists in these areas. Although their original promise has yet to be actualized, further research is necessary to better understand the potential role of these agents in the treatment of patients with AHFS.

References

1. American Heart Association. Heart Disease and Stroke Statistics—2004 Update. Dallas, TX: American Heart Association; 2003.

2. Krumholz HM, Parent EM, Tu N, et al. Readmission after hospitalization for congestive heart failure among Medicare beneficiaries. Arch Intern Med. 1997;157(1):99–104.
3. Dikshit K, Vyden JK, Forrester JS, Chatterjee K, Prakash R, Swan HJ. Renal and extrarenal hemodynamic effects of furosemide in congestive heart failure after acute myocardial infarction. N Engl J Med. 1973;288(21):1087–90.
4. The ADHERE® Registry. Second Quarter 2003 National Benchmark Report. http://www.adheregistry.com/national_BMR/Q2_03_National_ADHERE_BMR.pdf. Scios, Inc. Available at: http://www.adhereregistry.com/national_BMR/Q2_03_National_ADHERE_BMR.pdf.
5. Yanagisawa M, Kurihara H, Kimura S, et al. A novel potent vasoconstrictor peptide produced by vascular endothelial cells. Nature. 1988;332(6163):411–5.
6. Cernacek P, Stewart DJ. Immunoreactive endothelin in human plasma: marked elevations in patients in cardiogenic shock. Biochem Biophys Res Commun. 1989;161(2):562–7.
7. Margulies KB, Hildebrand FL Jr, Lerman A, Perrella MA, Burnett JC Jr. Increased endothelin in experimental heart failure. Circulation. 1990;82(6):2226–30.
8. Teerlink JR, Löffler BM, Hess P, Maire JP, Clozel M, Clozel JP. Role of endothelin in the maintenance of blood pressure in conscious rats with chronic heart failure. Acute effects of the endothelin receptor antagonist Ro 47-0203 (bosentan). Circulation. 1994;90(5):2510–8.
9. Aronson D, Burger AJ. Neurohumoral activation and ventricular arrhythmias in patients with decompensated congestive heart failure: role of endothelin. Pacing Clin Electrophysiol. 2003;26(3):703–10.
10. Aronson D, Burger AJ. Neurohormonal prediction of mortality following admission for decompensated heart failure. Am J Cardiol. 2003;91(2):245–8.
11. McNeill JR. Role of endothelin in regulation of resistance, fluid-exchange, and capacitance functions of the systemic circulation. Can J Physiol Pharmacol. 2003;81(6):522–32.
12. Gray GA, Löffler BM, Clozel M. Characterization of endothelin receptors mediating contraction of rabbit saphenous vein. Am J Physiol. 1994;266(3 pt 2):H959–H66.
13. Teerlink JR, Breu V, Sprecher U, Clozel M, Clozel JP. Potent vasoconstriction mediated by endothelin ETB receptors in canine coronary arteries. Circ Res. 1994;74(1):105–14.
14. Dohi Y, Hahn AW, Boulanger CM, Buhler FR, Luscher TF. Endothelin stimulated by angiotensin II augments contractility of spontaneously hypertensive rat resistance arteries. Hypertension. 1992;19(2):131–7.
15. Clozel M, Clozel JP. Effects of endothelin on regional blood flows in squirrel monkeys. J Pharmacol Exp Ther. 1989;250(3):1125–31.
16. Ekelund U, Albert U, Edvinsson L, Mellander S. In-vivo effects of endothelin-1 and ETA receptor blockade on arterial, venous and capillary functions in skeletal muscle. Acta Physiol Scand. 1993;148(3):273–83.
17. Ekelund U, Adner M, Edvinsson L, Mellander S. Effects of selective ETB-receptor stimulation on arterial, venous and capillary functions in cat skeletal muscle. Br J Pharmacol. 1994;112(3):887–94.
18. Filep JG, Fournier A, Foldes-Filep E. Acute proinflammatory actions of endothelin-1 in the guinea-pig lung: involvement of ETA and ETB receptors. Br J Pharmacol. 1995;115(2):227–36.
19. Hocher B, Thone-Reineke C, Rohmeiss P, et al. Endothelin-1 transgenic mice develop glomerulosclerosis, interstitial fibrosis, and renal cysts but not hypertension. J Clin Invest. 1997;99(6):1380–9.
20. Moreau P, Dao HH. Endothelin receptor antagonists: novel agents for the treatment of hypertension? Expert Opin Invest Drugs. 1999;8(11):1807–21.
21. Schiffrin EL. Role of endothelin-1 in hypertension and vascular disease. Am J Hypertens. 2001;14(6 pt 2):83S-9S.
22. Dao HH, Martens FM, Lariviere R, Yamaguchi N, Cernacek P, de Champlain J, Moreau P. Transient involvement of endothelin in hypertrophic remodeling of small arteries. J Hypertens. 2001;19(10):1801–12.
23. Loennechen JP, St<o/>ylen A, Beisvag V, Wisl<o/>ff U, Ellingsen O. Regional expression of endothelin-1, ANP, IGF-1, and LV wall stress in the infarcted rat heart. Am J Physiol Heart Circ Physiol. 2001;280(6):H2902–H10.
24. Tsutamoto T, Wada A, Maeda K, et al. Transcardiac extraction of circulating endothelin-1 across the failing heart. Am J Cardiol. 2000;86(5):524–8.
25. Yamamoto T, Kimura T, Ota K, et al. Central effects of endothelin-1 on vasopressin release, blood pressure, and renal solute excretion. Am J Physiol. 1992;262(6 pt 1):E856–E62.
26. Belloni AS, Rossi GP, Andreis PG, et al. Endothelin adrenocortical secretagogue effect is mediated by the B receptor in rats. Hypertension. 1996;27(5):1153–9.
27. Imai T, Hirata Y, Emori T, Yanagisawa M, Masaki T, Marumo F. Induction of endothelin-1 gene by angiotensin and vasopressin in endothelial cells. Hypertension. 1992;19(6 pt 2):753–7.

28. Yoshida K, Yasujima M, Kohzuki M, Kanazawa M, Yoshinaga K, Abe K. Endothelin-1 augments pressor response to angiotensin II infusion in rats. Hypertension. 1992;20(3):292–7.
29. Kaddoura S, Firth JD, Boheler KR, Sugden PH, Poole-Wilson PA. Endothelin-1 is involved in norepinephrine-induced ventricular hypertrophy in vivo. Acute effects of bosentan, an orally active, mixed endothelin ETA and ETB receptor antagonist. Circulation. 1996;93(11):2068–79.
30. MacCarthy PA, Grocott-Mason R, Prendergast BD, Shah AM. Contrasting inotropic effects of endogenous endothelin in the normal and failing human heart: studies with an intracoronary ET(A) receptor antagonist. Circulation. 2000;101(2):142–7.
31. Duru F, Barton M, Lüscher TF, Candinas R. Endothelin and cardiac arrhythmias: do endothelin antagonists have a therapeutic potential as antiarrhythmic drugs? Cardiovasc Res. 2001; 49(2):272–80.
32. Yorikane R, Shiga H, Miyake S, Koike H. Evidence for direct arrhythmogenic action of endothelin. Biochem Biophys Res Commun. 1990;173(1): 457–62.
33. Burrell KM, Molenaar P, Dawson PJ, Kaumann AJ. Contractile and arrhythmic effects of endothelin receptor agonists in human heart in vitro: blockade with SB 209670. J Pharmacol Exp Ther. 2000;292(1): 449–59.
34. Rabelink TJ, Kaasjager KA, Boer P, Stroes EG, Braam B, Koomans HA. Effects of endothelin-1 on renal function in humans: implications for physiology and pathophysiology. Kidney Int. 1994; 46(2):376–81.
35. Sorensen SS, Madsen JK, Pedersen EB. Systemic and renal effect of intravenous infusion of endothelin-1 in healthy human volunteers. Am J Physiol. 1994;266(3 Pt 2):F411–F8.
36. Silverberg D, Wexler D, Blum M, Schwartz D, Iaina A. The association between congestive heart failure and chronic renal disease. Curr Opin Nephrol Hypertens. 2004;13(2):163–70.
37. Dries DL, Exner DV, Domanski MJ, Greenberg B, Stevenson LW. The prognostic implications of renal insufficiency in asymptomatic and symptomatic patients with left ventricular systolic dysfunction. J Am Coll Cardiol. 2000;35(3):681–9.
38. Hess P, Clozel M, Clozel JP. Telemetry monitoring of pulmonary arterial pressure in freely moving rats. J Appl Physiol. 1996;81(2):1027–32.
39. Clozel M, Qiu C, Qiu CS, Hess P, Clozel JP. Short-term endothelin receptor blockade with tezosentan has both immediate and long-term beneficial effects in rats with myocardial infarction. J Am Coll Cardiol. 2002;39(1):142–7.
40. Filep JG. Endogenous endothelin modulates blood pressure, plasma volume, and albumin escape after systemic nitric oxide blockade. Hypertension. 1997;30(1 Pt 1):22–8.
41. Finsnes F, Skjonsberg OH, Tonnessen T, Naess O, Lyberg T, Christensen G. Endothelin production and effects of endothelin antagonism during experimental airway inflammation. Am J Respir Crit Care Med. 1997;155(4):1404–12.
42. Verma S, Li SH, Badiwala MV, Weisel RD, Fedak PW, Li RK, Dhillon B, Mickle DA. Endothelin antagonism and interleukin-6 inhibition attenuate the proatherogenic effects of C-reactive protein. Circulation. 2002;105(16):1890–6.
43. Lariviere R, Lebel M. Endothelin-1 in chronic renal failure and hypertension. Can J Physiol Pharmacol. 2003;81(6):607–21.
44. Hino A, Weir BK, Macdonald RL, Thisted RA, Kim CJ, Johns LM. Prospective, randomized, double-blind trial of BQ-123 and bosentan for prevention of vasospasm following subarachnoid hemorrhage in monkeys. J Neurosurg. 1995;83(3):503–9.
45. Kwan AL, Lin CL, Chang CZ, et al. Oral administration of an inhibitor of endothelin-converting enzyme attenuates cerebral vasospasm following experimental subarachnoid haemorrhage in rabbits. Clin Sci (Lond). 2002;103:414S-7S.
46. Ohnishi M, Wada A, Tsutamoto T, et al. Chronic effects of a novel, orally active endothelin receptor antagonist, T-0201, in dogs with congestive heart failure. J Cardiovasc Pharmacol. 1998;31(2): S236–S8.
47. Bauersachs J, Braun C, Fraccarollo D, et al. Improvement of renal dysfunction in rats with chronic heart failure after myocardial infarction by treatment with the endothelin A receptor antagonist, LU 135252. J Hypertens. 2000;18(10):1507–14.
48. Qiu C, Ding SS, Hess P, Clozel JP, Clozel M. Endothelin mediates the altered renal hemodynamics associated with experimental congestive heart failure. J Cardiovasc Pharmacol. 2001;38(2):317–24.
49. Ding SS, Qiu C, Hess P, Xi JF, Clozel JP, Clozel M. Chronic endothelin receptor blockade prevents renal vasoconstriction and sodium retention in rats with chronic heart failure. Cardiovasc Res. 2002;53(4):963–70.
50. Fleisch M, Sutsch G, Yan XW, et al. Systemic, pulmonary, and renal hemodynamic effects of endothelin ET(A/B)-receptor blockade in patients with maintained left ventricular function. J Cardiovasc Pharmacol. 2000;36(3):302–9.
51. Grover GJ, Dzwonczyk S, Parham CS. The endothelin-1 receptor antagonist BQ-123 reduces infarct size in a canine model of coronary occlusion and reperfusion. Cardiovasc Res. 1993;27(9):1613–18.

52. Burke SE, Nelson RA. Endothelin-receptor antagonist FR 139317 reduces infarct size in a rabbit model when given before, but not after, coronary artery occlusion. J Cardiovasc Pharmacol. 1997;29(1):87–92.
53. Sakai S, Miyauchi T, Kobayashi M, Yamaguchi I, Goto K, Sugishita Y. Inhibition of myocardial endothelin pathway improves long-term survival in heart failure. Nature. 1996;384(6607):353–5.
54. Mulder P, Richard V, Bouchart F, Derumeaux G, Münter K, Thuillez C. Selective ETA receptor blockade prevents left ventricular remodeling and deterioration of cardiac function in experimental heart failure. Cardiovasc Res. 1998;39(3):600–8.
55. Podesser BK, Siwik DA, Eberli FR, et al. ET(A)-receptor blockade prevents matrix metalloproteinase activation late postmyocardial infarction in the rat. Am J Physiol Heart Circ Physiol. 2001;280(3): H984–H91.
56. Spinale FG, Walker JD, Mukherjee R, Iannini JP, Keever AT, Gallagher KP. Concomitant endothelin receptor subtype-A blockade during the progression of pacing-induced congestive heart failure in rabbits. Beneficial effects on left ventricular and myocyte function. Circulation. 1997;95(7): 1918–29.
57. Nguyen QT, Cernacek P, Calderoni A, et al. Endothelin A receptor blockade causes adverse left ventricular remodeling but improves pulmonary artery pressure after infarction in the rat. Circulation. 1998;98(21):2323–30.
58. Hu K, Gaudron P, Schmidt TJ, Hoffmann KD, Ertl G. Aggravation of left ventricular remodeling by a novel specific endothelin ET(A) antagonist EMD94246 in rats with experimental myocardial infarction. J Cardiovasc Pharmacol. 1998;32(3): 505–8.
59. Moe GW, Albernaz A, Naik GO, Kirchengast M, Stewart DJ. Beneficial effects of long-term selective endothelin type A receptor blockade in canine experimental heart failure. Cardiovasc Res. 1998;39(3):571–9.
60. Clozel M, Breu V, Gray GA, et al. Pharmacological characterization of bosentan, a new potent orally active nonpeptide endothelin receptor antagonist. J Pharmacol Exp Ther. 1994;270(1):228–35.
61. Mulder P, Richard V, Derumeaux G, et al. Role of endogenous endothelin in chronic heart failure: effect of long-term treatment with an endothelin antagonist on survival, hemodynamics, and cardiac remodeling. Circulation. 1997;96(6):1976–82.
62. Fraccarollo D, Hu K, Galuppo P, Gaudron P, Ertl G. Chronic endothelin receptor blockade attenuates progressive ventricular dilation and improves cardiac function in rats with myocardial infarction: possible involvement of myocardial endothelin system in ventricular remodeling. Circulation. 1997;96(11):3963–73.
63. Oie E, Bjonerheim R, Grogaard HK, Kongshaug H, Smiseth OA, Attramadal H. ET-receptor antagonism, myocardial gene expression, and ventricular remodeling during CHF in rats. Am J Physiol Heart Circ Physiol. 1998;275(3 pt 2):H868–H77.
64. Iwanaga Y, Kihara Y, Inagaki K, et al. Differential effects of angiotensin II versus endothelin-1 inhibitions in hypertrophic left ventricular myocardium during transition to heart failure. Circulation. 2001;104(5):606–12.
65. Mishima T, Tanimura M, Suzuki G, et al. Effects of long-term therapy with bosentan on the progression of left ventricular dysfunction and remodeling in dogs with heart failure. J Am Coll Cardiol. 2000;35(1):222–9.
66. Clozel M, Ramuz H, Clozel JP, et al. Pharmacology of tezosentan, new endothelin receptor antagonist designed for parenteral use. J Pharmacol Exp Ther. 1999;290(2):840–6.
67. Qiu CB, Qiu CS, Hess P, Clozel JP, Clozel M. Additional effects of endothelin receptor blockade and angiotensin converting enzyme inhibition in rats with chronic heart failure. Acta Pharmacol Sin. 2001;22(6):541–8.
68. Seed A, Love MP, McMurray JJ. Clinical experience with endothelin receptor antagonists in chronic heart failure. Heart Fail Rev. 2001;6(4):317–23.
69. Kiowski W, Sutsch G, Hunziker P, et al. Evidence for endothelin-1-mediated vasoconstriction in severe chronic heart failure. Lancet. 1995;346(8977): 732–6.
70. Sütsch G, Kiowski W, Yan XW, et al. Short-term oral endothelin-receptor antagonist therapy in conventionally treated patients with symptomatic severe chronic heart failure. Circulation. 1998;98(21):2262–8.
71. Dingemanse J, Clozel M, van Giersbergen PL. Pharmacokinetics and pharmacodynamics of tezosentan, an intravenous dual endothelin receptor antagonist, following chronic infusion in healthy subjects. Br J Clin Pharmacol. 2002;53(4):355–62.
72. van Giersbergen PL, Dingemanse J. Effect of severe renal impairment on the pharmacokinetics and tolerability of the parenteral endothelin antagonist tezosentan. Int J Clin Pharmacol Ther. 2003;41(6): 261–6.
73. Schalcher C, Cotter G, Reisin L, et al. The dual endothelin receptor antagonist tezosentan acutely improves hemodynamic parameters in patients with advanced heart failure. Am Heart J. 2001; 142(2):340–9.

74. Torre-Amione G, Young JB, Durand J, et al. Hemodynamic effects of tezosentan, an intravenous dual endothelin receptor antagonist, in patients with class III to IV congestive heart failure. Circulation. 2001;103(7):973–80.
75. Torre-Amione G, Durand JB, Nagueh S, Vooletich MT, Kobrin I, Pratt C. A pilot safety trial of prolonged (48 h) infusion of the dual endothelin-receptor antagonist tezosentan in patients with advanced heart failure. Chest. 2001;120(2):460–6.
76. Cowburn PJ, Cleland JG, McArthur JD, MacLean MR, McMurray JJ, Dargie HJ. Short-term haemodynamic effects of BQ-123, a selective endothelin ET(A)-receptor antagonist, in chronic heart failure. Lancet. 1998;352(9123):201–02.
77. Spieker LE, Mitrovic V, Noll G, et al. Acute hemodynamic and neurohumoral effects of selective ET(A) receptor blockade in patients with congestive heart failure. ET 003 Investigators. J Am Coll Cardiol. 2000;35(7):1745–52.
78. Lüscher TF, Enseleit F, Pacher R, et al. Hemodynamic and neurohumoral effects of selective endothelin A (ET(A)) receptor blockade in chronic heart failure: the Heart Failure ET(A) Receptor Blockade Trial (HEAT). Circulation. 2002;106(21):2666–72.
79. Givertz MM, Colucci WS, LeJemtel TH, et al. Acute endothelin A receptor blockade causes selective pulmonary vasodilation in patients with chronic heart failure. Circulation. 2000;101(25):2922–7.
80. Ooi H, Colucci WS, Givertz MM. Endothelin mediates increased pulmonary vascular tone in patients with heart failure: demonstration by direct intrapulmonary infusion of sitaxsentan. Circulation. 2002;106(13):1618–21.
81. Smith W, Iteld B, LeJemtel T, et al. Improved hemodynamics with the ETA selective receptor antagonist BMS-193884 in patients with heart failure. J Am Coll Cardiol. 2000;35(2):241 (Abstract).
82. Chen HH, Salz LM, McKinley LJ, et al. Safety and efficacy of an orally active selective endothelin-A receptor antagonist in moderate-severe human chronic heart failure. J Cardiac Fail. 1999;5(3): 172(astr).
83. Cotter G, Kiowski W, Kaluski E, et al. Tezosentan (an intravenous endothelin receptor A/B antagonist) reduces peripheral resistance and increases cardiac power therefore preventing a steep decrease in blood pressure in patients with congestive heart failure. Eur J Heart Fail. 2001;3(4):457–61.
84. Teerlink JR, Torre-Amione G. A new strategy for a clinical development program in acute decompensated heart failure: The Randomized Intravenous TeZosentan (RTIZ) trials. J Cardiac Fail. 2000; 6(suppl 2):48(abstr).
85. Torre-Amione G, Young JB, Colucci WS, et al. Hemodynamic and clinical effects of tezosentan, an intravenous dual endothelin receptor antagonist, in patients hospitalized for acute decompensated heart failure. J Am Coll Cardiol. 2003;42(1):140–7.
86. Teerlink JR, Massie BM, Cleland JGF, Tzivoni D, for the RITZ-1 Investigators. A double-blind, parallel-group, multi-center, placebo-controlled study to investigate the efficacy and safety of tezosentan in reducing symptoms in patients with acute decompensated heart failure. Circulation. 2001;104: II-526(abstr).
87. Coletta AP, Cleland JG. Clinical trials update: highlights of the scientific sessions of the XXIII Congress of the European Society of Cardiology—WARIS II, ESCAMI, PAFAC, RITZ-1 and TIME. Eur J Heart Fail. 2001;3(6):747–50.
88. O'Connor CM, Gattis WA, Adams KF Jr, et al. Tezosentan in patients with acute heart failure and acute coronary syndromes: results of the Randomized Intravenous TeZosentan Study (RITZ-4). J Am Coll Cardiol. 2003;41(9):1452–7.
89. Kaluski E, Kobrin I, Zimlichman R, et al. RITZ-5: randomized intravenous TeZosentan (an endothelin-A/B antagonist) for the treatment of pulmonary edema: a prospective, multicenter, double-blind, placebo-controlled study. J Am Coll Cardiol. 2003; 41(2):204–10.
90. Cotter G, Kaluski E, Stangl K, et al. The hemodynamic and neurohormonal effects of low doses of tezosentan (an endothelin A/B receptor antagonist) in patients with acute heart failure. Eur J Heart Fail. 2004;6(5):601–9.
91. Teerlink JR, McMurray JJ, Bourge RC, et al. Tezosentan in patients with acute heart failure: design of the Value of Endothelin Receptor Inhibition with Tezosentan in Acute heart failure Study (VERITAS). Am Heart J. 2005;150(1):46–53.
92. McMurray JJ, Teerlink JR. Late-breaking clinical trials session: Value of Endothelin Receptor Inhibition With Tezosentan in Acute Heart Failure Studies (VERITAS). Paper presented at the American College of Cardiology Annual Scientific Session March 9, 2005, Orlando, FL.
93. Teerlink JR. Dyspnea as an end point in clinical trials of therapies for acute decompensated heart failure. Am Heart J. 2003;145(2 suppl):S26–33.

59 Antiplatelets and Anticoagulation in the Setting of Acute Heart Failure Syndrome

Nathalie Dervaux, Gilles Montalescot, and Alexandre Mebazaa

Acute heart failure (AHF) is the final common pathway for many cardiovascular diseases. Many of the common problems encountered in the clinical care of patient with AHF relate to thrombus formation (thrombogenesis).

Antithrombotics have played a key role in the prophylaxis, treatment, and surgical/interventional management of thrombotic events in cardiovascular disorders. Thrombosis can be treated effectively by three classes of pharmacologic agents: antiplatelets, anticoagulants, and thrombolytic drugs. The first two, which are discussed in this chapter, prevent the formation and growth of thrombi, whereas the third involves lyses of existing thrombi.

This chapter identifies the molecular targets of antiplatelets and anticoagulants, describes the rationale behind antithrombotic treatment, discusses the opportunities and clinical perspective for new drugs, and provides informed guidance on treatment decisions, assisting clinicians to make the optimal therapeutic choice for the adult patient with AHF.

ABCs of Antithrombotic Therapy: Updates in Acute Heart Failure

Antithrombotics in routine use include antiplatelets (aspirin, clopidogrel, and glycoprotein IIb/IIIa receptor antagonists) and anticoagulants (warfarin, unfractionated and low molecular weight heparin, fondaparinux, and direct thrombin inhibitors). The development of new anticoagulants to target specific clotting enzymes or steps in coagulation is expanding the list of drugs that can be used to treat thrombosis in AHF. New parenteral anticoagulants have been developed to overcome the limitations of heparin and low-molecular-weight heparin, whereas novel orally active anticoagulants have been designed to provide more streamlined therapy than the vitamin K antagonists. These advances have been possible because of an improved understanding of the molecular mechanisms underlying blood coagulation, the isolation and characterization of anticoagulants from hematophagous organisms, and advances in structure-based drug design.

Antiplatelet Drugs (Figs. 59.1 and 59.2)

Aspirin

Aspirin irreversibly inhibits platelet cyclooxygenase-1, thereby preventing the formation of thromboxane A_2, a platelet aggregant and potent vasoconstrictor. Inhibition occurs also in the megakaryocyte and because all budding platelets are unable to regenerate fresh cyclo-oxygenase, the effect of aspirin remains as long as the life span of the platelet (10 days). Aspirin has no effect on platelet aggregation induced by other pathways, and is therefore a relatively weak platelet inhibitor.

Platelet–Adenosine Diphosphate–Receptor Antagonists: Clopidogrel and Ticlopidine

These thienopyridines irreversibly inhibit platelet aggregation by preventing the binding of

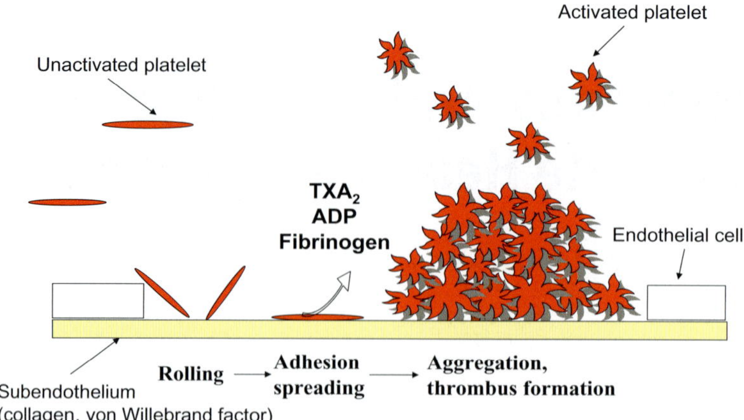

FIGURE 59.1. Antiplatelet drugs. Platelet adhesion, activation, aggregation, and thrombus formation on subendothelial surface at an injured blood vessel. Activated platelets release thromboxane A_2 (TXA_2), adenosine diphosphate (ADP), and fibrinogen pro-aggregated factors.

adenosine diphosphate (ADP) to platelet surface P2Y12 receptor, and also by impairing the platelet response to other platelet-activating factors (collagen, fibrinogen, and von Willebrand factor). The peak action on platelet function occurs after several days of oral dosing when no loading is used. For patients taking clopidogrel in whom surgery is planned, the drug should be withheld for at least 5 days, unless the surgery outweighs the risk of excess bleeding.

Thienopyridines are at least as effective in preventing platelet aggregation than aspirin and have fewer gastrointestinal side effects. Clopidogrel has fewer (if any) neutropenia side effects than ticlopidine.

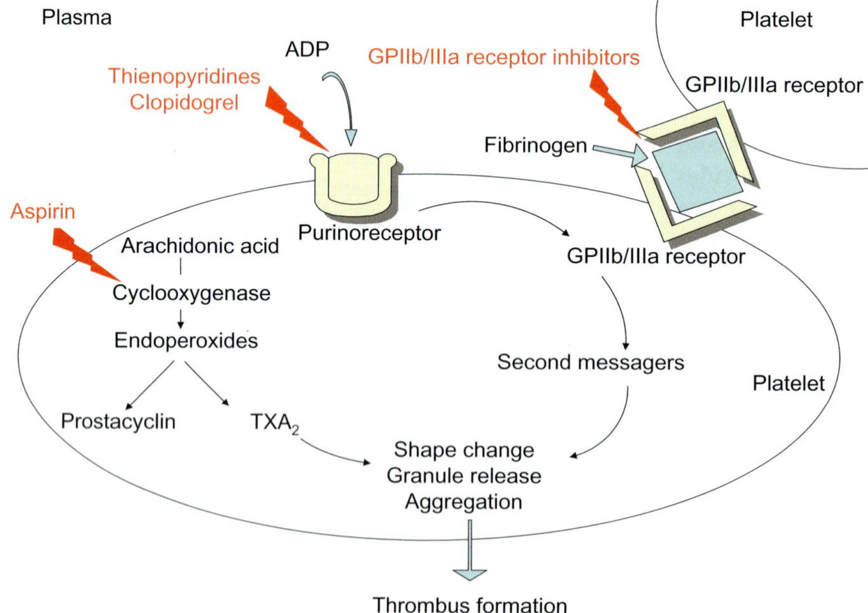

FIGURE 59.2. Routes to inhibiting platelet function. TXA_2, thromboxane A_2, ADP, adenosine diphosphate.

Glycoprotein IIb/IIIa Receptor Inhibitors (GPIIb/IIIa Inhibitors): Abciximab (ReoPro®), Tirofiban (Aggrastat®), Eptifibatide (Integrilin®)

Ligands bound on specific receptors on the surface of the platelet lead to structural modification of the final common pathway for platelet aggregation: the fibrinogen receptor, glycoprotein (GP) IIb/IIIa on the surface, resulting in cross-linking of platelets. Abciximab is a monoclonal antibody and the first GPIIb/IIIa inhibitor to have been developed. Both eptifibatide and tirofiban are small molecules, nonimmunogenic, and therefore suitable for repeat infusions. GPIIb/IIIa inhibitors are much more effective in preventing platelet aggregation than aspirin and thienopyridines. After intravenous bolus administration of abciximab, platelet aggregation is rapidly and fully inhibited (90%), with function recovered within a few days of infusion cessation. Because they are mainly renally cleared, the doses of the small molecules (eptifibatide and tirofiban) should be adjusted with renal impairment. Abciximab and eptifibatide are indicated as adjunctive antithrombotics in patients undergoing percutaneous coronary intervention (PCI), while eptifibatide and tirofiban are approved among patients presenting with non-ST elevation (NSTE) acute coronary syndrome (ACS).

Clinical trials with oral GPIIb/IIIa receptor inhibitors have been disappointing, with no beneficial effects seen, and even evidence of harm and excess of mortality.

Anticoagulant Drugs (Fig. 59.3)

Vitamin K Antagonists

Vitamin K antagonists (VKAs) inhibit the vitamin K–dependent synthesis of clotting factors II (prothrombin), VII, IX, X, and proteins C and S. Two drug classes are distinguished: coumarinic (acenocoumarol, Sintrom®; and warfarin, Coumadin®) and indanedione (fluindione, Previscan®) drugs. Warfarin and fluindione have a long half-life, so they have a more stable international normalized ratio (INR), in which the prothrombin time is compared with a standard) than acenocoumarol (Table 59.1). Warfarin is the most widely used anticoagulant. Because of a delayed reduction in some of the clotting factors, VKAs should be used concomitantly with rapidly acting anticoagulant agents in the initial days of therapy. Absorption of warfarin from the gastrointestinal tract is rapid, with high bioavailability. The VKAs are approximately 97% bound to albumin (only 3% of the molecule absorbed is active) with subsequent accumulation and are metabolized by

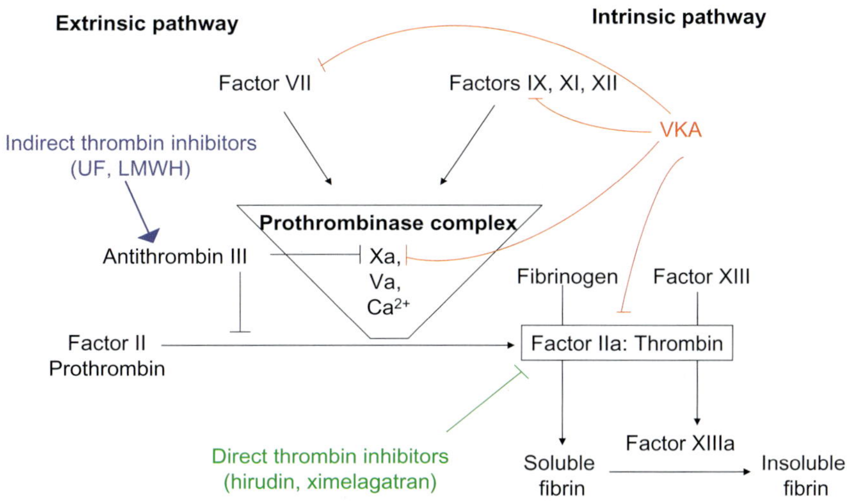

FIGURE 59.3. Effect of anticoagulants on simplified coagulation cascade: vitamin K antagonist (VKA); unfractionated heparin (UH); low molecular weight heparin (LMWH; e.g., fondaparinux); and direct thrombin inhibitors.

Table 59.1. Vitamin K agonists and half-life

Vitamin K agonists	Half-life (h)
Acenocoumarol (Sintrom®)	8
Fluindione (Previscan®)	31
Warfarin (Coumadin®)	40

liver via cytochrome P-450. Given the extent of drug interactions and range of genetic factors impacting drug disposition, interindividual and intraindividual variability in the VKAs' efficacy and safety is not surprising and demands frequent laboratory monitoring. The degree of anticoagulation required varies with clinical circumstance, but the target INR value usually ranges from 2 to 3. The main adverse event is major bleeding (2%/year). Two antidotes exist: vitamin K and the immediately active vitamin K–dependent factors.

Activators of Antithrombin: Heparins

Unfractionated heparin (UH) is a glycosaminoglycan whose major anticoagulant effect can be accounted for by a pentasaccharide with high affinity for antithrombin III, leading to accelerated inactivation of clotting factors IIa (thrombin) and Xa. Its short half-life and its extensive first-pass metabolism mean it must be given continuously and parentally. The effect on the intrinsic clotting cascade must be monitored carefully by measuring the activated partial thromboplastin time (aPTT); aPTT values >1.5 times the upper limit of control reduce the recurrence in venous thromboembolism and are sufficient in the context of left ventricular mural thrombus prophylaxis and the maintenance of coronary arterial patency following tissue-type plasminogen activator administration. Heparin is a heterogeneous mixture of molecules, only a fraction of which have anticoagulant activity. In some patients, heparin causes immunologic thrombocytopenia and, more disastrously, immune-mediated thrombosis.

Low molecular weight heparins (LMWH), synthetic heparinomimetics, are smaller pieces of the heparin molecule that preferentially inhibit clotting factor Xa over factor IIa. The newest synthetic agents (fondaparinux, idraparinux) are exclusive anti-Xa pentasaccharide drugs. The LMWHs have a longer half-life (enabling once-a-day subcutaneous administration), more predictable bioavailability and antithrombotic response without laboratory monitoring, and cause less immunologic thrombocytopenia than UH. The LMWHs have been extensively studied and are replacing UH in many clinical settings. The dose of LMWH is adjusted to weight but must be adjusted down in renal failure patients (creatinine clearance <30 mL/min) or used with caution and possibly monitoring of Xa activity in pregnancy, in obese patients, and in shock patients (resorption issues). Fondaparinux (Arixtra®) was first developed for indications where classical anticoagulants are poorly efficient (e.g., prophylaxis of postorthopedic indications) and recently studied in the management of coronary artery diseases (1). Idraparinux, a novel factor-Xa inhibitor with a longer half-life, can be given once weekly subcutaneously, and has been compared with warfarin in the AMADEUS study of patients with atrial fibrillation (AF) in stroke prevention, but this trial failed to demonstrate superiority of idraparinux.

Direct Thrombin Inhibitors: Pure Anti-IIa

Oral anticoagulation remains a laborious and poorly predictable therapy. Another approach to developing new oral anticoagulants took its cue from the medicinal leech, *Hirudo medicinalis,* which produces hirudin, a direct thrombin inhibitor. The direct thrombin inhibitors (hirudin, melagatran), initially developed for arterial indications, are approved as a substitute anticoagulant in patients with heparin-induced thrombocytopenia and PCI. Because of their liver and renal elimination, these direct antithrombins are contraindicated in cases of hepatic or renal failure. Since there is no available antidote at this time, their development is somewhat limited.

Melagatran is poorly absorbed, but chemically modified in the form of ximelagatran (Exanta®) is the first new oral anticoagulant since warfarin. Ximelagatran does not require systematic laboratory monitoring and was in the process of being tested in large-scale clinical studies but was withdrawn from the worldwide market for its liver toxicity [elevated liver enzymes in 5% of cases (2)]. There are other oral direct thrombin inhibitors in development that look promising for patients with thromboembolism in AF, pulmonary embolism, and ACS potentially complicated by AHF.

At this time it is safe to state that heparin and its LMWH derivatives will remain the anticoagulant of choice for cardiovascular indications until the newer agents that target factor Xa or thrombin have been validated in extended clinical trials in polytherapeutic settings. However, with the plethora of new anticoagulants under development, our list of agents to prevent and treat thrombosis in AHF is likely soon to be expanded.

Acute Heart Failure and Thrombogenesis

Virchow's Triad in Acute Heart Failure

Over 150 years ago, Virchow recognized three prerequisites for thrombogenesis: abnormal blood flow, blood constituent abnormalities, and vessel wall injury. This concept has been extended by modern knowledge of flow characteristics, blood constituents including hemorheologic factors, clotting factors, platelet physiology, and endothelial function.

Because heart failure is marked by low cardiac output, relative stasis of blood in the intracardiac chambers, poor contractility, regional wall motion abnormalities, the high prevalence of AF, various degrees of a hypercoagulable state, platelet abnormalities, and defects in hemostatic mediators and endothelial function, a reasonable pathophysiologic construct is created for using antithrombotics in patients with heart failure and high rates of thromboembolism. Severe heart failure can also induce multiorgan failure, which may be associated with thrombogenesis.

Underlying Thrombogenesis Causes in Acute Heart Failure

The underlying etiology of heart failure has important implications for prognosis and for treatment, including antithrombotics. With coronary artery disease (CAD) underlying 70% of heart failure today, the role of coronary thrombosis with platelet activation and atherosclerotic disease cannot be underestimated (3). Because arterial thrombi consist of platelet aggregates held together by small amounts of fibrin, strategies to inhibit arterial thrombogenesis focus mainly on drugs that block platelet function, but they often include anticoagulants to prevent fibrin deposition. In contrast, anticoagulants are the drugs of choice for prevention of cardioembolic events.

Atrial fibrillation, occurring either as a cause or a complicating factor in AHF, impairs hemodynamics. Disturbed blood flow in the fibrillating left atrium predisposes to the formation of thrombi (mostly in the left atrial appendage) and arterial embolism, especially in the presence of underlying heart disease. Although ischemic stroke and systemic arterial occlusion in AF are generally attributed to cardioembolism, the pathogenesis of thromboembolism is complex (4).

Venous thrombosis (composed mainly of fibrin and red blood cells) leads to pulmonary embolism (PE). Its effects on right heart function have been described (5).

Standard Antithrombotic Treatment in Acute Heart Failure

Anticoagulation therapy is particularly well established in ACS and in AF. There is less evidence for the antithrombotic strategies specifically in the acute phase of diseases causing AHF. Antithrombotics in AHF cannot be optimally managed without consideration of its underlying cause. Indeed, a large placebo-controlled trial of enoxaparin 40 mg subcutaneously in acutely ill and hospitalized patients including a major group of heart failure patients showed less venous thrombosis but no clinical improvement (6).

When an effective anticoagulation is required, the possibilities are limited to continuous infusion of UFH, full anticoagulant treatment with LMWH (e.g., enoxaparin 1 mg/kg b.i.d.), or warfarin. Association with antiplatelet therapy could also be discussed in specific cases.

Thus, antithrombotics should be administered based on the characteristics of the patient and the cause of the AHF.

Antithrombotics Management Adapted to the Context

Careful monitoring of the coagulation system is mandatory in AHF, as there is often concomitant liver and renal dysfunction (7). In patients taking anticoagulant drugs in whom AHF is present, the drug should be withheld and heparin used in the interim, while the liver is replenishing the normal vitamin K–dependent factors. In addition, warfarin interacts with a host of other drugs, often making anticoagulant control difficult to achieve.

Acute Heart Failure and Acute Coronary Syndrome

Based on evidence from clinical trial data covering the broad topic of CAD, the current recommendations concerning the management of antithrombotics are shown in Figure 59.4 (8,9). In ACSs complicated by AHF, especially in case of cardiogenic shock, revascularization should be performed promptly. Moreover, antithrombotics, in conjunction with intervention procedures, have become an essential component of management of patients with an ACS. The use of antithrombotics in ACS has reduced the incidence of death and Q wave myocardial infarction. Combined antithrombotics have decreased the major events with a good tolerance, because of the short duration of such aggressive strategy, and increased the benefit of an early invasive strategy including stent percutaneous coronary angioplasty.

Antiplatelets

In ACS patients with heart failure undergoing revascularization acutely, the recommended

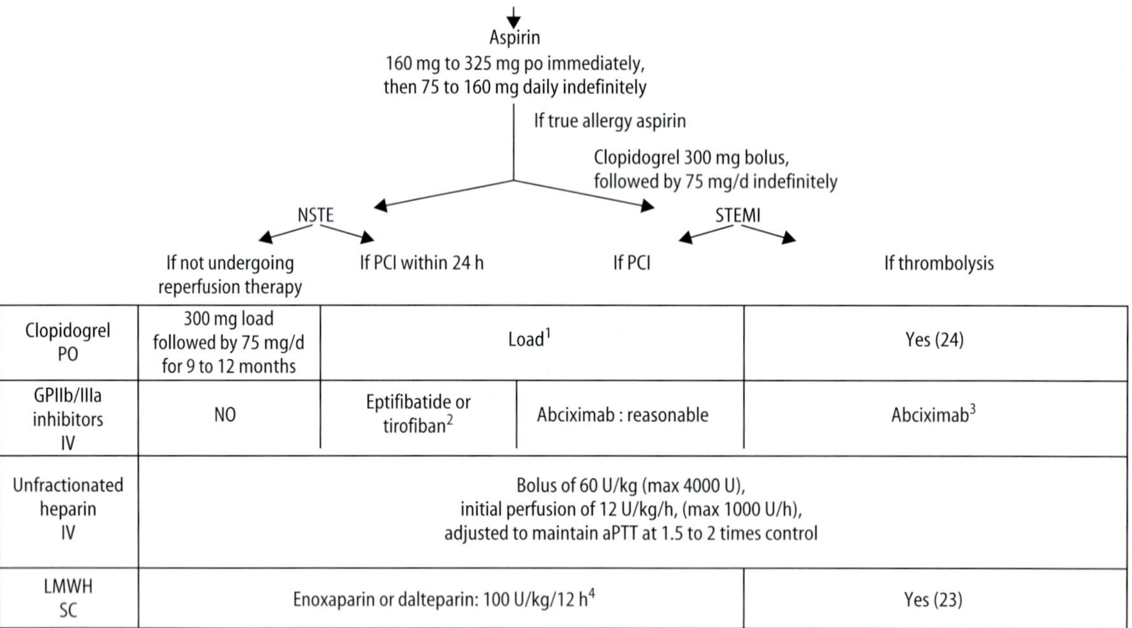

	If not undergoing reperfusion therapy (NSTE)	If PCI within 24 h (NSTE)	If PCI (STEMI)	If thrombolysis (STEMI)
Clopidogrel PO	300 mg load followed by 75 mg/d for 9 to 12 months	Load[1]		Yes (24)
GPIIb/IIIa inhibitors IV	NO	Eptifibatide or tirofiban[2]	Abciximab : reasonable	Abciximab[3]
Unfractionated heparin IV	Bolus of 60 U/kg (max 4000 U), initial perfusion of 12 U/kg/h, (max 1000 U/h), adjusted to maintain aPTT at 1.5 to 2 times control			
LMWH SC	Enoxaparin or dalteparin: 100 U/kg/12 h[4]			Yes (23)

Figure 59.4. Antithrombotic management in acute coronary syndrome. NSTE;non-ST elevation;STEMI, ST segment elevation myocardial infarction. [1]There are no safety data comparing 300 and 600 mg as loading doses for clopidogrel. Then, clopidogrel should be continued after bare metal stent implantation for at least 1 month, or after coated-stent, 3 months for sirolimus, 6 months for paclitaxel. [2]In moderate- to high-risk patients. [3]Reperfusion with abciximab and half-dose reteplase or tenecteplase may be considered for prevention of reinfarction and other complications of STEMI in selected patients: anterior location of MI, less 75 years, and no risk factors for bleeding. [4]For the acute treatment of NSTE ACS (including patients receiving GPIIb/IIIa inhibitors as upstream treatment), we recommend LMWH over UH and suggest continuing LMWHs during percutaneous coronary intervention (PCI) treatment. aPTT, activated partial thromboplastin time. [From Antman et al. (8), and Braunwald et al. (9).]

antithrombotic treatment is ruled by the treatment needed for the revascularization procedure, relying on one anticoagulant (LMWH or UFH) and two or three antiplatelet agents (acetylsalicylic acid [ASA], clopidogrel, and/or GPIIb-IIIa inhibitors). Aspirin is the cornerstone of the early treatment in all suspected ACS and chronic coronaropathy. It has been shown to reduce the mortality and myocardial infarction in patients with unstable angina. The beneficial effects of aspirin seem to be sustained for at least 2 years and regardless of the dose used. However, 75 to 150 mg daily may have a lower incidence of gastrointestinal side effects than higher doses used in some randomized studies.

In the large double-blind Clopidogrel in Unstable Angina to Prevent Recurrent Events (CURE) trial, patients with NSTE ACS received aspirin 75 to 325 mg and then were randomly assigned to additional clopidogrel (300 mg load followed by 75 mg daily) or placebo for 3 months to a year. Additional clopidogrel resulted in a significant relative risk reduction in the primary end point (cardiovascular death, myocardial infarction, or stroke)(10).

In a meta-analysis of all major randomized clinical trials with patients with ACS, the rate of death, reinfarction, and refractory angina was reduced when GPIIb/IIIa inhibitors were added to aspirin and heparin (11). Eptifibatide and tirofiban resulted in a significant reduction in death and myocardial infarction when given to patients with an NSTE ACS already receiving aspirin and heparin, which was maintained at 6 months (12, 13). The benefits of GPIIb/IIIa are greatest in patients with diabetes, dynamic ST-segment changes, or elevated levels of troponin (compared with heparin alone), indicating those most likely to benefit from treatment. Although using GPIIb/IIIa inhibitors for ACS in addition to conventional antithrombotics before revascularization procedures in ACS shows clear benefit, there is some uncertainty of benefit if these drugs are used only as "medical" management without revascularization (14). For the management of antithrombotics in the ST segment elevation myocardial infarction (STEMI), some large studies are expected. Regarding acute myocardial infarction (AMI) complicated by cardiogenic shock, there are few data. Indeed, the cardiogenic shock was an exclusion criterion in trials studying the primary angioplasty in AMI management. Only the ADMIRAL (Abciximab Before Direct Angioplasty and Stenting in Myocardial Infarction Regarding Acute and Long-Term Follow-Up) study has shown that abciximab was also efficient in the subgroup of patients presenting with cardiogenic shock for primary PCI of AMI (15).

Anticoagulant

A pooled analysis in ACS, the Antithrombotic Therapy in Acute Coronary Syndromes Research Group (ATACS) trial, yields a relative risk (RR) of 0.44 for death/MI with combination aspirin and UH therapy compared with aspirin alone (16). The Global Use of Strategies to Open Occluded Coronary Arteries (GUSTO-IIB) study evaluated the relationship between levels of systemic anticoagulation and clinical events among the patients with NSTE ACS (17).

The LMWHs (enoxaparin, Lovenox® and dalteparin, Fragmin®) are commonly used for the management of ACS. A pooled meta-analysis of the Efficacy and Safety of Subcutaneous Enoxaparin in Non–Q-Wave Coronary Events Study Group (ESSENCE) (18) and Thrombolysis in Myocardial Infarction (TIMI IIB) (19) trials, including 7081 patients with NSTE ACS, revealed a significant reduction in death, MI, and urgent revascularization with a benefit sustained through 1 year favoring enoxaparin over UH. It indicates that enoxaparin should be considered as a replacement for UH for NSTE ACS. Although LMWH administration provides an element of protection, those individuals should be treated aggressively (and early) whenever possible. If PCI is planned but delayed, continued therapy as a bridge to revascularization should be considered. Combined with a GPIIb/IIIa inhibitor in patients with NSTE ACS, LMWH is significantly associated with less urgent revascularization, major bleeding, and combined death or MI at 30 days than UH (20,21).

Fondaparinux use in patients with or without evolving ST-elevation ACS is limited to a single phase II trial; phase III trials are underway.

In the management of ACS, compared with UH, direct thrombin inhibitors were associated with a significant lower risk of death or MI but there was a nonsignificant increased rate of major bleeding (22).

Some major trials are expected to clarify the appropriate choice of antithrombotics with PCI (ADVANCE-MI, Addressing the Value of facilitated Angioplasty after Combination therapy or Eptifibatide monotherapy in cute Myocardial Infarction and FINESS, First International NIR Endovascular Stent Study) and with thrombolysis [enoxaparin in (EXTRACT, Enoxaparin and Thrombolysis Reperfusion for Acute myocardial infarction Treatment) EXTRACT-TIMI 25 (23) and clopidogrel in PCI-Clopidogrel as adjunctive reperfusion therapy (CLARITY) (24) seem to be promising], but it should be noted that mortality has not been selected as a primary end point.

Acute Heart Failure and Atrial Fibrillation (Table 59.2)

In parallel with the correction of the cause of the arrhythmias and of antiarrhythmic therapy, antithrombotics should be administered to all patients with AF, and managed for each patient based on the patient's intrinsic risk of thromboembolism (25).

The prognosis in terms of thromboembolism and mortality is related to coexistent cardiovascular disease and is most benign when applied to young individuals (less than 60 years) without cardiopulmonary disease. The risk factor for stroke increases if associated with a clinical risk factor: previous stroke (RR, 2.5); hypertension (RR, 1.6); heart failure (RR, 1.4); diabetes (RR, 1.7); coronaropathy (RR, 1.5); age ≥75 years and with an echocardiography risk factor, such as dilated left atrium (LA), thrombus or spontaneous contrast in left atrium, reduced LA appendage flow velocity, left ventricular systolic dysfunction, aortic plaque thickness >4 mm (26,27) has also a RR > 1.

The AF is associated with a particularly high risk of thromboembolism, mainly stroke (5% per year without antithrombotic), which is reduced respectively by about 60% and 20% by long-term treatment of VKA and by aspirin, respectively (28). Aspirin offers only a weak protection against thromboembolism and overall mortality. If there is a contraindication to anticoagulation, aspirin in a dose of 325 mg daily is an alternative treatment, but might be efficacious more for AF patients with hypertension or diabetes and for reducing the noncardioembolic versus cardioembolic ischemic strokes. The atrial fibrillation clopidogrel trial with irbesartan for prevention of vascular events (ACTIVE) trial, which compared the combination of aspirin plus clopidogrel with adjusted dose warfarin in the prevention of vascular events in high-risk patients with atrial fibrillation, failed to demonstrate superiority of the dual antiplatelet regimen.

Concerning the antithrombotic strategies in AF, more solid clinical evidence exists for prevention of embolism in the long term (using VKA versus

Table 59.2. Antithrombotic management in atrial fibrillation and pulmonary embolism

	Atrial fibrillation	Pulmonary embolism
Acute phase		
Unfractionated heparin	Initial IV bolus: 50 U/kg	80 U/kg
	Followed by a continuous infusion	
	Adjusted to maintain aPTT at 1.5 to 2 times control	
LMWH	Limited data:	Tinzaparin, INNOHEP©
	enoxaparin, dalteparin, 100 U/kg/12 h	175 U/kg/d SC[a]
Chronic phase		
VKA	Initiation recommended together with heparin on the first treatment day adjusted dose, target INR 2 to 3[b]	
	At least 3 to 4 weeks (if back in sinus rhythm) or for lif	At least 3 months
Aspirin	325 mg daily	
	(if contraindication of VKA)	

[a]In patients with acute nonmassive pulmonary embolism (PE), low molecular weight heparin (LMWH) is recommended over unfractionated heparin (UH). In patients with acute PE treated with LMWH, we recommend against routine monitoring with anti-factor Xa level measurements.
[b]International normalized ratio (INR) should be determined at least weekly during the initiation of oral anticoagulation and monthly when the patient is stable.
Sources: Fuster et al. (25); Buller et al. (35).

others drugs) than for the acute phase with severe AHF (studying heparin). When acute AF produces hemodynamic instability and immediate cardioversion is needed, atrial thrombus should be excluded first by transesophageal echocardiography and UH or LMWH administered. When cardioversion can be scheduled, anticoagulation should be given first for at least 3 to 4 weeks. In the Anticoagulation in Cardioversion using Enoxaparin (ACE) trial, Stellbrink et al. demonstrated in patients scheduled for cardioversion of AF of >48 hours and ≤1 year's duration that enoxaparin was not inferior to UH (followed by VKA) with regard to the incidence of embolic events, all-cause death, and major bleeding complications.

The open-label SPORTIF III (SPORTIE, stroke prevention using an oral thrombin inhibitor of atrial fibrillation) (29), along with the double-blind SPORTIF V trial, proved that ximelagatran, administered in fixed doses (36 mg twice daily) without coagulation monitoring, is at least as effective as dose-adjusted warfarin in preventing stroke and systemic embolic events, and at least as safe for bleeding complications. It is important to note that the control of warfarin anticoagulation in these studies was excellent, in comparison to usual practice. Consequently, these trials may overestimate the efficacy and safety of warfarin. From a practical standpoint, ximelagatran has the potential to greatly simplify the anticoagulant management and is an easier drug to use than warfarin, also because it does not have drug- and food-related interactions. However, because of elevated liver enzymes (even asymptomatic), ximelagatran has been withdrawn from the worldwide market.

Based on the results of the SPORTIF III and V trials, direct thrombin inhibitors are a promising alternative to warfarin for stroke prevention in patients with AF and may increase anticoagulant use in high-risk patients.

Acute Heart Failure and Hypertension

The impact of antithrombotics has never been investigated in the initial treatment of AHF with hypertension. In the long term, evidence about the benefits and possible risks of administering low-dose aspirin to hypertensive patients was obtained from the Hypertension Optimal Treatment (HOT) study (30), showing a significant reduction in myocardial infarction (with no effect on the incidence of stroke), but nonfatal major bleeds were twice as common. It is possible that blood pressure control was instrumental in avoiding an increment in intracerebral hemorrhage (practically all patients had diastolic blood pressure ≤90 mm Hg).

Because there is a graded association between each risk factor and overall cardiovascular risk, the contemporary approach to treatment is to determine the threshold based on the calculation of estimated cardiovascular risk over a defined, relatively short-term (e.g., 5- or 10-year) period. These observations are in line with a large meta-analysis (31) proving that low-dose aspirin reduces the risk of vascular events (stroke, myocardial infarction, and vascular death) when given to patients at high cardiovascular risk. It can be noted that high-risk patients are frequently selected in order to increase the power of the trial, so that the vast majority of uncomplicated and lower risk hypertensives are rarely represented.

In summary, recommendations may be given to use low-dose aspirin, 75 mg daily, in hypertensive patients older than 50 years with an even moderate increase in serum creatinine (>115 μmol/L), or in patients at high cardiovascular risk (with a 10-year total cardiovascular risk ≥20%) or with higher initial blood pressure values (32).

Acute Heart Failure and Valvular Disease

Acute heart failure can be caused by valvular conditions such as acute valve incompetence, stenosis, or thrombosis of a prosthetic valve. In patients with mechanical heart valves, Turpie et al. (33) reported that the addition of aspirin (100 mg per day) to warfarin therapy reduced mortality, particularly mortality from vascular causes, although there was some increase in bleeding.

Patients with mechanical heart valves require lifelong anticoagulation. Still to be determined are the utility of direct thrombin inhibitors in patients with mechanical heart valves. The management of AHF from prosthetic valve thrombosis (PVT) remains controversial. Thrombolysis is used for right-sided prosthetic valves and for high-risk surgical candidates. Surgery is preferred for left-sided PVT (34).

Acute Heart Failure and Pulmonary Embolism

The efficacy of unfractionated heparin in the treatment of PE in comparison to no treatment was first proved in 1960. Subsequent trials concentrated on the dose, duration of infusion, mode of administration, and combination with warfarin treatment. Unfractionated heparin, administered by continuous infusion adjusted to achieve an aPTT greater than 1.5, is effective as initial treatment and should be followed by long-term anticoagulation with oral anticoagulants for at least 3 months (adapted to the underlying context) (35).

Many later trials have reported that LMWH is at least as effective and safe for initial treatment of PE as dose-titrated UH (36). Its use is now firmly established, and LMWH is recommended over UH in symptomatic nonmassive PE. In massive PE, or where rapid reversal of the effect may be needed, UH should be considered as a first dose bolus. Because of the favorable results with anticoagulants, thrombolytics should usually be reserved for treatment of selected patients with hemodynamically unstable PE and at low risk of bleeding. In hemodynamically stable patients with echocardiographic evidence of right ventricular dysfunction, further studies are required to document a clinically relevant improvement in the benefit-risk ratio of thrombolytics over anticoagulants.

Initiation of VKA is recommended together with LMWH or UFH on the first treatment day, and discontinuation of heparin when the INR is stable and >2.0. In the initial treatment of acute symptomatic PE, a large open-label trial has also reported that the fondaparinux administered subcutaneous once daily without laboratory monitoring is at least as effective and as safe as adjusted-dose IV UH (37). In terms of costs, treatment with fondaparinux is more expensive than treatment with LMWH, but both drugs are undoubtedly less costly overall than UH because of savings in costs associated with hospitalization (in case of minor PE) and laboratory monitoring. The trial thrombin inhibition in venous thromboembolism (THRIVE) suggests, in patients with acute deep vein thrombosis (in whom one third had concomitant PE) that ximelagatran (36 mg twice daily) is as effective on rates of recurrent venous thromboembolism as conventional anticoagulation with enoxaparin (1 mg/kg twice daily) followed by warfarin (38). Since these new compounds (fondaparinux and ximelagatran) have not been registered, no recommendations are made.

Severe Chronic Heart Failure

The literature does not indicate whether the long-term effect of anticoagulants or antiplatelets contribute to mortality reduction in patients with left ventricular (LV) dysfunction. Evaluating patients for personal risk for emboli or for ischemic coronary artery events may affect the choice of therapies.

Recent observational data suggest that mild or moderate heart failure is associated with an annual risk of stroke of 1.2%. Anticoagulation reduces the rate of embolic events, but there is controversy about the mandatory use of antiplatelet or anticoagulant for all patients with ventricular dysfunction in sinus rhythm. The benefits and risks of warfarin may be increased as the ejection fraction (EF) worsens or heart failure functional class declines.

At present, anticoagulation is indicated only in high-risk subgroups of patients—those with AF, thrombi, or a recent history of thromboembolism. In post-STEMI patients with LV thrombus, warfarin should be prescribed for at least 3 months and indefinitely in patients without an increased risk of bleeding.

Large-scale, prospective randomized controlled trials of both antiplatelets and anticoagulation in heart failure include the recently reported Warfarin and Antiplatelet Therapy in Chronic Heart failure (WATCH) trial and the Warfarin Versus Aspirin in Reduced Cardiac Ejection Fraction (WARCEF) trial, which is currently underway. The WATCH trial failed to find significant differences among aspirin, warfarin, and clopidogrel in the primary composite end point of all-cause mortality, nonfatal MI, and nonfatal stroke. The pooled data may provide much information about the outcome differences between these agents to define optimal preventative measures for thromboembolism in patients with left ventricular systolic dysfunction and sinus rhythm. This would suggest that all patients with depressed LV function should be on some type of antithrombotic. The future appears promising due to the advent of direct thrombin inhibitors, unmonitored oral anticoagulant, with good efficacy and safety for the treatment and prevention of thromboembolism.

Acute Heart Failure and Mechanical Assist Devices

Patients with refractory AHF or end-stage heart failure should be considered for further circulatory support (as a temporary measure or as a bridge to heart transplantation) such as intraaortic balloon counterpulsation, implantable turbine pump (Hemopump), percutaneous cardiopulmonary bypass support (extracorporeal life support), right/left heart, biventricular assist devices placed by thoracotomy, or intra- and extrathoracic total artificial hearts.

Improvements in pump technology and the scarcity of donor organs have led to an increased use of mechanical assist devices, but the problem of thromboembolism has still not been solved. Thrombotic complication associated with mechanical assist devices have been reported but few trials have studied antithrombotics.

For cardiogenic shock or severe acute left heart frequently associated with multiorgan failure, the development of heparin-coated devices appears more promising than studying the high-risk systemic anticoagulation.

Case Report

A 75-year-old man with dyslipidemia, hypertension, and a history of myocardial infarction 4 years previously is admitted to the hospital with congestive heart failure. He reports dyspnea and palpitation for 3 days. He does not smoke. His father died suddenly at the age of 49 years. Echocardiography performed 15 months before admission revealed inferior and apical akinesis, thickening of the upper septum, and diastolic and systolic left ventricular dysfunction (left ventricular ejection fraction [LVEF] 42%). Medications include aspirin (160 mg daily), a beta-blocker, a statin, and an angiotensin-converting enzyme inhibitor.

Physical examination reveals a blood pressure of 155/90 mm Hg, an irregular heart rate, and pulmonary rales. The patient weighs 80 kg. Electrocardiographic testing reveals atrial fibrillation at an average rate of 130 beats per minute. A chest radiograph shows pulmonary edema and mild cardiomegaly. Laboratory tests and an echocardiography were performed.

Medical treatment of acute heart failure with atrial fibrillation is started including anticoagulation. The management of antithrombotic depends on three issues: the acute cause (including alcohol intake, surgery, sepsis, myocarditis, pulmonary embolism, and hyperthyroidism), the duration of AF, and the underlying associated cardiovascular disease. In this case, AF was the first-detected episode (lasting more than 48 hours), was associated with coronary artery disease, and the precipitating factor found was hypertension.

Enoxaparin 8000 UI/12 hours subcutaneous was administrated in the initial days of therapy. The patient was hemodynamically stable, so warfarin per os was started concomitantly in a dose adjusted to achieve a target intensity of INR 2 to 3. To restore sinus rhythm, a cardioversion was scheduled after 4 weeks of anticoagulation. The hypertension was treated, antiarrhythmic agent (sotalol) given and sinus rhythm maintained. The dose of aspirin was reduced (75 mg/d). A low dose of aspirin (less than 100 mg per day) or clopidogrel (75 mg per day) may be given concurrently with anticoagulation in patients with coronaropathy, but there are no solid data. The duration of anticoagulation after the cardioversion depends on the likelihood that AF will recur and on the patient's intrinsic risk of thromboembolism. In this aged patient with coronaropathy, hypertension, and heart failure, warfarin was continued for life.

Conclusion

As more is learned about the mechanisms of drug effects in different populations, physicians may be better able to direct appropriate therapies to reduce platelet aggregation or to interfere with the clotting process. The oral direct thrombin inhibitors (candidate for both acute and chronic therapy thanks to its fast onset of action and oral administration) and the synthetic Xa inhibitors may offer improved safety-efficacy profiles, without the need for hematologic monitoring. Both are appealing candidates for additional study.

Despite the wealth of reports on antithrombotics for many cardiovascular diseases leading to AHF, it is not possible to produce a simple algorithm, given the heterogeneity of patient profiles and availability of resources in various clinical settings. Clinicians must consider the risks and benefits of each drug (alone and in combination) for a patient based on the individual's risk for thrombosis if untreated weighed against the risk of bleeding if treated.

References

1. Yusuf S, Mehta SR, Chrolavicius S, et al. Effects of fondaparinux on mortality and reinfarction in patients with acute ST-segment elevation myocardial infarction: the OASIS-6 randomized trial. JAMA 2006;295:1579–80.
2. Olsson SB, Executive Steering Committee on behalf of the SPORTIF III Investigators. Stroke prevention with the oral direct thrombin inhibitor ximelagatran compared with warfarin in patients with non-valvular atrial fibrillation (SPORTIF III): randomised controlled trial. Lancet 2003;362:1691–8.
3. Fuster V, Badimon L, Badimon JJ, et al. The pathogenesis of coronary artery disease and the acute coronary syndromes. N Engl J Med 1992; 326:242–50.
4. Hart RG, Halperin JL, Pearce LA, et al. Stroke Prevention in Atrial Fibrillation Investigators. Lessons from the Stroke Prevention in Atrial Fibrillation trials. Ann Intern Med 2003;138:831–8.
5. Wood KE. Major pulmonary embolism: review of a pathophysiologic approach to the golden hour of hemodynamically significant pulmonary embolism. Chest 2002;121:877–905.
6. Samama MM, Cohen AT, Darmon JY, et al. A comparison of enoxaparin with placebo for the prevention of venous thromboembolism in acutely ill medical patients. Prophylaxis in Medical Patients with Enoxaparin Study Group. N Engl J Med 1999;341:793–800.
7. Nieminen MS, Bohm M, Cowie MR, et al.; ESC Committee for Practice Guideline (CPG). Executive summary of the guidelines on the diagnosis and treatment of acute heart failure: the Task Force on Acute Heart Failure of the European Society of Cardiology. Eur Heart J 2005;26:384–416.
8. Antman EM, Anbe DT, Armstrong PW, et al. ACC/AHA guidelines for the management of patients with ST-elevation myocardial infarction executive summary: a report of the American College of Cardiology/American Heart Association Task Force on Practice Guidelines (Writing Committee to Revise the 1999 Guidelines for the Management of Patients With Acute Myocardial Infarction). Circulation 2004;110:588–636.
9. Braunwald E, Antman EM, Beasley JW, et al. American College of Cardiology/American Heart Association Task Force on Practice Guidelines (Committee on the Management of Patients With Unstable Angina). ACC/AHA guideline update for the management of patients with unstable angina and non-ST-segment elevation myocardial infarction: summary article. Circulation 2002;106:1893–900.
10. Peters RJ, Mehta SR, Fox KA, et al. Effects of aspirin dose when used alone or in combination with clopidogrel in patients with acute coronary syndromes: observations from the Clopidogrel in Unstable angina to prevent Recurrent Events (CURE) study. Circulation 2003;108:1682–7.
11. Boersma E, Harrington RA, Moliterno DJ, et al. Platelet glycoprotein IIb/IIIa inhibitors in acute coronary syndromes: a meta-analysis of all major randomised clinical trials. Lancet 2002;359:189–98.
12. The PURSUIT Trial Investigators. Inhibition of platelet glycoprotein IIb/IIIa with eptifibatide in patients with acute coronary syndromes. Platelet glycoprotein IIb/IIIa in unstable angina: receptor suppression using integrilin therapy. N Engl J Med 1998;339:436–43.
13. The Platelet Receptor Inhibition in Ischemic Syndrome Management in Patients Limited by Unstable Signs and Symptoms (PRISM-PLUS) Study Investigators. Inhibition of the platelet glycoprotein IIb/IIIa receptor with tirofiban in unstable angina and non-Q-wave myocardial infarction. N Engl J Med 1998;338:1488–97.
14. Simoons ML;GUSTO IV-ACS Investigators. Effect of glycoprotein IIb/IIIa receptor blocker abciximab on outcome in patients with acute coronary syndromes without early coronary revascularisation: the GUSTO IV-ACS randomised trial. Lancet 2001;357:1915–24.
15. Montalescot G, Barragan P, Wittenberg O, et al.; ADMIRAL Investigators. Abciximab before Direct Angioplasty and Stenting in Myocardial Infarction Regarding Acute and Long-Term Follow-up. Platelet glycoprotein IIb/IIIa inhibition with coronary stenting for acute myocardial infarction. N Engl J Med 2001;344:1895–903.
16. Cohen M, Adams PC, Parry G, et al. Combination antithrombotic therapy in unstable rest angina and

non-Q-wave infarction in nonprior aspirin users. Primary end points analysis from the ATACS trial. Antithrombotic Therapy in Acute Coronary Syndromes Research Group. Circulation 1994;89: 81–8.

17. Gilchrist IC, Berkowitz SD, Thompson TD, et al. Heparin dosing and outcome in acute coronary syndromes: the GUSTO-IIb experience. Global Use of Strategies to Open Occluded Coronary Arteries. Am Heart J 2002;144:73–80.
18. Cohen M, Demers C, Gurfinkel EP, et al. A comparison of low-molecular-weight heparin with unfractionated heparin for unstable coronary artery disease. Efficacy and Safety of Subcutaneous Enoxaparin in Non-Q-Wave Coronary Events Study Group. N Engl J Med 1997;337:447–52.
19. Antman EM, McCabe CH, Gurfinkel EP, et al. Enoxaparin prevents death and cardiac ischemic events in unstable angina/non-Q-wave myocardial infarction. Results of the Thrombolysis in Myocardial Infarction (TIMI) IIB trial. Circulation 1999;100:1593–601.
20. Mahaffey KW, Cohen M, Garg J, et al. High-risk patients with acute coronary syndromes treated with low-molecular-weight or unfractionated heparin: outcomes at 6 months and 1 year in the SYNERGY trial. JAMA 2005;294:2594–600.
21. Goodman SG, Fitchett D, Armstrong PW, et al. Randomized evaluation of the safety and efficacy of enoxaparin versus unfractionated heparin in high-risk patients with non-ST-segment elevation acute coronary syndromes receiving the glycoprotein IIb/IIIa inhibitor eptifibatide. Circulation 2003;107:238–44.
22. Antman EM, Morrow DA, McCabe CH, et al. Enoxaparin versus unfractionated heparin with fibrinolysis for ST-elevation myocardial infarction. N Engl J Med 2006;354:1477–88.
23. Sabatine MS, Cannon CP, Gibson CM, et al. Addition of clopidogrel to aspirin and fibrinolytic therapy for myocardial infarction with ST-segment elevation. N Engl J Med 2005;352:1179–89.
24. Direct Thrombin Inhibitor Trialists' Collaborative Group. Direct thrombin inhibitors in acute coronary syndromes: principal results of a meta-analysis based on individual patients' data. Lancet 2002;359:294–302.
25. Fuster V, Ryden LE, Asinger RW, et al. ACC/AHA/ESC guidelines for the management of patients with atrial fibrillation: Executive Summary: A Report of the American College of Cardiology/American Heart Association Task Force on Practice Guidelines and the European Society of Cardiology Committee for Practice Guidelines and Policy Conferences (Committee to Develop Guidelines for the Management of Patients with Atrial Fibrillation) Developed in Collaboration with the North American Society of Pacing and Electrophysiology. Circulation 2001;104:2118–50.
26. Predictors of thromboembolism in atrial fibrillation: I. Clinical features of patients at risk. The Stroke Prevention in Atrial Fibrillation Investigators. Ann Intern Med 1992;116:1–5.
27. Predictors of thromboembolism in atrial fibrillation: II. Echocardiographic features of patients at risk. The Stroke Prevention in Atrial Fibrillation Investigators. Ann Intern Med 1992;116:6–12.
28. Hart RG, Benavente O, McBride R, et al. Antithrombotic therapy to prevent stroke in patients with atrial fibrillation: a meta-analysis. Ann Intern Med 1999;131: 492–501.
29. Albers GW;SPORTIF Investigators. Stroke prevention in atrial fibrillation: pooled analysis of SPORTIF III and V trials. Am J Manag Care 2004;10(14 suppl): S462–9.
30. Hansson L, Zanchetti A, Carruthers SG, et al. Effects of intensive blood-pressure lowering and low-dose aspirin in patients with hypertension: principal results of the Hypertension Optimal Treatment (HOT) randomised trial. Lancet 1998;351:1755–62.
31. Antithrombotic Trialists' Collaboration. Collaborative meta-analysis of randomised trials of antiplatelet therapy for prevention of death, myocardial infarction, and stroke in high risk patients. BMJ 2002;324:71–86.
32. Williams B, Poulter NR, Brown MJ, et al.; BHS guidelines working party, for the British Hypertension Society. British Hypertension Society guidelines for hypertension management 2004 (BHS-IV): summary. BMJ 2004;328:634–40.
33. Turpie AG, Gent M, Laupacis A, et al. A comparison of aspirin with placebo in patients treated with warfarin after heart-valve replacement. N Engl J Med 1993;329:524–9.
34. Alpert JS. The thrombosed prosthetic valve: current recommendations based on evidence from the literature. J Am Coll Cardiol 2003;41:659–60.
35. Buller HR, Agnelli G, Hull RD, et al. Antithrombotic therapy for venous thromboembolic disease: the Seventh ACCP Conference on Antithrombotic and Thrombolytic Therapy. Chest 2004;126(3 suppl):S401–28.
36. Quinlan DJ, McQuillan A, Eikelboom JW. Low-molecular-weight heparin compared with intravenous unfractionated heparin for treatment of pulmonary embolism: a meta-analysis of randomized, controlled trials. Ann Intern Med 2004;140: 175–83.

37. Buller HR, Davidson BL, Decousus H, et al. Matisse Investigators. Subcutaneous fondaparinux versus intravenous unfractionated heparin in the initial treatment of pulmonary embolism. N Engl J Med 2003;349:1695–702.

38. Fiessinger JN, Huisman MV, Davidson BL, et al.; THRIVE Treatment Study Investigators. X imelagatran vs low-molecular-weight heparin and warfarin for the treatment of deep vein thrombosis: a randomized trial. JAMA 2005;293:681–9.

2.5
Specific Intensive Care Unit Management of Acute Heart Failure Syndrome

60
Successful Analgesia and Sedation for Patients with Acute Heart Failure Syndromes

Nuala J. Meyer and Jesse B. Hall

Patients presenting with an acute heart failure syndrome (AHFS) report the rapid onset of symptoms referable to their abnormal heart function.[1] Their cardinal symptoms include dyspnea and fatigue, which are often accompanied by significant anxiety when the breathlessness is severe. Like the majority of critically ill patients, patients with acute heart failure commonly experience pain and discomfort, and relief of these symptoms is of paramount importance in their overall plan of care. This chapter provides an overview for the assessment of a patient's need for analgesia and sedation, reviews the common medications and strategies used to successfully provide comfort and relieve pain, and discusses potential complications of sedative therapy.

Assessment of Pain

As physicians we place a preeminent importance on the relief of our patients' suffering. In critical care settings, suffering is frequently twofold: that caused by pain and discomfort, and that caused by anxiety and fear.[2] Unfortunately, a typical hospitalization for acute heart failure is fraught with potentially noxious stimuli. Patients with AHFS may have pain related to their underlying heart failure or due to a comorbid condition, such as ischemic disease, diabetic neuropathy, or recent invasive procedures. Dyspnea itself is inherently uncomfortable and anxiety-provoking. In addition, some patients are distressed by routine monitoring or nursing devices, including catheters, telemetry wires, or ventilation equipment.[3,4] Among critically ill patients with congestive heart failure, one study found that 43% of patients reported pain, and 10% of patients with pain were dissatisfied with their pain control.[4] Untreated pain seems to trigger an inflammatory stress response, as evidenced by increased heart rate, myocardial oxygen consumption, and markers of coagulability and immunosuppression.[5] Pain also stimulates autonomic activity independent of the systemic inflammatory response, eliciting a sympathetic outpouring that is deleterious to the patient with impaired left ventricular function. Furthermore, appropriate perioperative treatment with analgesics and sedatives in patients undergoing coronary artery bypass grafting apparently modifies the stress response as measured by cortisol and catecholamine levels.[6] The importance of adequate pain control is thus widely accepted as a universal goal in the care of hospitalized patients, and receives close attention from such accrediting bodies as the Joint Commission on Accreditation of Healthcare Organizations (JCAHO) in the United States.[7]

Pain is an inherently subjective experience, and as such it can be difficult for even trained observers to appropriately gauge a patient's analgesic requirements. The most reliable and valid indication of pain is a patient's self-report.[8,9] Whenever the patient is able to communicate her level of pain, the following information should be routinely assessed and reevaluated: the pain's location, quality, intensity, and whether there are any aggravating or alleviating factors. The assessment of pain intensity may be facilitated by the use of tools such as a verbal rating scale (VRS), visual analogue scale (VAS), and numeric rating scale (NRS). Of these, the NRS, in which the patient is asked to rate the pain on a scale from 1 (minimal pain) to 10 (extremely severe pain), is generally preferred because the numerical scales have been shown to have the least variance.[10] Unfortunately, while we recognize that the patients themselves are the most reliable indicator of pain intensity, critically ill patients are frequently impaired in their ability to communicate effectively. It is therefore important to have tools that quantify pain intensity even for an unconscious patient. The FACES scale (Fig. 60.1), which has the observer—physician, nurse, or family member—rate the patient's pain based on her facial expression,[11] scored favorably against the VAS in postoperative intensive care unit (ICU) patients, although it performed less well as the pain intensity increased.[12] When even the FACES scale is problematic, clinicians must integrate patients' nonverbal communications with their behavior and physiologic information.[13] Increased heart rate, respiratory rate, and blood pressure, along with diaphoresis or restless motor activity, are appropriately interpreted as manifestations of discomfort, although relying on these markers alone is likely to underestimate the severity of a patient's pain experience.[14] Lastly, it is appropriate to include the patient's family members or surrogates in the assessment of a noncommunicative patient's discomfort. One study comparing family responses to the patient's assessment found that surrogates accurately estimated the presence or absence of pain in their loved one almost 75% of the time, although they were less accurate in describing the pain intensity.[15]

Assessment of Sedation

Even when pain is not a prominent feature of a patient's illness, the fear and anxiety associated with acute illness can be profoundly distressing. Fear may stem from a sense of threat to one's life, from unfamiliar surroundings, from isolation from family and loved ones—often compounded by an inability to communicate effectively—and replacement of one's individual routine with that imposed by the hospital. Agitation is frequently the physical manifestation of these fears, or as one clinician has described it, "the motor restlessness that accompanies anxiety."[2] Agitation is extremely common among critically ill patients; one study of a mixed medical-surgical ICU found that agitation was documented at least once in 71% of all patients, regardless of age.[16] Agitation may result from many different causes other than pain or anxiety, including hypoxemia, hypoperfusion, hypercapnia, hypoglycemia, pain, drug effect, and withdrawal from alcohol or other drugs. As such, it is imperative that the first priority in approaching the agitated patient be to seek and treat any underlying physiologic abnormality, before proceeding to sedation and anxiolysis. In addition, it is wise to remember that not all patients with anxiety will manifest agitation. Some patients

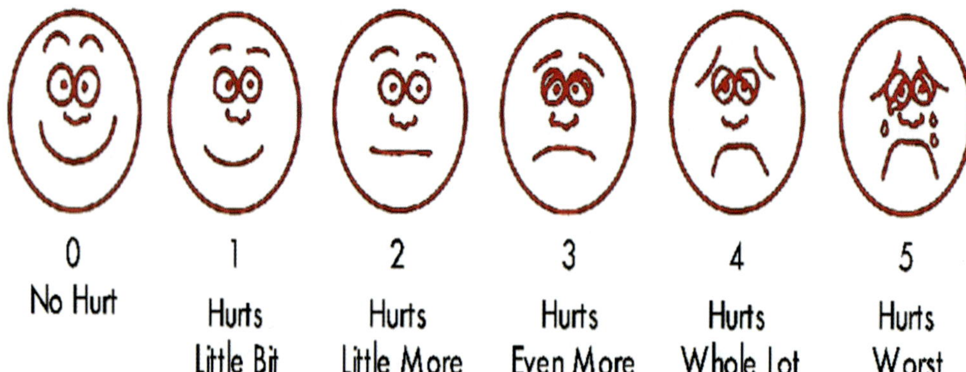

FIGURE 60.1. Wong-Baker FACES pain rating scale. (From Hockenberry et al.,[11] with permission.)

may instead appear fearful or withdrawn. Survivors of critical illness have reported that despite being assessed by their physicians and nurses as fully oriented and competent, they themselves recollect struggling with the distinction between reality and delusion, and with terrifying paranoia that their caregivers were plotting to harm them.[17–19]

Several other indications for sedation bear mention. Sedatives potentiate the analgesic effect of narcotics, in effect lowering the necessary dose of narcotic needed to achieve the desired pain control.[2] Rarely, sedatives may themselves possess analgesic qualities, an effect best described for α-agonists such as dexmedetomidine.[20] The use of neuromuscular blocking agents or other paralytics absolutely mandates the coadministration of adequate sedation to prevent the unpleasant sensation of awareness during therapeutic paralysis.[21,22] In addition, amnesia itself may occasionally be an explicit goal, especially during invasive procedures or while a patient's respiratory insufficiency is severe. Benzodiazepines possess the strongest amnestic qualities, with propofol approaching but not equaling their effectiveness. While the necessity of amnesia during surgical procedures and neuromuscular blockade is unquestioned, the role of amnesia during critical illness remains uncertain. Amnesia has never been proven beneficial to critically ill patients, and in fact may contribute to poor neuropsychological recovery. Several studies have shown a positive association between the development of posttraumatic stress disorder (PTSD) and the lack of awareness during the ICU experience,[23–25] and research suggests that preserving awareness during mechanical ventilation may mitigate the development of PTSD.[23,26]

Delirium, or acute brain dysfunction, may be another factor in choosing or modifying sedative therapy. Delirium seems to affect the majority of critically ill patients, and may accompany anxiety or any number of physiologic perturbations, such as sepsis, fever, encephalopathy, hepatic or renal failure, withdrawal syndromes, or medications.[27] In mechanically ventilated patients, delirium is an independent risk factor for mortality.[28] Hyperactive delirium, manifest by patient restlessness, agitation, and attempts to remove indwelling devices, may respond well to neuroleptic medication such as haloperidol or risperidone, as recommended by some consensus guidelines.[29] However, the most common type of delirium reported in the ICU is actually a hypoactive, withdrawn, "quiet" delirium, and to date no study testing whether neuroleptics improve outcomes from such delirium has been published. Further, use of sedating medications such as narcotics and benzodiazepines are the leading iatrogenic risk factors for delirium,[28] suggesting that physicians may need to modify sedative regimens based on patients' cognitive functioning. A tool named the Confusion Assessment Method for ICU Patients (CAM-ICU) has been validated as a rapid and reliable instrument to aid in the diagnosis of delirium in critically ill patients.[30]

Having established the indications for sedation, the clinician's next task is to appropriately target an individual level of sedation for each patient. Just as titrating pain control is best done by patient self-assessment, achieving the desired depth of sedation is best accomplished by the use of a validated scale. The Ramsay scale was published in 1974, and remains a frequently cited instrument in clinical investigations of sedation.[31] While the Ramsay scale manifests good interrater reliability and correlates well with the Glasgow Coma Scale,[32] in many ways it represents more of an assessment of consciousness than of sedation.[33] In recent years, several new tools such as the Sedation Agitation Scale (SAS), Richmond Agitation-Sedation Scale (RASS) (Table 60.1), and the Adaptation to Intensive Care Environment (ATICE) instrument have been developed and validated against the Ramsay scale for use in the ICU.[34–37] It is our practice to employ the RASS, for it is singular in being validated to detect changes in sedation status over time, as well as against constructs of level of consciousness and delirium. Both the RASS and the ATICE have been noted to correlate well with the amount of sedatives and analgesics given to patients. The ATICE may gain increased acceptance in the ICU, for it has the advantage of measuring not only awakeness and comprehension, but also features of tolerance of the ventilator, such as ventilator synchrony, facial relaxation, and calmness. Finally, regardless of the tool used to titrate sedation and the initial indication for sedation, we advocate a daily interruption of sedatives to reassess a patient's ongoing sedative

TABLE 60.1. Richmond Agitation-Sedation Scale (RASS)

Score	Term	Description
+4	Combative	Overtly combative/violent, danger to staff
+3	Very agitated	Pulls/removes tubes and catheters; aggressive
+2	Agitated	Nonpurposeful movement; asynchronous with ventilator
+1	Restless	Anxious, but movements not aggressive or violent
0	Alert and calm	
−1	Drowsy	Sustained awakening to voice with eye contact (>10 s)
−2	Light sedation	Briefly awakens to voice, with eye contact (<10 s)
−3	Moderate sedation	Movement or eye opening to voice, but no eye contact
−4	Deep sedation	No response to voice; movement to physical stimulation
−5	Unarousable	No response to voice or physical stimulation

Procedure:

1. Observe patient. If calm, score 0. If restless or agitated, score +1 to +4.
2. If not alert: speak name in a loud clear voice, and direct patient to look at speaker. Repeat once if necessary. Gauge response: score −1 to −3.
3. If no response to voice, then physically stimulate patient. Gauge response: score −4 to −5.

Adopted from Sessler et al.[36] and Hogarth and Hall, with permission.[86]

requirements and to permit a neurologic assessment.

Kress et al.[38] performed a study in which mechanically ventilated patients were randomized either to a daily interruption, whereby medications were held until the patient was awake enough to be able to follow simple commands or to the point of demonstrating agitation, versus management of sedation at the discretion of the ICU team. After holding sedation, patients who were deemed to have an ongoing need for sedation were reinitiated on their prior medications but at half the previous dose, and then titrated according to clinical goals. Perhaps unexpectedly, patients in the daily interruption group required 2 fewer ventilator days, 3 fewer ICU days, and more than a 15% reduction in tests to assess mental status, such as brain computed tomography (CT).[38] In addition, patients in the daily interruption group had no increase in complications such as unplanned extubations[38] or in long-term psychological problems such as PTSD.[23] We thus advocate the following guiding principles for any sedated patient in the ICU: individualize sedation using a validated instrument such as the RASS; seek the least sedation necessary to safely accomplish ventilatory and hemodynamic demands; and reassess sedation requirements daily with an interruption of medication to minimize accumulation of medication and to allow neurologic exams.

Analgesic Medications

In addition to considering pharmacologic analgesia, it is also appropriate to maximize nonpharmacologic pain-control strategies. Correct endotracheal tube positioning at least 2 cm above the carina, with the cuff below the vocal cords, can reduce coughing and gagging. Positioning patients in such a manner as to relieve pressure on wounds, chest tubes, or incisions can also relieve pain. However, pain in the critically ill should be considered omnipresent unless proven otherwise, and most patients will require some form of pharmacologic analgesic.

The mainstay of pain control for most ICU patients is narcotic analgesia. Even in the patient suffering from an acute coronary syndrome (ACS), where significant relief of chest pressure may be achieved with aspirin, nitroglycerin, and oxygen, morphine is often necessary to obliterate chest discomfort. While nonsteroidal antiinflammatory drugs (NSAIDs) are an important class of analgesics to treat pain in general, in the patient with acute heart failure, concern about preserving renal blood flow typically contraindicates use of this class of medication. Opiate receptors are widespread in both the central nervous system and the peripheral tissues, but their most relevant effects are mediated predominantly through the opiate mu and kappa receptors. Mu receptors occur as two subtypes; mu-1 receptors mediate analgesia, whereas mu-2 receptors are responsible for respiratory depression, nausea, emesis, constipation, and euphoria. Both mu-2 receptors and kappa receptors appear to mediate narcotic-induced cough suppression.[39] Despite the obvious desire to find a mu-1 selective agent, to date there is no such medication clinically available.

Morphine and fentanyl are the most commonly used narcotic agents. Table 60.2 lists the pharma-

Table 60.2. Properties of commonly used analgesics[29,39–42,47–52]

Agent	Onset after IV dose	$T_{1/2}$	Metabolism	Equianalgesic dose	Side effects	Starting dose	Cost
Morphine	10 min	3–7 h	Hepatic	10 mg	Histamine release	1–4 mg bolus; 2–5 mg/h gtts	¢
Hydromorphone	10 min	2–3 h	Hepatic	1.5 mg	No active metabolite	0.2–1 mg bolus; 0.2–2 mg/h gtts	$
Fentanyl	1 min	1.5–6 h	Hepatic Oxidation	200 μg	Chest wall rigidity	25–100 mcg bolus; 25–200 μg/h gtts	$$
Remifentanil	1–3 min	3–10 min	Plasma esterase	No data available	Fast offset → pain	0.6–15 μg/kg/h	$$$
Methadone	10–20 min IV; 30–60 min po	7–22 h	Hepatic, renal	10 mg	Prolonged elimination $T_{1/2}$ with repeat doses	10 mg po or IV q8–12 h	po: ¢ IV:$

cologic characteristics of commonly used opiates.[40,41] While comparative trials of narcotic agents have not been performed in a critically ill population, a physician's selection can be greatly aided by applying the knowledge of each agent's pharmacology and potential hazards. Fentanyl has the most rapid onset of action, typically within minutes, although with repeated dosing it may accumulate and cause prolonged effects. Morphine has a longer duration of action and can be used successfully as either a continuous drip or as an intermittent dosing regimen. Morphine's drawbacks include the potential for accumulation of an active metabolite in the setting of renal insufficiency, and excess histamine release causing flushing, bradycardia, or vasodilation.[42]

In clinical practice, we find significant histamine release to be a very rare occurrence. In addition, morphine may be the ideal analgesic for patients with acute heart failure in vasoconstrictive crisis, as it leads to venodilation as well as a slowed heart rate through sympatholytic activity and direct effects on the sinoatrial node.[43] While fentanyl and morphine account for the vast majority of narcotic agents used, hydromorphone—an agent with similar onset of action but slightly shorter duration of action than morphine—is occasionally chosen due to its lack of active metabolite.[29] Use of meperidine, another medium-onset narcotic, is discouraged for chronic analgesia as its active metabolite has neuroexcitatory properties that can lead to apprehension, tremors, and even seizures.[8,44–46]

One newer agent that is receiving attention of late is remifentanil, a narcotic derivative with an ester linkage that allows it to be metabolized by nonspecific esterases.[47] Due to this unique metabolism, remifentanil appears to have a very rapid onset and elimination, and it therefore may be of particular use for patients requiring frequent interruptions in medication for neurologic assessment.[29] Studies of remifentanil in the ICU setting include comparisons to morphine or fentanyl in intubated patients, and these investigations found no significant differences in hemodynamics or time to extubation.[48,49] Patients in the remifentanil group did report a higher incidence of pain, a potential disadvantage of remifentanil's rapid offset of action.[49] Remifentanil may accumulate in patients with renal insufficiency, with more variable time to offset in moderate to severe renal impairment.[50] As remifentanil is both more expensive than morphine and fentanyl and without a clear advantage over the older agents as regards time to extubation, it remains to be seen how widespread its use will become.

Another drug that warrants mention is methadone. Methadone is a synthetic opioid that can be given either enterally or parenterally and is much longer acting than morphine. It is similar to morphine both in its pain control and adverse effects, but is less sedating.[51] While methadone's long half-life makes it difficult to titrate in an acutely ill patient with fluctuating hemodynamics or analgesic requirements, it can be an excellent choice for a patient receiving narcotics for a prolonged period, or with a long recovery ahead.[51] In addition, methadone lacks active metabolites and does not accumulate in renal failure.[52]

All narcotics cause some degree of respiratory depression. This effect is centrally mediated and dose dependent, interacting with a patient's ability to metabolize the drug. The predominant mechanism by which narcotics induce respiratory depression is by blunting the response to hypercapnia and essentially obliterating the response to hypoxia. In mechanically ventilated patients with profound respiratory distress, hypoxemia, or refractory shock, clinicians may exploit these depressive properties, improving ventilator synchrony and reducing cough or patient effort. Narcotics typically have a minimal effect on a patient's hemodynamic parameters, provided that the patient is euvolemic. However, when a patient's blood pressure is sustained in part by endogenous catecholamine release, as is often the case for a distressed patient requiring emergent intubation or a patient in severe pain, hypotension following administration of any narcotic may be observed.

Our typical practice is to begin a low-dose, continuous IV infusion of morphine at induction of mechanical ventilation, which is titrated to patient comfort, synchrony with the ventilator, and the individual sedation goal chosen for the patient. A typical starting dose is 2 mg/h of morphine. Sedative medication is typically begun concurrently. In the heart failure patient not requiring mechanical ventilation, it is reasonable to use judicious morphine intermittently to allow adjustment to a noninvasive ventilation mask or merely to control pain. In these instances we prefer morphine to fentanyl due to the longer effect and the less potent immediate sedation.

Sedative Medications

Benzodiazepines

Benzodiazepines are sedative hypnotics that act by potentiating γ-aminobutyric acid (GABA) receptors, which inhibit central nervous system excitability. Through the GABA receptor, benzodiazepines regulate influx of chloride into the cell, which hyperpolarizes neurons and sets a higher excitability threshold. All members of the class are lipid soluble and thus widely distributed throughout body tissues, with the onset of action of each agent being proportional to its lipid solubility. Properties of commonly used sedative agents are listed in Table 60.3. As a class, benzodiazepines tend to have excellent sedative, hypnotic, and amnestic qualities, and they potentiate the

TABLE 60.3. Properties of commonly used sedating agents[20,29,51–70]

Agent	Onset p IV dose	$T_{1/2}$	Metabolism	Active metabolite	Unique side effect	Starting dose	Cost
Diazepam	2–5 min	20–120 h	Hepatic	Yes	Phlebitis	5–10 mg bolus q12–24 h No infusion	$
Lorazepam	5–20 min	8–15 h	Hepatic	No	Precipitation; solvent-induced acidosis; renal failure	2–5 mg bolus q4–12 h. No infusion	$
Midazolam	2–5 min	3–11 h	Hepatic	Yes	Prolonged sedation	1–3 mg bolus; 0.5–5 mg/h gtts	$$
Propofol	1–2 min	26–32 h	Oxidation	No	↑ triglycerides, ↑ pancreatic enzymes; lactic acidosis (esp. children)	10–15 μg/kg/min gtts No bolus	$$$
Dexmedetomidine	1–2 min	2 h	Hepatic	No	Approved for ICU sedation for <24 h; hypertension followed by hypotension, bradycardia	0.2–0.7 μg/kg/h No bolus	$$$

analgesic effects of narcotics.[2] Midazolam has the fastest onset of action, generally within 1 to 5 minutes, and has a short duration of action after one dose. Lorazepam has a lower lipid solubility, and thus a slightly longer onset of action, as well as a longer duration. Diazepam has a rapid onset but its metabolites are long-acting, causing a very prolonged sedative effect.

With all benzodiazepines, the pharmacokinetics in critically ill patients can be highly variable, especially when given by continuous infusion over long periods of time. Accumulation of the drug in peripheral tissues, where the drug cannot be metabolized, becomes commonplace, and after infusions are discontinued the peripheral tissue stores slowly release active drug back into the circulation, continuing the clinical effect.[53–55] Obese patients with large lipid stores and thus large volumes of distribution, as well as patients with renal and hepatic dysfunction, may be especially prone to prolonged effects. Because midazolam produces a pharmacologically active metabolite prone to accumulation whereas lorazepam does not, lorazepam is the preferred benzodiazepine for prolonged sedation. Lorazepam is best given as intermittent bolus rather than as a continuous infusion, both because its long half-life impairs one's ability to titrate a drip,[56] and because the drug may precipitate even when appropriately reconstituted due to its propylene glycol vehicle.[57] Rarely, lorazepam use in large doses has resulted in propylene glycol toxicity such as acute tubular necrosis, lactic acidosis, and hyperosmolality.[58]

Propofol

Propofol is a phenolic derivative whose mechanism of action is imprecisely understood but appears to involve modification of GABA receptors in the central nervous system (CNS). Propofol is recognized for its excellent sedative and hypnotic properties, and has some amnestic effect, although not as powerful as that of benzodiazepines. It provides no analgesia.[51] Prepared as an oil-in-water emulsion, it is highly lipophilic and thus rapidly crosses the blood–brain barrier, resulting in a rapid onset of action. Propofol also allows a rapid emergence from sedation, as its lipophilic nature permits a fast redistribution into peripheral tissues with metabolic clearance.[59] With bolus administration, propofol may cause a dose-dependent, transient hypotension associated with bradycardia, so slow initial infusions are generally recommended. Propofol has been characterized as both a negative inotrope and chronotrope[2]; however, in comparative studies, the hypotensive effect of propofol was not significantly different from that of midazolam during continuous infusions.[60,61] In fact, most sedative agents cause some degree of hypotension, likely due to the blunting of the body's endogenous catecholamine response, which accompanies most forms of respiratory distress (Fig. 60.2).[59,62] Propofol is a potent respiratory depressant, and thus is advocated for use only in intubated

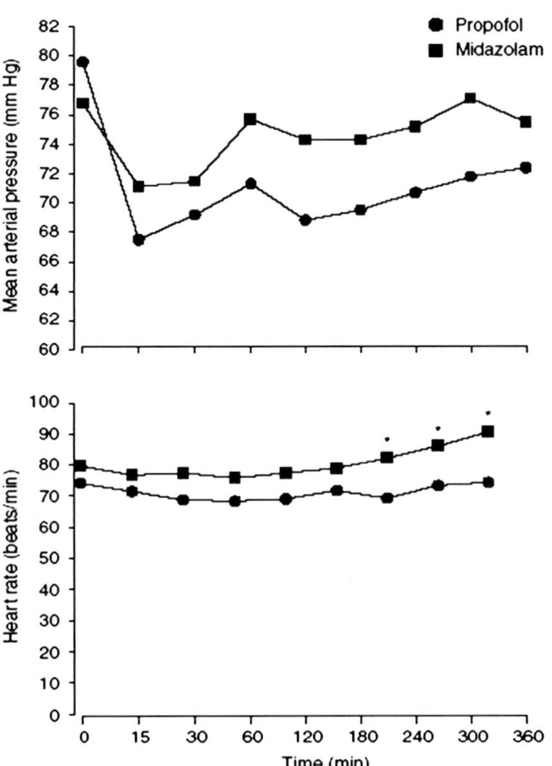

Figure 60.2. The comparative effects of propofol and midazolam on mean arterial blood pressure and heart rate. Patients were randomized to a propofol loading dose of 1 mg/kg followed by a mean infusion rate of 2.7 mg/kg/h ($n = 15$) or a midazolam loading dose of 0.07 mg/kg followed by a mean infusion rate of 0.092 mg/kg/h ($n = 15$) after coronary artery bypass graft surgery.[62] (*$p < .05$ vs. comparator.) (From McKeage and Perry,[59] with permission.)

patients, or if personnel trained to intubate are immediately on hand.

Several unique aspects of propofol concern its lipid formulation, which account for fat calories of 1.1 kcal/mL and mandate monitoring for hypertriglyceridemia and pancreatitis.[63] Its lipophilic emulsion is also considered a high risk for microbial contamination, and despite the addition of an antibacterial preservative to retard growth of microorganisms, propofol bottles and infusion tubing should be changed every 12 hours.[51] Lastly, the propofol infusion syndrome—a rare but often fatal syndrome involving severe lactic acidosis, rhabdomyolysis, renal failure, and cardiac dysrhythmias—has been reported in critically ill adults and children receiving high-dose propofol, often with corticosteroids and vasoactive support.[64–66] As such, most professional societies recommend against the use of propofol for ICU sedation in children under the age of 16. The risk of this catastrophic syndrome seems highest for patients who receive propofol at very high dose (>5 mg/kg/h or >80 μg/kg/min) for greater than 48 hours.[64]

Dexmedetomidine

Dexmedetomidine, a newer sedative agent, is an α_2-agonist that binds α_2-receptors eight times more avidly than clonidine, acting in the CNS to provide sedation and at the spinal cord to provide analgesia.[20] Attractive features of dexmedetomidine include marked sedation with relatively little respiratory depression, blunted hemodynamic response to intubation or other stressors, and potentiation of analgesia.[47,67–70] The agent was approved by the United States Food and Drug Administration (FDA) in 1999 for short-term—less than 24 hours—sedation in critically ill patients. It has yet to be approved for use in Europe. Patients receiving dexmedetomidine are described as appearing tranquil, but arousing easily and interactive if stimulated.[20] Potential adverse effects include hypertension, mediated by stimulation of α_2-receptors in the vasculature smooth muscle, followed by hypotension and bradycardia indicative of α_2-inhibition of sympathetic activity.[20] While dexmedetomidine has promise as an agent that may augment analgesia, blunt sympathetic overactivity, and prevent respiratory depression, its use in patients with acute heart failure remains unknown, and merits further study.

Analgesia and Sedation in the Context of Acute Heart Failure Syndrome

Specific to the patient with AHFS, there are several common scenarios that present themselves as the practitioner assesses for pain and anxiety. First, let us emphasize that the typical autonomic response to acute dyspnea and anxiety triggers a profound catecholamine release, which frequently exacerbates the AHFS patient's underlying left ventricular dysfunction. While this counterproductive response can mean that a patient will appear desperately ill upon presentation, much of the sympathetic overactivity is treated by appropriate control of the patient's dyspnea. As such, optimal control of dyspnea, pain, and anxiety greatly augment the success of concomitant medical therapy for AHFS.

We encounter three common scenarios when faced with a dyspneic patient with acute heart failure. In the least severe cases, patients may present with acute dyspnea and mild hypoxemia but without significant hypercapnia. Frequently, moderate anxiety accompanies this breathlessness. Within minutes of the administration of oxygen and appropriate medical therapy with diuresis, afterload reduction, and rate control, however, this group of patients reports considerable symptomatic relief. For such patients, it is reasonable to rapidly institute oxygen and medical therapy and to observe for a time before proceeding to analgesic or sedating medication. If the patient complains of chest discomfort, morphine would be a natural choice to mitigate both dyspnea and pain while attending to other potential etiologies of pain. Anxiolysis is rarely necessary once the patient's dyspnea has been properly managed.

The second common presentation is the patient with acute dyspnea but additional significant manifestations of acute heart failure, such as pulmonary edema on chest radiograph, moderate hypoxemia and hypercapnia, and severe anxiety.

For such patients, medical therapy alone is often ineffective at relieving dyspnea, and supplemental ventilatory assistance is required. As discussed in Chapter 45, noninvasive ventilation (NIV) is very effective for the majority of such patients and reduces the need for invasive ventilation.[71] Good candidates for NIV are those with competent mentation and normal intact airway reflexes.[72,73] Noninvasive ventilation is best reserved for patients without hemodynamic compromise, without need for transfer, and who will not require prolonged periods of lying supine for procedures. We advocate the use of judicious morphine for the treatment of pain and dyspnea associated with pulmonary edema and to help the patient adjust to NIV; many of the trials comparing NIV to oxygen in pulmonary edema used an average dose of 2 to 3 mg of morphine sulfate for patients whose $PaCO_2$ was below 50 mm Hg.[74,75] Patients receiving NIV for pulmonary edema must be closely monitored, as a failure to demonstrate an early improvement in gas exchange, respiratory rate, and heart rate should be viewed as probable indication for proceeding to mechanical ventilation.[72]

Finally, the patient with the most severe form of AHFS may present in cardiogenic shock, which necessitates intubation and mechanical ventilation. Other well-accepted indications for rapid intubation include patients who either require transfer to a higher level care facility or require a procedure, patients with impaired neurologic status, and patients with hypoxemia requiring high levels of positive end-expiratory pressure (PEEP). Most mechanically ventilated patients experience some discomfort related to the endotracheal tube,[76,77] which has led to the consensus opinion that pain and anxiety be aggressively controlled in such patients.[29] In general, successful strategies target both analgesia and anxiolysis.

In the critically ill patient with cardiogenic shock, sedation and analgesia often begin simultaneously with management of the airway. Once such a patient is deemed to require intubation and mechanical ventilation, we generally select morphine and propofol infusions and begin with very low dose administration of first morphine, at 2 mg/h, and subsequently propofol, at 5 to 10 μg/kg/min. The drips are then titrated with the aid of the bedside nurse to a targeted goal on the RASS, individualized for the patient's situation. If the patient's hemodynamics preclude use of any medication that may blunt sympathetic tone, we ask our anesthesiologists to attempt an awake intubation with ample local anesthetic, and then use a spontaneous mode of ventilation with abundant pressure support to match the patient's undoubtedly high minute ventilation until we have determined that an analgesic or anxiolytic is safe to use. We advocate continuous rather than bolus propofol, especially in patients with impaired cardiac reserve who may be more prone to the drug's cardiovascular suppressant effects. In patients who do manifest some hemodynamic reserve despite profound respiratory distress, we occasionally prescribe a bolus of low-dose fentanyl (50 to 100 μg) and/or midazolam (2 to 4 mg) immediately after intubation to help the patient accommodate to the ventilator while we begin low-dose infusions. In our experience, this has provided a smooth transition from bolus to continuous medication.

In practice, we have rarely found it necessary to use neuromuscular blocking drugs in order to achieve adequate sedation for the ventilated patient, and we caution against their routine use. Neuromuscular blockade can improve chest wall compliance, minimize a patient's respiratory muscle oxygen consumption, and in theory might facilitate a patient's adaptation to the ventilator,[78,79] but this comes at great risk to the patient. The chief complication of drug-induced paralysis in the intensive care unit is prolonged muscle weakness, which can occur in up to 10% of patients who receive neuromuscular blockade for more than 24 hours.[80] The resultant loss of power can be so pronounced as to resemble quadriparesis, and can impair the patient's ability to breathe spontaneously. Weakness is often multifactorial, but can take the form of myopathic, neuropathic, or neuromuscular junction abnormalities. Coadministration of agents with even weak effects at the neuromuscular junction, including magnesium sulfate, lidocaine, calcium channel blockers, or beta-blockers, can potentiate the neuromuscular blockade and compound the weakness.[78] In addition, practitioners have difficulty assessing the depth of sedation for patients who are paralyzed. Despite the widely accepted mantra that neuromuscular blockade mandates deep sedation

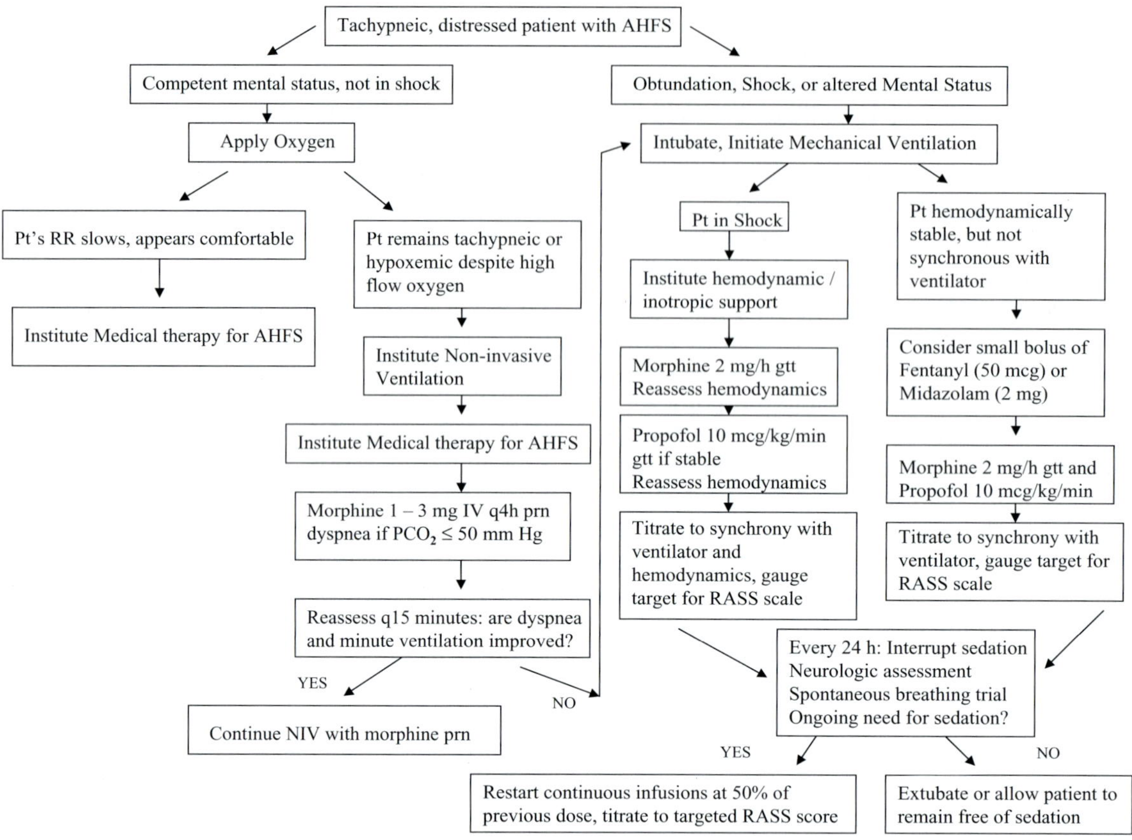

FIGURE 60.3. Algorithm to sedate the AHFS patient.

and analgesia to prevent awareness, one study found that 10% of patients receiving neuromuscular blockade and deep sedation recalled pain, discomfort, or anxiety.[22] We have rarely encountered such difficulty in achieving adequate sedation that paralytics become necessary, and advocate liberal use of narcotics and occasionally multiple sedative agents—propofol and a benzodiazepine—prior to considering neuromuscular blockade.

As the patient's medical therapy brings the AHFS slowly under control, we raise our targeted level of sedation for the patient toward "alert and calm," or RASS level 0.[35,36] We interrupt sedation daily to achieve this target, often combining this awakening with the patient's daily spontaneous breathing trial, and then make an assessment of whether the patient continues to require sedation or will be equally calm and stable without pharmacologic intervention. If we deem ongoing sedation necessary, we recommence the patient's previous continuous infusions at half of the prior dose, and again titrate to the desired level by the RASS scale. An algorithm depicting this approach to sedation in the distressed patient with severe AHFS is presented in Figure 60.3.

Complications of Sedation

As with any drug, the medications used for sedation and analgesia in the ICU may exhibit accumulation during organ failure, variable half-lives even in the same patient, and occasional drug–drug interactions. Even without dwelling on these issues, however, sedatives and narcotics are uniquely prone to accumulation, with persistent or protracted effect on the CNS or respiratory drive. Oversedation—when patients fails to arouse within the typical time period expected, given their hepatic function, renal function, and duration of medication use—can have measurable deleterious effects, such as prolonged stay on the ventilator and in the ICU, increased use in diagnostic procedures and imaging studies to explain altered mental status, and decreased reliability of the neurologic exam.[38,81] These observations have provided the impetus to better assess adequacy and depth of sedation, and to employ validated tools to individualize each patient's sedation.

Adaptation or physical dependence on narcotics or sedatives is another potential complication. While typically described as occurring after high-dose administration of narcotics and sedatives for longer than 1 week, withdrawal syndromes are occasionally observed in patients after as few as 3 to 5 days. The symptoms of withdrawal can range from discomfort—lacrimation, rhinorrhea, sweating, myalgias, agitation, anxiety—to the life-threatening, such as delirium and seizures.[82] A prospective study of infants—for whom there exists a validated opiate abstinence scoring system to objectify withdrawal—observed the frequency of withdrawal to be 57% in patients receiving intravenous fentanyl, and correlated the incidence of withdrawal both with total fentanyl dose and duration.[83] To date, all clinical investigations in adult critically ill populations have been retrospective; however, similar high-risk situations for opiate and sedative withdrawal have been established. One study found that the patients who experienced withdrawal were more likely to have received neuromuscular blocking agents or propofol during their ICU stay, and had received both higher mean daily doses and higher peak doses of opiates and benzodiazepines.[84] There was also an association between longer duration of mechanical ventilation and an increased rate of withdrawal.[84] Another study found a significant relationship between the rate of benzodiazepine and opiate taper and the occurrence of clinical withdrawal.[85]

While the retrospective nature of these studies makes it difficult to infer cause and effect, it seems clear that sedative withdrawal is associated with increased morbidity to the patient, and as such, practitioners must routinely screen for and treat withdrawal behaviors. To remedy this physical dependence, we advocate a multifaceted approach including a switch to longer acting forms of the offending medications—typically methadone and diazepam—in order to begin a slow titration downward in dose by 10% per day, concomitant use of clonidine to control sympathetic nervous system overactivity, and occasionally enlisting the help of a behavioral psychologist or psychiatrist to guide further pharmacologic management.[86]

Clinical Case

A 62-year-old woman with a history of ischemic cardiomyopathy and a reported left ventricular ejection fraction of 23% presents to the emergency department accompanied by her daughter. The daughter states that her mother called her to say that she awoke very short of breath that morning. When the daughter arrived, the patient's breathing appeared to be so labored that the daughter immediately called 911. The daughter reports that her mother had undergone bypass surgery 6 years earlier and an angioplasty 18 months ago, and she brings with her the following medications that she found in her mother's home: furosemide, carvedilol, spironolactone, lisinopril, aspirin, atorvastatin, and isosorbide mononitrate.

The patient is breathing 28 times a minute and appears fatigued. Vitals include a blood pressure of 176/98 mm Hg, pulse 114 beats per minute, temperature of 36.8°C, and pulse oximetry of 84% on room air. She is able to speak only in fragmented sentences, and despite being fully oriented, she is lethargic. Chest exam reveals crackles bilaterally to the mid-lung zone, and cardiac exam demonstrates thready pulses, delayed nailbed capillary return, tachycardia with an S_3 gallop, and jugular venous pulsation elevated to 11 cm. The patient has pitting edema confined to below the knees bilaterally.

The patient is immediately placed on oxygen at 10 L by face mask, which results in an improvement in oxygen saturation to 93%. She denies chest pain, and the electrocardiogram (ECG) reveals sinus tachycardia and evidence of an old infarction in the anterolateral leads, but no acute ST or T wave changes. She is given an intravenous dose of furosemide 120 mg, but the blood pressure remains elevated at 165/93 mm Hg, and her respiratory rate remains 28 breaths per minute. She is switched from face mask oxygen to noninvasive mask ventilation initially set at 6 cm H_2O continuous positive airway pressure (CPAP) with an FiO_2 of 60%. Her minute ventilation is high at 12 L/minute, but she adjusts well to the mask by having the respiratory therapist at her bedside, adjusting the fit and providing reassurance. The arterial blood gas (ABG) lab report, based on blood drawn while the patient was on face-mask ventilation, reveals pH of 7.29, PCO_2 of 54 mm Hg, PaO_2 of 66 mm Hg, and SaO_2 of 93%. Noting the acute respiratory acidosis, the physician adds inspiratory pressure to the patient's noninvasive ventilation, now with an inspiratory pressure of 14 cm H_2O over the expiratory pressure of 7 cm H_2O, and FiO_2 of 60%. On these settings, the patient's respiratory rate has slowed to 22 breaths per minute and she signals an improvement in her work of breathing. Repeat blood pressure is 136/88 mm Hg. Twenty minutes after the ventilator adjustment, the patient begins to pull at her mask and attempts to sit up off the bed. Her respiratory rate has climbed to 26 breaths per minute, but tidal volumes remain high at 500 mL. She is more alert, but appears panicked to her daughter. She continues to deny chest pressure, but reports, "I can't breathe." While a repeat ECG is performed, she is given morphine 2 mg intravenously, and within a few minutes is again breathing at a rate of 18 to 22 per minute and will lie back on the gurney. A repeat ABG shows a pH of 7.32, PCO_2 of 49 mm Hg, PaO_2 of 94 mm Hg, and SaO_2 of 96%.

A portable chest x-ray shows an enlarged cardiac silhouette with a wide vascular pedicle and air-space opacification in a gravity-dependent pattern, from both bases to almost two thirds of the way up her lungs. She has a moderate right pleural effusion. Her urine output has been 40 cc in the 30 minutes since her furosemide dose was given, but she still feels cool to touch and has thready pulses. Her blood pressure following a dose of captopril 12.5 mg is 96/80 mm Hg. Her mental status, initially improved on noninvasive ventilation with inspiratory pressure support, begins to worsen, and while she arouses in response to a loud voice or painful stimulus, she quickly drifts back to sleep. Her respiratory rate has begun to climb again and is now 26 breaths per minute on NIV, with a minute ventilation of 14 L/min. As her respiratory rate is increasing and a third ABG shows pH of 7.24, PCO_2 of 42 mm Hg, PaO_2 of 98 mm Hg, and SaO_2 of 95%, the patient's deteriorating mental status is correctly attributed to cardiogenic shock, rather than the small dose of narcotic. Dobutamine at 5 μg/kg/min is initiated, and she is intubated for cardiogenic shock.

Liberal administration of local anesthetic (4% viscous lidocaine jelly) to the base of the tongue and mouth allows an awake intubation by direct laryngoscopy; the patient does not struggle against the laryngoscope, and her immediate postintubation vitals include blood pressure of 98/76 mm Hg, heart rate of 123 beats per minute, and respiratory rate of 24 breaths per minute on a ventilator set with pressure support 20 cm H_20 over PEEP of 7 cm H_2O and 60% FiO_2. A morphine drip is begun at 2 mg/h and titrated slowly up to 6 mg/h for a targeted level of sedation of –3 (moderate sedation, some movement to sound) to –4 (deep sedation, movement only to physical stimuli) on the RASS scale. Propofol is begun simultaneously at 10 μg/kg/min by continuous infusion. With the secure airway, the patient is able to be transported out of the emergency department to the cardiac critical care unit. Fifteen minutes after the intubation, the patient's blood pressure is 88/71 mm Hg, respirations remain 22 breaths per minute with a minute ventilation of 14 L/minute, and heart rate is 96 beats per minute. Deep sedation facilitates expeditious placement of a right internal jugular venous catheter, which reveals a right atrial pressure of 18 cm H_2O. Central venous oxygen saturation drawn from the internal jugular vein is 42%. Chest radiograph confirms good placement of the endotracheal tube 3 cm above her carina, and shows the central line to be in good position. With the increase of dobutamine to 10 μg/kg/min, now administered through the central line, and norepinephrine 4 μg/min, the patient begins producing slightly more urine, 60 cc over the first hour and 80 cc in the next. Blood pressure remains low with a narrow pulse pressure, but the patient's urine output convinces her cardiologist to postpone an intraaortic balloon pump for the time being. Echocardiogram reveals left ventricular hypertrophy with globally reduced systolic function and anterior wall hypokinesis, and the left ventricular ejection fraction is reduced at 20%. There are no new regional wall motion abnormalities compared to an echocardiogram 18 months earlier. Cardiac enzymes have remained negative. The patient's creatinine is 2.3 mg/dL, whereas previously it had been 1.3 mg/dL. Bicarbonate is 19 mEq/L, and serum lactate is 1.2 mEq/L.

Over the next 24 hours, the patient's status slowly improves, with blood pressure now running 114/82 mm Hg on dobutamine alone. She has diuresed 4 L, for a net negative fluid balance of 2.6 L. Repeat central venous saturation is 65%. Her chest radiograph is considerably improved, showing air-space edema confined to the central medullary portions of her lungs, a vascular pedicle width that has diminished, and only a small right pleural effusion. She is tolerating 40% FiO_2 and PEEP of 5 cm H_2O, still with pressure support of 20 cm H_2O. Her most recent ABG is pH of 7.38, PCO_2 of 42 mm Hg, PaO_2 of 97 mm Hg, and SaO_2 of 96%. She remains deeply sedated, currently on propofol 30 μg/kg/min and morphine 6 mg/h. Sedatives are held to allow her to awaken, and within 60 minutes she has her eyes open and is squeezing her daughter's hand to command. She follows some simple commands such as "Stick out your tongue," but not "Show me two fingers." She is placed on a spontaneous breathing trial with 0 pressure support and 5 cm H_2O PEEP, and initially manifests a respiratory rate of 18 breaths per minute with tidal volumes of 450 mL, but breaths become successively more rapid and shallow over the next 45 minutes, so that at 60 minutes, her frequency to tidal volume ratio (F/V_T) is 120.[87] Central venous saturation at the end of the breathing trial had dropped to 58%, as has been described in some patients who fail to liberate from spontaneous ventilation.[88] As her breathing trial was unsuccessful, the physician opted to recommence sedation, but this time targeted to a RASS scale of −1 to −2 (light to moderate sedation), as the patient was no longer in extremis and seemed fairly well accommodated to the endotracheal tube. Morphine was reinitiated at 2 mg/h, and propofol at 10 μg/kg/min.

With further diureses of 4 L, titration off dobutamine, and reinitiation of her medical regimen of angiotensin-converting enzyme (ACE) inhibitor, nitrate therapy, and eventually carvedilol, the patient appears hemodynamically stable on the third hospital day. Again, sedation is interrupted to allow awakening, and as the sedation had been deliberately less deep than the previous day, the patient is awake within 15 minutes and following all commands. Another spontaneous breathing trial is performed, and this time the patient lasts 90 minutes breathing at a rate of 16 to 20 breaths per minute with a tidal volume of 420 mL (F/V_T 48). Central venous saturation was 69% at the outset of her spontaneous breathing trail, and is 68% at its completion. She is successfully extubated, and continues to receive aggressive medical management of her acute heart failure syndrome in the cardiac care unit (CCU) for 2 more days before being transferred to the cardiology floor.

Conclusion

Pain and anxiety are common among critically ill patients, and should be considered present unless the patient explicitly denies them. The most reliable indicator of pain is the patient herself. If a patient is unable to communicate her pain, the clinician must integrate nonverbal, behavioral, and physiologic clues in titrating analgesia.

Hospitalization for AHFS is inherently anxiety-provoking, and anxiety may manifest either as restless agitation or as quiet, hypoactive withdrawal. Acute dyspnea and discomfort in the patient with AHFS tends to trigger excessive sympathetic tone, which exacerbates the patient's heart function. By alleviating the patient's dyspnea, pain, and anxiety, providers greatly mitigate this counterproductive catecholamine surge, and often simultaneously improve heart function.

References

1. Nieminen MS, Bohm M, Cowie MR, et al. Executive summary of the guidelines on the diagnosis and treatment of acute heart failure: the Task Force on Acute Heart Failure of the European Society of Cardiology. Eur Heart J 2005;26:384–416.
2. Nasraway SA Jr. Use of sedative medications in the intensive care unit. Semin Respir Crit Care Med 2001;22:165–74.
3. Novaes MA, Knobel E, Bork AM, Pavao OF, Nogueira-Martins LA, Ferraz MB. Stressors in ICU: perception of the patient, relatives and health care team. Intensive Care Med 1999;25:1421–6.

4. Desbiens NA, Wu AW, Broste SK, et al. Pain and satisfaction with pain control in seriously ill hospitalized adults: findings from the SUPPORT research investigations. For the SUPPORT investigators. Study to Understand Prognoses and Preferences for Outcomes and Risks of Treatment. Crit Care Med 1996;24:1953–61.
5. Epstein J, Breslow MJ. The stress response of critical illness. Crit Care Clin 1999;15:17–33, v.
6. Parker SD, Breslow MJ, Frank SM, et al. Catecholamine and cortisol responses to lower extremity revascularization: correlation with outcome variables. Perioperative Ischemia Randomized Anesthesia Trial Study Group. Crit Care Med 1995;23: 1954–61.
7. Leddy KM, Wolosin RJ. Patient satisfaction with pain control during hospitalization. Jt Comm J Qual Patient Saf 2005;31:507–13.
8. Acute pain management: operative or medical procedures and trauma, Part 1. Agency for Health Care Policy and Research. Clin Pharm 1992;11:309–31.
9. Acute pain management: operative or medical procedures and trauma, Part 2. Agency for Health Care Policy and Research. Clin Pharm 1992;11:391–414.
10. Jensen MP, Karoly P, Braver S. The measurement of clinical pain intensity: a comparison of six methods. Pain 1986;27:117–26.
11. Hockenberry MJ, Wilson D, Winkelstein ML. Wong's Essentials of Pediatric Nursing, 7th ed. St. Louis: Mosby, 2005.
12. Terai T, Yukioka H, Asada A. Pain evaluation in the intensive care unit: observer-reported faces scale compared with self-reported visual analog scale. Reg Anesth Pain Med 1998;23:147–51.
13. Mularski RA. Pain management in the intensive care unit. Crit Care Clin 2004;20:381–401, viii.
14. Puntillo KA, Miaskowski C, Kehrle K, Stannard D, Gleeson S, Nye P. Relationship between behavioral and physiological indicators of pain, critical care patients' self-reports of pain, and opioid administration. Crit Care Med 1997;25:1159–66.
15. Desbiens NA, Mueller-Rizner N. How well do surrogates assess the pain of seriously ill patients? Crit Care Med 2000;28:1347–52.
16. Fraser GL, Prato BS, Riker RR, Berthiaume D, Wilkins ML. Frequency, severity, and treatment of agitation in young versus elderly patients in the ICU. Pharmacotherapy 2000;20:75–82.
17. Misak C. ICU psychosis and patient autonomy: some thoughts from the inside. J Med Philos 2005;30:411–30.
18. Misak CJ. The critical care experience: a patient's view. Am J Respir Crit Care Med 2004;170:357–9.
19. Schelling G, Stoll C, Haller M, et al. Health-related quality of life and posttraumatic stress disorder in survivors of the acute respiratory distress syndrome. Crit Care Med 1998;26:651–9.
20. Coursin DB, Maccioli GA. Dexmedetomidine. Curr Opin Crit Care 2001;7:221–6.
21. Johnson KL, Cheung RB, Johnson SB, Roberts M, Niblett J, Manson D. Therapeutic paralysis of critically ill trauma patients: perceptions of patients and their family members. Am J Crit Care 1999; 8:490–8.
22. Wagner BK, Zavotsky KE, Sweeney JB, Palmeri BA, Hammond JS. Patient recall of therapeutic paralysis in a surgical critical care unit. Pharmacotherapy 1998;18:358–63.
23. Kress JP, Gehlbach B, Lacy M, Pliskin N, Pohlman AS, Hall JB. The long-term psychological effects of daily sedative interruption on critically ill patients. Am J Respir Crit Care Med 2003;168:1457–61.
24. Jones C, Griffiths RD, Humphris G. Disturbed memory and amnesia related to intensive care. Memory 2000;8:79–94.
25. Jones C, Griffiths RD, Humphris G, Skirrow PM. Memory, delusions, and the development of acute posttraumatic stress disorder-related symptoms after intensive care. Crit Care Med 2001;29: 573–80.
26. Herridge MS, Cheung AM, Tansey CM, et al. One-year outcomes in survivors of the acute respiratory distress syndrome. N Engl J Med 2003;348:683–93.
27. Ely EW, Siegel MD, Inouye SK. Delirium in the intensive care unit: an under-recognized syndrome of organ dysfunction. Semin Respir Crit Care Med 2001;22:115–26.
28. Ely EW, Shintani A, Truman B, et al. Delirium as a predictor of mortality in mechanically ventilated patients in the intensive care unit. JAMA 2004; 291:1753–62.
29. Jacobi J, Fraser GL, Coursin DB, et al. Clinical practice guidelines for the sustained use of sedatives and analgesics in the critically ill adult. Crit Care Med 2002;30:119–41.
30. Ely EW, Inouye SK, Bernard GR, et al. Delirium in mechanically ventilated patients: validity and reliability of the confusion assessment method for the intensive care unit (CAM-ICU). JAMA 2001;286: 2703–10.
31. Ramsay MA, Savege TM, Simpson BR, Goodwin R. Controlled sedation with alphaxalone-alphadolone. Br Med J 1974;2:656–9.
32. De Jonghe B, Cook D, Appere-De-Vecchi C, Guyatt G, Meade M, Outin H. Using and understanding sedation scoring systems: a systematic review. Intensive Care Med 2000;26:275–85.

33. Hansen-Flaschen J, Cowen J, Polomano RC. Beyond the Ramsay scale: need for a validated measure of sedating drug efficacy in the intensive care unit. Crit Care Med 1994;22:732–3.
34. Riker RR, Picard JT, Fraser GL. Prospective evaluation of the Sedation-Agitation Scale for adult critically ill patients. Crit Care Med 1999;27:1325–9.
35. Ely EW, Truman B, Shintani A, et al. Monitoring sedation status over time in ICU patients: reliability and validity of the Richmond Agitation-Sedation Scale (RASS). JAMA 2003;289:2983–91.
36. Sessler CN, Gosnell MS, Grap MJ, et al. The Richmond Agitation-Sedation Scale: validity and reliability in adult intensive care unit patients. Am J Respir Crit Care Med 2002;166:1338–44.
37. De Jonghe B, Cook D, Griffith L, et al. Adaptation to the Intensive Care Environment (ATICE): development and validation of a new sedation assessment instrument. Crit Care Med 2003;31:2344–54.
38. Kress JP, Pohlman AS, O'Connor MF, Hall JB. Daily interruption of sedative infusions in critically ill patients undergoing mechanical ventilation. N Engl J Med 2000;342:1471–7.
39. Kamei J. Role of opioidergic and serotonergic mechanisms in cough and antitussives. Pulmon Pharmacol 1996;9:349–56.
40. Wagner BK, O'Hara DA. Pharmacokinetics and pharmacodynamics of sedatives and analgesics in the treatment of agitated critically ill patients. Clin Pharmacokinet 1997;33:426–53.
41. Barr J, Donner A. Optimal intravenous dosing strategies for sedatives and analgesics in the intensive care unit. Crit Care Clin 1995;11:827–47.
42. Rosow CE, Moss J, Philbin DM, Savarese JJ. Histamine release during morphine and fentanyl anesthesia. Anesthesiology 1982;56:93–6.
43. Hsu HO, Hickey RF, Forbes AR. Morphine decreases peripheral vascular resistance and increases capacitance in man. Anesthesiology 1979;50:98–102.
44. Danziger LH, Martin SJ, Blum RA. Central nervous system toxicity associated with meperidine use in hepatic disease. Pharmacotherapy 1994;14:235–8.
45. Hagmeyer KO, Mauro LS, Mauro VF. Meperidine-related seizures associated with patient-controlled analgesia pumps. Ann Pharmacother 1993;27:29–32.
46. Mauro VF, Bonfiglio MF, Spunt AL. Meperidine-induced seizure in a patient without renal dysfunction or sickle cell anemia. Clin Pharm 1986;5:837–9.
47. Maze M, Scarfini C, Cavaliere F. New agents for sedation in the intensive care unit. Crit Care Clin 2001;17:881–97.
48. Chinachoti T, Kessler P, Kirkham A, Werawatganon T. Remifentanil vs morphine for patients in intensive care unit who need short-term mechanical ventilation. J Med Assoc Thai 2002;85(suppl 3):S848–57.
49. Muellejans B, Lopez A, Cross MH, Bonome C, Morrison L, Kirkham AJ. Remifentanil versus fentanyl for analgesia based sedation to provide patient comfort in the intensive care unit: a randomized, double-blind controlled trial [ISRCTN43755713]. Crit Care 2004;8:R1–R11.
50. Breen D, Wilmer A, Bodenham A, et al. Offset of pharmacodynamic effects and safety of remifentanil in intensive care unit patients with various degrees of renal impairment. Crit Care 2004;8:R21–30.
51. Liu LL, Gropper MA. Postoperative analgesia and sedation in the adult intensive care unit: a guide to drug selection. Drugs 2003;63:755–67.
52. Davis MP, Walsh D. Methadone for relief of cancer pain: a review of pharmacokinetics, pharmacodynamics, drug interactions and protocols of administration. Support Care Cancer 2001;9:73–83.
53. Malacrida R, Fritz ME, Suter PM, Crevoisier C. Pharmacokinetics of midazolam administered by continuous intravenous infusion to intensive care patients. Crit Care Med 1992;20:1123–6.
54. Shelly MP, Mendel L, Park GR. Failure of critically ill patients to metabolise midazolam. Anaesthesia 1987;42:619–26.
55. Shelly MP, Sultan MA, Bodenham A, Park GR. Midazolam infusions in critically ill patients. Eur J Anaesthesiol 1991;8:21–7.
56. Pohlman AS, Simpson KP, Hall JB. Continuous intravenous infusions of lorazepam versus midazolam for sedation during mechanical ventilatory support: a prospective, randomized study. Crit Care Med 1994;22:1241–7.
57. McCollam JS, O'Neil MG, Norcross ED, Byrne TK, Reeves ST. Continuous infusions of lorazepam, midazolam, and propofol for sedation of the critically ill surgery trauma patient: a prospective, randomized comparison. Crit Care Med 1999;27:2454–8.
58. Laine GA, Hossain SM, Solis RT, Adams SC. Polyethylene glycol nephrotoxicity secondary to prolonged high-dose intravenous lorazepam. Ann Pharmacother 1995;29:1110–4.
59. McKeage K, Perry CM. Propofol: a review of its use in intensive care sedation of adults. CNS Drugs 2003;17:235–72.
60. Aitkenhead AR, Pepperman ML, Willatts SM, et al. Comparison of propofol and midazolam for sedation in critically ill patients. Lancet 1989;2:704–9.

61. Chamorro C, de Latorre FJ, Montero A, et al. Comparative study of propofol versus midazolam in the sedation of critically ill patients: results of a prospective, randomized, multicenter trial. Crit Care Med 1996;24:932–9.
62. Roekaerts PM, Huygen FJ, de Lange S. Infusion of propofol versus midazolam for sedation in the intensive care unit following coronary artery surgery. J Cardiothorac Vasc Anesth 1993;7:142–7.
63. Kumar AN, Schwartz DE, Lim KG. Propofol-induced pancreatitis: recurrence of pancreatitis after rechallenge. Chest 1999;115:1198–9.
64. Vasile B, Rasulo F, Candiani A, Latronico N. The pathophysiology of propofol infusion syndrome: a simple name for a complex syndrome. Intensive Care Med 2003;29:1417–25.
65. Koch M, De Backer D, Vincent JL. Lactic acidosis: an early marker of propofol infusion syndrome? Intensive Care Med 2004;30:522.
66. Perrier ND, Baerga-Varela Y, Murray MJ. Death related to propofol use in an adult patient. Crit Care Med 2000;28:3071–4.
67. Belleville JP, Ward DS, Bloor BC, Maze M. Effects of intravenous dexmedetomidine in humans. I. Sedation, ventilation, and metabolic rate. Anesthesiology 1992;77:1125–33.
68. Scheinin B, Lindgren L, Randell T, Scheinin H, Scheinin M. Dexmedetomidine attenuates sympathoadrenal responses to tracheal intubation and reduces the need for thiopentone and peroperative fentanyl. Br J Anaesth 1992;68:126–31.
69. Venn M, Newman J, Grounds M. A phase II study to evaluate the efficacy of dexmedetomidine for sedation in the medical intensive care unit. Intensive Care Med 2003;29:201–7.
70. Venn RM, Hell J, Grounds RM. Respiratory effects of dexmedetomidine in the surgical patient requiring intensive care. Crit Care 2000;4:302–8.
71. Agarwal R, Aggarwal AN, Gupta D, Jindal SK. Non-invasive ventilation in acute cardiogenic pulmonary oedema. Postgrad Med J 2005;81:637–43.
72. Pang D, Keenan SP, Cook DJ, Sibbald WJ. The effect of positive pressure airway support on mortality and the need for intubation in cardiogenic pulmonary edema: a systematic review. Chest 1998;114:1185–92.
73. Brochard L. Noninvasive ventilation for acute respiratory failure. JAMA 2002;288:932–5.
74. Lin M, Yang YF, Chiang HT, Chang MS, Chiang BN, Cheitlin MD. Reappraisal of continuous positive airway pressure therapy in acute cardiogenic pulmonary edema. Short-term results and long-term follow-up. Chest 1995;107:1379–86.
75. Bellone A, Vettorello M, Monari A, Cortellaro F, Coen D. Noninvasive pressure support ventilation vs. continuous positive airway pressure in acute hypercapnic pulmonary edema. Intensive Care Med 2005;31:807–11.
76. Puntillo KA. Pain experiences of intensive care unit patients. Heart Lung 1990;19:526–33.
77. Turner JS, Briggs SJ, Springhorn HE, Potgieter PD. Patients' recollection of intensive care unit experience. Crit Care Med 1990;18:966–8.
78. Murphy GS, Vender JS. Neuromuscular-blocking drugs. Use and misuse in the intensive care unit. Crit Care Clin 2001;17:925–42.
79. Hunter JM. New neuromuscular blocking drugs. N Engl J Med 1995;332:1691–9.
80. Murray MJ, Strickland RA, Weiler C. The use of neuromuscular blocking drugs in the intensive care unit: a US perspective. Intensive Care Med 1993;19(suppl 2):S40–4.
81. Kollef MH, Levy NT, Ahrens TS, Schaiff R, Prentice D, Sherman G. The use of continuous i.v. sedation is associated with prolongation of mechanical ventilation. Chest 1998;114:541–8.
82. George CF, Robertson D. Clinical consequences of abrupt drug withdrawal. Med Toxicol Adverse Drug Exp 1987;2:367–82.
83. Katz R, Kelly HW, Hsi A. Prospective study on the occurrence of withdrawal in critically ill children who receive fentanyl by continuous infusion. Crit Care Med 1994;22:763–7.
84. Cammarano WB, Pittet JF, Weitz S, Schlobohm RM, Marks JD. Acute withdrawal syndrome related to the administration of analgesic and sedative medications in adult intensive care unit patients. Crit Care Med 1998;26:676–84.
85. Brown C, Albrecht R, Pettit H, McFadden T, Schermer C. Opioid and benzodiazepine withdrawal syndrome in adult burn patients. Am Surg 2000;66:367–70;discussion 370–1.
86. Hogarth DK, Hall J. Management of sedation in mechanically ventilated patients. Curr Opin Crit Care 2004;10:40–6.
87. Yang KL, Tobin MJ. A prospective study of indexes predicting the outcome of trials of weaning from mechanical ventilation. N Engl J Med 1991;324:1445–50.
88. Jubran A, Mathru M, Dries D, Tobin MJ. Continuous recordings of mixed venous oxygen saturation during weaning from mechanical ventilation and the ramifications thereof. Am J Respir Crit Care Med 1998;158:1763–9.

61 Intraaortic Balloon Pump in the Management of Acute Heart Failure Syndromes

Eleftheria P. Tsagalou, Stavros G. Drakos, Elias Tsolakis, and John N. Nanas

Since its introduction by Moulopoulos et al. (1), the intraaortic balloon pump (IABP) has become essential for the treatment of cardiogenic shock. The flexible catheter with a polyurethane balloon mounted at its distal end is placed in the descending thoracic aorta from the femoral artery. Driven by a console, the balloon is deflated during cardiac systole, lowering left ventricular (LV) afterload, and inflated during diastole, increasing aortic diastolic pressure. Interactions between these effects explain the range of physiologic properties of the IABP. According to the Suga-Sagawa law, a linear relation exists between LV end-systolic pressure and end-systolic volume (ESV), if contractility remains unchanged (2,3). The increase in aortic compliance by balloon deflation during systole lowers the aortic and LV systolic pressures, which, according to the law, causes a proportionate decrease in ESV and, in the absence of change in LV end-diastolic volume (EDV), an increase in LV stroke volume and cardiac output. Blood ejected during diastole into the aorta receives additional energy by inflation of the balloon, resulting in greater blood flow and organ perfusion.

This chapter discusses the hemodynamic and metabolic effects of the IABP.

Hemodynamic Effects

Aortic Pressure

Deflation of the balloon at the end of diastole and during systole increases the aortic compliance during the systolic phase of the LV and so decreases the aortic pressure. The latter might also be due to changes in baroreceptor responses mediated by balloon pumping (4). The amount of decrease in systolic blood pressure depends mainly on the arterial compliance (5) and on LV stroke volume. The rapid inflation of the balloon immediately after closure of the aortic valve (onset of diastole) produces an additional pressure waveform known as aortic diastolic augmentation. The peak diastolic aortic pressure during optimal IABP support can be higher than the systolic aortic pressure, and the mean aortic pressure might remain unchanged or increase slightly (6).

Left Ventricular End-Diastolic Pressure

A decrease in left ventricular end-diastolic pressure (LVEDP) can occur by a shift of the LV pressure-volume curve to the left, decreasing the LVEDV. In severe LV failure, left ventricular ejection fraction (LVEF) and stroke volume might increase despite no change in LVEDP and LVEDV (7).

Left Ventricular Ejection Fraction

Because of a linear relationship, a decrease in end-systolic aortic pressure causes a proportionate decrease in LVESV (3). Thus, lowering of end-systolic pressure by IABP increases LVEF, provided that the preload, measured as LVEDV, is not lowered. In clinical studies, a greater increase in LVEF by IABP was observed in the presence of myocardial ischemia than in the presence of severe LV failure or large myocardial infarction (MI) (8,9).

Cardiac Output

In patients presenting with cardiogenic shock, the reported effects of IABP on cardiac output have varied from no change to increases ranging between 20% and 100% (10,11). This variability is attributable to individual variations in contractility and changes in preload induced by the IABP.

Tension-Time Index, Diastolic Pressure-Time Index, and Endocardial Viability Ratio

Tension-time index (TTI), the area under the LV systolic pressure curve within 1 minute, is strongly correlated with LV work and myocardial oxygen (O_2) demand (12). The IABP consistently decreases the TTI, indicating a proportionate decrease in myocardial O_2 demand.

The diastolic pressure-time index (DPTI), the sum of diastolic aortic pressures minus the corresponding LV pressure within 1 minute, is related to myocardial O_2 supply (13). This index is markedly increased by the IABP, mainly from augmentation of the diastolic aortic pressure, and secondarily from a decrease in LV diastolic pressure.

The endocardial viability ratio (EVR), equals to DPTI/TTI represents an index of balance between myocardial O_2 supply and demand in an individual patient (13). Values <0.7 indicate a severe shortage of myocardial O_2 supply. The IABP increases EVR by increasing DPTI and decreasing TTI. This increase is particularly important when myocardial ischemia or stunning contributes significantly to myocardial dysfunction, circumstances in which EVR can be used as an indication to apply IABP (14).

Effects of Balloon Counterpulsation on the Left Ventricular Isovolumetric Phase

The rapid deflation of the IABP decreases the end-diastolic aortic pressure and prompts an earlier opening of the aortic valve, shortening the isovolumetric phase of LV contraction and decreasing myocardial O_2 consumption (15). A 10% decrease in the peak rate of rise in LV pressure (dP/dT) also has been described (16).

Pulmonary Circulation

The decrease in pulmonary capillary wedge pressure (PCWP) by the IABP decreases intrapulmonary shunting, the amount of extravascular lung water, pulmonary vascular resistance, and the arterial-alveolar O_2 difference (17).

Effects of Balloon Counterpulsation on the Right Ventricle

The effects of the IABP on right ventricular function depend on the underlying cause of heart failure. It reduces RV afterload by decreasing PCWP and increases the pressure-dependent O_2 supply. A decrease in central venous and pulmonary pressures, and an increase in RV output have been observed in most clinical studies. However, data on the effects of the IABP in isolated RV failure are few. Experimental (18,19) and clinical (20) studies have shown hemodynamic improvements, which have been attributed to ventricular interdependence (18) or to a decrease in pulmonary arterial resistance (19).

Heart Rate and Rhythm

The heart rate usually decreases during IABP support, and ventricular premature activity is often suppressed as a result of improvements in myocardial O_2 supply versus demand, higher cardiac output, and a decrease in sympathetic activity (4).

Peripheral Vascular Resistance

In patients with cardiogenic shock and increased peripheral vascular resistance, improvements in hemodynamic function conferred by the IABP result in a decrease in peripheral vascular resistance (21). However, not all patients who develop MI-induced cardiogenic shock have an increased peripheral vascular resistance.

Metabolic Effects

Coronary Blood Flow

Coronary blood flow is directly related to the perfusion pressure, the presence of stenosis in the epicardial arteries, and the intramyocardial vascular resistance. The blood pressure at the origin of a coronary artery is similar to the aortic pressure. The coronary flow is mainly autoregulated in the intramyocardial arterial bed by changes in resistance in response to myocardial oxygen demand. Thus changes in perfusion pressure influence coronary blood flow only when associated with maximal coronary vasodilation as, for instance, in the presence of a critical coronary stenosis or severe hypotension. In animals with normal hearts, the IABP reduces coronary blood flow by lowering myocardial oxygen demand (22), while in patients in cardiogenic shock a prominent increase in coronary blood flow has been observed (23,24).

Peripheral Organ Perfusion

A >50% increase in carotid blood flow by the IABP was observed in an experimental study (25), while in patients its effects remain controversial (26–28). Likewise, data on the effects of the IABP on renal blood flow are conflicting (25,29–31), although renal function usually improves with or without improvement in cardiac function (32). Mesenteric and splanchnic perfusions are also improved by the IABP (26).

Effect in Acute Myocardial Infarction

The addition of IABP to thrombolysis enhanced myocardial salvage in animals (33,34), by LV unloading, improving the oxygen supply/demand ratio, increasing the coronary blood flow, and mitigating no-reflow phenomenon (34,35). Furthermore, the IABP accelerates the recovery of LV function after reperfusion (36).

Determinants of Balloon Counterpulsation Performance

Inflation and Deflation Timing

Proper timing of the balloon inflation and deflation is usually accomplished by using the electrocardiogram, a pacing signal, or the aortic pressure waveform. The optimal timing of deflation, before the aortic valve opens (37), strongly influences LV afterload. Early deflation may cause suboptimal diastolic augmentation and coronary and carotid flow reversal (28), while late deflation may result in late aortic valve opening and an increase in afterload and LV energy consumption (38).

Inflation of the balloon is timed to start at the onset of diastole, 40 ms before the dicrotic notch on the recorded aortic pressure waveform. Early inflation causes premature aortic valve closure and less LV unloading, and late inflation causes suboptimal aortic augmentation.

Balloon Size and Position

While the hemodynamic performance of the IABP is directly related to its stroke volume (39), balloon diameters >90% of the descending aorta diameter may cause trauma to the aorta and distal hypoperfusion, whereas small balloons do not effectively augment diastole (40). Placement of the balloon near the aortic valve increases the amount of diastolic augmentation (40,41). The tip of the catheter should be placed distal to the aortic arch branches, while a much lower placement causes poor performance and may occlude the splanchnic arteries (40).

Heart Rate

Optimal hemodynamics are reached at heart rates between 80 and 110 bpm (42). Rates >120 bpm may be associated with incomplete balloon inflation and deflation, low diastolic augmentation, and ineffective LV unloading. The long diastole associated with rates >80 bpm does not allow the achievement of optimal simultaneous diastolic augmentation and systolic unloading. Delaying balloon inflation away from the time of aortic valve closure while leaving deflation at its optimal timing will optimize systolic unloading against diastolic augmentation. The opposite result is reached by inflating the balloon near the time of aortic valve closure (40,43).

Other Factors

The effectiveness of IABP also depends on the LV stroke volume (40,44) and aortic blood pressure. In patients with a mean aortic pressure <40 mm Hg, the IABP is not effective (5). A low systemic vascular resistance and highly distensible aortic wall are causes of ineffective balloon function, whereas a stiff aortic wall results in a high aortic pressure during balloon inflation (21,26).

Results of Clinical Trials

Acute Myocardial Infarction Complicated by Hypotension and Acute Heart Failure

The Thrombolysis And Counterpulsation To Improve Cardiogenic shock Survival (TACTICS) trial (45) examined the benefits conferred by IABP added to thrombolytic therapy for MI complicated by sustained hypotension, acute heart failure, or cardiogenic shock. An IABP was inserted at a median of 30 minutes after thrombolysis and continued for a median of 34 hours. There was a trend toward lower 6-month mortality ($p = .23$) among patients randomly assigned to thrombolysis and IABP (34%) versus thrombolysis alone (43%). The difference was significant in the subgroup of patients with Killip class III or IV (39% vs. 80%; $p = .05$).

Acute Myocardial Infarction Associated with Severe Acute Heart Failure and Cardiogenic Shock

The incidence of cardiogenic shock, the most serious complication of acute MI, is 6% to 8%, with an approximately 50% 30-day mortality (46).

Prethrombolytic Era

In the early 1980s, two small randomized trials showed no benefit of IABP on infarct size or mortality in patients with cardiogenic shock (47,48). One trial, which compared IABP and intravenous (IV) nitroglycerin for 4 to 5 days versus routine management in patients with large amounts of myocardium at risk, observed no significant difference in mortality or clinical outcomes between 10 patients who received combined treatment versus 10 who were routinely managed (47). However, the afterload-lowering effects of combined IABP and nitroglycerin appeared to prevent dilation or remodeling of the noninfarcted segments during the first 2 weeks after MI.

In a second trial (48), 30 patients with early transmural MI complicated by cardiogenic shock were randomly assigned to IABP ($n = 14$) versus standard therapy ($n = 16$). Counterpulsation began at a mean of 7.1 hours (range 4.8 to 13.7 hours) after the onset of pain and was continued for up to 11 days (mean = 4.5). No difference was observed between the two groups in in-hospital or long-term mortality or in functional class among the 1- to 36-month survivors.

Thrombolytic Era

Although the effectiveness of thrombolytic therapy (TT) in the setting of post-MI cardiogenic shock is controversial (49–52), in various trials, IABP promoted thrombolysis, hastened the onset of coronary artery reperfusion, and salvaged considerable amounts of myocardium (24,33,53,54). Furthermore, one randomized and five observational studies (45,56–60) showed that TT plus IABP was associated with a significantly lower mortality than TT alone (Table 61.1).

Mechanical Revascularization Era

In the SHould we emergently revascularize Occluded Coronaries for cardiogenic shocK (SHOCK) trial (61), 302 patients with post-MI cardiogenic shock were randomly assigned to initial emergent revascularization versus medical management. An IABP was used in 86% of patients in both groups. Early revascularization resulted in a significant decrease in 6-month mortality (50.3% vs. 63.1%, $p = .027$). The low overall mortality in both arms, compared to historic controls, was attributed to intensive medical management, including a high rate of IABP utilization (61,62). Since the publication of the SHOCK trial results, rapid reperfusion of the infarct-related artery is

Table 61.1. Mortality of patients with cardiogenic shock treated with intraaortic balloon pump (IABP) versus controls in the thrombolytic era

	% Mortality		
	IABP	Control	p
National registry MI-2[56] ($n = 23{,}180$)*	49	67	<.05
GUSTO-I[57] ($n = 310$)†	47	60	.06
Waksman et al.[58] ($n = 85$)*	54	81	.001
Kovack et al[59] ($n = 46$)†	33	68	.019
SHOCK trial registry[60] ($n = 856$)*	47	63	<.001

*In-hospital mortality; †30-day mortality.

considered key in the management of post-MI cardiogenic shock (46,63–65), during hemodynamic support with the IABP.

Among 856 patients with post-MI cardiogenic shock included in the SHOCK trial registry (60) the in-hospital mortality was lowest (p <.0001) with TT plus IABP (47%), versus IABP only (52%), versus TT only (63%), versus neither TT nor IABP (77%). Coronary revascularization was performed during the same hospitalization in 68% and 70% of patients treated with TT plus IABP and IABP only, respectively, versus 20% and 18% of patients treated with TT only and neither TT nor IABP, respectively (p = .0001). Furthermore, in-hospital mortality was 39% among revascularized vs. 78% among nonrevascularized patients (p = .0001). Thus, the survival benefit observed among patients treated with the IABP was attributable to the higher rates of revascularization performed later during hospitalization. Similarly, in pooled data from the Global Utilization of Streptokinase and Tissue plasminogen activator for Occluded coronary arteries (GUSTO) I and III trials (66), 3396 patients in cardiogenic shock treated with IABP had a lower 30-day mortality (45%) than controls (58%, p = .001). Patients treated with IABP were more likely to undergo cardiac catheterization and coronary revascularization than patients who were not treated with the IABP. Bengtson et al. (67) studied 200 patients from the Duke Cardiovascular Databank who developed MI-induced cardiogenic shock. The in-hospital mortality was 53%, and its most important independent predictors were infarct-related artery patency, cardiac index, and peak creatine kinase. The in-hospital mortality in 99 patients (49.5%) who underwent IABP insertion was 48%, compared with 57% among patients who did not undergo IABP insertion (p = .23). In subgroup analysis, the mortality of patients who were treated with IABP in conjunction with percutaneous coronary revascularization was lower (38%) than that of patients who were treated with the IABP only (63%, p = .01).

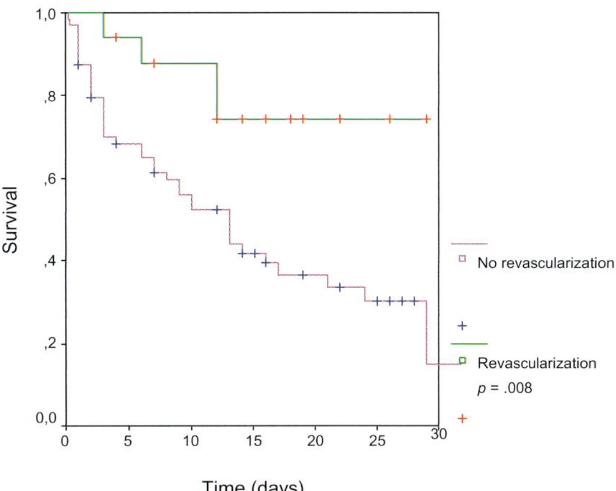

FIGURE 61.2. Impact of late revascularization on in-hospital survival.

We recently reviewed the records of 81 consecutive patients (mean age = 63 ± 11 years) referred to our institution in the last decade for management of post-MI cardiogenic shock (unpublished data). Cardiogenic shock developed at a mean of 13 ± 13 hours after the onset of chest pain, and the mean duration of IABP was 88 ± 83 hours. Mean systolic blood pressure at presentation was 74 ± 15 mm Hg, mean central venous pressure 17 ± 7 mm Hg, and one third of the patients were anuric for ≥24 hours. Thrombolysis was administered in 49% and mechanical ventilation in 46% of patients. The in-hospital mortality was 54.3% (Fig. 61.1). Over a follow-up of 85 ± 47 months (range 6 to 173 months) the postdischarge survival was 63.3% (83% at 1 year), and nearly half of the deaths were due to noncardiac causes. As observed by others, the patients who underwent revascularization during the initial hospitalization had significantly higher in-hospital (76.5%) and 6-month (60.0%) survival than the patients in whom no coronary revascularization attempt was made (36.5% and 25.4%, p = .008 and p = .01, respectively; Figs. 61.2 and 61.3).

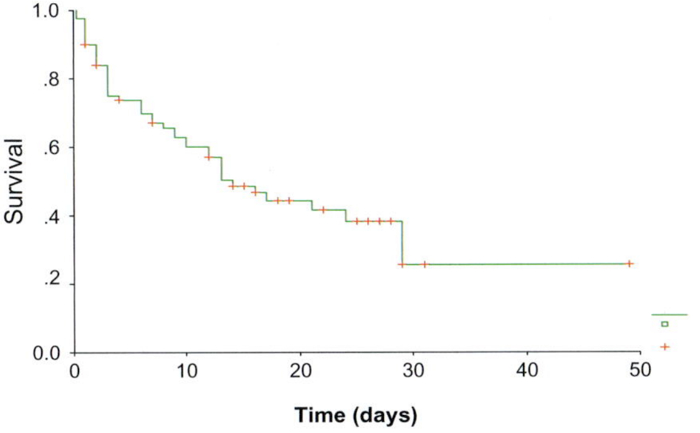

FIGURE 61.1. In-hospital actuarial survival (Kaplan-Meier method) among 81 patients in cardiogenic shock treated with intraaortic balloon pump (IABP).

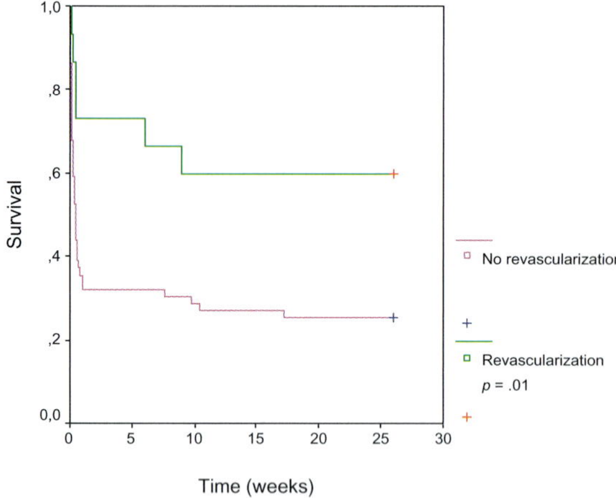

Figure 61.3. Impact of late revascularization on 6-month survival.

In conclusion, the benefits conferred by IABP when used to stabilize the patient with a view to proceeding with coronary revascularization explain the discordant results of studies of post-MI cardiogenic shock performed before versus after the introduction of coronary reperfusion techniques. In the pre-reperfusion era, the advantage conferred by the IABP was limited to initial hemodynamic stabilization (47,48), whereas in the reperfusion era, patients with post-MI cardiogenic shock treated with the IABP are stabilized with a view to proceeding with cardiac catheterization and revascularization (60,62,68).

Postoperative Acute Heart Failure

Cardiothoracic surgeons use IABP as first-line circulatory support for complicated weaning of patients from cardiopulmonary bypass (69–71). Naunheim et al. (69) reported their experience with 6856 adults who underwent cardiac surgical procedures, of whom 580 (8.5%) had an IABP inserted preoperatively ($n = 107$), intraoperatively ($n = 419$), or postoperatively ($n = 54$). Operations included 376 coronary artery bypass grafts (CABG), 85 aortic valve replacements with or without CABG, and 32 miscellaneous procedures. Operative mortality in patients supported by IABP was 44%, and was independently predicted by preoperative New York Heart Association functional class, transthoracic insertion of an intraaortic balloon, preoperative administration of IV nitroglycerin, age, female gender, and preoperative IABP.

Decompensation of Chronic Heart Failure: Bridge to Cardiac Transplantation

The IABP has also been used as a bridge to transplantation in patients with decompensated end-stage heart failure (72–74). Cochran et al. (72) described four patients managed with ambulatory IABP inserted through the left axillary artery without complication. They were able to ambulate soon after the insertion procedure, and optimized their rehabilitation for 12 to 70 days before undergoing successful transplantations. Compared with standard ventricular assist devices, ambulatory IABP, including multiple replacement procedures, represented a 10- to 50-fold saving for each patient.

Rosenbaum et al. (73) evaluated 43 patients who presented with end-stage heart failure due to nonischemic ($n = 27$) or ischemic ($n = 16$) cardiomyopathy, and required IABP while awaiting transplantation. Hemodynamics improved within 15 to 30 minutes after IABP insertion in both groups, with a significantly greater improvement in cardiac index and a trend toward greater reduction in filling pressures in the nonischemic group. Systemic vascular resistance fell similarly in both groups. During support ranging between 0.13 and 38 days in the nonischemic group, and 1 to 54 days in the ischemic group, all hemodynamic changes persisted in both groups, with a significantly larger decrease in systemic vascular resistance and increase in cardiac index among patients with nonischemic disease. The fall in filling pressures, however, tended to be greater in patients with ischemic cardiomyopathy, while renal and hepatic functions improved similarly in both groups. Rates of complications and clinical outcomes during IABP were also similar in both groups, with 33% of patients with ischemic and 44% with nonischemic disease successfully weaned from treatment.

Acute Heart Failure Due to Rejection of Cardiac Allograft

In five patients suffering from cardiac allograft rejection and acute predominantly right ventricular failure, Arafa et al. (20) observed significant hemodynamic improvement at 12 hours after onset of IABP. They suggested that allograft rejection might be another indication for IABP since LV unloading and increasing perfusion of the right ventricle might improve outcomes.

Myocarditis

The successful application of IABP as first-line circulatory support has been described in a few isolated cases or in small series of patients suffering from fulminant myocarditis complicated by severe acute heart failure (75–79).

Treatment Recommendations

Choice of Proper Instrumentation and Insertion of the Balloon Catheter

The polyurethane intraaortic balloon is mounted on the flexible shaft of a 7- to 11-French (F) double-lumen catheter. The central lumen allows the advancement of the catheter to the descending aorta over a 0.021-inch-wide, 150-cm-long, stiff guidewire, and monitoring of the aortic pressure during mechanical assistance. The size of the polyurethane balloon ranges between 30 and 50 cc.

The balloon catheter is inserted percutaneously through the common femoral artery. In rare cases of severe aortoiliac disease, a subclavian or transaortic insertion of the balloon catheter (for surgical patients) has been proposed (80,81). A history of claudication or prior peripheral vascular surgery should be elicited, physical examination performed, and platelet count and coagulation studies should be obtained. The femoral artery with the most prominent pulse should be selected for balloon insertion, and the examination of the distal pulses will serve as a reference for the monitoring of possible circulatory compromise by the balloon catheter, although oxymetry is more accurate and easily applied.

The balloon can be inserted either through a 7.5F to 11F sheath, or without a sheath. Since the balloon shaft is approximately 1.5F smaller than the outer diameter of the sheath, a sheathless insertion causes less circulatory obstruction, enabling the delivery of IABP to a larger number of patients, including small adults, diabetics, and patients with peripheral vascular disease.

Before its insertion, the balloon catheter is prepared by flushing the guidewire lumen with heparin solution, and evacuating the air from the balloon lumen with a 50-cc syringe attached to a one-way valve, keeping the lowest profile during balloon insertion. Using the Seldinger technique, a 0.021-inch-wide, 150-cm-long stiff guidewire is advanced to the aortic arch and, after predilatation with a 7F to 8F dilator, the sheath or a sheathless balloon catheter is introduced. The balloon is advanced in the descending aorta and positioned approximately 2 cm distal to the left subclavian artery. The guidewire is removed, and its lumen aspirated, flushed, and connected to a pressurized flushing device. The one-way valve attached to the gas lumen is removed and the lumen connected to the console by an appropriate connector. Fluoroscopic observation should be carried out; when fluoroscopy is not available, serial x-rays and corrective movements should be obtained to confirm the device's optimal placement before the balloon's shaft is sewn to the skin.

Timing of the Counterpulsation

Once the balloon catheter has been positioned, the central lumen is connected with a 3 mL/h continuous infusion system pressurized to 300 mm Hg. Regular manual syringe aspirations and flushing, tight connections, and elimination of unnecessary catheter extensions optimize the quality of the central pressure tracing. Counterpulsation is initiated with the timing cycle of the balloon initially at 1:2, using the central arterial pressure tracing from the guidewire lumen. The console is synchronized from the ECG or the pressure tracing to inflate the balloon in early diastole (at the time of aortic dicrotic notch, or T wave on the ECG) and to deflate, the balloon just before systole (before the QRS) to produce the maximum reduction in aortic systolic pressure. The IABP can also be synchronized to atrioventricular (AV) pacing stimuli or to an internal rate. Timing can be problematic when the rate is >120 beats/min or the rhythm is irregular, though refined software automates the recognition of trigger sources and optimizes the signal utilization.

In patients with systolic blood pressures <60 mm Hg before IABP, the diastolic aortic augmentation might be the only pressure curve displayed on the monitor, with two pressure peak deflections appearing later, after hemodynamic improvement. However, in patients with systolic blood pressures >80 mm Hg before IABP, peak systolic aortic pressure and diastolic aortic augmentation are usually both displayed on the monitor after the onset of IABP. Timing errors produce characteristic pressure waveform changes that need to be rapidly identified since they can be life threatening or cause ineffective hemodynamic support.

Daily chest radiographs and continuous monitoring of the aortic pressure are necessary to verify the optimal position and function of the IABP. Peripheral pulses should be examined at least hourly for the first 6 hours and every 3 hours thereafter.

Anticoagulation

Few studies have examined the need for intravenous anticoagulation during IABP. A randomized trial in 153 patients observed no difference in vascular complications or laboratory end points in patients undergoing IABP with versus without continuous heparin anticoagulation (82). Manufacturers of intraaortic balloon pumps do not recommend anticoagulation, particularly when used at a 1 : 1 ratio. In absence of contraindications however, we recommend anticoagulation with a goal of maintaining an activated clotting time between 150 and 200 seconds, when IABP is used for >24 hours, or at assist ratios below 1 : 1.

Weaning and Removal

A gradual weaning in assist ratio from 1 : 1 to 1 : 2 and to 1 : 3 over several hours is recommended. If a 1 : 3 ratio is tolerated, the IABP can be removed. The gas line should be disconnected and exposed to room air. The tubing should not be placed to negative pressure, and the balloon and sheath, if used, should be slowly removed as a unit. While removing the balloon and sheath, pressure should be applied distal to the insertion site and washout blood flow is allowed for a few seconds. Pressure should also be applied simultaneously on the contralateral femoral artery. These maneuvers help prevent distal embolization of clots that might have formed at the insertion site or on the tip of the balloon. Manual pressure or a mechanical/pneumatic clamp device can then be applied to the artery, slightly above the insertion site, until hemostasis is achieved. The peripheral pulses should be examined regularly and the patient kept supine for at least 6 hours to limit the risk of bleeding complications.

Contraindications

Absolute contraindications to IABP include patient refusal and more than mild aortic valve regurgitation, since the increase in diastolic aortic pressure increases the amount of regurgitation. Relative contraindications include, though are not limited to, severe peripheral arterial disease, aortic aneurysm, and active bleeding.

Complications

The IABP is associated with serious complications, the most common being bleeding and arterial injury (83). A history of claudication, femoral bruit, or absent pulses are the most reliable predictors of complications (84). In over 22,000 patients included in the Benchmark Registry, the rates of major bleeding, amputation, and death attributed to the IABP were 1.4%, 0.1%, and 0.05%, respectively (85,86). In selected patients, the sheathless percutaneous insertion technique may further lower the rate of ischemic complications (87).

Acute Heart Failure Postmyocardial Infarction

Despite the absence of definite proof of the beneficial effect of IABP in acute heart failure or cardiogenic shock complicating acute MI, observational studies have consistently found that its use in high-risk patients as an adjunct to reperfusion therapy, decreases rates of ischemic events (88), episodes of heart failure (89,90), and vascular and hemorrhagic complications (85,86). Therefore, prophylactic IABP should be considered in patients >70 years of age with a history of heart failure, left main or three-vessel disease, large myocardial infarctions, and sustained hypotension or Killip class III. A strategy of standby versus elective initiation of IABP can be adopted, although there is increasing evidence that early initiation is beneficial. Furthermore, primary or rescue percutaneous revascularization is more likely to be successful in a hemodynamically stable patient. To minimize complications, the duration of counterpulsation should be limited to 24 hours whenever possible.

Guidelines from professional societies for management of patients with acute MI formulate a class I recommendation for the use of IABP in patients with cardiogenic shock refractory to medical therapy (64). Following thrombolysis there is no reason to postpone IABP since in both the SHOCK (61) and TACTICS trial (45), where IABP was instituted at an average of 3 hours and 30 minutes after thrombolysis, respectively, it did not increase the rates of hemorrhagic complications.

The IABP is also a class I indication for mechanical complications of acute MI, such as ventricular septal rupture or acute mitral insufficiency due to papillary muscle dysfunction or rupture (64) since the improvement in hemodynamics is especially prominent in these cases. The IABP support should be continued until definite surgical treatment can be performed.

Low-Output Acute Heart Failure

Left ventricular unloading by IABP can be beneficial in low output heart failure due to right ventricular dysfunction. It should be considered in the setting of cardiogenic shock secondary to right ventricular infarction (19), and in early postoperative low cardiac output syndrome due predominantly to right ventricular failure after cardiac transplantation (20).

Reversible Causes of Severe Acute Heart Failure

The IABP should also be used as a supportive measure for patients suffering from severe acute heart failure secondary to reversible LV dysfunction. In the case of acute fulminant myocarditis (75–78), IABP can be offered either as a bridge to recovery in responders, or to left ventricular assist device (LVAD) in nonresponders. Likewise, patients in severe heart failure due to acute or chronic valvular heart disease (acute or decompensated mitral valve regurgitation, critical aortic valve stenosis) can be effectively supported with the IABP until definite surgical management can be offered.

Finally, IABP might play a role in the management of chronic heart failure for patients suffering from intractable symptoms despite maximal medical therapy, and can be used as a bridge to transplantation, to LVAD, or to a conventional operation (72–74).

Clinical Case

A 72-year-old hypertensive man is admitted to the hospital after he was found confused and profoundly weak. He had experienced substernal chest pain associated with nausea and vomiting few hours earlier.

Upon admission to the hospital the patient is confused. His skin is cold and clammy, the blood pressure is 65/30 mm Hg, the pulse is faint, regular at a rate of 140 bpm, and the jugular veins are distended. The electrocardiogram shows left bundle branch block, and the chest radiograph shows bilateral pulmonary infiltrates consistent with pulmonary edema.

Question: What are the initial steps in this patient's management?

Answer: Since the patient is hemodynamically unstable, immediate hemodynamic support should be initiated with vasopressors, including noradrenalin, 0.05 to 0.3 μg/kg/min, and dopamine, 6 to 20 μg/kg/min. A central venous catheter is placed and right heart catheterization is performed to measure the pulmonary capillary wedge pressure (PCWP), and guide the administration of diuretics and fluids.

Question: The central venous pressure is 9 mm Hg, mean pulmonary pressure 40 mm Hg, PCWP 25 mm Hg, and cardiac index 1.6 L/min/m^2. The patient remains hypotensive despite maximal vasopressor therapy. What is the next treatment option?

Answer: Since the patient is in cardiogenic shock, additional support with an IABP is indicated to unload the failing ventricle and augment diastolic coronary blood flow. The femoral artery with the most prominent pulse should be selected for a sheathless introduction of the balloon, the proximal end of which must be placed at the second intercostal space under fluoroscopic surveillance. Anticoagulation with intravenous unfractionated heparin shoud be initiated. Synchronized 1:1 counterpulsation is best accomplished with the electrocardiogram.

Question: The systemic blood pressure rises to 90/60 mm Hg, with a peak diastolic aortic augmentation of 120 mm Hg. What is the next step?

Answer: After achievement of temporary hemodynamic stability, the patient should be taken to the cardiac catheterization laboratory for a primary percutaneous coronary intervention.

Question: Left main artery disease is diagnosed and primary stenting is successfully performed. The patient returns to the cardiac care unit in stable condition. When should the IABP be removed?

Answer: The IABP should be removed as soon as the patient's condition allows, past the first 24 hours. Inotropic support should be gradually withdrawn first. If the patient remains stable, weaning off the IABP should be undertaken by reducing the counterpulsation ratio. If stability persists for 2 to 3 hours at a ratio of 1:3, the IABP can be safely removed.

References

1. Moulopoulos SD, Topaz S, Kolff WJ. Diastolic balloon pumping (with carbon dioxide) in the aorta: a mechanical assistance to the failing circulation. Am Heart J 1962;63:669–75.
2. Suga H, Sagawa K. Instantaneous pressure-volume relationships and their ratio in the excised, supported canine left ventricle. Circ Res 1974;35:117–26.
3. Sagawa K, Suga H, Shoukas AA, End-systolic pressure/volume ratio: a new index of ventricular contractility. Am J Cardiol 1977;40:748–53.
4. Normann NA, Kennedy JH. Arterial baroreceptor responses to intraaortic balloon assistance. J Surg Res 1971;11:396–400.
5. Papaioannou TG, Mathioulakis DS, Stamatelopoulos KS, et al. New aspects on the role of blood pressure and arterial stiffness in mechanical assistance by intra-aortic balloon pump: in-vitro data and their application in clinical practice. Artif Organs 2004;28:717–27.
6. Mullins CB, Sugg WL, Kennelly BM, Jones DC, Mitchell JH. Effect of arterial counterpulsation on left ventricular volume and pressure. Am J Physiol 1971;220:694–8.
7. Nanas JN, Mason JW, Yoshiyuki T, Chiang BY, Olsen DB. Hemodynamic effects of an implanted abdominal aortic counterpulsation device designed for chronic use in graded heart failure. Life Support Syst 1985;3(suppl 1):245–9.
8. Weiss AT, Engel S, Gotsman CJ, et al. Regional and global left ventricular function during intra-aortic balloon counterpulsation in patients with acute myocardial infarction shock. Am Heart J 1984; 108:249–54.
9. Iskandrian AS, Colby J, Hakki AH, Boston B, Kane SA. Effect of intra-aortic balloon pumping on left ventricular function: evaluation by radionuclide ventriculography. Clin Cardiol 1984;7:211–6.
10. Scheidt S, Wilner G, Mueller H, et al. Intra-aortic balloon counterpulsation in cardiogenic shock. Report of a cooperative clinical trial. N Engl J Med 1973;288:979–84.
11. Chatterjee S, Rosensweig J. evaluation of intraaortic balloon counterpulsation. J Thorac Cardiovasc Surg 1971;61:405–10.
12. McDonald RH Jr, Taylor RR, Cingolani HE. Measurement of myocardial developed tension and its relation to oxygen consumption. Am J Physiol 1966;211:667–73.
13. Buckberg GD, Fixler DE, Archie JP, Hoffman JI. Experimental subendocardial ischemia in dogs with normal coronary arteries. Circ Res 1972; 30:67–81.
14. Philips PA, Bergman D. intraoperative application of intraaortic balloon counterpulsation determined by clinical monitoring of the endocardial viability ratio. Ann Thorac Surg 1977;23:45.
15. Schipke JD, Burkhoff D, Kass DA, Alexander J Jr, Schaefer J, Sagawa K. Hemodynamic dependence of myocardial oxygen consumption indexes. Am J Physiol 1990;258:H1281–91.
16. Matloff JM, Parmley WW, Manchester JH, Berkovits B, Sonnenblick EH, Harken DE. Hemodynamic effects of glucagon and intraaortic balloon counterpulsation in canine myocardial infarction. Am J Cardiol 1970;25:675–82.
17. Sugita Y, Emoto H, Morita K, et al. The effect of intraaortic balloon pumping (IABP) on pulmonary circulation. Trans Am Soc Artif Intern Organs 1985;31:389–94.
18. Darrah WC, Sharpe MD, Guiraudon GM, et al. Intraaortic balloon counterpulsation improves right ventricular failure resulting from pressure overload. Ann Thorac Surg 1997;64:1718–24.

19. Nordhaug D, Steensrud T, Muller S, Husnes KV, Myrmel T. Intraaortic balloon pumping improves hemodynamics and right ventricular efficiency in acute ischemic right ventricular failure. Ann Thorac Surg 2004;78:1426–32.
20. Arafa OE, Geiran OR, Andersen K, Fosse E, Simonsen S, Svennevig JL. Intraaortic balloon pumping for predominantly right ventricular failure after heart transplantation. Ann Thorac Surg 2000;70: 1587–93.
21. Kim SY, Euler DE, Jacobs WR, et al. Arterial impedance in patients during intraaortic balloon counterpulsation. Ann Thorac Surg 1996;61:888–94.
22. Tsolakis E, Ntalianis A, Drakos S, et al. Intra-aortic balloon counterpulsation facilitates coronary microcirculation during myocardial reperfusion: experimental study. Circ Res 2005;97(2):e41.
23. Katz ES, Tunick PA, Kronzon I. Observations of coronary flow augmentation and balloon function during intraaortic balloon counterpulsation using transesophageal echocardiography. Am J Cardiol 1992;69:1635–9.
24. Kern MJ, Aguirre FV, Tatineni S, et al. Enhanced coronary blood flow velocity during intraaortic balloon counterpulsation in critically ill patients. J Am Coll Cardiol 1993;21:359–68.
25. Bhayana JN, Scott SM, Sethi GK, Takaro T. Effects of intra-aortic balloon pumping on organ perfusion in cardiogenic shock. J Surg Res 1979;26:108.
26. Shimamoto H, Kawazoe K, Kito Y, et al. Influences of intra-aortic balloon pumping on peripheral hemodynamics. Respir Circ 1991;39:73–8.
27. Gee W, Smith RL, Perline RK, Gallagher HS. Assessment of intra-aortic balloon pumping by ocular pneumoplethysmography. Am Surg 1986;52:489–91.
28. Brass LM. Reversed intracranial blood flow in patients with an intra-aortic balloon pump. Stroke 1990;21:484–7.
29. Oster H, Stanley TH, Olsen DB, Nielsen M, Kolff WJ. Regional blood flow after intra-aortic balloon pumping before and after cardiogenic shock. Trans Am Soc Artif Intern Organs 1974;20B:721–3.
30. Nichols WW, Pepine CJ. Left ventricular afterload and aortic input impedance: implications of pulsatile blood flow. Prog Cardiovasc Dis 1982;24: 293–306.
31. Swartz MT, Sakamoto T, Arai H, et al. Effects of intraaortic balloon position on renal artery blood flow. Ann Thorac Surg 1992;53(4):604–10.
32. Koterazawa T, Okada M, Nakamura K. Effect of the intra-aortic balloon pumping on renal function. Nippon Kyobu Geka Gakkai Zasshi (J Jpn Assoc Thorac Surg) 1989;37:1908–16.
33. Nanas JN, Nanas SN, Kontoyannis DA, et al. Myocardial salvage by the use of reperfusion and intraaortic balloon pump: experimental study. Ann Thorac Surg 1996;61:629–34.
34. Bonios M, Ntalianis A, Stavrakis S, et al. Intraaortic balloon counterpulsation during myocardial reperfusion increases coronary blood flow and myocardial salvage: experimental study. J Am Coll Cardiol 2005;45(suppl 1):253A(abstr).
35. Amado LC, Kraitchman DL, Gerber BL, et al. Reduction of "no-reflow" phenomenon by intraaortic balloon counterpulsation in a randomized magnetic resonance imaging experimental study. J Am Coll Cardiol 2004;43:1291–8.
36. Azevedo CF, Amado LC, Kraitchman DL, et al. The effect of intra-aortic balloon counterpulsation on left ventricular functional recovery early after acute myocardial infarction: a randomized experimental magnetic resonance imaging study. Eur Heart J 2005;26(12):1235–41.
37. Sakamoto T, Suzuki A, Kazama S, Komatsu S, Sasaki S, Shoji Y. Effects of timing on ventriculoarterial coupling and mechanical efficiency during intraaortic balloon pumping. ASAIO J 1995;41(3): M580–3.
38. Schottler M, Schaefer J, Schwarzkopf HJ, et al. Experimentally induced changes of arterial mean and aortic opening pressure by controlled variation of diastolic augmentation. Basic Res Cardiol 1974;69:59–607.
39. Nanas JN, Nanas SN, Charitos CE, et al. Hemodynamic effects of a counterpulsation device implanted on the ascending aorta in severe cardiogenic shock. ASAIO Trans 1988;34(3):229–34.
40. Sun Y. Modeling the dynamic interaction between left ventricle and intra-aortic balloon pump. Am J Physiol 1991;261(4 pt 2):H1300–11.
41. Furman S, Whitman R, Stewart J, Parker B, McMullen M. Proximity to aortic valve and unidirectionality as prime factors in counterpulsation effectiveness. Trans Am Soc Artif Intern Organs 1971;17:153–9.
42. Papaioannou TG, Terrovitis J, Kanakakis J, et al. Heart rate effect on hemodynamics during mechanical assistance by the intraaortic balloon pump. Int J Artif Organs 2002;25:1160–5.
43. Bolooki H. Physiology of balloon pumping. In: Clinical Application of the Intraaortic Balloon Pump, 3rd ed. New York: Futura, 1998:109–61.
44. Feola M, Haiderer O, Kennedy JH. Intra-aortic balloon pumping (IABP) at different levels of experimental acute left ventricular failure. Chest 1971;59(1):68–76.
45. Ohman EM, Nanas J, Stomel RJ, et al. Thrombolysis and counterpulsation to improve survival in

myocardial infarction complicated by hypotension and suspected cardiogenic shock or heart failure: results of the TACTICS trial. J Thromb Thrombolysis 2005;19(1):33–9.
46. Sanborn TA, Feldman T. Management strategies for cardiogenic shock. Curr Opin Cardiol 2004;19: 608–12.
47. Flaherty JT, Becker LC, Weiss JL, et al. Results of a randomized prospective trial of intraaortic balloon counterpulsation and intravenous nitroglycerin in patients with acute myocardial infarction. J Am Coll Cardiol 1985;6:434–46.
48. O'Rourke MF, Norris RM, Campbell TJ, Chang VP, Sammel NL. Randomized controlled trial of intraaortic balloon counterpulsation in early myocardial infarction with acute heart failure. Am J Cardiol 1981;47:815–20.
49. Gruppo Italiano per lo Studio della Streptochinasi nell'Infarto Miocardico (GISSI). Effectiveness of intravenous treatment in acute myocardial infarction. Lancet 1986;1:397–402.
50. Fibrinolytic Therapy Trialists' (FTT) Collaborative Study Group. Indications for fibrinolytic therapy in suspected acute myocardial infarction: collaborative overview of mortality and major morbidity results from all randomised trials of more than 1000 patients. Lancet 1994;343:311–22.
51. The International Study Group. In-hospital mortality and clinical course of 20,891 patients with suspected acute myocardial infarction randomised between alteplase and streptokinase with or without heparin. Lancet 1990;336:71–5.
52. Holmes DR Jr, Bates ER, Kleiman NS, et al., for the GUSTO-I Investigators. Contemporary reperfusion therapy for cardiogenic shock: the GUSTO-I trial experience. J Am Coll Cardiol 1995;26:668–7.
53. Prewitt RM, Gu S, Schick U, Ducas J. Effect of a mechanical vs a pharmacologic increase in aortic pressure on coronary blood flow and thrombolysis induced by IV administration of a thrombolytic agent. Chest 1997;111:449–53.
54. Gurbel PA, Anderson RD, MacCord CS, et al. Arterial diastolic pressure augmentation by intra-aortic balloon counterpulsation enhances the onset of coronary artery reperfusion by thrombolytic therapy. Circulation 1994;89:361–5.
55. Nanas JN, Moulopoulos SD. Counterpulsation: historical background, technical improvements, hemodynamic and metabolic effects. Cardiology 1994;84:156–67.
56. Barron HV, Every NR, Parsons LS, et al. The use of intraaortic balloon counterpulsation in patients with cardiogenic shock complicating acute myocardial infarction: data from the National Registry of Myocardial Infarction 2. Am Heart J 2001;141: 933–9.
57. Anderson RD, Ohman EM, Holmes DR Jr, et al. Use of intraaortic balloon counterpulsation in patients presenting with cardiogenic shock: Observations from the GUSTO-I study. J Am Coll Cardiol 1997;30:708–15.
58. Waksman R, Weiss AT, Gotsman MS, Hasin Y. Intra-aortic counterpulsation improves survival in cardiogenic shock complicating acute myocardial infarction. Eur Heart J 1993;14:1–74.
59. Kovack PJ, Rasak MA, Bates ER, Ohman EM, Stomel RJ. Thrombolysis plus aortic counterpulsation: improved survival in patients who present to community hospitals with cardiogenic shock. J Am Coll Cardiol 1997;29:1454–8.
60. Sanborn TA, Sleeper LA, Bates ER, et al. Impact of thrombolysis, intra-aortic balloon pump counterpulsation, and their combination in cardiogenic shock complicating acute myocardial infarction: a report from the SHOCK trial registry. J Am Coll Cardiol 2000;36:1123–9.
61. Hochman JS, Sleeper LA, Webb JG, et al. for SHOCK Investigators. Early revascularization in acute myocardial infarction complicated by cardiogenic shock. Should we emergently revascularize occluded coronaries for cardiogenic shock? N Engl J Med 1999;341:625–34.
62. Santa-Cruz RA, Cohen MG, Ohman EM. Aortic counterpulsation: a review of the hemodynamic effects and indications for use. Catheter Cardiovasc Intervent 2006;67:68–77.
63. Duvernoy CS, Bates ER. Management of cardiogenic shock attributable to acute myocardial infarction in the reperfusion era. J Intensive Care Med 2005;20:188–98.
64. Antman EM, Anbe DT, Armstrong PW, et al. ACC/AHA guidelines for the management of patients with ST-elevation myocardial infarction: a report of the American College of Cardiology/American Heart Association Task Force on Practice Guidelines. J Am Coll Cardiol 2004;44:E1–211.
65. Hochman JS. Cardiogenic shock complicating acute myocardial infarction. Expanding the paradigm. Circulation 2003;107:2998–3002.
66. Hudson MP, Granger CB, Stebbins AL, et al. Cardiogenic shock survival and use of intra-aortic balloon counterpulsation: results from the GUSTO I and III trials. Circulation 1999;100(suppl): I370.
67. Bengtson JR, Kaplan AJ, Pieper KS, et al. Prognosis in cardiogenic shock after acute myocardial infarction in the interventional era. J Am Coll Cardiol 1992;20:1482–9.

68. Ohman EM, Hochman JS. Aortic counterpulsation in acute myocardial infarction: Physiologically important but does the patient benefit? Am Heart J 2001;141:879–92.
69. Naunheim KS, Swartz MT, Pennington DG, et al. Intraaortic balloon pumping in patients requiring cardiac operations. Risk analysis and long-term follow-up. J Thorac Cardiovasc Surg 1992;104:1654–60.
70. Baldwin RT, Slogoff S, Noon GP, et al. A model to predict survival at time of postcardiotomy intraaortic balloon pump insertion. Ann Thorac Surg 1993; 55:908–13.
71. Christenson JT, Buswell L, Velebit V, et al. The intraaortic balloon pump for postcardiotomy heart failure. Experience with 169 intraaortic balloon pumps. Thorac Cardiovasc Surg 1995;43:129–33.
72. Cochran RP, Starkey TD, Panos AL, Kunzelman KS. Ambulatory intraaortic balloon pump use as bridge to heart transplant. Ann Thorac Surg 2002;74: 746–52.
73. Rosenbaum AM, Murali S, Uretsky BF. Intra-aortic balloon counterpulsation as a 'bridge' to cardiac transplantation. Effects in nonischemic and ischemic cardiomyopathy. Chest 1994;106: 1683–8.
74. Peric M, Frazier OH, Macris M, Radovancevic B. Intra-aortic balloon pump as a bridge to transplantation. J Heart Transplant 1986;5:380.
75. Chen YS, Yu HY, Huang SC, et al. Experience and result of extracorporeal membrane oxygenation in treating fulminant myocarditis with shock: what mechanical support should be considered first? J Heart Lung Transplant 2005;24:81–7.
76. Sauvant G, Bossart W, Kurrer MO, Follath F. Diagnosis and course of myocarditis: a survey in the medical clinics of Zurich University Hospital 1980 to 1998. Schweiz Med Wochenschr 2000;130: 1265–71.
77. Kato S, Morimoto S, Hiramitsu S, et al. Risk factors for patients developing a fulminant course with acute myocarditis. Circ J 2004;68:734–9.
78. Yoshikawa J, Yanagihara K, Asaka T, et al. Treatment of cardiogenic shock and medically refractory left ventricular failure in acute myocardial infarction and acute myocarditis by intraaortic balloon counterpulsation. J Cardiogr Suppl 1984;3:93–7.
79. Yamaguchi K, Iwaoka K. Effectiveness of intraaortic balloon pumping for fulminant myocarditis. Nippon Geka Hokan 1988;57:92–6.
80. Murai N, Kaneko T, Oobayashi T, et al. Left subclavian artery approach for insertion of IABP. Kyobu Geka 1998;51:579–82.
81. Santini F, Mazzucco A. Transthoracic intraaortic counterpulsation: a simple method for balloon catheter positioning. Ann Thorac Surg 1997;64: 859–60.
82. Jiang CY, Zhao LL, Wang JA, Mohammod B. Anticoagulation therapy in intra-aortic balloon counterpulsation: does IABP really need anti-coagulation? J Zhejiang Univ Sci 2003;4:607–11.
83. Alderman JD, Gabliani GI, McCabe CH, et al. Incidence and management of limb ischemia with percutaneous wire-guided intraaortic balloon catheters. J Am Coll Cardiol 1987;9:524–30.
84. Cohen M, Dawson MS, Kopistansky C, McBride R. Sex and other predictors of intra-aortic balloon counterpulsation-related complications: prospective study of 1119 consecutive patients. Am Heart J 2000;139:282–7.
85. Ferguson JJ 3rd, Cohen M, Freedman RJ Jr, et al. The current practice of intra-aortic balloon counterpulsation: results from the Benchmark Registry. J Am Coll Cardiol 2001;38:1456–62.
86. Stone GW, Ohman EM, Miller MF, et al. Contemporary utilization and outcomes of intra-aortic balloon counterpulsation in acute myocardial infarction: the benchmark registry. J Am Coll Cardiol 2003;41:1940–5.
87. Tatar H, Cicek S, Demirkilic U, et al. Vascular complications of intraaortic balloon pumping: unsheathed versus sheathed insertion. Ann Thorac Surg 1993;55:1518–21.
88. van't Hof AW, Liem AL, de Boer MJ, Hoorntje JC, Suryapranata H, Zijlstra F. A randomized comparison of intra-aortic balloon pumping after primary coronary angioplasty in high risk patients with acute myocardial infarction. Eur Heart J 1999;20: 659–65.
89. Ohman EM, George BS, White CJ, et al. for the Randomized IABP Study Group. Use of aortic counterpulsation to improve sustained coronary artery patency during acute myocardial infarction. Results of a randomized trial. Circulation 1994; 90:792–9.
90. Ohman EM, Califf R, Topol E, et al. Aortic counterpulsation with thrombolysis for myocardial infarction: salutary effect on reocclusion of the infarct related artery. J Am Coll Cardiol 1992;19(suppl A): 381A(abstr).

62
Cardiac Resynchronization Therapy in Acute and Chronic Heart Failure Syndromes

Paul Milliez, Abdeddayem Haggui, Fabrice Extramiana, Olivier Thomas, and Antoine Leenhardt

Despite recent advances in drug treatment, congestive heart failure (CHF) remains a major health care issue associated with a poor quality of life and a severe prognosis. In the last decade, cardiac resynchronization therapy (CRT) has been assessed as a new therapy option in patients with severe left ventricular (LV) dysfunction. Hence, CRT has become a challenging and an efficient treatment in patients in New York Heart Association (NYHA) class III or IV with a left ventricular ejection fraction (LVEF) of less than 35%, wide QRS, or echocardiographic ventricular dyssynchrony.[1–6] Recently, CRT has demonstrated a significant reduction in both overall and cardiac mortality and great improvement in various functional parameters.[6] It is now a validated treatment for severe CHF patients in NYHA class III or IV despite an optimal medical therapy. This chapter summarizes the history of CRT since preliminary reports have been published, and addresses a challenging question about the usefulness of CRT in unstable overt CHF patients.

Rationale for Cardiac Resynchronization Therapy in Chronic Congestive Heart Failure Patients

In normal heart, electrical conduction takes birth in the sinus node tissue located in the high right atrium, midway between the superior vena cava and the right atrial appendage. The electrical impulse reaches the atrioventricular (AV) node tissue using atrial connection pathways. This impulse walks along to the AV node, goes through the His bundle and simultaneously to its left and right bundle branch and to the Purkinje system. Hence, in normal heart there no conduction delays between the sinus and AV nodes, within the AV node, as well as between the two His bundle branches. As a result, there is no mechanical dyssynchrony related to electrical asynchrony within the electrical conduction system.

In patients with CHF, two electrical conduction defects can be observed and considered deleterious for cardiac function: prolongation of QRS and large PR interval. Prolongation of QRS (QRS ≥120 ms) happens in approximately 30% of CHF patients with predominantly a left bundle branch block (LBBB) pattern.[7] QRS prolongation (QRS ≥120 ms) is known to be a significant predictor of LV dysfunction.[7] In patients with CHF, a negative correlation between QRS duration and left LVEF has been observed.[7] Furthermore, the incidence of QRS ≥120 ms increased from 10% to 53% when patients moved from NYHA functional class I to class III.[8] However, in addition to these observations, epidemiologic studies have shown that patients with CHF and QRS prolongation have higher overall mortality as well as sudden cardiac death than those with narrowed QRS.[9] In a prospective study, mortality at 36 months increased from 20% to 36% to 58% when QRS duration was <120 ms, between 120 and 160 ms, and >160 ms, respectively.[10] All these data suggest that QRS prolongation is particularly observed in patients with severe LV dysfunction and seems to be correlated with a poor prognosis.

However, does QRS prolongation in these patients represent only a marker of LV impairment, or could it be deleterious itself, when observed, to LV function? QRS prolongation with an LBBB pattern is a marker of electrical conduction delay, an "electrical dyssynchrony," between right and left ventricles, called ventriculoventricular (VV) dyssynchrony, as well as within the left ventricle, called LV dyssynchrony. In LBBB, the activation sequence for LV contraction is modified, as observed with apical RV pacing ("pseudo"-LBBB induced by right ventricular [RV] pacing). In 1989, Grines et al.[11] showed in an echocardiographic and isotopic study of patients with a normal heart, an electrical dyssynchrony of LV compared to RV contraction when a pseudo-LBBB was present. As a consequence of this electrical dyssynchrony, an increase in the systolic time was observed that was detrimental for the LV filling time, and as a consequence, the LVEF dropped from 62% ± 5% to 54% ± 7% ($p < .005$) in patients with LBBB. In addition, another study has shown that LBBB was also harmful for diastolic LV function (Table 62.1).

Hence, QRS prolongation with a LBBB pattern underlies an "electrical-mechanical dyssynchrony" of the heart that has deleterious hemodynamic consequences with cardiac output impairment related to the following:

- LV contraction dyssynchrony (V-V dyssynchrony) compared to the RV with LV/RV delay moving from 40 ms (physiologic) to 150 ms
- Inversion of the activation sequence of LV contraction (LV dyssynchrony): RV apex → LV apex → lateral and posterior free wall.

However, independently of the presence of a VV or LV dyssynchrony related to QRS prolongation, it has been observed that further impairment of cardiac hemodynamic when an AV conduction delay occurs, represented by PR prolongation, is associated in CHF patients. Several acute hemodynamic studies have shown that AV dyssynchrony related to PR prolongation increases both mitral and tricuspid regurgitations and decreases both diastolic LV filling time and cardiac output.[12] As a consequence of these observations, CRT has been proposed to correct AV, VV, and LV dyssynchrony related to both PR and QRS prolongation, in order to counteract and maybe reverse progressive chronic impairment of cardiac function.

Implantation of Cardiac Resynchronization Therapy Devices

All procedures are performed in pre-sedated patients and under full supervision of anesthesiologists. A light sedation under noninvasive ventilation might be given during the implantation as well as a permanent monitoring of blood pressure using an intraarterial catheter. All leads are implanted transvenously. The atrial lead (in patients in sinus rhythm) is placed high in the right atrium. The right ventricular lead is positioned in all patients as far as possible from the left ventricular lead. The left ventricular lead is placed within the coronary sinus after a venogram is performed with right and left anterior oblique views during the procedure in order to spot the best lateral site. This target site is preferably the lateral wall, midway between the base and the apex, but if this vein is absent, other postero- or anterolateral veins can be used (Fig. 62.1). In the

Table 62.1. QRS prolongation with a left bundle branch block (LBBB) pattern and LV diastolic function

	LBBB ($n = 14$)	Normal QRS ($n = 16$)	p
E-wave max. (cm/s)	60 ± 15	81 ± 17	.001
E-wave integral (cm)	8.5 ± 2.6	11.5 ± 2.7	.006
A-wave max. (cm/s)	78 ± 27	82 ± 26	NS
A-wave integral (cm)	9.0 ± 3.0	8.3 ± 1.8	NS
E/A max.	0.8 ± 0.2	1.0 ± 0.2	.02
E/A integral	1.0 ± 0.3	1.4 ± 0.3	.002
Deceleration time of E wave (ms)	131 ± 60	178 ± 62	.04
Deceleration velocity of E wave (cm/s^2)	267 ± 104	380 ± 100	.009
Heart rate	70 ± 7	71 ± 10	NS

case of nonaccessible lateral veins, the great cardiac vein or the middle cardiac vein can be used. The CRTs used are either a standard dual-chamber technology devices with built-in adapters to synchronize the pacing of the two ventricles, or a current CRT device with separate exits for each leads. Hence, we are able to program AV as well as VV conduction in order to reduce AV delay and to restore synchronization of both right and left ventricles thanks to the lead placed in the lateral wall of the LV.

However, such procedures must be performed by extremely well-experienced cardiologist, as there is a steep learning curve to perform a successful implantation. Technical problems are encountered in almost 15% of the patients, and can lead to an unsuccessful procedure. Among these problems are unsuccessful catheterizations of the coronary sinus, the risk of coronary dissection with pericardial effusion, the absence of lateral veins, LV lead dislodgment, and phrenic stimulation. Despite these technical problems, the rate of successful procedure reaches 90%. Also, because patients are very ill (very low LVEF, stage NYHA III/IV), they can die during the procedure, although it becomes exceptional with shorter and well-monitored procedures.

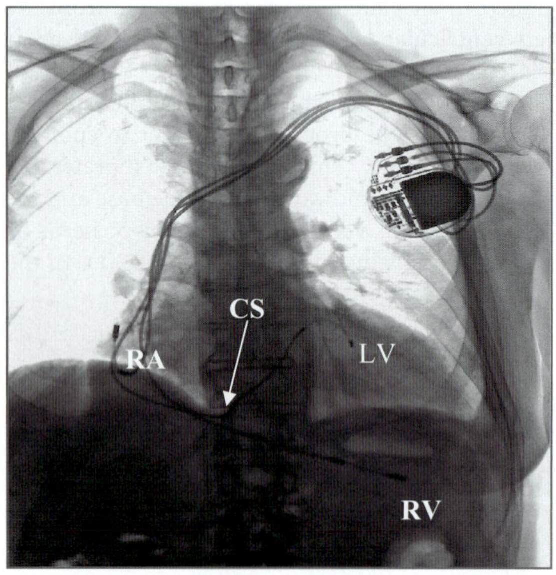

FIGURE 62.1. Cardiac resynchronization therapy (CRT) device with an atrial lead in the right atrium (RA) laterally, an apical right ventricle (RV) lead, and a left ventricle (LV) lead within the coronary sinus (CS), midway between base and apex of the lateral vein. (Paul Milliez personnal unpublished data.)

Initial reports of Cardiac Resynchronization Therapy in Congestive Heart Failure Patients: Acute Hemodynamic Studies

Several preliminary reports had suggested that patients with dilated cardiomyopathy with CHF may benefit from dual-chamber pacing with AV-delay optimization. Such beneficial results have been observed in patients with long PR interval (first-degree AV block) and a subsequent diastolic mitral regurgitation in whom shortening of AV delay had improved LV filling. A study published in 1992 included 12 patients with idiopathic dilated cardiomyopathy with functional mitral and tricuspid regurgitations. Echocardiographic criteria assessed LV/RV filling times, cardiac output, and mitral and tricuspid regurgitation. All the echocardiographic parameters were significantly improved (increased filling time and cardiac output, decreased valve regurgitations) while the AV delay was shortened.[13] A second publication was an acute hemodynamic study comprising 15 patients with dilated cardiomyopathy and severe LV dysfunction. The results showed that pacing with a short AV delay had (1) reversed diastolic mitral regurgitation in patients with first-degree AV block, and (2) restored a more physiologic AV delay with improvement of LV hemodynamic.

In addition to the beneficial effects of AV resynchronization, it has been proposed to correct not only AV but also VV and LV dyssynchrony in patients with dilated cardiomyopathy and associated LBBB. To counteract such VV and LV dyssynchrony, a biventricular pacing approach, so-called CRT, has been developed as technically described above. The first report in 1998 assessed the acute effects of biventricular pacing in patients with severe dilated cardiomyopathy and an LBBB.[14] There were three groups of patients: (1) control patients with right atrial pacing; (2) patients with apical RV pacing, and (3) biventricular pacing patients. Results showed that biventricular pacing acutely improved the cardiac index and decreased pulmonary capillary wedge pressure compared to both apical RV and atrial control pacing patients. More recently, another acute hemodynamic study of 27 patients has confirmed that CRT with AV delay optimization in patients with severe dilated cardiomyopathy and LBBB improved the same hemodynamic parameters, particularly in patients with QRS >140 ms. In addition, the authors observed stronger improvement when both AV and VV/LV dyssynchrony were corrected. Also, Nelson et al.[15] demonstrated that maximal improvement of dP/dt after CRT was independent of the peak oxygen consumption, while peak oxygen consumption increased with dP/dt improvement in patients on dobutamine.

Recent reports on Cardiac Resynchronization Therapy: Chronic Prospective Clinical Studies

These preliminary encouraging results, however, needed to be confirmed in clinical and prospective studies. To confirm the efficacy of CRT in CHF patients, data must be published on persistent improvement of various functional parameters, as well as an actual beneficial effect on mortality. All the prospective studies that have assessed functional parameters are summarized in Table 62.2. The first significant clinical and prospective study was the MUltisite STimulation In Cardiomyopathy (MUSTIC) trial,[2] in which patients with dilated cardiomyopathy and LVEF <35%, in NYHA class III, and with wide QRS were assessed in a single-blind, randomized, crossover study, both before and after CRT, on various functional parameters (6-minute walking test, VO_2 max, quality of life questionnaire, hospitalizations for CHF). When patients were on CRT, significant improvement of all these parameters was observed, with a large decrease in hospitalization (↓60%) for CHF compared to the period without CRT. All these data have been confirmed by three other studies—Pacing Therapies in Congestive Heart Failure (PATH-CHF), Multicenter InSync Randomized Clinical Evaluation (MIRACLE),[3] and CONTAK-CD[5]—showing beneficial effects on the

Table 62.2. Cardiac resynchronization therapy in randomized clinical trials

Trials	Patients	Design	End points	Results summary
PATH-CHF[1]	41	Crossover	*Primary* 6MWT, peak VO_2 *Secondary* NYHA functional class QOL, hospitalizations	*Improvement in:* 6MWT, QOL NYHA functional class Fewer hospitalizations
MUSTIC-SR[2]	58	Crossover	*Primary* 6MWT *Secondary* NYHA functional class QOL, Peak VO_2 LV volumes, MR, hospitalizations Total mortality	*Improvement in:* 6MWT NYHA functional class QOL Peak VO_2 LV volumes, MR Hospitalizations
MIRACLE[3]	453	Parallel arms	*Primary* 6MWT, QOL NYHA functional class *Secondary* Peak VO_2, LVEF, LVEDD, MR Clinical composite response	*Improvement in:* 6MWT NYHA functional class QOL, LVEF, LVEDD, MR
CONTAK-CD[5]	490	Crossover, parallel controlled	*Primary* 6MWT, QOL NYHA functional class *Secondary* LVEF, LV volumes Composite mortality, hospitalizations, VT/VF	*Improvement in:* 6MWT, QOL NYHA functional class LVEF, LV volumes

6MWT, 6-minute walk test; QOL, quality of life; MR, mitral regurgitation; NYHA, New York Heart Association; LVEF, left ventricular ejection fraction; LV, left ventricle; LVEDD, left ventricular end diastolic diameter; VT, ventricular tachycardia; VF, ventricular fibrillation.

same functional parameters. Hence, after the acute studies, clinical trials gave further insight into the positive effects of CRT.

However, until last year, no data were available about a potential reduction of mortality with CRT. In 2004, the Comparison of Medical Therapy, Pacing, and Defibrillation in Heart Failure (COMPANION) trial has provided interesting information about the use of CRT in severe CHF patients in a randomized and prospective study.[4] The COMPANION trial assessed the beneficial effects of CRT alone or combined with a defibrillator in patients with dilated cardiomyopathy in NYHA class III or IV with an LVEF <35% and a QRS >120 ms, compared to a control group under optimal medical therapy. There were three groups with a primary combined end point of total mortality and hospitalizations. Secondary end points were total mortality, combined cardiac mortality, and cardiac hospitalizations, and combined CHF mortality and hospitalizations for CHF. Cardiac resynchronization therapy alone was able to reduce significantly the primary end point compared to the control group, while CRT failed to significantly reduce total mortality. However, when CRT was combined with the defibrillator, total mortality was significantly reduced compared to the control group. Hence, the beneficial effect on total mortality was still an unanswered question after the COMPANION trial.

Fortunately, the Cardiac Resynchronization-Heart Failure (CARE-HF) trial, published in 2005, reported for the first time a significant beneficial effect of CRT on total mortality.[6] The trial comprised 813 patients in NYHA class III or IV with an LVEF <35% and a QRS >120 ms randomized to either medical optimal therapy or to CRT, with a mean follow-up of 29 months. All primary and secondary end points were significantly reduced by CRT. Hence, CRT has significantly reduced the combined end point of total mortality and hospitalizations from any cause (37%), total mortality (36%), and the combined criterion of total mortality and hospitalizations for CHF (46%). In addition, significant improvement of various functional parameters, such as LVEF and LV remodeling, was observed in patients with CRT. There were a 16% absolute reduction for the primary end point and 10% absolute reduction for total mortality related to the CRT group. The CARE-HF trial has demonstrate, as COMPANION has previously roughed out, that CRT can save lives in addition to improve patients' quality of life. Hence, CRT is now a validated treatment of patients with severe CHF in whom optimal medical therapy failed to improve their morbidity and mortality.

Is There a Future for Cardiac Resynchronization Therapy in Acute Heart Failure Syndromes?

In clinical practice, unstable overt CHF patients in whom infusion of inotropic agents failed to improve the hemodynamic with persistent low cardiac output are candidates for ventricular assist devices or heart transplantation. However, such alternatives are not recommended in elderly patients, and several patients are ineligible because of severe associated diseases. As a consequence, no other options are available, and unfortunately patients have died from end-stage heart failure within a few days despite repetitive infusion of inotropic agents. Since the earliest reports of the potential beneficial effects of CRT have been assessed in acute hemodynamic studies, one might postulate that in patients with persistent low cardiac output, despite drugs that usually improved cardiac function, CRT may be helpful.

In our department, we have assessed the feasibility, safety, and efficacy of CRT in patients with refractory CHF with no medical alternative. In our study, dependence from inotropic agents was defined by the recurrence after three attempts of these clinical signs of cardiogenic shock, despite correction of preload, as soon as the infusion was stopped or decreased. These data (under submission) showed that CRT in these patients is beneficial. In our study we were able to successfully implant all patients without any complications during the procedure. Permanent monitoring of the hemodynamics with both central venous and arterial pressures, under light sedation and oxygen and under the supervision of an anesthesiologist during the procedure, was mandatory for the management of such unstable patients. In addition, once patients have been discharged from the hospital, we found that the benefit of CRT observed acutely was sustained, with 88% of these particularly severe patients surviving 6 months after successful implantation.

Clinical Case

A 76-year-old man with dilated cardiomyopathy, LVEF of 20%, and QRS >120 ms presented with refractory overt CHF despite being on dobutamine (10 μg/kg/min). He had both severe pulmonary and renal insufficiency. As a consequence, he was not a candidate for heart transplantation. The dobutamine could not be stopped because of an immediate recurrence of clinical and biologic signs of low cardiac output with permanent low systolic blood pressure (under 80 mm Hg), hypoxemia, tachycardia, low urine output with renal failure (<0.5 mL/kg/h), and liver failure, as soon as the intravenous drug was decreased. After considering our inability to control the hemodynamic status of the patient despite optimal medical treatment orally and intravenously, we performed a CRT implantation after the family was informed of the severe clinical situation and was told that there was no other medical alternative. The implantation was performed (<2 hours) without any complications during and after the procedure, with a significant shortening of the QRS duration (Fig. 62.2). Before the end of the procedure, blood pressure increased as soon as the CRT was turned

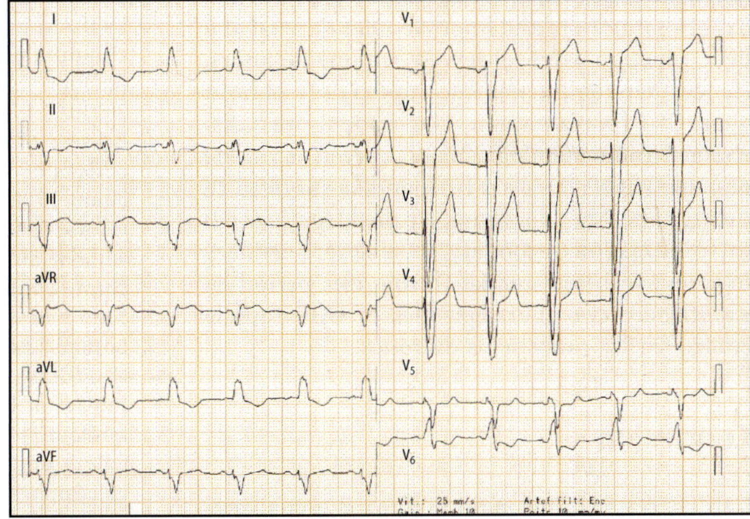

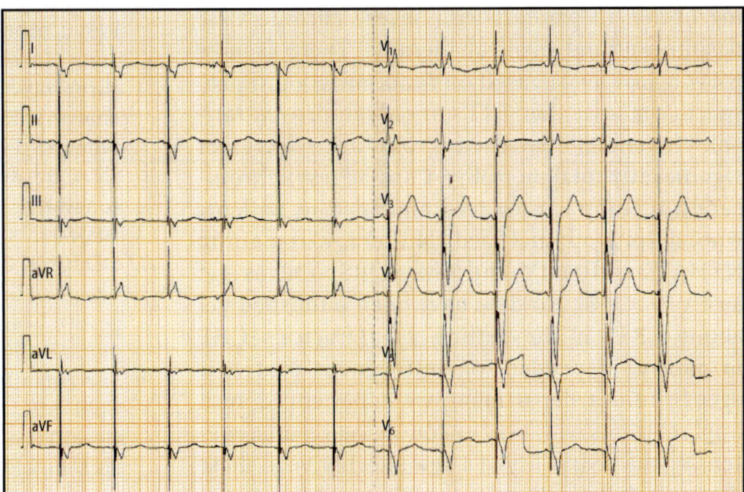

FIGURE 62.2. A 12-lead electrocardiogram of the patient with a left bundle branch block (LBBB) pattern before (top) and after CRT (bottom). CRT narrowed QRS duration with a right bundle branch block (RBBB) pattern right axis related to a LV pacing from a left lateral vein.

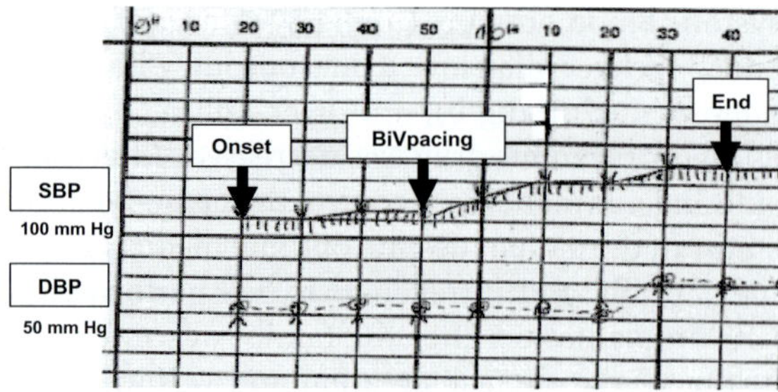

Figure 62.3. Permanent blood pressure monitoring along the implantation procedure showing an immediate increased of blood pressure as soon as the CRT was turned on. BiV, biventricular pacing; DBP, diastolic blood pressure; SBP, systolic blood pressure.

on (Fig. 62.3). After CRT implantation, resumption of dieresis (5 L), increased blood pressure and oxygen saturation, and improvement of renal and liver function were observed within 24 hours. Hence, dobutamine was interrupted only 24 hour after CRT implantation. The patient was discharged from our department a week later. He remained in NYHA class II/III and he survived 28 months after the procedure. He died from electrical dissociation secondary to a severe urinary infection with septicemia. During this period he experienced two short episodes of CHF rapidly controlled by intravenous diuretics.

Conclusion

Cardiac resynchronization therapy is a challenging option in patients with severe chronic CHF despite optimal medical therapy. There is now growing evidence based on randomized and prospective studies that CRT not only improves variable functional parameters but also decreases significantly total mortality. Cardiac resynchronization therapy is now recommended in patients who, despite optimal medical therapy, remain in NYHA class III or IV, and have a QRS >130 ms and an LVEF <35%. No data have been published yet about CRT in the setting of refractory CHF in patients dependent on intravenous inotropic agents. In our department, we experienced such implantations with very encouraging results, presenting the possibility of a new alternative in these particularly severe patients with rapid bad prognosis. However, our data must be confirmed in a larger cohort of patients in order to validate such an indication.

References

1. Auricchio A, Stellbrink C, Sack S, et al. Pacing Therapies in Congestive Heart Failure (PATH-CHF) Study Group. Long-term clinical effect of hemodynamically optimized cardiac resynchronization therapy in patients with heart failure and ventricular conduction delay. J Am Coll Cardiol 2002;39:2026–33.
2. Cazeau S, Leclercq C, Lavergne T, et al. Effects of multisite biventricular pacing in patients with heart failure and intraventricular conduction delay. N Engl J Med 2001;344:873–80.
3. Abraham WT, Fisher WG, Smith AL, et al. Multicenter InSync Randomized Clinical Evaluation (MIRACLE) Study Group. Effect of cardiac resynchronization therapy on left ventricular size and function in chronic heart failure. Circulation 2003;107:1985–90.
4. Bristow MR, Saxon LA, Boehmer J, et al. Comparison of Medical Therapy, Pacing, and Defibrillation in Heart Failure (COMPANION) Investigators. Cardiac-resynchronization therapy with or without an implantable defibrillator in advanced chronic heart failure. N Engl J Med 2004;350:2140–50.
5. Lozano I, Bocchiardo M, Achtelik M, et al. VENTAK CHF/CONTAK CD Investigators Study Group. Impact of biventricular pacing on mortality in a randomized crossover study of patients with heart failure and ventricular arrhythmias. Pacing Clin Electrophysiol 2000;23:1711–2.
6. Cleland J, Daubert JC, Erdmann E, et al. Cardiac Resynchronization-Heart Failure (CARE-HF) Study Investigators. The effect of cardiac resynchronization on morbidity and mortality in heart failure. N Engl J Med 2005;352:1539–49.
7. Iuliano S, Fisher SG, Karasik PE, Fletcher RD, Singh SN. QRS duration and mortality in patients with congestive heart failure. Am Heart J 2002;143:1085–91.
8. Stellbrink C, Auricchio A, Diem B, et al. Potential benefit of biventricular pacing in patients with congestive heart failure and ventricular tachyarrhythmia. Am J Cardiol 1999;83:143D–50D.
9. Silverman ME, Pressel MD, Brackett JC, Lauria SS, Gold MR, Gottlieb SS. Prognostic value of the signal-averaged electrocardiogram and a prolonged QRS in ischemic and nonischemic cardiomyopathy. Am J Cardiol 1995;75:460–4.

10. Shamim W, Francis DP, Yousufuddin M, et al. Intraventricular conduction delay: a prognostic marker in chronic heart failure. Int J Cardiol 1999;70:171–8.
11. Grines CL, Bashore TM, Boudoulas H, et al. Functional abnormalities in isolated left bundle branch block. The effect of interventricular asynchrony. Circulation 1989;79:845–53.
12. Nishimura RA, Hayes DL, Holmes DR, et al. Mechanism of hemodynamic improvement by dual-chamber pacing for severe left ventricular dysfunction: an acute Doppler and catheterization hemodynamic study. J Am Coll Cardiol 1995;25:281–8.
13. Brecker SJD, Xiao HB, Sparrow J, et al. Effects of dual chamber pacing with short atrioventricular delay in dilated cardiomyopathy. Lancet 1992;340: 1308–12.
14. Leclercq C, Cazeau S, Le Breton H, et al. Acute hemodynamic effects of biventricular DDD pacing in patients with end-stage heart failure. J Am Coll Cardiol 1998;32:1825–31.
15. Nelson GS, Berger RD, Fetics BJ, et al. Left ventricular or biventricular pacing improves cardiac function at diminished energy cost in patients with dilated cardiomyopathy and left bundle-branch block. Circulation 2000;102:3053–9.

63
Acute Heart Failure Treatment and Brain Protection

Nicolas Deye, Bruno Mégarbane, and Frédéric J. Baud

Brain damage and heart failure may coexist if terminal heart failure or arrhythmias induce cerebral hypoperfusion. Another frequent situation of heart failure–induced brain damage is represented by cardiac arrest, which remains a major public health problem and a leading cause of death. Cardiac arrest either occurs during the course of a known cardiopathy or suddenly reveals an unknown underlying cardiac disease. Following refractory shock or multiorgan failure, and after experiencing cardiac arrest, irreversible brain damages remain the major cause of death. Thus, several therapies are commonly used to reduce brain injuries, including hypothermia, which remains to date the most convincing treatment for brain protection.

Pathophysiology

Acute heart failure outcome is determined by the underlying cardiac disease. Successfully resuscitated cardiac arrest outcome is also dependent on the post-resuscitation syndrome (e.g., ischemia-reperfusion syndrome). The pathogenesis of post-ischemic encephalopathy is multifactorial and still not completely understood (1,2). Following cardiac arrest, brain ischemia results in cell membrane depolarization with an increase in intracellular calcium, a loss of phosphate compounds, and a release of glutamate (3). During reperfusion these mechanisms initiate multiple independent biochemical cascades, resulting in mitochondrial damages, neuronal cell necrosis and apoptosis. Thus, only a multifaceted treatment strategy appears able to allow survival without brain damage (4). To date, mild hypothermia is the most efficient treatment to achieve this goal. Hypothermia benefit is related to the reduction in the brain metabolism, with a 5% to 7% decrease in oxygen consumption for each 1°C decrease (5). Hypothermia also inhibits several deleterious reactions, such as caspase activation, excitatory amino acid release, calcium intracellular shift, and free-radical production (3). Hypothermia moderates the ischemia-induced inflammatory response and limits alteration in membrane permeability and its resulting intracellular acidosis. Hypothermia reduces the disruption in the blood–brain barrier and vascular permeability, decreasing cerebral edema and hemoglobin extravasation. Hypothermia is clearly effective in controlling intracranial hypertension. Several injured brain areas may reach significantly higher temperatures than the measured core temperature. Therapeutic hypothermia may thus prevent this thermo-pooling. In contrast to pharmacological agents, hypothermia seems to act on the whole destructive mechanisms.

Hypothermia for Neuroprotection

Definitions

Hypothermia is defined as a reduction in the body temperature below the normal core temperature (36.6° ± 0.4°C) and usually as ≤35°C (95°F) (3). Accidental hypothermia induces deleterious defense mechanisms such as shivering and increased oxygen consumption and cell metabolism. Different degrees of therapeutic hypothermia are defined: mild (≤35°C and >32°C [90°F]), moderate (<32°C and ≥28°C), deep (<28°C and >10°C), profound (≤10°C and >5°C), and ultra-profound (≤5°C and >0°C) (1,6). Accidental hypothermia is uncontrolled and induces deleterious defense mechanisms such as shivering and increased oxygen consumption and cell metabolism. In contrast, therapeutic hypothermia is induced by artificial and controlled cooling and commonly used in cardiac surgery, neurosurgery, or resuscitation.

Historical View of Resuscitative Hypothermia

The therapeutic interest of hypothermia is not a new concept: it was described by the ancient Egyptians, the Greeks, and the Romans, and in the 19th century by Napoleon's Surgeon General Larrey (3). Clinical interest in hypothermia increased in the 1940s when successful outcomes were reported with profound accidental hypothermia. In the 1950s, the beneficial outcome from hypothermia was related to a protective-preservative mechanism against cerebral ischemia. Moderate hypothermia was then used during open-heart surgical procedures, intracerebral aneurysm repair, and focal brain ischemia. However, systemic complications were observed, including shivering, vasospasm, increased hematocrit and plasma viscosity, hypocoagulation, severe arrhythmias, and decreased resistance to infection (6). Therapeutic hypothermia was consequently discontinued because of its uncertain benefits and its difficult management. In the 1980s, animal studies showed that mild hypothermia was as protective as moderate hypothermia, even when delayed after cardiac arrest, with fewer and less severe side effects. When minimal delay after cardiac arrest was relevant in animal models, prolonged duration of mild hypothermia was of major importance. The renewed interest in hypothermia was then facilitated with improvements in intensive care and the ability to control potential artificial cooling side effects, resulting in promising clinical trials (3).

Clinical Trials with Hypothermia After Cardiac Arrest

In the late 1990s, a nonrandomized study demonstrated that induced mild hypothermia increases significantly the number of patients with good functional outcome in comparison to a matched historic control group, with a reduced mortality rate (7). Surface cooling with ice packs was used for 12 hours. Despite a limited number of patients, this study pointed out the potential benefits of therapeutic hypothermia in comatose survivors of nonventricular fibrillation arrest. Another study evaluated cardiac arrest survivors cooled to a core temperature between 33° and 34°C over 48 hours, using water-filled cooling blankets in combination with alcohol (8). Three of 13 patients in the hypothermia group survived without disabilities as compared to one of 15 patients in the historical control group. However, a higher rate of nonlethal pulmonary infection was observed in the hypothermia group. In a European multicenter pilot study, 27 comatose patients were cooled after successful resuscitation of ventricular fibrillation using surface cooling and a water-filled blanket (9). The target temperature (33° ± 1°C) was maintained for 24 hours. Neurologic outcome was evaluated using the cerebral performance category (CPC) score, subdivided into good outcome (CPC 1 or 2), poor outcome (CPC 3 or 4), or death (CPC 5) at 6 months (Table 63.1). This was a twofold improvement in neurologic outcome

Table 63.1. Glasgow-Pittsburgh Outcome Categorization of Brain Injury: the cerebral performance categories (CPCs)

1. Good cerebral performance. Conscious, alert, and able to work and lead a normal life. Might have psychological or neurologic deficits (mild dysphasia, non-incapacitating hemiparesis, or minor cranial nerve abnormalities).
2. Moderate cerebral disability. Conscious; sufficient cerebral function for part-time work in a sheltered environment or independent activities of daily life (dress, travel by public transportation, food preparation). Such patients may have hemiplegia, seizures, ataxia, dysarthria, dysphasia, or permanent memory or mental changes.
3. Severe cerebral disability. Conscious; patient dependent on others for daily support (in an institution or at home with exceptional family effort) because or impaired brain functions. Has at least limited cognition. This category includes a wide range of cerebral abnormalities, from patients who are ambulatory but have severe memory disturbances or dementia precluding independent existence, to those who are paralyzed and can communicate only with their eyes, as in the locked-in syndrome.
4. Coma/vegetative state. Not conscious, unaware of surroundings, no cognition. No verbal and/or psychological interaction with the environment.
5. Brain death. Certified brain death or death established using traditional criteria.

compared to historic controls. No harmful side effects or major complications related to mild hypothermia were detected.

Encouraged by these positive results, prospective randomized clinical trials were initiated. The first randomized trial included 30 patients with asystole and pulseless electrical activity successfully resuscitated after out-of-hospital cardiac arrest (10). A helmet device around the head and neck was used to induce mild hypothermia. When the bladder temperature reached 34°C or when cooling extended over 4 hours, the patient was passively rewarmed spontaneously over the next 8 hours. Favorable neurologic recovery and survival rate were similar in the normothermia and the hypothermia groups. No complications were reported. This study documented significant improved metabolic end points (lactate and O_2 extraction) for the comatose patients cooled after return of spontaneous circulation (ROSC) when compared with the noncooled patients.

In 2002, two randomized prospective trials were published (11,12). An Australian study randomized 77 patients with ROSC after cardiac arrest from cardiac origin (ventricular fibrillation or pulseless ventricular tachycardia) to receive either hypothermia treatment (33°C core temperature over 12 hours using ice packs) either normothermia (11). The primary end point was survival to hospital discharge with sufficient good neurologic function to be discharged to home or to a rehabilitation unit. Mild hypothermia improved significantly neurologic outcomes in comatose patients compared to normothermia (49% for hypothermic patients vs. 26% for normothermic patients). After adjustment for baseline differences, the odds ratio for a good neurologic outcome was 5.25 (95% confidence interval, 1.47 to 18.76; $p = .011$) for patients treated with hypothermia when compared to patients treated with normothermia. There was no difference in the frequency of adverse events, but hypothermia was associated with a lower cardiac index, higher systemic vascular resistance, and higher hyperglycemia.

The European trial included 273 patients with ROSC after cardiac arrest of cardiac origin (ventricular fibrillation or pulseless ventricular tachycardia) randomly assigned either to therapeutic hypothermia (32–34°C bladder temperature, using cold air mattress devices) during a 24-hour period or to standard treatment with normothermia (12). This study also included a small subset of patients with in-hospital cardiac arrest. All patients received standard intensive care according to a detailed protocol for 32 hours, including sedatives, analgesics, and muscle paralysis to prevent shivering. The primary end point was a favorable neurologic outcome within 6 months after cardiac arrest defined as CPC 1 or 2. Secondary end points were mortality within 6 months and complications within 7 days. A favorable neurologic outcome was obtained in 55% for the hypothermia group as compared to 39% for the normothermia group (risk ratio, 1.40; 95% confidence interval, 1.08 to 1.81). Mortality at 6 months was 41% in the hypothermia group as compared to 55% in the normothermia group (risk ratio, 0.74; 95% confidence interval, 0.58 to 0.95). The rate of complications observed in the two groups was not significantly different.

These two randomized trials showed improved outcome in adults who remained comatose after initial resuscitation from out-of-hospital ventricular fibrillation cardiac arrest and who were cooled within minutes to hours after ROSC. However, both studies were conducted in highly selected populations with the exclusion up to 92% of the patients with out-of-hospital cardiac arrest assessed for eligibility. Inclusion criteria explain the apparent good survival in the controlled normothermic groups as compared to the high mortality rates described in the literature for out-of hospital cardiac arrest patients.

A recent meta-analysis including individual patient data of the three randomized trials testing mild therapeutic hypothermia after cardiac arrest showed that significantly more patients in the hypothermia group were discharged with favorable neurologic recovery (risk ratio, 1.68; 95% confidence interval 1.29–2.07) (13). The 95% confidence interval of the number needed to treat to allow one additional patient to leave the hospital with favorable neurologic recovery was 4 to 13. This translates to a number-needed-to treat of 6. Additionally, being alive at 6 months with favorable functional neurologic recovery was more likely when patients were treated with mild hypothermia (risk ratio, 1.44; 95% confidence interval, 1.11–1.76).

Interestingly, therapeutic hypothermia interest was recently enhanced in neonates, although its use is not yet routinely recommended (14). In 2005, three studies of mild hypothermia in asphyxiated newborns pointed out its significant positive effect in reducing long-term disability or death.

Hypothermia Management

Prevention and Treatment of Hyperthermia and Therapeutic Hypothermia

A period of hyperthermia after the first 48 hours following a cardiac arrest is common (15). The risk of unfavorable neurologic outcome increases for each degree of body temperature >37°C after brain injury (3,15). Fever is an independent factor of adverse outcome, morbidity, mortality, and more severe neurologic impairment in patients with various neurologic injuries. This difference persists when patients are matched for other confounding factors such as infection (3). A causal relationship has been demonstrated in animal experiments. Prevention of fever is recommended for traumatic brain injured patients or after stroke (class II level of evidence). Animal and preliminary clinical studies suggest the effectiveness of hypothermia in stroke with severe middle cerebral artery infarction, but hypothermia is still experimental in these clinical indications. However, hyperthermia should be avoided and protective normothermia applied for all ventilated patients with brain damage including cardiac arrest patients, within the first 24 to 48 hours, after searching rigorously for infections or deep thrombosis (3,15).

According to international guidelines, unconscious adult patients with spontaneous circulation after out-of-hospital cardiac arrest should be cooled to 32° to 34°C for 12 to 24 hours when the initial rhythm is a ventricular fibrillation or a pulseless ventricular tachycardia (protective hypothermia) (15,16). Such cooling may be considered for unconscious adult patients with spontaneous circulation after out-of-hospital cardiac arrest from any other rhythm or in-hospital cardiac arrest. Numerous studies in animals documented the importance of initiating cooling as soon as possible and for an adequate duration. However, the optimal characteristics for cooling, including precise onset, depth, and duration of cooling, are unknown. Cooling should probably be initiated as soon as possible and continued for 12 to 24 hours.

Cooling Methods

Numerous external or internal cooling techniques can be used to initiate cooling within minutes to hours (Table 63.2) (5,15,16). The only studies demonstrating improved outcome with therapeutic hypothermia after cardiac arrest used external cooling methods. Including hypothermia using surface cooling is simple but slow, needing up to 8 hours to reach target temperatures. Other cooling techniques based on invasive procedures are more efficient in decreasing core temperature. However, these techniques have not been proven superior in comparison to external ones to improve prognosis or mortality. One study in cardiac arrest patients and three studies in the neurologic intensive care unit and in neurosurgery established that intravascular cooling enables better control of core temperature than external methods.

A delay in cooling can negate the beneficial effects of protective hypothermia (6). Thus, a

Table 63.2. Available methods or devices for inducing hypothermia

Peripheral cooling (from the most simple to sophisticated methods)
Control of ambient temperature
Exposure of skin (remove clothes)
Sponge baths
Water and alcohol sprays
Ice packs (avoid direct contact between ice and skin)
Fans
Cooling caps
Air-circulating cooling blankets
Water-circulating cooling blankets
Helmet device
Ice-water nose cooling and selective brain cooling
Immersion
Specially designed beds
Core cooling
Antipyretic agents (often ineffective if hyperthermia is caused by impaired thermoregulation: central fever)
Infusion of ice-cold (4°C) fluids (saline, Ringer's solution)
Intravascular cooling catheters
Peritoneal or pleural lavage (not generally used)
Extracorporeal circulation (venovenous or arteriovenous)

feasible method to induce rapid hypothermia seems mandatory in the prehospital setting. Invasive cooling techniques are more powerful to induce hypothermia but are not practical at the prehospital scene and could result in further delay. Venovenous extracorporeal pump cooling is efficient to rapidly induce hypothermia, but it requires devices such as a double-lumen venous catheter with a miniaturized pump, a heat exchanger, and a cold source. Endovascular cooling devices, using central venous catheter with balloons filled with temperature-controlled cold fluid, are clinically already used for cardiac arrest, acute myocardial infarction, or neurologic pathologies (5,6,15,16). This approach may be safe and advantageous in heart failure patients because no fluid enters the circulation, but the cooling rate is limited to 0.8° ± 0.3°C/h. However, whether faster cooling could result in a better outcome remains to be determined.

Recently intravenous infusion of 30 mL/kg ice-cooled (4°C) saline solution over 30 minutes (or at a rate of 100 mL/min in adult patients) was proposed in the prehospital setting or thereafter, after successful resuscitation of nontraumatic cardiac arrest and hemodynamic stabilization. It decreased cardiac arrest survivors' core temperature of approximately 1.5°C without providing important side effects. Infusion of intravenous ice-cold fluid in healthy humans changed core temperature only from 0.6°C with moderate volume to 2.5°C with very large volume (40 mL/kg) (6). However, in the absence of large randomized studies, this procedure should be used with caution for heart failure patients.

Temperature Measurement and Monitoring During Mild Hypothermia

Several side effects are possible during hypothermia (Table 63.3). The incidence of complications increases if the core temperature falls considerably or if rewarming is performed too quickly (5). Careful monitoring of body temperature is thus recommended during the cooling and rewarming phases (15,16). Adapted thermometers for <35°C or internal devices (central venous or rectal temperatures, bladder or esophageal probes) are needed. The oral and most of the tympanic thermometers should be avoided because they can

Table 63.3. The main side effects of ≤35°C hypothermia

The temperature thresholds where these effects appear and their intensity are variable from a patient to another. They are markedly influenced by age, degree of hypothermia, and comorbidities, especially cardiovascular diseases.
Physiological attempts to maintain normal temperature
In awake patients: generation of heat (shivering, peripheral vasoconstriction, increased muscle activity, increased oxygen consumption, increased rate of metabolism), but if temperature <30°C, hibernation (shivering ceases, marked decrease in rate of metabolism)
Hemodynamic effects
Bradycardia, mild arrhythmias, tachyarrhythmias, as atrial fibrillation, ECG modifications
Slight increase in blood pressure (average 10 mm Hg)
Increases in central venous pressure
Increase in mixed venous saturation
Decrease in cardiac output
Myocardial ischemia
Renal effects
Hypothermia-induced diuresis: increased diuresis leading to hypovolemia
Tubular dysfunction and electrolytes disorders: loss and decreased levels of potassium, magnesium, phosphate, calcium
Neurologic
Decreased consciousness, lethargy, coma
Metabolic effects
Decreases in oxygen consumption, carbon dioxide production, and overall metabolism except for "fat metabolism"; increase in serum lactate levels, metabolic acidosis and increased production of free fatty acids, ketones, and glycerol
Decrease in insulin sensitivity and secretion: insulin resistance and rise in serum glucose levels
Increases of levels of endogenic adrenaline, noradrenaline, and cortisol
Immunohematologic effects
Thrombocytopenia
Coagulation disorders: increase in bleeding time, activated partial thromboplastin time (aPTT), and partial thromboplastin time (PTT)
Bleeding
Leukocytopenia
Impaired coagulation cascade and impaired platelet, leukocyte, neutrophil and macrophage functions
Suppression of proinflammatory mediator release
Increased risk of infection (pneumonia or wound principally)
Miscellaneous
Impaired bowel function and intestinal motility (ileus)
Pancreatitis, increase in serum amylase levels
Increase in liver enzymes (particularly aminotransferases)
Pharmacokinetics
Changes in drug effects and drug metabolism: altered clearance of various medications (muscle paralyzers, propofol, fentanyl, phenytoin, pentobarbital, verapamil, propanol and volatile anesthetics, etc.)

accurately record temperatures only as low as 35°C. Cooling methods such as air mattress, water cover, or endovascular catheters can be connected to the device used to measure continuously the core temperature.

Seizures or myoclonii occurs after brain damage and may produce heat. A combination of sedation and neuromuscular blockade is needed to avoid shivering in ventilated patients (Table 63.4) (5,15,16). However, as these therapies may mask seizures, closed clinical and electroencephalographic monitoring is required. For noncardiac arrest and nonventilated patients, shivering can be controlled with oral buspirone or intravenous meperidine (but meperidine-related nausea has to be prevented).

Electrocardiogram Findings in Hypothermic Patients

Increasing hypothermia progressively decreases cardiac conduction, slows depolarization and repolarization, and causes atrioventricular and nodal blocks or atrioventricular dysrhythmias (17). The usual ECG manifestations of hypothermia include the presence of Osborn J waves, PR, QRS or QT interval prolongations, sinus bradycardia, and atrial or ventricular arrhythmias. With moderate hypothermia, junctional rhythms and atrial reentrant dysrhythmias may occur. More than 50% of patients with moderate hypothermia develop atrial fibrillation. However, routine anticoagulation for atrial fibrillation is not recommended because of the likelihood of its spontaneous conversion and the risk of hypothermia-induced coagulopathy. Ventricular arrhythmias are more likely to occur when core temperature falls below 30°C. The risk of asystole increases significantly with deeper hypothermia (<25°C).

Osborn wave is a positive deflection in the terminal portion of the QRS complex and elevation of the J point, resembling a domed T wave (small humps after the QRS complex, late delta wave following the QRS or small secondary R' wave). The J waves are commonly found in the anterior and lateral precordial leads. Their size usually inversely correlates with the body temperature. They are most prominent in II, III, aVF, aVR, and V_3 to V_6 leads. They may sometimes be present in only a single lead. They have no prognostic value. They

Table 63.4. Summary for the treatment of heart failure patients with brain injury (for instance, cardiac arrest patients)

- Temperature management: control of normothermia in the first 24–48 hours (upper limit ≈37.5°C)
  Mild therapeutic hypothermia for comatose patients after cardiac arrest from cardiac origin (ventricular fibrillation) with respect to nonindications (pregnancy, trauma, severe bleeding, intracerebral bleeding, terminal disease or previous coagulopathy), initiated as soon as possible (necessary time between sustained return of spontaneous circulation and initiation of cooling <240 min), targeting 32–34°C for 12–24 hours, associated with closed core temperature monitoring (bladder or esophageal probes) and with a controlled rewarming phase (0.5°C/h max)
- Treatments of hypothermia side effects (shivering, arrhythmias)
- Treatment of associated complications (infections, deep thrombosis)
- Control of seizures and myoclonii (from benzodiazepines such as lorazepam to barbiturates such as thiopental for refractory status epilepticus) with clinical and electroencephalographic monitoring
- Initial sedation (such as midazolam 0.5 to 3.6 μg/kg/min; barbiturates can decrease intracranial pressure) with strict monitoring of the sedation level and of its potential side effects (hypotension); early interruption of sedatives (following rewarming, and according to the respiratory and hemodynamic status)
- Analgesia (morphinomimetics such as fentanyl 0.02 to 0.1 μg/kg/min with titration)
- Neuromuscular blockade (intermittent or continuous paralyzation such as rocuronium 0.7 mg/kg bolus, and 0.3 to 0.6 mg/kg/h) for hypothermia-induced shivering in ventilated patients (with closed monitoring and discontinuation of paralysis when temperature >35°C); for nonventilated non–cardiac arrest patients, buspirone or meperidine can prevent shivering (with prevention of meperidine-related nausea by intravenous ondansetron or otherwise)
- Normoxia: initial controlled mechanical ventilation is mandatory for severe cardiac and brain damages and cardiac arrest patients with no excessive end expiratory pressure and with FiO_2 level to obtain SpO_2 >90% and PaO_2 >60 mm Hg (especially when endotracheal suctioning is performed)
- Normocarbia (range >36 and ≤40 mm Hg and no hyperventilation without intracranial pressure control)
- Blood pressure (and cerebral blood flow) control and monitoring with euvolemia and normotension (systolic blood pressure >90 mm Hg and mean blood pressure >65 mm Hg): fluid loading (in case of proved hypovolemia), catecholamines (dobutamine in case of heart failure, noradrenaline in case of vasoplegia); vasodilators should initially be used with caution
- Normonatremia (saline 0.9% is isotonic when compared to hypotonic ringer lactate or glucose solutions)
- Normoglycemia with insulin protocol: range 80–110 mg/dL (4.4–6.1 mmol/)L if a strict glycemic monitoring is achieved to avoid hypoglycemia; in other cases, glucose level maintained <215 mg/dL (<11.9 mmol/L)
- Semirecumbent position (30 degrees) in the bed
- Prevention of complications (prophylactic thromboembolic treatment, continuation of an antiarrhythmic drug that successfully restored a stable rhythm during resuscitation)

are highly specific but have been reported in nonhypothermic patients (subarachnoid hemorrhage, acute cardiac ischemia). They usually occur in patients with temperatures less than 32°C and are detectable in 80% of patients below a temperature of 30°C.

Other ECG findings associated with hypothermia should be recognized, such as myocardial ischemia-like signs (flat or inverted T waves). ST elevation may sometimes accompany J waves or the J wave may be mistaken for ST segment elevation related to an acute myocardial infarction. ST segment elevation spontaneously resolved following rewarming. Thus, inappropriate administration of thrombolytics is not useful and could be catastrophic. Hyperkalemia is often associated with acidosis, rhabdomyolysis, and renal failure. However, subtle peaked T waves may be misdiagnosed and could delay hyperkalemia treatment.

Future Perspectives: Suspended Animation with Hypothermia

In the 1980s, Peter Safar (4) introduced the concept of suspended animation for delayed resuscitation, meaning the "preservation of the organism during transport under prolonged controlled clinical death, followed by delayed resuscitation to survival without brain damage." Preservative hypothermia, induced and reversed with cardiopulmonary bypass before cardiac arrest, has been shown to preserve the organism for up to 15 minutes by mild hypothermia, for up to 20 minutes by moderate hypothermia, for up to 30 minutes by deep hypothermia, and for up to 60 minutes by profound hypothermia (4,6). This concept is based on the possible complete recover of nonresuscitated patients after experiencing cardiac arrest treated with prolonged cardiopulmonary bypass. To rapidly preserve the brain, aortic cold saline flush via a balloon catheter has been proposed until cardiopulmonary bypass can restore circulation (6). The induction of suspended animation in a cardiac arrest dog model by the use of cold (4°C) aortic flush within the first 5 minutes of cardiac arrest preserved brain viability for a 15 to 120 minutes of cardiac arrest. The aortic flush was followed by a period of hypothermic no-flow, and then animals were resuscitated with cardiopulmonary bypass. This approach to allow organ preservation needs further evaluation. Hypothermia should find a new place in these cases of impossibility to quickly restore spontaneous circulation. Thus cooling to achieve the lowest possible temperatures to preserve the brain and heart should be the main prehospital goal, leaving patients in cardiac arrest and transporting them to the emergency department where cardiopulmonary bypass will be initiated.

Hypothermia for Acute Myocardial Infarction and Surgery

Therapeutic hypothermia may reduce or delay myocardial cell necrosis, decreasing reperfusion injury (18). In animal studies, hypothermia succeeded in reducing myocardial infarct size when performed during the ischemia phase but failed at the reperfusion time. A preliminary report in patients undergoing cooling via a catheter placed into the inferior vena cava before angioplasty showed no overall reduction in acute myocardial infarction size. However, another study in patients with anterior wall acute myocardial infarction cooled to temperatures less than 35°C at the time of reperfusion had significantly smaller left ventricular infarcts (9.3%) versus controls (18.2%). The investigators observed that core temperatures were not cooled quickly enough before angioplasty, while angioplasty was accomplished rather quickly. Early therapeutic hypothermia should be promising if cooling can be achieved more rapidly before coronary artery reperfusion. The feasibility of inducing mild hypothermia in acute ST elevation myocardial infarction and percutaneous coronary angioplasty was recently documented by several pilot studies using endovascular or noninvasive surface cooling (19,20).

Intraoperative hypothermia is widely used in neurosurgical procedures, cardiac surgery, and major vascular surgery (5,21). Usually the aim is to increase the time available for specific surgical procedures. Thus the cooling treatment is initiated before and during the insult. However, randomized controlled trials are still lacking, or are conflicting for cardiac surgery. These controversial results obtained with cooling during bypass may be due to the duration and the depth of cooling, the risk of hemorrhage induced by hypothermia during surgery, the differences in cardioplegia techniques, the speed of rewarming with the risk of deleterious hyperthermia, and the selection for the best sites for temperature monitoring (the brain temperature can exceed rectal and esophageal temperatures by 1.2 to 1.9°C after rewarming). There is a class IIb level of evidence to support the use of intraoperative hypothermia for intracerebral aneurysm surgery (5). For cerebral and spinal cord protection during thoracoabdominal aortic aneurysm repair and for neuroprotection during cardiac surgery, hypothermia is supported by class III evidence. In any of these studies, no harmful effects have been observed with mild hypothermia.

Other Medical Treatments for Brain Protection

Interesting neuroprotective effects were found in experimental and animal studies concerning the use of barbiturates, calcium channel blockers, and corticosteroids. Unfortunately, human trials performed in the 1980s with these treatments (thiopenthal, lidoflazine, nipodipine) failed to show neuroprotective effects for brain resuscitation after cardiac arrest.

Neuroprotection in acute heart failure or cardiac arrest could be base on some therapies used in traumatic brain-injured patients (22,23). Specific neurosurgical tools and treatments (e.g., Glasgow Coma Scale as an outcome predictor, intracranial pressure measurement and control, prehospital management such as the rapid sequence induction for oral endotracheal intubation, SjO_2 monitoring, and transcranial Doppler evaluations) will not be detailed thereby. However, the usual associated means of decreasing cerebral pressure include the semirecumbent position in bed (30 degrees), controlled mechanical ventilation with no excessive end-expiratory pressure, sedatives, barbiturates or neuromuscular blockers, and $PaCO_2$ control (within the 36 to 40 mm Hg range). Hyperthermia, hyperglycemia, hypotension, hypercapnia, deep hyperventilation ($PaCO_2$ <30 mm Hg), hypoxemia, and hyponatremia are deleterious and must be avoided. Thus, associated treatments should target normoxia and normocarbia, normal blood pressure level, and normoglycemia with no metabolic disorders.

Based on international guidelines for post-resuscitation management after cardiac arrest, interventions detailed elsewhere in the volume are categorized into four areas: (1) ventilation, (2) temperature control, (3) seizure control and sedation, and (4) other supportive therapies (Table 63.4) (15).

Control of Arterial Carbon Dioxide

Five studies in humans and numerous animal studies documented the harmful effects of hypocapnia (inducing cerebral ischemia) after cardiac arrest (15). There are no data supporting a specific $PaCO_2$ target after resuscitation. However, normocarbia is appropriate in traumatic brain injury patients (22,23). Thus, routine hyperventilation may be detrimental and should be avoided for brain-damaged patients.

Prevention and Control of Seizures

No study assessed the use of prophylactic anticonvulsant drugs after cardiac arrest (15). Seizures could be prevented principally for the most severe traumatic brain-injured patients (22,23). Some data indicate that seizures increase the oxygen requirements of the brain, can cause life-threatening arrhythmias and respiratory arrest, and can precipitate cardiac arrest (15). Therefore, brain damage– or cardiac arrest–induced seizures should be detected and promptly treated.

Sedation and Paralysis

There are no data supporting or refuting the use of sedation and neuromuscular blockade for a defined period of ventilation after cardiac arrest (15). One observational study documented increased incidence of pneumonia when sedation was prolonged beyond 48 hours after prehospital or in-hospital cardiac arrest. Daily interruption of sedative infusions in critically ill patients undergoing mechanical ventilation reduces intensive care unit length of stay and decreases the incidence of complications associated with prolonged intubation and mechanical ventilation (24). Thus, neuromuscular blockades and sedatives should be interrupted as soon as possible after shivering control, and after respiratory, neurologic, and hemodynamic stabilization.

Blood Glucose Control

In a surgical intensive care unit, tight control of blood glucose (range 80 to 110 mg/dL or 4.4 to 6.1 mmol/L) with insulin improved the outcome and reduced the hospital mortality rate in undifferentiated critically ill patients, including patients with cardiopulmonary bypass or hemodynamic failure. However, the effect of this strict therapy is unknown in post–cardiac arrest or brain-injured patients and continues to be debated (15). Control of hyperglycemia in acute heart failure patients seems important. Several studies documented a positive association between high blood glucose after resuscitation and poor neurologic outcome. Persistent hyperglycemia after stroke is also associated with a worse neurologic outcome. In diabetic patients with acute myocardial infarction, therapy to maintain blood glucose at a level below 215 mg/dL (11.9 mmol/L) improved the long-term outcome. This should be taken into account, as therapeutic hypothermia can be associated with hyperglycemia (3,5). Hyperglycemia or insulin resistance may lead to complications, such as increased susceptibility to infections, multiple organ failure, or polyneuromyopathy. Sustained blood-glucose control should prevent the cellular damage and the immune dysfunction, reduce the systemic inflammation, and protect the endothelium and mitochondrial function induced by hyperglycemia. The optimal blood glucose target in critically ill patients has not been determined.

A recent study of the tight control of the glucose level in a medical intensive care unit was inconclusive: side effects (fatal hypoglycemia) were more frequent in the first 3 days of hospitalization, although there was a decreasing mortality rate when hospitalization duration was longer than 3 days (25). The risk of hypoglycemia increases as the target blood glucose concentration is lowered. Furthermore, comatose patients were at particular risk for unrecognized hypoglycemia (15). Thus continuous or strict glucose monitoring must be considered before intensive insulin therapy for medical critically ill patients.

The benefit of a treatment with glucose, insulin, and potassium (GIK) to improve cardiac dysfunction or prognosis is still debated (26). These GIK infusions have been safely administered to acute stroke patients with mild to moderate hyperglycemia producing a physiologic but attenuated glucose response to acute stroke. However, its possible effectiveness remains to be elucidated.

Coagulation Control

Excluding strokes and myocardial infarctions, no study evaluated the role of curative anticoagulation to improve cardiac arrest outcome. In several reports using fibrinolytics combined with heparin after prolonged cardiac arrest, ROSC, but not 24-hour survival rates, was significantly better (15). However, the deeper the level of hypothermia, the more frequent are the coagulation disorders, with a hypothetic risk of intracranial bleeding, leading to a prophylactic coagulation control approach.

Clinical Case

An out-of-hospital first call was received from a railway station for a 51-year-old man who had suddenly complained of chest pain and then presented generalized seizures while becoming unresponsive. The witnesses did not performed basic life support (BLS). A team including an emergency medicine physician arrived at the scene after an estimated no-flow interval of 9 minutes (interval from witnessed cardiac arrest to initiation of CPR). His previous medical history was unremarkable. Standard advanced cardiac life support (ACLS) was immediately performed as recommended by the International Liaison Committee on Resuscitation (ILCOR). The initial electrocardiogram showed ventricular fibrillation. After one defibrillation (200 J with a biphasic model defibrillator), the patient experienced a return of spontaneous circulation (ROSC). The electrocardiogram showed sinusal rhythm with signs of acute anterior myocardial infarction. The initial blood pressure was 70/40 mm Hg and the heart rate was 82 beats/min. There were no signs of left ventricular failure. Circulation became stable (blood pressure, 105/50 mm Hg; heart rate, 115 beats/min) with cold fluid loading (1.5 L of 0.9% saline solution stored at 4°C) and continuous epinephrine infusion (1.5 mg/h).

The patient was transferred to the hospital. A coronary angiography was performed immediately upon arrival at the catheter lab and showed a single acute main left coronary artery occlusion. Successful angiographic result was obtained using a coated stent insertion (final coronary flow was normal), while glycoprotein IIb/IIIa inhibitor was infused and intraaortic balloon counterpulsation inserted. Body temperature and heart rate were initially 35.2°C and 90 beats/minute, respectively. Initial laboratory tests revealed metabolic lactic acidosis and serum troponin Ic elevation. A specific central venous catheter was inserted to allow continuous infusions and endovascular mild hypothermia (33°C for a 24-hour period). An esophageal probe was inserted to measure the patient central temperature (Fig. 63.1). Electrocardiograms showed correction of the ST elevation myocardial infarction (STEMI) and discrete hypothermia signs without reocclusion evidence (bradycardia). Sedation (midazolam) and muscle paralysis (discontinuous pancuronium) were induced during the hypothermia period and the controlled rewarming phase (0.5°C/h to achieve 37°C).

During the first 10 hours in the intensive care unit (ICU), the patient experienced cardiac failure (Killip class 2 with marked PaO_2/FiO_2 ratio decrease), which required up to 15 μg/kg/min dobutamine and 2 mg/h norepinephrine. Fluid loading was secondary, guided by repeated echocardiographic examinations (left ventricular ejection fraction: 40%). Laboratory tests showed decreased cardiac enzymes. Blood glucose concentration was closely controlled using an intravenous insulin protocol. Arterial blood gases were regularly monitored for a strict PaO_2 and $PaCO_2$ control. Daily chest x-ray demonstrated an improvement in the initial bilateral infiltrates, while cultures of pulmonary secretions remained negative. Diastolic counterpulsation was maintained for 4 days. Intravenous norepinephrine and dobutamine were stopped at day 4 and 7, respectively. Renal function remained stable during the whole ICU stay, allowing the introduction of small doses of angiotensin-converting enzyme inhibitor. After sedation discontinuation,

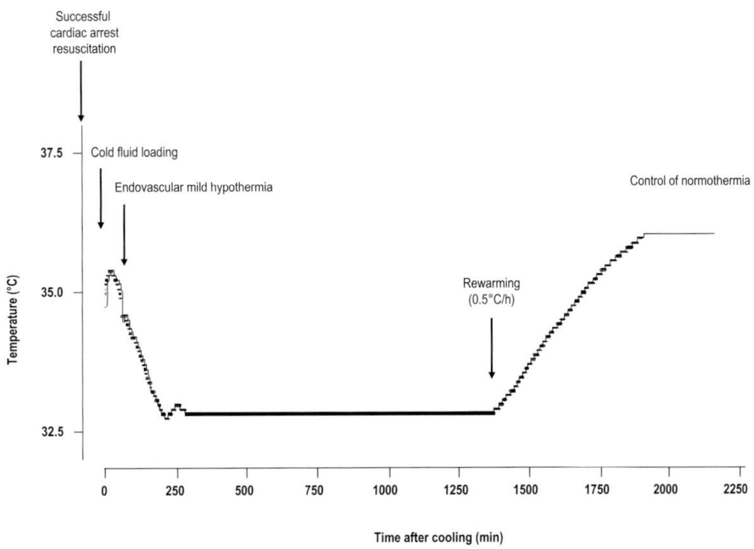

FIGURE 63.1. Central temperature measurements in time after the cardiac arrest resuscitation.

the patient awakened (Glasgow Coma Scale score of 10 on day 3). The patient was extubated on day 5. He achieved a neurologic recovery except for significant memory loss, including a complete amnesia of the recent events. Central venous and arterial catheters were removed on day 6. No infection occurred during the hospitalization. The highest Pittsburgh Cerebral Performance Category during his ICU stay was 2 out of 5. He was discharged from the ICU 8 days after the cardiac arrest onset and was transferred to the cardiologic ward for further investigation, medication adjustment, and rehabilitation.

Conclusion

Several medical interventions may be useful for neuroprotection in heart failure patients. Controlled temperature (therapeutic hypothermia or hyperthermia prevention), sedation, control of ventilation, seizures, and of blood glucose levels are beneficial. Therapeutic mild induced hypothermia (32° to 34°C) is currently the most advanced medical concept to prevent neuronal damage after cardiac arrest and is recommended by international guidelines. It remains to be precisely determined whether mild hypothermia is also beneficial for patients experiencing cardiac arrest from asystole or pulseless electrical activity, for in-hospital cardiac arrest patients, for severe cardiogenic shock, for life-threatening arrhythmia, for angioplasty in acute myocardial infarction, for stroke from cardiac origin, or during cardiac surgery.

References

1. Safar P. Resuscitation of the ischemic brain. In: Albin MS, ed. Textbook of Neuroanesthesia with Neurosurgical and Neuroscience Perspectives. New York: McGraw-Hill, 1997:557–93.
2. Safar P, Behringer W. Brain resuscitation after cardiac arrest. In: Layon AJ, Gabrielli A, Friedman WA, eds. Textbook of Neurointensive Care. Philadelphia: WB Saunders, 2003:457-98.
3. Polderman K. Application of therapeutic hypothermia in the intensive care unit. Opportunities and pitfalls of a promising treatment modality. Part 1: indications and evidence. Intensive Care Med. 2004;30:556–75.
4. Safar P. Resuscitation from clinical death: pathophysiologic limits and therapeutic potentials. Crit Care Med. 1988;16:923–41.
5. Polderman K. Application of therapeutic hypothermia in the intensive care unit. Opportunities and pitfalls of a promising treatment modality. Part 2: practical aspects and side effects. Intensive Care Med. 2004;30:757–9.
6. Sterz F, Behringer W, Holzer M. Global hypothermia for neuroprotection after cardiac arrest. Acute Cardiac Care. 2006;8:25–30.
7. Bernard SA, Jones BM, Horne MK. Clinical trial of induced hypothermia in comatose survivors of out-of hospital cardiac arrest. Ann Emerg Med. 1997;30:146–53.
8. Yanagawa Y, Ishihara S, Norio H, et al. Preliminary clinical outcome study of mild resuscitative hypothermia after out-of hospital cardiopulmonary arrest. Resuscitation. 1998;39:61–6.
9. Zeiner A, Holzer M, Sterz F, et al. Mild resuscitative hypothermia to improve neurological outcome after cardiac arrest. A clinical feasibility trial. Hypothermia After Cardiac Arrest (HACA) Study Group. Stroke. 2000;31:86–94.
10. Hachimi-Idrissi S, Corne L, Ebinger G, et al. Mild hypothermia induced by a helmet device: a clinical feasibility study. Resuscitation. 2001;35:275–81.
11. Bernard SA, Gray TW, Buist MD, et al. Treatment of comatose survivors of out-of-hospital cardiac arrest with induced hypothermia. N Engl J Med. 2002;346:557–63.
12. The Hypothermia After Cardiac Arrest Group. Mild therapeutic hypothermia to improve the neurologic outcome after cardiac arrest. N Engl J Med. 2002;346:549–56.
13. Holzer M, Bernard SA, Hachimi-Idrissi S, et al. Hypothermia for neuroprotection after cardiac arrest: systematic review and individual patient data meta-analysis. Crit Care Med. 2005;33:414–8.
14. 2005 American Heart Association Guidelines for Cardiopulmonary Resuscitation and Emergency Cardiovascular Care of Pediatric and Neonatal Patients: Neonatal Resuscitation Guidelines. American Heart Association, American Academy of Pediatrics. Pediatrics. 2006;117;1029–38.
15. International Liaison Committee On resuscitation, European Resuscitation Council and American Heart Association. Part 4: Advanced Life Support. Resuscitation. 2005;67:213–47.
16. Nolan JP, Morley PT, Vanden Hoek TL, Hickey RW. Therapeutic hypothermia after cardiac arrest. An advisory statement by the Advancement Life Support Task Force of the International Liaison Committee On Resuscitation. Circulation. 2003;108: 118–21.

17. Mattu A, Brady WJ, Perron AD. Electrocardiographic manifestations of hypothermia. Ann J Emerg Med. 2002;20:314–26.
18. Kloner RA, Rezkalla SH. Cardiac protection during acute myocardial infarction: where do we stand in 2004? J Am Coll Cardiol. 2004;44:276–86.
19. Kandzari DE, Chu A, Brodie BR, et al. Feasibility of endovascular cooling as an adjunct to primary percutaneous coronary intervention (results of the LOWTEMP pilot study). Am J Cardiol. 2004; 93:636–9.
20. Ly HQ, Denault A, Dupuis J, et al. A pilot study: The noninvasive surface cooling thermoregulatory system for mild hypothermia induction in acute myocardial infarction (The NICAMI study). Am Heart J. 2005;150:933.e9–13.
21. Ali MS, Harmer M, Kirkham F. Cardiopulmonary bypass temperature and brain function. Anaethesia. 2005;60:365–72.
22. Guidelines for the management of severe head injury. Brain Trauma Foundation, American Association of Neurological Surgeons, Joint Section on Neurotrauma and Critical Care. J Neurotrauma. 1996;13:641–734.
23. The Brain Trauma Foundation: The American Association of Neurological Surgeons, The Joint Section on Neurotrauma and Critical Care. Resuscitation of blood pressure and oxygenation. J Neurotrauma. 2000;17:641–734.
24. Schweickert WD, Gehlbach BK, Pohlman AS, Hall JB, Kress JP. Daily interruption of sedative infusions and complications of critical illness in mechanically ventilated patients. Critical Care Med. 2004;32:1272–6.
25. Van den Berghe G, Wilmer A, Hermans G, et al. Intensive Insulin therapy in the medical ICU. N Engl J Med. 2006;354:449–61.
26. The CREATE-ECLA trial Group Investigators. Effect of Glucose-Insulin-Potassium infusion on mortality in patients with acute myocardial infarction. The CREATE-ECLA randomized controlled trial. JAMA. 2005;293:437–46.

64
End-of-Life Care for Critically Ill Patients with Heart Failure: A Multidisciplinary Viewpoint from the Intensive Care Unit

Thomas Fassier and Elie Azoulay

Abstract

Care near the end of life (EOL) for critically ill patients is emerging as an essential task in cardiology and heart failure (HF) management. Professional recommendations were recently published on this topic and a consensus exists that research and debate in this area need further progress. In the field of critical care medicine, development of research about EOL care was substantial during the last decade. The growing incidence of decisions to forgo life-sustaining therapies (DFLSTs) stimulated ethical debates and led to official statements of European and American intensive care medicine societies. This chapter discusses the interdisciplinary aspects of EOL care by reviewing the critical care medicine literature concerning EOL care in the intensive care unit (ICU), for the benefit of physicians involved in EOL care for critically ill patients with HF. First, EOL decisions in the ICU, their incidence, and the legal/ethical background of the decision-making process leading to DFLSTs are reviewed, with comparison with data available about patients with HF. Then, three ways of optimizing EOL care in the ICU are explored (incorporation of palliative care skills into critical care medicine, strengthening of communication with families, improvement of multidisciplinary approach), with a discussion about how they can be used in EOL care for HF patients. Finally, future prospects in the development of EOL care for critically ill patients are reviewed, focusing on palliative and intensive medicine, interdisciplinary cooperation, professional training, and research in EOL care.

Introduction

Heart failure is a paramount public health issue affecting 1% to 2% of the general population in Western industrialized countries and 6% to 10% of the elderly population (1–3). Despite pharmacologic, surgical, and technological advances in the last decades, its prognosis remains poor, with a high mortality rate, reaching 24%, 37%, and 75% at 1, 2, and 6 years after diagnosis (4–6). In addition, HF is associated with increasing high treatment costs, which have been estimated at between 1% to 2% of the total annual health care expenditure in several developed countries (7–9). In November 2005, the American College of Chest Physicians published an official position statement to encourage the development of palliative care and EOL care for patients with HF (10), and other reviews appealed for more integration of palliative care into cardiology (3,11–13). Nevertheless, apart from review articles published in the last 5 years, a lot is yet to be done for this challenging task.

In the field of intensive care medicine, however, debates and research about EOL care were stimulated during the 1990s by the growing incidence of do-not resuscitate (DNR) orders in the ICU. Studies focused on two main questions: the DFLSTs, including withholding and withdrawal, and the optimization of comfort care near the end of life. The DFLSTs for patients near the end of life in the ICU have been described worldwide (14,15) and are nowadays recommended by European and North American intensive care medicine societies, which settled an international consensus conference in April 2003 (16). Concurrently, strategies to improve EOL care have emphasized the transition from curative care to comfort care with considerable attention to the development of palliative and patient/family-centered care in the ICUs (17).

As intensivists, why should we write a chapter about EOL care for patients with HF? The project reported in this chapter emerged during our resident rotation in a medical ICU. Confronted with several problematic cases of patients near the end of life with terminal HF, the fruitful experience of cooperation and discussions with colleagues and cardiologists highlighted the great benefit of sharing our respective knowledge of the research and literature in the field of EOL care. Thus, this chapter proposes a multidisciplinary point of view about the development of EOL care for patients with HF, based on the experience of ICU caregivers in the field of EOL care for critically ill patients.

We provide here insight into the intensive care medicine literature concerning EOL care that will be useful for physicians involved in the development of EOL care for critically ill patients with HF. This chapter is based on a previous review about EOL care in European ICUs conducted by interrogating the Medline database with the keywords *end of life*, *DNR order*, and *ethics*, combined with *intensive care* (18). The research was then broadened with the keywords *heart failure* and *cardiac failure*, allowing the selection of additional papers after careful examination of the references.

Decisions to Forgo Life-Sustaining Treatments Near the End of Life

Incidence of Decisions to Forgo Life-Sustaining Treatments and Do Not Resuscitate Orders in the Intensive Care Unit

Important data about the incidence of DFLSTs in the ICUs were provided by international and nationwide multicenter and single-center studies conducted in Europe and in North America since the concept emerged in the late 1980s (15,19–23). The key finding of this research is that DFLSTs are common in the ICUs, with a diverse incidence rate worldwide. In North America, it was initially observed that DFLSTs affected 50% of the patients dying in the ICUs, but the incidence dramatically increased over the last 10 years, now affecting 80% to 90% of patients dying in ICUs (14,24). In European ICUs, recently described in the Ethicus study, DFLSTs are also common, used by 76% of patients, representing 9.8% of admissions, who die after the withdrawal or withholding of life sustaining treatment (15). In France, according to the LATAREA study, (Limitations et Arrêts des Thérapeutiques Actives en RÉAnimation: DFLSTs in the ICU) occurred in 53% of the patients who died in 1997 (11% of ICU admissions) (19), but this incidence has probably increased since that time. Nevertheless, DFLSTs and EOL decisions are diverse from one country to another and even in the same country, with treatment withdrawal less common in Southern European countries than in Northern ones (15) and with wide variations of use of treatment withdrawal and withholding among ICUs in the United States (14). Although epidemiologic questionnaire surveys are less accurate than descriptive studies, findings from both are consistent: European physicians working in ICUs report that they regularly withdraw and withhold life-sustaining treatments from patients near the end of life, and there are important differences in attitudes between northern and southern countries, where fewer physicians report using DNR orders or DFLSTs (25–27).

The DFLST Decision-Making Process in the ICU: Legal Frameworks and Ethical Debates

The decision-making process resulting in DFLSTs is a major topic in EOL care, and ICU caregivers have made a large contribution to it. They search for variant decision-making modalities, through advance care planning (ACP) and promotion of surrogates, because of many patients' inability to make decisions near the EOL in the ICU (14,19). Furthermore, the attitude of ICU physicians toward EOL discussions and decisions raises questions about ethics, highlighting the importance of legal and cultural issues in DFLSTs.

Legal Frameworks

Legal frameworks for ACP and surrogate designation vary from country to country, and the development of EOL care is changing in keeping with local laws and case precedents. A detailed presentation of national legal systems is beyond the scope of this chapter, but one should keep in mind that a traditional divide used to exist between the U.S., where the patients' decisions are given primary consideration, according to the Patient Self-Determination Act, and most European countries, where ACP is less developed and the medical decisions are primary.

Nevertheless, it is worth noting that several European countries recently changed their laws, reflecting the European population's desire for greater autonomy. Although these laws did not deal until now with the specific issue of patients receiving life support in the ICU, advance directives were acknowledged as legally valid in several countries in the last decade, and most European countries now allow individuals to designate a surrogate decision maker, though this legal authority varies among countries (28,29).

However, despite these changes in the legal framework, supporting the promotion of ACP and surrogate designation, it is unclear if they will help the decision-making process for DFLSTs in the ICU (30). Though interesting in theory, ACP appears to be limited in practice; observational studies found that patients' wishes were known in only 10% of ICU admissions, in Europe and in the U.S. (16,19,21). This finding may mean that ACP is not developed enough and needs to be promoted in the general population, but also that ACP is not efficient for ICU patients. Thus, limitations of this concept have been pointed out; notably, it fails to improve quality of life or to reduce hospitalization costs in the ICU (31–33). Surrogate designation is also subject to question, with doubts raised about the ability of family members to express the wishes of unconscious patients (32,34).

In addition to legal framework, professional working habits certainly influence the decision-making process at the EOL. Several descriptive studies observed that the involvement of proxies in DFLSTs varies widely from 17% to 77% in European countries to 90% in the U.S. (14,19). European intensivists responding to questionnaire surveys seem to consider themselves the sole decision maker for DLFSTs (26,27), and most European intensive care medicine societies, though promoting the respect of patients' and families' wishes, consider that DFLSTs remain a medical responsibility (16).

Ethical Debates

Ethical debates among intensivists about EOL decisions underlie the differences in legal frameworks and the physicians' attitudes described above. There used to be two main ways of thinking about the EOL decision-making process: the American autonomist attitude and the European paternalist attitude. But paramount ethical issues of EOL decisions are far more complex and should not be summarized as a transatlantic quarrel between autonomists and paternalists, for several reasons.

First, the relatively rare involvement of families in DFLSTs in European ICUs may be in part explained by proxies' unwillingness to participate in such decisions. In France, for instance, although most patients in emergency departments and ICUs want to designate surrogates and even if 90% of the general population would like their family to share care decisions (35,36), a recent study showed that half the family members of ICU patients did not want to be involved in the decision-making process (37).

Second, paternalism is based on the fundamental ethical principal of nonmalfeasance, seeking to avoid causing pain. It remains unclear until now if involving relatives in EOL decisions is harmful or beneficial to them. On the one hand, a recent multicenter randomized trial in France found that relatives involved in DFLSTs exhibited higher levels of stress disorders and anxiety (38). On the other hand, a Canadian study showed a high degree of satisfaction of families with their involvement in the decision-making process (39). Family needs may vary across cultures, and a balance is still to be found between physician–patient–family relationship models that exist on either side of the Atlantic.

Third, paternalism is no longer the dogma in European countries. Recent changes in legal frameworks about EOL, in accordance with public opinion, as well as recent studies about DFLSTs and families in the ICU provide arguments suggesting that intensivists are more willing to respect families' and patients' needs in EOL care (18).

Fourth, rather than a theoretic debate opposing dogmas, a balanced attitude on a case-by-case approach is recommended for DFLSTs in order to tailor the involvement of patients and families in the decision-making process to their wishes and needs (40,41). This requires a full awareness of nuances in the communication with the critically ill patients and their families. This is why we consider communication to be the core of ethical involvement in EOL care, not only for intensivists in the design of DFLSTs in the ICU but also for any physician at the bedside of patients near the end of life.

DFLSTs with Heart Failure Patients: Incidence and Disease-Related Specificities

Data about the incidence of DNR orders and DFLSTs among patients with HF are more difficult to find in the literature and several reasons may explain why. First, DFLSTs were developed initially in the ICUs, and research about EOL in cardiology is more recent, with a lack of epidemiologic data. Second, the EOL of patients affected by HF is certainly difficult to describe because they are treated in various health care facilities and because HF is a multifaceted disease with different and sometimes unexpected causes of death. Third, studies of DFLSTs in the ICUs concern a wide spectrum of patients, including patients with HF, but it is difficult to describe their specific characteristics from these data because many of them have many comorbidities. Despite these difficulties, partial data obtained from previous descriptive studies lead to the estimate that DNR orders may affect 25% to 45% of patients dying with congestive HF (42,43). Other studies report that DNR orders are less frequently used in heart failure than in other diseases such as dementia, AIDS, lung cancer, and cirrhosis (44,45), and the reasons for such differences are still to be explained (46).

End-of-life care for patients with HF has the same legal framework as EOL care in the ICU. Nevertheless, ethical issues about the decision-making process are different because the patient is more often able to be involved in the discussion. Thus, the relationship with the physician of a patient suffering from HF may be more comparable with a patient affected by cancer or chronic respiratory failure than with an ICU patient. Nevertheless, each of these medical conditions can result in the patient's being admitted in the ICU and in the patient's possibly losing consciousness. Furthermore, in outpatient clinics and in the wards, families and proxies are also often involved in EOL discussions, supporting the patient. Thus, even if differences exist between ICU patients and HF patients as far as EOL decisions are concerned, the shared decision-making process used in the ICU could be useful in HF care. More multidisciplinary debates are needed to identify disease-related specificities in ethical discussions with critically patients, and cooperation between cardiologists and intensivists could also contribute to promote EOL care in this field.

Care Near the End of Life for Patients and Families

The two key principles for development of EOL care in the ICU—a balanced decision-making process for DFLST and patient/family-centered care—can be discussed separately for the sake of clarity but should be dealt with simultaneously in clinical practice (16,17,47). We now address the challenging question of improving EOL care. We focus on three ways explored in critical care medicine that may be relevant to developing EOL care for HF patients: incorporating palliative care into critical care, strengthening communication with families, and improving multidisciplinary care.

Palliative Care

For EOL care in the ICU, the need for developing palliative care has been pointed out, with the aim of promoting a holistic approach, taking into account the emotional, social, spiritual, and physical needs of dying patients and their families (47). Integration of palliative caregivers' experience with symptom and pain management, a multidisciplinary approach, communication, and support skills appears to be relevant to improving EOL care in the ICU (48). Several options were tried, from proactive interventions by palliative care physicians (49), which were found to improve EOL management in a single-center study (50), to academic exchanges and education and training of nurses and residents (48).

Although pain and symptom management is traditionally one of the palliative caregivers' well-recognized areas of expertise, cooperation between palliative and critical care medicine is often lacking in pain control strategies. Most patients dying in the ICUs are under analgesia and sedation at the end stage of their disease, and one might think that analgesia is managed more appropriately there than anywhere else, even if further progress still needs to be made. Thus, in challenging the integration of palliative care in the ICU, emphasis is placed on improving the communication skills, particularly with family members, considering the high-level experience of palliative care teams in communicating with dying patients and supporting proxies and caregivers for terminal care and bereavement (51,52).

In the field of HF care, the integration of palliative care is also a challenging task, promoted by recent official statements and reviews (10,11,13). In cardiology, unlike in critical care medicine, it is the need for better pain and symptom management that initially led to more integration of palliative medicine. Two observational studies found disconcerting results about the discomfort of many patients dying from HF and cardiac diseases, initiating the debate of EOL care for those patients. Breathlessness, pain, depression, and anorexia were reported as being inadequately addressed by approximately 60% of dying patients (43,53). Mental disturbance, including low mood, insomnia, and anxiety, were also found in 30% to 60% of cases, and depression in about 50% of the older patients with congestive heart failure, with no specific treatment or specialized assessment by a psychiatrist (54). Since then, few studies have been published on this topic. The current development of palliative care in HF includes a research agenda addressing strategies for improving symptom control and militating in favor of a growing awareness that more can be done to relieve patients dying from HF (12).

Communication and Information

Communication with family members of critically ill patients is a major task of ICU caregivers, and this mission is of special importance for EOL patients (52). Several research studies were conducted in this field during the last 10 years, notably in France and in the U.S. Defending the concept that proxies are more than visitors in the ICUs, a research agenda was settled by the French FAMIREA ICU network (FAMIlles en RÉanimation: families in the ICU) with the goal of assessing relatives' needs in the critical setting of the ICU and promoting communication with families (55). Although this research was centered on family members, because most dying patients are unconscious in the ICU, it is also useful in finding ways to increase communication with HF patients at the EOL and with their relatives.

Assuming that information and communication are essential components of the needs of critically ill patients' families, the FAMIREA investigators sought to evaluate the communication with families in the ICU, using information comprehension, anxiety, and depression as quality markers. Half of the family members of ICU patients felt they received inadequate communication, resulting in poor comprehension of diagnosis, prognosis, and treatment (56). Poor comprehension and inadequate communication with caregivers were associated with less satisfaction of family members (56). At the same time, anxiety or depression were found among 72% of family members and 84% of spouses of ICU patients, and poor communication was independently associated with higher risk of these symptoms (57).

If communication is important for EOL care in the ICU, especially for patients' relatives, it is also crucial in EOL care in HF, for both patients and families. Results of observational studies of patients dying from HF indicate the need for more communication about the illness, its prognosis, and the hospice options (13,58). Barriers and difficulties in communication with patients near the end of life have been identified (59) and include disease symptoms for patients dying from HF (60). Recent recommendations and statements highlighted the importance of this core component in the development of EOL care in the field of HF (3,10,61).

By improving their communication skills, caregivers create important opportunities to improve the quality of EOL care (52), and guidelines provided by professional societies and research in this field conducted in the ICU can help them to achieve this goal. Useful data have been published about barriers to communication, criteria for assessing the quality of communication, efficacy of an information leaflet, performance of junior physicians in dealing with families, and specific needs of families of patients dying in the ICU (55,62–64). These results may be useful as well in dealing with patients with HF, and further research is needed to evaluate them in this disease.

The lack of information and poor communication with family members and within the caregivers' team are major obstacles to appropriate EOL management. Appropriate information and communication are prerequisites to sharing the decision-making process, allowing ethical DFLSTs for terminally ill patients in the ICUs (51,65). Furthermore, poor communication within the team and with non-ICU professionals is an obstacle to multidisciplinary management that generates frustration and conflicts (66–68).

Coming from palliative medicine and imported into the ICU by researchers, family conferences constitute a simple, inexpensive, and effective tool for improving communication with families (69,70). We encourage the development of this structured communication modality that can be simply used by caregivers concerned with improving their communication skills. They should then keep in mind key research findings of the studies conducted using family conferences: families do need to be listened to, and their satisfaction is associated with greater communication from the family (71,72). Thus, intensive communication within the ICU team before, during, and after the dying process provides multiple opportunities for a multidisciplinary decision-making process, effective communication with family members, and improved satisfaction of caregivers (73,74).

Multidisciplinary Care

Multidisciplinary management, one of the key concepts of palliative medicine, is strongly advocated by intensive care medicine societies to provide EOL care in the ICU (16,47). The core of this multidisciplinary approach in the ICU is the close partnership between nurses and physicians, which should be reinforced for well-structured communication and high-quality EOL care.

The evidence of the central role of nurses in DFLSTs and EOL care is supported by daily practice and by descriptive studies. Nurses' professional expertise is essential not only for pain and symptom management but also for EOL discussion and family support and information (75). Their close proximity to the patient, inherent in the nurse–patient relationship, provides them with knowledge of his wishes and of his family network, which are crucial data in the decision-making process. Furthermore, studies suggest that the lack of communication between nurses and physicians in the ICU can lead to misunderstandings, divergent practices, and conflicts regarding EOL management, which may translate into a worse prognosis for the patients (66–68). Thus, nurses' communication within the ICU team and with families should be encouraged, so as to improve EOL care.

Nevertheless, difficulties in team cooperation exist in EOL care. Despite a culture of communication and teamwork in ICU, limited involvement of nurses in EOL discussions is still common, especially in European countries, where nurse involvement in DFLSTs has ranged from 13% to 54%, far less than in the U.S., where nurse integration seem to be more systematic (19,27). Thus, it is not surprising if huge gaps between nurses and physicians satisfaction with the EOL decision-making process can be observed in the ICU (76).

Beyond the nurse–physician interaction, the multidisciplinary approach in EOL care can include the participation of consultants, such as attending physicians, psychologists, or ethics committee members. Despite some evidence supporting the interest of ethics consultations in improving communication and decreasing conflicts and length of ICU stay for dying patients, they are still rarely used in daily practice (77,78). Nevertheless, cooperation with non-ICU professionals is still difficult even if things are improving and one can imagine more interdisciplinary interactions in the future (79).

We believe that a true interdisciplinary approach is essential to improve EOL care in the ICU, and not only in the ICU but also on the wards, especially before the ICU admission. On the one hand, during a hospitalization in the ICU, accurate information about the patient's disease, history, and lifestyle is often provided by the general practitioner, the attending physician, and the social workers, who have to be consulted before DFLST.

On the other hand, before the ICU admission, a collegial discussion can take place to assess different care options, including a potential nonadmission in the ICU, for patients with potentially critical worsening condition. In practice, the collegial decision should then be written in the medical chart to foster communication among caregivers and to avoid an unnecessary transfer to the ICU. We believe that such multidisciplinary collaboration of attending physicians and intensivists, organized on a case-by-case basis, can help to tailor EOL care to the needs of each patient, including patients with heart failure.

Future Prospects in the Development of EOL Care for Critically Ill Patients

Palliative and Intensive Medicines: A Cooperation to Be Defined

One of the main difficulties in developing EOL care in the ICU, but also one of the most challenging opportunities, is the still-unclear interaction between palliative medicine and intensive medicine. This raises the question of the specific place of palliative caregivers with regard to their colleagues and specialists in the care of critically ill patients. In practice, collaboration between palliative care teams and the ICU staff is still often more a concept than a reality. Two problems are commonly met: first, many consider that palliative care and intensive care are two contradictory approaches that cannot be reconciled. Second, there is a widespread belief that intensivists have little to learn from their colleagues working in palliative care units.

Concerning the first point, we are confident that opinions are changing. Recent official statements, joint symposia, and publications reflect the increasing awareness among intensivists and palliative medicine physicians that their specialties are complementary in some situations (16,80,81). Concerning the second point, it is worth noting that palliative medicine teams are experiencing difficulties not only with intensivists, but also with many physicians in other specialties, including cardiologists (82). The status and boundaries of palliative medicine are still emerging, and the place of this newly recognized specialty still needs to be defined in the ICU as in the cardiology ward (11,82,83).

Development of EOL care for HF patients provides an excellent opportunity to tackle the question of cooperation between palliative medicine and cardiology. Different options are taking shape, from clinical cooperation at the bedside and clinical case discussions, to academic exchange and research. Whatever the option, one of the most important obstacle is currently being overcome with the emergence of the concept of duality of care, meaning that comfort care and curative care are not exclusive of each other but rather can be associated for the same patient at the same time (3,11). This concept led specialists to plead for an early and timely introduction of comfort care, without waiting for the terminal stage of HF, and for a balanced use of different means for the best care of patients (13).

Professional Open-Mindedness and Training

Integration of palliative medicine principles into EOL care for critically ill patients is a concept currently gaining credibility among intensivists and cardiologists, as mentioned above, but its development still requires more open-mindedness on the part of medical staff and more training. A better understanding of barriers to multidisciplinary collaboration, such as professional working habits, is an important step. We believe that a "culture gap" exists between an organ failure–oriented strategy, with the "rule of rescue" culture of most cardiologists and intensivists, and a patient comfort–centered strategy, with a comfort care culture promoted by palliative physicians. To develop true multidisciplinary management of dying patients requires an open mind from caregivers coming from different backgrounds to integrate their differences (79,82).

Another barrier to integration of palliative medicine into intensive care medicine, cardiology, and other specialties is the frequent lack of palliative medicine training in medical schools and residency programs (79). Nevertheless, the recent introduction of palliative medicine into medical school curricula can be expected to improve the ability of physicians to provide EOL care in a multidisciplinary approach and to use the shared decision-making model (48,79,84).

New technologies and new teaching tools also offer opportunities that could be developed in the future to spread palliative medicine skills among medical staff (85,86).

Research

Research in the area of EOL care is challenging, and several interesting approaches have been suggested recently, including descriptive studies about DFLSTs and interventional studies about communication with family members cited above. Another step will be the development of indicators for assessing the quality of EOL care, including patient- and family-centered decision making and communication. A few indicators were described with suggestions for interventions aimed at generating improvements (87–89). Concurrently, a research agenda has been suggested for EOL care in the ICU (90).

In the field of EOL care for patients with HF, there is a special need of research about clinical practices, pain and symptom management, benefit-to-risk, and cost-effectiveness evaluation. Concerning pain and symptom management, an important effort is being made to estimate the utility of morphine (12,91,92) and dobutamine for end-stage patients with HF (93). Another need in research about EOL care for HF patients concerns the evaluation of the benefit-to-risk ratio of invasive, potentially harmful, and expensive procedures for patients with advanced HF, especially among the elderly. For instance, the benefits of cardiac pacemakers or implantable cardioverters defibrillators are controversial near the EOL (94). In the same spirit, physicians caring for patients with HF should keep in mind that new options derived from pharmacologic advances do not really "save" lives but at the most modify the natural history of the disease, delaying the time to deterioration (95). Moreover, most patients in severe condition are usually disqualified from trials, so evidence-based results are not necessarily usable for end-stage HF patients. Thus, more specific research is needed to provide data about the best therapeutic strategies to improve the quality of life for patients with advanced and terminal HF.

Another critical point that needs further research in EOL care for HF patients is the evaluation of prognosis in a disease that remains often unpredictable with numerous pathologic scenarios and a high-incidence of sudden death (12). Because determining when comfort care should be substituted for curative care is a major difficulty for clinicians, most of patients do not receive comfort care until the very end stage of the disease. Although a host of parameters with clinical, biochemical, functional capacity, and echocardiographic markers has been developed, the assessment of prognosis for a single patient remains often unreliable (96). Additional work is required to appreciate how to better integrate the prognosis evaluation into clinical strategies that may improve the quality of care provided to patients with HF.

However, development of research in the field of EOL care faces difficulties, notably in methodology and fund-raising. Traditional quantitative research, descriptive studies, and interventional trials fail to fully capture the complexity of the dying process. Despite a few original studies reporting evaluation of palliative medicine integration in HF care, a lot is yet to be done (97,98). Furthermore, difficulties in providing a multidisciplinary approach in EOL care are also faced in research. Lack of experience in cooperation with other specialties and differences in scientific background may explain the rarity of research gathering palliative teams and other specialists (99,100). Lastly, funding for research in this field is difficult to obtain, in part because improving EOL care has no potential for generating earnings in the health care industry (90).

Conclusion

As heart failure is a major health care issue affecting a growing population of aging patients with a poor prognosis, the development of end-of-life care in this area is of crucial importance. Consulting the data provided by research about end-of-life care for critically ill patients in the intensive care medicine literature can help in meeting this challenging task with a multidisciplinary approach.

Research about decisions to forgo life-sustaining therapies provides insight into the legal framework, the ethical debates sustaining the decision-making process, and the patient-family-caregiver interactions involved in the EOL context. The ways explored by ICU caregivers to improve EOL care for critically ill patients can be used in HF care: development of palliative medicine skills, intensive communication with family members, and multidisciplinary care.

The concept of palliative/intensive medicine interaction, the training of physicians in palliative care, and the need for further research and discussion on EOL care are important issues in treating critically ill patients. Heart failure care provides a very interesting opportunity to gather caregivers, notably cardiologists and intensivists, in a multidisciplinary approach to care and research.

References

1. Cowie MR, Wood DA, Coats AJ, et al. Incidence and aetiology of heart failure; a population-based study. Eur Heart J 1999;20(6):421–8.
2. McMurray JJ, Stewart S. Epidemiology, aetiology, and prognosis of heart failure. Heart 2000;83(5): 596–602.
3. Pantilat SZ, Steimle AE. Palliative care for patients with heart failure. JAMA 2004;291(20):2476–82.
4. Senni M, Tribouilloy CM, Rodeheffer RJ, et al. Congestive heart failure in the community: trends in incidence and survival in a 10-year period. Arch Intern Med 1999;159(1):29–34.
5. Ho KK, Anderson KM, Kannel WB, Grossman W, Levy D. Survival after the onset of congestive heart failure in Framingham Heart Study subjects. Circulation 1993;88(1):107–15.
6. Havranek EP, Masoudi FA, Westfall KA, Wolfe P, Ordin DL, Krumholz HM. Spectrum of heart failure in older patients: results from the National Heart Failure project. Am Heart J 2002;143(3): 412–47.
7. Stewart S, MacIntyre K, Capewell S, McMurray JJ. Heart failure and the aging population: an increasing burden in the 21st century? Heart 2003; 89(1):49–53.
8. Malek M. Health economics of heart failure. Heart 1999;82(suppl 4):IV11–13.
9. McMurray JJ, Petrie MC, Murdoch DR, Davie AP. Clinical epidemiology of heart failure: public and private health burden. Eur Heart J 1998;19(suppl P):P9–16.
10. Selecky PA, Eliasson CA, Hall RI, Schneider RF, Varkey B, McCaffree DR. Palliative and end-of-life care for patients with cardiopulmonary diseases: American College of Chest Physicians position statement. Chest 2005;128(5):3599–610.
11. Hauptman PJ, Havranek EP. Integrating palliative care into heart failure care. Arch Intern Med 2005;165(4):374–8.
12. Ward C. The need for palliative care in the management of heart failure. Heart 2002;87(3):294–8.
13. Gibbs JS, McCoy AS, Gibbs LM, Rogers AE, Addington-Hall JM. Living with and dying from heart failure: the role of palliative care. Heart 2002; 88(suppl 2):ii36–9.
14. Prendergast TJ, Claessens MT, Luce JM. A national survey of end-of-life care for critically ill patients. Am J Respir Crit Care Med 1998;158(4):1163–7.
15. Sprung CL, Cohen SL, Sjokvist P, et al. End-of-life practices in European intensive care units: the Ethicus Study. JAMA 2003;290(6):790–7.
16. Carlet J, Thijs LG, Antonelli M, et al. Challenges in end-of-life care in the ICU. Statement of the 5th International Consensus Conference in Critical Care: Brussels, Belgium, April 2003. Intensive Care Med 2004;30(5):770–84.
17. Thompson BT, Cox PN, Antonelli M, et al. Challenges in end-of-life care in the ICU: statement of the 5th International Consensus Conference in Critical Care: Brussels, Belgium, April 2003: executive summary. Crit Care Med 2004;32(8):1781–4.
18. Fassier T, Lautrette A, Ciroldi M, Azoulay E. Care at the end of life in critically ill patients: the European perspective. Curr Opin Crit Care 2005;11(6): 616–23.
19. Ferrand E, Robert R, Ingrand P, Lemaire F. Withholding and withdrawal of life support in intensive-care units in France: a prospective survey. French LATAREA Group. Lancet 2001;357(9249): 9–14.
20. Wunsch H, Harrison DA, Harvey S, Rowan K. End-of-life decisions: a cohort study of the withdrawal of all active treatment in intensive care units in the United Kingdom. Intensive Care Med 2005;31(6):823–31.
21. Esteban A, Gordo F, Solsona JF, et al. Withdrawing and withholding life support in the intensive care unit: a Spanish prospective multi-centre observational study. Intensive Care Med 2001;27(11): 1744–9.
22. Holzapfel L, Demingeon G, Piralla B, Biot L, Nallet B. A four-step protocol for limitation of treatment in terminal care. An observational study in 475 intensive care unit patients. Intensive Care Med 2002;28(9):1309–15.

23. Eidelman LA, Jakobson DJ, Pizov R, Geber D, Leibovitz L, Sprung CL. Foregoing life-sustaining treatment in an Israeli ICU. Intensive Care Med 1998;24(2):162–6.
24. Prendergast TJ, Luce JM. Increasing incidence of withholding and withdrawal of life support from the critically ill. Am J Respir Crit Care Med 1997;155(1):15–20.
25. Vincent JL. Forgoing life support in western European intensive care units: the results of an ethical questionnaire. Crit Care Med 1999;27(8):1626–33.
26. Sjokvist P, Nilstun T, Svantesson M, Berggren L. Withdrawal of life support—who should decide? Differences in attitudes among the general public, nurses and physicians. Intensive Care Med 1999; 25(9):949–54.
27. Giannini A, Pessina A, Tacchi EM. End-of-life decisions in intensive care units: attitudes of physicians in an Italian urban setting. Intensive Care Med 2003;29(11):1902–10.
28. Lemaire FJ. A law for end of life care in France? Intensive Care Med 2004;30(11):2120.
29. Damas F, Damas P, Lamy M. Euthanasia: a law in Belgium? Intensive Care Med 2001;27(10):1683.
30. Baker DW, Einstadter D, Husak S, Cebul RD. Changes in the use of do-not-resuscitate orders after implementation of the Patient Self-Determination Act. J Gen Intern Med 2003;18(5): 343–9.
31. Prendergast TJ. Advance care planning: pitfalls, progress, promise. Crit Care Med 2001;29(2 suppl): N34–9.
32. Thompson T, Barbour R, Schwartz L. Adherence to advance directives in critical care decision making: vignette study. BMJ 2003;327(7422):1011.
33. A controlled trial to improve care for seriously ill hospitalized patients. The study to understand prognoses and preferences for outcomes and risks of treatments (SUPPORT). The SUPPORT Principal Investigators. JAMA 1995;274(20):1591–8.
34. Booth MG, Doherty P, Fairgrieve R, Kinsella J. Relatives' knowledge of decision making in intensive care. J Med Ethics 2004;30(5):459–61; discussion 61–2.
35. Ferrand E, Bachoud-Levi AC, Rodrigues M, Maggiore S, Brun-Buisson C, Lemaire F. Decision-making capacity and surrogate designation in French ICU patients. Intensive Care Med 2001; 27(8):1360–4.
36. Azoulay E, Pochard F, Chevret S, et al. Opinions about surrogate designation: a population survey in France. Crit Care Med 2003;31(6):1711–14.
37. Azoulay E, Pochard F, Chevret S, et al. Half the family members of intensive care unit patients do not want to share in the decision-making process: a study in 78 French intensive care units. Crit Care Med 2004;32(9):1832–8.
38. Azoulay E, Pochard F, Kentish-Barnes N, et al. Risk of post-traumatic stress symptoms in family members of intensive care unit patients. Am J Respir Crit Care Med 2005;171(9):987–94.
39. Heyland DK, Cook DJ, Rocker GM, et al. Decision-making in the ICU: perspectives of the substitute decision-maker. Intensive Care Med 2003;29(1): 75–82.
40. Tonelli MR. Waking the dying: must we always attempt to involve critically ill patients in end-of-life decisions? Chest 2005;127(2):637–42.
41. Manisty C, Waxman J. Doctors should not discuss resuscitation with terminally ill patients: for. BMJ 2003;327(7415):614–15.
42. Krumholz HM, Phillips RS, Hamel MB, et al. Resuscitation preferences among patients with severe congestive heart failure: results from the SUPPORT project. Study to Understand Prognoses and Preferences for Outcomes and Risks of Treatments. Circulation 1998;98(7):648–55.
43. Levenson JW, McCarthy EP, Lynn J, Davis RB, Phillips RS. The last six months of life for patients with congestive heart failure. J Am Geriatr Soc 2000;48(5 suppl):S101–9.
44. Wachter RM, Luce JM, Hearst N, Lo B. Decisions about resuscitation: inequities among patients with different diseases but similar prognoses. Ann Intern Med 1989;111(6):525–32.
45. Haydar ZR, Lowe AJ, Kahveci KL, Weatherford W, Finucane T. Differences in end-of-life preferences between congestive heart failure and dementia in a medical house calls program. J Am Geriatr Soc 2004;52(5):736–40.
46. Wenger NS, Pearson ML, Desmond KA, et al. Epidemiology of do-not-resuscitate orders. Disparity by age, diagnosis, gender, race, and functional impairment. Arch Intern Med 1995;155(19):2056–62.
47. Truog RD, Cist AF, Brackett SE, et al. Recommendations for end-of-life care in the intensive care unit: The Ethics Committee of the Society of Critical Care Medicine. Crit Care Med 2001;29(12):2332–48.
48. Danis M, Federman D, Fins JJ, et al. Incorporating palliative care into critical care education: principles, challenges, and opportunities. Crit Care Med 1999;27(9):2005–13.
49. Albert NM, Davis M, Young J. Improving the care of patients dying of heart failure. Cleve Clin J Med 2002;69(4):321–8.

50. Campbell ML, Guzman JA. Impact of a proactive approach to improve end-of-life care in a medical ICU. Chest 2003;123(1):266–71.
51. Friedrichsen MJ, Strang PM, Carlsson ME. Receiving bad news: experiences of family members. J Palliat Care 2001;17(4):241–7.
52. Azoulay E, Pochard F. Communication with family members of patients dying in the intensive care unit. Curr Opin Crit Care 2003;9(6):545–50.
53. McCarthy M, Lay M, Addington-Hall J. Dying from heart disease. J R Coll Physicians Lond 1996; 30(4):325–8.
54. Koenig HG. Depression in hospitalized older patients with congestive heart failure. Gen Hosp Psychiatry 1998;20(1):29–43.
55. Azoulay E, Pochard F, Chevret S, et al. Meeting the needs of intensive care unit patient families: a multicenter study. Am J Respir Crit Care Med 2001;163(1):135–9.
56. Azoulay E, Chevret S, Leleu G, et al. Half the families of intensive care unit patients experience inadequate communication with physicians. Crit Care Med 2000;28(8):3044–9.
57. Pochard F, Azoulay E, Chevret S, et al. Symptoms of anxiety and depression in family members of intensive care unit patients: ethical hypothesis regarding decision-making capacity. Crit Care Med 2001;29(10):1893–7.
58. McCarthy M, Hall JA, Ley M. Communication and choice in dying from heart disease. J R Soc Med 1997;90(3):128–31.
59. Curtis JR, Patrick DL, Caldwell ES, Collier AC. Why don't patients and physicians talk about end-of-life care? Barriers to communication for patients with acquired immunodeficiency syndrome and their primary care clinicians. Arch Intern Med 2000;160(11):1690–6.
60. Rogers AE, Addington-Hall JM, Abery AJ, et al. Knowledge and communication difficulties for patients with chronic heart failure: qualitative study. BMJ 2000;321(7261):605–7.
61. Goodlin SJ, Hauptman PJ, Arnold R, et al. Consensus statement: Palliative and supportive care in advanced heart failure. J Card Fail 2004; 10(3):200–9.
62. Azoulay E, Sprung CL. Family-physician interactions in the intensive care unit. Crit Care Med 2004;32(11):2323–8.
63. Azoulay E, Pochard F, Chevret S, et al. Impact of a family information leaflet on effectiveness of information provided to family members of intensive care unit patients: a multicenter, prospective, randomized, controlled trial. Am J Respir Crit Care Med 2002;165(4):438–42.
64. Moreau D, Goldgran-Toledano D, Alberti C, et al. Junior versus senior physicians for informing families of intensive care unit patients. Am J Respir Crit Care Med 2004;169(4):512–17.
65. Abbott KH, Sago JG, Breen CM, Abernethy AP, Tulsky JA. Families looking back: one year after discussion of withdrawal or withholding of life-sustaining support. Crit Care Med 2001;29(1): 197–201.
66. Asch DA. The role of critical care nurses in euthanasia and assisted suicide. N Engl J Med 1996; 334(21):1374–9.
67. Baggs JG, Schmitt MH, Mushlin AI, et al. Association between nurse-physician collaboration and patient outcomes in three intensive care units. Crit Care Med 1999;27(9):1991–8.
68. Studdert DM, Mello MM, Burns JP, et al. Conflict in the care of patients with prolonged stay in the ICU: types, sources, and predictors. Intensive Care Med 2003;29(9):1489–97.
69. Curtis JR, Patrick DL, Shannon SE, Treece PD, Engelberg RA, Rubenfeld GD. The family conference as a focus to improve communication about end-of-life care in the intensive care unit: opportunities for improvement. Crit Care Med 2001;29 (2 suppl):N26–33.
70. Curtis JR. Communicating about end-of-life care with patients and families in the intensive care unit. Crit Care Clin 2004;20(3):363–80, viii.
71. McDonagh JR, Elliott TB, Engelberg RA, et al. Family satisfaction with family conferences about end-of-life care in the intensive care unit: increased proportion of family speech is associated with increased satisfaction. Crit Care Med 2004;32(7): 1484–8.
72. Curtis JR, Engelberg RA, Wenrich MD, Shannon SE, Treece PD, Rubenfeld GD. Missed opportunities during family conferences about end-of-life care in the intensive care unit. Am J Respir Crit Care Med 2005;171(8):844–9.
73. Pronovost P, Berenholtz S, Dorman T, Lipsett PA, Simmonds T, Haraden C. Improving communication in the ICU using daily goals. J Crit Care 2003;18(2):71–5.
74. Halcomb E, Daly J, Jackson D, Davidson P. An insight into Australian nurses' experience of withdrawal/withholding of treatment in the ICU. Intensive Crit Care Nurs 2004;20(4):214–22.
75. Puntillo KA. The role of critical nurses in providing and managing end-of-life care. In: Managing death in the ICU: the transition from cure to comfort. Oxford: Oxford University Press, 2001:149–64.

76. Ferrand E, Lemaire F, Regnier B, et al. Discrepancies between perceptions by physicians and nursing staff of intensive care unit end-of-life decisions. Am J Respir Crit Care Med 2003;167(10):1310–15.
77. Dowdy MD, Robertson C, Bander JA. A study of proactive ethics consultation for critically and terminally ill patients with extended lengths of stay. Crit Care Med 1998;26(2):252–9.
78. Schneiderman LJ, Gilmer T, Teetzel HD, et al. Effect of ethics consultations on nonbeneficial life-sustaining treatments in the intensive care setting: a randomized controlled trial. JAMA 2003;290(9):1166–72.
79. Mularski RA, Bascom P, Osborne ML. Educational agendas for interdisciplinary end-of-life curricula. Crit Care Med 2001;29(2 suppl):N16–23.
80. Nelson JE, Danis M. End-of-life care in the intensive care unit: where are we now? Crit Care Med 2001;29(2 suppl):N2–9.
81. Curtis JR, Rubenfeld GD. Managing death in the ICU: the transition from cure to comfort. Oxford: Oxford University Press, 2001.
82. Hibbert D, Hanratty B, May C, Mair F, Litva A, Capewell S. Negotiating palliative care expertise in the medical world. Soc Sci Med 2003;57(2): 277–88.
83. Higginson IJ, Finlay I, Goodwin DM, et al. Do hospital-based palliative teams improve care for patients or families at the end of life? J Pain Symptom Manage 2002;23(2):96–106.
84. Stevens L, Cook D, Guyatt G, Griffith L, Walter S, McMullin J. Education, ethics, and end-of-life decisions in the intensive care unit. Crit Care Med 2002;30(2):290–6.
85. Ogle K, Greene DD, Winn B, Mishkin D, Bricker LG, Lambing AK. Completing a life: development of an interactive multimedia CD-ROM for patient and family education in end-of-life care. J Palliat Med 2003;6(5):841–50.
86. http://www.promotingexcellence.org.
87. Clarke EB, Curtis JR, Luce JM, et al. Quality indicators for end-of-life care in the intensive care unit. Crit Care Med 2003;31(9):2255–62.
88. Clarke EB, Luce JM, Curtis JR, et al. A content analysis of forms, guidelines, and other materials documenting end-of-life care in intensive care units. J Crit Care 2004;19(2):108–17.
89. Steinhauser KE, Clipp EC, Bosworth HB, et al. Measuring quality of life at the end of life: validation of the QUAL-E. Palliat Support Care 2004; 2(1):3–14.
90. Rubenfeld GD, Randall Curtis J. End-of-life care in the intensive care unit: a research agenda. Crit Care Med 2001;29(10):2001–6.
91. Johnson MJ, McDonagh TA, Harkness A, McKay SE, Dargie HJ. Morphine for the relief of breathlessness in patients with chronic heart failure—a pilot study. Eur J Heart Fail 2002;4(6):753–6.
92. Farncombe M, Chater S, Gillin A. The use of nebulized opioids for breathlessness: a chart review. Palliat Med 1994;8(4):306–12.
93. Rich MW, Shore BL. Dobutamine for patients with end-stage heart failure in a hospice program? J Palliat Med 2003;6(1):93–7.
94. Harrington MD, Luebke DL, Lewis WR, Aulisio MP, Johnson NJ. Cardiac pacemakers at end of life #111. J Palliat Med 2005;8(5):1055–6.
95. Malkin CJ, Channer KS. Life-saving or life-prolonging? Interpreting trial data and survival curves for patients with congestive heart failure. Eur J Heart Fail 2005;7(2):143–8.
96. Pocock SJ, Wang D, Pfeffer MA, et al. Predictors of mortality and morbidity in patients with chronic heart failure. Eur Heart J 2006;27(1):65–75.
97. Johnson MJ, Houghton T. Palliative care for patients with heart failure: description of a service. Palliat Med 2006;20(3):211–14.
98. Paes P. A pilot study to assess the effectiveness of a palliative care clinic in improving the quality of life for patients with severe heart failure. Palliat Med 2005;19(6):505–6.
99. Lewis C, Stephens B. Improving palliative care provision for patients with heart failure. Br J Nurs 2005;14(10):563–7.
100. Davis MP, Albert NM, Young JB. Palliation of heart failure. Am J Hosp Palliat Care 2005;22(3): 211–22.

2.6
Anesthesia and Surgical Management of Acute Heart Failure Syndrome

65
Anesthesia for Patients with Acute Heart Failure Syndromes

Dan Longrois and Paul Michel Mertes

This chapter provides a conceptual framework for anesthesia for cardiac surgery, and discusses selected practical issues concerning anesthesia for patients with acute heart failure syndromes (AHFSs). We first develop the conceptual framework by selectively presenting recent knowledge (including definitions and pathophysiology) relevant for anesthesia and postanesthesia care of patients with AHFS. We then discuss diagnosis, treatment decisions, and procedures. Finally, a case report is presented.

Conceptual Framework

The definitions of acute heart failure syndromes (AHFSs) used in this chapter are those recently published by the European Society of Cardiology (ESC) guidelines (1): acute decompensated heart failure (de novo or as decompensated congestive heart failure [CHF]), hypertensive acute heart failure, pulmonary edema, cardiogenic shock, and high output failure (1). Cardiogenic shock is defined in the ESC guidelines as a syndrome characterized by evidence of tissue hypoperfusion induced by heart failure after correction of preload (1). This definition constitutes a change from previous criteria that were mainly based on values of cardiac index and arterial blood pressure (see below).

The causes of AHFS have been detailed in the ESC guidelines (1). The search for a cause should be done rapidly. When a correctable causes (surgical or nonsurgical) is not found, therapy should be aimed at correction of the precipitating factor(s) and symptomatic therapy.

A frequent cause of cardiogenic shock is acute myocardial infarction (AMI). In this context, the mechanism of cardiogenic shock is related mainly to isolated left ventricular systolic dysfunction (79% of cases), but also to isolated right ventricular systolic dysfunction (2.8%), severe mitral regurgitation (6.8%), ventricular septal rupture (3.9%), and tamponade (1.4%) (2). Thus, the mechanism of cardiogenic shock is not isolated left ventricular systolic dysfunction in 20% of patients presenting with AMI. Hemodynamic signs are not helpful for recognizing these 20% of cases, nor is the presence or absence of pulmonary congestion. Understanding the mechanisms of cardiac dysfunction in patients with AHFS is necessary in order to provide adequate therapy but also in order to anticipate, prevent, and correct the potential effects of anesthetic drugs.

New Pathophysiologic Paradigms and Therapeutic Approaches

There are two new pathophysiologic paradigms that are relevant for this chapter. The first is the paradigm of a therapeutic window for all shock states; the second is the interaction between cardiogenic shock and the inflammatory response.

Therapeutic Window of Shock States

Whatever the initial cause of shock, its persistence for prolonged periods of time leads to vital organ dysfunction that will evolve by itself to multiple organ failure even if the initial cause of shock is successfully corrected. The duration of "prolonged" depends on the type of shock. It is minutes for anaphylactic shock (3), and a few hours for hemorrhagic, cardiogenic, and septic shock. Therefore, there is a therapeutic window for each type of shock when adequate therapy decreases the probability of subsequent occurrence of multiple organ failure. Compliance with the therapeutic window paradigm has been shown to decrease mortality in patients with severe sepsis (4). All shock states therefore represent an acceleration of the symptom/sign-diagnosis-therapy cycle.

Interaction Between Cardiogenic Shock and the Inflammatory Response

Cardiogenic shock was classically defined by the presence of arterial hypotension (systolic blood pressure <90 mm Hg for at least 30 minutes or the need for supportive pharmacologic or mechanical measures to maintain a systolic blood pressure >90 mm Hg) and end-organ hypoperfusion (e.g., cool extremities or a urine output of <30 mL/h). The hemodynamic criteria were a cardiac index (CI) of no more than 2.2 L/min/m^2 and a pulmonary capillary wedge pressure (PCWP) of at least 15 mm Hg.

This canonical clinical and hemodynamic presentation can be complicated by clinical and biologic signs that usually define systemic inflammatory response syndrome SIRS (e.g., fever >38.5°C, leukocytosis). In a recently published substudy of the SHOCK (SHould we emergently revascularize Occluded Coronaries for cardiogenic shocK) trial, it was shown that of the 302 enrolled patients, 59 (20%) presented with signs of SIRS (out of which two had signs of SIRS before the onset of cardiogenic shock and three that could not be properly evaluated) (5). Of the remaining 54 patients, 40 had documented infection by positive cultures (mostly blood cultures) and 14 had negative bacterial cultures (5). Median (interquartile range [IQR]) systemic vascular resistance values expressed as dyne/s/cm^5 were significantly (p = 0.006) lower for patients with cardiogenic shock and SIRS [i.e., 1051 (862–1486), $n = 31$ for patients with SIRS and positive bacterial cultures, and 1174 (705–1370), $n = 11$ for patients with SIRS and negative bacterial cultures] as compared to patients with cardiogenic shock without SIRS [1402 (1088–1807), $n = 168$]. Duration of stay in the intensive care unit (ICU) and in the hospital was significantly longer for the patients with SIRS. The mortality of patients with SIRS and positive bacterial cultures, after adjustment for age and use of coronary artery bypass grafting, was significantly higher than for controls (no SIRS) (odds ratio 2.2; 95% confidence interval [CI] 1.32–3.76; p = 0.008) (5). Three parameters predicted the occurrence of positive bacterial cultures in patients with cardiogenic shock: younger age, the use of CABG, and lower initial systemic vascular resistance (SVR) (5). For each decrease in SVR of 200 dyne/s/cm^5 upon the initial hemodynamic evaluation, the odds ratio of subsequent culture-positive SIRS was 1.21 (95% CI, 1.04–1.40; $p <$ 0.05) (5). The unifying hypothesis proposed by the authors is that in patients with SIRS, low SVR predisposes to endothelial damage and a leakage syndrome in which normal barriers against infection are disrupted (5).

This study confirmed previous reports and demonstrates that in up to 20% of patients with cardiogenic shock following AMI, SIRS, most frequently a consequence of bacterial infection, significantly increases mortality (5). The mediators that contribute to the reduced SVR are probably cytokines and excessive production of nitric oxide due to deregulated activation of the inducible isoform of the nitric oxide synthase (NOS_2) in both cardiac tissue (6) and vascular bed (7). An interaction between NOS and cyclooxygenase isoforms could contribute to the cardiovascular abnormalities of SIRS (8).

There are several relevant implications of the new cardiogenic shock and inflammation paradigm: (1) Clinical and hemodynamic signs of inadequately low vascular resistance can be a presentation of cardiogenic shock complicated by SIRS. (2) A vasoconstrictor is probably part of the therapeutic armamentarium because it could improve left-ventricular to aorta coupling and increase coronary perfusion pressure. Nevertheless, vasoconstrictors could decrease mesenteric blood flow and result in bowel ischemia. (3) When hypnotics and opioids are prescribed for the sedation and anesthesia of patients with inadequately low SVR, they can result in further vasodilatation and reduced cardiac preload and arterial hypotension. This may require either volume expansion to optimize preload or increased doses of vasoconstrictors. (4) Bacterial cultures should be prescribed routinely in such patients. The diagnosis of infection could probably be enforced by high values (>2 ng/mL) of procalcitonin (PCT), although it has been suggested that much higher PCT concentrations (>10 ng/mL) are predictive of infection in patients with cardiogenic shock (9). (5) If a bacterial infection is suspected, probabilistic antiinfectious therapy should be instituted rapidly (4), given the fact that mortality was significantly increased in culture-positive SIRS as compared to negative-culture SIRS and no SIRS patients, all with cardiogenic shock (5).

New Therapeutic Approaches

The most important therapeutic approach, in the authors' opinion, relevant for patients with AHFS who must undergo anesthesia, is the more and more frequent use of percutaneous cardiopulmonary support (PCPS) devices. Uni- or biventricular assist devices have been developed for different indications (bridge to transplantation, destination therapy in patients with contraindications to transplantation, and in a smaller number of patients as bridge-to-recovery). For many years they were inserted nearly exclusively by thoracotomy and were mainly intended for cardiac surgery patients. More recently, the use of PCPS devices has been extended to other situations such as cardiogenic shock due to a variety of causes, including acute intoxications and cardiopulmonary arrest (10). Results of PCPS devices in terms of survival are particularly encouraging in patients with cardiogenic shock as compared with patients with cardiovascular arrest. In a recently published randomized study in patients with cardiogenic shock after AMI, it was shown that the use of PCPSs resulted in improved hemodynamic and metabolic status as compared with the classic intraaortic balloon pump (IABP) counterpulsation (11). Nevertheless, the improved hemodynamic status with PCPS was associated with a higher incidence of severe complications and did not translate into improved 30 days survival (11). This observation suggests the requirement for additional studies in this field in order to improve survival in patients with PCPS.

The anesthetic and sedation techniques for the insertion and follow-up of PCPS have not been standardized. A whole array of anesthetic regimens has been reported (12). Anesthesiologists familiar with cardiac surgery and cardiopulmonary bypass techniques will not encounter any specific difficulties in the management of such patients and the PCPS devices, except that in many cases these patients undergo procedures outside the cardiac surgery operating room. For anesthesiologists unfamiliar with the above-mentioned situations, it is necessary to acquire the basic knowledge and skills in cardiopulmonary bypass, cannulas, pumps, oxygenators, anticoagulation, weaning from cardiopulmonary bypass (CPB), and the risk of bleeding. It is beyond the aims of this chapter to review the literature on PCPS devices. Nevertheless, their availability in an institution can dramatically change the management of patients with cardiogenic shock. The key to their success is early insertion. Ideally, algorithms for their insertion, according to specific clinical situations, should be implemented in order to respect the therapeutic window paradigm. One such algorithm is proposed in Figure 65.1. It has been suggested that recovery of cardiac function in such patients could be predicted by simple parameters such as increased end-tidal CO_2 concentrations and decreased arterial lactate.

Practical Issues Concerning Anesthesia for Patients with Acute Heart Failure Syndromes

There are several clinical situations in patients with AHFS that may require the intervention of the anesthesia team: (1) emergent cardiac surgery; (2) emergent nonsurgical myocardial revascularization procedures (such as percutaneous transluminal coronary angioplasty [PTCA]) with or without prior insertion of a PCPS device; and (3) emergent noncardiac surgery. Anesthesia for emergent cardiac surgery is discussed in major textbooks of cardiac anesthesia and will not be covered here. The two latter situations (items 2 and 3 on the above list) are the subject of this chapter because they are rarely discussed in textbooks. There are no evidence-based

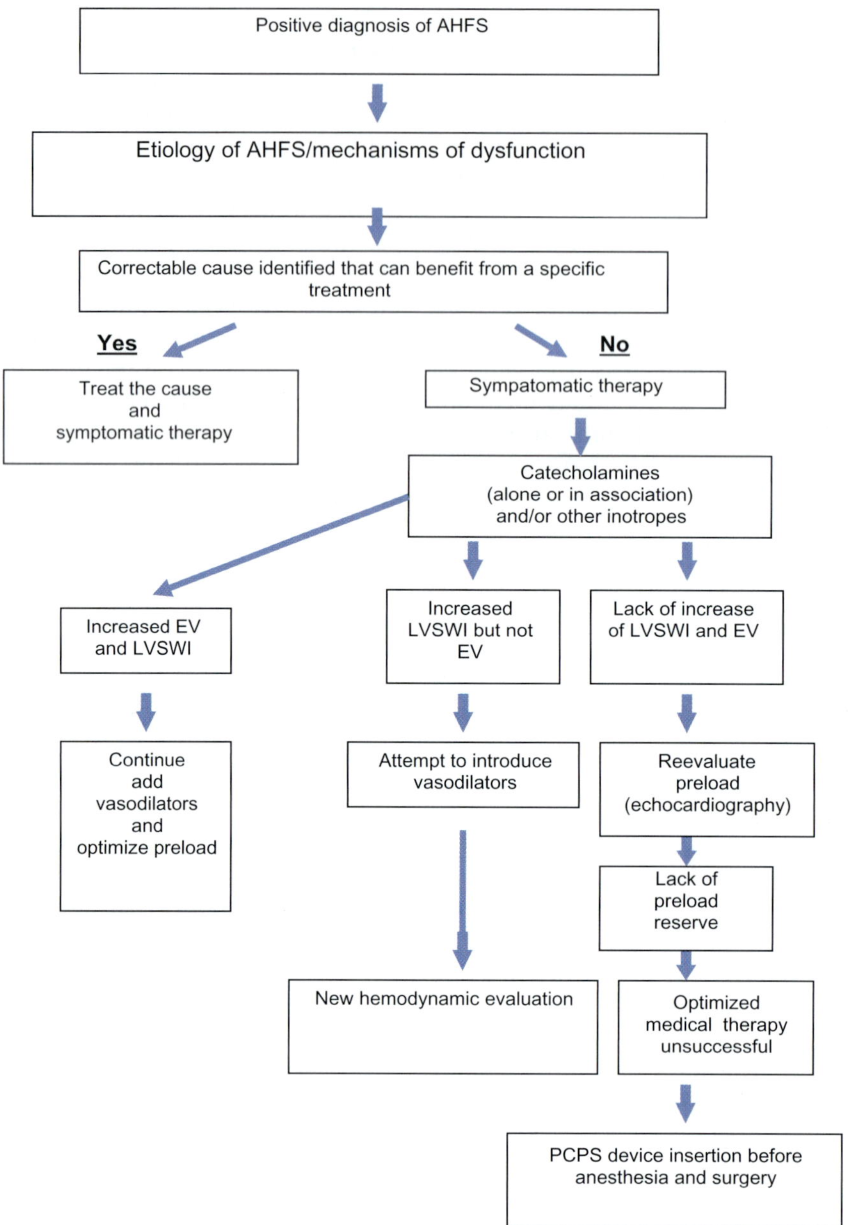

FIGURE 65.1. Algorithm for insertion of percutaneous cardiopulmonary support (PCPS) device in patients with acute heart failure syndromes. EV, ejection volume; LVSWI, left ventricular stroke work index.

recommendations concerning anesthesia for patients with AHFS, and therefore this chapter is based on the authors' interpretation of the literature and on their clinical experience.

Providing anesthesia for patients with AHFS should be integrated in a continuum of care that includes three periods: (1) preoperative evaluation, resulting in the anesthesia plan; (2) the anesthesia procedure per se, which includes resuscitation during the nonsurgical procedure; and (3) postoperative care and follow-up.

Preoperative Evaluation

The time devoted to preoperative evaluation is short. The goals are to gather information concerning the positive and differential diagnosis of the AHFS, its causes and mechanisms, the therapy already instituted, and the response to therapy. A brief medical and surgical history should focus on chronic cardiovascular problems and medications as well as frequently associated comorbidities. These pieces of information are essential in order to anticipate, prevent, and correct (1) possible further alterations of cardiovascular performance by anesthetic drugs (Fig. 65.2); (2) changes in vital organ (lung, kidney, central nervous system, gut) function induced by the AHFS and its therapy; and (3) possible correctable factors that could increase oxygen transport.

Details concerning the onset of the AHFS should include therapy (inotropes, vasodilators, diuretics) as well as the time of the last oral intake in conscious patients without tracheal intubation. In patients already sedated and with tracheal intubation, the occurrence of cardiorespiratory arrest and external cardiac massage should be documented. The conditions of tracheal intubation could suggest the possibility of inhalation. Obtaining information on recent medication is important. Early (day 0 to day 1) administration of β-adrenergic antagonists in patients presenting with AMI has been reported to significantly increase the early risk of cardiogenic shock despite delayed beneficial effects through reduction of the rate of reinfarction. The increased risk of cardiogenic shock upon early administration of β-adrenergic blocking drugs in patients with

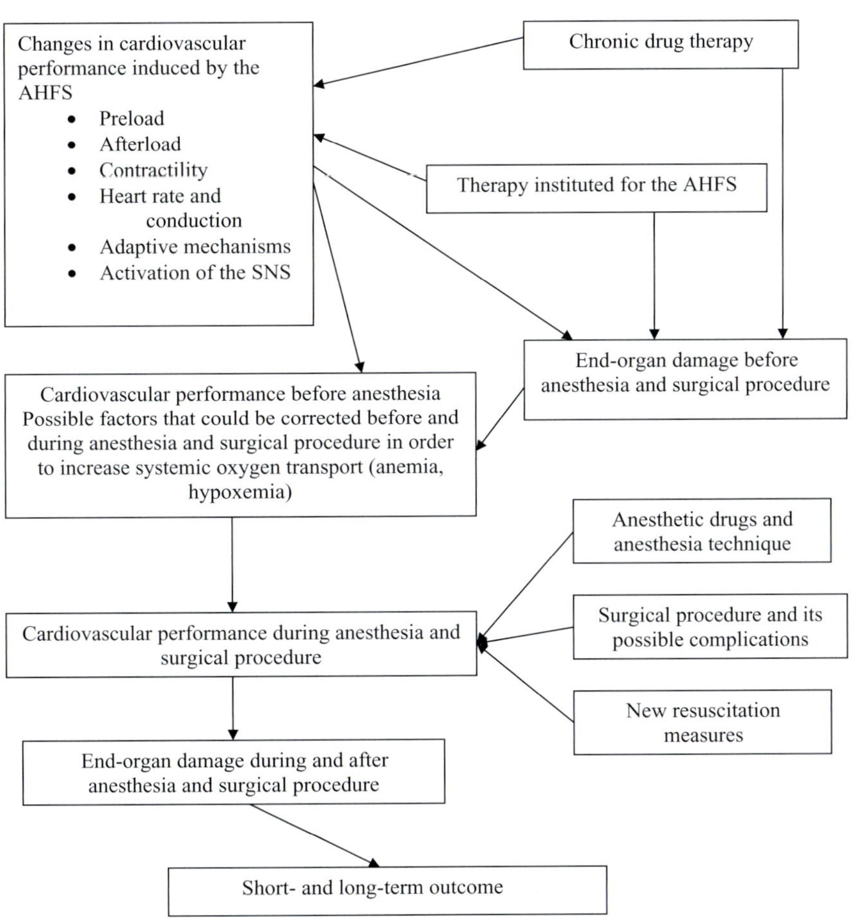

FIGURE 65.2. Impact of anesthesia and surgical procedure on short- and long-term outcomes. SNS, sympathetic nervous system.

AMI has triggered a recommendation to use β-adrenergic antagonists only in patients with AMI and stable hemodynamics. The occurrence of cardiogenic shock in patients with chronic or acute administration of β-adrenergic blocking drugs decreases the effects of β-adrenergic agonists and is an accepted indication for the use of positive inotropes such as levosimendan or phosphodiesterase inhibitors that have effects independent of the β-adrenergic receptor (13,14). Knowing the types and total amount of volume expanders already infused will help in interpreting the concentration of hemoglobin and plasma proteins.

Clinical examination should include vital signs such as noninvasive measurement of arterial blood pressure in both arms (even in the presence of a radial artery catheter), heart rate, respiratory rate in patients with spontaneous ventilation, temperature, and diuresis if a Foley catheter is in place. The neurologic examination is performed by taking into consideration the medication already used (hypnotics, opioids, neuromuscular blocking drugs). Conditions of lung ventilation (tidal volume, rate, positive end-expiratory pressure [PEEP], peak and plateau pressure values) should be recorded. Vascular access should be checked (caliber, location, back flow when possible for central venous catheters because vascular access could have been performed under substandard conditions).

The medical workup should focus on (1) systemic consequences of the AHFS such as acidosis (pH on blood gas, lactic acidosis), hemostasis abnormalities due to hemodilution or to disseminated intravascular coagulation (DIC) (prothrombin time (PT), activated partial thromboplastin time (APTT), fibrinogen, platelets, D-dimers), rhabdomyolysis (creatine phosphokinase [CPK], myoglobin); (2) myocardial damage (troponin Ic); (3) alteration of vital organ function such as lung (PaO_2/FiO_2, $PaCO_2$); kidney (creatinine, BUN), liver (aspartate aminotransferase [ASAT], alanine aminotransferase [ALAT], bilirubin, coagulation factors), bowel (intraabdominal pressure); and (4) possible signs of infection (blood, urine and tracheal aspiration cultures, C-reactive protein, procalcitonin). Blood grouping and detection of irregular antierythrocyte antibodies are routine.

Imaging is usually limited to echocardiography and chest radiography, which provide helpful information on the cardiac silhouette, lung edema, and the proper location of central venous catheters and tracheal tube.

The preoperative evaluation in patients who must undergo anesthesia despite the presence of an AHFS is challenging. The short symptoms/signs-diagnosis-therapy cycle must be translated into diagnoses, treatment decisions, and procedures.

Diagnoses

At the end of the preoperative evaluation, the anesthesiologist should be able to estimate the following: (1) The severity of the AHFS, which is demonstrated by the impairment of hemodynamic parameters (cardiac index, left ventricular stroke work, estimators of preload), and its consequences on oxygen transport and consumption (SvO_2, lactic acidosis) as well as the amount of support (pharmacologic, mechanical) required to maintain those values. (2) The mechanisms of the AHFS should be documented as carefully as possible by preoperative and, if not detailed enough, by intraoperative echocardiography. Understanding the causes and mechanisms of the AHFS is mandatory in order to provide adequate therapy within the therapeutic window. It is essential to understand whether the patient has extracardiac (tamponade; pulmonary embolism) versus cardiac dysfunction, or myocardial versus valvular dysfunction. If myocardial dysfunction is the cause of the AHFS, then it is important to document systolic versus diastolic dysfunction, and left ventricular versus right ventricular versus biventricular failure. (3) The alterations of end-organ function due to the AHFS and its therapy (neurological, lung, renal, liver, bowel, metabolic) should be documented. (4) The occurrence of problems such as inhalation upon tracheal intubation should be documented. (5) The possible factors that could be corrected in order to increase oxygen transport such as preload, afterload, atrioventricular (AV) asynchrony, and anemia should be documented. (6) Major electrolyte (potassium, calcium, magnesium) and metabolic abnormalities (hyperglycemia) should be documented.

Treatment Decisions

The severity of the impairment and the mechanism of AHFS should allow the anesthesiologist to address two issues. The first is whether the cardiac dysfunction is reversible in the short term, that is, in minutes (e.g., cardiac tamponade), potentially reversible after a period of hours to days (myocardial revascularization, acute valvular dysfunction that can be corrected by cardiac surgery), or probably not reversible (a history of recurrent myocardial infarction in a patient with chronic heart failure). If the cardiac dysfunction is not rapidly reversible, the second issue is whether the pharmacologic support is sufficient to avoid vital organ dysfunction and multiple organ failure, or whether the patient should receive a PCPS device before the index surgery or procedure. There are no widely accepted criteria for the institution of PCPS in this context. Other decisions concern strategies for transportation to the operating room, anesthesia induction (rapid sequence if the patient is not already intubated), maintenance of anesthesia, and postoperative care.

Procedures

Procedures done before induction of anesthesia will depend on the balance between, on the one hand, the necessity to rapidly correct the cause of AHFS (e.g., rapid myocardial revascularization by PTCA) and, on the other hand, the necessity to stabilize the hemodynamic and metabolic status of the patient before the procedure. When time is available, procedures include implementation of monitoring (cardiovascular, respiratory, temperature). There is a lack of consensus about the choice of a specific cardiovascular monitoring strategy (invasive versus noninvasive). Frequently, arterial and central venous catheters are required. There are no proved benefits of pulmonary artery catheters on mortality. Also, when time is available, preanesthesia improvement of vascular access should be attempted. The lack of sufficient and secure intravascular lines should be anticipated. The intravenous lines for inotropes and anesthetic drugs administration should be separated. A Y-type trifurcated intravenous extension set with a low (<0.5 mL) priming volume is helpful to simultaneously infuse several anesthetic drugs with the lowest possible dead volumes. In addition, intravascular access for rapid volume expansion should be available.

The Anesthesia Procedure

The therapeutic goals upon induction of anesthesia are as follows: (1) preserve life through maintenance of the cerebral and coronary perfusion pressure; (2) avoid further worsening of preload and afterload conditions; (3) minimize changes in heart rate that could worsen myocardial ischemia or valvular dysfunction; (4) avoid complications such as inhalation if the patient's trachea is not already intubated; (5) avoid explicit awareness upon tracheal intubation due to inadequately low effect site concentrations of hypnotics and opioids; (6) avoid worsening of end-organ function (lung, renal) by inadequate volume expansion. The therapeutic goals for maintenance are as follows: (7) continue to provide hemodynamic stability as well as "cardioprotection"; (8) avoid anesthetic drugs over- and underdosing by monitoring depth of anesthesia; (9) maintain homeostasis (temperature, hemoglobin, glycemia, electrolytes); (10) prevent and correct hemostasis abnormalities to avoid excessive bleeding during surgery.

For most AHFS patients who require anesthesia, recovery will take place in an ICU. Tracheal extubation is delayed until cardiopulmonary and other vital organs functions have stabilized. Pain therapy is usually administered in the context of postoperative sedation of a patient with intubated trachea, mechanical ventilation, and in the most severe cases multiple organ dysfunction or failure.

Providing Hemodynamic Stability (Goals 1 to 3 and 7)

The main immediate concerns when choosing anesthetic drugs for induction and maintenance of anesthesia are preservation of (nearly) physiologic cerebral and coronary perfusion pressure together with minor changes in heart rate. Such hemodynamic stability is often, but not always, associated with preserved myocardial oxygen balance and no electrocardiogram (ECG) signs of myocardial ischemia (usually estimated by changes of the ST segment). Other, less immediate concerns are anesthetic drug-mediated myocardial protection, especially in patients who will be confronted with myocardial ischemia/reperfusion sequences such as those who will undergo cardiac surgery.

These general considerations require several comments. First, in addition to the intrinsic effects of anesthetic drugs on cardiovascular function, their integrated effects in a given patient depend on chronic and acute preoperative medication (β-adrenergic receptor antagonist for instance) as well as on their effects on the autonomic nervous system. Second, in most, if not all, published studies, any mean differences in terms of hemodynamic effects between anesthetic regimens are lower than interpatient variability within the same regimen. In other words, whatever the choice of anesthetic drugs, the main challenge, yet unsolved in the literature, is the titration of anesthesia for an individual patient. Two algorithms for titration of anesthetic drugs upon anesthesia induction have been proposed in patients without AHFS and could partially be extrapolated to patients with AHFS (15,16). Third, in the most difficult cases, hemodynamic stability is a secondary goal, just after avoidance of inhalation by rapid sequence induction. In these cases, once the airway is secured, correction, rather than prevention of hemodynamic instability, is the only choice.

For induction of anesthesia, the hypnotic drug with the highest therapeutic index on hemodynamic stability is etomidate because it preserves sympathetic outflow and autonomic reflexes. This has been demonstrated in prospective randomized clinical studies and in studies analyzing thousands of patients in routine clinical practice. Experimental data also suggest that in contrast to other hypnotics, the pharmacokinetic and pharmacodynamic effects of etomidate are not altered by shock states. Several studies have raised concerns for an effect of etomidate, even given in single bolus infusion, on cortisol metabolism and subsequent infraclinical adrenal insufficiency. Supplementation with low-dose corticosteroids could be helpful in the postoperative period in patients with cardiogenic shock who received etomidate for anesthesia induction.

For maintenance of anesthesia, it has been shown in patients undergoing coronary artery bypass graft surgery that inhaled (sevoflurane and desflurane) as compared to intravenous (propofol and midazolam) hypnotics resulted in better postoperative myocardial function (17). Although sevoflurane and desflurane have not been specifically investigated in patients with AHFS, clinical experience suggests that these two drugs could be a reasonable choice for these patients during maintenance of anesthesia mainly because their hemodynamic effects are no worse than those of other drugs such as propofol and because of their clinically relevant cardioprotective effects. Sevoflurane has been shown to better preserve left ventricular function in elderly patients as compared to propofol. Sevoflurane has also been shown to have cardiac sympatholytic effects, whereas propofol does not. This effect could be beneficial in patients with myocardial ischemia in order to avoid further tachycardia. Inhaled anesthetics are mainly used in the operating room. For patients who require anesthesia in the catheter laboratory, intravenous anesthetics are the first choice.

The choice of opioid is also based on hemodynamic stability upon induction and maintenance. From a pharmacokinetic point of view, the most interesting drug is remifentanil, especially when administration by target-controlled infusion (TCI) through commercially available devices (in Europe) allows more reproducible titration. The advantages of remifentanil are its short onset time and short contextual half-life that allows rapid decrease of plasma and effect site concentrations, even in the presence of liver or renal dysfunction. The main concern with remifentanil upon induction, when given by bolus, is the occurrence of severe bradycardia and even asystolia especially when patients receive preoperative β-adrenergic receptor antagonists or calcium channel blockers such as diltiazem. Administration with TCI devices by targeting plasma and not the effect compartment results in lower plasma concentrations and less severe bradycardia.

If muscle relaxation is required during the procedure, the choice of the neuromuscular blocking during maintenance of anesthesia should be based on its effects on heart rate, especially through interaction with the opioids. Vecuronium as opposed to pancuronium and suxamethonium, when associated with etomidate and fentanyl, results in the highest incidence of bradycardia requiring atropine. It also should be based on the pharmacokinetic properties and the possible alterations induced by renal and hepatic impairment.

Avoiding Perioperative Awareness (Goals 5 and 8)

Many anesthesiologists, when providing anesthesia for patients with AHFS, focus their attention and efforts on hemodynamic stability. Although this is an accepted proof of quality of anesthesia for patients with AHFS, providing comfort and avoiding explicit awareness are also necessary. The occurrence of explicit perioperative awareness is reported by most patients as being one of the worst possible personal experiences (18).

Recent evidence from observational and prospective (18) trials have shown that patients with altered cardiovascular reserve are at increased risk of perioperative awareness because of inadequately low concentrations of hypnotics and opioids for a given intensity and duration of nociceptive stimulation. Interestingly, it was shown that an interval of inadequately "shallow" anesthesia as short as 1 to 2 minutes was probably sufficient to result in explicit awareness. Risk factors of perioperative explicit awareness, in addition to reduced cardiovascular reserve, were cardiac, abdominal/thoracic, or orthopedic surgery (versus all other types of surgery) (18).

There are several complementary methods of preventing or dealing *a posteriori* with explicit awareness that have recently been recommended in a "sentinel event alert" of the Joint Commission on Accreditation of Healthcare Organization (October 6, 2004, issue 32; available at www.jcaho.org). Among other methods, this document, together with a document from the American Society of Anesthesiology (ASA) (available at www.asahq.org) suggests that in patients at risk of perioperative explicit awareness, the use of depth of anesthesia monitors can reduce by approximately 80% the incidence of such episodes. These recommendations are based on observational and randomized-controlled trials. In addition to the decrease in the incidence of perioperative explicit awareness, monitoring depth of anesthesia is probably helpful in avoiding anesthetic drugs overdose in such patients. Anesthesia overdose has been incriminated (although no formal proof was provided) in increasing long-term mortality after surgery (19). We think that the above-cited studies and the recommendations of JCAHO and ASA are arguments in favor of monitoring depth of anesthesia in all patients with AHFS who must undergo general anesthesia. This is a financial and organizational challenge, especially for patients who require anesthesia outside of the operating room. A few algorithms for titration of anesthesia in order to avoid under- and overdosing of anesthetic drugs have been published (15,16).

Other Concerns for the Perioperative Period, Not Specific of Patients with Acute Heart Failure Syndromes

In all patients undergoing anesthesia, maintenance of homeostasis is a routine goal. This means avoiding hypothermia, severe anemia, and hyperglycemia.

End of Surgery, and Transfer to the Recovery Area or Intensive Care Unit

Part of the anesthesia plan is the choice of the recovery unit and the transfer from the operating room. This requires the choice of a sedation regimen. Continuation of the opioid infusion at a lower concentration than that used during surgery is reasonable. An effect site remifentanil concentration of 1 to 2 ng/mL is adequate in most situations in the absence of nociceptive stimulation. If an inhaled anesthetic was used during maintenance, an intravenous hypnotic should be started in the operating room sufficiently early to provide adequate hypnosis during transfer to and installation in the recovery unit. Propofol, given by TCI, at 1 to 1.5 μg/mL is a reasonable choice. Defining such a sedation regimen in each institution is useful for patients with AHFS who are frequently transferred between several locations of the hospital.

Clinical Case

A 78-year-old man with a history of chronic arterial hypertension, tobacco use, old myocardial infarction, peripheral vascular disease, and abdominal aorta aneurysm was scheduled for angiography with possible percutaneous iliac angioplasty without the supervision of the anesthesia team. The patient was taken to the operating room, and positioned on the operation table after insertion of one intravenous cannula. Oxygen ($FiO_2 = 0.5$) was given through a face mask. After the first attempt of femoral artery cannulation, the patient became agitated and complained of severe shortness of breath, and the anesthesia team was asked to intervene.

Upon arrival of the anesthesia team, the patient was conscious and complained of worsening shortness of breath. His respiratory rate was 60/min and he was cyanotic. Pulse oxymetry revealed that oxygen saturation was 73%. Arterial blood pressure was 245/130 mm Hg and heart rate was 110 bpm. Lung auscultation revealed fine crackles in the two lung fields. The FiO_2 was increased to 1, and the patient was given two intravenous bolus injections of 2 mg of nicardipine, 20 mg of furosemide, and 2 mg of isosorbide dinitrate. Arterial blood pressure decreased to 160/95 mm Hg without changes in heart rate and there was no improvement in the shortness of breath. Oxygen saturation decreased to 34% and the patient did not respond anymore to verbal commands.

The patient was administered 0.5 mg/kg of etomidate, 15 μg of sufentanil, and 30 mg of atracurium, and tracheal intubation was performed without problems and manual ventilation was performed for 5 minutes with oxygen. Anesthesia was maintained with 2% sevoflurane. Oxygen saturation increased to 95%. Mechanical ventilation was instituted with a tidal volume of 8 mL/kg, a respiratory rate of 12/min, and a PEEP of 8 cm H_2O. Lung auscultation revealed crackles in the two lung fields and symmetric breath sounds. Blood pressure decreased to 120/75 mm Hg and heart rate was 110 bpm. A second intravenous cannula was inserted with a three-way device and anesthesia was maintained with TCI (Base Primea®, Fresenius Vial, Brézins, France), remifentanil (3 ng/mL), and sevoflurane 2%. Depth of anesthesia was monitored with a BIS XP® monitor (Aspect Medical System, Newton, MA, USA) and sevoflurane concentrations were adapted to maintain BIS values between 50 and 55. Pulse oxymetry revealed oxygen saturation of 99%, the FiO_2 was decreased to 0.6, and the surgical and anesthesia team decided to continue the procedure. After 2 hours, oxygen saturation was stable, arterial blood pressure was 130/80 mm Hg, and the patient was taken to the ICU under propofol sedation (TCI, Diprifusor®, 2 μg/mL). A Foley catheter was inserted and a chest x-ray was performed and revealed acute pulmonary edema. Transthoracic echocardiography revealed a left ventricular ejection fraction of 0.5 and an undilated right ventricle. The propofol infusion was stopped; 30 minutes later, the remifentanil infusion was stopped. The patient was weaned from the mechanical ventilation 2 hours after arrival in the ICU and received oxygen through a face mask for the following 12 hours.

This clinical case concerns anesthesia in a patient with AHFS, diagnosed as hypertensive acute heart failure (signs and symptoms of AHF in the presence of high arterial blood pressure and preserved left ventricular systolic function). Because respiratory and hemodynamic functions were rapidly stabilized, it was possible to continue the procedure. Therapy to reduce arterial blood pressure was instituted according to the ESC guidelines (1). Anesthesia was induced and maintained by taking into account the above-described goals.

Conclusion

Providing anesthesia for patients presenting with AHFS is challenging for anesthesiologists not familiar with cardiac surgery. This field is uncharted territory because there are no evidence-based recommendations. The easiest way to adopt an anesthesia plan in such patients, in our opinion, is to define goals that should include, but not be limited, to hemodynamic stability. Through careful titration of anesthetic drugs, it is often possible to provide both hemodynamic stability and to avoid anesthetic drug over- and underdose.

References

1. Nieminen MS, Bohm M, Cowie MR, et al. Executive summary of the guidelines on the diagnosis and treatment of acute heart failure: the Task Force on Acute Heart Failure of the European Society of Cardiology. Eur Heart J 2005;26(4):384–416.

2. Hochman JS, Buller CE, Sleeper LA, et al. Cardiogenic shock complicating acute myocardial infarction—etiologies, management and outcome: a report from the SHOCK Trial Registry. SHould we emergently revascularize Occluded Coronaries for cardiogenic shocK? J Am Coll Cardiol 2000;36(3 suppl A):1063–70.
3. Dewachter P, Jouan-Hureaux V, Franck P, et al. Anaphylactic shock: a form of distributive shock without inhibition of oxygen consumption. Anesthesiology 2005;103(1):40–9.
4. Gao F, Melody T, Daniels DF, Giles S, Fox S. The impact of compliance with 6-hour and 24-hour sepsis bundles on hospital mortality in patients with severe sepsis: a prospective observational study. Crit Care 2005;9(6):R764–70.
5. Kohsaka S, Menon V, Lowe AM, et al. Systemic inflammatory response syndrome after acute myocardial infarction complicated by cardiogenic shock. Arch Intern Med 2005;165(14):1643–50.
6. Balligand JL, Ungureanu-Longrois D, Smith TW. Role of cytokine-inducible nitric oxide synthase in the control of myocardial contractile state. Heart Failure Rev 1996;1:193–201.
7. Mebazaa A, De Keulenaer GW, Paqueron X, et al. Activation of cardiac endothelium as a compensatory component in endotoxin-induced cardiomyopathy: role of endothelin, prostaglandins, and nitric oxide. Circulation 2001;104(25):3137–44.
8. Devaux Y, Seguin C, Grosjean S, et al. Lipopolysaccharide-induced increase of prostaglandin E(2) is mediated by inducible nitric oxide synthase activation of the constitutive cyclooxygenase and induction of membrane-associated prostaglandin E synthase. J Immunol 2001;167(7):3962–71.
9. Geppert A, Steiner A, Delle-Karth G, Heinz G, Huber K. Usefulness of procalcitonin for diagnosing complicating sepsis in patients with cardiogenic shock. Intensive Care Med 2003;29(8):1384–9.
10. Asaumi Y, Yasuda S, Morii I, et al. Favourable clinical outcome in patients with cardiogenic shock due to fulminant myocarditis supported by percutaneous extracorporeal membrane oxygenation. Eur Heart J 2005;26(20):2185–92.
11. Thiele H, Sick P, Boudriot E, et al. Randomized comparison of intra-aortic balloon support with a percutaneous left ventricular assist device in patients with revascularized acute myocardial infarction complicated by cardiogenic shock. Eur Heart J 2005;26(13):1276–83.
12. Burkle CM, Nuttall GA, Rihal CS. Cardiopulmonary bypass support for percutaneous coronary interventions: what the anesthesiologist needs to know. J Cardiothorac Vasc Anesth 2005;19(4):501–4.
13. Alhashemi JA. Treatment of cardiogenic shock with levosimendan in combination with beta-adrenergic antagonists. Br J Anaesth 2005;95(5): 648–50.
14. Follath F, Franco F, Cardoso JS. European experience on the practical use of levosimendan in patients with acute heart failure syndromes. Am J Cardiol 2005;96(6A):80G–85G.
15. Lambert P, Junke E, Fuchs-Buder T, Meistelman C, Longrois D. Inter-patient variability upon induction with sevoflurane estimated by the time to reach predefined end-points of depth of anaesthesia. Eur J Anaesthesiol 2006;23(4):311–18.
16. Forestier F, Hirschi M, Rouget P, et al. Propofol and sufentanil titration with the bispectral index to provide anesthesia for coronary artery surgery. Anesthesiology 2003;99(2):334–46.
17. De Hert SG, Cromheecke S, ten Broecke PW, et al. Effects of propofol, desflurane, and sevoflurane on recovery of myocardial function after coronary surgery in elderly high-risk patients. Anesthesiology 2003;99(2):314–23.
18. Sebel PS, Bowdle TA, Ghoneim MM, et al. The incidence of awareness during anesthesia: a multicenter United States study. Anesth Analg 2004;99(3): 833–9, table.
19. Monk TG, Saini V, Weldon BC, Sigl JC. Anesthetic management and one-year mortality after noncardiac surgery. Anesth Analg 2005;100(1):4–10.

66
Mechanical Circulatory Support for Management of Cardiogenic Shock Beyond Intraaortic Balloon Pump Support and Inotropes

Aly El-Banayosy, Reiner Koerfer, and Dagmar Cobaugh

The use of ventricular assist devices (VADs) has become a widely accepted therapeutic option in end-stage cardiac failure. Most commonly, VADs are indicated as a bridge to transplantation in chronic heart disease. A variety of cardiovascular conditions such as myocardial infarction, dilatative cardiomyopathy, and myocarditis can lead to severe acute heart failure, which, in some cases, results in persistent cardiogenic shock. Irrespective of the etiology and despite new intervention measures, morbidity and mortality rates of cardiogenic shock patients remain unacceptably high. For patients who remain in cardiogenic shock despite optimal medical therapy and intraaortic balloon pumping (IABP), implantation of a VAD might be the last lifesaving therapeutic option. The longer end-organ malperfusion persists, the poorer the chance of survival. Ventricular assist device therapy can provide hemodynamic support, allowing cardiac function to recover while peripheral perfusion is maintained at adequate levels. Patients with acute cardiogenic shock are mostly primarily treated in local hospitals, which may not be able to offer assist device implantation or cardiac transplantation. Contact and transport to specialized centers might be required. For the success of VAD therapy, a multidisciplinary network approach might be beneficial.

Definition of Cardiogenic Shock in Acute Heart Failure Syndrome

Cardiogenic shock is defined as tissue hypoxia resulting from severe impairment of ventricular pump function after correction of preload. According to the SHOCK (SHould we emergently revascularize Occluded Coronaries for cardiogenic shocK) trial (1), clinical criteria for cardiogenic shock are a systolic blood pressure less than 90 mm Hg for 30 minutes before inotropes/vasopressors, the requirement for vasopressors or IABP to maintain systolic blood pressure at 90 mm Hg or more, evidence of decreased organ perfusion, and heart rate of 60 beats per minute or less. Hemodynamic criteria for cardiogenic shock are pulmonary capillary wedge pressure of 15 mm Hg or more and a cardiac index of 2.2 $L\,min^{-1}\,m^{-2}$ or less (1).

Etiology

One major cause of cardiogenic shock is acute myocardial infarction (AMI). Cardiogenic shock occurs in only 7% of AMI patients (2). Despite aggressive support the mortality rate for cardiogenic shock following AMI remains high. The SHOCK registry reported a mortality rate of 47%

for AMI patients treated with IABP support and thrombolytics and a mortality rate of 77% for patients who received neither of those therapies. In patients who were revascularized early in addition to receiving IABP and thrombolytic therapy, the death rate was reduced to 37% (1). There is no consensus regarding the management of patients who remain in cardiogenic shock after delivering the appropriate above-mentioned therapeutic measures.

Other diseases that can cause severe persistent cardiogenic shock are acute fulminate myocarditis or end-stage cardiomyopathies. The acute heart failure syndrome (AHFS) registries (Acute Decompensated Heart Failure National Registry [ADHERE], the EuroHeart Failure Survey [EHFS], and the Organized Program to Initiate Lifesaving Treatment in Hospitalized Patients with Heart Failure [OPTIMIZE-HF]) have so far shown that the incidence of worsening chronic heart failure in AHFS is about 70%. It is not clear in how many cases cardiogenic shock or refractory heart failure occurs that is not responsive to therapy. According to the above-mentioned registries, 2% of patients had a cardiogenic shock (3). In another two-center European study in 312 patients who were hospitalized for AHFS, 4% suffered from cardiogenic shock (3). There are no reliable data in the literature regarding incidence of cardiogenic shock for acute fulminate myocarditis.

For these few selected patients suffering persistent cardiogenic shock with the imminent risk of dying, the use of VAD offers more circulatory support than IABP counterpulsation. Rapid intervention, though, is required not only to limit myocardial injury but also to restore adequate circulation in order to prevent further systemic hypoperfusion and reduce end-organ damage. The rapid mechanical circulatory support intervention is usually associated with the significant reduction of high doses of inotropic support agents, thus eliminating their toxic effects. The ultimate goal is a reduction of the high mortality rates.

Ventricular Assist Device Options

Ventricular assist devices are mechanical pumps that partially replace the mechanical work of the ventricle. They decrease myocardial work through unloading of the ventricle and pumping blood into the arterial system, which leads to increased peripheral and end-organ flow. Over the past two decades a variety of VADs have been developed. Since the most critical heart damage is usually found in the left ventricle, most patients can be managed with a left ventricular assist device (LVAD). In some cases with extensive cardiac damage, a biventricular assist device (BiVAD) might be necessary. In a few selected patients with a massive myocardial infarction the destruction of the myocardium is so extensive that for technical or surgical reasons a BiVAD cannot be implanted (left ventricle apical cannulation is not possible). These patients can only be salvaged with removal of the native heart and implantation of a total artificial heart (TAH).

Which Ventricular Assist Device Is Indicated When?

Several aspects have to be taken into account for the decision about which VAD system is indicated in AHFS patients suffering from persistent cardiogenic shock. Since this work is dealing with severe persistent cardiogenic shock patients in disastrous condition, who usually require VAD as rescue therapy, inexpensive, short-term, less-invasive devices are ideal for these patients. Thus, in this chapter we concentrate on these devices, which are mainly suitable for bridge to bridge (BTB), until the initial shock state is under control. They are mainly a bridge to the next therapy (bridge to transplantation, bridge to recovery, destination therapy, or cardiac transplantation HTX). For more VAD indications, see Table 66.1.

In a primary care hospital, the cardiologist should be aware of the possibility of a VAD implantation. Early contact with a specialized VAD center is advisable. Ideal is the establishment of a network between the primary care hospitals of one region and a specialized center. This allows a multidisciplinary approach, not limited to one institution. If the patient seems not to be stable enough for transfer to another hospital, institution of a simple, short-term assist device should be done in the primary care hospital. This also gives more time for further assessment of the patient. The patient's situation should be reassessed regularly if possible according to a

TABLE 66.1. Available ventricular assist device (VAD) systems with regard to duration of support and the intention to treat

Assist device	Duration of support	Type of possible support	Indication to treat BTB; BTR; BTT; DT
ECMO extracorporeal	Short-term	BiVAD	BTB, BTR
Centrifugal pump extracorporeal	Short-term	LVAD, RVAD, BiVAD	BTB, BTR
CentriMag	Short-term	LVAD, RVAD, BiVAD	BTB, BTR
Impella intracorporeal	Short-term	LVAD, RVAD, BiVAD	BTB, BTR
Medos paracorporeal	Short-term	LVAD, RVAD, BiVAD	BTB, BTR
Abiomed BVS 5000 extracorporeal	Short-term	LVAD, RVAD, BiVAD	BTB, BTR
Novacor LVAD Partially implantable	Mid-term, long-term	LVAD	BTT, BTR, DT
Thoratec (PVAD) paracorporeal	Mid-term, long-term	LVAD, RVAD, BiVAD	BTT, BTR, DT
HeartMateI Partially implantable	Mid-term, long-term	LVAD	BTT, BTR, DT
BerlinHeart paracorporeal	Mid-term, long-term	LVAD, RVAD, BiVAD	BTT, BTR
Thoratec IVAD Partially implantable	Mid-term, long-term	LVAD, RVAD, BiVAD	BTT, BTR, DT
CardioWest TAH Partially implantable	Mid-term, long-term	BiVAD	BTT, DT
Axial flow pumps Partially implantable	Mid-term, long-term	LVAD	BTT, BTR
Miniaturized centrifugal pumps DuraHeart, CorAide Partially implantable	Mid-term, long-term	LVAD	BTT, BTR, DT

Short-term: <1 month; mid-term support: 30 days to 1 year; long-term support: >1 year.
BTB, bridge to bridge; BTR, bridge to recovery; BTT, bridge to transplantation; DT, destination therapy.

standard protocol. During this time contact with a VAD specialized center is desirable.

Different Types of Ventricular Assist Device Support

The simplest form for short-term mechanical support can be provided by percutaneous cardiopulmonary bypass. This can be done with centrifugal pumps, such as the Biomedicus pump (Medtronic Inc., Minneapolis, MN, USA), which are easy to implant but should be considered only for short-term use (up to 7 to 10 days), as they are associated commonly with bleeding problems, thromboembolic complications, hemolysis, or the risk of limb ischemia. A novel magnetically levitated centrifugal pump is the CentriMag pump (Levitronix LLC, Waltham, MA, USA), which is constructed without bearings and rotating seals, and therefore reduces shear stress and minimizes the risk of hemolysis and thrombosis. It can also be applied percutaneously as femerofemoral bypass or as cardiopulmonary bypass from right atrium to aorta after sternotomy.

The Abiomed 5000 BVS (Abiomed, Danvers, MA, USA) can provide right/left or biventricular support, but requires sternotomy for implantation. Thus it is not recommended for primary care centers.

Other systems that can be used are the Impella Recover Pump (Impella Cardiosystems AG, Aachen, Germany) or the Tandem Heart (CardiacAssist Inc., Pittsburgh, PA, USA). Our own experience has shown that in patients with severe shock, biventricular heart failure might be present, which can be sufficiently controlled by the CentriMag pump, as it achieves a high cardiac (pump) output and does not produce hemolysis. Some of these short-term support pumps may include extracorporeal membrane oxygenation.

Another advantage of these easy to implant pumps is that they allow transferring the patient from a primary care hospital to a VAD experienced center.

The short-term support requires constant assessment of cardiac function to observe the progress of recovery, which usually is expected to happen within 7 to 14 days. Also, the neurologic situation of the patient needs to be reassessed. In case of insufficient cardiac recovery on a short-term device, further decision making is necessary about whether the patient needs to be switched to a long-term device. This should be considered only if the patient is a candidate for heart transplantation, and these devices should be used only in a specialized center with a full VAD institutional program.

The most common problems associated with mechanical circulatory support are thromboembolism, bleeding, and infections. Also hemolysis and device malfunction can occur. The risk of these events happening is not as high as the risk of death for patients with persistent cardiogenic shock.

Experience of Cardiogenic Shock Patients at the Heart Center, North-Rhine Westphalia

We performed a retrospective study of the data of 50 cardiogenic shock patients who were treated in our hospital from January 1998 to December 2000. They were referred to our center from surrounding hospitals, which belong to a network we have established in our area since 1994 (4). Only severe, persistent cardiogenic shock patients who had already been treated with multiple medications, including at least three different inotropes on high dosage and who had already received intervention measures in the primary care hospital were accepted for further treatment in our center. If they were sufficiently hemodynamically stable, they were transferred to our hospital by ambulance or helicopter. For unstable patients, we have a mobile mechanical circulatory support team that is responsible for the transport of these unstable patients. The team consists of a cardiac surgeon, an emergent interventional cardiologist, an intensivist, and a VAD coordinator. Once the patient is admitted to our intensive care unit (ICU), we apply our evaluation and decision-making protocol (5).

Evaluation and Decision-Making Protocol

Directly after admission of the patient, we try to stabilize the hemodynamics. Our aim is to achieve a cardiac index >2.4 L/m/m^2, a mean arterial pressure >60 mm Hg, and a urine output >30 mL/h. We try to achieve this by adjusting the inotropic support agents and other vasoactive drugs; IABP support is initiated in case the patient had not previously received the IABP. At the same time, the patient is evaluated for further VAD therapy and transplantation. All patients are thoroughly checked for concomitant diseases. Since all admitted patients are on extremely high doses of inotropes and vasoactive drugs, we aim to reduce the dosages during the first 12 hours after admission. If we fail to realize our aim, an emergent VAD system is applied (Fig. 66.1).

Patients in Our Retrospective Study

Of our 50 patients included in the retrospective study, 38 were male and 12 female. Mean age was 49 ± 14 years. The etiology of the cardiogenic shock was acute myocardial infarction in 22 patients (44%), followed by idiopathic dilatative cardiomyopathy, fulminate myocarditis, and ischemic cardiomyopathy. Fifteen of the 22 AMI patients had undergone rescue percutaneous transluminal coronary angioplasty (PTCA). Commonly found concomitant diseases were hypertension, insulin-dependent diabetes mellitus, and stroke. Several patients had previously been treated with a defibrillator or coronary artery bypass surgery. Most patients required ventilatory support and 50% IABP support, 38% needed continuous venovenous hemofiltration, and 16% depended on coronary artery bypass grafting. Four patients (8%) had cardiopulmonary resuscitation in the primary care hospital. Twenty-one patients (42%) needed to be transported to our center by our mobile mechanical support team. Mean doses of inotropes on admission were as follows: adrenaline 0.33 $\mu g\,kg^{-1}\,min^{-1}$ (standard deviation [SD] 0.24 $\mu g\,kg^{-1}\,min^{-1}$), dopamine 8.8 $\mu g\,kg^{-1}\,min^{-1}$ (SD 5.5 $\mu g\,kg^{-1}\,min^{-1}$), dobutamine 8.6 $\mu g\,kg^{-1}\,min^{-1}$ (SD 4.2 $\mu g\,kg^{-1}\,min^{-1}$), and noradrenaline 0.25 $\mu g\,kg^{-1}\,min^{-1}$ (SD 0.34 $\mu g\,kg^{-1}\,min^{-1}$). Echocardiography revealed a mean left ventricular end-diastolic diameter of 66 mm Hg (SD 12 mm Hg) in our patients on admission. Mean systolic arterial blood pressure was found to be just 83 mm Hg (SD 13 mm Hg), and mean arterial blood pressure was only 60 mm Hg (SD 12 mm Hg). Mean left ventricular ejection fraction was 24% (SD 13%), mean pulmonary artery pressure was 33 mm Hg (SD 11 mm Hg), pulmonary artery wedge pressure was 20 mm Hg (SD 7 mm Hg), and cardiac index was 2.6 L/min/m^2 (SD 1.0 L/min/m^2).

Our main interest was to investigate outcome. Moreover, we tried to assess variables that might potentially influence outcome (5).

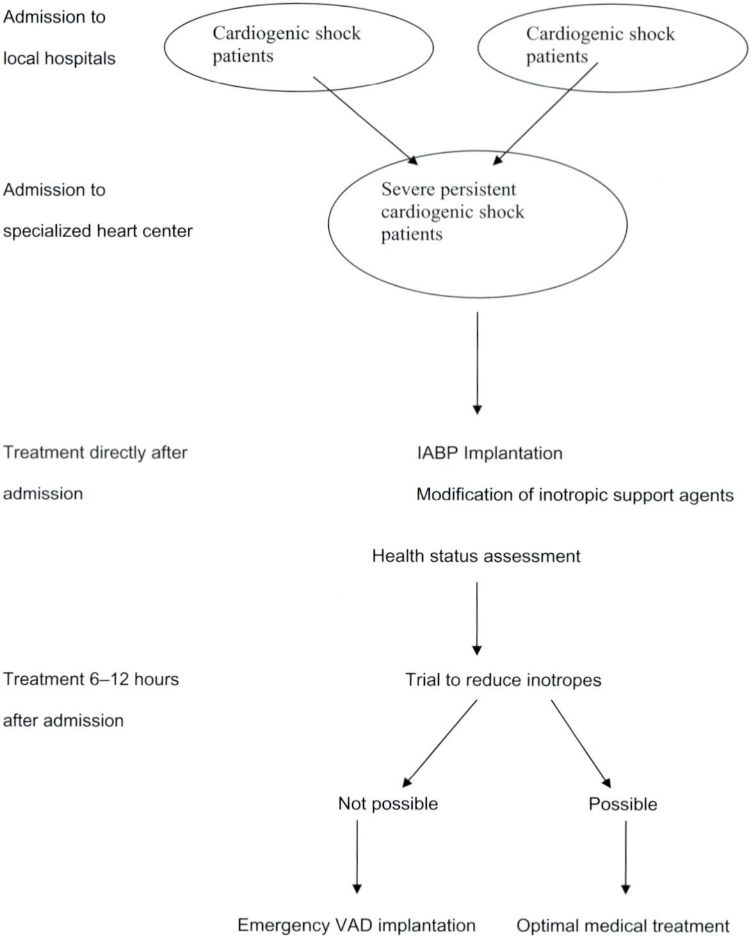

FIGURE 66.1. Management protocol for severe, persistent cardiogenic shock patients.

Results

Of the 50 patients, six required initial emergency VAD support. Four of these patients died, while two could be discharged and transplanted later on. The other 44 patients were initially stabilized by optimal medical treatment. Of this group, nine patients died. Sixteen patients could be weaned from inotropic support and discharged without further invasive therapy. Six patients who remained dependent on inotropes were transplanted on an emergency basis; five of them could be discharged, and one patient died after transplantation. Mean waiting time until HTX was 54 ± 30 days.

Thirteen patients who remained dependent on inotropes required urgent VAD therapy. Mean time until VAD implantation was 6 ± 6 days. Of these 13 patients, five could be weaned and discharged later, four patients were later transplanted successfully and discharged after HTX, and the remaining four VAD patients died on support. Of the 13 patients, VAD support was delivered as LVAD in six patients (mostly we used the Novacor left ventricular assist system [LVAS]), but five patients required biventricular support, and two needed a total artificial heart (TAH); we use the Syncardia CardioWest TAH (SynCardia Systems Inc., Tucson, AZ, USA).

Early in-hospital mortality of all 50 patients was 36% (18 patients). Sixteen patients died due to multiple organ failure and two due to mesenteric ischemia. With just optimized medical treatment 16 patients survived and could be discharged;

Table 66.2. Relative risks and 95% confidence intervals (CI) for 12-month mortality according to absence of sinus rhythm and age

Variable	Relative risk	95% CI	*p* value
Sinus rhythm (No.)	3.18	1.127–8.95	.029
Age (per year)	1.071	1.024–1.12	.003

also 16 patients of the VAD group plus the HTX group survived. Late mortality (postdischarge, after HTX and after VAD) was 10% (five patients). Causes of deaths in this group were persistent heart failure (two patients), pneumonia (one patient), renal failure (one patient), and gastrointestinal bleeding (one patient). Overall survival at 1, 6, and 12 months was 70%, 56%, and 52%, respectively. Without counting transplanted patients, the 12-month survival rate is still 50%.

In a multivariate Cox proportional hazard analysis, age and the absence of sinus rhythm were the only risk factors of 12-month mortality. The relative risk of death during the 12-month follow-up period was two times higher if sinus rhythm was absent, and increased 7.1% with each year of age (Table 66.2).

Discussion

The disastrous condition of patients with prolonged severe cardiogenic shock is a challenge for doctors treating these patients. Cardiogenic shock remains the leading cause of death for patients hospitalized with an AMI. Any patient with decompensated, acute severe heart failure requires immediate diagnostic evaluation and care and frequent resuscitative measures to improve symptoms and survival (6). If the initial treatment fails and the patient has refractory acute heart failure, further support must be considered. The simplest form of circulatory support, the IABP, often does not provide enough support. For these selected patients support with a VAD needs to be considered, preferably in a specialized center. Cardiologists should be aware of the possibility of transferring severe cardiogenic shock patients to a specialized center that has the facilities for HTX and VAD implantation. A multidisciplinary approach through a network that includes intensivists, cardiologists, and cardiac surgeons from primary care centers and specialized hospitals is desirable. The responsibilities of this team imply not only regular updates of new developments in the VAD area, but also training of ICU nursing staff; communication with patients, relatives, or other caregivers; and close communication within the team. Such a network can raise the awareness of VAD therapy as an option even for general practitioners or other doctors referring patients to hospitals.

The data from our retrospective study are, in our view, encouraging, as they show that even from these very sick patients several could be saved by VAD therapy. Our patients were in a worse state than those of the SHOCK trial. One inclusion criteria in that study was a systolic blood pressure of <90 mm Hg for 30 minutes before inotropes/vasopressors, or vasopressors or IABP were required to maintain systolic blood pressure at 90 mm Hg or higher. In our study, however, mean systolic blood pressure was only 83 ± 13 mm Hg despite high doses of three different inotropes. Moreover, 86% of our patients required mechanical ventilation and 38% needed continuous venovenous hemofiltration as renal replacement therapy before VAD therapy.

In the SHOCK trial, overall survival at 1, 6, and 12 months of follow-up was found to be 53%, 50%, and 47%, respectively, in the emergency revascularization group; in the group that could be stabilized with medical therapy, survival rates were 44%, 37%, and 34%, respectively (1,7). Compared to that, our overall survival rates at the same time points of 70%, 56%, and 52%, respectively, were encouraging, particularly as the state of our patients seems to have been even more critical. Eleven of our patients survived after successful emergency or urgent VAD implantation; 11 other patients survived because heart transplantation became available. Thus, we conclude that survival might indeed be better if patients are treated in a specialized heart center, offering HTX and VAD therapy. Moreover, from the referred 50 patients, 16 could be saved with optimal medical treatment.

We do not advocate VAD implantation for every cardiogenic shock patient, but rather for carefully selected patients. The selection process requires a lot of experience, and consequently an experienced, specialized center might be a better treatment place for these critically ill patients than a primary care hospital. For our network with the local surrounding hospitals, we plan to use our experience and teach the doctors of the local hospitals about the management of cardiogenic shock patients. Early treatment is essential and will also provide more time for decision making and picking the best therapeutic strategy. The survival rate of >50% after 12 months justifies the employment of immense financial and staff resources. As we could identify age as a risk factor for mortality, the application of VAD or transplantation should be limited to younger patients. Organ recovery is more likely in younger patients.

In 2001 in Germany, 12,000 patients younger than 65 years died from cardiogenic shock following myocardial infarction. This is an incidence of 0.015% in the general population (8). In our retrospective study we observed no difference in outcome between patients with acute myocardial infarction and those with other causes of shock. In consequence we conclude that our network and multidisciplinary approach is justified for all patients with severe persistent cardiogenic shock, regardless of the etiology.

The patients in our study who suffered an early in hospital death mostly died due to preexisting multiple organ failure or due to toxic catecholamine-induced ischemia. Moreover, late death was also caused by other reasons than cardiac failure in three of the five patients. Of our cohort of 50 patients, 21 could be discharged with their own, native heart. Once again this demonstrates that experience with this kind of patient at a specialized center might be lifesaving.

The absence of sinus rhythm as a risk factor for mortality is currently unclear and requires further evaluation and clarification.

Conclusion

Persistent cardiogenic shock is still associated with unacceptably high mortality rates. To improve outcome, a multidisciplinary and network approach might be beneficial. Prompt recognition of cardiogenic shock that is unresponsive to conventional therapy should lead to referral to a specialized center offering HTX and VAD implantation. The establishment of an early diagnosis, as well as further improvement of medical treatment and finding an optimal time and management schedule after admission until VAD implantation, needs to be investigated to further reduce the mortality rates.

References

1. Menon V, Fincke R. Cardiogenic shock: a summary of the randomized SHOCK trial. Congest Heart Fail 2003;9:35–9.
2. Duvernoy CS, Bates ER. Management of cardiogenic shock attributable to acute myocardial infarction in the reperfusion era. J Intensive Care Med 2005;20:188–98.
3. Nieminen MS, Veli-Pekka H. Definition and epidemiology of acute heart failure syndromes. Am J Cardiol 2005;96 (suppl):5G–10G.
4. El-Banayosy A, Posival H, Hartmann D, et al. Transport of patients in cardiogenic shock with mobile femoral-femoral cardiopulmonary bypass. J Cardiothorac Vasc Anesth 1995;9:301–3.
5. El Banayosy A, Cobaugh D, Zittermann A, et al. A multidisciplinary network to save the lives of severe, persistent cardiogenic shock patients. Ann Thorac Surg 2005;80:543–7.
6. Nieminen MS, et al., for the Task Force on Acute Heart Failure of the European Society of Cardiology. Executive summary of the guidelines on the diagnosis and treatment of acute heart failure. Eur Heart J 2005;26:384–416.
7. Hochman JS, Sleeper LA, Webb JG, et al. Early revascularization in acute myocardial infarction complicated by cardiogenic shock. Shock Investigators. Should we emergently revascularize occluded coronaries for cardiogenic shock? N Engl J Med 1999;341:34–65.
8. Statistisches Bundesamt. Statistisches Jahrbuch für die Bundesrepublik Deutschland 2003, Fa. Baden Baden: Wesel Kommunikation, 2003:442–3.

67 Role of Left Ventricular Assist Devices in Acute Heart Failure Syndrome and the Future of the Replacement Heart

José A. Tallaj, Salpy V. Pamboukian, and Robert C. Bourge

Historical Perspective

The first attempts to artificially sustain the circulation in modern times occurred with the development of the cardiopulmonary bypass machine by John Gibbon and later modified by John Kirklin in the mid-1950s[1,2]. These early machines revolutionized the field of cardiac surgery, allowing complex repairs to be done while sustaining the circulation with cardiopulmonary bypass. About a decade later, the first pulsatile pumps were being used to assist the failing left ventricle, especially in patients with cardiogenic shock postcardiotomy[3,4]. These early reports encouraged scientists of the time, like Dr. Michael DeBakey, in a crusade to produce a device intended for long-term ventricular support[5]. By the late 1960s, with the birth of heart transplantation[6], interest in mechanical assist devices waned. As the limitations of heart transplantation became apparent, especially the lack of adequate immunosuppression early on, renewed interest in mechanical ways of supporting the failing heart surged in the mid-1970s. In 1975, the first intraabdominally placed, pneumatically powered left ventricular device was used for patients who could not be weaned from cardiopulmonary bypass[7]. The same device was used extracorporeally to support a patient for 6 days until heart transplantation. Unfortunately, the patient died shortly after transplantation from massive infection[8].

The field of mechanical support devices received a major boost in 1980 when the National Institutes of Health issued a request for proposals (RFP) for the development of a long-term left ventricular assist device (LVAD) capable of supporting the patient for at least 2 years. This proposal was largely responsible for the development of the Novacor and HeartMate left ventricular assist systems (LVASs). The Novacor LVAS was the first device to be used successfully in a patient as a bridge to transplantation[9]. These two devices are currently approved by the U.S. Food and Drug Administration (FDA) as a bridge to transplantation. More recently, based on the results of the REMATCH trial[10], the HeartMate LVAD was also approved as destination therapy in patients with end-stage heart disease (see below).

Because of the limitations of the current devices, including the need for an external power sources connected through a percutaneous drive line and concerns regarding the ability of the pulsatile pumps to sustain patients for over 2 years, a completely new concept of chronic support in the form of axial flow technology has emerged. These devices are smaller and achieve circulatory support without the need of a compliance chamber or ventricle. The prototype of these devices, the Hemopump, was a catheter-based device positioned in the ascending aorta for patients who could not be weaned from cardiopulmonary bypass[11]. Even though this device was not introduced clinically, largely due to design problems, it led to further development in the axial flow technology for surgical implantation. Several of these devices are currently under clinic investigation, including the Jarvik 2000, MicroMed DeBakey, and HeartMate II. In addition, the concept of a temporary assist device placed percutaneously under fluoroscopic guidance has

Table 67.1. Current ventricular assist devices in use

Class	Device	Long term	BiVAD capable	Hospital D/C	No AC	FDA	Advantage(s)	Disadvantage(s)
TAH	SynCardia CardioWest	+	+			+	Greatest TAH clinical experience	Fitting required, immobility, infection (10–90%), emboli (12%)
TAH	Abiomed	+	+	+			Totally implantable	Fitting required; limited experience, emboli common
Centrifugal	Biomedicus		+			+	Simple, easy, inexpensive, widely available.	Bleeding (45%), embolus (2–63%), device failure (15%), RF (35%), bed-bound, bedside perfusionist required
External pneumatic	Abiomed		+			+	Easy, most common	Flow limit 6 L, bleeding (40%), hospital-bound
External pneumatic	Thoratec	+	+			+	Relatively simple device, RV support possible, external	Hospital-bound, BSA limitation, bleeding (42%), infection (36%), RF (36%), embolus (8%)
Pusher plate	Berlin Heart	+	+	+			Low BSA-compatible; different sizes	Pump cleaning required
Pusher plate	HeartMate VE	+		+	+	+	Low CVA rate, minimal anticoagulation; Only one approved for DT.	Infection rate; BSA >1.5
Pusher plate	Novacor	+		+		+	Reliable (0.8%)	Infection (30–50%), BSA limit, CVA (12–26%)
Axial flow	Jarvik-2000	+		+			Small size, small drive line	? Nonpulsatile, AI with pump failure, RPM only
Axial flow	HeartMate II (Nimbus)	+		+			Small size, small drive line	? Nonpulsatile, AI with pump failure
Axial flow	MicroMed DeBakey	+		+			Small size, small drive line, flow probe	? Nonpulsatile, AI with pump failure, fixed pump speed; aggressive anticoagulation required
Percutaneous	Impella Recover 100						Small size, percutaneously placed	? Nonpulsatile; short-term support only; requires aggressive anticoagulation
Percutaneous	Tandem Heart						Small size, percutaneously placed	? Nonpulsatile; short-term support only; requires aggressive anticoagulation
Epicardial compression	CTI		+		+		Weanable, defibrillation option	? Myocardial trauma, unproven durability
Epicardial compression	Abiomed		+		+		Weanable, defibrillation option	? Myocardial trauma, unproven durability

TAH, total artificial heart; VAD, ventricular assist device; D/C, discharge; AC, anticoagulation; FDA, Food and Drug Administration; RF, renal failure; BSA, body surface area; VE, vented electric; DT, destination therapy; CVA, cerebrovascular accident; AI, aortic insufficiency; RPM, revolutions per minute.

Source: Adapted from DiGiorgi et al.[56]

been readdressed, and several of these devices are under development and investigation. The physiologic effects of axial flow, as opposed to normal pulsatile blood flow, on autoregulation of the circulatory system and vital organ perfusion is still being elucidated.

Concomitant with the evolution and improvement in the technology of ventricular assist devices, there has been a parallel development of a total artificial heart capable of assuming all cardiac functions after diseased heart explantation. Dr. Denton Cooley implanted the first such device in 1969, just 2 years after the first heart transplantation[12]. A second and modified total artificial heart (TAH) was implanted 2 years later. Both patients survived until heart transplantation 64 and 55 hours after placement but subsequently died due to infection and multiorgan failure shortly after transplantation[3].

By the early 1980s, a second artificial heart was developed in Salt Lake City by Dr. William DeVries for destination therapy, the Jarvik-7 TAH. It was used in five patients, supported for a range of 10 to 620 days, all of whom were confined to the hospital due to the large pneumatic console required to operate the system. Eventually all succumbed to complications related to either emboli or infection[13].

As the field of heart transplantation evolved, especially the development of better immunosuppressive agents, the use of the Jarvik-7 TAH (later renamed Symbion) proved to be an adequate device for bridge to transplantation, with 66% of patients undergoing successful transplantation while on the device[14]. The Jarvik-7 technology was subsequently purchased and refined, and the device was named the CardioWest TAH and subsequently the SynCardia CardioWest TAH. The results with this device continue to be quite impressive, with more recent data indicating that almost 80% of patients survive to transplantation[15]. As impressive as these results are, the large pneumatic console required by the system, restricting patients to the hospital until transplantation and the associated cost, limits the use of this technology for long-term support (a smaller console is under development). Early results with the totally contained AbioCor Implantable Replacement Heart System in patients in cardiogenic shock, not eligible for transplantation, with an overall survival measured in days, has also been encouraging, with two of seven patients surviving discharge from the hospital[16]. As the technology advances, and new long-term devices are developed, we are getting closer to finding a device that may last long-term, and be reliable and safe and easy to operate for out-of-hospital independent living. Current devices that are available either clinically or through clinical investigation, and their main advantages and disadvantages, are summarized in Table 67.1.

Left Ventricular Assist Devices in Heart Failure

The earliest cases of mechanical support consisted of prolonged cardiopulmonary bypass in patients with postcardiotomy shock[17]. That was followed by the development of a pulsatile pump that was able to sustain the left or both ventricles for short periods of time until a more definitive therapy was instituted. The Thoratec ventricular assist device is another pump, relatively easy to insert, that has been used since the early 1980s. Its main advantage is its ability to provide reliable, long-term uni- or biventricular support[18] for up to 200 days, allowing either recovery of the native heart or as a bridge to transplantation[19]. These early models, still widely used today, are primarily used for the short-term support of patients in cardiogenic shock. The need for aggressive anticoagulation and lack of portability led to the development of more long-term pulsatile devices, like the Novacor and HeartMate LVAD, in patients considered to be transplant candidates (bridge to transplant)[20,21]. Both of these devices are now FDA approved as a bridge to transplantation in patients with advanced heart failure.

Recent data from the REMATCH trial suggest that highly selected patients with refractory heart failure may be candidates for implantable mechanical support as an alternative, rather than bridge to transplantation, the so-called destination therapy indication[10]. Patients with New York Heart Association (NYHA) class IV heart failure, most of them inotrope dependent, were randomized to received a HeartMate ventricular assist device (VAD) versus optimal medical management. There was a significant improvement in the

1-and 2-year survival in the group assigned to the HeartMate VAD. However, the 1- and 2-year survival in this group was only 52% and 23%. Most of the patients in this group succumbed to complications of bearing wear in the device or infection. Despite the high mortality seen at 2 years, a postapproval registry and subsequent analyses of the study suggest that outcomes are improving with device modification and with better surgical technique and prevention of infection[22].

Mechanical Circulatory Support for Acute Heart Failure

The initial therapy for acute heart failure, in addition to inotropic support, is usually the use of an intraaortic balloon pump (IABP). Such devices primarily support the circulation by decreasing afterload but improve the diastolic filling of the coronary arteries. They are therefore of important use in patients with myocardial ischemia. Unfortunately, these devices have limited use in very young patients (due to the relatively compliant aorta), smaller patients, and those with severe recurrent arrhythmias[23].

The major use of direct circulatory support devices (VADs) that directly pump blood is in the management of acute heart failure are in patients with postcardiotomy shock, cardiogenic shock from acute myocardial infarction, or from other forms of acute heart failure, including acute myocarditis. Another patient group of interest is in the support of patients with critically low cardiac output from progression of chronic heart failure.

Mechanical Support in Postcardiotomy Shock

With the growing era of heart surgery, the need for adequate support devices followed. Although these devices have been used for postcardiotomy shock for many years, the initial overall results were disappointing. During the early years of use, it became apparent that both timing of implantation and the type of support provided by these devices were the main factors in determining the success of such application. Inability to wean from extracorporeal circulation support of the left ventricle alone, without a right ventricular support device, contributed to the very high mortality[24]. Excessive bleeding was also a major contributor to the early mortality, possibly due to the late timing of placement of these devices, with resultant severe coagulopathy[25]. As the selection of surgical patients improved and our understanding of postcardiotomy shock increased, better results were obtained in randomized trials. The Abiomed BVS 5000, a uni- or biventricular support system, was the first to receive FDA approval for the short-term support of postcardiotomy patients, with a survival rate of about 50% in the post-operative period[26]. The main disadvantage of this system is its short-duration of support, in the range 5 to 9 days, usually necessitating transfer of a very ill patient to a transplant center for a trial of device weaning, or a switch to a more durable system to await transplantation[27]. The Thoratec VAD can be used in the perioperative period, providing reliable uni- or biventricular support[28] for over 200 days, allowing either recovery of the native heart or as a bridge to transplantation[29]. The main disadvantages of the Thoratec VAD are the need for long-term anticoagulation with its associated bleeding complications and its limited portability, usually restricting the patient to the hospital setting until transplantation. Currently, the use of either device is acceptable in clinical practice. Smaller and more durable devices are undergoing clinical evaluation for use in this setting.

Mechanical Support in Cardiogenic Shock from Acute Myocardial Infarction

Cardiogenic shock resulting from acute myocardial infarction has been recognized for years. A minority of patients have an initial presentation of cardiogenic shock, but most cases occur within 48 hours of admission[30]. The prognosis in these patients is quite poor, with a 30-day mortality of up to 50%, despite aggressive medical management and early coronary revascularization[31]. Clinical predictors of poor outcome include increased age, peripheral hypoperfusion, or elevated pulmonary artery wedge pressure[32]. Given this poor outcome, there has been an increase use of mechanical support devices in this setting. Aggressive salvage efforts are initially needed to maintain vital organ function and prevent irreversible end-organ damage, especially neurologic or renal dysfunction. Some of these patients may then be eligible for coronary intervention, coronary artery bypass surgery, or switched to a more durable device as a bridge to transplantation. The Abiomed BVS 5000 was the first VAD to be used in this setting, with a 64% success rate in bridging patients to transplantation[33]. Of note, all of these patients were transplanted while still on the device, in less than 12 days, something that is not easy to achieve in most transplant programs in the U.S. The Thoratec VAD has also been used in cardiogenic shock complicating acute myocardial infarction with variable results[34]. Given these data, a patient with post–myocardial infarction shock should be evaluated for short- or long-term mechanical support, allowing either institution of definitive treatment or bridging to additional therapy, such as cardiac transplantation.

In recent years, a new and exciting method of mechanical support has been developed, especially for use in patients with cardiogenic shock complicating myocardial infarction. The new devices, called percutaneous VAD, are the Tandem Heart (approved by the FDA) and Impella Recover 100 (currently investigational in the U.S.) systems. These axial-flow devices are implanted percutaneously under fluoroscopic guidance in the catheterization laboratory and provide adequate support of up to 4 L/min, unloading the LV, allowing for recovery of LV function, or simply sustaining the patient during high-risk coronary intervention[35,36]. Proliferation in the use of such devices is likely to be seen in the near future.

Mechanical Support in Acute Heart Failure Due to Myocarditis

Patients with myocarditis pose a major challenge to the treating physician. Most patients present with an indolent and chronic course, but some patients may present with a fulminant and frequently lethal disease. Interestingly, the prognosis for patients with fulminant disease is better than for patients presenting with a more indolent form of the disease[37]. Therefore, aggressive hemodynamic support is warranted to support patients during the acute event. It has been known that patients could be safely weaned off of mechanical support, even months after the placement of an assist device[38].

In recent years, there has been an increase in the use of such devices as a lifesaving therapy in patients with fulminant myocarditis. Clinical experience with bridge to recovery in myocarditis has been described by multiple investigators[39,40,41,42,43,44]. In these series, patients were supported with various devices (pulsatile, and then most recently axial flow) either as LVAD or a biventricular assist device for short- to medium-term use with documented improvement or recovery in EF. The overall survival of patients with fulminant myocarditis treated with an assist device in these series, either by recovery and weaning off of the mechanical support or as a bridge to transplantation, is excellent, ranging between 70% and 100%[45]. Extracorporeal membrane oxygenation (ECMO) has also supported infants and children with cardiac failure secondary to acute myocarditis[46] with similarly excellent short-term results. It is reasonable, then, to use ECMO in children as the first line of therapy, beyond inotropic support and intraaortic balloon pump. In our institution, we routinely use ECMO in pediatric patients with acute myocarditis in cardiogenic shock. After several days of stabilization, if there is no irreversible end-organ damage or meaningful recovery of LV function, then switch to a long-term device like the Thoratec or Berlin Excor Heart is undertaken. The Berlin Heart has the advantage of having several different sizes available that can be tailored for use in patients ranging from neonates to large adults[47].

Giant cell myocarditis, another rare form of acute myocarditis, also progresses rapidly to a fulminant outcome, often to lethal ventricular arrhythmias. As opposed to fulminant lymphocytic myocarditis, these patients do not seem to respond as well to medical therapy, and the chances of recovery of myocardial function are minimal. Therefore, mechanical support allows a bridge to transplantation with fairly good results[48]. There have been several case reports of other forms of myocarditis, unresponsive to medical therapy, that are treated with mechanical support until a definitive therapy like transplantation or aggressive immunosuppression is instituted.

Mechanical Support in Patients with Critically Low Cardiac Output from Exacerbation of Chronic Heart Failure

Most of the current experience with mechanical support in patients with low cardiac output from progression or acute exacerbation of chronic heart failure are as bridge to transplantation[10,21]. The patient with once-stable heart failure decompensates to a critically low output state, with its associated end-organ damage.

Challenges in Implementing Mechanical Support in Patients with Acute Heart Failure

Caring for patients with acute, decompensated heart failure can be quite challenging and complicated. If a patient is in extremis, the acute situation must be stabilized. Aggressive use of inotropic agents, in combination with vasopressors, should be instituted to keep a normal oxygenation and adequate perfusion and blood pressure. A rapid assessment of volume status by exam should be performed prior to any invasive procedures, with measurement. Figure 67.1 illustrates an approach to the categorization of the volume and perfusion status of patients based on signs and symptoms. Figure 67.2 shows an algorithm published by the European Society of Cardiology for the selection of candidates for LV assist device[49]. In our experience, most patients with acute decompensated heart failure are "warm and wet," with an excess volume or hypervolemia being the major problem. These patients may be successfully treated with diuretics and vasodilators (and, in some cases, inotropes).

Most patients with NYHA class IV heart failure can be restored to NYHA class III with intensive medical management, with an expected short- and intermediate-term survival superior to that observed in the REMATCH trial[50]. On the other hand, patients who cannot be weaned from intravenous inotropic therapy[51] or in whom angiotensin-converting enzyme inhibitors have to be discontinued due to hypotension or renal insufficiency[52], may also benefit from mechanical support, as their 6-month and 1-year survival is more than 50%, worse than that observed in the REMATCH trial. The Acute Physiology and Chronic Health Evaluation (APACHE II) score system has also been used in an attempt to select patients with a very high short-term mortality who may benefit from long-term mechanical support[53]. It is the minority of

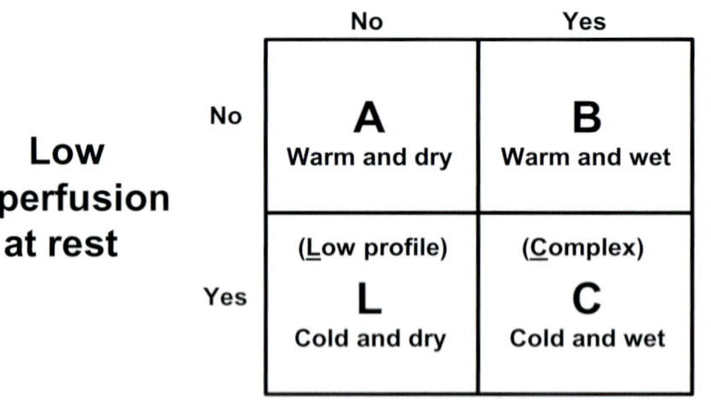

FIGURE 67.1. Rapid assessment of hemodynamic status in heart failure. Abdominal; ACE, angiotensin-converting enzyme; JV, jugular vein; PA, pulmonary artery; PND, paroxysmal nocturnal dyspnea. (Adapted from Stevenson LW. Tailored therapy to hemodynamic goals for advanced heart failure. Eur J Heart Failure 1999;1:251–7. Copyright 1999, with permission from the European Society of Cardiology.)

patients who are still in cardiogenic shock despite maximal medical management who may require mechanical support in the acute setting.

Figure 67.3 summarizes the mortality of the different heart failure populations in relationship to the reported mortality with VADs[54]. It may be prudent to stabilize the patient acutely, with inotropic and vasopressors agents, intraaortic balloon pump before being considered for an assist device. The outcome of patients who arrive in the operating room in cardiogenic shock, hypotensive, or in impending cardiac arrest is dismal. The timing of VAD placement is of utmost importance and may be the primary differentiator between a favorable or poor outcome.

In addition to these other considerations, we cannot underestimate the vital contribution of the right ventricle. The status of the right ventricle is important when making a decision regarding mechanical support. Unloading the left ventricle, with its subsequent decrease in the filling pressure

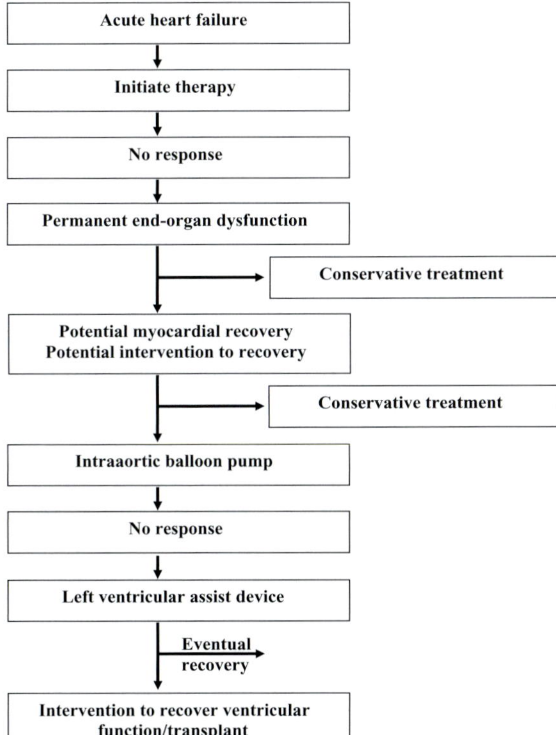

FIGURE 67.2. Selection of candidates for left ventricular assist devices. (Adapted from Nieminen et al., for the European Society of Cardiology.[49])

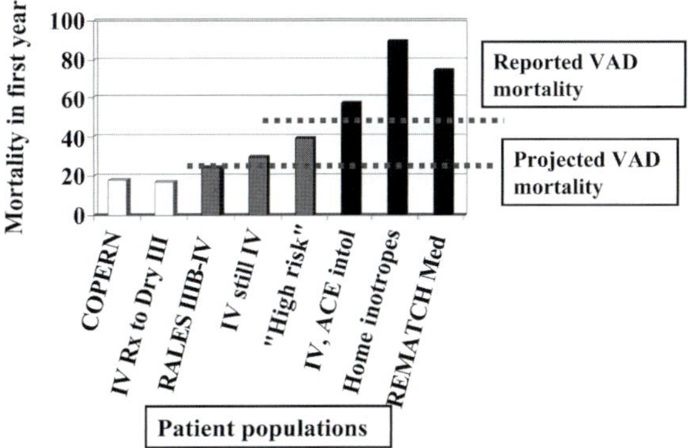

FIGURE 67.3. Comparison of estimated 1-year mortality of different heart failure populations. ACE, angiotensin-converting enzyme; IV, intravenous; VAD, ventricular assist device. (Adapted from Stevenson and Shekar.[54])

and secondary pulmonary hypertension, leads to beneficial effects on the right ventricle. However, this beneficial effect may take days to weeks to become apparent; therefore, RV failure needs to be treated aggressively perioperatively. The outcome of patients with the placement of a right ventricular assist device at the time of LVAD placement have not been favorable, with a very high perioperative and short-term mortality[55]. Although trying to stabilize the patient is important, we should not "pull the trigger" too late, when irreversible end-organ damage (primarily renal and liver) has occurred. Moreover, early consideration for an LV assist device should be given to patients who are potential transplant candidates or who have the potential for recovery of myocardial function, such as those with proven or presumed acute myocarditis. If recovery from the acute heart failure decompensation or cardiac transplantation is not possible, then the use of mechanical support is not advised. One caveat to this point would be in situations where placement of LVAD is done for possible destination therapy. Such patients are usually evaluated extensively to evaluate their psychological and social support prior to consideration for destination VAD placement, if possible.

Device Selection

There are six FDA-approved assist devices, with several more in clinical trials (Table 67.1). Considering the clinical scenario, the heart failure

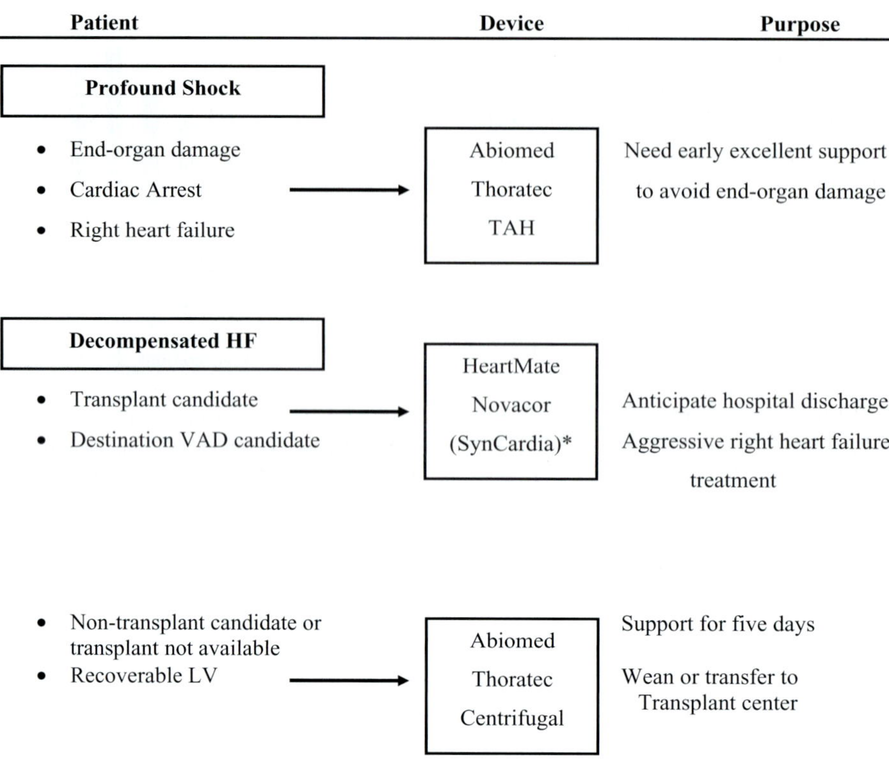

FIGURE 67.4. Device selection. TAH, total artificial heart. (Adapted from DiGiorgi et al.[56])

cardiologist, cardiovascular surgeon, and sometimes the patient and the patient's family are faced with several decisions regarding which device to use for acute heart failure, when to implant the device, and how to do it. A patient's size, the patient's clinical condition, and the major indication for which the device is being used influence the device selection. A Thoratec device, for example, might be appropriate for a heart transplant candidate in cardiogenic shock, requiring biventricular support, whereas the same device would not be appropriate for a patient who is not a transplant candidate, as use of this device is restricted to the hospital setting. Similarly, in emergent situations, it may be more appropriate to use a Thoratec LVAD or Abiomed BVS 5000, which are easily and rapidly placed, rather than a HeartMate XVE or a Novacor, which may take longer to place. Moreover, currently, biventricular devices or the TAH should only be used in patients as a bridge to transplantation (other than in investigational circumstances), as these are generally not portable devices or approved by the FDA for discharge from the hospital. Figure 67.4 provides a helpful algorithm for the application of VAD technology, depending on the various clinical scenarios[56].

Future of Mechanical Circulatory Support

The field of circulatory support is progressing fast. New devices are being developed everyday. Most of these devices are initially evaluated in patients awaiting transplantation. If favorable and effective, then these devices may be used to provide more prolonged support, and as the final or destination therapy for this group of patients. The Berlin Heart is the only pulsatile VAD in development, which may be especially useful in small children and pediatric patients because of the sizing options. Most VADs currently under development are axial or centrifugal pumps. The advantage of the centrifugal over the axial flow devices is their smaller size and potentially total implantability. The new HeartMate II trial, an axial flow pump, as destination therapy, is progressing rapidly and may gain FDA approval in the near future. The DeBakey and Jarvik-2000 axial pumps are also undergoing evaluation. We believe that the use of the percutaneous VADs will increase significantly in the near future, especially to provide support for patients in cardiogenic shock and acute heart failure.

A new form of device being developed is the cardiac compression device, which supports the circulation by compressing the failing heart from its epicardial surface. The force generated by the device is triggered by the electrocardiogram (ECG), and adds to the ventricular pressure generated by the contracting myocardium, therefore increasing the volume of blood ejected from the left ventricle[57]. Two such devices are currently under development.

The field of a total artificial heart has developed slowly, largely due to technology limitations and the problem of the blood–device interface leading to clot formation. The AbioCor TAH shows some promise, given the potential for full implantability, but preliminary data from the first few implants showed a very high risk of stroke and thrombus formation within the device[58]. We believe that we are still years away from a reliable, long-lasting, and portable total artificial heart, which could be used for patients with severe end-stage heart failure.

Conclusion

There is a role for mechanical support in the treatment of patients with acute heart failure. Selecting the correct device depends on the clinical scenario and institutional preferences. New devices are undergoing clinical testing and new and exciting new technology is under development. As technology improves, the survival and quality of life of patients suffering from acute and severe heart failure will continue to improve.

References

1. Gibbon JH Jr. Application of a mechanical heart and lung apparatus to cardiac surgery. Minn Med 1954;37:171–80.
2. Kirklin JW, DuShane JW, Patrick RT, et al. Intracardiac surgery with the aid of a mechanical pump-oxygenator system (Gibbon type): report of eight cases. Staff Meetings Mayo Clin 1955;30:201–6.
3. Frazier OH. Ventricular assist devices and artificial hearts. A historical perspective. Cardiol Clin 2003; 21:1–13.
4. Hall CW, Liotta D, Henry WS, et al. Development of artificial intrathoracic circulatory pumps. Am J Surg 1964;108:685–92.
5. DeBakey ME. Left ventricular bypass pump for cardiac assistance: clinical experience. Am J Cardiol 1971;27:3–11.
6. Barnard CN. A human cardiac transplant: an interim report of a successful operation performed at Groote Schuur Hospital, Cape Town. S Afr Med J 1967;41:1271–4.
7. Norman JC, Duncan JM, Frazier OH, et al. Intracorporeal (abdominal) left ventricular assist devices or partial artificial hearts: a five year clinical experience. Arch Surg 1981;116:1441–5.
8. Norman JC, Brook MI, Cooley DA, et al. Total support of the circulation of a patient with post-cardiotomy stone-heart syndrome by a partial artificial heart (ALVAD) for 5 days followed by heart and kidney transplantation. Lancet 1978;1(8074): 1125–7.
9. Portner PM, Oyer PE, McGregor CGA, et al. First human use of an electrically powered implantable ventricular assist system. Artif Organs 1985;9: 36.
10. Rose EA, Gelijns AC, Moskowitz AJ, et al. Long-term use of a left ventricular assist device for end-stage heart failure. N Engl J Med 2001;345: 1435–43.
11. Frazier OH, Wampler RK, Duncan JM, et al. First human use of the Hemopump, a catheter-mounted ventricular assist device. Ann Thorac Surg 1990; 49:299–304.
12. Cooley DA, Liotta D, Hallman GL, et al. Orthotopic cardiac prosthesis for two-staged cardiac replacement. Am J Cardiol 1969;24:723–30.

13. DeVries WC, Anderson JL, Joyce LD, et al. Clinical use of the total artificial heart. N Engl J Med 1984;310:273–8.
14. Johnson KE, Prieto M, Joyce LD, et al. Summary of the clinical use of the Symbion total artificial heart: a registry report. Ann Surg 1995;222:327–36.
15. Copeland JG, Smith RG, Arabia FA, et al. Cardiac replacement with a total artifical heart as a bridge to transplantation. N Engl J Med 2004;351:859–67.
16. Dowling RD, Gary LA Jr, Etoch SW, et al. Initial experience with the AbioCor implantable replacement heart system. J Thorac Cardiovasc Surg 2004; 127:131–41.
17. Spencer FC, Eiseman B, Tinkle JK, Rodd NP. Assisted circulation for cardiac failure following intracardiac surgery with cardiopulmonary bypass. J Thorac Cardiovasc Surg 1965;49:56–73.
18. Pennington DG, Bernhard WF, Golding LR, et al. Long-term follow-up of postcardiotomy patients with profound cardiogenic shock treated with ventricular assist devices. Circulation 1985;72:II216–26.
19. Farrar DJ, Hill JD. Univentricular and biventricular Thoratec VAD support as a bridge to transplantation. Ann Thorac Surg 1993;55:276–82.
20. Dasse KA, Frazier OH, Lesniak JM, Myers T, Burnett CM, Poirier VL. Clinical responses to ventricular assistance versus transplantation in a series of bridge to transplant patients. ASAIO J 1992;38: M622–6.
21. Portner PM, Oyer PE, Pennington DG, et al. Implantable electrical left ventricular assist device: bridge to transplantation and the future. Ann Thorac Surg 1989;47:142–50.
22. Park SJ, Tector A, Piccioni W, et al. Left ventricular assist devices as destination therapy: a new look at survival. J Thorac Cardiovasc Surg 2005;129:9–17.
23. Trost JC, Hillis LD. Intra-aortic balloon counterpulsation. Am J Cardiol 2006;97:1391–8.
24. Wolner E, Deutsch M, Losert U, et al. Clinical application of the ellipsoid left heart assist device. Artif Organs 1978;2:268–72.
25. Olsen EK, Pierce WS, Donachy JH, et al. A two and one half year clinical experience with a mechanical left ventricular assist pump in the treatment of profound postoperative heart failure. Int J Artif Organs 1979;2:197–206.
26. Guyton RA, Schonberger JP, Everts PA, et al. Postcardiotomy shock: clinical evaluation of the BVS 5000 biventricular support system. Ann Thorac Surg 1993;56:346–56.
27. Helman DN, Morales DL, Edwards NM, et al. Left ventricular assist device bridge-to-transplant network improves survival after failed cardiotomy. Ann Thorac Surg 1999;1187–94.
28. Pennington DG, Bernhard WF, Golding LR, et al. Long-term follow-up of postcardiotomy patients with profound cardiogenic shock treated with ventricular assist devices. Circulation 1985;72:II216–26.
29. Farrar DJ, Hill JD. Univentricular and biventricular Thoratec VAD support as a bridge to transplantation. Ann Thorac Surg 1993;55:276–82.
30. Holmes DR Jr, Bates ER, Kleiman NS, et al. Contemporary reperfusion therapy for cardiogenic shock: the GUSTO-1 trial experience. The GUSTO-1 Investigators. J Am Coll Cardiol 1995;26:668–74.
31. Hochman JS, Sleeper LA, Webb JG, et al., for the SHOCK Investigators. Early revascularization in acute myocardial infarction complicated by cardiogenic shock. N Engl J Med 1999;341:625–34.
32. Hasdai D, Holmes DR Jr, Califf RM. Cardiogenic shock complicating acute myocardial infarction: predictors of death. GUSTO Investigators. Am Heart J 1999;138:21–31.
33. Castells E, Calbet JM, Saura E, et al. Acute myocardial infarction with cardiogenic shock: treatment with mechanical circulatory assistance and heart transplantation. Transplant Proc 2003;35:1940–1.
34. McBride LR. Naunheim KS. Fiore AC. Moroney DA. Swartz MT. Clinical experience with 111 Thoratec ventricular assist devices. Ann Thorac Surg 1999;67:1233–8.
35. Meyns B, Dens J, Sergeant P, et al. Initial experiences with the Impella device in patients with cardiogenic shock—Impella support for cardiogenic shock. Thorac Cardiovasc Surgeon 2003;51:312–7.
36. Thiele H, Sick P, Boudriot E, et al. randomized comparison of intra-aortic balloon support with a percutaneous left ventricular assist device in patients with revascularized acute myocardial infarction complicated by cardiogenic shock. Eur Heart J 2005;26:1276–83.
37. McCarthy RE, Boehmer JP, Hruban RH, et al. Long term outcome of fulminant myocarditis as compared with acute (nonfulminant) myocarditis. N Engl J Med 2000;343:690–5.
38. Holman WL, Bourge RC, Kirklin JK. Case report: circulatory support for seventy days with resolution of acute heart failure. J Thorac Cardiovasc Surg 1991;102:932–4.
39. Rockman HA, Adamson RM, Dembitsky WP, Bonar JW, Jaski BE. Acute fulminant myocarditis: long-term follow-up after circulatory support with left ventricular device. Am Heart J 1991;121: 922–6.

40. Kesler KA, Pruitt AL, Turrentine MW, Heimansohm A, Brown JW. Temporary left-sided mechanical cardiac support during acute myocarditis. J Heart Lung Transplant 1994;13:268–70.
41. Marelli D, Laks H, Amsel B, et al. Temporary mechanical support with BVS 5000 assist device during treatment of acute myocarditis. J Card Surg 1997;12:55–59.
42. Reinhartz O, Hill JD, Al-Khaldi A, Pelletier MP, Robbins RC, Farrar DJ. Thoratec ventricular assist devices in pediatric patients: update on clinical results. ASAIO J 2005;51:501–3.
43. Grinda JM, Chevalier P, D'Attellis N, et al. Fulminant myocarditis in adults and children: biventricular assist device for recovery. Eur J Cardio-Thorac Surg 2004;26:1169–73.
44. Duncan BW, Bohn DJ, Atz AM, French JW, Laussen PC, Wessel DL. Mechanical circulatory support for the treatment of children with acute fulminant myocarditis. J Thorac Cardiovasc Surg 2001;122: 440–8.
45. Acker MA. Mechanical circulatory support for patients with acute fulminant myocarditis. Ann Thorac Surg 2001;71:S73–6.
46. Chen, YS, Yu HY, Huang SC, et al. Experience and result extracorporeal membrane oxygenation in treating fulminant myocarditis with shock—what mechanical support should be considered first? J Heart Lung Transplant 2005;24:81–7.
47. Hetzer R, Potapov EV, Stiller B, et al. Improvement in survival after mechanical circulatory support with pneumatic pulsatile ventricular assist devices in pediatric patients. Ann Thorac Surg 2006;82:917–24.
48. Davies RA, Veinot JP, Smith S, Struthers C, Hendry P, Masters R. Giant cell myocarditis: clinical presentation, bridge to transplantation with mechanical circulatory support, and long-term outcome. J Heart Lung Transplant 2002;21:674–9.
49. Nieminen MS, Bohm M, Cowie R, et al., for the European Society of Cardiology. Executive summary of the guidelines on the diagnosis and treatment of acute heart failure. Eur Heart J 2005;26: 384–416.
50. Lucas C, Johnson W, Hamilton MA, et al. Freedom from congestion predicts good survival despite previous class IV symptoms of heart failure. Am Heart J 2000;140:840–7.
51. Stevenson LW, Miller LW, Desvigne-Nickens P, et al. Left ventricular assist device as destination for patients undergoing intravenous inotropic therapy: a subset analysis from REMATCH (Randomized Evaluation of Mechanical Assistance in Treatment of Chronic Heart Failure). Circulation 2004;110: 975–81.
52. Kittleson M, Hurtzwitz S, Shah MR, et al. Development of circulatory-renal limitations to angiotensin-converting enzyme inhibitors identifies patients with severe heart failure and early mortality. J Am Coll Cardiol 2003;41:2029–35.
53. Gracin N, Johnson MR, Spokas D, et al. The use of the APACHE II scores to select candidates for left ventricular assist device placement. Acute Physiology and Chronic Health Evaluation. J Heart Lung Transplant 1998;17:1017–23.
54. Stevenson LW, Shekar P. Ventricular assist devices for durable support. Circulation 2005;112:e111–5.
55. Deng MC, Edwards LB, Hertz MI, et al. Mechanical circulatory Support Device Database of the International Society for Heart and Lung Transplantation: third annual report—2005. J Heart Lung Transplant 2005;24:1182–7.
56. DiGiorgi PL, Rai V, Naka Y, Oz M. Which patient, which pump? J Heart Lung Transplant 2003;22: 221–35.
57. Artrip JH, Yi GH, Burkhoff D, Wang J. Physiological and hemodynamic evaluation of non-uniform direct cardiac compression. Circulation 1999;100: II236–43.
58. Dowling RD, Gray LA Jr, Etoch SW, et al. Initial experience with the AbioCor implantable replacement heart system. J Thorac Cardiovasc Surg 2004; 127:131–41.

2.7
Management of Organ Dysfunction Associated with Acute Heart Failure Syndrome

68
Kidney in Acute Heart Failure

Guido Boerrigter, Fernando L. Martin, and John C. Burnett, Jr.

The hallmark of symptomatic heart failure (HF) is sodium and water retention, leading to congestion and symptoms of edema. Indeed, Starling in the 19th century asked provocatively, "What, if anything, does the heart have to do with heart failure?" He also advanced the theory that "humors" must be released in HF that lead to leakiness of capillaries and edema formation, a concept that is not opposed to our current understanding of the complex activation of diverse neurohumoral systems that characterize symptomatic HF and contribute to renal dysfunction. Key epidemiologic studies have refocused our attention on the role of the kidney in this syndrome, as they have established that renal dysfunction is one of the most robust predictors of mortality and morbidity in the setting of ventricular dysfunction and HF. Specifically, in two retrospective analyses, impaired renal function was identified as a major predictor of mortality in human HF, more powerful even than New York Heart Association (NYHA) class or left ventricular ejection fraction.[1,2] These studies underscore the importance of considering renal function in the treatment of HF, especially in acute decompensated HF (ADHF), in which worsening renal function, congestion, and poor outcomes predominate.

This seminal role of the kidney in HF is not surprising. As the kidney fails in chronic renal failure, sodium and water retention increase myocardial preload and lead to pressure overload secondary to hypertension. This cardiac overload contributes to further cardiac remodeling and worsening HF, underscoring a common heart and kidney connection in organ failure of either cardiac or renal origin. Further, we also have come to realize the importance of renal perfusion pressure—mean arterial pressure minus right atrial pressure—as a key determinant of renal function in HF. Evidence suggests that the venous pressure may be as important as arterial pressure; increasing venous pressure decreases the glomerular filtration rate (GFR), especially in the presence of excessive arterial hypotension.[3,4]

This chapter reviews the relevant structure and function of the kidney, its temporal and complex adjustments to progressive HF, and the conventional and innovative therapies that target the kidney to enhance GFR as well as improve sodium and water homeostasis, serving to address the need for more effective natriuretic and aquaretic agents in HF, especially in ADHF and the cardiorenal syndrome.

The Single Nephron and the Cardiorenal Axis

Optimal cardiovascular homeostasis crucially depends on the kidney in its regulation of intravascular volume and arterial pressure via the control of sodium and water excretion and the renin-angiotensin-aldosterone system (RAAS). We now appreciate that the kidney integrates inputs of multiple physiologic variables, which include hemodynamic, neurohormonal, and metabolic factors. Under normal conditions, approximately a quarter of the cardiac output is directed to the kidneys. Figure 68.1 illustrates the single nephron, the basic functional and structural unit

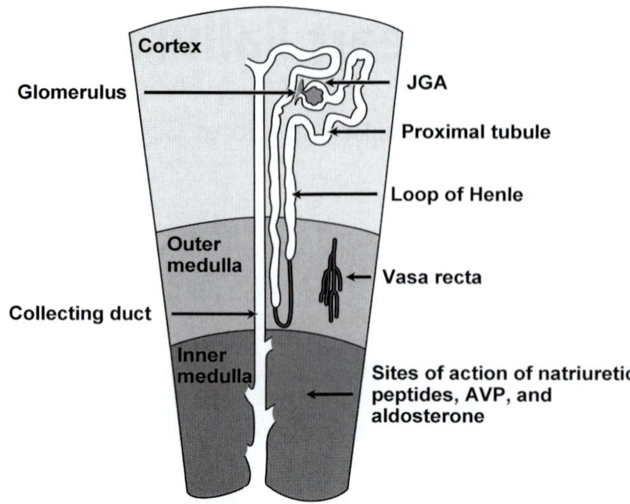

FIGURE 68.1. Schematic of a single nephron, the basic functional unit of the kidney, with major sites of physiologic regulation. AVP, arginine vasopressin.

of the kidney. Blood enters the glomerulus via the afferent arteriole, and plasma is filtered via endothelial cells, a basement membrane, and podocytes into the tubular space. Blood that is not filtered leaves the glomerulus via the efferent arteriole and subsequently flows through the peritubular vessels to the veins and back to the heart. The GFR is the amount of plasma over time that is filtered in the glomerulus. Determinants of GFR are filtration pressure, which depends on the hydrostatic and oncotic pressure gradients across the membrane, and the coefficient for ultrafiltration (K_f) of the glomerular membrane. From the glomerulus, the ultrafiltrate flows through the proximal tubule, the loop of Henle, the distal tubule, and the collecting duct.

It is now well recognized that the different segments of the tubule vary in permeabilities for water and solutes and are regulated by neurohumoral factors. As illustrated in Figure 68.1, the collecting duct is the final determinant of sodium and water excretion. Some of the most important humoral regulators of salt and water excretion—the natriuretic peptides atrial and B-type natriuretic peptide (ANP and BNP, respectively), arginine vasopressin (AVP), and aldosterone—all target this terminal nephron. Furthermore, the interstitial solute content is important also in dictating sodium and water excretion in the terminal nephron with the highest osmotic pressures occurring in the renal medulla. Indeed, the tonicity of the renal medulla is increased in response to a decrease in vasa recta flow (i.e., medullary plasma flow) as occurs in HF.

An important intrarenal modulator of GFR is the juxtaglomerular apparatus, a structure that connects the distal tubule with the afferent arteriole. An increase in sodium delivery to the distal tubule is sensed in the juxtaglomerular apparatus and leads to vasoconstriction of the afferent arteriole, decreasing blood flow into the glomerulus and effective filtration pressure, thus reducing GFR. This feedback mechanism is called "tubuloglomerular feedback" (TGF). A potential mediator of this feedback is adenosine.[5] It is well recognized that increased sodium delivery to the distal tubule leads to increased activation of adenosine triphosphate (ATP)-dependent ion pumps with a subsequent increase in adenosine. In addition, the hypoxic kidney may also increase adenosine production, the plasma concentration of which is increased in HF.[6] This TGF phenomenon has important implications for the use of diuretic agents. As most conventional diuretics inhibit the tubular reabsorption of sodium and thus increase the tubular sodium concentration, TGF will reduce GFR and thus limit the efficacy of the diuretic. This may be further complicated by diuretic activation of aldosterone, which enhances sodium reabsorption in the inner medullary collecting duct. Of interest, the cardiac natriuretic peptide ANP inhibits TGF in experimental congestive heart failure (CHF), which may in part explain some of its renoprotective actions.[7] We will discuss later the therapeutic promise of agents that antagonize adenosine in the kidney.

Another important determinant for renal dysfunction in HF is what can be termed the cardiorenal axis, specifically the balance of the RAAS versus the natriuretic peptides ANP and BNP. If renal perfusion is low, the kidney increases renin secretion. Renin cleaves angiotensinogen to angiotensin I, which in turn is cleaved by the angiotensin converting enzyme (ACE) to angiotensin II. Angiotensin II promotes vasoconstriction, sodium and water retention, and secretion of the mineralocorticoid aldosterone. In contrast, if the cardiac chambers are stretched, such as in volume overload with increased cardiac filling pressures, the heart secretes ANP and BNP, which promote vasodilation and sodium and water excretion together with suppression of aldosterone. Under physiologic conditions, these two systems complement each other and contribute to optimal sodium and water homeostasis. With excessive sodium intake ANP and BNP are increased, while the RAAS is suppressed. In contrast, in volume depletion the RAAS is activated, while ANP and BNP are not.

In the natural history of progressive HF, ANP and BNP are activated in early asymptomatic left ventricular dysfunction (ALVD) secondary to atrial stretch, which studies suggest is responsible for suppression of the RAAS.[8] As cardiac impairment worsens with the reduction in blood pressure, decrease in cardiac output, and increase in cardiac filling pressures, there is transition to overt HF as discussed below with simultaneous activation of the natriuretic peptides, the RAAS, and AVP. It is here that the kidney becomes less responsive to ANP and BNP, and secondary to neurohumoral systems such as the RAAS and AVP the balance tips to sodium and water retention.

The precise mechanisms that make the kidney retain sodium and water in progressive HF, thus fundamentally contributing to the evolution from asymptomatic to symptomatic ventricular dysfunction, are not fully understood. The kidney has a substantial capability for autoregulation, that is, keeping glomerular perfusion pressure constant even as systemic arterial pressure changes. However, in HF compensatory mechanisms are not enough and the decrease in renal perfusion pressure results in GFR reduction and renal water and sodium retention.

A hallmark of overt symptomatic HF as we discussed above is a global activation of various neurohumoral systems, which can be divided upon their impact on renal sodium and water handling. Major neurohumoral systems that promote sodium and water reabsorption include the RAAS, the sympathetic nervous system (SNS), AVP, and the endothelin system. As mentioned, ANP and BNP are important promoters of renal sodium and water excretion. Given the importance of electrolyte and volume homeostasis, it is no wonder that there is an extensive crosstalk between the heart and the kidney. When high pressure arterial baroreceptors in the aortic arch and carotid arteries detect arterial underfilling, such as after hemorrhage, sodium and water retaining systems, including AVP and the RAAS, are activated by the SNS to maintain or restore circulating volume and blood pressure.[9] In contrast, in conditions of cardiac overload, the cardiac peptides ANP and BNP are secreted and lead to enhanced sodium and water excretion. Under physiologic conditions, renin and the natriuretic peptides should not be activated simultaneously. However, as HF is characterized by low renal perfusion and high cardiac filling pressures, there is simultaneous activation of sodium retaining and natriuretic systems, resulting in conflicting input to the kidney. Thus, with progression of HF, the sodium and water retaining systems overpower the capacity of the NPS to compensate, and symptoms ensue. Indeed, even diuretic therapy used in severe CHF may via activation of the RAAS attenuate the renal response to the natriuretic peptides.

We now focus on one of the challenging renal complications of end-stage HF, the cardiorenal syndrome, which is often associated with ADHF.

The Cardiorenal Syndrome

There are differing definitions of the term *cardiorenal syndrome*. In a broad sense it can be defined as a syndrome in which either the heart or the kidney fails to compensate for the functional impairment of the respective other organ, resulting in a vicious cycle that ultimately leads to decompensation of the entire cardiorenal system. More specifically, the cardiorenal syndrome can be defined as worsening renal function in patients hospitalized for HF who may be resistant to diuretics. Importantly, studies have reported predictive characteristics for such patients who are at high risk for worsening renal function while in the hospital.[10,11] The prognostic characteristics include (1) a history of HF or diabetes mellitus, (2) admission creatinine ≥1.5 mg/dL, and (3) systolic blood pressure >160 mm Hg.[11] A recent nested case-control study analyzed 382 subjects who were hospitalized with HF, half of whom demonstrated worsening renal function, which was defined as a rise in serum creatinine of >0.3 mg/dL. In addition to the factors mentioned above, the use of calcium channel blockers (25% vs. 10%) and loop diuretic dose (199 ± 195 mg vs. 143 ± 119 mg) were higher in patients with worsening renal function.[12]

Most recently, the combination of increased N-terminal pro-BNP (NT-pro-BNP) and reduced calculated GFR emerged as the strongest predictor of 60-day mortality in ADHF.[13] In this study, 720 patients were dichotomized according to NT-pro-BNP concentration and baseline GFR. The study found that the combination of a GFR <60 mL/min/1.73 m^2 with an NT-pro-BNP >4647 pg/mL was the best predictor of 60-day mortality. Among subjects with an NT-pro-BNP above the median, those with a GFR <60 mL/min/1.73 m^2 or creatinine rise ≥0.3 mg/dL had the worst prognosis, whereas in subjects with a NT-pro-BNP below the median, prognosis was not influenced by either impaired renal function at presentation or the development of renal impairment during admission.

While hospitalization for ADHF continues to rise, a major question has been whether the incidence of the cardiorenal syndrome has been increasing as well. This was addressed in a recent study that compared the secular trends in renal dysfunction in 6440 unique patients hospitalized for HF between 1987 and 2002.[14] During this period, admission creatinine increased, as did age and the prevalence of diabetes and hypertension. In contrast, the incidence of worsening renal function was stable, and the mortality of HF decreased. As this study was performed at a single major academic medical center with extensive medical expertise in HF, it remains to be established if this experience can be extended to community hospitals.

To date, there are few studies on which to base treatment recommendations for the cardiorenal syndrome. Indeed, many HF trials exclude patients with reduced renal function.[15] In the subsequent sections we first discuss some conventional therapeutic strategies directly targeting the kidney, and then we review some innovative novel strategies that could target the cardiorenal syndrome in ADHF. Device-based treatments such as dialysis, ultrafiltration, and catheter-based intrarenal drug infusions are beyond the scope of this discussion.

Conventional Strategies

Loop Diuretics

Loop diuretics are the hallmark of therapy for HF. The major site of action is the ascending limb of the loop of Henle. The dose of a loop diuretic must be defined for each patient, which will be higher in the presence of renal insufficiency. Loop diuretics have a relatively short half-life (a few hours) leading to postdiuretic sodium retention, and their action can be offset by increased sodium reabsorption in more distal nephron segments. More frequent administrations or continuous intravenous infusions can limit the first, while addition of a thiazide diuretic can address the second concern. While loop diuretics can be very effective in patients with ADHF, it should be noted that chronic administration of furosemide in a porcine model of experimental HF significantly accelerated the development of contractile and metabolic features of HF.[16] Indeed, mortality was higher in the presence of chronic diuretic therapy as well in this experimental animal study. The authors implicated furosemide-induced activation of aldosterone with its adverse myocardial actions as the mechanism for accelerated ventricular dysfunction and increased mortality.

Further, we have documented in human HF the decrease in GFR to acute furosemide, which can be attenuated with an angiotensin receptor antagonist.[17] Further studies have demonstrated other deleterious actions of furosemide on the kidney. One could speculate that excessive loop diuretic therapy in patients with the cardiorenal syndrome may actually contribute to the decline in renal function. Finally, in a retrospective analysis of the Studies of Left Ventricular Dysfunction (SOLVD) trial, investigators found that the use of potassium-sparing diuretics in HF patients is associated with a reduced risk of death from, or hospitalization for, progressive HF or all-cause or cardiovascular death, compared with patients taking only non–potassium-sparing diuretics.[18] Taken together, while diuretics may provide acute symptomatic benefit, evidence from studies with long-term use raises concerns regarding adverse outcomes requiring further investigation.

B-Type Natriuretic Peptide (Nesiritide)

Nesiritide (Natrecor®) is a recombinant form of BNP and in 2001 was the first new drug in 14 years to be approved in the United States for the treatment of patients hospitalized with HF. It is a balanced vasodilator that has recently been reported to release nitric oxide in patients with pulmonary hypertension, and in human HF it has been observed at low doses to suppress the SNS.[19–21] In HF, there may occur a resistance to endogenous BNP levels, which can at least partially be overridden by the administration of exogenous BNP. In addition, posttranslational modification of BNP may occur in human HF in which the biologically active BNP 1–32 is not present, producing a state of actual BNP deficiency despite increased plasma BNP immunoreactivity with conventional assays.[22]

B-type natriuretic peptide is unique in that it has a variety of beneficial actions. It reduces cardiac preload by venodilation and natriuretic actions, it decreases cardiac afterload by vasodilation, it is lusitropic, and it suppresses the SNS as well as renin and aldosterone secretion.[23–25] In the Vasodilatation in the Management of Acute CHF (VMAC) trial, BNP was more effective than nitroglycerin in reducing pulmonary capillary wedge pressure.[19] B-type natriuretic peptide is a less powerful diuretic in HF than loop diuretics, but importantly it inhibits TGF and can enhance renal function, especially in combination with conventional diuretics.[26] A subgroup analysis of the VMAC trial suggested that nesiritide was safe and had similar beneficial actions in patients with and without renal insufficiency (defined as serum creatinine ≥2.0 mg/dL).[27] In a separate trial, patients who received BNP required less diuretics than patients treated with standard therapy.[28] Similarly, BNP in experimental HF potentiated the diuretic effect of furosemide while at the same time preventing a furosemide-induced increase in plasma aldosterone.[26]

Nonetheless, controversy exists over the use of BNP in human HF. In a small crossover study of 15 patients who appeared resistant to diuretic therapy, nesiritide did not improve renal function (urinary sodium excretion, urine flow, GFR, effective renal plasma flow) as compared to placebo.[29] A possible explanation is that the dose of the nesiritide infusion (0.01 μg/kg/min) was too low to overcome the renal resistance to nesiritide. Furthermore, the lack of a renal response contrasts with the beneficial hemodynamic effects of patients with renal dysfunction, as mentioned above. Nonetheless, ANP resistance is well known and in experimental HF thought to be mediated by both receptor and postreceptor dysfunction.[30] As the natriuretic peptide degrading enzyme neutral endopeptidase 24.11 (NEP) is especially abundant in the proximal tubule in the kidney, additional NEP inhibition might enhance the renal actions of exogenous BNP and will be addressed below. It also should be stated that a meta-analysis of nesiritide studies reported that nesiritide may increase mortality in HF.[31] This important issue will be addressed in an international multicenter trial involving 7000 patients with ADHF. Results should be available in 2008 or 2009.

Relevant, however, to an important renal resistance to BNP and therapeutic strategies is the report that renal phosphodiesterases (PDEs) may be increased at the level of the glomerulus in experimental HF.[32] It is well established that generation of cyclic guanosine monophosphate (cGMP) mediates the biologic effects of natriuretic peptides such as ANP, BNP, CNP, and DNP. PDE5, which hydrolyzes and thus inactivates cGMP, is abundant in the kidney and vasculature and was found recently in the heart. Sildenafil is a PDE5 inhibitor that is used clinically for erectile dysfunction. We recently hypothesized that chronic inhibition of PDE5 would enhance the renal actions of exogenous BNP by potentiating renal cGMP.[33] Cardiorenal and humoral function was determined at baseline in two groups of dogs with experimental HF in which one group received chronic sildenafil. The response to acute subcutaneous BNP administration was compared in both groups. We found PDE5 inhibition enhanced GFR and sodium excretion consistent with the concept of excessive PDE5 activation in overt HF in the kidney. Further human studies are needed to investigate the benefit of maximizing the renal cGMP system by combined PDE5 inhibition and natriuretic peptide administration in human HF including the cardiorenal syndrome.

It also should be noted that ANP (carperitide) was approved for the treatment of ADHF in Japan in 1995.[34,35] Importantly, Sward et al.[36] reported that ANP enhanced renal excretory function, decreased the probability of dialysis, and improved dialysis-free survival in early, ischemic acute renal dysfunction after complicated cardiac surgery. It remains to be established which natriuretic peptide has the best pharmacodynamic and pharmacokinetic profile for HF. Possibly, other naturally occurring natriuretic peptides or designer peptides such as the recently identified peptide DNP may turn out to be superior.[37] Furthermore, different patients may benefit from different peptides. Indeed, the recent report of a polymorphism for the ANP gene rendering a relative deficiency of ANP in humans may prompt the co-measurement of both ANP and BNP in human HF, resulting in targeted therapy.[38] Furthermore, chronic administration of BNP, for example in the form of chronic subcutaneous injection, intermittent intravenous infusion on an outpatient basis, and now even oral BNP are potential new strategies that clearly warrant further clinical research efforts.[39–41]

Emerging Therapeutic Strategies

Vasopressin Antagonists

Arginine vasopressin is a nonapeptide and its release is stimulated by hyperosmolality, hypotension, and hypovolemia. It is vasoconstrictive via V1a receptors and promotes free water reabsorption in the renal collecting duct via V2 receptors, the activation of which induces the translocation of the water channel aquaporin-2 into the apical membrane. Nonosmotic release of AVP in HF can lead to water retention and dilutional hyponatremia, which is associated with prolonged hospitalization and increased mortality in HF patients. Both selective V2 antagonists as well as dual V1a/V2 antagonists are in clinical development.[42,43] While most of the conventional diuretics are "saluretics," V2 receptor blockers act essentially as "aquaretics"; that is, they promote free water excretion without (or with less) electrolyte loss. This could be especially useful in patients with hyponatremia, a condition that limits the efficacy of conventional diuretics. In a seminal clinical trial (Acute and Chronic Therapeutic Impact of a Vasopressin antagonist [ACTIV] in Chronic Heart Failure [CHF]), the V2 receptor antagonist tolvaptan resulted in a larger weight reduction at discharge in patients admitted to the hospital with ADHF.[44] During a 60-day follow-up period, tolvaptan treatment tended to improve mortality, which was significant in the subgroup with hyponatremia, renal dysfunction, or peripheral edema.

The cardiorenal actions of tolvaptan were compared with furosemide (80 mg) in a single-dose, crossover study in 14 patients with NYHA class II to III HF.[45] Fluid losses were replaced at intervals with distilled water. Neither treatment changed mean arterial pressure or GFR compared to placebo. Tolvaptan induced a diuresis similar to furosemide, but without natriuresis and kaliuresis, thus acting as an aquaretic. Furosemide reduced renal blood flow compared to placebo and tolvaptan, which could be explained by TGF. Similarly, furosemide increased plasma renin activity compared to placebo and tended to increase it compared to tolvaptan. Of note, the patients HF medications were discontinued for the duration of the study.

Currently, a large randomized placebo-controlled clinical trial evaluating tolvaptan added to standard therapy is being conducted, the Efficacy of Vasopressin Antagonism in Heart Failure: Outcome Study with Tolvaptan (EVEREST) trial.[46] Results, including effects on mortality, were expected in early 2007 (but too late for inclusion in this chapter). Another orally available, selective V2-antagonist in clinical development is lixivaptan, which in NYHA class II to III patients dose-dependently increased urine flow, solute-free water excretion, serum osmolality, and serum sodium without neurohumoral activation or increasing sodium, potassium, chloride, magnesium, or urea nitrogen excretion.[47]

Given that the relevance of V1a activation by displaced AVP with selective V2 receptor antagonism is currently unknown, it remains to be established whether combined V1a/V2 receptor antagonism is more beneficial in HF.

Neutral Endopeptidase Inhibitors

Neutral endopeptidase is involved in the degradation of the natriuretic peptides. It has been thought that this enzyme limits the renal actions of the natriuretic peptides and there is evidence that NEP is upregulated in human HF. Therefore, therapeutic targeting of NEP with specific and selective inhibitors could enhance renal function by potentiating endogenous ANP and BNP. Chronic oral NEP inhibition was studied in a canine model that progresses from early to moderate and finally severe HF over a 38-day period.[48] In this model ANP increased progressively and significantly as HF evolved (Fig. 68.2). Urinary sodium excretion decreased in the moderate phase of chronic HF with an even more profound decline in the severe HF period, accompanied by an increase in plasma aldosterone in this late phase. In contrast, chronic oral NEP inhibition delayed the onset of reduction of sodium excretion during the transition from early to severe HF, while enhancing ANP and suppressing aldosterone activation. Therefore, this study with its demonstration of a selective renal and adrenal action of chronic NEP inhibition in HF underscores a therapeutic potential for this pharmacological strategy.

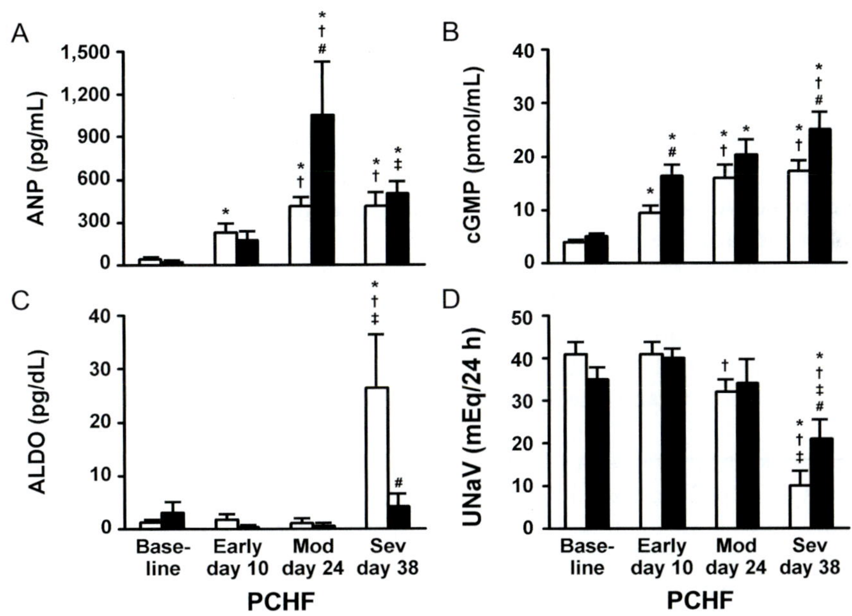

FIGURE 68.2. Neurohumoral and sodium excretion data in control (open bars) and neutral endopeptidase inhibition with a neutral endopeptidase (NEP) inhibitor (closed bars). (A) Plasma atrial natriuretic peptide (ANP). (B) Plasma cyclic guanosine monophosphate (cGMP). (C) Aldosterone (ALDO). (D) Urinary sodium excretion (UNaV). PCHF, progressive chronic heart failure. (From Martin et al.,[48] with permission.)

Adenosine Antagonists

As discussed above, adenosine plays a key role in renal regulation, including mediating TGF. Recently, studies reported that the selective A1 adenosine antagonist BG9719 increased GFR, urine flow, and urinary sodium excretion in a pig model of pacing induced HF.[49] In addition, BG9719 increased diuresis when added to furosemide and prevented furosemide-induced declines in GFR in patients with HF.[50]

Adenosine antagonism with KW-3902 was recently evaluated in 34 patients with ADHF refractory to diuretics.[51] All doses of KW-3902, administered as 2-hour infusions, increased hourly urine volume compared to placebo, with the greatest increase taking place between hours 1 and 3 in the 30-mg group. The antagonist also increased creatinine clearance compared to baseline in the 3- to 9-hour period after start of drug infusion. The study investigators concluded that these initial results suggest that the adenosine receptor antagonist KW-3902 may prove beneficial in facilitating diuresis in ADHF patients refractory to conventional pharmacologic therapy while simultaneously potentiating renal function. Clearly, these data need to be confirmed in larger studies.

Ryanodine Receptor Antagonists

Recent investigations have revealed antiarrhythmic and cardioprotective properties of a newly developed 1,4-benzothiazepine derivative, K201 (JTV519), via stabilization of the ryanodine receptor-calcium release channel in the heart.[52] Importantly, studies have also reported that chronic administration of this molecule in experimental HF improves cardiac function and attenuates HF progression.

Currently, three known ryanodine receptor (RyR) isoforms (RyR1, RyR2, and RyR3), encoded by separate genes, have been identified. RyR1 is the predominant isoform in skeletal muscle and RyR2 in heart. RyR3 is expressed at low levels in various tissues, including myocardium, but its presence is not essential. With regard to the kidney, studies have demonstrated that the RyR-2 isoform is present in the rabbit kidney cortex and that calcium influx through voltage-dependent calcium channels triggers periodic calcium release through the RyRs in the afferent preglomerular arterioles, which leads to afferent arteriolar rhythmic contraction.[53–55] As these latter studies suggest that the RyRs in the kidney may play an important role in the control of renal hemodynamics, we defined for the first time the renal actions of this novel new drug class (i.e., of K201). K201 was potently natriuretic and diuretic, and enhanced GFR and renal blood flow.[56] The excretory responses to K201 administration were associated with decreases in distal tubular reabsorption of sodium despite a mild decrease in mean arterial pressure, which returned to baseline levels after K201 discontinuation. Therefore, K201 possesses natriuretic, diuretic, GFR-enhancing, and vasodilating properties that go beyond myocardial actions and may support its therapeutic role in treatment of HF.

Direct Soluble Guanylate Cyclase Stimulators

Renal vasoconstriction characterizes severe overt HF and contributes to the cardiorenal syndrome. This vasoconstriction may in part be a consequence of reduced nitric oxide (NO). Soluble guanylate cyclase (sGC) is a heterodimeric heme protein and the main target of NO. Via the generation of the second messenger cGMP, sGC has vasorelaxing, antiaggregatory, antiinflammatory, growth-inhibiting, and antifibrotic properties. Importantly, NO-sGC-cGMP signaling is frequently impaired in cardiovascular disease states ("endothelial dysfunction"), which can be due to oxidative and nitrosative stress. This pathway can be augmented by the administration of exogenous nitrovasodilators, such as nitroglycerin or sodium nitroprusside; however, these can be associated with tachyphylaxis, nitrosative stress, and cyanide toxicity. Importantly, a novel class of direct, that is, NO-independent, sGC stimulators has been identified that is not associated with the development of tolerance or the cGMP-independent actions of cGMP. BAY 41-2272 is a NO-independent but heme-dependent sGC stimulator and in experimental tachypacing-induced HF has been shown to reduce systemic and renal vascular resistance and increase cardiac output and renal blood flow, while maintaining GFR (Fig. 68.3).[57] BAY 58-2667, a NO- and hemeindependent sGC

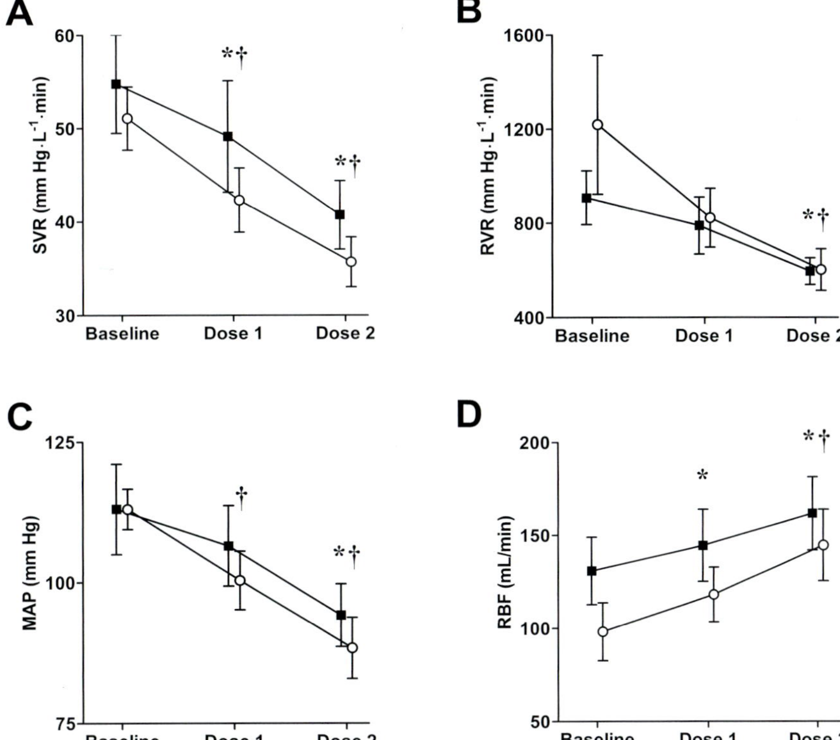

FIGURE 68.3. Effect of BAY 41–2272 (filled-in boxes) as compared to nitroglycerin (open circles) on (A) systemic vascular resistance, (B) renal vascular resistance, (C) mean arterial pressure, and (D) renal blood flow in experimental canine congestive heart failure. Dose 1: BAY 41–2272: 2 μg/kg/min; nitroglycerin: 1 μg/kg/min. Dose 2: BAY 41–2272: 10 μg/kg/min; nitroglycerin: 5 μg/kg/min. *,†$p < .05$ compared to baseline for the BAY 41–2272 and nitroglycerin group, respectively. (Adapted from Boerrigter et al.,[57] with permission.)

activator, which preferentially activates NO-insensitive oxidized or heme-free sGC, had similar actions and also decreased cardiac preload by reducing right atrial pressure.[58–60] Both compounds attenuated renal remodeling and improved renal function in animal models of chronic renal disease.[61–63] Clinical studies in patients with BAY 58-2667 in ADHF are currently being conducted, and it will be seen whether the beneficial hemodynamic and renoprotective actions of direct sGC stimulation in preclinical studies will translate into beneficial actions in human HF.

Conclusion

The kidney plays a key role in HF and may indeed dictate the progression of this syndrome via the regulation of intravascular volume and arterial pressure as well as via neurohumoral systems affecting myocardial function and structure. The cardiorenal syndrome has become an important focus of research in HF and remains a very high priority and challenge for the practicing clinician. The mechanism of the cardiorenal syndrome is clearly multifactorial but appears to involve three important mechanisms—hemodynamic, neurohumoral, and metabolic—which respectively involve renal perfusion pressure, multiple hormones, and adenosine. Several potential new therapeutic strategies for this serious disorder have emerged, which have to be evaluated in prospective clinical trials as well as in both basic and clinical research. If successful, we can expect important changes in the management of HF in the future, which, recognizing the importance of the heart–kidney connection, are focused on renoprotection in order to improve the heart. As presumably the best way to deal with the cardiorenal syndrome is to prevent it, additional studies should specifically investigate the impact of chronic therapeutic strategies on renal function in order to preserve and enhance renal function, thus, it is hoped, also delaying the progression of HF.

References

1. Hillege HL, Girbes AR, de Kam PJ, et al. Renal function, neurohormonal activation, and survival in patients with chronic heart failure. Circulation 2000;102:203–10.
2. Dries DL, Exner DV, Domanski MJ, et al. The prognostic implications of renal insufficiency in asymptomatic and symptomatic patients with left ventricular systolic dysfunction. J Am Coll Cardiol 2000;35:681–9.
3. Burnett JC, Knox FG. Renal interstitial pressure and sodium excretion during renal vein constriction. Am J Physiol 1980;238:F279–82.
4. Firth JD, Raine AE, Ledingham JG. Raised venous pressure: a direct cause of renal sodium retention in oedema? Lancet 1988;1:1033–5.
5. Thomson S, Bao D, Deng A, et al. Adenosine formed by 5′-nucleotidase mediates tubuloglomerular feedback. J Clin Invest 2000;106:289–98.
6. Funaya H, Kitakaze M, Node K, et al. Plasma adenosine levels increase in patients with chronic heart failure. Circulation 1997;95:1363–5.
7. Margulies KB, Burnett JC, Jr. Atrial natriuretic factor modulates whole kidney tubuloglomerular feedback. Am J Physiol 1990;259:R97–101.
8. Stevens TL, Burnett JCJ, Kinoshita M, et al. A functional role for endogenous atrial natriuretic peptide in a canine model of early left ventricular dysfunction. J Clin Invest 1995;95:1101–8.
9. Schrier RW, Abraham WT. Hormones and hemodynamics in heart failure. N Engl J Med 1999;341: 577–85.
10. Krumholz HM, Chen YT, Vaccarino V, et al. Correlates and impact on outcomes of worsening renal function in patients > or = 65 years of age with heart failure. Am J Cardiol 2000;85:1110–3.
11. Forman DE, Butler J, Wang Y, et al. Incidence, predictors at admission, and impact of worsening renal function among patients hospitalized with heart failure. J Am Coll Cardiol 2004;43:61–7.
12. Butler J, Forman DE, Abraham WT, et al. Relationship between heart failure treatment and development of worsening renal function among hospitalized patients. Am Heart J 2004;147:331–8.
13. van Kimmenade R, Januzzi J, Baggish A, et al. Amino-terminal pro-brain natriuretic peptide, renal function, and outcomes in acute heart failure. J Am Coll Cardiol 2006;48:1621–7.
14. Owan TE, Hodge DO, Herges RM, et al. Secular trends in renal dysfunction and outcomes in hospitalized heart failure patients. J Card Fail 2006; 12:257–62.
15. Coca SG, Krumholz HM, Garg AX, et al. Underrepresentation of renal disease in randomized controlled trials of cardiovascular disease. JAMA 2006;296:1377–84.
16. McCurley JM, Hanlon SU, Wei SK, et al. Furosemide and the progression of left ventricular dysfunction in experimental heart failure. J Am Coll Cardiol 2004;44:1301–7.
17. Chen HH, Redfield MM, Nordstrom LJ, et al. Angiotensin II AT1 receptor antagonism prevents detrimental renal actions of acute diuretic therapy in human heart failure. Am J Physiol Renal Physiol 2003;284:F1115–19.
18. Domanski M, Norman J, Pitt B, et al. Diuretic use, progressive heart failure, and death in patients in the Studies Of Left Ventricular Dysfunction (SOLVD). J Am Coll Cardiol 2003;42:705–8.
19. Publication Committee for the VMAC Investigators (Vasodilatation in the Management of Acute CHF). Intravenous nesiritide vs nitroglycerin for treatment of decompensated congestive heart failure: a randomized controlled trial. JAMA 2002;287:1531–40.
20. Brunner-La Rocca HP, Kaye DM, Woods RL, et al. Effects of intravenous brain natriuretic peptide on regional sympathetic activity in patients with chronic heart failure as compared with healthy control subjects. J Am Coll Cardiol 2001;37:1221–7.
21. Khush KK, De Marco T, Vakharia KT, et al. Nesiritide acutely increases pulmonary and systemic levels of nitric oxide in patients with pulmonary hypertension. J Card Fail 2006;12:507–13.
22. Hawkridge AM, Heublein DM, Bergen HR, III, et al. Quantitative mass spectral evidence for the absence of circulating brain natriuretic peptide (BNP-32) in severe human heart failure. Proc Natl Acad Sci U S A 2005;102:17442–7.
23. Yamamoto K, Burnett JCJ, Redfield MM. Effect of endogenous natriuretic peptide system on ventricular and coronary function in failing heart. Am J Physiol 1997;273:H2406–14.
24. Elkayam U, Akhter MW, Singh H, et al. Comparison of effects on left ventricular filling pressure of intravenous nesiritide and high-dose nitroglycerin

in patients with decompensated heart failure. Am J Cardiol 2004;93:237–40.
25. Akabane S, Matsushima Y, Matsuo H, et al. Effects of brain natriuretic peptide on renin secretion in normal and hypertonic saline-infused kidney. Eur J Pharmacol 1991;198:143–8.
26. Cataliotti A, Boerrigter G, Costello-Boerrigter LC, et al. Brain natriuretic peptide enhances renal actions of furosemide and suppresses furosemide-induced aldosterone activation in experimental heart failure. Circulation 2004;109:1680–5.
27. Butler J, Emerman C, Peacock WF, et al. The efficacy and safety of B-type natriuretic peptide (nesiritide) in patients with renal insufficiency and acutely decompensated congestive heart failure. Nephrol Dial Transplant 2004;19:391–9.
28. Colucci WS, Elkayam U, Horton DP, et al. Intravenous nesiritide, a natriuretic peptide, in the treatment of decompensated congestive heart failure. Nesiritide Study Group. [Erratum appears in N Engl J Med 2000;343(20):1504; and N Engl J Med 2000;343(12):896]. N Engl J Med 2000;343:246–53.
29. Wang DJ, Dowling TC, Meadows D, et al. Nesiritide does not improve renal function in patients with chronic heart failure and worsening serum creatinine. Circulation 2004;110:1620–5.
30. Margulies KB, Heublein DM, Perrella MA, et al. ANF-mediated renal cGMP generation in congestive heart failure. Am J Physiol 1991;260:F562–8.
31. Sackner-Bernstein JD, Kowalski M, Fox M, et al. Short-term risk of death after treatment with nesiritide for decompensated heart failure: a pooled analysis of randomized controlled trials. JAMA 2005;293:1900–5.
32. Supaporn T, Sandberg SM, Borgeson DD, et al. Blunted cGMP response to agonists and enhanced glomerular cyclic 3′,5′-nucleotide phosphodiesterase activities in experimental congestive heart failure. Kidney Int 1996;50:1718–25.
33. Chen HH, Huntley BK, Schirger JA, et al. Maximizing the renal cyclic 3′-5′-guanosine monophosphate system with type v phosphodiesterase inhibition and exogenous natriuretic peptide: a novel strategy to improve renal function in experimental overt heart failure. J Am Soc Nephrol 2006;17:2742–7.
34. Mizuno O, Onishi K, Dohi K, et al. Effects of therapeutic doses of human atrial natriuretic peptide on load and myocardial performance in patients with congestive heart failure. Am J Cardiol 2001;88:863–6.
35. Kikuchi M, Nakamura M, Suzuki T, et al. Usefulness of carperitide for the treatment of refractory heart failure due to severe acute myocardial infarction. Jpn Heart J 2001;42:271–80.
36. Sward K, Valsson F, Odencrants P, et al. Recombinant human atrial natriuretic peptide in ischemic acute renal failure: a randomized placebo-controlled trial. Crit Care Med 2004;32:1310–5.
37. Lisy O, Lainchbury JG, Leskinen H, et al. Therapeutic actions of a new synthetic vasoactive and natriuretic peptide, dendroaspis natriuretic peptide, in experimental severe congestive heart failure. Hypertension 2001;37:1089–94.
38. Rubattu S, Bigatti G, Evangelista A, et al. Association of atrial natriuretic peptide and type a natriuretic peptide receptor gene polymorphisms with left ventricular mass in human essential hypertension. J Am Coll Cardiol 2006;48:499–505.
39. Chen HH, Redfield MM, Nordstrom LJ, et al. Subcutaneous administration of the cardiac hormone BNP in symptomatic human heart failure. J Card Fail 2004;10:115–19.
40. Yancy CW, Saltzberg MT, Berkowitz RL, et al. Safety and feasibility of using serial infusions of nesiritide for heart failure in an outpatient setting (from the FUSION I trial). Am J Cardiol 2004;94:595–601.
41. Cataliotti A, Schirger JA, Martin FL, et al. Oral human brain natriuretic peptide activates cyclic guanosine 3′,5′-monophosphate and decreases mean arterial pressure. Circulation 2005;112:836–40.
42. Gheorghiade M, Niazi I, Ouyang J, et al. Vasopressin V2–receptor blockade with tolvaptan in patients with chronic heart failure: results from a double-blind, randomized trial. Circulation 2003;107:2690–6.
43. Udelson JE, Smith WB, Hendrix GH, et al. Acute hemodynamic effects of conivaptan, a dual V(1A) and V(2) vasopressin receptor antagonist, in patients with advanced heart failure. Circulation 2001;104:2417–23.
44. Gheorghiade M, Gattis WA, O'Connor CM, et al. Effects of tolvaptan, a vasopressin antagonist, in patients hospitalized with worsening heart failure: a randomized controlled trial. JAMA 2004;291:1963–71.
45. Costello-Boerrigter LC, Smith WB, Boerrigter G, et al. Vasopressin-2–receptor antagonism augments water excretion without changes in renal hemodynamics or sodium and potassium excretion in human heart failure. Am J Physiol Renal Physiol 2006;290:F273–8.
46. Gheorghiade M, Orlandi C, Burnett JC, et al. Rationale and design of the multicenter, randomized, double-blind, placebo-controlled study to evaluate

the Efficacy of Vasopressin antagonism in Heart Failure: Outcome Study with Tolvaptan (EVEREST). J Card Fail 2005;11:260–9.
47. Abraham WT, Shamshirsaz AA, McFann K, et al. Aquaretic effect of lixivaptan, an oral, non-peptide, selective V2 receptor vasopressin antagonist, in New York Heart Association functional class II and III chronic heart failure patients. J Am Coll Cardiol 2006;47:1615–21.
48. Martin FL, Stevens TL, Cataliotti A, et al. Natriuretic and antialdosterone actions of chronic oral NEP inhibition during progressive congestive heart failure. Kidney Int 2005;67:1723–30.
49. Lucas DG, Jr., Hendrick JW, Sample JA, et al. Cardiorenal effects of adenosine subtype 1 (A1) receptor inhibition in an experimental model of heart failure. J Am Coll Surg 2002;194:603–9.
50. Gottlieb SS, Brater DC, Thomas I, et al. BG9719 (CVT-124), an A1 adenosine receptor antagonist, protects against the decline in renal function observed with diuretic therapy. Circulation 2002; 105:1348–53.
51. Givertz MM, Tansey M, Pearson L, et al. Effect of the adenosine A1 receptor antagonist, KW-3902, on diuresis and renal function in patients with acute decompensated heart failure refractory to maximum doses of conventional diuretics: a randomized, double-blind, placebo controlled, dose escalation study. J Card Fail 2006;12:S82:266.
52. Wehrens XH, Lehnart SE, Reiken SR, et al. Protection from cardiac arrhythmia through ryanodine receptor-stabilizing protein calstabin2. Science 2004;304:292–6.
53. Tunwell RE, Lai FA. Ryanodine receptor expression in the kidney and a non-excitable kidney epithelial cell. J Biol Chem 1996;271:29583–8.
54. Fellner SK, Arendshorst WJ. Ryanodine receptor and capacitative Ca2+ entry in fresh preglomerular vascular smooth muscle cells. Kidney Int 2000; 58:1686–94.
55. Takenaka T, Ohno Y, Hayashi K, et al. Governance of arteriolar oscillation by ryanodine receptors. Am J Physiol Regul Integr Comp Physiol 2003;285: R125–31.
56. Lisy O, Burnett JC, Jr. New cardioprotective agent K201 is natriuretic and glomerular filtration rate enhancing. Circulation 2006;113:246–51.
57. Boerrigter G, Costello-Boerrigter LC, Cataliotti A, et al. Cardiorenal and humoral properties of a novel direct soluble guanylate cyclase stimulator BAY 41–2272 in experimental congestive heart failure. Circulation 2003;107:686–9.
58. Stasch JP, Schmidt P, Alonso-Alija C, et al. NO- and haem-independent activation of soluble guanylyl cyclase: molecular basis and cardiovascular implications of a new pharmacological principle. Br J Pharmacol 2002;136:773–83.
59. Stasch JP, Schmidt PM, Nedvetsky PI, et al. Targeting the heme-oxidized nitric oxide receptor for selective vasodilatation of diseased blood vessels. J Clin Invest 2006;116:2552–61.
60. Boerrigter G, Costello-Boerrigter L, Cataliotti A, et al. Cardiorenal and humoral actions of the new heme-independent direct soluble guanylate cyclase activator BAY 58–2667 in experimental congestive heart failure. Circulation 2003;108: IV–398.
61. Wang Y, Kramer S, Loof T, et al. Stimulation of soluble guanylate cyclase slows progression in anti-thy1-induced chronic glomerulosclerosis. Kidney Int 2005;68:47–61.
62. Wang Y, Kramer S, Loof T, et al. Enhancing cGMP in experimental progressive renal fibrosis: soluble guanylate cyclase stimulation vs. phosphodiesterase inhibition. Am J Physiol Renal Physiol 2006;290: F167–76.
63. Kalk P, Godes M, Relle K, et al. NO-independent activation of soluble guanylate cyclase prevents disease progression in rats with 5/6 nephrectomy. Br J Pharmacol 2006;148:853–9.

69
Acute Hypoxic Hepatitis and Hepatic Consequences of Acute Heart Failure Syndrome

Alain Cohen Solal and François Durand

Acute hypoxic hepatitis, also termed shock liver, acute ischemic hepatitis, or liver hypoxia, is generally defined on the basis of histologic findings including liver cell necrosis and congestion predominating in centrilobular areas (1), both resulting from circulatory changes or profound hypoxemia. Most often, it results from severe circulatory failure. However, severe liver necrosis may occasionally follow mild circulatory and transient circulatory changes. Controversy remains about the respective roles of decreased hepatic blood flow ("forward failure"), venous congestion ("backward failure"), and hypoxemia in its pathophysiology. Whether or not two or more of these mechanisms have to coexist for acute hypoxic hepatitis to occur also represents an unresolved issue (2–4). The prognosis of hypoxic hepatitis is variable, depending on the severity of the underlying circulatory or respiratory disorder rather than the extent of liver cell damage.

Liver Lesions

The effects of cardiac dysfunction on the liver seem to greatly depend on how acutely the hemodynamic changes occur and whether or not they are predominantly affecting the right or left side of the circulation (5). In most instances, there is a combination of events affecting the entire circulation occurring over a variable period of time. Additionally, the impact of cardiac dysfunction may be significantly influenced by underlying chronic liver lesions. On a theoretical basis, three distinct mechanisms may lead to hypoxic liver cell necrosis: (1) decreased blood supply (both portal and arterial), (2) congestion (due to impaired suprahepatic venous outflow), and (3) profound ischemia. It is thought, but not clearly demonstrated, that extensive liver cell necrosis occurs only when two or three of these mechanisms coexist. A number of heart diseases can lead to either decreased liver blood flow via decreased cardiac output or congestion via right heart insufficiency. Hypoxemia resulting from pulmonary edema may also be a contributing factor. However, it is worth noting that patients with severe pulmonary hypertension and markedly dilated right heart chambers may not have evidence of liver cell damage unless an acute precipitating factor (such as arrhythmia) coexists. Similarly, the majority of patients with advanced left ventricular failure have normal liver function tests.

Pathophysiology

Significant left heart failure leading to decreased cardiac output and decreased arterial pressure is characterized by liver cell necrosis, predominating in centrilobular areas. Liver lesions predominate in centrilobular areas because hepatocytes located in this zone of the lobule are the most distant from portal tracts and, as a consequence, the most distant from arterial and portal blood supply. In parallel, hepatocytes surrounding centrilobular veins are more exposed to congestion than periportal hepatocytes.

Besides left heart failure, liver parenchyma can be significantly damaged due to shock resulting from a variety of causes. Liver lesions similar to those observed during left heart failure can result from massive bleeding, profound hypovolemia, septic shock, and major burns. These lesions are uncommon if shock is transitory (less than 10 hours). Conversely, they are almost constant if the duration of shock exceeds 24 hours. However, severe liver cell necrosis may occasionally result from transient and self-resolving cardiac arrhythmias (6).

Because the liver receives a dual blood supply, from the hepatic artery and the portal vein, liver infarction is especially rare, including in patients with massive shock. Liver infarction occurs only when both hepatic and venous supply are compromised. Patients who acutely develop complete portal vein thrombosis (a condition that is generally associated with hypercoagulable states) only present with transient and spontaneously resolving liver ischemia, provided the hepatic artery remains patent.

Etiology

Hepatocyte necrosis is coagulative rather than cytolytic in aspect. Lobular or periportal inflammatory infiltrates, a common finding during acute and chronic hepatitis due to viral infections or drug toxicity, are typically absent. However, some patients have mild inflammatory infiltrates consisting of polymorphonuclear cells and/or lymphocytes. Again, liver cell necrosis predominates in centrilobular areas. Necrosis may appear to be asymmetric within zone 3 (the parenchymal area surrounding centrilobular veins), depending on the variability of blood flow through the acini. Generally, the extent of centrilobular necrosis correlates with the severity of hypotension, whatever sustained or transient. However, overt clinical shock is not an absolute prerequisite for extensive liver cell necrosis to occur. Interestingly, most patients with significant hepatocyte necrosis have evidence of coexisting right-sided failure, including prominent congestive changes. As necrosis progresses, hepatocytes may be replaced by accumulated red blood cells within centrilobular zone of the acini. Preserved hepatocytes in the vicinity of necrosis may contain periodic acid-Schiff (PAS)-positive spherical inclusions. Toxic drug-induced liver lesion, those resulting from paracetamol overdose in particular, are also characterized by centrilobular liver cell necrosis without significant inflammatory infiltrates. In the absence of congestion, these lesions can be indistinguishable from those resulting from liver hypoxia.

Superimposed congestion is characterized by the accumulation of red cells within sinusoids. Congestion also predominates in centrilobular areas. Sinusoids are enlarged and adjacent hepatocytes become atrophic.

With prolonged congestion, liver cell necrosis and congestion are associated with fibrotic transformation of central veins. Central veins appear enlarged with thickened walls. In the most severe cases, bridging fibrosis may extend between central veins. On macroscopic examination of cut sections, there is a classic nutmeg appearance with deep brown centrilobular zones alternating with yellowish periportal zones.

Cardiac cirrhosis, with a nodular transformation of liver parenchyma and extensive fibrosis has become highly uncommon. It is only observed in patients with especially long-standing congestion.

Manifestations

The diagnosis of shock liver or hypoxic hepatitis is often considered to be easy (the topic is generally not addressed in cardiology texts). This is generally true when hypoxic hepatitis is a complication of overt heart failure or shock. Hypoxic hepatitis, however, may be much more difficult to recognize when hepatic changes predominate over circulatory changes (7). Hypoxic hepatitis represents a pitfall in patients without clear evidence of acute heart failure and no past history of heart disease, a situation that is not uncommon. In such a situation, hypoxic hepatitis may closely resemble acute liver failure due to primary liver disease, viral hepatitis, and toxic or drug-induced liver injury in particular.

Most investigators agree that a diagnosis of hypoxic hepatitis can be considered when five conditions are met: (1) a typical clinical setting of severe cardiac or circulatory failure, (2) a massive but rapidly reversible rise in serum aminotransferase level, (3) normal or moderately elevated serum bilirubin, (4) concomitant impairment of renal function with prerenal characteristics, and (5) the exclusion of other causes of acute liver injury. When these five conditions are met, liver biopsy is not mandatory for the diagnosis. Patients without overt cardiac insufficiency or shock and predominating hepatic manifestations are frequently referred to hepatologists or intensivists. Even in the absence of any obvious manifestation suggesting an underlying circulatory disorder, hypoxic hepatitis should always be suspected in case of (1) an abrupt rise in serum aminotransferase over 100 times the upper limit of normal, (2) aspartate aminotransferase (AST) level markedly exceeding alanine aminotransferase (ALT) level, (3) normal or near-normal serum bilirubin, (4) concomitant deterioration of renal function, and (5) no other cause of acute liver injury. Right upper quadrant pain is uncommon. It only occurs in cases of severe congestion with an abrupt distention of the liver capsule, due to hepatic outflow obstruction. Serum alkaline phosphatases and γ-glutamyl transpeptidases are normal or moderately elevated. Low platelet count can also be observed. None of the abnormalities in liver function tests is specific of hypoxic hepatitis.

Acute cardiomyopathy and acute decompensation of previously unrecognized chronic heart disease represent the main causes of "occult" hypoxic hepatitis. In this context, attention should focus on the recent onset of breathlessness on effort, cardiac enlargement on chest radiograph, dilated jugular veins, tachycardia, low arterial pressure, cardiac murmur, and lower extremities edema. Abnormalities in cardiac plasma biomarkers—B-type natriuretic peptide (BNP), troponin—may orient to the cardiac origin of the clinical picture, with raised levels suggesting increased cardiac wall stress and myocytic necrosis respectively. Emergency echocardiography is the clue for an appropriate diagnosis. Transjugular liver biopsy makes it possible to obtain histologic evidence of hypoxic (or congestive) hepatitis and, at the same time, to perform invasive hemodynamic measurements, providing further evidence for circulatory disorders. Dilated hepatic veins or inferior vena cava on abdominal ultrasonography is an inconstant finding, although suggestive. A rapid response to specific therapy (inotropes and diuretics in most cases) also represents a strong argument for this diagnosis.

Other causes of acute liver injury, including acute viral hepatitis A, B, or E, drug-induced hepatitis, paracetamol intoxication, autoimmune disease, and obstruction of the hepatic veins (Budd-Chiari syndrome) have to be ruled out.

A decrease in coagulation factors (prothrombin index and factor V) as well as increased international normalized ratio (INR) may occur in patients with massive liver cell necrosis, as a reflection of the profound alteration of liver function. Intravascular coagulation can participate in the decrease in coagulation factors. The occurrence of hepatic encephalopathy, defining the acute liver failure syndrome is highly uncommon in patients with hypoxic hepatitis. Indeed, patients either improve rapidly due to the correction of the causative circulatory change or die due to refractory circulatory failure.

General Course and Prognosis

As indicated above, the course of hypoxic hepatitis is marked by an abrupt rise in serum transaminases, AST level being initially superior to ALT level (Fig. 69.1). Serum transaminases peak 24 to 48 hours after the causative circulatory event. If circulatory changes are efficiently treated (and if the patient does not have an underlying chronic liver disease), improvement is rapid with a drop in serum transaminases. The decrease in serum AST is more rapid than that of ALT. Therefore, an ALT level that is higher than the AST level is a frequent finding 48 hours or more after admission (7). In contrast to most patients with paracetamol overdose, serum creatinine is increased as early as at admission. In patients with evidence of liver insufficiency and decreased coagulation factors at admission, recovery is marked by a rapid rise in prothrombin index and factor V. Usually, coagulation returns to normal within 1 week after the initial event.

In patients with an unfavorable outcome, death is due to refractory circulatory failure rather than the proper complications of liver failure. Patients with hypoxic hepatitis are unlikely to develop progressive encephalopathy and, eventually, brain edema, in contrast to patients with other causes of acute liver failure such as fulminant hepatitis B.

The prognosis essentially depends on the outcome of the causative condition. However, the

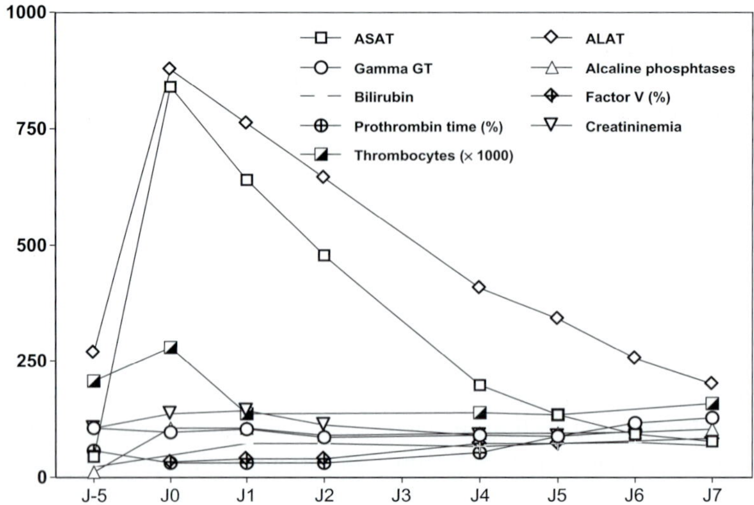

Figure 69.1. Evolution of biologic parameters in a recent series of patients. ALAT, alanine aminotransferase; ASAT, aspartate aminotransferase; GT, gamma-glutamyl transpeptidase.

presence of any underlying chronic liver disease also represents a determinant prognostic factor. While liver regeneration is a rapid process in patients with normal liver status who experience acute hypoxic (or congestive) liver cell necrosis, those with extensive fibrosis or even cirrhosis, whatever the cause, have very limited regeneration capacities. Therefore, cirrhotic patients with severe hypoxic hepatitis and a massive decrease in coagulation factors are unlikely to have sufficient regeneration. Mortality is especially high in this group. However, whether patients with an underlying chronic liver disease are especially at risk of developing hypoxic hepatitis after a given circulatory event is unclear.

Management

There is no specific treatment of hypoxic hepatitis. Basically, the treatment is based on the correction of the hemodynamic process having resulted in hypoxic hepatitis. An increase in cardiac output and blood pressure by inotropes or a decrease in right heart pressures by diuretics is generally required, depending on the causal mechanisms. As for any patients with early acute liver insufficiency, factors that may precipitate encephalopathy (administration of sedative agents, hypoglycemia) or further deteriorate renal function (aminoglycosides, nonsteroidal antiinflammatory agents, imaging with infusion of contrast media) should be avoided.

Patients who have ingested paracetamol, even at therapeutic doses, within the days preceding admission and who have a significant decrease in coagulation factors (prothrombin index below 50% of normal or INR over 1.7) should receive *N*-acetylcysteine on a prophylactic basis.

Emergency liver transplantation is an efficacious option in patients with the most severe forms of acute liver failure. However, transplantation is hardly justified in patients with hypoxic hepatitis unless on exceptional occasions (namely, in patients with a severe underlying chronic liver disease). Again, the prognosis essentially depends on the cause of hypoxic hepatitis and liver regeneration rapidly occurs after the cause has been corrected.

Conclusion

Acute hypoxic hepatitis ("shock liver") can still be a major diagnostic pitfall and may have a poor prognosis according to its cause. It is important to consider, in the context of the intensive care unit, that a major (even more than 100-fold) increase in transaminases may be due not only to acute viral or toxic hepatitis, but also to acute hypoxic hepatitis. This latter diagnosis should be seriously considered in patients with (1) past or present cardiac disease (even minimal); (2) electrocardiographic abnormalities (an ECG must be done systematically; our findings suggest that a normal ECG virtually eliminates the diagnosis of acute hypoxic hepatitis); (3) radiographic pulmonary abnormalities (found in about half of all patients with acute hypoxic hepatitis); (4) classic hepatic biochemical abnormalities (marked increase in transaminase activity, contrasting with less severe signs of cholestasis); and (5) early renal impairment, rare in other causes of hepatitis.

In the vast majority of such cases, two examinations rapidly provide the correct diagnosis: (1) abdominal echography is virtually pathognomonic when it shows dilation of the inferior vena cava and suprahepatic veins, and (2) Doppler echocardiography yields the diagnosis. They therefore should be done nearly systematically in every patient in whom a diagnosis of fulminant hepatitis is suspected, in particular before liver biopsy.

References

1. Henrion J, Luxaert R, Colin L, Schmitz A, Schapira M, Heller F. Hépatite hypoxique. Gastroenterol Clin Biol. 1990;14:836–41.
2. Bernuau J. Ischémie hépatique aiguë. La Presse Med. 1986;2:80–6.
3. Fuchs S, Bogomolski-Yahalom V, Partiel O, Ackerman Z. Ischemic hepatitis. J Clin Gastroenterol. 1998;28:183–6.
4. Henrion J, Minette P, Colin L, Schapira M, Delannoy A, Heller F. Hypoxic hepatitis caused by acute exacerbation of chronic respiratory failure: a case-controlled, hemodynamic study of 17 consecutive cases. Hepatology. 1999;29(2):427–33.
5. Seeto R, Fenn B, Rockey D. Ischemic hepatitis: clinical presentation and pathogenesis. Am J Med. 2000;109:109–13.
6. Shovman O, George J, Shoenfeld Y. [Ischemic hepatitis in congestive heart failure after an episode of hypotension]. Harefuah. 1997;132(7):459–60, 527.
7. Denis C, De Kerguennec C, Bernuau J, Beauvais F, Cohen Solal A. Acute hypoxic hepatitis ("liver shock"): still a frequently overlooked cardiological diagnosis. Eur J Heart Fail. 2004;6(5):561–5.

70 Lactate and Acute Heart Failure Syndrome

Carole Ichai, Xavier Leverve, and Jean-Christophe Orban

This chapter discusses the different pathways of lactate metabolism and the mechanisms by which hyperlactatemia could appear during acute heart failure. The clinical practical interpretation of hyperlactatemia requires repeated lactate measurement. In all cases, it must be compared with the clinical situation and other biologic parameters. Hyperlactatemia entails a poor prognosis, especially if it is persistent. But even though it has been considered deleterious for a long time, recent data show that lactate is probably a key metabolic intermediate substrate during acute energetic crisis. Thus, hyperlactatemia, and more precisely a high lactate turnover, may be viewed as an adaptive or protective response to acute illness. Neither low pH nor hyperlactatemia requires a specific treatment (1).

Lactate Metabolism

Plasma lactate concentration, or lactatemia, results from a stable equilibrium between both lactate production and elimination (1–3).

Metabolic Pathways of Lactate (1–4)

Lactate is produced in the cytosol from pyruvate, which is reduced by the lactate dehydrogenase (LDH) enzyme. This reversible reaction may be summarized as follows:

$$\text{Pyruvate} + \text{NADH} + \text{H}^+ \leftrightarrow \text{Lactate} + \text{NAD}$$

where NADH is reduced nicotinamide adenine dinucleotide and NAD is nicotinamide adenine dinucleotide. According to the law of the action of mass:

$$\text{Lactate} = \text{K} \cdot \text{Pyruvate} \cdot \text{NADH} + \text{H}^+/\text{NAD}^+$$

where K is the equilibrium constant.

Thus, the cell concentration of lactate depends on three elements: pyruvate, NADH/NAD ratio, and the proton concentration.

Cellular Concentration of Pyruvate

Lactate synthesis increases when the production of pyruvate in cytosol exceeds its consumption. Pyruvate is essentially issued from glycolysis. Glycolytic flux depends on several enzymes. Two of them play an important role. Phosphofructokinase (PFK) catalyzes the conversion of fructose-6P to fructose-1,6P, and pyruvate kinase (PK) induces the conversion of phosphoenolpyruvate to pyruvate. Both have a tight allosteric regulation. Thus, PFK is stimulated by adenosine diphosphate (ADP) and OH^- ions, and in contrast inhibited by adenosine triphosphate (ATP) and H^+ ions. This explains why a mild hyperlactatemia frequently accompanies alkalosis, which stimulates glycolysis.

Pyruvate has four possible metabolic pathways (Fig. 70.1); two are intramitochondrial (oxidation and carboxylation) and two are cytosolic (gluconeogenesis and transamination). The most important is the intramitochondrial aerobic oxidation via the Krebs' cycle, which is stimulated by the pyruvate dehydrogenase enzyme (PDH):

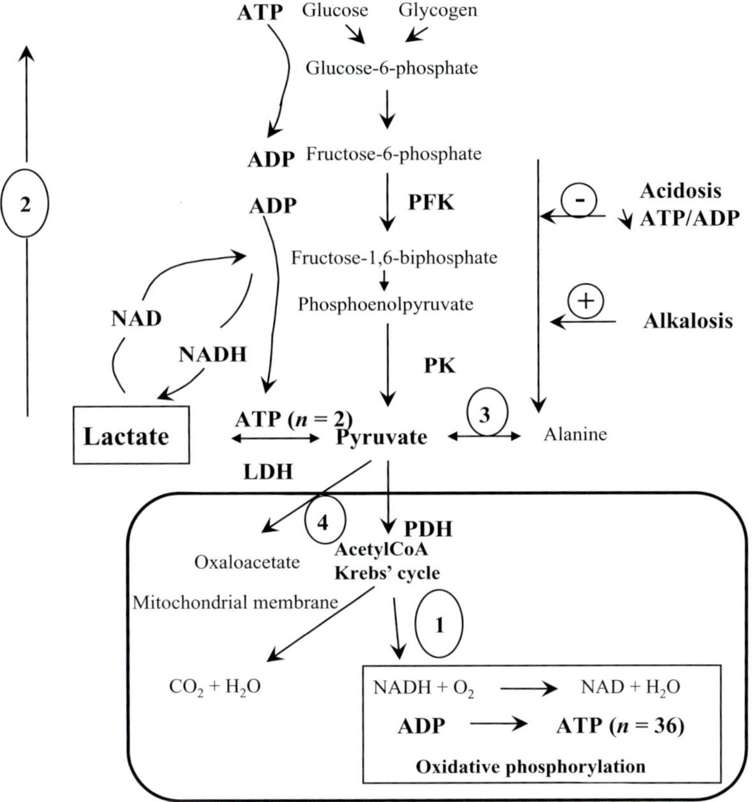

FIGURE 70.1. The possible metabolic pathways for pyruvate. 1, intramitochondrial oxidation; 2, cytosolic gluconeogenesis; 3, cytosolic transamination; 4, intramitochondrial carboxylation. ADP, adenosine diphosphate; ATP, adenosine triphosphate; LDH, lactate dehydrogenase; NAD, nicotinamide adenine dinucleotide; NADH, reduced nicotinamide adenine dinucleotide; PFK, phosphofructokinase.

$$\text{Pyruvate} + \text{CoA} + \text{PDH} \leftarrow \text{Acetyl-CoA} + \text{NADH} + \text{H}^+ + \text{CO}_2$$

where CoA is coenzyme A, PDH is pyruvate dehydrogenase.

Reduced equivalents use the respiratory chain leading to ATP, H_2O, and CO_2 synthesis with oxygen consumption; this is the oxidative phosphorylation. The activity of PDH depends on a reversible reaction of phosphorylation; the phosphorylated form, which is catalyzed by a kinase, is inactive, whereas the dephosphorylated form, which is catalyzed by a phosphorylase, is active.

Redox Potential (NADH/NAD)

The NADH/NAD ratio tightly controls the intracellular concentration of pyruvate, by regulating both glycolysis and pyruvate oxidation into acetyl-CoA or pyruvate reduction into lactate.

(H^+) or pH

The variations in proton concentration lead to complex modifications. Acidemia favors the conversion of pyruvate to lactate, but at the same time it decreases pyruvate production by a inhibition of PFK, which inhibits glycolysis.

Lactate Turnover

The global lactate production is 1300 to 1500 mmol per day. It is issued from so-called producer organs during classically anaerobic work (2). Among the most important, we found erythrocytes, gut, brain, skin, and muscles, especially during physical exercise. In normal conditions, this production is totally compensated by "consumer organs" such as the liver, kidneys, and heart. The liver plays a major role because it may eliminate up to 70% of lactate produced. Only a decrease in hepatic blood flow reaching 20% to 25% of the basal value may impair the hepatic clearance capacities. If hepatic blood flow is under this value, the liver becomes a producer of lactate. Impairment of hepatic clearance, such as in cirrhosis, may decrease lactate clearance, leading to a longer half-life. In contrast, only high levels of lactate above 5 mmol/L may saturate the hepatic enzymatic system. The kidney is a secondary actor because lactate elimination is near 0. Indeed, lactate is totally reabsorbed in the tubules until lactatemia reaches 10 mmol/L. In special conditions, the kidney may eliminate up to 30% of lactate. However, during shock, the kidney becomes a producer of lactate due to the redistribution of blood flow from the cortex to the medulla. Other organs such as the skeletal muscles or brain have a complex action in the turnover of lactate. Usually they are producers of lactate, but under some situations, skeletal muscles (5) and brain (6, 7) may become consumer organs.

Thus, in physiologic conditions, lactate production equals its elimination, leading to a stable lactate plasma concentration of 0.5 to 1.5 mmol/L in adults. Its mean plasma half-life is about 10 minutes. In this view, it is easy to understand that lactatemia cannot be an accurate reflection of lactate turnover. Thus, hyperlactatemia always indicates a disequilibrium between lactate production and elimination. In contrast, lactatemia may be quite normal, whereas lactate metabolism may be multiplied by 2 or 3.

Energy Metabolism in the Healthy Heart

Under normal working conditions, the healthy heart uses approximately two thirds of the ATP hydrolyzed for contractile working, and the remaining one third for ion pumps (8, 9). In the presence of oxygen, ATP is issued at 98% from oxidative phosphorylation in the mitochondria, whereas only 2% comes from glycolysis. About 60% to 90% of the ATP generated in the mitochondria comes from β-oxidation of fatty acids, and 10% to 40% comes from pyruvate (issued from glycolysis or lactate). In terms of quantity, fatty acids represent the most important store of substrates. However, in terms of oxygen, lactate and glucose are more efficient than fatty acids. Indeed, the molar ratio of ATP to oxygen is 11% higher with glucose and lactate than with fatty acids. In other words, for a given rate of ATP production, fatty acids oxidation requires a greater rate of oxygen consumption than carbohydrate oxidation. In humans, 80% of free fatty acids uptake is rapidly oxidized in the cardiac mitochondria (10). The rate of free fatty acids uptake is essentially dependent on the plasma concentration of free fatty acids, and the content of the specific fatty acids transport protein in the sarcolemmal membrane. The healthy heart is also able to oxidize lactate and glucose. This metabolic pathway is regulated by insulin, so that cardiac tissue is considered as an insulin-dependent tissue. Thus, the uptake of extracellular glucose by the heart is dependent on insulin concentration, which regulates the numbers of the specific glucose transporter GLUT-4. Lactate uptake appears also as a major source of pyruvate formation. It contributes 50% of pyruvate oxidation in the healthy heart (11). Lactate uptake is mainly related to the arterial lactate concentration.

Thus, lactate must be viewed as a key metabolic intermediate between the cell organs that are useful during a metabolic crisis (12–14). This phenomenon is illustrated during physiologic exercise. Lactate production by the working skeletal muscles increases. The resulting increased plasma lactatemia facilitates lactate uptake by the heart, so that lactate becomes the preferential fuel for the heart (9, 11).

Mechanisms of Hyperlactatemia in Heart Failure

Blood lactate reflects only a steady state. Thus, for it to occur, hyperlactatemia needs an imbalance between production and consumption. In practice, both disturbances contribute to induce hyperlactatemia. Many alterations in metabolic pathway are implicated in the occurrence of hyperlactatemia. These modifications have been largely studied during sepsis (2, 13–17). All these studies confirmed that hyperlactatemia reflects not only an anaerobic metabolism. Although they are less studied in heart failure, the same mechanisms are involved in the occurrence of hyperlactatemia.

Hyperlactatemia as a Marker of Hypoxia

In physiologic situations, energy metabolism in humans is produced for 90% of the aerobic ATP production issued from mitochondrial oxidative phosphorylation. Anaerobic metabolism produces only 10% of ATP synthesis. In anaerobic conditions, only glycolysis, consuming glucose and producing lactate, permits the production of ATP (12). Thus, hyperlactatemia has long been interpreted exclusively as a marker of hypoxia, the degree of hyperlactatemia being related to the severity of the oxidative deficit. For a long time, the sole responsibility of tissue hypoxia in the development of hyperlactatemia has been admitted in cardiac surgery (18–22). Some authors have found a relationship between O_2 delivery (DO_2) and hyperlactatemia (23). However, hypoxia is associated with complex metabolic modifications, which cannot be attributed solely to increased lactate synthesis. Hypoxia induces a shift in the cellular redox state (increase of NADH/NAD ratio) and a decrease in the ATP to ADP ratio, which stimulates glycolysis via an activation of PFK. At the same time, pyruvate carboxylase and PDH activity are inhibited, leading to enhanced pyruvate accumulation. In these conditions, hyperlactatemia results from pyruvate accumulation, but above all from an increased conversion of pyruvate into lactate due to the modification in the redox state.

Thus, hyperlactatemia may be considered as a marker of anaerobic metabolism if it is associated with other metabolic disturbances including an increased glucose consumption, an absence of cellular respiration, and an oxidative deficit expressed by an increase in the lactate-to-pyruvate ratio.

Hyperlactatemia without Hypoxia

During heart failure, many factors may contribute to the development of hyperlactatemia irrespective of tissue hypoxia.

Energy Metabolism Related to Heart Failure

Recent data suggest that myocardial substrate utilization is different in normal hearts and in heart failure (8, 9). The specific hormonal and neurohormonal modifications observed in chronic heart failure may account for the metabolic changes. The role of chronic activation of the endogenous neurohormonal system is supported by several reports showing a significant relationship between neurohormonal status and mortality rate (24, 25). Moreover, abnormalities in metabolic pathway are related to the severity of heart failure and the hormonal environment (26, 27).

Metabolism in moderate heart failure is characterized by an increase in the rate of fatty acid oxidation and a decrease in carbohydrate oxidation (8, 9, 28). Paolissimo et al. (26) found a decrease in glucose uptake with a corresponding 60% decrease in carbohydrate oxidation in patients with New York Heart Association (NYHA) class II or III congestive heart failure. In contrast, in decompensated heart failure, free fatty acids oxidation is switched toward a preferential carbohydrate oxidation (27). Not only lactate production but also impaired lactate elimination contribute to hyperlactatemia. Indeed, several studies have shown that mitochondrial function in cardiac tissue from the failing heart is reduced when compared with the normal heart (29–31). Di Lisa et al. (32) have found in cardiomyopathic animals a decrease in the activity of PDH, which was related to the severity of impaired left ventricular contractility.

Inflammatory Syndrome and Heart Failure

Numerous studies conducted in patents with sepsis or systemic inflammatory response syndrome (SIRS) have demonstrated that proinflammatory mediators are responsible for huge metabolic changes (33, 34), including hyperlactatemia, which results partly from an acceleration of aerobic glycolysis. In hemodynamically stable septic patients, Gore et al. (34) reported that lactate and pyruvate were markedly increased and related to a higher glucose turnover. During inflammatory syndrome, hyperlactatemia may also partly result from a decrease in lactate clearance (35, 36). The mechanism by which lactate elimination is impaired is not clear. Several studies suggest that only major hepatic failure can impair hepatic lactate clearance and leads to hyperlactatemia (36–38). Despite major hepatectomy, lactate and glucose metabolisms are well maintained without any increase in plasma lactate concentration (37). In a model of endotoxinic rats, hyperlactatemia was attributed to an impaired lactate clearance without any increase in production (36). However, the decrease in lactate clearance was associated with an increase in hepatic lactate uptake. Moreover, for a similar degree of hepatic insufficiency, hyperlactatemia is higher in septic patients (38). Decrease in lactate clearance may also be explained by an inhibition in pyruvate oxidation. Cytokines are responsible for an inhibition in PDH activity, which prevents pyruvate from entering into the Krebs' cycle. As a consequence of pyruvate accumulation, lactate synthesis increases (39).

Even as described essentially during sepsis, all of these metabolic disturbances, that is, acceleration in glycolytic flux and decreased lactate clearance, are probably present in heart failure. Indeed, recent data have shown that the pathogenesis of heart failure not only entails muscular illness but also is often associated with SIRS (40–48). Systemic inflammatory response syndrome, expressed by evident clinical signs such as fever, elevated white blood cell count, C-reactive protein, interleukins, activation of complement, and low systemic vascular resistances, can be present in patients presenting with acute myocardial infarction (AMI). A release of cytokines by the heart has been reported in patients after AMI, especially when reperfusion was obtained (49). In experimental models, high inducible nitric oxide synthase (iNOS) and nitric oxide (NO) levels have been described after AMI and subsequent reperfusion. Elevated concentrations of endotoxin and cytokines have also been found in patients with chronic heart failure, especially during the decompensation period (45). Moreover, the degree of this inflammatory response seems to be related to the severity of heart failure (42, 43). Its pharmacologic inhibition is able to improve myocardial contractile function and survival of patients with cardiogenic shock (44).

Finally, the presence of a SIRS in heart failure is probably involved in the occurrence of hyperlactatemia via an increased glycolytic flux and a decreased lactate clearance. The relationship between hyperlactatemia and the inflammatory status has been well documented during cardiac surgery, especially with cardiopulmonary bypass. Some studies have shown that endotoxins actually come from the circulation via the inferior vena cava during cardiopulmonary bypass, supporting the view that the gut was probably the source of endotoxins (22, 50–52). This may be the consequence of a splanchnic area hypoperfusion, which could increase gut permeability, leading finally to endotoxin or bacterial translocation (22, 51, 52).

Several studies performed during cardiopulmonary bypass support also the development of hyperlactatemia without any tissue hypoxia (53–55). Chiolero et al. (53) have found in patients presenting with cardiogenic shock after cardiac surgery that hyperlactatemia was mainly related to an increase in tissue lactate endogenous production, whereas hepatic lactate clearance was not impaired. Moreover, exogenous lactate was normally oxidized. Hyperlactatemia, hyperglycemia, and stimulation of glycolysis has been also observed during the early phase of shock induced by cardiac tamponade (55). On the other hand, a minor decrease in lactate clearance has been found in patients after pump coronary artery surgery, but not after an off-pump surgical procedure (56). In all patients, basal lactatemia was slightly elevated and the alteration in lactate clearance was only revealed by exogenous infusion. All of these data suggest that in uncomplicated postoperative patients, hyperlactatemia is mainly related to increased lactate production associated with increased lactate oxidation. The decrease in lactate clearance may contribute to enhance hyperlactatemia only in cases of complications (shock, hypoxia).

Role of Catecholamines

Energy metabolism including glycolysis, is compartmentalized in the cell. The plasma membrane–linked cellular adenosine triphosphatase (ATPase) activities are supported by glycolytic ATP, leading to lactate formation even in fully aerobic experimental conditions (15, 57–59). Moreover, the administration of Na^+-K^+–ATPase inhibitor decreases lactatemia (15). Studies have offered evidence that hyperlactatemia may be the result of catecholamine stimulation that activates the membrane Na^+-K^+–ATPase activity coupled with aerobic glycolysis (15, 58). In fact, β-adrenergic stimulation activates adenylate cyclase, which catalyzes the conversion of ATP to cyclic adenosine monophosphate (cAMP). In turn, cAMP via an activation of protein kinase A stimulates the Na^+-K^+–ATPase activity.

The relationship among adrenaline, Na^+-K^+–ATPase stimulation, and hyperlactatemia is largely demonstrated in experimental models of septic (15, 58, 60) or hemorrhagic shock (59), with fully aerobic conditions of incubation. In a recent study, Bungaard et al. (57) have evaluated the metabolic effects of endotoxemia in healthy human subjects. They found that both lactate and endogenous adrenaline plasma concentrations increased. In rats, both perfusion of adrenaline and hemorrhage increase lactate production by muscle (59). Administration of ouabain, which blocks the Na^+-K^+–ATPase pump, reverses these effects. All of these results have been recently confirmed in patients with septic shock (61).

Thus, there is strong evidence that β-adrenergic–stimulated Na^+-K^+–ATPase activity that is coupled with aerobic glycolytic ATP production can lead to hyperlactatemia in fully aerobic conditions. Even if not specifically studied in acute heart failure, increased lactate plasma levels of endogenous catecholamines or exogenous administration of catecholamines probably contributes to hyperlactatemia irrespective of tissue hypoxia.

Special Mechanisms

Thiamine deficiency, which is called beriberi, is a rare cause of lactic acidosis. Thiamine as a precursor of thiamine pyrophosphate is a coenzyme for pyruvate dehydrogenase. As a result, thiamine deficiency blocks pyruvate oxidation. In turn, pyruvate accumulation favors its conversion into lactate (62).

Congestive heart failure requiring a pharmaceutical treatment represents a risk of metformin-associated lactic acidosis development (63–66). The mechanism by which metformin induces lactic acidosis remains largely controversial. In most situations, patients presented with collapse, so that the toxic role of metformin is difficult to distinguish from that of hypoxia. In all cases, congestive heart failure is still a relative contraindication for prescribing this medication.

Practical Interpretation of Hyperlactatemia

The diagnosis of hyperlactatemia is very easy based on the lactate plasma concentration measurement. Anion gap calculation is a poor tool for the diagnosis of hyperlactatemia (67, 68). On the other hand, hyperlactatemia's relationship with tissue hypoxia and its exact cause is more difficult to establish. Generally, hyperlactatemia is multifactorial, resulting from an overproduction of lactate, a decreased lactate clearance, or both (Fig. 70.2).

An elevated lactate level cannot be considered in isolation. The history and the complete clinical evaluation of the patient must be taken into account. Lactatemia is associated with other parameters and thus requires multimodal metabolic and hemodynamic monitoring. Lactate variation obtained by repeated measures provides better information and facilitates the interpretation of hyperlactatemia.

Causes of Hyperlactatemia in Acute Heart Failure

Despite a possible aerobic or anaerobic lactate accumulation, tissue hypoxia must always be evoked first. During acute heart failure, tissue hypoxia, when present, is global due to systemic low flow. When low cardiac output is associated with an evident cardiogenic shock or hemodynamic failure, anaerobic lactate production is easy to diagnose (18, 23, 55, 69–71). However, when hypoperfusion is present only in microcirculation, the relationship between hyperlactatemia and tissue hypoxia may not be so evident. Indeed, hyperlactatemia may be present in patients with normal arterial blood pressure and arterial blood oxygenation (72, 73). It has been found to be an indicator of AMI in patients without any circulatory failure (72). So, it is clear that hyperlactatemia alone cannot be a good indicator of anaerobic metabolism. It must be associated with other hemodynamic and metabolic abnormal parameters. Hypoxic hyperlactatemia is then usually associated with metabolic acidosis and hyperglycemia (74).

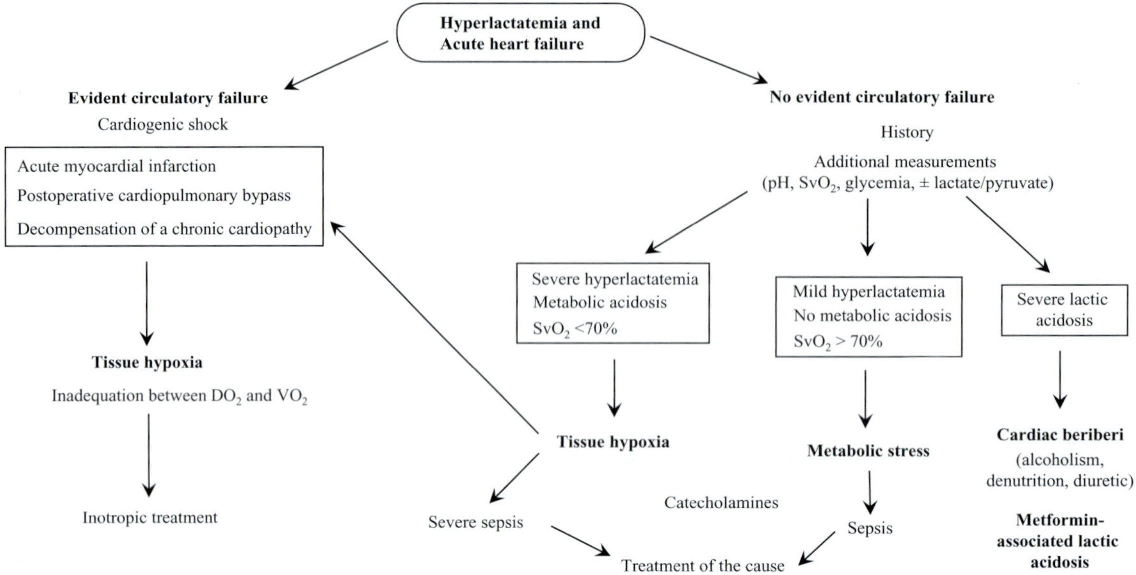

FIGURE 70.2. Guidelines for interpreting hyperlactatemia during heart failure.

The lactate-to-pyruvate ratio, which reflects the cytosolic redox state, could be one of the most accurate bedside tools used to assess the deficit in oxidative energy metabolism (70). Levy et al. (75) have demonstrated that, for the same level of hyperlactatemia, the lactate-to-pyruvate ratio was significantly higher in patients with cardiogenic shock than in those with septic shock. Anaerobic metabolism can also be suggested by an imbalance between O_2 demand (VO_2) and DO_2. A decrease in O_2 venous saturation (SvO_2) below 70% indirectly reflects this situation (70). Unfortunately, all of these parameters only reflects the whole-body metabolic status. Nevertheless, a simultaneous determination of lactatemia with arterial pH, the lactate-to-pyruvate ratio, and SvO_2 permits strongly supporting the relationship between hyperlactatemia and tissue hypoxia.

A persistent hyperlactatemia, despite hemodynamic optimization, indicates that tissue hypoxia is no longer responsible of the trouble. The presence of SIRS must be recognized. Moderate hyperlactatemia after cardiopulmonary bypass is very frequent and partly related to the activation of proinflammatory mediators induced by the extracorporeal circulation (18, 50, 53). Acute heart failure may be present as a complication of severe sepsis (76–80). Only 10% to 20% of patients with severe sepsis present with myocardial depression requiring inotropic treatment. In this situation, heart failure is characterized by a biventricular decreased ejection fraction and dilatation (78, 79). Myocardial depression occurs early, during the first 2 days after the beginning of sepsis, and reverses in 5 to 10 days in survivors (78). Low cardiac output with an SvO_2 less than 70% associated with hyperlactatemia indicates a very severe sepsis with a severe myocardial dysfunction. In this situation, an adequate DO_2 may be obtained by an inotropic treatment. If lactatemia partially decreases with a parallel increased SvO_2, hyperlactatemia may be partly related to tissue hypoxia.

Mild hyperlactatemia may be associated in severe sepsis with a high or normal cardiac output, low systemic vascular resistances, and an SvO_2 >70%. In this frequent situation, hyperlactatemia indicates a normoxic metabolic stress that is due to an accelerated glycolytic pathway (74). Catecholamine administration, by stimulating the Na-K-ATPase pump, may also contribute to maintain a mild hyperlactatemia.

Lactic acidosis may be observed in two special situations. The first is cardiac beriberi, which is related to thiamine deficiency. Patients classically present with a high cardiac output heart failure, neurologic deficit, and a severe lactic acidosis (62, 81–84). It may be manifested by other symptoms such as fatigue, irritability, loss of appetite, constipation, and cramps. A less classic presentation is "shoshin beriberi," which corresponds to an acute form of low cardiac output and cardiovascular collapse, leading to death within a few days (83, 84). Shoshin beriberi may have two clinical presentations: (1) a low cardiac output with cardiovascular collapse, cardiomegaly, hepatomegaly, and cyanosis; and (2) acute sudden death without clear-cut signs of cardiomegaly (84, 85). Even considered as a rare cause of lactic acidosis with acute heart failure, cardiac beriberi occurs only in special clinical conditions such as alcoholism, total parenteral nutrition, and diuretic therapy (82, 86, 87). Thus, the diagnosis must be rapidly suspected in these high-risk populations, and the empiric treatment initiated immediately, permitting a complete recovery.

Metformin-associated lactic acidosis is the second special condition associated with heart failure. The diagnosis must be systematically suspected (63, 64, 66). It may be confirmed by the determination of plasma and intra-erythrocyte metformin concentration. In this context, the respective contribution of hemodynamic failure with an anaerobic metabolism and the toxic effect of metformin without hypoxia for the development of lactic acidosis is generally difficult to determine.

Hyperlactatemia Is a Marker of Poor Prognosis

There is no doubt that whatever the cause, hyperlactatemia still correlates with illness severity and the patient's outcome (23, 69, 71, 73, 88–93). Hyperlactatemia above 5 mmol/L on admission is associated with a high level of mortality: 59% at 3 days and 83% at 30 days (17). The course of hyperlactatemia has a better prognostic value (89, 90, 94). Toraman et al. (95) have demonstrated that hyperlactatemia after coronary artery bypass grafting, is associated with an adverse outcome. In patients suffering from cardiogenic shock treated with an intraaortic balloon, a high lactate level, greater than 2.5 mmol/L, appears to be a good marker of poor prognosis with a high level of mortality (96, 97).

Hyperlactatemia Is an Adapted Metabolic Answer

Lactate per se is not a toxic compound. Indeed, the significance of hyperlactatemia depends on the metabolic surroundings. For example, after exhaustive physical exercise, subjects presented with a severe lactic acidosis, but their prognosis is generally quite good. Infusion of lactate results in high lactate levels without any deleterious effect (53, 98, 99). Thus hyperlactatemia is not the cause but rather the consequence of a metabolic and energy crisis. Moreover, lactatemia is a poor indicator of lactate metabolism. In fact, recent work supports the fact that acidosis and hyperlactatemia are at least an adapted if not a protective response to an acute injury.

Lactate participates greatly in metabolic organ balance and interorgan cooperation (4, 12, 13, 70). In physiologic situations, due to the lack of mitochondria, erythrocytes only produce ATP via glycolysis without O_2 consumption, leading to lactate production. Under steady-state conditions, lactate released by erythrocytes is then metabolized by other organs under fully aerobic conditions, entering either the oxidative phosphorylation or the gluconeogenic pathways. Lactate, which is a reduced equivalent, permits energetic exchanges between organs via a redox shuttle lactate-pyruvate. In this view, lactate must be considered as a key metabolic intermediate between cells or organs, especially during acute situations with energy crisis. After ischemia-reperfusion, because of a decreased ATP/ADP ratio, glucose cannot be metabolized at the initial phase of reperfusion. Thus, oxygen without substrate could exacerbate the oxidative stress. It is proposed that lactate, by supplying pyruvate, actually could be a preferred substrate for aerobic energy production during the initial stage of recovery from ischemia. This has already been demonstrated in a model of ischemia-reperfusion in rats (6, 7). Experimental studies performed in heart failure found that shifting the energy substrate preference of the heart toward glucose and lactate ameliorates hemodynamic and biochemical alterations (8, 9, 27). Mustafa et al. (98) compared the effects of hypertonic saline and lactate solutions in patients after cardiac pulmonary bypass. Although both solutions produced increases in cardiac index and oxygen delivery, there was a decreased in oxygen extraction only in patients receiving lactate. Moreover, lactate was normally metabolized in all patients.

All of these data support a possible protective effect of lactate as a preferential energy substrate in critical situations. Indeed, lactate, which is initially excreted by some cells, is oxidized by others. In this view, the higher the lactate turnover, the more the energy metabolism of injured cells or tissues is supported by the rest of the body (100). Indeed, in septic patients with a normal or mild hyperlactatemia, it has been shown survivors presented a higher lactate metabolism than those who did not survive (99). In this study, the increased lactate metabolism was characterized by both an increased lactate production and a decreased lactate clearance.

Treatment of Hyperlactatemia

This section addresses the question of whether there is any rationale to treat hyperlactatemia and metabolic acidosis, if present. As lactate is not toxic, decreasing lactatemia must not be an objective of treatment. Dichloroacetate, which leads to lactate elimination by the activation of pyruvate dehydrogenase, has no benefit in lactic acidosis (101). As hyperlactatemia is only a marker of metabolic crisis, treatment addresses only its cause, such as hemodynamic optimization in cases of shock, or antibiotherapy in cases of sepsis. As soon as the critical situation improves, the lactate concentration will normalize at the same time. Thus, the course of the lactate level is a good way of appreciating the efficacy of the treatment.

Are There Indications for Treating a Low pH?

For several years, many deleterious effects, especially cardiovascular effects such as myocardial depression and rhythm abnormalities, have been attributed to acidosis (102). However, all of them have been reported only in experimental studies with a very low pH (<7) and isolated organs. Results from these studies do not translate to most clinical situations where acidosis is not so severe. On the other hand, theoretical data strongly suggest that acidosis may be considered a protective response. Acidosis, by inhibiting glycolysis, precludes rapid glycogenic substrate exhaustion. This metabolic-sparing beneficial effect can be viewed as the same that is obtained with hypothermia. Some experimental studies have demonstrated the beneficial effects of acidosis on death cells after ischemia-reperfusion (103, 104). Moreover, several clinical trial have shown that alkalinization of lactic acidosis does not produce any beneficial effect (105, 106). Alkalinization may be justified only when pH is very low (<7) and persists for a long time.

Conclusion

The relationship between tissue hypoxia and hyperlactatemia has been recognized for several years. However, recent knowledge about lactate metabolism enhances the complex role of lactate during acute situations with energy crisis, such as acute heart failure. Of course, hypoxia first must be evoked to interpret hyperlactatemia during heart failure. However, many studies confirmed in humans that hyperlactatemia may occur irrespective of tissue hypoxia. Hyperlactatemia may result from an excessive production of lactate related to an anaerobic or aerobic increase in glycolytic flux or a decrease in lactate clearance. The administration of catecholamines, the presence of a systemic inflammatory response with or without sepsis during acute heart failure, partly contributes to the development of hyperlactatemia. Persistent hyperlactatemia remains a poor prognosis marker but is not deleterious. The modern concept seems to be that lactate is a major oxidizable substrate during critical metabolic situations. Finally, as hyperlactatemia is a consequence rather than a cause of the illness, neither specific correction of acidosis nor normalization of lactatemia must be a therapeutic goal.

References

1. Cohen RD, Woods HF. Lactic acidosis revisited. Diabetes 1983;32:181–91.
2. Gutierrez G, Wulf M. Lactic acidosis in sepsis: a commentary. Intensive Care Med 1996;22:6–16.
3. Vincent JL. Lactate levels in critically ill patients. Acta Anaesth Scand 1995;107(suppl):261–6.

4. Leverve X. Lactic acidosis. A new insight. Minerva Anesthesiol 1999;65:205–9.
5. Pagano C, Granzotto M, Giaccari A, et al. Lactate infusion to normal rats during hyperglycemia enhances in vivo muscle glycogen synthesis. Am J Physiol 1997;273:R2072–9.
6. Schurr A, Payne RS, Miller JJ, Rigor BM. Brain lactate is an obligatory aerobic energy substrate for functional recovery after hypoxia: further in vitro validation. J Neurochem 1997;69: 423–6.
7. Schurr A, Payne RS, Miller JJ, Rigor BM. An increase in lactate output by brain tissue serves to meet the energy needs of glutamate-activated neurons. J Neurosci 1999;19:34–9.
8. Stanley WC, Chandler MP. Energy metabolism in the normal and failing heart: potential for therapeutic interventions. Heart Fail Rev 2002;7:115–30.
9. Stanley WC, Lopaschuk GD, Hall JL, et al. Regulation of myocardial carbohydrate metabolism under normal and ischaemic conditions: potential for pharmacological interventions. Cardiovasc Res 1997;33:243–57.
10. Wineski JA, Gertz EW, Neese RA, et al. Myocardial metabolism of free fatty acids: studies with ^{14}C-labeled substrates in humans. J Clin Invest 1987; 79:359–66.
11. Stanley WC. Myocardial lactate metabolism during exercise. Med Sci Sport Exerc 1991;23:920–4.
12. Leverve XM, Mustafa I, Peronnet F. Pivotal role of lactate in aerobic metabolism. In: Vincent JL, ed. Yearbook of Intensive Care and Emergency Medicine. Berlin: Springer-Verlag, 1998:588–96.
13. Brook G. Lactate production under fully aerobic conditions: the lactate shuttle during rest and exercise. Fed Proc 1986;45:2924–9.
14. Gladden LB. Lactate metabolism: a new paradigm for the third millennium. J Physiol 2004;558: 5–30.
15. James JH, Luchette FA, Mc Carter FD, Fischer JE. Lactate is an unreliable indicator of tissue hypoxia in injury or sepsis. Lancet 1999;354:505–8.
16. Silverman H. Lack of a relationship between induced changes in oxygen consumption and changes in lactate levels. Chest 1991;100:1012–5.
17. Stacpoole PW, Wright EC, Baumgartner S, Curry SH. Natural history and course of acquired lactic acidosis in adults. Am J Med 1994;97:47–54.
18. Takala J, Uusaro A, Parviainen I, et al. Lactate metabolism and regional lactate exchange after cardiac surgery. New Horiz 1996;4:483–92.
19. Ballinger WF, Vollenweider H, Pierucci L, et al. Anaerobic metabolism and metabolic acidosis during cardiopulmonary bypass. Ann Surg 1961;153:499–506.
20. Aziza M, Gothard JWW, Macnaughton P, et al. Blood lactate and mixed venous-arterial PCO_2 gradient as indices of poor peripheral perfusion following cardiopulmonary bypass. Intensive Care Med 1991;17:320–4.
21. Litwin MS, Panico FG, Rubini C, et al. Acidosis and lactacidemia in extracorporeal circulation: the significance of perfusion flow rate and the relation to preperfusion respiratory alkalosis. Ann Surg 1959;149:188–99.
22. Landow L. Splanchnic lactate production in cardiac surgery patients. Crit Care Med 1993;21: S84–91.
23. Raskhin MC, Bosken C, Baughman RP. Oxygen delivery in critically ill patients: relationship to blood lactate and survival. Chest 1985;87:580–4.
24. Packer M. The neurohormonal hypothesis: a theory to explain the mechanism of disease progression in heart failure. J Am Coll Cardiol 1992;20: 248–54.
25. Cohn JN, Levine TB, Olivari MT, et al. Plasma norepinephrine as a guide to prognosis in patients with chronic congestive heart failure. N Engl J Med 1984;311:819–23.
26. Paolissimo G, Gambardella A, Galzerano D, et al. Total body and myocardial substrate oxidation in congestive heart failure. Metabolism 1994;43:174–9.
27. Recchia FA, McConnell PI, Bernstein RD, Vogel TR, Xu X, Hintze TH. Reduced nitric oxide production and altered myocardial metabolism during the decompensation of pacing-induced heart failure in the conscious dog. Circ Res 1998;83:969–79.
28. Swan JW, Walton C, Godsland IF, et al. Insulin resistance in chronic heart failure. Eur Heart J 1994;15:1528–32.
29. Bashore TM, Magorien DJ, Letterio J, Shafer P, Unverferth DV. Histologic and biochemical correlates of left ventricular chamber dynamics in man. J Am Coll Cardiol 1987;9:734–42.
30. Sanbe A, Tanonake K, Kobayasi R, Takeo S. Effect of long-term therapy with ACE inhibitors on myocardial energy metabolism in rats with heart failure following myocardial infarction. J Mol Cell Cardiol 1995;27:2209–22.
31. Sabbah HN, Sharov VG, Riddle JM, Kono T, Lesch M, Goldstein S. Mitochondrial abnormalities in myocardium of dogs with chronic heart failure. J Mol Cell Cardiol 1992;24:1333–47.
32. Di Lisa F, Chong-Zu F, Gambassi G, Hogue GA, Kudryashova I, Hansford RG. Altered pyruvate

dehydrogenase control and mitochondrial and free Ca^{2+} in hearts of cardiomyopathic hamsters. Am J Physiol 1993;264:H2188–97.
33. Widnell CC, Baldwin SA, Danies A, Martin S, Pasternak CA. Cellular stress induces a redistribution of the glucose transporter. FASEB J 1990;4:1634–7.
34. Gore D, Jahoor F, Hibbert J, DeMaria E. Lactic acidosis during sepsis is related to increased pyruvate production, not deficits in tissue oxygen availability. Ann Surg 1996;224:97–102.
35. Levraut J, Ciebiera JP, Chave S, et al. Mild hyperlactatemia in stable septic patients is due to impaired lactate clearance rather than overproduction. Am J Respir Crit Care Med 1998;157:1021–6.
36. Severin PN, Uhing MR, Beno DW, Kimura RE. Endotoxin-induced hyperlactatemia results from decreased lactate clearance in hemodynamically stable rats. Crit Care Med 2002;30:2509–14.
37. Chioléro R, Tappy L, Gillet M, et al. Effect of a major hepatectomy on glucose and lactate metabolism. Ann Surg 1999;4:505–13.
38. Kruse JA, Zaidi SA, Carlson SW. Significance of blood lactate levels in critically ill patients with liver disease. Am J Med 1987;83:77–82.
39. Vary TC. Sepsis-induced alterations in pyruvate dehydrogenase complex activity in rat skeletal muscle: effects on plasma lactate. Shock 1996;6: 89–94.
40. Hochman JS. Cardiogenic shock complicating acute myocardial infarction: expanding the paradigm. Circulation 2003;107:2998–3002.
41. Sabatine MS, Morrow DA, Cannon CP, et al. Relationship between baseline white blood cell count and degree of coronary artery disease and mortality in patients with acute coronary syndromes: a TACTICS-TIMI 18. J Am Coll Cardiol 2002;40: 1761–8.
42. Lange LG, Schreiner GF. Immune mechanisms of cardiac disease. N Engl J Med 1994;330:1129–35.
43. Blum A, Miller H. Pathophysiological role of cytokines in congestive heart failure. Annu Rev Med 2001;52:15–27.
44. Cotter G, Kaluski E, Milo O, Blatt A, et al. LINCS: L-NAME (a NO synthase inhibitor) in the treatment of refractory cardiogenic shock: a prospective randomized study. Eur Heart J 2003;24:1287–95.
45. Niebauer J, Volk HD, Kemp M, et al. Endotoxin and immune activation in chronic heart failure: a prospective cohort study. Lancet 1999;353:1838–42.
46. Neumann FJ, Ott I, Gawaz M, et al. Cardiac release of cytokines and inflammatory responses in acute myocardial infarction. Circulation 1995;92:748–55.
47. Liuzzo G, Buffon A, Biasucci LM, et al. Enhanced inflammatory response to coronary angioplasty in patients with severe unstable angina. Circulation 1998;98:2370–6.
48. Feng O, Lu X, Jones DL, et al. Increased inducible nitric oxide synthase expression contributes to myocardial dysfunction and higher mortality after myocardial infarction in mice. Circulation 2001; 104:700–4.
49. Alexander RW. Inflammation and coronary artery disease. N Engl J Med 1994;331:417–24.
50. Wan S, LeClerc JL, Schmartz D, et al. Hepatic release of interleukin-10 during cardiopulmonary bypass in steroid-pretreated patients. Am Heart J 1997;133:335–9.
51. Wan S, DeSmet JM, Barvais L, et al. Myocardium is a major source of proinflammatory cytokines in patients undergoing cardiopulmonary bypass. J Thorac Cardiovasc Surg 1996;112:806–11.
52. Ohri SK, Somasundaram S, Koak Y, et al. The effect of intestinal hypoperfusion on intestinal absorption and permeability during cardiopulmonary bypass. Gastroenterology 1994;106:318–23.
53. Chiolero RL, Revelly JP, Leverve X, et al. Effects of cardiogenic shock on lactate and glucose metabolism after heart surgery. Crit Care Med 2000;28:3 784–91.
54. Raper R, Cameron G, Walker D, et al. Type B lactic acidosis following cardiopulmonary bypass. Crit Care Med 1997;25:46–51.
55. Daniel AM, Taylor ME, McLean LD. Metabolism of prolonged shock. Adv Shock Res 1983;9: 19–30.
56. Mustafa I, Roth H, Hanafiah A, et al. Effect of cardiopulmonary bypass on lactate metabolism. Intensive Care Med 2003;29:1279–85.
57. Bungaard H, Kjeldsen K, Suarez Krabbe K, et al. Endotoxemia stimulates skeletal muscle NA^+-K^+-ATPase and raises blood lactate under aerobic conditions in humans. Am J Physiol Heart Circ Physiol 2003;284:H100–28–34.
58. James JH, Fang CH, Schranz SJ, Hausselgren PO, Paul RJ, Fischer JE. Linkage of aerobic glycolysis to sodium-potassium transport in rat skeletal muscle. Implications for increased muscle lactate production in sepsis. J Clin Invest 1996;98:2288–97.
59. Luchette FA, Friend LA, Brown CC, Upputori RK, James JH. Increased skeletal muscle Na^+, K^+-ATPase activity as a cause of increased lactate

production after hemorrhagic shock. J Trauma 1998;44:796–803.
60. Day NP, Phu NH, Bethell DP, et al. The effects of dopamine and adrenalin infusion on acid-base balance and systemic haemodynamics in severe infection. Lancet 1996;348:219–23.
61. Levy B, Gibot S, Franck P, Cravoisy A, Bollaert PE. Relation between muscle Na^+ K^+ ATPase activity and raised lactate concentrations in septic shock: a prospective study. Lancet 2005;365:871–5.
62. Naito E, Ito M, Yokota I, Saijo T, Matsuda J, Kuroda Y. Thiamine-responsive lactic acidaemia: role of pyruvate dehydrogenase complex. Eur J Pediatr 1998;157:648–52.
63. Emslie-Smith AM, Boyle DI, Evans JM, Sullivan F, Morris AD, DARTS/MEMO Collaboration. Contraindications to metformin therapy in patients with type 2 diabetes—a population-based study of adherence to prescribing guidelines. Diabet Med 2001;18:483–8.
64. Chan NN, Fauvel NJ, Feher MD. Non-steroidal anti-inflammatory drugs and metformin: a cause for concern? Lancet 1998;352:201.
65. Franzetti I, Paolo D, Marco G, Emanuela M, Elisabetta Z, Renato U. Possible synergistic effect of metformin and enalapril on the development of hyperkaliemic lactic acidosis. Diabetes Res Clin Pract 1997;38:173–6.
66. Holstein A, Nahrwold D, Hinze S, Egberts EH. Contra-indications to metformin therapy are largely disregarded. Diabet Med 1999;16:692–6.
67. Levraut J, Bounatirou T, Ichai C, Ciais JF, Jambou P, Grimaud D. Reliability of anion gap as an indicator of blood lactate level in critically ill patients. Intensive Care Med 1997;23:417–22.
68. Adams BD, Bonzani TA, Hunter CJ. The anion gap does not accurately screen for lactic acidosis in emergency department patients. Emerg Med J 2006;23:179–82.
69. Vincent JL. End-points of resuscitation: arterial blood pressure, oxygen delivery, blood lactate, or . . . ? Intensive Care Med 1996;22:3–5.
70. Leverve XM. From tissue perfusion to metabolic marker: assessing organ competition and cooperation in critically ill patients. Intensive Care Med 1999;25:890–2.
71. Bakker J, Coffernils M, Leon M, Gris P, Vincent JL. Blood lactate levels are superior to oxygen derived variables in predicting outcome in human septic shock. Chest 1991;99:956–62.
72. Rahimi AR, Marzano PM 3rd, Richard CM. Evaluation of lactate and C-reactive protein in the assessment of acute myocardial infarction. South Med J 2003;96:1107–12.
73. Meregalli A, Oliveira RP, Friedman G. Occult hypoperfusion is associated with increased mortality in hemodynamically stable, high-risk, surgical patients. Crit Care 2004;8:96–8.
74. Mizock BA. Significance of hyperlactatemia without acidosis during hypermetabolic stress. Crit Care Med 1997;25:1780–1.
75. Levy B, Sadoune LO, Gelot AM, Bollaert PE, Nabet P, Larcan A. Evolution of lactate/pyruvate and arterial ketone body ratios in the early course of catecholamine-treated septic shock. Crit Care Med 2000;28:114–9.
76. Parker MM, Shetlander J, Bacharach SL, et al. Profound but reversible myocardial depression in patients with septic shock. Ann Intern Med 1987;100:483–90.
77. Parker MM, McCarthy KE, Ognibene FP, Parrillo JE. Right ventricular dysfunction and dilatation, similar to left ventricular changes, characterize the cardiac depression of septic shock in humans. Chest 1990;97:126–31.
78. Parrillo JE. Pathogenetic mechanisms of septic shock. N Engl J Med 1993;328:1471–7.
79. Mebazaa A, Karpati P, renaud E, Algotsson L. Acute right ventricular failure-from pathophysiology to new treatments. Intensive Care Med 2004;30:185–96.
80. Rivers E, Nguyen B, Havstad S, et al. Early goal-directed therapy collaborative group. Early goal-directed therapy in the treatment of severe sepsis and septic shock. N Engl J Med 2001;345:1368–77.
81. Ozawa H, Homma Y, Arisawa H, Fukuuchi F, Handa S. Severe metabolic acidosis and heart failure due to thiamine deficiency. Nutrition 2001; 17:351–2.
82. Nakasaki H, Ohta M, Soeda J, et al. Clinical and biochemical aspects of thiamin treatment for metabolic acidosis during total parenteral nutrition. Nutrition 1997;13:100–3.
83. Klein M, Weksler N, Gurman GM. Fatal metabolic acidosis caused by thiamine deficiency. J Emerg Med 2004;26:301–3.
84. Naidoo DP, Gathiram V, Sadhabiriss A, Hassen F. Clinical diagnosis of cardiac beriberi. S Afr Med J 1990;77:125–7.
85. Shilvalkhar B, Engelmann I, Carp L, De Raedt H, Daelemans R. Shoshin syndrome: two cases reports representing opposite ends of the same disease spectrum. Acta Cardiol 1998;53:195–9.
86. Centers for disease control and prevention. Lactic acidosis traced to thiamine deficiency related to nationwide shortage of multivitamins for total

parenteral nutrition: United States. JAMA 1997; 218:109–4.
87. Suter PM, Vetter W. Diuretics and vitamin B1: are diuretics a risk factor for thiamine malnutrition? Nutr Rev 2000;58:319–23.
88. Marecaux G, Pinsky M, Dupont E, Kahn R, Vincent JL. Blood lactate levels are better prognostic indicators than TNF and IL-6 levels in patients with septic shock. Intensive Care Med 1996;22:404–8.
89. Bernardin G, Pradier C, Tiger F, Deloffre P, Mattei M. Blood pressure and arterial lactate level are early indicators of short-term survival in human septic shock. Intensive Care Med 1996;22:17–25.
90. Manikis P, Jankowski S, Zhang H, Khan R, Vincent JL. Correlation of serial blood lactate levels to organ failure and mortality after trauma. Am J Emerg Med 1995;13:619–22.
91. Singhal R, Coghill JE, Bradbury AW, Adam DJ, Scriven JM. Serum lactate and base deficit as predictors of mortality after ruptured abdominal aortic aneurysm repair. Eur J Endovasc Surg 2005;30:263–6.
92. Cerovic O, Golubovic V, Spec-Marn A, Kremzar B, Vidmar G. Relationship between injury severity and lactate levels in severely injured patients. Intensive Care Med 2003;29:1300–5.
93. Bakker J, de Lima AP. Increased blood lactate levels: an important warning signal in surgical practice. Crit Care 2004;8:96–8.
94. Bakker J, Gris P, Coffernils M, Khan R, Vincent JL. Serial blood lactate levels can predict the development of multiple organ failure. Am J Surg 1996;171: 221–6.
95. Toraman F, Evrenkaya S, Yuce M, et al. Lactic acidosis after cardiac surgery is associated with adverse outcome. Heart Surg Forum 2004;7: E155–9.
96. Davies AR, Bellomo R, Raman JS, Gutteridge GA, Buxton BF. High lactate predicts the failure of intraaortic balloon pumping after cardiac surgery. Ann Thorac Surg 2001;71:1415–20.
97. Dens J, Dubois C, Ector H, Desmet W, Janssens S. Survival of patients treated wit intra-aortic balloon counterpulsation for cardiogenic shock in a tertiary centre: variables correlated with death. Eur J Emerg Med 2003;10:213–8.
98. Mustafa I, Leverve XM. Metabolic and hemodynamic effects of hypertonic solutions: sodium-lactate versus sodium chloride infusion in postoperative patients. Shock 2002;18:306–10.
99. Levraut J, Ichai C, Petit I, Ciebiera JP, Perus O, Grimaud D. Low exogenous lactate clearance as an early predictor of mortality in normolactatemic critically ill patients. Crit Care Med 2003;31:705–10.
100. Leverve XM. Energy metabolism in critically ill patients: lactate is a major oxidizable substrate. Curr Opin Clin Nutr Metab Care 1999;2:165–9.
101. Stacpoole PW, Lorenz AC, Thomas RG, Harman EM. Dichloroacetate in the treatment of lactic acidosis. Ann Intern Med 1998;108:58–63.
102. Orchard C, Cingolani H. Acidosis and arrhythmias in cardiac muscle. Cardiovasc Res 1994;28: 1312–9.
103. Morimoto Y, Kemmotsu O, Alojado ES. Extracellular acidosis delays cell death against glucose-oxygen deprivation in neuroblastoma X glioma hybrid cells. Crit Care Med 1997;25:841–7.
104. Xu L, Glassford AJ, Giaccia AJ, Giffard RG. Acidosis reduces neuronal apoptosis. Neuroreport 1998; 9:875–9.
105. Mathieu D, Nevière R, Billard V, Fleyfel M, Wattel F. Effects of bicarbonate therapy on hemodynamics and tissue oxygenation in patients with lactic acidosis: a prospective, controlled clinical study. Crit Care Med 1991;1:1352–6.
106. Cooper DJ, Walley KR, Wiggs BR, Russel JA. Bicarbonate does not improve hemodynamics in critically ill patients who have lactic acidosis: a prospective, controlled clinical study. Ann Intern Med 1990;112:492–8.

71
Glucose Disturbance and Acute Heart Failure Syndrome

Dirk Vlasselaers and Greet Van den Berghe

Acute heart failure syndrome (AHFS) is a common clinical syndrome in the intensive care setting. It can be caused by primarily cardiac pathology such as acute coronary syndromes (ACSs), acute myocarditis, acute endocarditis with severe valvular insufficiency, and several other cardiac diseases. In the cardiac surgical intensive care unit, acute heart failure, eventually leading to cardiogenic shock, is a well-described problem, often referred to as postcardiotomy heart failure. Besides these single organ failure syndromes, acute or chronic heart failure is often part of the multiorgan failure syndrome and accompanies sepsis, septic shock, and the systemic inflammatory response syndrome. Each of these clinical entities has its proper causal and supportive therapy.

A common biochemical feature of these acute heart failure syndromes is the frequent occurrence of hyperglycemia (i.e., blood glucose above 110mg/dL). This type of hyperglycemia is traditionally described as a physiologic endocrine response of the human body to acute and chronic stress. Prolonged stress causes disturbances in glucose homeostasis, resulting in insulin resistance and hyperglycemia. These natural adaptive responses have always been interpreted as normal and beneficial. Admission to an intensive care unit (ICU) with AHFS is associated with both acute and chronic stress inflicted on the body. The associated hyperglycemia is often perceived as an adequate stress response reflecting the severity of the underlying disease or medical problem. Thus the sustained hyperglycemia is often left untreated, or treated only if blood glucose exceeds 200 to 220 mg/dL for several hours. For many years it has been known that in patients hospitalized for stroke (1) and acute myocardial infarction (2), this stress-induced hyperglycemia is associated with adverse outcome and increased hospital mortality. Nevertheless, very often this disturbance of blood glucose is left untreated or undertreated. Treating the elevations in blood glucose became a major therapeutic target in critically ill patients only in 2001, after a publication reported that tight glycemic control with intensive insulin therapy significantly reduced the risk of organ failure and death (3), and was brought into the spotlight again in 2006 after confirmation of the beneficial effects of tight glycemic control in medical ICU patients (4).

Hyperglycemia, Insulin, Myocardial Ischemia, and Reperfusion

Glucose–insulin–potassium (GIK) is thought to produce beneficial effects in the setting of myocardial ischemia and reperfusion. Increasing potassium flux inward in the myocardium reduces the risks of malignant arrhythmias. Optimizing substrate utilization in the ischemic myocardium by shifting from consumption of free fatty acids to anaerobic glycolysis theoretically reduces oxygen consumption and therefore could protect the vulnerable (post)ischemic myocardial cells by restoring the myocardial oxygen supply and consumption balance, resulting in improved ventricular contractility. Additional to the direct metabolic effects on glucose metabolism, more recently insulin has been assumed to be the primary component of GIK therapy by modulating intracellular survival pathways favoring cardioprotection (5) and by decreasing generation and accumulation of toxic free radicals in the ischemic myocardium.

Nearly half a century after the introduction of metabolic modulation with the GIK concept by Sodi-Pallares et al. (6) and after many studies and publications in different clinical and experimental settings of myocardial ischemia and reperfusion, the clinical role of GIK is still not determined. Both study design and scientific reasons are responsible for this matter still being in abeyance. Until recently, the accumulated data of randomized placebo-controlled studies of GIK therapy in acute myocardial infarction (AMI) are promising overall and suggest a reduction in hospital mortality, in particular with high-dose GIK treatment (7,8). Two recent large trials (9,10), however, could not confirm the beneficial effect of GIK therapy versus usual care on cardiac mortality and morbidity in AMI. Before drawing inappropriate conclusions about the futility of GIK therapy, one should consider the observation that persistent hyperglycemia (blood glucose >110 mg/dL) was present in all study groups and that the degree of improvement of glycemic control was minimal and maybe insufficient. A post hoc analysis of the tight glycemic control study in ICU patients indicated that it was the tight blood glucose control and not the amount of insulin administered that explained the mortality benefit of intensive insulin therapy in the population of ICU patients (11). Hence, avoiding toxic hyperglycemia, especially at the time of reperfusion and the beneficial action of insulin on intracellular survival pathways in the window of reperfusion are two important aspects to consider when interpreting the GIK studies and designing new studies.

Ischemic preconditioning is a well-known cardioproctective mechanism that can limit the myocardial infarct size in patients with a history of angina. In animal experiments, acute hyperglycemia in clinical relevant ranges has been shown to abolish the protective effects of ischemic preconditioning and to neutralize the favorable effects on myocardial infarct size, resulting in larger extent of myocardial infarction (12,13). The activity of the cardiac mitochondrial K_{ATP} channel, an important effector of endogenous cardioprotective signal transduction, is impaired by hyperglycemia, resulting in more extensive myocardial damage (14). Furthermore, high glucose upregulates inducible nitric oxide synthase (iNOS) gene expression and raises nitric oxide (NO) production and release, which together with increased superoxide generation may generate peroxynitrite that can induce cardiac cell apoptosis (15).

In addition to the role of glucose and the toxic effects of hyperglycemia in the setting of myocardial ischemia and reperfusion, insulin itself has, besides its blood glucose lowering effect, cardioprotective properties through activation of pro-survival kinases at the time of reperfusion of the ischemic myocardium. Reperfusion injury is characterized by reperfusion-induced myocyte loss beyond that evoked by ischemia per se, and is caused by apoptosis. Data from different experimental conditions have shown that insulin, administered at the time of reperfusion, attenuates the apoptotic processes, reduces the degree of apoptosis, and enhances myocardial cell viability (16–18). These antiapoptotic and prosurvival properties of insulin are mediated through phosphoinositide-3-kinase and Akt signaling. Finally, as shown in animal experiments, the cardioprotective properties of insulin, mediated by K_{ATP} channel activation, are abolished when hyperglycemia is present at the onset of ischemia (19).

Recommendations for Blood Glucose Management in the Setting of Acute Heart Failure Syndromes

These recommendations are partially based on the statements of the Diabetes in Hospitals Writing Committee of the American Diabetes Association as published in 2004 (20):

1. *Acute coronary syndrome:* In the setting of acute myocardial infarction (AMI) there is evidence for a blood glucose threshold for increased mortality in AMI. The meta-analysis by Capes et al. (2) and the Diabetes Mellitus, Insulin Glucose Infusion in Acute Myocardiol Infarction (DIGAMI-1) trial (21) point out that in nondiabetic and diabetic patients, the mortality risk in AMI patients increases with higher blood glucose values. Hyper-

glycemia, defined as blood glucose above 200 mg/dL, at admission was associated with a higher 1-year mortality rate compared to normoglycemia (44% versus 19.3%) (22). Finally, tight glycemic control in surgical and medical ICU patients has been shown to decrease mortality and morbidity (3,4). *Recommendation*: Based on the current data, we recommend avoiding hyperglycemia (fasting and random blood glucose: ≥126 and ≥200 mg/dL, respectively). Implementing tight glycemic control (target blood glucose: 80 to 110 mg/dL) in patients admitted to the cardiac ICU with diagnosis of AMI is strongly advocated.

2. *Cardiac surgery:* Cardiac surgical procedures are characterized by periods of myocardial ischemia and reperfusion during the operation. Many measures, such as cardioplegia and temperature management, are taken attempting to reduce the extent of myocardial damage caused by ischemia and reperfusion. Nevertheless, permanent or temporary myocardial dysfunction provoked by ischemia-reperfusion injury leading to myocardial infarction or stunning still threatens the postoperative course. In view of the experimental data, on the one hand, about the harmful and toxic effects of hyperglycemia and, on the other hand, the beneficial effects of insulin in the setting of myocardial ischemia-reperfusion injury, the encouraging results of studies applying perioperative glycemic control are not surprising. High peak serum glucose level during cardiopulmonary bypass is an independent risk factor for death and morbidity in diabetic and nondiabetic patients (23). Continuous insulin infusion to achieve perioperative normoglycemia in diabetic patients undergoing coronary artery bypass graft (CABG) eliminates the incremental increase in hospital mortality associated with CABG in diabetes patients and improves perioperative outcomes (24,25). In contrast with data indicating that lower glucose levels are beneficial in heart surgery patients, there are several studies showing improved outcomes in nondiabetic cardiac surgical patients receiving high-dose GIK infusions resulting in hyperglycemia (26,27). Although data support the use of GIK solutions during and after cardiac surgery to enhance myocardial performance, to decrease the need for inotropic support and to decrease the incidence of atrial fibrillation despite the occurrence of hyperglycemia, no prospective data are available comparing GIK therapy with or without tight glycemic control. *Recommendation*: Based on the current data, there is sufficient evidence that hyperglycemia is obsolete and should be avoided in diabetic patients undergoing cardiac surgery. Furthermore, there are indications that GIK therapy exerts beneficial properties in nondiabetic cardiac surgical patients. Whether GIK therapy combined with tight glycemic control is superior to tolerating hyperglycemia is unanswered, but in view of the current knowledge about the toxic effects of hyperglycemia and the beneficial action of insulin in attenuating reperfusion injury, we recommend aiming for normoglycemia.

3. *Postoperative cardiac surgery:* In a properly designed and large clinical study in surgical ICU patients with a majority of cardiac surgical patients, Van den Berghe et al. (3) reported that tight glycemic control (range: 80 to 110 mg/dL) with intensive insulin therapy significantly reduced mortality and morbidity (3). *Recommendation*: We strongly recommend implementing tight glycemic control (target blood glucose range: 80 to 110 mg/dL) with continuous insulin infusion in all adult patients admitted to the ICU after cardiac surgery.

4. *Critical care patients:* Hyperglycemia is a common feature in critically ill patients admitted to the ICU. Many of them suffer from multiorgan failure syndrome, and very often the cardiovascular system is involved, requiring inotropic and vasopressor support. Both landmark studies by Van den Berghe et al. (3,4) in surgical and medical ICU patients show a significant benefit of tight glycemic control with intensive insulin therapy. Krinsley (28) reported a similar beneficial effect of glycemic control on morbidity and mortality. *Recommendation*: Based on the current evidence provided by proper designed studies, we strongly advocate implementing tight glycemic control (target blood glucose range: 80 to 110 mg/dL) in all patients admitted to the ICU.

References

1. Capes SE, Hunt D, Malmberg K, et al. Stress hyperglycemia and prognosis of stroke in nondiabetic and diabetic patients: a systematic overview. Stroke 2001;32:2426–32.

2. Capes SE, Hunt D, Malmberg K, et al. Stress hyperglycaemia and increased risk of death after myocardial infarction in patients with and without diabetes: a systematic overview. Lancet 2000; 355:773–8.
3. Van den Berghe G, Wouters P, Weekers F, et al. Intensive insulin therapy in critically ill patients. N Engl J Med 2001;345:1359–67.
4. Van den Berghe G, Wilmer A, Hermans G, et al. Intensive insulin therapy of medical intensive care patients. N Engl J Med 2006;354:449–61.
5. Sack MN, Yellon DM. Insulin therapy as an adjunct to reperfusion after acute coronary ischemia. A proposed direct myocardial cell survival effect independent of metabolic modulation. J Am Coll Cardiol 2003;41:1404–7.
6. Sodi-Pallares D, Testelli MR, Fishleder BL, et al. Effects of an intravenous infusion of a potassium-glucose-insulin solution on the electrocardiographic signs of myocardial infarction. A preliminary clinical report. Am J Cardiol 1962;9: 166–81.
7. Fath-Ordoubadi F, Beat KJ. Glucose-insulin-potassium therapy for treatment of acute myocardial infarction. An overview of randomized placebo-controlled trials. Circulation 1997;96:1152–56.
8. Gnaim CI, McGuire DK. Glucose-insulin-potassium therapy for acute myocardial infarction: What goes around comes around. Am Heart J 2004;148: 924–30.
9. The CREATE-ECLA Trial Group Investigators. Effect of glucose-insulin-potassium infusion on mortality in patients with acute ST-segment elevation myocardial infarction. The CREATE-ECLA randomized controlled trial. JAMA 2005;293:437–46.
10. Malmberg K, Rydén L, Wedel H, et al. Intense metabolic control by means of insulin in patients with diabetes mellitus and acute myocardial infarction (DIGAMI 2): effects on mortality and morbidity. Eur Heart J 2005;26:650–61.
11. Van den Berghe G, Wouters PJ, Bouillon R, et al. Outcome benefit of intensive insulin therapy in the critically ill: insulin dose versus glycemic control. Crit Care Med 2003;31:359–66.
12. Kersten JR, Schmeling TJ, Orth KG, et al. Acute hyperglycemia abolishes ischemic preconditioning in vivo. Am J Physiol Heart Circ Physiol 1998;275: H721–5.
13. Kersten JR, Toller WG, Gross ER, et al. Diabetes abolishes ischemic preconditioning: role of glucose, insulin, and osmolality. Am J Physiol Heart Circ Physiol 2000;278:H1218–24.
14. Kersten JR, Montgomery MW, Ghassemi T, et al. Diabetes and hyperglycemia impair activation of mitochondrial K_{ATP} channels. Am J Physiol Heart Circ Physiol 2001;280:H1744–50.
15. Ceriello A, Quagliaro L, D'Amico M, et al. Acute hyperglycemia induces nitrotyrosine formation and apoptosis in perfused heart from rat. Diabetes 2002;51:1076–82.
16. Jonassen AK, Brar BK, Mjøs OD, et al. Insulin administered at reoxygenation exerts a cardioprotective effect in myocytes by a possible anti-apoptotic mechanism. J Mol Cell Cardiol 2000;32: 757–64.
17. Jonassen AK, Sack MN, Mjøs OD, et al. Myocardial protection by insulin at reperfusion requires early administration and is mediated via Akt and p70s6 kinase cell-survival signaling. Circ Res 2001;89: 1191–8.
18. Gao F, Gao E, Yue T-L, et al. Nitric oxide mediates the antiapoptotic effect of insulin in myocardial ischemia-reperfusion. The roles of P13-kinase, Akt and endothelial Nitric Oxide Synthase phosphorylation. Circulation 2002;105:1497–1502.
19. LaDisa JF, Krolikowski JG, Pagel PS, et al. Cardioprotection by glucose-insulin-potassium: dependence on K_{ATP} channel opening and blood glucose concentration before ischemia. Am J Physiol Heart Circ Physiol 2004;287:H601–7.
20. Clement S, Braithwaite SS, Magee MF, et al. Management of diabetes and hyperglycemia in hospitals. Diabetes Care 2004;27:553–91.
21. Malmberg K. Prospective randomised study of intensive insulin treatment on long term survival after acute myocardial infarction in patients with diabetes mellitus. BMJ 1997;314:1512–5.
22. Bolk J, van der Ploeg T, Cornel JH, et al. Impaired glucose metabolism predicts mortality after a myocardial infarction. Int J Cardiol 2001;79:207–14.
23. Doenst T, Wijeysundera D, Karkouti K, et al. Hyperglycemia during cardiopulmonary bypass is an independent risk factor for mortality in patients undergoing cardiac surgery. J Thorac Cardiovasc Surg 2005;130:1144–50.
24. Furnary AP, Gao G, Grunkemeier GL, et al. Continuous insulin infusion reduces mortality in patients with diabetes undergoing coronary artery bypass grafting. J Thorac Cardiovasc Surg 2003; 125:1007–21.
25. Lazar HL, Chipkin SR, Fitzgerald CA, et al. Tight glycemic control in diabetic coronary artery bypass graft patients improves perioperative outcomes and decreases recurrent ischemic events. Circulation 2004;109:1497–1502.

26. Bothe W, Olschewski M, Beyersdorf F, et al. Glucose-insulin-potassium in cardiac surgery: a meta-analysis. Ann Thorac Surg 2004;78:1650–8.
27. Quinn DW, Pagano D, Bonser RS, et al. Improved myocardial protection during coronary artery surgery with glucose-insulin-potassium: a randomized controlled trial. J Thorac Cardiovasc Surg 2006;131:34–42.
28. Krinsley JS. Effect of an intensive glucose management protocol on the mortality of critically ill adult patients. Mayo Clin Proc 2004;79:992–1000.

72
Hyponatremia in the Setting of Acute Heart Failure Syndrome

Carole Ichai and Diane Lena

Hyponatremia is usually defined as a decrease in plasma sodium to a level ≤135 mEq/L. It is the most frequent electrolyte disorder occurring in hospitalized patients.[1–3] Its actual incidence depends on the defined level of hyponatremia: 20% for natremia ≤136 mEq/L and 1% to 4% for natremia <130 mEq/L. This chapter discusses the pathophysiology, diagnosis and principles of treatment of hyponatremia, and suggests specific considerations for hyponatremia occurring in patients with heart failure.

Hyponatremia: General Considerations

Pathophysiology

Cell Volume: Osmolarities

Total body water (TBW) represents in an adult 50% to 70% of body weight, which is distributed in two compartments[4–7]:

- Intracellular fluid compartment (ICF), which represents two thirds of TBW, that is, 40% to 50% of body weight, a high concentration of potassium, and a low concentration of sodium.
- Extracellular fluid compartment (ECF), which represents the remaining third of TBW, that is, 20% to 25% of body weight. The ECF is subdivided in two other volumes: (1) plasma volume or effective volemia corresponds to water circulating in vessels, that is, about 5% of TBW with a high sodium and proteins contents; (2) the interstitial compartment equals 10% to 20% of TBW, and its ion concentration is very close to plasma volume, except for proteins, which are normally absent (Gibbs-Donan equilibrium).

The movement of water between interstitial and plasma volume depends on both hydrostatic and oncotic pressures. Water freely crosses the semipermeable cell membrane. Consequently, under steady-state conditions transcellular movements of water are passive and the concentration of particles in the ECF and the ICF is identical. Water shifts between ECF and ICF depends on the osmotic gradient between these two compartments. According to their ability for distribution among cell membrane, two types of solute particles are present:

- Ineffective or diffusive osmoles (e.g., urea, methanol, ethanol, ethylene glycol) are readily permeable to cell membranes. They do not create any osmotic gradient and consequently no movement of water between ECF and ICF.
- Effective or active osmoles are impermeable to cell membrane. Their accumulation in ICF or ECF leads to an osmotic gradient, and therefore obligates the movement of water until reaching the same osmotic forces between both compartments. In this way, an increase in ECF particle concentration such as sodium, glucose, mannitol, or glycerol is responsible for a movement of water from the ICF to the ECF, that is, intracellular dehydration.

Based on these physiologic principles, three types of plasma osmolarities are defined:

- Plasma osmolality is defined by the concentration of all solutes per kilogram of plasma water (mOsm/kg). It is measured directly by an osmometer (delta cryoscopic).
- Plasma osmolarity is defined by the concentration of all solutes per liter of plasma (mOsm/L). As sodium, glucose, and urea are the major osmotic particles of ECF, it can be easily calculated at bedside using the following formula: (Sodium × 2) + Glucose + Urea (mEq/L) = 280 to 295 mOsm/L.
- Plasma tonicity is defined by the concentration of effective osmoles alone per liter of plasma (mOsm/L). As urea is the only substantial ineffective osmole in the plasma, it is not taken into account for the calculation of plasma tonicity, which is as follow: (Sodium × 2) + Glucose (mEq/L) = 275 to 290 mOsm/L.

In most situations, plasma osmolality and osmolarity are close because 1 L of plasma contains 93% of water, the remaining 7% being constituted by proteins and lipids. Only severe hyperprotidemia or hyperlipidemia can lead to subsequent differences between plasma osmolarity and osmolality. If nonionic abnormal solutes accumulate in the plasma (methanol, ethanol, ethylene glycol, mannitol), measured plasma osmolality will largely exceed calculated plasma osmolarity, leading to a high osmolar gap (>12 mOsm/L). This parameter is clinically useful to detect the presence of such toxic substances.

Regulation of Water Balance

Water intake and excretion vary largely during the day. However, ICF and electrolytes concentrations remain unchanged thanks to an equilibrium in the water balance (Fig. 72.1). The regulation of water balance depends especially on two major mechanisms: arginine vasopressin (AVP) secretion and thirst.[4–9]

Regulation of Arginine Vasopressin Secretion

Arginine vasopressin or antidiuretic hormone (ADH) is synthesized by the supraoptic and paraventricular nuclei of hypothalamus. Osmoreceptors are stimulated by several factors (Fig. 72.2):

- Osmotic stimulus: Hypothalamic receptors are highly sensitive to changes in plasma tonicity. This is the most powerful stimulus, because only 1% of the change in plasma tonicity induces AVP release. Plasma hypertonicity stimulates the release of AVP and vice versa. When plasma tonicity range between 280 and 295 mOsm/L, the release of AVP is linearly related to the increase in plasma tonicity. At a plasma tonicity less than 280 mOsm/L, plasma AVP concentration is undetectable. Above 295 mOsm/L, despite the elevation of plasma AVP concentration, urine reaches its maximal concentration (1200 mOsm/L).
- Nonosmotic stimulus: Hypovolemia and arterial hypotension stimulate the release of AVP

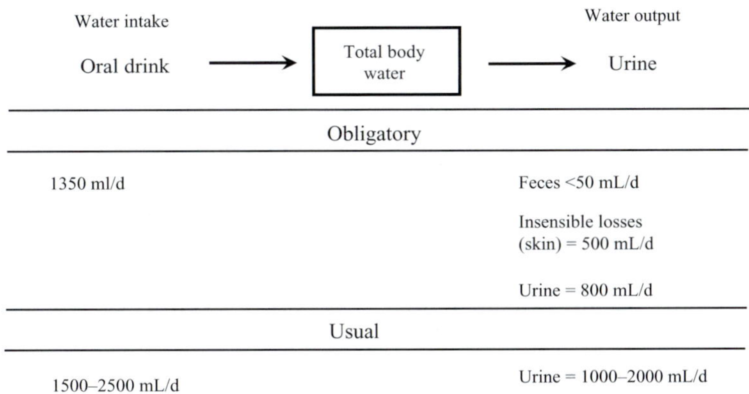

FIGURE 72.1. Water balance (standard intake of 70 g of proteins and 4 g of sodium per day).

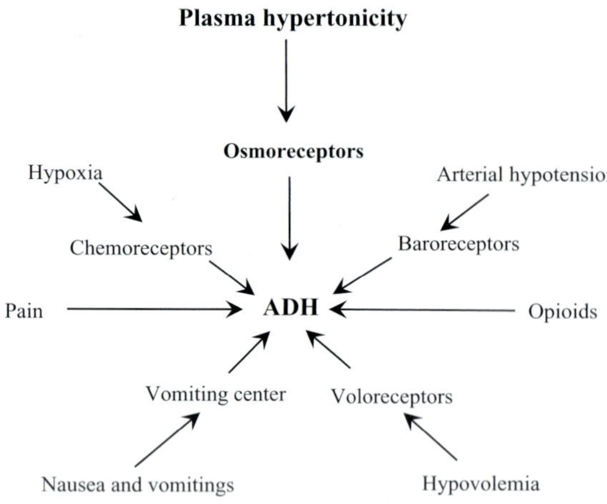

Figure 72.2. Major factors responsible for antidiuretic hormone (ADH) release.

via volo- and baroreceptors. Activation of these receptors is less sensitive than osmoreceptors, as they require at least a reduction of 8% to 10% of the ECF volume. The release of AVP may be activated by a variety of other stimuli: nausea and vomiting, pain, opioids, and hypoxia.

The effects of AVP result from the activation of four types of receptors: V1a, V1b (or V3), V2, and V4[5,10–14]:

- V1a receptors are located on vascular smooth muscles, myocardium, hepatocytes, and platelets. Their activation, which is cyclic adenosine monophosphate (cAMP)-mediated phosphorylation, results in vasoconstriction, glycogenolysis in the liver, and platelet aggregation. They also have a positive inotropic effect and promote myocyte hypertrophy.
- V1b receptors are found in the anterior pituitary, and they activate the release of adrenocorticotropin via a phosphoinositide pathway.
- V2 receptors are located in the collecting duct cells. They mediate renal water retention by the kidney and are predominantly responsible for the antidiuretic effect of AVP. Binding of AVP on V2 receptors activates adenylate cyclase, which stimulates cAMP, resulting finally in the release of protein kinase. This latter induces the translocation of aquaporins (water channels) from intracellular vesicles to the apical membrane, thereby allowing water retention.
- V4 receptors are present in the glial cell membranes. They contribute to the activation of aquaporin-4 water channel in the brain and could have a role in the development of brain edema.

Regulation of Thirst

Thirst is targeted by plasma hypertonicity, hypovolemia, and arterial hypotension,[4–7] and is suppressed by hypotonicity and hypervolemia. Thirst is mediated by osmoreceptors, which are located in the hypothalamus, but distinct from those responsible of AVP release. The osmotic threshold for thirst is greater than AVP (290 to 295 mOsm/L).

Cerebral Osmoregulation

Because it is contained in a rigid skull, the brain is particularly vulnerable to osmotic shift. Thus, plasma hypotonicity may be responsible for cerebral swelling and thereby for intracranial hypertension. Fortunately, the brain is not a perfect osmometer, and it is able to regulate its volume. This phenomenon, so-called cerebral osmoregulation, is mediated by modifications in the cerebral content of intracellular osmotically active particles.[15–18] Two types of such protective osmoles are involved in this mechanism:

- Inorganic osmoles are electrolytes (sodium, potassium, chloride)
- Organic osmolytes or idiogenic osmoles are essentially represented by amino acids, polyols, and triethylamines.

The efficacy of cerebral osmoregulation depends on the rapidity of the development of tonicity variation. In fact, cellular loss of electrolytes occurs in response to acute hypotonicity. It begins in the first hour by sodium extrusion and persists for 24 hours aided by potassium extrusion. The delayed response to chronic hypotonicity is characterized by a decrease in intracellular organic osmolyte content. Acute osmoregulation due to changes in electrolytes content is very rapid but not complete, so that the osmotic gradient is only attenuated and moderate changes in cerebral volume appear. In cases of chronic changes in plasma tonicity, the modifications of organic osmolytes permit obtaining an osmotic equilibrium between ECF and ICF, and thus avoiding modifications in cerebral volume. Converse phenomenon develops in case of plasma hypertonicity. Beside the rapidity of variation in tonicity, gender may influence the efficacy of cerebral osmoregulation. Estrogen and progesterone, which inhibit the activity of NA-K-adenosine triphosphatase (ATPase), reduce the cerebral volume regulation. Thus, menstruating women have a higher risk of brain damage during hyponatremia.[18–22] Hypoxia, by the same mechanism, alters cerebral osmoregulation and must be considered a risk factor of brain injury during variations of plasma tonicity.

Classification and Treatment of Hyponatremia

Hyponatremia may be present with normal, decreased, or increased osmolality. Thus according to plasma tonicity, hyponatremia may be associated with normal ICF, intracellular dehydration, or hyperhydration.

Hyponatremia with Normal or Increased Plasma Osmolality

Both severe hyperprotidemia and hyperlipidemia may coexist with hyponatremia. As sodium is only dissolved in this aqueous phase, the sodium concentration measured per liter of plasma will be low, but normal if measured per liter of plasma water. These factitious hyponatremias are isotonic and have no effect on ICF volume.[4–7,23] Hyperglycemia creates plasma hypertonicity and thereby water shift from ICF to ECF. This movement is responsible for both ICF dehydration and a dilutional hyponatremia in ECF. In this situation, hyponatremia accompanies plasma hypertonicity.[4–7,23] Such hypertonic hyponatremia is also reported with hypertonic mannitol treatments.

Hypotonic Hyponatremia

Diagnosis and Classification

Only hypotonic hyponatremia induces intracellular hyperhydration. The first step is to evaluate the severity of the trouble, which determines the therapeutic management and the prognosis.[4–7,24] Classically, the degree of severity of hyponatremia was based on the value of sodium concentration; severe hyponatremia is defined by a plasma sodium concentration <110 to 120 mEq/L. However, more than an absolute value, severity of hyponatremia depends on the efficacy of cerebral volume regulation, that is, the rapidity of development of hyponatremia, gender, and age. Although hyponatremia is also often classified as acute or chronic, it is more clinically relevant to distinguish symptomatic from asymptomatic hyponatremia. Indeed, the severity of hyponatremic encephalopathy reflects the severity of cerebral edema, which is the result of the individual efficacy of cerebral osmoregulation. Neurologic symptoms are not specific and variable.

Sodium concentration is the primary determinant of ICF volume, whereas total body sodium content determines ECF volume. Therefore, plasma tonicity may vary independently of ECF volume, and hyponatremia may develop with a normal, increased, or decreased ECF volume. This classification is the second step in diagnosing the cause of hyponatremia (Table 72.1).

Principles of Nonspecific Treatment

Whatever the cause, the actual management of hyponatremia is based on the absence or presence and severity of neurologic symptoms. This enables deciding between a passive, slow treatment and an active, rapid one. This decision must be made because an inappropriate rate (too rapid or not rapid enough) of correction of sodium concentration may lead to the death of the patient. In cases of severe symptomatic hyponatremia, brain death resulting from cerebral edema may occur if natremia does not rapidly reach a safe level. In contrast, a rapid correction of asymptomatic hyponatremia may be responsible for severe brain damage, for example, osmotic demyelination lesions. Central pontine and extrapontine myelinolysis is the classic severe complication of a rapid correction of hyponatremia.[4,11,12,25–28] This syndrome appears after an initial improvement of the patient followed by a free period of some days. Finally, at days 4 to 7, the neurologic status of the patient worsens progressively. Manifestations are

Table 72.1. Major causes of hypotonic hyponatremia according to the variation of the extracellular fluid volume

Euvolemia	Hypervolemia	Hypovolemia
Water retention	Water and Na^+ retention	Water and Na^+ losses
Syndrome of inappropriate ADH secretion (SIADH)	Natriuresis >20 mEq/L	Natriuresis >20 mEq/L
Potomania	Oliguric acute renal failure	Renal losses:
Endocrinologic illnesses:	Iatrogenous causes:	Renal salt wasting
Adrenal insufficiency	Abundant infusions of hypotonic solutions	Hypoaldosteronism
Hypothyroidism	Natriuresis <20 mEq/L	Loop diuretics (furosemide)
Thiazides	Edema states: congestive heart failure, cirrhosis, nephrotic syndrome, sepsis	Cerebral salt wasting
		Natriuresis <20 mEq/L
	Severe denutrition	Gastrointestinal losses :
	Pregnancy	Vomiting, diarrhea, gastrointestinal fistulas or suctioning
		Skin losses
		Burns

variable, beginning with a simple stupor, but the evolution is often severe, characterized by a pseudobulbar paralysis, dysphagia, dysarthria, quadriparesis, locked-in syndrome, or death. All of these complications must be prevented by treatment (Fig. 72.3). Symptomatic hyponatremia requires an active therapeutic intervention with hypertonic saline solution associated if necessary with the treatment of vital function. The rate of increase in sodium concentration must be rapid (4 to 5 mEq/L/h) until neurologic signs disappear, and slower in the following hours. Infusion of hypertonic saline should be discontinued when natremia achieves 130 mEq/L to avoid a rebound effect.[9,12,25–30] Intravenous furosemide may be added, but is never sufficient alone. Repeated clinical examinations and electrolytes concentration determinations are always necessary. Water restriction combined with a loop diuretic is usually sufficient to treat asymptomatic hyponatremia.

Hyponatremia During Heart Failure

Pathophysiological Mechanisms

Hyponatremia as a Consequence of Heart Failure

The pathophysiologic mechanisms of heart failure (HF) are complex. Heart failure is usually characterized by decreased cardiac output associated with impaired left ventricular function and decreased arterial pressure. These modifications lead to the compensatory activation of vasoactive neurohormonal systems including the sympa-

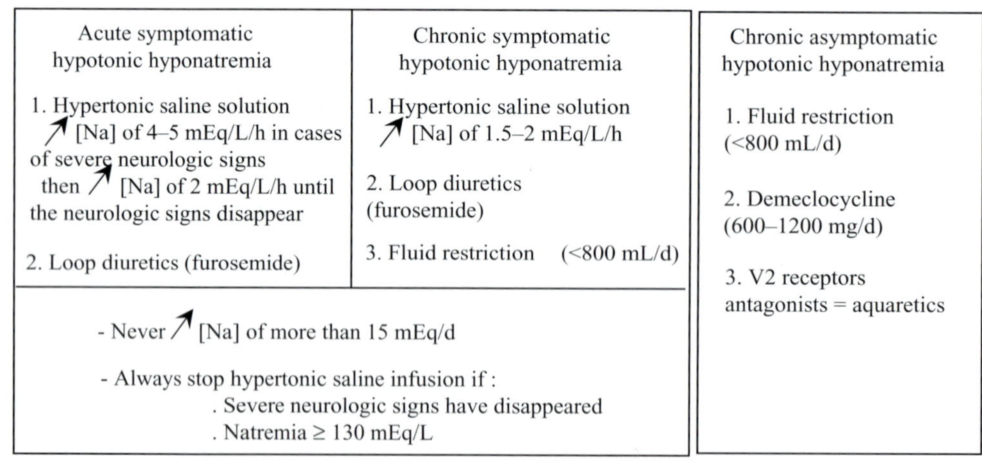

Figure 72.3. General principles of treatment of hypotonic hyponatremia according to their severity.

thetic nervous system, the renin-angiotensin-aldosterone system (RAAS), and the AVP hormone.[30–36] All of them may initially help to maintain blood flow to vital organs. However, in both acute and chronic situations, these systems lead finally to adverse effects and to the development of a vicious circle. The activation of RAAS induces vasoconstriction, sodium and water renal retention, and AVP overproduction. In addition to these classic effects, RAAS produces inflammatory reactions (cytokines production) and remodeling processes, which aggravate myocardial hypertrophy and cell apoptosis. The nonosmotic AVP secretion during HF seems to play a major role in the pathogenesis and severity of HF.[18,34–37] Indeed, AVP aggravates the progression of HF by several mechanisms. The V1 receptor activation could induce vasoconstriction and lead to increase left ventricular afterload and cardiac remodeling. The V2 receptors stimulation could also induce volume expansion and increase cardiac preload. Plasma AVP levels are inappropriately high in both acute and chronic HF.[30–42] Moreover, AVP levels seem to be related to the severity of HF.

Hyponatremia during HF is mostly due to the excessive AVP secretion resulting from nonosmotic stimulation. AVP secretion increases from free-water absorption, leading to a hypervolemic hyponatremia.[4–7,12]

Hyponatremia as a Consequence of Diuretic Treatments

Even though they are widely prescribed, the use of diuretics in patients with HF remains debated.[43] Diuretic therapy has a large number of side effects, including worsening renal function and electrolyte disturbances.[44,45] Among them, thiazides are the most often implicated in the occurrence of hyponatremia.[45–49] Sonnenblick et al.[50] have found that diuretic-induced hyponatremia was related in 73% of cases to thiazides, but only in 6% and 1% of cases, respectively, to furosemide and spironolactone. Thiazides act by blocking sodium chloride cotransport in the distal convoluted tubule, which is the major site for diluting urine. Loop diuretics may also impair free-water clearance on the loop site, but to a lesser extent. Thiazide-induced hyponatremia usually appears 2 weeks after initiation of treatment, whereas it develops after a longer delay with furosemide. Hyponatremia occurs preferentially in women (80% of cases) and in elderly patients.[45,46,50,51] In this situation, hyponatremia may cause severe neurologic symptoms and severe brain damages. Consequently, thiazides in elderly women should be used with great caution and a close sodium level monitoring.

Hyponatremia: A Risk Factor During Heart Failure

Hyponatremia occurs approximately in 5% of patients with HF.[33] The relationship between hyponatremia and the importance of neurohormonal disturbances support the fact that hyponatremia is a marker of the severity of HF. However, several studies demonstrated that hyponatremia is an independent factor of poor prognosis in patients with HF.[52–56] Hyponatremia has been found to be a predictor of 30-day and 1-year mortality in patients hospitalized for congestive heart failure (CHF).[52] Hyponatremia is also an independent factor of readmission in hospital, and of major complications.[52–56] Klein et al.[56] have shown that hyponatremia was associated with a higher number of days hospitalized for cardiovascular causes and a twofold higher in-hospital and 60-day mortality. Interestingly, the improvement in sodium level during hospitalization was associated with an improved postdischarge mortality. Finally, hyponatremia in HF may interact with the administration of diuretics.[46]

Hyponatremia and Heart Failure: Treatment

General principles of treatment of hyponatremia are the same in HF. However, most of the conventional treatments of HF may induce or aggravate hyponatremia, and most of the treatments of hyponatremia may worsen HF. Thus, correction of hyponatremia in HF is more complicated than in other situations.

Conventional Treatments

Fluid Restriction

The restriction of water intake remains the first nonaggressive treatment of asymptomatic hypervolemic hyponatremia.[4–7,12,25] However, its efficacy to increase natremia is limited: a fluid intake <80 mL/d increases natremia by only 1 to 2 mEq/L.[9] Thus, this therapy is not appropriate in severe symptomatic hyponatremia. Moreover, adherence to strict fluid restriction is often difficult because of the obligatory fluid infusions in hospitalized patients. Thirst and decrease in blood volume, which are aggravated by diuretics, make this therapy difficult in chronic patients too.

Hypertonic Saline Solutions

Hypertonic saline intravenous infusion remains the best treatment of severe symptomatic hyponatremia. However, beside the previous risk of osmotic demyelination, this treatment could be poorly tolerated in patients with CHF. Indeed, hypertonic saline solutions, by increasing the ECF volume, could precipitate pulmonary edema. If necessary, this therapy must be cautiously administered in association with diuretics and controlled by a strict hemodynamic monitoring. A recent randomized study conducted in 1047 patients with a refractory CHF has compared one group receiving high-dose furosemide alone with another one receiving the same dose of furosemide associated with a small infusion of hypertonic saline.[57,58] The study found that serum sodium levels were corrected only in the group receiving hypertonic saline infusion. Interestingly, the survival rate during a 4-year follow-up period was 55% and 13%, respectively, in the group treated with hypertonic saline and the group treated with furosemide alone. This result strongly supports hyponatremia as an independent risk factor in CHF.

Diuretics

Diuretic therapy represents an essential treatment of CHF. But diuretics are responsible for many electrolyte disorders, especially hyponatremia. Thiazides must be stopped in cases of acute hyponatremia. Loop diuretics, even possibly inducing hyponatremia, may be combined with hypertonic saline infusion if necessary. Other diuretics aside from thiazides do not often lead to severe hyponatremia, which is precipitated by other factors such as a prolonged sodium intake restriction, thirst, hypovolemia, and AVP secretion.

Hemofiltration and Ultrafiltration

Hemofiltration and ultrafiltration offer some substantial advantages in treating acute and chronic CHF. These techniques enable an appropriate fluid regulation, permitting obtaining large losses from the ECF while maintaining the effective circulating volume.[58–63] Because of isotonic losses, these techniques also enable correcting electrolytes disturbances in a safe way, especially hyponatremia. Several studies have confirmed the beneficial effects of hemofiltration in patients with acute HF resistant to diuretics: persistent weight loss, improvement in renal function and diuresis, and correction of hyponatremia.[58–63] If continuous hemofiltration is the most appropriate technique in acute patients, intermittent ultrafiltration could be efficient in less severe patients with CHF.

Vasopressin Antagonists

Considering the pathophysiology of CHF, vasopressin antagonists appear as theoretical appropriate molecules. Several nonpeptide vasopressin receptors antagonists, so-called vaptan, have been developed. Their action depends on their relative selectivity for the different vasopressin receptors subtypes. Blockade of the V1a receptor induces vasodilation, and decrease in systemic vascular resistance, which may improve cardiac and renal hemodynamic. To date, for pharmaceutical reasons, no clinical study has been performed with such antagonists. In contrast to salidiuretics, V2 receptor antagonists, "aquaresis," induce diuresis (positive free-water clearance) without any change in electrolytes. Moreover, by decreasing preload, they do not activate the RAAS. Unlike conventional diuretic treatments with their side effects and their limited efficacy, vasopressin antagonists seem to offer prolonged efficacy without worsening HF.[1,39]

V2 Antagonists

Tolvaptan, an oral specific and selective V2 receptor antagonist, has been studied in two large controlled trials in patients with CHF.[64–66] The first double-blind trial was conducted in 221 patients with moderate CHF. Three doses of daily tolvaptan for 25 days were compared to the usual treatment.[64] A significant decrease in edema, body weight, increase in diuresis, and correction of hyponatremia were found in all patients receiving tolvaptan. These beneficial effects were observed from day 1 and persisted in the following days. No severe side effect related to tolvaptan was observed. The second trial was performed using a similar methodology, but including more severe patients presenting an acute CHF with clinical congestion and a left ventricular fraction <40%.[66] Two doses of intravenous tolvaptan were administered in addition to standard therapy for 60 days. The same beneficial effects were found and a trend toward a lower mortality was observed.

Combined V1a/V2 Antagonists

Conivaptan has been evaluated in humans by intravenous administration. Udelson et al.[67] compared the effect of two single intravenous doses of conivaptan versus placebo in 142 patients with advanced CHF. They found that conivaptan significantly reduced pulmonary wedge pressure and right atrial pressure at 3 and 6 hours after administration, without any effect on cardiac index, systemic vascular resistance, and blood pressure. Moreover, diuresis increased during the first 4 hours in a dose-dependent manner.

Association of Vasopressin Antagonists and Other Treatments

As both AVP and RAAS are involved in the pathophysiology of CHF and hyponatremia, coadministration of AVP antagonists and angiotensin-converting enzyme inhibitor could induce an effective management of vasoconstriction while treating overload and hyponatremia. An experimental randomized trial has confirmed that the administration of conivaptan alone significantly decreases body weight, whereas a combination of conivaptan and captopril decrease blood pressure, natriuretic peptide level, and ventricular mass.[68]

Gheorghiade et al.[69], in a recent randomized controlled trial, compared the efficacy of fluid restriction with or without the addition of tolvaptan to treat hyponatremia in euvolemic or hypervolemic states. A significant increase in serum sodium level was observed rapidly, 4 hours after the first dose of tolvaptan. In both groups, the increase in natremia reached a plateau at day 5, but it was higher with tolvaptan (+5.2 ± 4.5 vs. +1 ± 4.7 mEq/L, $p = .019$). Correction of hyponatremia was associated with a significant increase in urine output and positive free-water clearance, but no change in body weight.

Conclusion

Hyponatremia mostly occurs as a consequence of neurohormonal activation during CHF. High AVP levels and RAAS activation usually lead to a hypervolemic asymptomatic hyponatremia. Diuretic treatments, especially thiazides, may induce severe euvolemic or hypovolemic hyponatremia in patients at risk, such as elderly women. Rules and risks of the treatment of hyponatremia are the same whatever the cause. Hypertonic saline infusion is necessary in severe symptomatic disorder to avoid brain edema. A slow increase in serum sodium level is recommended in asymptomatic hyponatremia to prevent central nervous myelinolysis.

Hyponatremia occurring during HF represents not only a marker of severity, but also an independent factor of poor prognosis. Thus, correction of hyponatremia is widely recommended, but it represents a real challenge. Indeed, conventional treatments of HF have some limitations due to a possible worsening of hyponatremia and vice versa. The new molecules, AVP antagonists, which act as aquaretic agents, could be the most appropriate treatment in the future, and recent clinical data are promising.

References

1. De Luca L, Klein L, Udelson JE, et al. Hyponatremia in patients with heart failure. Am J Cardiol 2005; 96(suppl):19L–23L.
2. Anderson RJ, Chung H, Kluge R, Schrier RW. Hyponatremia: a prospective analysis of its epidemiology and the pathogenic role of vasopressin. Ann Intern Med 1985;102:164–8.
3. Anderson RJ. Hospital-associated hyponatremia. Kidney Int 1986;29:1237–47.
4. Adrogue HJ, Madias NE. Hyponatremia. N Engl J Med 2000;342:1581–9.
5. Gennari FJ. Hypo- and hypernatremia: disorders of water balance. In: AM Davidson, JS Cameron, JP

Grünfeld, DN Ken, E Ritz, CG Winearls, eds. Oxford Textbook of Clinical Nephrology. Oxford: Oxford University Press, 1998:175–200.
6. Kumar S, Berl T. Sodium. Lancet 1998;352:220–8.
7. Sterns RH, Schrier RW, Narins RG. Hyponatremia: physiopathology, diagnosis and therapy. In: Narins RG, ed. Clinical Disorders of Fluid and Electrolyte Metabolism. New York: McGraw-Hill, 1994:583–613.
8. Zerbe R, Robertson GL. Osmotic and non osmotic regulation of thirst and vasopressin secretion. In: Narins RG, ed. Clinical Disorders of Fluid and Electrolyte Metabolism. New York: McGraw-Hill, 1994:81–100.
9. Fraser CL, Arieff AI. Epidemiology, pathophysiology and management of hyponatremic encephalopathy. Am J Med 1997;102:67–77.
10. Preston GM, Carroll TP, Guggino WB, Agre P. Appearance of water channels in Xenopus oocytes expressing red cell CHIP28 protein. Science 1992; 256:385–7.
11. Cadnapaphornchai MA, Schrier RW. Pathogenesis and management of hyponatremia. Am J Med 2000; 109:688–92.
12. Adrogue HJ. Consequences of inadequate management of hyponatremia. Am J Nephrol 2005;25: 240–9.
13. Goldsmith SR. Current treatments and novel pharmacologic treatments for hyponatremia in congestive heart failure. Am J Cardiol 2005;95(suppl): 14B–23B.
14. Nielsen S, Kwon TH, Christensen BM, Promeneur D, Froklaer J, Marples D. Physiology and pathophysiology of renal aquaporins. J Am Soc Nephrol 1999;10:647–63.
15. Ichai C, Fenouil E, Grimaud D. Osmolalité et cerveau. Ann Fr Anesth Réanim 1994;13:68–79.
16. Melton JE, Patlak CS, Pettigrew KD, Cserr HF. Volume regulatory loss of Na, Cl and K from rat brain during acute hyponatremia. Am J Physiol 1987;252:F661–9.
17. Trachman H. Cell volume regulation: a review of cerebral adaptation mechanisms and implications for clinical treatment of osmolal disturbances: II. Pediatr Nephrol 1992;6:104–12.
18. Fraser CL, Swanson RA. Female sex hormones inhibit volume regulation in rat brain astrocyte culture. Am J Physiol 1994;267:C909–14.
19. Ayus JC, Arieff AI. Brain damage and postoperative hyponatremia: the role of gender. Neurology 1996;46:323–8.
20. Ayus JC, Arieff AI. Chronic hyponatremic encephalopathy in postmenopausal women: association of therapies with morbidity and mortality. JAMA 1999;281:2299–304.
21. Arieff AI, Kozniewska E, Roberts TP, Vexler ZS, Ayus JC, Kucharczyk J. Age, gender and vasopressin affect survival and brain adaptation in rats with metabolic encephalopathy. Am J Physiol 1995;268: R1143–52.
22. Arieff AI. Hyponatremia, convulsions, respiratory arrest, and permanent brain damage after elective surgery in healthy women. N Engl J Med 1986; 314:1529–35.
23. Yeates KE, Singer M, Morton AR. Salt and water: a simple approach to hyponatremia. Can Med Assoc J 2004;170:365–9.
24. Verbalis JG. Hyponatremia and hypoosmolar disorders. In: A Greenberg, ed. Primer on Kidney Diseases. San Diego: Academic Press, 1998:57–63.
25. Han DS, Chu BS. Therapeutic approach to hyponatremia. Nephron 2002;92(suppl):9–13.
26. Ellis SJ. Severe hyponatraemia: complications and treatment. Q J Med 1995;88:905–9.
27. Laureno R, Karp BI. Myelinolysis after correction of hyponatremia. Ann Intern Med 1997;126:57–62.
28. Decaux G, Soupart A. Treatment of symptomatic hyponatremia. Am J Med Sci 2003;326:25–30.
29. Sterns RH. Severe symptomatic hyponatremia: treatment and outcome. A study of 64 cases. Ann Intern Med 1987;107:656–64.
30. Lauriat SM, Berl T. The hyponatremic patient: practical focus on therapy. J Am Soc Nephrol 1998;8:1599–607.
31. Thibonnier M. Vasopressin receptors antagonists in heart failure. Curr Opin Pharmacol 2003;3: 683–7.
32. Jessup M, Brozena S. Heart failure. N Engl J Med 2003, 348:2007–18.
33. Oren RM. Hyponatremia in congestive heart failure. Am J Cardiol 2005;95(suppl):2B–7B.
34. DeLuca L, Orlandi C, Udelson JE, Fedele F, Gheorghiade M. Overview of vasopressor receptor antagonists in heart failure resulting in hospitalization. Am J Cardiol 2005;96(suppl):24L–33L.
35. Goldsmith SR. Congestive heart failure: potential role of arginine vasopressin antagonists in the therapy of heart failure. Congest Heart Fail 2002;8: 251–6.
36. Goldsmith SR, Francis GS, Cowley AW, Levine TB, Cohn JN. Increased plasma arginine vasopressin levels in patients with congestive heart failure. J Am Coll Cardiol 1983;1:1385–90.
37. Chatterjee K. Neurohormonal activation in congestive heart failure and the role of vasopressin? Am J Cardiol 2005;95(suppl):8B–13B.
38. Lee CR, Watkins ML, Patterson JH, et al. Vasopressin: a new target for the treatment of heart failure. Am Heart J 2003;146:9–18.

39. Goldsmith SR, Gheorghiade M. Vasopressin antagonism in heart failure. J Am Coll Cardiol 2005;46:1785–91.
40. Francis GS, Benedicte C, Johnstone DE, et al. Comparison of neuroendocrine activation in patients with left ventricular dysfunction with and without congestive heart failure. A substudy of the Studies of Left Ventricular Dysfunction (SOLVD). Circulation 1990;82:1274–9.
41. Rouleau JL, Packer M, Moye L, et al. Prognostic value of neurohumoral activation in patients with an acute myocardial infarction: effect of captopril. J Am Coll Cardiol 1994;24:583–91.
42. Swedberg K, Eneroth P, Kjekshus J, Wilhelmsen L. Hormones regulating cardiovascular function in patients with severe congestive heart failure and their relation to mortality. Circulation 1990;82: 1730–6.
43. Gupta S, Neyses L. Diuretic usage in heart failure: a continuing conundrum in 2005. Eur Heart J 2005;26:644–9.
44. Anand I, Florea VG. Diuretics in chronic heart failure: benefits and hazards. Eur Heart J 2001; 3(suppl G):G18.
45. Greenberg A. Diuretic complications. Am J Med Sci 2000;319:10–24.
46. Brater C. Diuretic therapy in congestive heart failure. Congest Heart Fail 2000;6:197–201.
47. Chow KM, Szeto CC, Wong TY, Leung CB, Li PK. Risk factors for thiazide-induced hyponatremia. Q J Med 2003;96:911–7.
48. Kramer BK, Schweda F, Riegger AJ. Diuretic treatment and resistance in heart failure. Am J Med 1000;106:90–6.
49. Spital A. Diuretic-induced hyponatremia. Nephrology 1999;19:447–52.
50. Sonnenblick M, Friedlander Y, Rosin AJ. Diuretic-induced severe hyponatremia. Review and analysis of 129 reported patients. Chest 1993;103:601–6.
51. Clark BA, Shannon RP, Rosa RM, Epstein FH. Increased susceptibility to thiazide-induced hyponatremia in the elderly. J Am Soc Nephrol 1994;5: 1106–11.
52. Lee D, Austin PC, Rouleau JL. Predicting mortality among patients hospitalized for heart failure: derivation and validation of a clinical model. JAMA 2003;290:2581–7.
53. Chin MH, Goldman L. Correlates of major complications or death in patients admitted to the hospital with congestive heart failure. Arch Intern Med 1996;156:1814–20.
54. Chen MC, Chang HW, Cheng CI, Chen YH, Chai HT. Risk stratification of in-hospital mortality in patients hospitalized for chronic congestive heart failure secondary to non-ischemic cardiomyopathy. Cardiology 2003;100:136–42.
55. Klein L, Gattis WA, Leimberger JD, Pina IL, O'Connor CM, Gheorghiade M. Prognostic value of hyponatremia in hospitalized patients with worsening heart failure: insights from the outcome of a prospective trial of intravenous milrinone for exacerbations of chronic heart failure (OPTIME-CHF). J Card Fail 2003;9(suppl):S83.
56. Klein L, O'Connor CM, Leimnerger JD, et al. Lower serum sodium is associated with increased short-term mortality in hospitalized patients with worsening heart failure: results from the OPTIME-CHF study. Circulation 2005;111:2454–60.
57. Licata G, Di Pasquale P, Parrinello G, et al. Effects of high-dose furosemide and small-volume hypertonic saline solution infusion in comparison with a high-dose of furosemide as bolus in refractory congestive heart failure: long term effects. Am Heart J 2003;145:459–66.
58. Bart BA, Boyle A, Bank AJ, et al. Ultrafiltration versus usual care for hospitalized patients with heart failure. J Am Coll Cardiol 2005;46:2043–6.
59. Sharma A, Hermann DD, Mehta RL. Clinical benefit and approach of ultrafiltration in acute heart failure. Cardiology 2001;96:144–54.
60. Brause M, Deppe C, Hollenbeck M, et al. Congestive heart failure as an indication for continuous renal replacement therapy. Kidney Int 1999;72(suppl): S95–8.
61. Simonelli R, Saltarelli G, Violo F. Daily hemofiltration in severe heart failure. Miner Electrolyte Metab 1999;25:38–42.
62. Marenzi G, Agostino P. Hemofiltration in heart failure. Int J Artif Organs 2004;27:1070–6.
63. Costanzo MR, Salteberg M, O'Sullivan J, Sobotka P. Early ultrafiltration in patients with decompensated heart failure and diuretic resistance. J Am Coll Cardiol 2005;46:2047–51.
64. Gheorghiade M, Niazi I, Ouyang J, et al. Vasopressin V2-receptor blockade with tolvaptan in patients with chronic heart failure: results from a double-blind, randomized trial. Circulation 2003;107: 2690–6.
65. Gheorghiade M, Gattis WA, Barbagelata A, et al. Rationale and study design for multicenter, randomized, double-blind, placebo-controlled study of the effect of tolvaptan on the acute and chronic outcomes of patients hospitalized with worsening congestive heart failure. Am J Heart 2003;145: S51–4.
66. Gheorghiade M, Gattis WA, O'Connor CM, et al., for the Acute and Chronic Therapeutic Impact of a Vasopressin Antagonist in Congestive Heart Failure (ACTIV in CHF) Investigators. Effects of

tolvaptan, a vasopressin antagonist, in patients hospitalized with worsening heart failure: a randomized controlled trial. JAMA 2004;291:1963–71.

67. Udelson JE, Smith WB, Hendrix GH, et al. Acute hemodynamic effects of conivaptan, a dual V1a and V2 vasopressin receptor antagonist, in patients with advanced heart failure. Circulation 2001;104:2417–23.

68. Naitoh M, Risvanis J, Balding LC, Johnston CI, Burrell LM. Neurohormonal antagonism in heart failure: beneficial effects of vasopressin V1a and V2 receptor blockade and ACE inhibition. Cardiovasc Res 2002;46:375–81.

69. Gheorghiade M, Gottlieb SS, Udelson JE, et al. Vasopressin V2 receptor blockade with Tolvaptan versus fluid restriction in the treatment of hyponatremia. Am J Cardiol 2006;97:1064–7.

73
Pulmonary Disease in the Setting of Acute Heart Failure Syndrome

Damien Roux and Jean-Damien Ricard

It has often been suggested that patients with acute heart failure (AHF) were particularly susceptible to pulmonary infections, the reason being that congested lungs had diminished capacity to clear respiratory secretions and ensure rapid bacterial clearance. To the best of our knowledge, this point has never been clearly investigated. Nonetheless, in AHF, bacterial growth may be favored in injured lungs, in the same way as in the acute respiratory distress syndrome (1). Indeed, experimental studies have shown that cardiogenic hydrostatic pulmonary edema may be accompanied by a certain degree of permeability-type lung edema with cellular damage and capillary stress failure (2–4), enabling erythrocytes to reach the alveolar space (4) and rendering the edema fluid an appropriate milieu for bacterial growth. This is in agreement with the clinical observation that lung infection may precipitate, accompany, or follow AHF and cardiogenic pulmonary edema. Three situations can be distinguished: community-acquired pneumonia that precipitates cardiac failure, lung infection that is unmasked when cardiogenic pulmonary edema resolves, and, in the most severe patients, lung infection that complicates the intensive care unit (ICU) course of AHF that required invasive mechanical ventilation. The questions that then face the clinician are when to suspect lung infection, how to confirm it, which pathogens must be suspected, and which treatment should be given. Paradoxically, these questions may be more easily answered in the most critical patients—those whose management has required invasive mechanical ventilation. Indeed, once the patient is intubated, lung parenchyma is directly available for bacteriologic sampling, enabling confirming or ruling out lung infection, ascertaining the pathogen involved, and guiding antibiotherapy according to the pathogen's susceptibility to antibiotics. In the other two circumstances, empiric antibiotic treatment will be given if the clinical suspicion is high enough and according to epidemiologic data and guided when possible by bacteriological data.

Community-Acquired Pneumonia and Lower Respiratory Tract Infection

Respiratory diseases are major noncardiac comorbidities associated with AHF (5, 6), with respiratory tract infection being a common cause of cardiac decompensation (7–9), which may, in some studies, represent the major precipitating factor in both systolic and diastolic heart failure (8). Not surprisingly, congestive heart failure is identified as one of the five comorbid conditions associated with community-acquired pneumonia (CAP), and as a major risk factor for death in cases with CAP (10).

The most common etiologic agent identified in almost all studies of CAP is *Streptococcus pneumoniae*. Other pathogens are listed in Table 73.1. Enteric gram-negative bacteria are not common in CAP, but may be present in up to 10% of non-ICU-hospitalized patients with underlying comorbid illnesses such as cardiac disease (11).

In published guidelines (12), patients are commonly stratified to highlight particular bacterial etiologies or potential drug-resistant bacteria.

Table 73.1. Initial empiric antibiotic therapy for community-acquired pneumonia (CAP) in the setting of acute heart failure (AHF)

Place of therapy	Microorganisms	Therapy[a]
Outpatients	*Streptococcus pneumoniae* (including penicillin-resistant pneumococcus) *Mycoplasma pneumoniae* *Chlamydia pneumoniae* *Haemophilus influenzae*	Oral B-lactam (high-dose amoxicillin, amoxicillin/clavulanate, cefuroxime, oral cefpodoxime) *plus* Oral macrolide (azithromycin, clarithromycin) or doxycycline *or* Oral antipneumococcal fluoroquinolone alone
Inpatients, not in ICU	Enteric gram-negative bacilli *Legionella* spp. Mixed infection (bacteria plus atypical pathogen) Respiratory viruses Miscellaneous (*Moraxella catarrhalis*, anaerobes, *Mycobacterium tuberculosis*, endemic fungi)	Intravenous β-lactam (cefotaxime, ceftriaxone, ampicillin/sulbactam) *plus* Intravenous or oral macrolide (azithromycin, clarithromycin) *or* Intravenous antipneumococcal fluoroquinolone alone
ICU-admitted patients	All of the above pathogens plus *Staphylococcus aureus*	Intravenous β-lactam[b] (cefotaxime, ceftriaxone) *plus either* Intravenous macrolide (clarithromycin, erythromycin) *or* Intravenous fluoroquinolone
ICU-admitted patients and risk factors for *Pseudomonas aeruginosa* (structural lung disease such as bronchiectasis, corticosteroid therapy >10 mg/d, broad-spectrum antibiotic therapy for >7 days in the past month, malnutrition, leukopenic immune suppression)	All of the above pathogens plus *Pseudomonas aeruginosa*	Selected intravenous antipseudomonal β-lactam[b] (cefepime, ceftazidime piperacillin/tazobactam, imipenem) *plus* intravenous antipseudomonal quinolone (ciprofloxacin) *or* Selected antipseudomonal β-lactam[b] *plus* intravenous aminoglycoside *plus either* Intravenous macrolide or intravenous nonpseudomonal fluoroquinolone

ICU, intensive care unit.
[a]Antibiotic regimen is detailed in Table 73.5.
[b]β-lactam allergy: fluoroquinolone ± clindamycin.
Source: Adapted from ATS and IDSA guidelines (10, 12).

Stratification takes into account the place of treatment (outpatient, hospital ward, or ICU), the presence of coexisting cardiopulmonary disease (chronic obstructive pulmonary disease [COPD], congestive heart failure); and the presence of modifying factors, which include the presence of risk factors for drug-resistant pneumococcus, the presence of risk factors for gram-negative infection (including nursing home residence), and the presence of risk factors for *Pseudomonas aeruginosa* (specifically in patients requiring ICU admission) (12).

Patients with heart failure presenting with CAP are considered at risk of having (in addition to the pathogens listed in Table 73.1) penicillin-resistant pneumococcus, anaerobes, and enteric gram-negative bacteria. These considerations directly impact on the antibiotic regimen that will be administered (Table 73.1).

Diagnosis

Clinical diagnosis of CAP in AHF is difficult because both conditions are accompanied by dyspnea, fever, and pulmonary crackles. Nevertheless, purulent sputum, temperature above 38°C, chills, or asymmetrical crackles are evocative of lung infection. Community-acquired pneumonia should be systematically evoked during decompensated cardiac insufficiency of the elderly, given the fact that fever may be absent and that risk factors for both diseases are often present in these patients (12). Chest x-ray confirms the diagnosis of congestive heart failure and may help evoke pneumonia in case of lobar involvement or lung abscess. Pleural effusions are difficult to interpret in the context of AHF, but may be related to pneumonia if unilateral (parapneumonic effusion). Hyperleukocytosis or leukopenia, and increased C-reactive protein (CRP) provide additional evidence for the diagnosis of pneumonia. Recently, procalcitonin, a serum marker of bacterial infections, has gained interest in the management of CAP; a recent study found that discouraging antibiotic prescription when its value was below 0.25 μg/L reduced antibiotic use without altering outcome (13).

Microbiological Examination

Once CAP is suspected, efforts should be made to precisely identify the pathogen involved, keeping in mind that studies evaluating the causes of CAP in adults have failed to identify a causative agent in 40% to 60% of cases of CAP (10).

Two sets of blood cultures should be systematically drawn before administration of antibiotic therapy. Because less than one third of cases of CAP due to *S. pneumonia* are bacteremic (and because this pathogen accounts for two thirds of bacteremic cases of CAP), infective endocarditis should be scrupulously looked for and ruled out in acute heart failure syndrome (AHFS) with positive blood culture.

Obtaining bacteriologic sampling of the lung, although desirable, is difficult in the context of acute respiratory distress and should not delay antibiotherapy.

The need for a sputum Gram stain and culture is debated (10, 12). Sputum Gram stain has shown the following limitations: not all patients can provide an adequate sample, especially if they are very dyspneic; and interpretation is observer dependent and difficult because of the contamination by the flora of the upper airways, the flora may include potential pathogens (leading to false-positive cultures), and the normal flora often overgrow the true pathogen (leading to false-negative cultures), especially with fastidious pathogens such as *S. pneumoniae.* Atypical pathogens (which are common either singly or as co-infecting agents) cannot be seen. The definition of "positive" varies from study to study, and a positive result for pneumococcus is poorly predictive of the ability to recover that organism from a sputum or blood culture. Moreover, correlating data from a Gram stain of expectorated sputum with cultures of alveolar material in large numbers of patients with CAP are lacking. In addition, the following points warrant consideration: (1) Patients with AHF and CAP often have, as stated above, underlying respiratory disease, mainly COPD. The upper respiratory tract of these patients is often chronically colonized, making it very difficult to ascertain if the pathogen recovered in the sputum is the one involved in the acute infection. (2) These patients often receive antibiotics before reaching the hospital, and prior antibiotic therapy may reduce the yield of common respiratory pathogens in cultures of respiratory tract specimens from any source and is often associated with false-positive cultures for upper airway contaminants, such as gram-negative bacilli or *Staphylococcus aureus.*

If performed, a properly collected sputum should show fewer than 10 squamous epithelial cells and greater than 25 neutrophils per low-power field. The main aim of this test is to visualize an organism that was not anticipated rather than to narrow initial empiric antibiotic therapy. Bacterial cultures of sputum are relevant when drug-resistant pathogens or pathogens that are not covered by the usual empiric antibiotic therapy are suspected. Measurement of urinary antigen can be of great interest for diagnosis of *Legionella* spp., keeping in mind that this test detects only *Legionella pneumophila* serogroup 1.

Interpretation of pleural effusion in patients with AHF may be difficult. Nevertheless, abundant unilateral or loculated pleural effusion should be sampled, before starting antibiotic therapy, in order to rule out empyema or complicated parapneumonic effusion. Samples of pleural effusion should be evaluated for protein, lactate dehydrogenase, pH, glucose, and white blood cell. A Gram stain and an acid-fast stain should be done followed by culture for bacteria, mycobacteria, and fungi. In addition, some fluid should also be cultured in blood culture bottles so as to increase sensitivity.

Serologic testing should not be routinely performed as it will not modify antibiotic therapy. It may occasionally be useful for retrospective confirmation of a suspected diagnosis or to provide data useful for epidemiologic surveillance.

Invasive diagnostic methods such as protected specimen brush (PSB), bronchoalveolar lavage (BAL), or plugged telescopic protected catheter (PTC) through bronchoscopy should be performed in patients who require intubation and mechanical ventilation, especially in case of underlying disease such as COPD. In patients without chronic respiratory tract colonization, Gram stain examination and culture of tracheal aspiration just following intubation may be an alternative.

Laboratory Testing

Usual laboratory testing of pulmonary, cardiac, liver, and renal function should also be performed.

Hospitalization Decision and Intensive Care Unit Admission

In most instances, CAP associated with AHFS requires hospitalization. An ICU admission is indicated if there is a need for mechanical ventilation, if the patient has septic shock, or for the presence of two of the following three criteria: systolic blood pressure <90 mm Hg, multilobar disease, and PaO_2/FiO_2 ratio <250.

Treatment Recommendations

Table 73.1 displays the antibiotic therapy recommendations adapted from the American Thoracic Society (ATS) guidelines and the Infectious Diseases Society of America (IDSA) (10, 12). First-dose antibiotic therapy should be administered immediately after microbiologic sampling. Delaying administration longer than 8 hours has been shown to be associated with poorer outcome.

If anaerobes are present on microbiologic culture, or in cases of lung abscess, metronidazole or clindamycin should be added to the antibiotic regimen.

In most patients with good response to antibiotic therapy, CAP should be treated for 7 to 10 days, even in bacteremic patients. Community-acquired pneumonia due to *Mycoplasma pneumoniae, Chlamydia pneumoniae*, and *Legionella* spp. should be treated for 10 to 14 days. A good response to antibiotic therapy is revealed by an improvement in clinical (resolution of fever, dyspnea, arterial oxygen saturation) and biologic data (white blood cell count, CRP) by day 3. Absence of a complete response to the treatment can result from unadapted antibiotic therapy (drug-resistant pathogen, pathogen not covered by initial empiric antibiotic regimen), pulmonary complication (empyema, lung abscess), metastatic infection (meningitis, arthritis, endocarditis), or mistaken or associated diagnosis (congestive heart failure, intrapulmonary hemorrhage, inflammatory lung disease, pulmonary infarction). Amelioration in chest x-ray abnormalities is slower. Antibiotic therapy should not be modified before day 3, except in severe CAP with clinical and radiologic deterioration and after microbiologic reevaluation. However, antibiotic therapy spectrum should be narrowed if a specific pathogen has been identified. Patients can be switched to oral treatment in cases of favorable evolution, in order to reduce costs and shorten hospital stay.

Prevention

Pneumococcal and influenza vaccine have proved to be effective in patients with coronary artery disease or congestive heart failure and is therefore recommended for all patients with cardiovascular disease. In addition, cessation of cigarette smoking should be strongly encouraged, being a major risk factor for both cardiovascular and respiratory diseases.

Aspiration Pneumonia

As indicated above, it is not unusual for patients hospitalized for AHF to develop fever and pulmonary infiltrates while cardiac symptoms improve. Because the injured lung is more susceptible to bacterial infection (1), and because patients may have silently aspirated at the worst moment of their respiratory distress, lung superinfection and aspiration pneumonia should be suspected at this stage. Aspiration pneumonia is the presumed cause of nearly all cases of anaerobic pulmonary infection, and consequently, microaerophiles and anaerobes from the mouth flora are the anticipated pathogens.

The basal segments of the lower lobes are usually affected after aspiration in an upright or semirecumbent position, whereas posterior segments of the upper lobes and the apical segments of the lower lobes are involved when aspiration occurs in recumbent position.

Treatment with amoxicillin-clavulanate for a maximum of 7 days is effective in aspiration pneumonia unless risk factors for multidrug-resistant pathogens (recent or current hospitalization, nursing home residency, recent antibiotic therapy) are present.

Ventilator-Associated Pneumonia

Epidemiology

Intubation increases the risk of developing nosocomial pneumonia by 6- to 21-fold and up to 30% of ventilated patients develop ventilator-associated pneumonia (VAP) (14), which is responsible for increased length of stay, morbidity, and mortality. Regarding the causative pathogens, VAP can be divided into early-onset (pneumonia occurring within the first 4 days of hospitalization) and late-onset VAP.

Early Onset

Early-onset VAP usually carries a better prognosis than late-onset VAP, and is more likely to be caused by antibiotic-sensitive bacteria. These include *S. pneumoniae, Haemophilus influenzae*, methicillin-sensitive *S. aureus*, and antibiotic-sensitive enteric gram-negative bacilli (*Escherichia coli, Klebsiella pneumoniae, Enterobacter* sp., *Proteus* sp., *Serratia marcescens*). However, patients who have received prior antibiotics or have had prior hospitalization within the past 90 days are at greater risk for colonization and infection with multidrug resistant pathogens.

Late Onset

Multidrug-resistant pathogens are usually responsible for late-onset VAP. Most frequent bacteria isolated during late-onset VAP are resistant gram-negative bacilli (*P. aeruginosa*, Enterobacteriaceae, *Acinetobacter* sp.) and methicillin-resistant *S. aureus* (MRSA).

Diagnosis and Management of Ventilator-Associated Pneumonia

Clinical, radiologic, and biologic abnormalities that should lead clinicians to suspect VAP are listed in Table 73.2. To help clinicians decide whether or not ongoing lung infection is involved, the clinical pulmonary infection score (CPIS) has been developed (15), based on six variables: body temperature, blood leukocytes, abundance and purulence of tracheal secretions, oxygenation, pulmonary radiography, and culture of endotracheal aspirates. Each variable is given a value ranging from 0 to 2 depending on its association with pneumonia. A CPIS >6 has a good positive predictive value for pneumonia. Adjustments of this score have been made to take into account gram stain examination of PTC or BAL (16).

Table 73.2. Clinical, biologic, and radiologic features of ventilator-associated pneumonia (VAP) suspicion

Clinical findings	Persistent fever or new febrile episode
	Abundant and purulent respiratory secretions
	Oxygen desaturation
	Tachycardia
	Hemodynamic instability or septic shock
Biologic findings:	hypoxemia
	Hyperleukocytosis
Radiologic findings:	Persistent or new pulmonary infiltrate

Microbiological Diagnosis

Because a majority of patients mechanically ventilated for AHF harbors many of the risk factors for multidrug resistant pathogens (Table 73.3, part D), efforts should be made to identify causative pathogen, even in cases of early-onset VAP. Respiratory tract cultures can be obtained from endotracheal aspirate, BAL, PSB, or PTC. Contrary to endotracheal aspirates, the invasive methods (BAL, PSB, and PTC) prevent contamination of the distal airway specimens by the proximal flora. In addition, quantitative cultures of these samples help distinguish colonization from true pulmonary infection. Local expertise and availability guide the choice of the method; however, invasive bronchoscopic methods have been found to improve outcome and reduce antibiotic use (17).

Initial Empiric Treatment

As soon as bacterial samples are obtained, antibiotic therapy must be started or modified. Antibiotic recommendations depend on the time of VAP occurrence (i.e., early- versus late-onset VAP) and

Table 73.3. Initial empiric antibiotic therapy for VAP

Ventilator-associated pneumonia		
Type	Microorganisms	Therapy[a]
A: Early-onset VAP *And* No risk factor for multidrug-resistant bacteria	*Streptococcus pneumoniae* *Haemophilus influenzae* Sensitive enteric gram-negative bacilli Methicillin-sensitive *Staphylococcus aureus*	Mono-antibiotic IV therapy ampicillin/sulbactam *Or* Third-generation cephalosporin (cefotaxime, ceftriaxone) *Or* Fluoroquinolone (levofloxacin, moxifloxacin)
B: Late-onset VAP *Or* Risk factor for multidrug-resistant bacteria	*Pseudomonas aeruginosa* Methicillin-resistant *Staphylococcus aureus** Resistant enteric gram-negative bacilli *Acinetobacter baumanii*	Combination IV therapy Selected antipseudomonal β-lactam (cefepime, ceftazidime piperacillin/tazobactam, imipenem or meropenem) *Plus* Aminoglycoside (amikacin or tobramycin) *Or* Antipseudomonal quinolone (ciprofloxacin or levofloxacin) *Plus* Vancomycin[b] *or* linezolid[b]
C: Late-onset VAP *And* Gram-negative bacilli on Gram stain of protected distal airway specimen	*Pseudomonas aeruginosa* Resistant enteric gram-negative bacilli *Acinetobacter baumanii*	*Combination IV therapy* Selected antipseudomonal β-lactam (cefepime, ceftazidime piperacillin/tazobactam, imipenem or meropenem) *Plus* Aminoglycoside (amikacin or tobramycin) *Or* Antipseudomonal quinolone (ciprofloxacin or levofloxacin)
D: Risk factors for multidrug-resistant bacteria • Recent hospitalization or residence in a nursing home or extended-care facilities • Current hospitalization of more than 4 days • Recent antibiotic therapy • Immunosuppression (disease or therapy)		

[a]Antibiotic regimen is detailed in Table 73.5.
[b]Only if risk factor for MRSA or high local incidence.
Source: Adapted from ATS and IDSA joint guidelines (18).

on the presence of risk factors for multidrug-resistant pathogens (18).

In cases of early-onset VAP and absence of any disease severity or risk factor for multidrug-resistant pathogens, a monoantibiotic therapy is usually sufficient (Table 73.3, part A). Clinicians may choose among ampicillin-sulbactam, third-generation cephalosporin (cefotaxime, ceftriaxone), fluoroquinolone (levofloxacin, moxifloxacin), and ertapenem. The β-lactam (penicillin or cephalosporin) should be preferred, as the two other antibiotic classes more readily select resistant pathogens in intensive care unit.

In the other cases (Table 73.3, parts B and C), empiric intravenous antibiotic therapy should also cover *P. aeruginosa*, Enterobacteriaceae, and *Acinetobacter* sp. Moreover, MRSA should be suspected in the presence of risk factors (namely MRSA colonization) or high local incidence. In cases where patients are clinically stable, and clinical suspicion of pneumonia is low (and even more so if direct examination of a respiratory tract specimen is negative), antibiotic administration can be delayed until results of the culture are received. The initial antibiotic (Table 73.3, part B) therapy should combine (1) an antipseudomonal β-lactamin; (2) either an antipseudomonal fluoroquinolone or an aminoglycoside; and (3) vancomycin or linezolid if MRSA is suspected (18).

If available, direct specimen examination of the respiratory tract sample enables focusing antibiotic therapy on the suspected pathogens (for instance, no use of vancomycin or linezolid if only gram-negative bacilli are observed, Table 73.3, part C). If the patient received antimicrobial molecules within the past 2 weeks, the antibiotic therapy should not include agents from the same antibiotic class.

Aminoglycosides are usually injected once a day and should not be used more than 3 to 5 days in responding patients. Vancomycin can be injected twice a day or continuously (19). A trough level of 20 to 30 μg/mL should be the aim.

TABLE 73.4. Microbiological culture thresholds for the diagnosis of VAP

	Endotracheal aspirate	Bronchoalveolar lavage	Protected specimen brush	Plugged telescopic catheter
Quantitative culture threshold (cfu/mL)	10^6	10^4	10^3	10^3

Treatment Adjustment According to Culture Results

The predictive negative value of those cultures is very high, so a negative culture can rule out VAP. But a positive culture alone cannot distinguish between true pneumonia and airway colonization, justifying the need for quantitative cultures. Table 73.4 shows the different thresholds for each technique above which VAP is confirmed. Cultures below the threshold represent colonization or contamination.

After identification of the etiologic pathogen, antibiotic therapy should be de-escalated or adjusted, taking into account antibiotic susceptibility of the causative pathogen. In cases of negative culture and clinical improvement on day 2 or 3, antibiotic therapy should be stopped as diagnosis of VAP is unlikely. In cases of negative culture and absence of clinical improvement, other pathogens or diagnoses (extrapulmonary site of infection, empyema, noninfectious diseases) must be evoked.

The duration of therapy tends to be shortened in order to decrease colonization and superinfection with antibiotic-resistant bacteria. If initial antibiotic therapy is appropriate and clinical response is good, the duration of therapy should not exceed 8 days (20). In cases of a complicated course of VAP, particularly with *P. aeruginosa*, the duration of therapy may be longer, such as 14 days.

TABLE 73.5. Antibiotic regimen: adult doses of antibiotics for initial intravenous therapy (based on normal renal and hepatic function)

β-lactam inhibitor	
Amoxicillin	1–2 g every 8 h
Piperacillin	4.5 g every 6 h
Third-generation cephalosporin	
Cefotaxime	1 g every 8 h
Ceftriaxone	1 g once a day
Antipseudomonal cephalosporin	
Cefepime	1–2 g every 8–12 h
Ceftazidime	2 g every 8 h
Carbapenem	
Imipenem-cilastatin	500 mg every 6 h
Meropenem	1 g every 8 h
Aminoside	
Gentamycin	7 mg/kg once a day
Amikacin	15–20 mg/kg once a day
Tobramycin	7 mg/kg once a day
Fluoroquinolone	
Levofloxacin	750 mg once a day
Moxifloxacin	400 mg once a day
Ciprofloxacin	400 mg every 8 h
Glycopeptide	
Vancomycin	15 mg/kg every 12 hours *or* 30 mg/kg/24 h continuously after loading dose of 15 mg/kg over 60 min
Oxazolidinone	
Linezolid	600 mg every 12 h

Practical Steps in the Diagnosis of Pneumonia in Ventilated Patients

- Step 1: Daily monitoring of body temperature, arterial blood gas, chest x-ray, and tracheal secretions.
  Satisfactory evolution, stay on Step 1.
  In case of suspicion of VAP (Table 73.2), go to Step 2.
- Step 2: Immediate protected distal airway specimen (BAL, PBS, or PTC) and go to Step 3 (invasive strategy);
  or
  Immediate endotracheal aspirate and go to Step 4 (clinical strategy).
- Step 3, invasive strategy:
  - In case of clinical instability, immediate antibiotic therapy following guidelines, if possible adapted to the direct examination of distal airway specimen.
  - In case of clinical stability and positive direct examination of BAL, PBS, or PTC, immediate adapted antibiotic therapy.
  - In case of clinical stability and negative direct examination of BAL, PBS, or PTC, wait and

start antibiotic therapy if culture is above the specific threshold.
  - Reevaluation after 48 to 72 hours and adjust antibiotic therapy based on culture results, antimicrobial susceptibility, and clinical response.
- Step 4, clinical strategy:
  - Immediate antibiotic therapy following recommendations, if possible adapted to the endotracheal aspiration Gram-stain examination.
  - If endotracheal aspirate culture is negative and in the absence of severe sepsis, VAP is unlikely and antibiotic therapy is stopped.
  - Reevaluation after 48 to 72 hours and adjust antibiotic therapy based on culture results, antimicrobial susceptibility, and clinical response.

Clinical Case

A 59-year-old man was intubated and ventilated for a severe acute decompensated heart failure (ADHF). He has a history of hypertension and ischemic cardiopathy with stenting of the anterior interventricular and circumflex arteries 5 years ago. Other antecedents are a right carotid endarterectomy and an aortofemoral bypass.

Upon his arrival, a coronarography ruled out an acute coronary syndrome. Because of severe hypoxemia, he was initially ventilated with FiO_2 = 1 and positive end-expiratory pressure (PEEP) = 15 cm H_2O. The patient received intravenous furosemide and salt restriction. On the second day, respiratory condition improved and FiO_2 was decreased to 0.5 with a PEEP at 6 cm H_2O.

On the third day, FiO_2 had to be progressively increased to 0.7 and PEEP to 10 cm H_2O because of arterial oxygen desaturation. The hemodynamics were stable. Body temperature was 38.2°C. Lung auscultation revealed crackles mainly in the lower right lobe. Nurses reported that tracheal secretions were more abundant.

How Should This Patient Be Managed?

Worsening of oxygenation may be related either to the underlying cause of initial respiratory failure (in the present case, cardiogenic pulmonary edema) or to early complications of mechanical ventilation. These would mainly include—apart from ventilator-related problems—barotrauma, atelectasis, aspiration pneumonia (which could have occurred during intubation) or early-onset ventilator-associated pneumonia. Fever, unilateral crackles, and abundant tracheal secretions suggest lung infection. A chest x-ray should be taken, and arterial blood gas and complete blood count should be done.

New Laboratory Data

Chest x-ray: new infiltrates in the lower right lobe with a great diminution of the left alveolar infiltrate

CBC: hemoglobin 11 g/dL, leukocytes 21,000/μL (19,500 neutrophils), platelets 450,000/μL

Blood gas (FiO_2 = 0.7, PEEP = 10 cmH_2O): pH 7.41, $PaCO_2$ 45, PaO_2 95, HCO_3^- 28

Na 133 mM, K 4.1 mM, Cl 95 mM, creatinine 84 μM

This patient presented signs of infection with fever, and hyperleukocytosis. Worsening of hypoxemia and the presence of a new lung infiltrate suggest VAP.

How Can This Diagnosis Be Confirmed?

Lung sample is desirable for the diagnosis of VAP because airways of ventilated patients become rapidly colonized by pathogens. Thus, a quantitative culture of a bronchial specimen may help distinguish between airway colonization and bacterial pneumonia. Blind techniques (nonfibroscopic techniques) can be used. The easiest method is endotracheal aspiration but this methods lacks specificity and sensitivity. Endotracheal aspiration culture's threshold to retain the diagnosis of pneumonia is 10^6 colony-forming units (cfu)/mL. A blind plugged telescopic catheter can be used to sample the right lower lung because the catheter will preferably take its direction. In case of left infiltrates, fibroscopic techniques are preferred. A protected-specimen brush culture above 10^3 cfu/mL, a plugged telescopic catheter culture above 10^3 cfu/mL, or a BAL fluid culture above 10^4 cfu/mL is required for the diagnosis of VAP. *S. pneumoniae* and *H. influenzae* are the two main bacteria responsible for early-onset VAP.

In this patient, direct examination of the blind plugged telescopic catheter sample showed gram-positive diplococcus. Thus, *S. pneumoniae* early-onset VAP was suspected and antimicrobial therapy was immediately started (amoxicillin 1 g × 3 daily). The quantitative culture recovered 10^6 cfu/mL of *S. pneumoniae,* which confirmed the diagnosis of VAP. Minimal inhibitory concentration (MIC) for amoxicillin was 0.023 mg/L. Duration of antimicrobial therapy should not exceed 7 days.

Five days after the beginning of amoxicillin, weaning of mechanical ventilation was withheld because of a rapid decrease in oxygenation. The patient became febrile again, and tracheal secretions were noted to be purulent. The patient was hemodynamically unstable.

How Should This Patient Be Managed?

Among other diagnoses, a new episode of VAP (in this case late-onset VAP) must be evoked. A chest x-ray showed new infiltrates of the left upper lobe. An echocardiogram ruled out worsening heart failure.

A new protected lung sample is essential before any antibacterial treatment. As infiltrates are in the left lung, a bronchoscopic technique was preferred to a blind plugged telescopic catheter to obtain lung sample. The hemodynamic instability and worsening of respiratory status rendered immediate empiric antimicrobial compulsory. Treatment was immediately started after the lung sample, with intravenous broad-spectrum antibiotics.

The main bacteria responsible for late-onset VAP are *Pseudomonas aeruginosa* and methicillin-resistant *Staphylococcus aureus*, but many other pathogens can be involved. Before identification of the causative pathogen, antibacterial treatment should cover nonfermenting gram-negative bacilli, enterobacteriae, and methicillin-resistant *S. aureus*.

Direct examination of the lung sample may help orient treatment when positive. Antibiotherapy should be adjusted once the pathogen is identified and its susceptibility to antibiotics known.

In the present case, direct examination of the plugged telescopic catheter showed numerous gram-negative bacilli. Thus, the patient received intravenous ceftazidime (2 g × 3/d) with amikacin once a day; 48 hours later, a wild-type *P. aeruginosa* grew at 10^4 cfu/mL. Ceftazidime was substituted for piperacillin for 7 more days and amikacin was stopped. The patient's condition improved and he was extubated a week later.

Conclusion

Pneumonia frequently complicates the ICU course of ventilated patients and therefore should be easily evoked. Determining the presence of VAP is based on two important points: (1) immediate sampling of the lower respiratory tract before any changes in the antibiotic regimen, and (2) absence of delay in initiating an adapted antibiotic regimen following published guidelines. Conversely, efforts should be made to avoid the overuse of antibiotic therapy in order to limit the emergence of multidrug-resistant pathogens. Those efforts include invasive pulmonary sampling, de-escalation of the antibiotic regimen by using a monotherapy effective on the identified pathogen after 3 to 5 days, and shortening the duration of therapy.

References

1. Dreyfuss D, Ricard JD. Acute lung injury and bacterial infection. Clin Chest Med 2005;26:105–12.
2. Bachofen H, Schurch S, Weibel ER. Experimental hydrostatic pulmonary edema in rabbit lungs. Barrier lesions. Am Rev Respir Dis 1993;147:997–1004.
3. Bachofen H, Schurch S, Michel RP, et al. Experimental hydrostatic pulmonary edema in rabbit lungs. Morphology Am Rev Respir Dis 1993;147: 989–96.
4. Tsukimoto K, Mathieu-Costello O, Prediletto R, et al. Ultrastructural appearances of pulmonary capillaries at high transmural pressures. J Appl Physiol 1991;71:573–82.
5. Cleland JGF, Swedberg K, Follath F, et al. The EuroHeart Failure survey programme—a survey on the quality of care among patients with heart failure in Europe: Part 1: patient characteristics and diagnosis. Eur Heart J 2003;24:442–63.
6. Braunstein JB, Anderson GF, Gerstenblith G, et al. Noncardiac comorbidity increases preventable

hospitalizations and mortality among medicare beneficiaries with chronic heart failure. J Am Coll Cardiol 2003;42:1226–33.
7. Ghali JK, Kadakia S, Cooper R, et al. Precipitating factors leading to decompensation of heart failure. Traits among urban blacks. Arch Intern Med 1988;148:2013–6.
8. Erk O. Precipitating factors for systolic and diastolic heart failure: a four-year follow-up of 192 patients. Hong Kong Med J 2004;10:97–101.
9. Sarmento PM, Fonseca C, Marques F, et al. Acutely decompensated heart failure: characteristics of hospitalized patients and opportunities to improve their care. Rev Port Cardiol 2006;25:13–27.
10. Bartlett JG, Dowell SF, Mandell LA, et al. Practice guidelines for the management of community-acquired pneumonia in adults. Infectious Diseases Society of America. Clin Infect Dis 2000;31:347–82.
11. Ruiz M, Ewig S, Marcos MA, et al. Etiology of community-acquired pneumonia: impact of age, comorbidity, and severity. Am J Respir Crit Care Med 1999;160:397–405.
12. Niederman MS, Mandell LA, Anzueto A, et al. Guidelines for the management of adults with community-acquired pneumonia. Diagnosis, assessment of severity, antimicrobial therapy, and prevention. Am J Respir Crit Care Med 2001;163:1730–54.
13. Christ-Crain M, Jaccard-Stolz D, Bingisser R, et al. Effect of procalcitonin-guided treatment on antibiotic use and outcome in lower respiratory tract infections: cluster-randomised, single-blinded intervention trial. Lancet 2004;363:600–7.
14. Chastre J, Fagon JY. Ventilator-associated pneumonia. Am J Respir Crit Care Med 2002;165:867–903.
15. Pugin J, Auckenthaler R, Mili N, et al. Diagnosis of ventilator-associated pneumonia by bacteriologic analysis of bronchoscopic and nonbronchoscopic "blind" bronchoalveolar lavage fluid. Am Rev Respir Dis 1991;143:1121–9.
16. Fartoukh M, Maitre B, Honore S, et al. Diagnosing pneumonia during mechanical ventilation: the clinical pulmonary infection score revisited. Am J Respir Crit Care Med 2003;168:173–9.
17. Fagon JY, Chastre J, Wolff M, et al. Invasive and noninvasive strategies for management of suspected ventilator-associated pneumonia. A randomized trial. Ann Intern Med 2000;132:621–30.
18. Guidelines for the management of adults with hospital-acquired, ventilator-associated, and healthcare-associated pneumonia. Am J Respir Crit Care Med 2005;171:388–416.
19. Wysocki M, Delatour F, Faurisson F, et al. Continuous versus intermittent infusion of vancomycin in severe Staphylococcal infections: prospective multicenter randomized study. Antimicrob Agents Chemother 2001;45:2460–7.
20. Chastre J, Wolff M, Fagon JY, et al. Comparison of 8 vs 15 days of antibiotic therapy for ventilator-associated pneumonia in adults: a randomized trial. JAMA 2003;290:2588–98.

2.8
Rescue Management in Acute Heart Failure Syndrome

74
Mechanical Devices to Improve Circulation During Cardiopulmonary Resuscitation

Keith G. Lurie, Anja K. Metzger, and Demetris Yannopoulos

Even with the widespread practice of basic and advanced life support, the vast majority of patients in cardiac arrest never survive to hospital discharge. Each year over one million Europeans and Americans die from sudden cardiac arrest. The waste of human potential is enormous. Contrary to popular opinion, many of the victims die in their prime. Survival rates for out-of-hospital cardiac arrest vary geographically from 1% to 18%, while the in-hospital cardiac arrest survival rates vary from 5% to 25%. Differences in outcomes between geographic regions are due to many factors, but the intrinsic mechanical inefficiencies of standard cardiopulmonary resuscitation (sCPR) limit the potential of even the most highly skilled rescuers. Since the description of sCPR by Kouwenhoven and colleagues in 1960, several new cardiopulmonary resuscitation (CPR) techniques and a number of different CPR adjunctive devices have been described. These new approaches were developed based on insights into the mechanisms of blood flow during CPR. This chapter focuses on CPR devices and techniques that offer an improvement over sCPR and may improve the chances of survival after cardiac arrest. The reader is referred to the 2005 American Heart Association (AHA)[1] guidelines for further information on the devices and techniques discussed and to a comprehensive review article by Lars Wik[2] for a complete history of all mechanical CPR devices invented and studied since the 1960s.

The purpose of CPR is to propel blood from the heart to the brain and other vital organs during the compression phase and to enhance cardiac and cerebral perfusion as well as the return of blood back into the coronary arteries and cardiac chambers during the chest wall recoil or decompression phase. During sCPR, chest compression results in an elevation of intrathoracic pressure and direct cardiac compression. Both of these mechanisms result in forward blood flow out of the chest. The effectiveness of this pumping mechanism is largely determined by the amount of blood that returns to refill the heart after each compression phase. Blood flow back to the heart as well as blood flow to the brain is highly dependent on the degree of chest wall recoil and the integrity and functionality of the cardiac valves. When the chest recoils, intrathoracic pressures fall relative to extrathoracic pressures, venous blood returns to the right heart, and blood flows to the coronary and cerebral beds. In addition, when intrathoracic pressure falls below subatmospheric pressure, there is an immediate decrease in intracranial pressure. This reduction in intracranial "afterload" also facilitates forward blood flow to the brain. Devices that optimize this physiology are helpful adjuncts and have been shown to improve outcomes after cardiac arrest. Conversely, there are several common mistakes in sCPR techniques that result in suboptimal CPR quality: not allowing full chest wall recoil, inadequate compression force, incorrect compression rate, and hyperventilation. The devices and techniques discussed in this chapter have been designed to prevent these mistakes.

Allowing Full Chest Wall Recoil

Standard CPR by itself is inherently inefficient, in large part due to the lack of adequate blood return to the thorax during the chest wall recoil phase.[3] Moreover, the coronary and cerebral perfusion pressures are only marginally adequate, as the respective pressure gradients among the aorta, the right atrium, and the left ventricle, as well as the aorta and intracranial pressures are far from optimal. Typically sCPR provides <20% of the normal blood flow to the heart, ~25% of the normal blood flow to the brain, and <20% of the normal cardiac output. This low flow state results in ongoing ischemia and an often irreversible downward spiral. Devices that improve hemodynamics and perfusion during CPR have been developed based on an understanding of the complex physiology of this low flow state. Recently, investigations have focused on the decompression phase of CPR, where the refilling of the heart occurs. During the decompression (or passive relaxation) phase of CPR, a small decrease in intrathoracic pressure (relative to atmospheric pressure) develops; this promotes blood flow back to the heart. Myocardial perfusion predominantly occurs during the decompression phase. The difference between the diastolic aortic pressures and the diastolic right atrial pressures (coronary perfusion pressure) is thought to be the critical determinant of CPR efficacy. More recently it has been discovered that a small decrease in intrathoracic pressure also results in a decrease in intracranial pressure, thereby enhancing the cerebral perfusion pressure, calculated as the mean arterial pressure minus the intracranial pressure. The AHA and the European Resuscitation Council (ERC) recognized the inefficiencies of sCPR in 2000 when they issued a new guideline in performing sCPR. This guideline reinforces the importance of the chest decompression phase in its teaching on the performance of CPR: "Release the pressure on the chest to allow blood to flow into the chest and heart. You must release the pressure completely and allow the chest to return to its normal position after each compression."[4]

Despite these recommendations, recent studies have documented that when CPR is performed by professional rescuers, there is often incomplete chest wall recoil.[5] Failure to allow the chest to fully recoil results in significantly less blood flow back to the heart and brain.[6] Correction of this basic flaw (incomplete chest wall recoil) through rigorous training or by relying on a device that ensures full chest wall recoil has the potential to significantly improve the chances for survival after cardiac arrest. Full chest wall recoil can be achieved by a slight modification of the standard hand position so that the palms of the hand come completely off the chest wall after each compression as illustrated in Figure 74.1. Alternatively, active compression decompression (ACD) CPR increases the naturally occurring negative intrathoracic pressure by physically lifting the chest wall and helping it return to its resting decompressed position. Active compression decompression CPR ensures that the chest expands to generate the negative intrathoracic pressure needed to allow passive filling of the heart. Both of these alternatives still require considerable

A 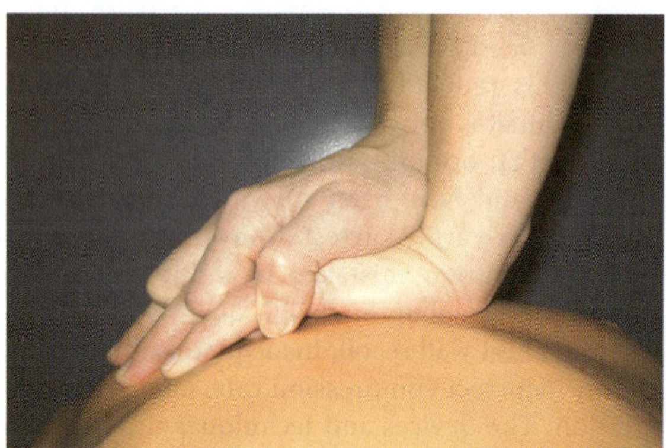

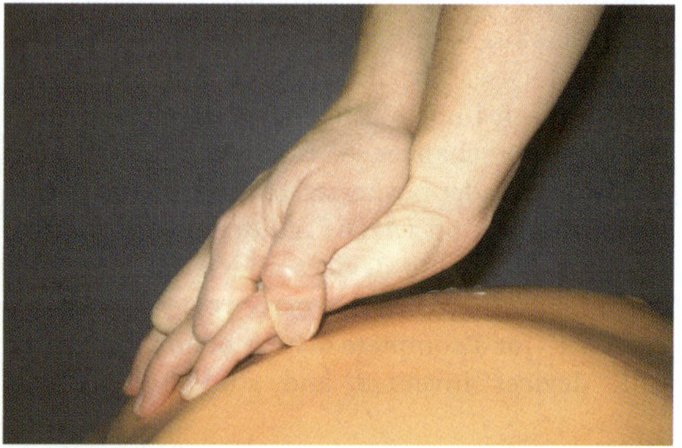 B

Figure 74.1. (A) Compression hand position. (B) Decompression hand position.

manual work to optimize the bellows-like action of the thorax during CPR.

Active compression decompression CPR was first inspired by the case of a patient who was resuscitated by family members with a common household plunger.[7] While ACD CPR does increase vital organ perfusion when compared with sCPR, it has been difficult to show a consistent benefit from one city to the next when evaluating the clinical benefit of this technique in patients in cardiac arrest. In St. Paul, Minnesota, and Paris, France, the use of ACD CPR significantly increased the chances for resuscitation acutely.[8,9] In the Minnesota trial, a higher percentage of ACD CPR patients than sCPR patients had a return of spontaneous circulation and were admitted to the intensive care unit (ICU) (45% vs. 31%, and 40% vs. 26%, respectively), but these trends were not statistically significant ($p < .10$ for both). Return of spontaneous circulation, ICU admission, and neurologic recovery in both CPR groups were highly correlated with downtime (time from collapse to emergency medical system personnel arrival to the scene in witnessed arrests). With less than 10 minutes downtime, survival to the ICU was 59% with ACD CPR and 33% with sCPR ($p < .02$), return to baseline neurologic function was 31% with ACD CPR and 20% with sCPR ($p = .27$), and hospital discharge rate was 38% with ACD CPR and 20% with sCPR ($p = .17$). In Paris, use of ACD CPR more than doubled the 1-year survival rate compared with sCPR (5% vs. 2%, $p = .03$). However, results with ACD CPR in other cities were similar to those observed with sCPR.[10,11]

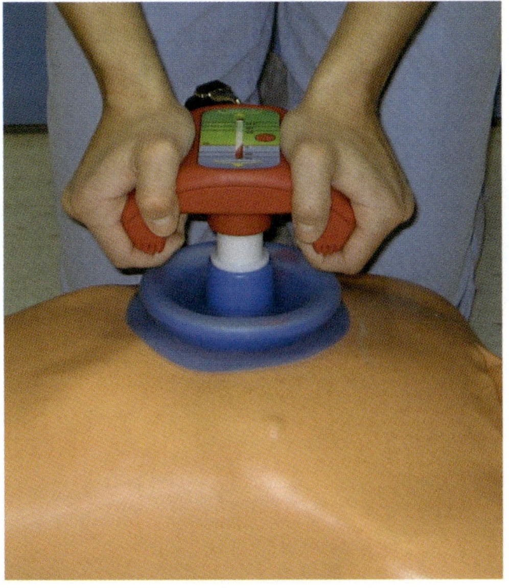

FIGURE 74.2. Active compression decompression (ACD) cardiopulmonary resuscitation (CPR) device.

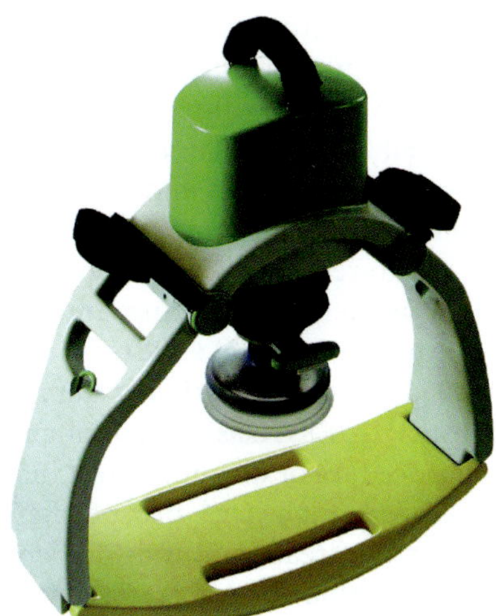

FIGURE 74.3. Automated ACD device.

The ACD CPR device called the CardioPump (Fig. 74.2) is not available in the United States, but it is currently being used in out-of-hospital cardiac arrest in Europe, China, Israel, and Japan. In addition to providing ACD CPR, the CardioPump has a compression force gauge that is used by the rescuer to ensure that adequate compression forces are being delivered and an audible metronome that ensures that the rescuer is performing an adequate number of compressions. In this manner, this device addresses three of the most common mistakes made when performing CPR. It ensures complete chest wall recoil, adequate compression force, and correct compression rate.

An automated ACD CPR device (LUCAS™, manufactured by Jolife, Lund, Sweden) shown in Figure 74.3 is currently being sold and used in Europe. Instead of relying on the physical endurance of the rescuer for proper technique, this pneumatically powered device provides consistent continuous compressions with active recoil of the chest to the baseline chest position following each compression. To date, the device is not commercially available in the United States. A recent study in Europe demonstrated patients with out-of-hospital witnessed cardiac arrest receiving LUCAS-CPR within 15 minutes of the ambulance call had a 30-day survival of 25% in ventricular fibrillation (VF) and 5% in asystole.[12] Active compression decompression CPR was given a class IIb recommendation for in-hospital CPR and an indeterminate rating (more research needed) for out-of-hospital CPR by the AHA and ERC in 2005. To put this rating system into perspective, the AHA/ERC class I recommendation is given to a procedure or diagnostic test that should be administered; high-level prospective clinical trials support the treatment and the benefit outweighs the potential for harm. In class IIa, the treatment is considered reasonable to perform and clinical trials support the usefulness. Class IIb recommendations are considered optional treatments or recommended by experts despite the absence of high-level supporting evidence. Indeterminate recommendations are given when there are not enough data to recommend for or against the technology. Class III ratings are treatments that should not be performed.[1]

Enhancing Venous Return During Cardiopulmonary Resuscitation

Complete chest wall recoil or ACD CPR creates a vacuum within the thorax during each chest wall decompression. However, much of the potential hemodynamic benefit of this vacuum is lost by the instantaneous influx of inspiratory gas. The impedance threshold device (ITD) contains pressure-sensitive valves that regulate the influx of inspiratory gas during chest wall decompression, augmenting the amplitude and duration of the vacuum within the thorax during the recoil phase. This greater and more sustained vacuum draws more venous blood back into the heart, resulting in increased cardiac preload and lower intracranial pressures. This combination of mechanisms results in improved cardiac output, increased cerebral perfusion pressure, and vital organ perfusion.

The ITD (ResQPod®) (Fig. 74.4) was first conceptualized when measuring intrathoracic pressures in patients undergoing ACD CPR. It was realized that if the endotracheal tube was transiently occluded during the active decompression phase, intrathoracic pressures became markedly more negative. This led to the idea of impeding inspiratory gas exchange during the chest wall decompression phase of CPR to create a greater pressure differential between the thorax and the rest of the body, thereby enhancing blood flow back into the thorax. As such, the impedance device harnesses the kinetic energy of the chest wall recoil, thereby augmenting the "bellows-like" action of the chest with each compression-decompression cycle.[13] Use of the ITD during sCPR in animals doubles the cardiac perfusion, increases brain flow, and increases 24-hour neurologically intact survival rates. In humans the

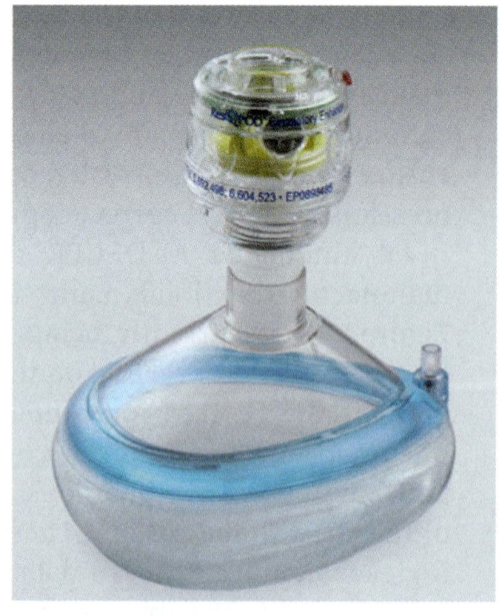

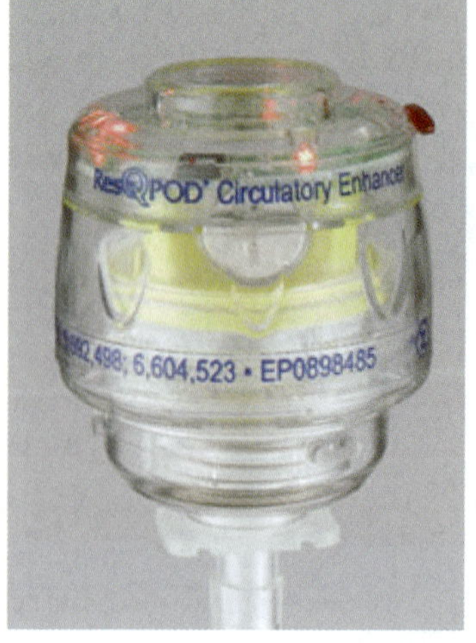

FIGURE 74.4. (A) Impedance threshold device (ITD) on face mask. (B) ITD on endotracheal (ET) tube.

ITD enhances circulation, doubles blood pressure, and in pulseless electrical activity increases 24-hour survival rates (27% for the ITD groups vs. 11% for the sham ITD group (p = .037).[14,15] The ITD has been given a Class IIa recommendation by the AHA/ERC as a device to increase circulation and return of spontaneous circulation.

The combination of ACD CPR plus the ITD has been evaluated in three randomized studies resulting in improved return of spontaneous circulation (ROSC) and 24-hour survival rates when compared to sCPR.[16–18] In a prospective, controlled trial performed in Mainz, Germany, patients with out-of-hospital arrest were sequentially randomized to ACD + ITD CPR or sCPR by the advanced life support team after intubation. An early study in that city failed to show a difference between sCPR and ACD CPR alone. The primary end point of that study was 1-hour survival. With ACD + ITD CPR (n = 103), 1- and 24-hour survival rates were 51%, and 37% versus 32% and 22% with S-CPR (n = 107) (p = .006 and .033), respectively. One- and 24-hour survival rates in witnessed arrests were 55% and 41% with ACD + ITD CPR versus 33% and 23% in control subjects (p = .011 and .019), respectively. One- and 24-hour survival rates in patients with a witnessed arrest in ventricular fibrillation were 68% and 58% after ACD + ITD CPR versus 27% and 23% after S-CPR (p = .002 and .009). Hospital discharge rates were 18% after ACD + ITD CPR versus 13% in control subjects (p = .41). Overall neurologic function trended higher with ACD + ITD CPR (14.6% for witnessed arrest) versus sCPR (5.3%) (p = .07). Importantly, patients randomized >10 minutes after the call for help to the ACD + ITD CPR had a three times higher 1-hour survival rate than control subjects (p = .002) and time-related benefits were observed regardless of presenting rhythm.

A second large randomized prospective blinded trial in which all patients received ACD CPR compared an active versus sham ITD. Results were similar: 24-hour survival rates were increased by 50% with the active ITD, and there was a similarly strong trend toward improved neurologic function in the survivors when the active ITD was used.[17] These clinical data emphasize the importance of an ACD device or complete chest wall decompression in addition to an ITD. At the time of this writing a multisite clinical trial is underway in the United States to determine whether the ResQPump (synonymous with the CardioPump) plus an ITD will significantly increase long-term survival rates compared with sCPR.

Most recently, an intrathoracic pressure regulator (ITPR) was described that is an improved version of the ITD. Following each positive pressure ventilation, the ITPR is used to generate a continuous negative intrathoracic pressure of between −5 and −10 mm Hg while chest compressions are being performed. This negative intrathoracic pressure enhances venous return, increases circulation and survival rates, and has been shown in animal models to be effective in the setting of cardiac arrest secondary to ventricular fibrillation and blood loss.[19,20]

Another method of CPR designed to enhance venous return and thus CPR efficacy is termed interposed abdominal counterpulsation (IAC) CPR. With this technique, one person compresses on the chest and a second person compresses, in an alternating fashion, on the abdomen. A third person ventilates the patient. With abdominal counterpulsation venous blood is pushed into the chest from the abdomen, thereby increasing the stroke volume of blood out of the chest with each subsequent chest compression. Clinical studies during in-hospital cardiac arrest have shown improved ROSC, short-term survival, and survival to hospital discharge.[21–23] This method has been given a level IIb recommendation for in-hospital resuscitation. Studies with IAC CPR in the prehospital arena have not shown a similar benefit.[24] A device, the LifeStick, was developed to try to perform IAC CPR: first compress the chest, and then simultaneously actively decompress the chest and compress the abdomen. Despite promising animal studies,[25] clinical data with this device showed no benefit and possible harm.[26] The reason for this failed effort and the lack of IAC in some studies may relate to the timing of the abdominal compression phase. The interposed abdominal counterpulsation increases intracranial pressures and right atrial pressures during the chest recoil phase, thereby actually decreasing the effective coronary and cerebral perfusion pressures. In 1992 Christenson et al.[27] showed in animals that increasing right atrial pressure immediately after delivering a chest compression may reduce coronary perfusion pressure. They demonstrated that a three-phase approach, wherein the chest was compressed and then allowed to recoil, followed by an abdominal counterpulsation, resulted in significantly better coronary and cerebral perfusion than a two-phase IAC approach. At the time of this writing, there are no devices that have been shown to successfully use abdominal counterpulsation as a means to enhance venous blood flow to the heart in patients.

Preventing Hyperventilation During Cardiopulmonary Resuscitation

Ventilations during CPR provide oxygenation. However, positive pressure ventilation also increases the pressures in the thorax and the brain. Positive pressure ventilation impedes blood from returning to the heart, thereby reducing cardiac output, and increases intracranial pressures, thus decreasing cerebral perfusion. Changing the compression/ventilation ratio from 15:2 to 15:1 results in higher coronary and cerebral perfusion pressures.[28] Recent data suggest that hyperventilation occurs frequently during CPR and that it can be harmful, if not deadly.[29] As such, it is fundamentally important to avoid hyperventilation during CPR. New AHA/ERC guidelines recommend a compression/ventilation ratio of 30:2 when performing CPR with an unsecured airway, and at a rate of 8 to 10 with a secured airway. Those performing CPR should be rigorously trained to comply with these recommendations. In addition to regulating gas exchange into the lungs during the chest recoil phase of CPR, the ITD noted above also provides visual guidance to the rescuer related to the proper ventilation and compression rate: it contains lights that flash at 10 times per minute. By providing a positive pressure ventilation each time the light flashes and compressing the chest 10 times for every light flash, rescuers can use the timing lights to help maintain proper CPR technique.

Providing Adequate Compression Forces and Rates Automatically and Mechanically

Standard CPR is a physically demanding task. The quality of CPR quickly deteriorates when the rescuer becomes fatigued. Several devices have been designed in an effort to provide consistent compression forces and rates. These devices have been automated to provide consistent compressions at a specified rate during CPR.

Mechanical piston devices like the Thumper® (Grand Rapids, MI) (Fig. 74.5), manufactured by Michigan Instruments, depress the sternum via a piston mounted to a baseplate that moves up and down by a compressed gas cylinder. Clinical studies have shown improved end-tidal CO_2 and mean arterial pressure in patients in cardiac arrest, but it is important to emphasize that no study has ever shown an improvement in short- or long-term survival rates.[30–32] With automated mechanical CPR devices, securing the airway, defibrillation, and placing intravenous lines can be performed concurrently with CPR, and thus chest compressions are continuous. However, until very recently the Thumper did not allow for full chest wall recoil, but rather relied on the intrinsic recoil action of the chest to push the compression surface and piston upward. This prevented full chest wall recoil, and these authors believe limited the value of the device.

In an effort to harness the bellows-like action of the thorax by increasing intrathoracic pressure and thus propel blood out of the heart, a circum-

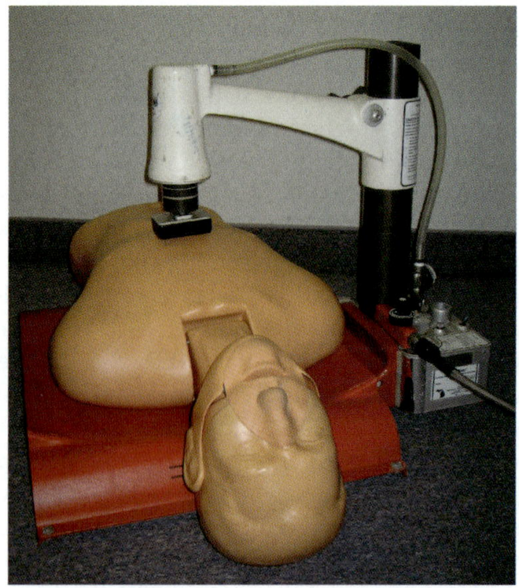

FIGURE 74.5. Automated mechanical device.

ferential vest device (vest CPR) was developed. With this approach, a circumferential band-like device is wrapped around the thorax and pneumatically inflated and deflated 60 times per minute. This increases intrathoracic pressure and squeezes blood out of the thorax. In animals and humans, vest CPR increases blood pressure and vital organ perfusion.[33,34] To date, regulatory and manufacturing challenges have prevented the successful clinical introduction of vest CPR. However, similar to vest CPR, a load-distributing band (LDB) CPR device was recently developed and has been successfully deployed clinically. This technology was recently embodied in a device called AutoPulse (Zoll Corporation, Chelmsford, MA) (Fig. 74.6). It consists of a portable backboard, a chest band, and a rechargeable battery pack. Two clinical studies have demonstrated improved hemodynamics and ROSC when compared to sCPR.[35,36] In a study of in-hospital cardiac arrest, it was shown in 31 patients that the coronary perfusion pressures generated by the AutoPulse were 33% higher than those generated by sCPR ($p < .015$). In the second study, a retrospective chart review of 162 patients demonstrated a 39% ROSC rate by the patients revived with the AutoPulse compared to a 29% ROSC when sCPR was used ($p = .003$). However, a recent multisite clinical trial, the ASPIRE trial, was stopped prematurely when the Data Safety Monitoring Board observed an increased mortality rate with the AutoPulse compared with sCPR. No prospective study has shown an increase in survival rates with the AutoPulse. At the time of this writing it is not clear if there are intrinsic flaws with this new device and/or whether the clinical studies suffered from a failure of proper implementation.

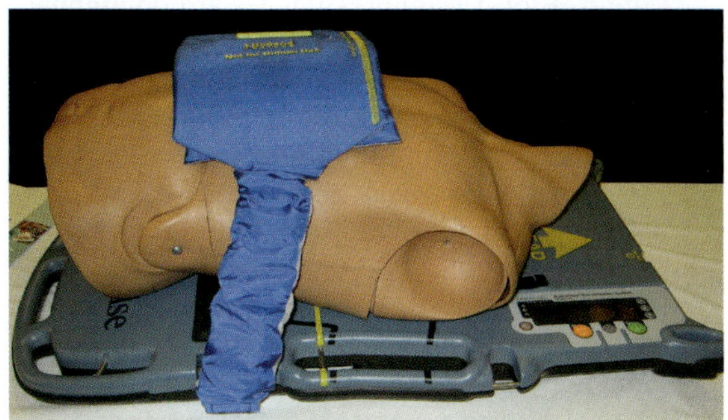

FIGURE 74.6. Automated load-distributing band CPR.

Minimally invasive direct cardiac massage (MIDCM) was developed in 1997 to allow internal cardiac massage without the need for a thoracotomy. The MIDCM is inserted into a 4-cm skin incision in the medial aspect of the left fourth intercostals space. Actuating the device compresses the heart against the vertebrae. Human studies have demonstrated higher perfusion pressures and flows when compared to sCPR.[37,38] Serious complications are possible and no large clinical trials have been completed to date.

Extracorporeal membrane oxygenation (ECMO) can be combined with prolonged CPR, which results in a technique called extracorporeal membrane oxygenation during CPR (ECPR). Several clinical studies have concluded that ECPR can be successfully utilized to treat some victims of cardiac arrest.[39–41] With this approach manual CPR is performed while the ECMO circuit is introduced in the patient. This invasive heart–lung perfusion system is then activated and circulates blood in the arrested patient. This approach has significant merit based on a number of successful anecdotal cases but is underutilized and not well evaluated at present. It was not evaluated in the recent AHA/ERC guidelines.

Simultaneous sternothoracic cardiopulmonary resuscitation (SST-CPR) can be performed with a device that simultaneously compresses the sternum while constricting the thoracic cavity. Bellows on sternum resuscitation cardiopulmonary resuscitation (BSR-CPR) allows a single rescuer to perform compressions and ventilations without changing position. During decompression, the device reservoir (Cardiovent™, Germany) fills with air, which is automatically delivered to the patient after each compression via tubing that is connected to the device on the chest and the endotracheal tube of the patient. Both SST-CPR and BSR-CPR have shown promise in small preclinical studies. However, no clinical studies have been performed to date.

The current devices and techniques that have shown clinical promise and that are recognized for their ability to improve upon the common mistakes made when performing manual conventional sCPR are summarized in Table 74.1. Research is ongoing to improve the chances

TABLE 74.1. Cardiopulmonary resuscitation (CPR) devices and techniques

Device and technique comparison	CPR devices: ACD CPR (ResQPump, LUCAS)	CPR devices: ITD (ResQPOD)	CPR devices: Thumper	CPR devices: AutoPulse	CPR techniques: IAC CPR
Allows full chest wall recoil	✔		✔	✔	
Ensures adequate compression depth	✔		✔	✔	
Ensures adequate compression rate	✔		✔	✔	
Minimizes hyperventilation		✔			
Available in the U.S.		✔	✔	✔	
AHA/ERC recommendation	Class IIb	Class IIa	Class IIb	Class IIb	Class IIb
Human data demonstrates improved survival	Mixed	Yes	No	No	Mixed

ACD, active compression decompression; AHA, American Heart Association; ERC, European Resuscitation Council; IAC, interposed abdominal counterpulsation; ITD, impedance threshold device.

of meaningful survival after cardiac arrest and should lead to additional novel techniques and devices in the near future.

Conclusion

A number of new devices have been recently evaluated to enhance circulation and ultimately survival rates during CPR. The ITD, either with sCPR or ACD CPR, regulates airway pressures during CPR to increase blood flow to the heart and brain. It has been studied extensively and recently given the highest level of recommendation of any device in the 2005 AHA and ERC guidelines as a means to enhance circulation and the return of spontaneous circulation. Other devices, including manual and automated compression and decompression devices, are also a step in the right direction. It is anticipated that over the next decade fully automated noninvasive circulatory assist systems will be developed and deployed to further improve the chances for long-term survival after cardiac arrest.

References

1. 2005 American Heart Association Guidelines for Cardiopulmonary Resuscitation and Emergency Cardiovascular Care. Circulation. Dec 13 2005;112 (24 suppl):IV1–203.
2. Wik L. Automatic and manual mechanical external chest compression devices for cardiopulmonary resuscitation. Resuscitation. Sep 2000;47(1):7–25.
3. Niemann JT. Cardiopulmonary resuscitation. N Engl J Med. Oct 8 1992;327(15):1075–80.
4. Guidelines 2000 for Cardiopulmonary Resuscitation and Emergency Cardiovascular Care. Part 2: ethical aspects of CPR and ECC. Circulation. Aug 22 2000;102(8 suppl):I12–21.
5. Aufderheide TP, Pirrallo RG, Yannopoulos D, et al. Incomplete chest wall decompression: a clinical evaluation of CPR performance by EMS personnel and assessment of alternative manual chest compression-decompression techniques. Resuscitation. Mar 2005;64(3):353–62.
6. Yannopoulos D, McKnite S, Aufderheide TP, et al. Effects of incomplete chest wall decompression during cardiopulmonary resuscitation on coronary and cerebral perfusion pressures in a porcine model of cardiac arrest. Resuscitation. Mar 2005;64(3): 363–72.
7. Lurie KG, Lindo C, Chin J. CPR: the P stands for plumber's helper. JAMA. Oct 3 1990;264(13):1661.
8. Lurie KG, Shultz JJ, Callaham ML, et al. Evaluation of active compression-decompression CPR in victims of out-of-hospital cardiac arrest. JAMA. May 11 1994;271(18):1405–11.
9. Plaisance P, Lurie KG, Vicaut E, et al. A comparison of standard cardiopulmonary resuscitation and active compression-decompression resuscitation for out-of-hospital cardiac arrest. French Active Compression-Decompression Cardiopulmonary Resuscitation Study Group. N Engl J Med. Aug 19 1999;341(8):569–75.
10. Mauer DK, Nolan J, Plaisance P, et al. Effect of active compression-decompression resuscitation (ACD-CPR) on survival: a combined analysis using individual patient data. Resuscitation. Aug 1999; 41(3):249–56.
11. Stiell IG, Hebert PC, Wells GA, et al. The Ontario trial of active compression-decompression cardiopulmonary resuscitation for in-hospital and prehospital cardiac arrest. JAMA. May 8 1996;275(18): 1417–23.

12. Steen S, Sjoberg T, Olsson P, et al. Treatment of out-of-hospital cardiac arrest with LUCAS, a new device for automatic mechanical compression and active decompression resuscitation. Resuscitation. Oct 2005;67(1):25–30.
13. Lurie KG, Mulligan KA, McKnite S, et al. Optimizing standard cardiopulmonary resuscitation with an inspiratory impedance threshold valve. Chest. Apr 1998;113(4):1084–90.
14. Aufderheide TP, Pirrallo RG, Provo TA, et al. Clinical evaluation of an inspiratory impedance threshold device during standard cardiopulmonary resuscitation in patients with out-of-hospital cardiac arrest. Crit Care Med. Apr 2005;33(4):734–40.
15. Pirrallo RG, Aufderheide TP, Provo TA, et al. Effect of an inspiratory impedance threshold device on hemodynamics during conventional manual cardiopulmonary resuscitation. Resuscitation. Jul 2005;66(1):13–20.
16. Plaisance P, Lurie KG, Payen D. Inspiratory impedance during active compression-decompression cardiopulmonary resuscitation: a randomized evaluation in patients in cardiac arrest. Circulation. Mar 7 2000;101(9):989–94.
17. Plaisance P, Lurie KG, Vicaut E, et al. Evaluation of an impedance threshold device in patients receiving active compression-decompression cardiopulmonary resuscitation for out of hospital cardiac arrest. Resuscitation. Jun 2004;61(3):265–71.
18. Wolcke BB, Mauer DK, Schoefmann MF, et al. Comparison of standard cardiopulmonary resuscitation versus the combination of active compression-decompression cardiopulmonary resuscitation and an inspiratory impedance threshold device for out-of-hospital cardiac arrest. Circulation. Nov 4 2003;108(18):2201–5.
19. Yannopoulos D, Nadkarni VM, McKnite SH, et al. Intrathoracic pressure regulator during continuous-chest-compression advanced cardiac resuscitation improves vital organ perfusion pressures in a porcine model of cardiac arrest. Circulation. Aug 9 2005;112(6):803–11.
20. Yannopoulos D, Aufderheide TP, McKnite S, et al. Hemodynamic and respiratory effects of negative tracheal pressure during CPR in pigs. Resuscitation. Jun 2006;69(3):487–94.
21. Babbs CF. Interposed abdominal compression CPR: a comprehensive evidence based review. Resuscitation. Oct 2003;59(1):71–82.
22. Sack JB, Kesselbrenner MB, Bregman D. Survival from in-hospital cardiac arrest with interposed abdominal counterpulsation during cardiopulmonary resuscitation. JAMA. Jan 15 1992;267(3):379–85.
23. Sack JB, Kesselbrenner MB, Jarrad A. Interposed abdominal compression-cardiopulmonary resuscitation and resuscitation outcome during asystole and electromechanical dissociation. Circulation. Dec 1992;86(6):1692–700.
24. Mateer JR, Stueven HA, Thompson BM, et al. Prehospital IAC-CPR versus standard CPR: paramedic resuscitation of cardiac arrests. Am J Emerg Med. Mar 1985;3(2):143–6.
25. Tang W, Weil MH, Schock RB, et al. Phased chest and abdominal compression-decompression. A new option for cardiopulmonary resuscitation. Circulation. Mar 4 1997;95(5):1335–40.
26. Arntz HR, Agrawal R, Richter H, et al. Phased chest and abdominal compression-decompression versus conventional cardiopulmonary resuscitation in out-of-hospital cardiac arrest. Circulation. Aug 14 2001;104(7):768–72.
27. Christenson JM, Hamilton DR, Scott-Douglas NW, et al. Abdominal compressions during CPR: hemodynamic effects of altering timing and force. J Emerg Med. May-Jun 1992;10(3):257–66.
28. Yannopoulos D, Tang W, Roussos C, et al. Reducing ventilation frequency during cardiopulmonary resuscitation in a porcine model of cardiac arrest. Respir Care. May 2005;50(5):628–35.
29. Aufderheide TP, Lurie KG. Death by hyperventilation: a common and life-threatening problem during cardiopulmonary resuscitation. Crit Care Med. Sep 2004;32(9 suppl):S345–51.
30. Dickinson ET, Verdile VP, Schneider RM, et al. Effectiveness of mechanical versus manual chest compressions in out-of-hospital cardiac arrest resuscitation: a pilot study. Am J Emerg Med. May 1998;16(3):289–92.
31. McDonald JL. Systolic and mean arterial pressures during manual and mechanical CPR in humans. Ann Emerg Med. Jun 1982;11(6):292–5.
32. Ward KR, Menegazzi JJ, Zelenak RR, et al. A comparison of chest compressions between mechanical and manual CPR by monitoring end-tidal PCO2 during human cardiac arrest. Ann Emerg Med. Apr 1993;22(4):669–74.
33. Halperin HR, Guerci AD, Chandra N, et al. Vest inflation without simultaneous ventilation during cardiac arrest in dogs: improved survival from prolonged cardiopulmonary resuscitation. Circulation. Dec 1986;74(6):1407–15.
34. Halperin HR, Tsitlik JE, Gelfand M, et al. A preliminary study of cardiopulmonary resuscitation by circumferential compression of the chest with use

of a pneumatic vest. N Engl J Med. Sep 9 1993; 329(11):762–8.
35. Casner M, Andersen D, Isaacs SM. The impact of a new CPR assist device on rate of return of spontaneous circulation in out-of-hospital cardiac arrest. Prehosp Emerg Care. Jan-Mar 2005;9(1):61–7.
36. Timerman S, Cardoso LF, Ramires JA, et al. Improved hemodynamic performance with a novel chest compression device during treatment of in-hospital cardiac arrest. Resuscitation. Jun 2004; 61(3):273–80.
37. Eynon CA. Minimally invasive direct cardiac massage and defibrillation. Resuscitation. Nov 2000;47(3):325–8.
38. Rozenberg A, Incagnoli P, Delpech P, et al. Prehospital use of minimally invasive direct cardiac massage (MID-CM): a pilot study. Resuscitation. Sep 2001;50(3):257–62.
39. Dalton HJ, Rycus PT, Conrad SA. Update on extracorporeal life support 2004. Semin Perinatol. Feb 2005;29(1):24–33.
40. Kelly RB, Porter PA, Meier AH, et al. Duration of cardiopulmonary resuscitation before extracorporeal rescue: how long is not long enough? ASAIO J. Sep–Oct 2005;51(5):665–7.
41. Younger JG, Schreiner RJ, Swaniker F, et al. Extracorporeal resuscitation of cardiac arrest. Acad Emerg Med. Jul 1999;6(7):700–7.

75
Pharmacology in Cardiopulmonary Resuscitation

Patrick I. Plaisance, Claire Broche, and Karima Mezaïb

The number of drugs available for cardiopulmonary resuscitation (CPR) is limited, and there are few data regarding their use. Furthermore, no drug should be administered before performing electric shocks when indicated and before starting chest compressions. A recent large study performed by Stiell et al. (1) showed that advanced cardiac life support is a less important parameter that positively influences outcome of patients in cardiac arrest.

Vasopressors

Despite the historical use of epinephrine in cardiac arrest and despite several studies using vasopressin, there are no randomized studies versus placebo proving that the routine use of vasopressor improves hospital discharge rates of patients with cardiac arrest. There is insufficient scientific evidence to indicate or counterindicate the systematic use of a specific vasopressor and to propose a rational therapeutic sequence. Nevertheless, despite the lack of scientific data in humans, it is necessary to keep using vasopressors in the treatment of cardiac arrest patients in order to improve cerebral and coronary perfusion pressures during CPR.

Epinephrine

Epinephrine has been used in cardiac arrest for more than 40 years. Its efficacy comes from its α-agonist properties inducing an increase in coronary and cerebral perfusion pressures secondary to systemic vasoconstriction. The standard intravenous dose of epinephrine is 1 mg repeated every 5 minutes. The use of higher doses in patients in refractory cardiac arrest never showed an improvement in hospital discharge rate, but a dose of 5 mg did show an improvement in return of spontaneous circulation (2). This improvement also includes reduced admission rates in the subgroup with asystole as initial cardiac rhythm, while there is no difference in survival rate in the subgroup with ventricular fibrillation.

Vasopressin

The β-agonist effect of epinephrine induces chronotropic and inotropic positive actions and contributes to increased coronary and cerebral perfusion pressures. However, these actions simultaneously increase myocardial oxygen consumption, enhance the risk of ventricular arrhythmia (specially in acidotic myocardium), and may induce transitory hypoxia by increasing pulmonary arteriovenous shunt. This potentially deleterious β-agonist effect leads authors to search for alternative medications.

Vasopressin is a hypothalamic polypeptide hormone whose physiologic action is antidiuretic and vasopressive due to its effect on vascular V1 receptors. The role of vasopressin in CPR was initially demonstrated in prehospital cardiac arrest studies showing that patients successfully resuscitated had higher levels of vasopressin concentrations in the blood than patients who did not survive (3,4). Most experimental studies showed an improvement in hemodynamics when vasopressin was administered instead of epinephrine (5–7). At the same time, the first clinical study in 1996 using vasopressin in CPR was promising. In this study, in a population of cardiac arrest patients refractory to standard therapy with epinephrine, vasopressin induced return of spontaneous circulation in the eight patients studied, three of whom had no neurologic sequelae (8).

The same authors published another small randomized study of cardiac arrest patients in ventricular fibrillation for whom the rate of return of spontaneous circulation and 24-hour survival were significantly higher in the patients treated with vasopressin as compared with those treated with epinephrine. Consequently, the American Heart Association recommended vasopressin as an alternative to epinephrine in ventricular fibrillation refractory to electric shocks (9). Since then, two important in-hospital (10) and out-of-hospital (11) prospective randomized studies comparing vasopressin to epinephrine were performed. The in-hospital study compared one intravenous injection of each vasopressor (1 mg epinephrine versus 40 UI vasopressin), while the out-of-hospital study compared two successive intravenous injections of epinephrine and vasopressin with the same doses. For both studies, the complementary treatment in cases of protocol inefficacy consisted of repeated injections of epinephrine in accordance with international guidelines. The in-hospital study of 200 patients did not find any difference between the two groups in terms of return of spontaneous circulation as well as hospital admission and hospital discharge rates (10). The out-of-hospital study of 1186 patients found no significant difference (p = .06) in the overall population in the two groups regarding hospital admission. The secondary analysis of subgroups showed that vasopressin significantly improved the hospital admission and hospital discharge rates in patients with asystole as the initial cardiac rhythm (11). In the same study, in the 732 patients who did not reach a return of spontaneous circulation after the two injections, the supplemental treatment with epinephrine induced an increase in hospital admission and hospital discharge rates in the vasopressin group as compared to the epinephrine group.

In a study using pigs, the combination of epinephrine and vasopressin significantly improved animal survival and coronary perfusion pressure (whatever the doses used) as compared to administration of each drug alone (12). The benefit of this combination was also found by the same research team using piglets (13).

A recent meta-analysis of five randomized studies showed that there is no significant difference between vasopressin and epinephrine in terms of return of spontaneous circulation, 24-hour survival, and hospital discharge (14).

Despite the lack of controlled studies versus placebo, epinephrine remains the standard vasopressor indicated in the treatment of cardiac arrest. There are insufficient scientific data for proposing or for discontinuing the use of vasopressin as an alternative or in combination with epinephrine in cardiac arrest. Epinephrine is still the first-line medication to use in cardiac arrest whatever the etiology. It must be administered every 3 to 5 minutes during CPR, following the universal algorithm. The initial advocated dose is 1 mg. If intravenous or intraosseous access is not immediately available, 2 to 3 mg of epinephrine diluted in 10 mL of sterile water may be administered through the endotracheal tube. If repeated doses of 1 mg epinephrine are insufficient in refractory asystole, it is possible to increase the doses up to 5 mg per injection despite the risk of inducing tachycardia, ventricular arrhythmia, or myocardial ischemia.

α-Methyl Norepinephrine

One clinical study has shown an equivalent effect of norepinephrine as compared with epinephrine (15). Other preliminary experimental studies also found a beneficial effect of norepinephrine in short-term outcome after cardiac arrest with ventricular fibrillation (16). In practice, due to the lack of subsequent studies, norepinephrine is not recommended as an alternative medication to epinephrine.

Endothelin

In several experimental studies, endothelin-1 has been shown to improve coronary perfusion pressure. Nevertheless, in the absence of clinical data, endothelin is not recommended.

Antiarrhythmic Drugs

There is no scientific evidence that antiarrhythmic medications improve hospital discharge rates after cardiac arrest. However, compared to placebo (17) and lidocaine (18), the use of amiodarone in ventricular fibrillations refractory to electric shocks improves resuscitation rates and hospital admission. Consequently, despite any significant data on long-term survival, it seems reasonable to keep using an antiarrhythmic drug in the treatment of ventricular fibrillation resistant to shocks.

Amiodarone

Amiodarone is an antiarrhythmic medication that stabilizes membranes and increases the auricular and ventricular period of he potential of action as well as the refractory period. The atrioventricular conduction is slowed down as well as conduction of appended bundles. Amiodarone has a negative inotropic effect and is responsible for peripheral vasodilation due to its nonspecific α-blocking action. In two prospective double-blind clinical trials in adults victims of out-of-hospital ventricular fibrillation refractory to two electric shocks, administration of 300 mg (5 mg/kg) by paramedics increased admission rates as compared to placebo (19), or to lidocaine (1.5 mg/kg) (18). Subsequent animal and human studies also found that amiodarone improved the response to defibrillation (20–23). On the other hand, there are no scientific data determining the optimal period to administer amiodarone. Up to now, clinical studies were performed with one injection of amiodarone administered after three shocks. For this reason, and in the absence of alternatives, amiodarone is recommended in this specific indication. Amiodarone must be ideally diluted in 20 mL of dextrose 5%. Peripheral intravenous injection of amiodarone may induce thrombophlebitis. Thus, this drug should be administered from a central intravenous line or at least from a large peripheral catheter.

Lidocaine

Since the international guidelines published in 2000, lidocaine is no longer the first-line antiarrhythmic in cases of ventricular fibrillation refractory to shocks. At present, lidocaine is not recommended, even when amiodarone is not available.

Magnesium

Magnesium is an important component of numerous enzymatic systems, particularly in adenosine triphosphate synthesis in muscle tissue. Magnesium improves contractile response in cases of stunned myocardium and potentially limits myocardial infarction size by an unknown mechanism (24). Hypomagnesemia is often associated with hypokalemia and may participate in the genesis of arrhythmias and in cardiac arrest. Furthermore, hypomagnesemia increases myocardial sensitivity to digitalis and decreases the adenosine triphosphate activity of the myocardial cell. The benefit of magnesium in patients with hypomagnesemia is well known, but the benefit of magnesium in cardiac arrest has not been proved. Clinical studies performed in adults with out-of-hospital or in-hospital cardiac arrest never demonstrated any improvement in return of spontaneous circulation after the administration of magnesium, except for one case report (25–31). The new guidelines recommend magnesium sulfate in the following situations:

- Patients with suspected hypomagnesemia who are in ventricular fibrillation refractory to shocks
- Patients with torsades de pointes
- Patients with digitalis poisoning

In these cases, an initial intravenous dose of 2 g is administered within 1 or 2 minutes. This dose may be repeated once after 10 to 15 minutes.

Other Medications

There is no scientific evidence justifying the routine use of other drugs.

Atropine

Atropine is an antagonist of acetylcholine acting on muscarinic receptors. It blocks the effect of the vagal nerve on the atrial sinus and the atrioventricular bond. It increases the automaticity of the sinus and facilitates atrioventricular conduction. Five prospective nonrandomized controlled studies have shown no benefit from atropine in the treatment of out-of-hospital and in-hospital cardiac arrest (32–36). Consequently, atropine is not systematically indicated in the treatment of asystole. It can be considered on a case-by-case basis in pulseless electrical activity appearing after an initially efficient bradycardia and must be administered as a unique bolus of 3 mg intravenously.

Aminophylline

Aminophylline is a phosphodiesterase inhibitor that increases cyclic adenosine monophosphate (cAMP) tissue concentration and facilitates adrenergic secretion from the suprarenal glands. Its acts as a positive chronotropic and inotopic drug. The few studies analyzing the effects of aminophylline in cardiac arrest with asystole secondary to bradycardia did not find any improvement in short-term survival (37–40). Aminophylline is not indicated in the treatment of cardiac arrest except in bradycardia preceding cardiac arrest or refractory to atropine.

Calcium

Calcium plays an essential role in the intracellular mechanism of myocardial contraction. But elevated plasma concentrations after intravenous injection of calcium may be deleterious in terms of myocardial ischemia and neurologic outcome. Thus, calcium is not recommended routinely in the treatment of cardiac arrest. The only indications are those that induce pulseless electrical activity: hyperkalemia, hypocalcemia, and calcium blocker poisoning. The initial intravenous dose is 10 mL of 10% calcium chloride.

Buffers

Cardiac arrest induces a mixed respiratory and metabolic acidosis induced by alveolocapillary mismatching and by anaerobic cellular metabolism. The best treatment is chest compressions and adequate ventilation. There are no high-level studies focusing on the potential benefit of the use of sodium bicarbonate during CPR. The only available studies did not find any benefit versus placebo (41) or any improvement in outcome (42–46), except for one study that suggests an improvement in outcome (47). Sandeman et al. (48) found a benefit by infusing sodium bicarbonate in cardiac arrests secondary to tricyclic or calcium antagonists poisoning. Then, systematic infusion of sodium bicarbonate during CPR or after return of spontaneous circulation is not recommended. Specific indications are cardiac arrest with severe hyperkalemia or with preexisting metabolic acidosis, and tricyclic poisoning; 50 mmol of sodium bicarbonate can be administered intravenously. This dose can be repeated if necessary 10 minutes later.

Fibrinolysis in Cardiopulmonary Resuscitation

Sudden cardiac arrest in adults is often due to acute myocardial ischemia secondary to occlusion of a coronary artery by a thrombus. The use of thrombolytic medications in CPR has been shown to be efficient particularly in cases of high suspicion of pulmonary embolism. Studies have shown improvement of cerebral prognosis when a thrombolytic agent is used during experimental (49) and clinical (50) trials. Two other studies found an improvement in return of spontaneous circulation after thrombolysis with no increase in hospital discharge rates (51,52). Case reports found an improvement in hospital discharge rates in patients with ventricular fibrillation or pulseless electrical activity (53). On the other hand, a large clinical prospective trial enrolling 233 patients with pulseless electrical activity did not find any improvement in outcome after thrombolysis (54).

Several clinical studies have shown clinical benefit with no hemorrhagic complications in cardiac arrest caused by pulmonary embolism (51,52,54,55). But clinical data are insufficient to routinely recommend thrombolysis in nontraumatic cardiac arrests. This therapy may be considered on a case-by-case basis when initial CPR is unfruitful and when an acute coronary etiology is suspected. Thrombolysis is indicated when pulmonary embolism is suspected or acknowledged. Due to its onset of action and the delay before efficacy, thrombolysis entails prolonging CPR for 60 to 90 minutes (56).

Fluids

Systematic fluid loading during CPR is controversial. There are no clinical studies in normovolemic cardiac arrest showing any benefit. Hypovolemia is a potentially reversible cause of cardiac arrest. In cases of hypovolemia, rapid fluid loading must be performed. Normal saline infusion is the first-line solution to administer in this specific indication.

Alternative Routes to Administer Medications in Cardiopulmonary Resuscitation

The main route to administer fluids and drugs in CPR is the intravenous one. The intravenous peripheral route is as effective as the central route (57). Because of a higher blood flow induced by chest compressions during CPR in the superior vena cava territory, the intravenous line should be put in this territory instead of the inferior vena cava territory.

The Intraosseous Route

If an intravenous line is not rapidly available, administration of drugs by the intraosseous route must be considered because plasma concentrations of drugs are adequate. Numerous studies have shown that the intraosseous route is safe and efficient for the distribution of drugs as well as solution infusions (58,59). Traditionally, the intraosseous route is largely used in children but may also be effective in adults.

The Endotracheal Route

Drugs may also be administered through an endotracheal tube, but plasma concentration obtained from this route is variable and significantly lower than the one obtained from the intravenous or intraosseous routes. To obtain equivalent plasma concentrations, doses of epinephrine must be tripled (60). In a nonrandomized study, return of spontaneous circulation and admission rates were higher when drugs (epinephrine and atropine) were administered intravenously instead of endotracheally (61). Furthermore, epinephrine plasma concentrations are higher when the drug is diluted in distilled water than in normal saline (62). During CPR, pulmonary perfusion does not exceed 10% to 30% of its normal value. This induces stagnation of the endobronchial distilled epinephrine. When spontaneous cardiac activity is reached after high doses of epinephrine administered from the endotracheal route, a prolonged epinephrine reabsorption from the lungs to pulmonary circulation may occur. This may induce hypertension, arrhythmias, or ventricular fibrillation recurrence (60). Lidocaine, atropine, and vasopressin can also be administered through the endotracheal tube, but plasma concentrations obtained are also variable (63). Amiodarone cannot be used by this route. There is no benefit to practice distal endobronchial injection of the drugs from a catheter connected to the syringe as compared with direct proximal injection into the endotracheal tube.

Conclusion

Even though the delivery of drugs has not been shown to increase survival to hospital discharge after cardiac arrest, it is still a part of advanced cardiac life support intervention. The first-line drug remains epinephrine whatever the initial cardiac rhythm. Lidocaine and vasopressin are second-line treatments, after epinephrine and amiodarone, for ventricular fibrillation.

References

1. Stiell IG, Wells GA, Field B, et al.: Ontario Prehospital Advanced Life Support Study Group: Advanced cardiac life support in out-of-hospital cardiac arrest. N Engl J Med 2004;351:647–56.
2. Gueugniaud PY, Mols P, Goldstein P, et al.: A comparison of repeated high doses and repeated standard doses of epinephrine for cardiac arrest outside the hospital. European Epinephrine Study Group. N Engl J Med 1998;339:1595–601.
3. Lindner KH, Strohmenger HU, Ensinger H, Hetzel WD, Ahnefeld FW, Georgieff M: Stress hormone response during and after cardiopulmonary resuscitation. Anesthesiology 1992;77:662–8.
4. Lindner KH, Haak T, Keller A, Bothner U, Lurie KG: Release of endogenous vasopressors during

and after cardiopulmonary resuscitation. Heart 1996;75:145–50.

5. Lindner KH, Brinkmann A, Pfenninger EG, Lurie KG, Goertz A, Lindner IM: Effect of vasopressin on hemodynamic variables, organ blood flow, and acid-base status in a pig model of cardiopulmonary resuscitation. Anesth Analg 1993;77:427–35.
6. Lindner KH, Prengel AW, Pfenninger EG, et al.: Vasopressin improves vital organ blood flow during closed-chest cardiopulmonary resuscitation in pigs. Circulation 1995;91:215–21.
7. Wenzel V, Lindner KH, Prengel AW, et al.: Vasopressin improves vital organ blood flow after prolonged cardiac arrest with postcountershock pulseless electrical activity in pigs. Crit Care Med 1999;27:486–92.
8. Lindner KH, Prengel AW, Brinkmann A, Strohmenger HU, Lindner IM, Lurie KG: Vasopressin administration in refractory cardiac arrest. Ann Intern Med 1996;124:1061–4.
9. American Heart Association in collaboration with International Liaison Committee on Resuscitation. Guidelines 2000 for Cardiopulmonary Resuscitation and Emergency Cardiovascular Care: International Consensus on Science: Section 6. Pharmacology II: agents to Optimize Cardiac Output and Blood Pressure. Circulation 2000; 102(suppl I):I129–35.
10. Stiell IG, Hebert PC, Wells GA, et al.: Vasopressin versus epinephrine for inhospital cardiac arrest: a randomised controlled trial. Lancet 2001;358:105–9.
11. Wenzel V, Krismer AC, Arntz HR, Sitter H, Stadlbauer KH, Lindner KH: A comparison of vasopressin and epinephrine for out-of-hospital cardiopulmonary resuscitation. N Engl J Med 2004;350: 105–13.
12. Mayr VD, Wenzel V, Voelckel WG, et al.: Developing a vasopressor combination in a pig model of adult asphyxial cardiac arrest. Circulation 2001; 104:1651–6.
13. Voelckel WG, Lurie KG, McKnite S, et al.: Effects of epinephrine and vasopressin in a piglet model of prolonged ventricular fibrillation and cardiopulmonary resuscitation. Crit Care Med 2002;30: 957–62.
14. Aung K, Htay T: Vasopressin for cardiac arrest: a systematic review and meta-analysis. Arch Intern Med 2005;165:17–24.
15. Callaham M, Madsen CD, Barton CW, Saunders CE, Pointer J: A randomized clinical trial of high-dose epinephrine and norepinephrine vs standard-dose epinephrine in prehospital cardiac arrest. JAMA 1992;268:2667–72.
16. Klouche KWM, Sun S, Tang W, Zhao DH: A comparison of alpha-methylnorepinephrine, vasopressin and epinephrine for cardiac resuscitation. Resuscitation 2003;57:93–100.
17. Hilwig RW, Berg RA, Kern KB, Ewy GA: Endothelin-1 vasoconstriction during swine cardiopulmonary resuscitation improves coronary perfusion pressures but worsens postresuscitation outcome. Circulation 2000;101:2097–102.
18. Dorian P, Cass D, Schwartz B, Cooper R, Gelaznikas R, Barr A: Amiodarone as compared with lidocaine for shock-resistant ventricular fibrillation. N Engl J Med 2002;346:884–90.
19. Kudenchuk PJ, Cobb LA, Copass MK, et al.: Amiodarone for resuscitation after out-of-hospital cardiac arrest due to ventricular fibrillation. N Engl J Med 1999;341:871–8.
20. Somberg JC, Timar S, Bailin SJ, et al.: Lack of a hypotensive effect with rapid administration of a new aqueous formulation of intravenous amiodarone. Am J Cardiol 2004;93:576–81.
21. Skrifvars MB, Kuisma M, Boyd J, et al.: The use of undiluted amiodarone in the management of out-of-hospital cardiac arrest. Acta Anaesthesiol Scand 2004;48:582–7.
22. Petrovic T, Adnet F, Lapandry C: Successful resuscitation of ventricular fibrillation after low-dose amiodarone. Ann Emerg Med 1998;32:518–9.
23. Levine JH, Massumi A, Scheinman MM, et al.: Intravenous amiodarone for recurrent sustained hypotensive ventricular tachyarrhythmias. Intravenous Amiodarone Multicenter Trial Group. J Am Coll Cardiol 1996;27:67–75.
24. Matsusaka T, Hasebe N, Jin YT, Kawabe J, Kikuchi K: Magnesium reduces myocardial infarct size via enhancement of adenosine mechanism in rabbits. Cardiovasc Res 2002;54:568–75.
25. Thel MC, Armstrong AL, McNulty SE, Califf RM, O'Connor CM: Randomised trial of magnesium in in-hospital cardiac arrest. Lancet 1997;350:1272–6.
26. Allegra J, Lavery R, Cody R, et al.: Magnesium sulfate in the treatment of refractory ventricular fibrillation in the prehospital setting. Resuscitation 2001;49:245–9.
27. Fatovich D, Prentice D, Dobb G: Magnesium in in-hospital cardiac arrest. Lancet 1998;351:446.
28. Hassan TB, Jagger C, Barnett DB: A randomised trial to investigate the efficacy of magnesium sulphate for refractory ventricular fibrillation. Emerg Med J 2002;19:57–62.
29. Miller B, Craddock L, Hoffenberg S, et al.: Pilot study of intravenous magnesium sulfate in refractory cardiac arrest: safety data and recommendations for future studies. Resuscitation 1995;30:3–14.

30. Longstreth WT Jr, Fahrenbruch CE, Olsufka M, Walsh TR, Copass MK, Cobb LA: Randomized clinical trial of magnesium, diazepam, or both after out-of-hospital cardiac arrest. Neurology 2002;59: 506–14.
31. Baraka A, Ayoub C, Kawkabani N: Magnesium therapy for refractory ventricular fibrillation. J Cardiothorac Vasc Anesth 2000;14:196–9.
32. Stiell IG, Wells GA, Hebert PC, Laupacis A, Weitzman BN: Association of drug therapy with survival in cardiac arrest: limited role of advanced cardiac life support drugs. Acad Emerg Med 1995;2: 264–73.
33. Engdahl J, Bang A, Lindqvist J, Herlitz J: Can we define patients with no and those with some chance of survival when found in asystole out of hospital? Am J Cardiol 2000;86:610–4.
34. Engdahl J, Bang A, Lindqvist J, Herlitz J: Factors affecting short- and long-term prognosis among 1069 patients with out-of-hospital cardiac arrest and pulseless electrical activity. Resuscitation 2001;51:17–25.
35. Dumot JA, Burval DJ, Sprung J, et al.: Outcome of adult cardiopulmonary resuscitations at a tertiary referral center including results of "limited" resuscitations. Arch Intern Med 2001;161:1751–8.
36. Dumot J, Burva LD, Sprung J, et al.: Outcome of adult cardiopulmonary resuscitations at a tertiary referral center including results of "limited" resuscitations. Arch Intern Med 2001;161:1751–8.
37. Viskin S, Belhassen B, Roth A, et al.: Aminophylline for bradyasystolic cardiac arrest refractory to atropine and epinephrine. Ann Intern Med 1993;118: 279–81.
38. Mader TJ, Gibson P: Adenosine receptor antagonism in refractory asystolic cardiac arrest: results of a human pilot study. Resuscitation 1997;35:3–7.
39. Mader TJ, Smithline HA, Gibson P: Aminophylline in undifferentiated out-of-hospital asystolic cardiac arrest. Resuscitation 1999;41:39–45.
40. Mader TJ, Smithline HA, Durkin L, Scriver G: A randomized controlled trial of intravenous aminophylline for atropine-resistant out-of-hospital asystolic cardiac arrest. Acad Emerg Med 2003;10: 192–7.
41. Dybvik T, Strand T, Steen PA: Buffer therapy during out-of-hospital cardiopulmonary resuscitation. Resuscitation 1995;29:89–95.
42. Aufderheide TP, Martin DR, Olson DW, et al.: Prehospital bicarbonate use in cardiac arrest: a 3-year experience. Am J Emerg Med 1992;10:4–7.
43. Delooz HH, Lewi PJ: Are inter-center differences in EMS-management and sodium-bicarbonate administration important for the outcome of CPR? The Cerebral Resuscitation Study Group. Resuscitation 1989;17 (suppl):S161–72.
44. Roberts D, Landolfo K, Light RB, Dobson K: Early predictors of mortality for hospitalized patients suffering cardiopulmonary arrest. Chest 1990;97: 413–9.
45. Suljaga-Pechtel K, Goldberg E, Strickon P, Berger M, Skovron ML: Cardiopulmonary resuscitation in a hospitalized population: prospective study of factors associated with outcome. Resuscitation 1984;12:77–95.
46. Weil MH, Trevino RP, Rackow EC: Sodium bicarbonate during CPR. Does it help or hinder? Chest 1985;88:487.
47. Bar-Joseph G, Abramson NS, Kelsey SF, Mashiach T, Craig MT, Safar P: Improved resuscitation outcome in emergency medical systems with increased usage of sodium bicarbonate during cardiopulmonary resuscitation. Acta Anaesthesiol Scand 2005;49:6–15.
48. Sandeman DJ, Alahakoon TI, Bentley SC: Tricyclic poisoning—successful management of ventricular fibrillation following massive overdose of imipramine. Anaesth Intensive Care 1997;25:542–5.
49. Fischer M, Bottiger BW, Popov-Cenic S, Hossmann KA: Thrombolysis using plasminogen activator and heparin reduces cerebral no-reflow after resuscitation from cardiac arrest: an experimental study in the cat. Intensive Care Med 1996;22:1214–23.
50. Ruiz-Bailen M, Aguayo de Hoyos E, Serrano-Corcoles MC, Diaz-Castellanos MA, Ramos-Cuadra JA, Reina-Toral A: Efficacy of thrombolysis in patients with acute myocardial infarction requiring cardiopulmonary resuscitation. Intensive Care Med 2001;27:1050–7.
51. Bottiger BW, Bode C, Kern S, et al.: Efficacy and safety of thrombolytic therapy after initially unsuccessful cardiopulmonary resuscitation: a prospective clinical trial. Lancet 2001;357:1583–5.
52. Lederer W, Lichtenberger C, Pechlaner C, Kroesen G, Baubin M: Recombinant tissue plasminogen activator during cardiopulmonary resuscitation in 108 patients with out-of-hospital cardiac arrest. Resuscitation 2001;50:71–6.
53. Tiffany PA, Schultz M, Stueven H: Bolus thrombolytic infusions during CPR for patients with refractory arrest rhythms: outcome of a case series. Ann Emerg Med 1998;31:124–6.
54. Abu-Laban RB, Christenson JM, Innes GD, et al.: Tissue plasminogen activator in cardiac arrest with pulseless electrical activity. N Engl J Med 2002;346: 1522–8.
55. Lederer W, Lichtenberger C, Pechlaner C, Kinzl J, Kroesen G, Baubin M: Long-term survival and

neurological outcome of patients who received recombinant tissue plasminogen activator during out-of-hospital cardiac arrest. Resuscitation 2004; 61:123–9.

56. Bottiger BW, Martin E: Thrombolytic therapy during cardiopulmonary resuscitation and the role of coagulation activation after cardiac arrest. Curr Opin Crit Care 2001;7:176–83.
57. Gueugniaud PY, Theurey O, Vaudelin T, Rochette M, Petit P: Peripheral versus central intravenous lines in emergency cardiac care. Lancet 1987;2: 573.
58. Guy J, Haley K, Zuspan SJ: Use of intraosseous infusion in the pediatric trauma patient. J Pediatr Surg 1993;28:158–61.
59. Macnab A, Christenson J, Findlay J, et al.: A new system for sternal intraosseous infusion in adults. Prehosp Emerg Care 2000;4:173–7.
60. Hornchen U, Schuttler J, Stoeckel H, Eichelkraut W, Hahn N: Endobronchial instillation of epinephrine during cardiopulmonary resuscitation. Crit Care Med 1987;15:1037–9.
61. Niemann JT, Stratton SJ, Cruz B, Lewis RJ: Endotracheal drug administration during out-of-hospital resuscitation: where are the survivors? Resuscitation 2002;53:153–7.
62. Naganobu K, Hasebe Y, Uchiyama Y, Hagio M, Ogawa H: A comparison of distilled water and normal saline as diluents for endobronchial administration of epinephrine in the dog. Anesth Analg 2000;91:317–21.
63. Prengel AW, Rembecki M, Wenzel V, Steinbach G: A comparison of the endotracheal tube and the laryngeal mask airway as a route for endobronchial lidocaine administration. Anesth Analg 2001;92:1505–9.

76 Role of Automated External Defibrillators in Acute Heart Failure Patients

Jane G. Wigginton, Paul E. Pepe, and Thomas R. Aversano

A lethal complication associated with acute heart failure syndrome (AHFS) is out-of-hospital cardiac arrest due to a sudden ventricular arrhythmia, either ventricular fibrillation (VF) or ventricular tachycardia (VT) deteriorating into VF (1–6). However, the unique morbidity of AHFS makes management more of a challenge. One potential intervention that should be considered is evolving technology for automated external defibrillation, the main focus of this chapter.

Pathophysiology

From a pathophysiologic perspective, the VF/VT associated with AHFS may be the consequence of an acute ischemic coronary syndrome that simultaneous leads to both pump failure and conductive dysfunction (1,5,6). The VF may also be the consequence of acute ventricular dysfunction, conduction abnormalities, or acute heart wall distention that leads to inadequate perfusion, distorted conduction, or reentrant phenomenon (2,5). It also may result from a myriad of miscellaneous mechanisms such an associated acute left atrial distention and a secondary sudden rapid tachycardia that deteriorates into VF/VT (5).

Management

Defibrillation in Acute Heart Failure Syndrome

While patients with chronic heart failure may have an acute exacerbation complicated by VF/VT, cardiac arrest may also be the first overt symptom of an AHFS event (5,6). In general, most cases of sudden VF, even in the out-of-hospital setting, are readily reversible when a defibrillator is immediately available and used rapidly (6–9). Given the complicated pathophysiologic pathways of AHFS, however, the onset of VF/VT and the respective response to therapy may be harder to predict (4,5). For example, the predisposition to the ventricular arrhythmia may make therapy for the AHFS more difficult and the AHFS presumably decreases the chance of rapidly achieving and sustaining a return of spontaneous circulation (ROSC) in an acute cardiac arrest event. Therefore, the confounding factors may pose a vicious cycle that can complicate the resuscitation effort.

Clearly, patients presenting first with apparent cardiogenic shock manifested by deteriorating blood pressure and other ostensible signs of shock are less likely to be resuscitated and survive. Studies of paramedics caring for patients who have a VF/VT cardiac arrest, after the paramedics have arrived on the scene, have demonstrated outstanding outcomes if blood pressures were greater than 120 mm Hg systolic versus those who presented with lower or unobtainable pressures before the onset of VF/VT (10). Presumably, even with immediate application of basic cardiopulmonary resuscitation (CPR) and defibrillation within seconds under such circumstances, the predominance of apparent severe pump failure leading to secondary VF is the likely underlying mechanism of the arrest. Therefore, the VF/VT is less likely to be reversible than VF/VT occurring in patients with better hemodynamics prior to the arrest.

Nevertheless, beyond such rudimentary studies, there are no definitive guidelines to determine which sudden death patients have an AHFS other than the crude history obtained under duress by responding emergency medical services (EMS) personnel at the scene of a VF/VT arrest. More importantly, even if the history of heart failure is known prospectively, it is not always clear which patients with AHFS will have a favorable prognosis (4,5).

Therefore, recognizing that VF is essentially untreatable in the absence of a defibrillator, it should be assumed for now that attempts at defibrillation should be the priority in all AHFS patients presenting with VF/VT, and the sooner the better. Irrespective of cerebral ischemia and evolving cardiovascular collapse, when a person with heart failure has the additional ischemic insult of cardiac arrest, it is intuitive that the longer the VF persists, the harder it will be to resuscitate the patient.

Rationale for Implanted Defibrillators

Given the assumption that a patient with known heart failure has a risk for VF/VT arrest and the earliest possible treatment is beneficial, an increasing number of patients with known coronary artery disease or heart failure have become recipients of automated implantable cardiac defibrillators (AICDs). Although AICDs have associated high costs and some morbidity, and may need replacement from time to time, evolving data support their insertion (1–5). In addition to overall survival advantages across study populations, they also provide some reassurances that, despite a predicted poor prognosis, even the sickest patients receive the most aggressive opportunity to survive (1–5).

As a result, many patients with heart failure may be provided with an AICD, particularly those with low ejection fractions after a myocardial infarction (3–5). At the same time, however, many patients are not provided this intervention immediately after their myocardial infarction or, for various reasons, they may not receive it at all. More importantly, as stated previously, many unidentified patients with AHFS may first present with VF/VT. Therefore, other considerations to provide immediate defibrillation must be entertained.

Effectiveness of the Automated External Defibrillator

Many of the lifesaving efforts now being studied in out-of-hospital cardiac arrest situations have begun to focus on how the average person can save lives through evolving technology and, in turn, even spare precious intensive care unit (ICU) resources (7,11,12). The relevant example of such technology has been the development and widespread deployment of the automated external defibrillator (AED). In the original study of public AED use conducted in the late 1990s at the Chicago airports, the AEDs were deployed throughout the airline terminals for emergency use by persons witnessing a collapse in those areas (7). Not only did random bystanders on the concourses save an extremely high percentage of cardiac arrest patients with the AEDs, the majority of patients rapidly awakened, even before the arrival of professional rescuers. As such, this technology-assisted intervention, performed by an average person, preempted the need for many other critical care interventions and the prolonged ICU stay usually required for persons resuscitated from out-of-hospital cardiac arrest (7,13,14) (Fig. 76.1).

Automated External Defibrillator in Acute Heart Failure Syndrome

Despite the clear efficacy of AEDs in VF/VT cardiac arrest, it is unknown from the available data whether or not the public AED studies and other similar investigations have specifically involved patients with AHFS and whether or not those subpopulations of patients with cardiac arrest benefited from the AED. However, until delineated otherwise, we must assume that this early intervention is beneficial for patients with AHFS because the lack of such early defibrillation would result in death, regardless of the underlying pathophysiology.

Just as empiric in-hospital experience has demonstrated, rapid defibrillation coupled with rapid treatment of AHFS will lead to resuscitation and eventual successful discharge of many patients, neurologically intact (15). Until proven otherwise, the application of this same philosophy should be applied in the out-of-hospital setting as well.

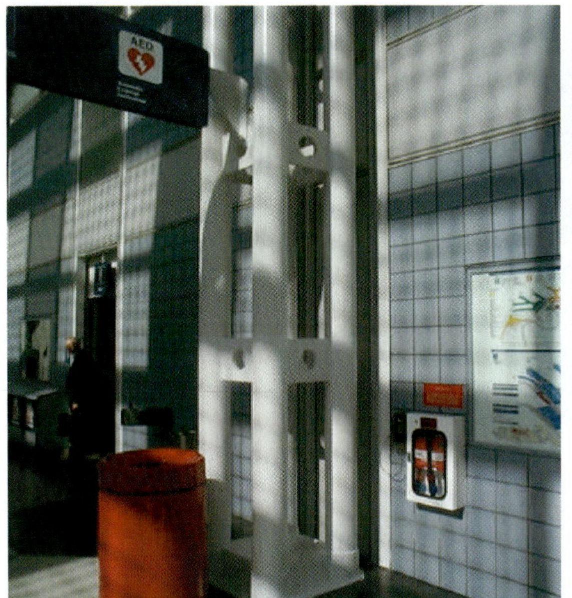

A

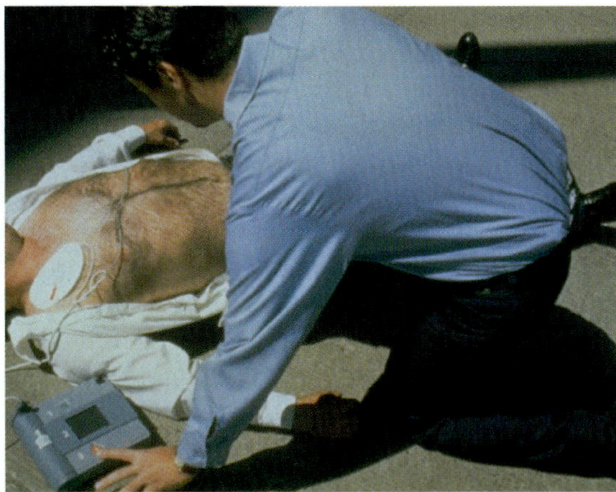

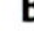

B

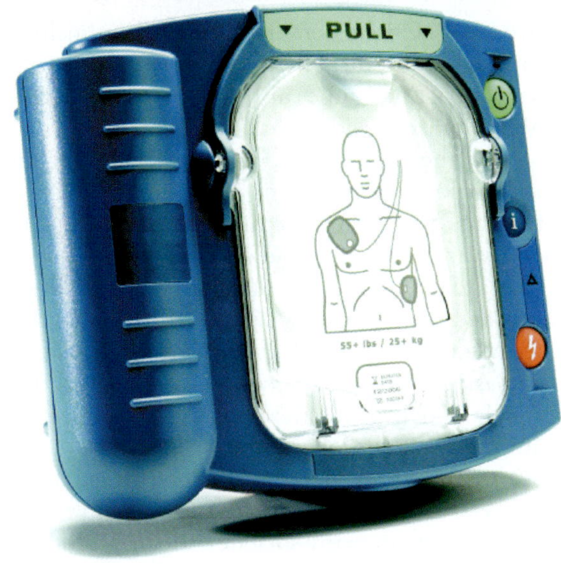

C

FIGURE 76.1. Automated external defibrillators (AED). (A) AED signs are increasingly seen in public places (here, Chicago's O'Hare Airport). (B,C) AEDs are easy to use.

Portability and Ease of Use of Automated External Defibrillator

Today's AEDs, typically weighing about 1500 g, and are so portable and so easy to use that even schoolchildren can operate them easily with no prior instruction (16). Today, the AED has become a standard part of basic CPR training for the average person, and public access to defibrillation has become an encouraged practice, at least within certain guidelines (6–9,12) (Fig. 76.1).

Special Clinical Features

It had been previously established that AEDs could be used successfully by specially targeted, specially trained laypersons such as flight attendants and casino security guards, especially because of the high likelihood of witnessed cardiac arrest and rapid, nearby availability of the AED (17,18). The results of the Chicago airport study were even more striking. In this case, random public bystanders without a duty to act successfully operated the AEDs, even though the majority of rescuers had never been specifically trained to operate an AED (7). More than three quarters of the patients collapsing in the concourses survived neurologically intact.

This higher rate of survival in the airport study may simply reflect the populations and the settings that were studied, namely an ambulating traveling public at large in the airport terminals versus a casino gambler or a passenger in the unique conditions of flight. For example, just for the purposes of speculation, the casinos may have included a greater number of patients with AHFS or some other comorbidity. Still, in all of these rapid defibrillation studies, survival rates were quite high regardless of the setting and the patients studied, thus emphasizing the central theme here of providing the most rapid AED application.

Taking this emphasis a step further, it should be noted that the majority of the patients at the Chicago airports were already awakening before the arrival of traditional EMS units (7). In contrast to the traditional experience with most out-of-hospital cardiac arrest survivors who often have remained in a coma for significant periods of time (13,14), these rapidly wakening patients clearly did not experience the usual need for endotracheal intubation, mechanical ventilation, and various intravenous pharmacologic infusions (7).

Therefore, with the rapid use of AEDs by bystanders, the usual scenario—aggressive intensive care, invasive assessments, and a myriad of consultations—was preempted for a large percentage of those patients who, traditionally, would have required them. These findings intuitively demonstrate strong evidence of a lesser global ischemic insult with rapid defibrillation. Although there are no hard data to support the claim explicitly, it is still logical that these findings would apply to patients with AHFS as well. Even if the chances of ROSC were to be less than those without a heart failure component, with a lesser global ischemic insult, they would be more likely to achieve ROSC and, ultimately, long-term, neurologically intact survival.

There are other considerations that support this concept. One of the complications of a cardiac arrest is systemic loss of tissue perfusion. That loss of oxygen delivery includes a resulting lack of energy substrate for the peripheral vasculature. The consequential loss of peripheral vascular tone can lead to severely diminished coronary artery perfusion over a matter of minutes. Even with an adequate heartbeat, there may be less of chance of ROSC because of the secondary severe drop in aortic diastolic pressures (19,20). Therefore, from this perspective as well, the shorter the duration of global ischemia, the better the chance of a good outcome, including a more effective coronary artery perfusion in the face of acute heart failure.

Feasibility of Automated External Defibrillator Use for Acute Heart Failure Syndrome

Feasibility of Layperson Use

Beyond a definitive demonstration of diminishing morbidity and mortality overall for patients with VF/VT, existing studies also supported the potential feasibility of widespread deployment of AEDs (7,8). In the Chicago airport study, many of the random persons witnessing the patients' collapse, and who stopped to help and operate the AEDs, had never been trained how to use them (7).

Regardless of manufacturer, the built-in directions and voice prompts of most AEDs make this lifesaving technology extremely easy to use. It enables the average person to become readily capable of delivering lifesaving critical care, even with little or no prior training (7,16).

Considering the fact that sudden cardiac death due to VF is one of the greatest causes of premature mortality in many societies, the magnitude of the public health impact of AEDs is potentially dramatic, both in terms of lifesaving and saving critical care resources (5,7,8). If ultimately adopted in a widespread manner and further honed by technologic advances, the use of AEDs by the average person could eventually be considered one of the greatest modern advances in medical care.

Assimilating the previous discussion and assumptions, widespread deployment of AEDs would theoretically be beneficial for AHFS, particularly for those AHFS patients who may have been considered candidates for AICDs or those who initially present with a VF/VT arrest. Although early (1980s) studies of AEDs deployed in the homes of at-risk persons did not find them to be as useful as expected (21), today's models may be much easier to operate, and the new techniques are easier to learn. The results of a more recent home AED program found that patients who had survived a previous sudden cardiac arrest event had a high acceptance of the placement of the AEDs as well as the related training, as did their families (22). While this study demonstrated confidence about their ability to use the AED if an actual emergency were to arise, survival studies have yet to be performed.

The Home Automated-Defibrillator Trial (HAT) is a 7000-patient randomized, multicenter trial designed to test the hypothesis that an in-home AED, in addition to the standard CPR training of potential in-home responders, reduces mortality in patients with prior anterior wall myocardial infarction considered at high risk for sudden death (http://www.clinicaltrials.gov/show/nct00047411).

Importance of Basic Cardiopulmonary Resuscitation Skills

Despite the clear effectiveness of the AED, the device by itself should not be considered a panacea. Specifically, AEDs should be considered one component of basic CPR techniques. Although the AED clearly enhances the effectiveness of traditional CPR, it may be ineffective without the other components of adequate chest compressions and ventilations (9,11,12).

Investigators in successful early defibrillation studies have noted that all treated patients received basic CPR interventions, even if for a brief period, before their AED application (7). In some cases, following defibrillation, the basic CPR techniques had to be continued to sustain the person before the return of spontaneous pulses (7). Moreover, recent data confirm the importance of providing aggressive chest compressions prior to defibrillation attempts if the elapsed time of cardiac arrest has extended beyond 4 or 5 minutes (12,23,24).

Likewise, studies have confirmed the importance of limiting the hands-off period between interruption of compressions and delivery of the shock. An interval as short as 15 to 20 seconds between the interruption of chest compressions until delivery of the shock may uniformly predict ineffectiveness in terms of achieving ROSC (12,25,26). On the other hand, limiting that interval to 5 seconds or less may dramatically improve the odds of ROSC. In essence, the lifesaving effectiveness of the AED may also depend on the proper use and appropriate integration of other basic CPR techniques as well. Today's AED algorithms are being amended to effect these considerations.

Facilitating Future Cardiopulmonary Resuscitation and Automated External Defibrillator Training

Half-Hour Courses

The majority of laypersons who know how to perform basic CPR and AED learned those techniques in schools or at their jobs because they were a "captured audience" and were provided the 3 to 4 hours it traditionally takes to learn the skills. Therefore, many of the persons who should be targeted to learn CPR (the spouses of older persons) are not trained, because of either a lack of easy access to a training venue or the inability to make the time commitment required to acquire CPR skills in the traditional courses. Even if they took a course in the distant past, the logistics and time commitment generally inhibit retraining. That same population of elderly spouses and partners are also the patients most likely to have AHFS as well.

Fortunately, recent innovative educational research efforts have produced video-based self-instruction (VSI) techniques that are not only highly portable but also just as effective as traditional courses, even though they are only a half-hour or less in duration (27,28). A study by Lynch et al. (27) demonstrated that a 22-minute American Heart Association (AHA) VSI course resulted in better overall CPR performance compared to the standard AHA Heartsaver® course (27). A subsequent study by Roppolo et al. (28) demonstrated not only equal effectiveness of the short VSI course but also long-term retention of those CPR skills. This abbreviated course also included the key skills of first aid for the choking victim and

5-minute training in AED use. Likewise, in formal follow-up testing, the 5-minute AED instruction was found to be just as effective as the traditional lengthy courses, not only at the time of completion of training, but 6 months later as well (29).

Technology to Improve Cardiopulmonary Resuscitation Performance

In addition to abbreviating and making CPR courses more portable, technology has also enhanced the quality of basic CPR. More recently, the quality of basic CPR techniques has come center stage in resuscitation research efforts (12). Recent investigations using innovative monitoring devices have demonstrated that current CPR performance is generally inadequate in most circumstances, both in and out of the hospital (30,31). At the same time, utilizing the same monitoring devices, rescuers can now be prompted and instructed, during an actual CPR event, to modify their actions, and, in turn, significantly improve outcomes (30–33). Combining these concepts with evolving AED technology, the effectiveness of layperson defibrillation may be enhanced even further, thus further improving survival chances for AHFS patients as well.

Key Caveats

Reliability

With the recent impetus to provide widespread proliferation of AEDs, particularly in public settings, there has been a similar growth in manufacturers and related vendors. In fact, between 1996 and 2005, the number of AED devices being purchased increased steadily (34). By 2005, the annual number of AEDs sold was tenfold that of 1996 (34). Consequently, there also has been an increasing number of reports regarding potential device flaws. Despite the initial demonstration of safety and efficacy among the original generation of AED manufacturers (8), recent reports have raised some concerns about the universal reliability of AEDs.

Specifically, during the decade between 1996 and 2005, there were a significant degree of device recalls, usually for software algorithm concerns (34). However, it was also noted that these recalls centered around potential, not actual, AED malfunctions. Considering that these recalls were generally preemptive, one could also consider these actions part of the reliability of the devices (34,35). Despite the widespread growth of manufacturers and propagation of AEDs, and although underreporting still remains a concern, the actual malfunction rate identified in available databases continues to remain less than 1 in 1000 (34,35). Therefore, given the available data and the tremendous success rates of AEDs, the reliability of the device remains impressively high.

Cost Barriers

The only remaining barrier to widespread AED deployment for AHFS patients and cases of out-of-hospital sudden death patients at large is cost. The AEDs are currently priced at about $1000 or more. While these costs are less than the cost of an AICD insertion and maintenance, the AEDs may still not be as effective in terms of the instantaneous defibrillation of an AICD. Despite the relative portability, logistically, they are not easy to bring everywhere that a person may go. It also requires that a would-be (trained) rescuer be near the patient at all times in order to immediately recognize a sudden cardiac arrest.

Nevertheless, even the temporary availability of an AED before AICD placement (or the decision to provide one is made) would be a viable consideration for the AHFS patient at high-risk for experiencing VF/VT, particularly in the early period after a myocardial infarction.

In addition, AEDs may be a good option for hospital, rehabilitation facility, or clinic use. Even with nearby accessibility of a so-called crash cart, the AED is so portable and so simple that any health care worker could use it immediately with little need for refresher in-service training. In turn, this simplicity further diminishes the interval of global ischemia before defibrillation can be provided, and empirically improves the chances for survival for the inpatient who unexpectedly has a VF/VT-associated cardiac arrest on a noncritical care ward or another facility where patients with AHFS may be found.

Clinical Case

A 67-year-old man, a previous smoker with a 10-year history of mild chronic hypertension treated with a combination of lisinopril and hydrochlorothiazide, is at a local hotel restaurant 1 month following an acute myocardial infarction involving the posterior wall of the left ventricle. He has been at the restaurant for more than 2 hours conversing at length with his wife and friends. He has had several alcoholic beverages and several courses of food including a tomato soup, a cured ham appetizer, and a beefsteak with an accompanying sauce. After arising from the dining table late in the evening and walking into the hotel lobby with his wife, he suddenly says that he feels faint, leans against his wife and suddenly collapses to the floor. After a brief period of seizure-like activity, he reportedly has turned "blue" and is unresponsive.

A passerby goes to the front desk to alert the staff, and EMS personnel are called to respond. In the meantime, a hotel manager brings one of the hotel's AED devices to the patient's side while the very upset wife attempts to explain about his heart condition between tears and outbursts of fear. Another hotel employee, a waiter, begins to perform basic CPR using 30 compressions at a time interspersed with two quick breaths in accordance with a new half-hour video-based self-instruction CPR course that focused heavily on practicing proper skills. He had taken the course at the time of his employment 4 months earlier.

Further History

At the time of the initial heart attack a month earlier, the patient had not sought medical attention immediately. Arriving at the hospital by private automobile 6 hours after the onset of his feeling ill, exhausted, and a sense of vague thoracic tightness, he was immediately found to have electrocardiographic findings indicative of a posterior wall ischemic event. Cardiac catheterization confirmed total thrombotic occlusion of the left circumflex coronary artery with an additional significant lesion in the proximal left anterior descending (LAD) artery and minimal coronary artery disease (CAD) in the right coronary circulation. Primary percutaneous coronary intervention (PCI) was performed immediately upon admission, which included deployment of a drug-eluting stent in the circumflex coronary artery. Two days later he was returned to the catheterization laboratory for elective PCI of the LAD lesion, again with deployment of a drug-eluting stent.

After the primary PCI the catheterization, the patient was free of symptoms and did not complain of shortness of breath or chest pain. However, following the second elective LAD PCI, the patient began ambulating and experienced some fatigue and dyspnea on exertion. An echocardiogram demonstrated an ejection fraction of about 28%. Vital signs throughout the admission remained stable with a systemic blood pressure of 122 to 128 mm Hg systolic and 86 to 99 mm Hg diastolic, with a heart rate of 88 to 96 per minute, respiratory rate 20 to 25 per minute, and afebrile. Discharge medications included lisinopril, hydrochlorothiazide, low-dose beta-blockade, aspirin, clopidogrel, and atorvastatin. Over the next month, his exercise tolerance remained low, but he still attempted to perform mild exercise and brief walks.

Current Attack

Now, within 2 minutes of his collapse, the patient begins to take gasping respirations as the hotel waiter performs the CPR skills that he had learned 4 months earlier. In fact, he is performing the CPR extremely well with appropriate rate, depth, and recoil techniques. The patient's shirt is removed, and the hotel manager applies the defibrillator pads as the waiter continues the compressions.

Turning on the AED, the waiter continues compressions based on the new AED algorithm, which can now distinguish the cardiac rhythm from the compressions. The AED then advises a shock and begins to charge itself. When it advises the rescuers to deliver the shock, the waiter pulls away and the manager immediately delivers the shock. The waiter immediately resumes compressions for another two cycles of 30 compressions and two breaths when he notices the patient beginning to flush in his face, taking larger breaths, and beginning to cough. Another passerby in the lobby is a nurse, who leans forward and finds a pulse in the lateral neck and wrist and a new AED analysis indicates that no shock is advised.

The patient continues to breathe more regularly and begins to have spontaneous eye opening from time to time followed by nonspecific movement of the arms and legs with searching head movements. After a very large breath and cough, he begins to speak. At that time, EMS personnel arrive with their monitors and advanced cardiac care equipment.

The patient is found to have a blood pressure of 142/92 mm Hg and an irregular pulse, later shown to be atrial fibrillation with only a moderate ventricular response of 130 per minute. The 12-lead electrocardiograph shows only the atrial fibrillation with nonspecific ST-T wave abnormalities and slightly prolonged QRS complexes that narrow over the next 15 minutes. The EMS personnel establish intravascular access and infuse a dose of intravenous amiodarone. En route to the hospital, the patient becomes fully conversant and the blood pressure diminishes to 105/88 mm Hg with continued atrial fibrillation and the ventricular response of 110 per minute.

He is brought to a teaching hospital where he arrives alert and oriented and has the same cardinal signs. The initial electrocardiograph is fairly similar to the prehospital tracing except for normal QRS complexes and clearing of most of the ST-T wave changes. Laboratory studies show a slight elevation of troponin and normal creatine phosphokinase (CPK), as well as elevated levels of B-type natriuretic peptide. The chest x-ray reveals cardiomegaly and some perihilar congestion.

After a single dose of intravenous furosemide ordered by the resident physician, the patient is admitted to the ICU, where he spontaneously converts to normal sinus rhythm. After an otherwise uneventful hospital course, he is found to have a 31% ejection fraction by echocardiogram. Prior to transfer to a monitored telemetry floor from the ICU, he is scheduled to have an automatic implantable cardiac defibrillator (AICD) placed and undergoes a review of his medication regimen with specialists.

Conclusion

Until demonstrated otherwise, it should be emphasized that the immediate availability of AEDs can be considered a key adjunct in the management of AHFS, especially for those at greatest risk of sudden cardiac arrest. Since AEDs should be available for the public at large, current strategies for public access deployment should help the patient with AHFS as well.

More importantly, patients with low ejection fractions following an acute myocardial infarction or who otherwise meet criteria for implantable defibrillators are at high risk of sudden death from VF/VT. Therefore, they would presumably benefit from immediate use of an AED either before insertion of the AICD or as a potential alternative medical care strategy. Extrapolating from both AICD and public AED programs, the availability of AEDs would probably enhance survival for most categories of patients with AHFS.

Based on available data, despite confounding morbidity factors and thus a lesser chance of surviving compared to those experiencing VF/VT without accompanying heart failure, AEDs should be used as soon as possible, even in those with known severe heart failure.

Nevertheless, widespread deployment of AEDs in public and private settings should not be done without accompanying training in basic CPR and a philosophy that AED operation is one key component of CPR. In fact, CPR may need to be performed aggressively before defibrillation attempts in certain circumstances.

Fortunately, new advances in CPR and AED education now increase the portability of such courses and dramatically decrease the time commitments for acquiring these skills. Consequently, the potential for saving lives has increased dramatically, even for the patient with AHFS.

References

1. Moss AJ, Zareba W, Hall WJ, et al. Prophylactic implantation of a defibrillator in patients with myocardial infarction and reduced ejection fraction. N Engl J Med 2002;346:877–83.
2. Kadish A, Dyer A, Daubert JP, et al. Prophylactic defibrillator implantation in patients with non-

ischemic dilated cardiomyopathy. N Engl J Med 2004;350:2151–6.

3. Hohnloser SG, Kuck KH, Dorian P, et al. Prophylactic use of an implantable cardioverter-defibrillator after acute myocardial infarction. N Engl J Med 2004;351:2481–8.
4. Bardy GH, Lee KL, Mark DB, et al. Amiodarone or an implantable cardioverter-defibrillator for congestive heart failure. N Engl J Med 2005;352:225–37.
5. Zipes DP, Camm AJ, Borggreffe M. American College of Cardiology/American Heart Association/European Society of Cardiology guidelines for management of patients with ventricular arrhythmias and the prevention of sudden cardiac death. Circulation 2006;114;1088–132.
6. The 2005 American Heart Association guidelines for cardiopulmonary resuscitation and emergency cardiovascular care, Part 8: Stabilization of the patient with acute coronary syndromes. Circulation 2005;112:IV-89–IV-110.
7. Caffrey SL, Willoughby PJ, Pepe PE, Becker LB. Public use of automated external defibrillators. N Engl J Med 2002;347(16):1242–7.
8. The Public Access Defibrillation Trial Investigators. Public-access defibrillation and survival from out-of-hospital cardiac arrest. N Engl J Med 2004; 351:637–46.
9. Caffrey-Villari S, Pepe PE. Public use of automated external defibrillators. N Engl J Med 2003;348(8): 755–6.
10. Pepe PE. Current standard and future directions of advanced cardio-pulmonary resuscitation. In: Update in Emergency and Intensive Care. Vincent JL (ed). Springer-Verlag, Berlin, 1990:565–85.
11. Pepe PE, Wigginton JG. Key advances in critical care in the out-of-hospital setting: the evolving role of laypersons and technology. Critical Care 2006;10:119 (electronic publication doi:10.1186/cc4838).
12. The 2005 American Heart Association guidelines for cardiopulmonary resuscitation and emergency cardiovascular dare Committee. Adult basic life support. Circulation 2005;112:IV-19–IV-34.
13. Longstreth WT Jr, Diehr P, Inui TS. Prediction of awakening after out-of-hospital cardiac arrest. N Engl J Med 1983;308:1378–82.
14. The Hypothermia After Cardiac Arrest Study Group. Mild therapeutic hypothermia to improve the neurological outcome after cardiac arrest. N Engl J Med 2002;346:546–9.
15. Peberdy MA, Kaye W, Ornato JP, et al. Cardiopulmonary resuscitation of adults in hospital: a report of 14,720 cardiac arrests from the National Registry of Cardiopulmonary Resuscitation. Resuscitation 2003;58:297–308.
16. Gundry JW, Comess KA, DeRook FA, Jorgenson D, Bardy GH. Comparison of naïve sixth-grade children with trained professionals in the use of an automated external defibrillator. Circulation 1999; 100:1703–7.
17. Valenzuela TD, Roe DJ, Nichol G, Clark LL, Spaite DW, Hardman RG. Outcomes of rapid defibrillation by security officers after cardiac arrest in casinos. N Engl J Med 2000;343:1206–9.
18. Page RL, Joglar JA, Kowal RC, Zagrodzky JD, Nelson LL, Ramaswamy K. Use of automated external defibrillators by a U. S. airline. N Engl J Med 2000;343:1210–6.
19. Lee SK, Vaageres P, Safar P, Stezoski SW, Scanlon M. Effect of cardiac arrest time on cortical cerebral blood flow during subsequent standard external cardiopulmonary resuscitation in rabbits. Resuscitation 1989;17:105–17.
20. Niemann J, Cairns C, Sharma J, Lewis R. Treatment of prolonged ventricular fibrillation. Immediate countershock versus high-dose epinephrine and CPR preceding countershock. Circulation 1992; 85(1):281–7.
21. Cummins RO, Ornato JP, Thies WH, Pepe PE. Improving survival from sudden cardiac arrest: the "chain of survival" concept. Circulation 1991;83: 1832–47.
22. Haugk, Robak O, Sterz, F, et al. High acceptance of a home AED programme by survivors of sudden cardiac arrest and their families. Resuscitation 2006;70:263–74.
23. Wik L, Hansen TB, Fylling F, et al. Delaying defibrillation to give basic cardiopulmonary resuscitation to patients with out-of-hospital ventricular fibrillation: a randomized trail. JAMA 2003;289: 1389–95.
24. Cobb LA, Fahrenbruch CE, Walsh TR, et al. Influence of cardiopulmonary resuscitation prior to defibrillation in patients with out-of-hospital ventricular fibrillation. JAMA 1999;281;1182–8.
25. Koster RW. Limiting "hands-off" periods during resuscitation. Resuscitation 2003;58(3):275–6.
26. Eftestol T, Sunde K, Steen PA. Effects of interrupting precordial compressions on the calculated probability of defibrillation success during out-of-hospital cardiac arrest. Circulation 2002; 105(19):2270–3.
27. Lynch B, Einspruch EL, Nichol G, Becker LB, Aufderheide TP, Idris A. Effectiveness of a 30-min CPR self-instruction program for lay responders: a controlled randomized study. Resuscitation 2005;67: 31–43.

28. Roppolo LP, Ohman K, Pepe PE, Idris AH. The effectiveness of a short cardiopulmonary resuscitation course for laypersons. Circulation 2005;112 (suppl II):325–6(abstr 1627).
29. Idris AH, Roppolo LP, Ohman K, Pepe PE. A five minute training program for automated external defibrillator use is more effective than a 4-hour course. Circulation 2005;112(suppl II):326 (abstr 1628).
30. Wik L, Kramer-Johansen J, Myklebust H, et al. Quality of cardiopulmonary resuscitation during out-of-hospital cardiac arrest. JAMA 2005;293:299–304.
31. Abella BS, Alvarado JP, Myklebust H, et al. Quality of cardiopulmonary resuscitation after in-hospital cardiac arrest. JAMA 2005;293:305–10.
32. Kern KB, Sanders AB, Raife J, Milander MM, Otto CE, Ewy GA. A study of chest compression rates in humans: the importance of rate-directed chest compressions. Arch Intern Med 1992;152:145–9.
33. Aufderheide TP, Pirallo RG, Yannopoulos D, et al. Incomplete chest wall compressions: a clinical evaluation of CPR performance by EMS personnel and assessment of alternate manual chest compression-decompression techniques. Resuscitation 2005;64:353–62.
34. Shah JS, Maisel WH. Recalls and safety alerts affecting automated external defibrillators. JAMA 2006;296:655–60.
35. Estes NAM. Automated external defibrillators—device reliability and clinical benefits. JAMA 2006;296:700–2.

77
Post–Cardiopulmonary Resuscitation Management in the Intensive Care Unit

Christophe Adrie, Ivan Laurent, and Mehran Monchi

Since the introduction of modern cardiopulmonary resuscitation (CPR) and emergency cardiovascular care 50 years ago, considerable progress has been achieved in the management of cardiac arrest patients (1). Nevertheless, patients admitted to the intensive care unit (ICU) after successful resuscitation are at high risk for postresuscitation disease (2), a condition of multiple life-threatening disorders, including neurologic failure. Despite advances in cardiac arrest resuscitation, neurologic impairments and other organ dysfunctions cause considerable mortality and morbidity after restoration of spontaneous cardiac activity. Community-wide studies found mortality rates ranging from 4% to 33% depending on the chain of survival. Reports of higher survival rates in patients treated with mild hypothermia (3, 4) after successful cardiac arrest resuscitation confirm that the outcome is determined not only by the time to circulation recovery, but also by pathogenic processes that are triggered by the cardiac arrest but continue to evolve subsequently, causing damage to the nervous system and other organs. The mechanisms underlying this postresuscitation disease probably involve myocardial dysfunction and whole-body ischemia/reperfusion syndrome responsible for a systemic inflammatory response that shares many features with severe sepsis (5). Improved understanding of these pathogenic processes can be expected to open up new avenues for research and treatment aimed at preventing both death from early refractory shock with multiple organ dysfunction and the secondary development of brain damage during the ICU stay.

Clinical Case

An out-of-hospital first-response team including an emergency medicine physician was called for a 72-year-old man who had complained of shortness of breath and subsequently become unresponsive. The patient had a history of hypertension. After an estimated "no-flow" interval of 5 minutes (interval from cardiac arrest to initiation of CPR), advanced life support was started on scene. The initial electrocardiogram showed ventricular fibrillation. After three defibrillations (200, 300, and 360 J), the patient experienced ventricular tachycardia and asystole in succession. Standard advanced cardiac life support (ACLS) was performed as recommended by the European Resuscitation Council and was continued for 25 minutes (low-flow interval). It required a total of four defibrillations and 5 mg of epinephrine to restore spontaneous circulation. The initial blood pressure was 70/40 mm Hg and the heart rate was 82 beats/minute. The hemodynamics became stable (blood pressure 150/70 mm Hg and heart rate 121 beats/minute) under epinephrine infusion (1 mg/h), and the patient was then transferred to the hospital. A coronary angiogram performed immediately upon arrival at the hospital showed dilated cardiomyopathy without significant coronary artery disease. During the first 12 hours in the ICU, the patient experienced severe cardiac failure, which required up to 1.2 mg per hour of epinephrine and large amounts of intravenous fluids. Intravenous epinephrine was then stopped and the patient was extubated 9 days after the cardiac arrest. He achieved a full neurologic recovery and was discharged from the ICU 14 days after the cardiac arrest. On days 2 and 8, we performed a load-independent assessment of left ventricular contractility, using a validated clinical bedside tool (6) that accurately measures end-systolic elastance (E'es). The results showed transient ventricular dysfunction (Fig. 77.1; unpublished data), a common finding in this clinical setting.

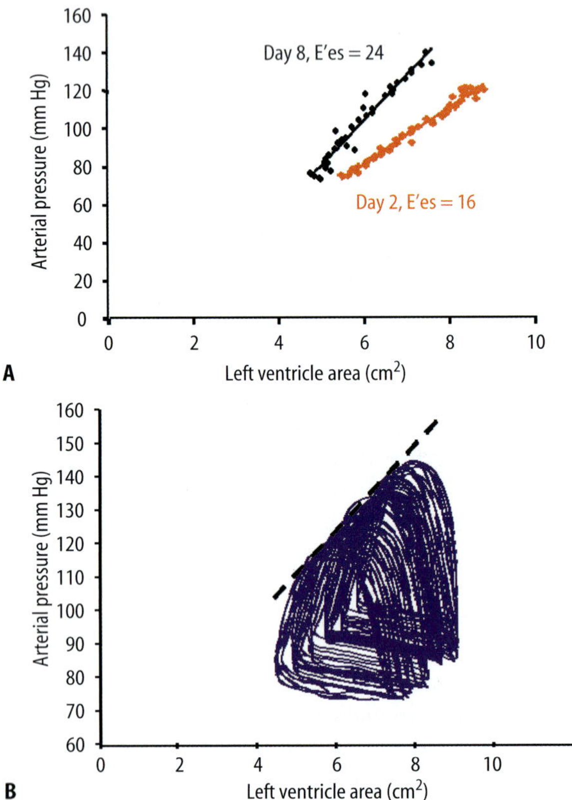

FIGURE 77.1. Transient ventricular dysfunction following cardiac arrest in the patient described in the clinical case report. We obtained a load-independent assessment of left ventricle (LV) contractility using a validated clinical bedside tool that accurately assesses end-systolic elastance (E'es) via echocardiographic measurement of LV cavity area as a surrogate for LV volume and femoral artery pressure measurement as a surrogate for LV ejection pressure, after a bolus of sodium nitroprusside (6). (A) Since this technique uses LV area, as opposed to LV volume, it is referred to as E'es. (B) Contractility improved dramatically between day 2 and day 8 (unpublished data).

Pathophysiology

Systemic Inflammatory Response Syndrome

Ischemia-Reperfusion Syndrome

Although prolonged ischemia results in severe tissue and organ damage, reperfusion-induced injury defined as tissue damage directly related to revascularization may be even more harmful. In cardiac arrest patients, successful resuscitation leads to whole-body ischemia-reperfusion injury. During the ischemic phase, hypoxia per se induces tissue damage. Blood reflow at the reperfusion phase may lead to further damage, a phenomenon known as the "oxygen paradox" and apparently related to the production of oxygen-free radicals, with coagulation activation and release of complement-activation products and cytokines.

As early as 3 hours after cardiac arrest, the concentrations of various cytokines, soluble receptors, and endotoxin rise in the bloodstream, more sharply in nonsurvivors than in survivors (5). Interestingly, hyporesponsiveness of circulating leukocytes, as assessed ex vivo, has been extensively documented in patients with systemic inflammatory response syndrome related to sepsis, trauma, or recovery from cardiac arrest. This phenomenon, known as endotoxin tolerance, seems to affect not only lymphocytes but also monocytes and neutrophils, and to be dependent on the activating signal. Although it may afford protection against overwhelming dysregulation of the proinflammatory process, it may also induce immune paralysis (or endogenous immunosuppression) with a potential increase in the risk of subsequent nosocomial infection.

Coagulation/anticoagulation and fibrinolysis/antifibrinolysis systems are activated in patients undergoing CPR, particularly those who return to spontaneous circulation (7). Anticoagulant factors such as antithrombin, protein S, and protein C are decreased, whereas endogenous activated protein C increases very transiently just after the cardiac arrest–resuscitation event (7). Contrary to severe sepsis in humans, cardiac arrest represents an acute event occurring at a well-defined time, so that early changes in systemic biomarkers can be detected. Early endothelial stimulation and thrombin generation may be responsible for the tremendous increase in protein C activation, which is followed rapidly by a phase of endothelial dysfunction, during which the endothelium may be unable to generate an adequate amount of activated protein C. Disseminated intravascular coagulation results in widespread microvascular thrombosis, which in turn causes multiple organ failures including neurologic impairments.

In a recent pilot study, fairly high baseline cortisol levels were found, contrasting with a 42% prevalence of relative adrenal insufficiency defined as failure to respond to corticotropin (i.e., cortisol increase <9 μg/mL) (8). The response to corticotropin was not associated with the usual markers for disease severity or with the cause of death (early refractory shock or neurologic dysfunction). However, baseline cortisol levels measured within 6 to 36 hours after the onset of cardiac arrest were lower in patients who subsequently died from early refractory shock than in patients who died later from neurologic failure, suggesting adrenal insufficiency in the former group (8).

Myocardial Dysfunction

Animal studies support the concept that postresuscitation hemodynamic instability is related to acute myocardial dysfunction characterized by impaired contractile function, decreased work capacity, and variable diastolic dysfunction, which resolve within hours or days after the return to spontaneous circulation. Transient hemodynamic instability and myocardial dysfunction have also been investigated in humans (9). For instance, in three patients younger than 40 years of age who survived cardiac arrest due to ventricular fibrillation, idiopathic dilated cardiomyopathy was diagnosed immediately after the cardiac arrest. However, follow-up investigations showed normal or near-normal function 2 weeks later. These findings suggest that myocardial stunning due to hypoperfusion during ventricular fibrillation or to the effects of transthoracic electrical shocks may result in profound but reversible myocardial depression. The underlying mechanisms were investigated recently in a large cohort of patients resuscitated after cardiac arrest presumably caused by cardiac disease. Postresuscitation myocardial dysfunction was a consistent finding, even in patients without hemodynamic instability or coronary heart disease. The onset of hemodynamic instability was often delayed, occurring 4 to 7 hours after admission, and full recovery was seen in survivors within 72 hours (9). Postresuscitation hemodynamic instability was more common in patients with acute coronary occlusion as the cause of cardiac arrest, high-dose epinephrine therapy, or longer duration of CPR. Interestingly, mortality from early refractory shock (13.5%) after successful angioplasty compared favorably to mortality (19.1%) from refractory shock in patients without acute myocardial infarction (10). Furthermore, successful angioplasty improved survival in patients who were resuscitated after cardiac arrest. This beneficial effect may be related to myocardial salvage with a lower rate of arrhythmia recurrence and better reversal of myocardial dysfunction.

Interestingly, although cardiac output increased rapidly in patients receiving vasoactive drugs, a large amount of volume expanders was required initially (cumulative crystalloid volume, 5000 [3500–6500] mL at 24 hours) to maintain filling pressures just above 12 mm Hg (a rather low value considering the myocardial dysfunction), resulting in hemodilution (9). Together with the sharp increases in cytokines and the presence of endotoxin in plasma, the need for large amounts of fluids suggests that vasoplegia may occur after cardiac arrest, as in severe sepsis, and may play a key role in hemodynamic instability. Conceivably, the acute myocardial dysfunction may be induced in part by circulating depressant factors, including the cytokines tumor necrosis factor-α and interleukin-1β beta, as observed in sepsis.

Post–Intensive Care Unit Management

The main treatment goal in the postresuscitation phase is to completely restore regional organ and tissue perfusion. Restoration of blood pressure alone (although a prerequisite) and improvements in tissue gas exchange do not necessarily improve survival. In addition to standard critical care aimed at supporting failing organs, we will discuss the specific features of the postresuscitation phase depending on the cause of the cardiac arrest.

Standard Supportive Care

Cardiovascular Management

The hemodynamic and inflammatory profiles after cardiac arrest share many similarities with those seen in severe sepsis. Early aggressive fluid resuscitation is the first step in maintaining adequate blood pressure (mean arterial blood pressure >60 to 65 mm Hg). Fluid challenges are followed by the administration of vasopressor and inotropic agents. Because systolic dysfunction associated with vasodilation is common and often profound initially, epinephrine may be the best agent, as it exerts both vasopressor and inotropic effects. The need for pulmonary artery catheterization has been challenged recently (11). Techniques for central monitoring are improving, and less invasive alternatives for hemodynamic evaluation such as transesophageal Doppler or echocardiography are being investigated. Although these technologies showed promise in terms of performance during trials, their ability to influence clinical outcomes is unknown.

Ventilatory Settings

Low airway pressures should be used to avoid an increase in cerebral venous pressure and intracranial pressure. However, in clinical practice, gas exchanges are often impaired, sometimes severely. In our experience, this impairment was not related to cardiogenic edema, since occlusion pulmonary artery pressure was consistently below 18 mm Hg. A more likely mechanism is ischemia-reperfusion syndrome and gastric aspiration, a common event in this clinical setting, leading to pulmonary capillary leak syndrome with acute respiratory distress syndrome or acute lung injury depending on the PaO_2/FiO_2 ratio impairment.

Specific Management

Antiarrhythmic Agents

All electrolyte disturbances such as aberrations in potassium, magnesium, calcium, and sodium levels must be treated aggressively. Amiodarone has been found to be more effective than placebo or lidocaine in out-of-hospital cardiac arrest due to shock-refractory ventricular fibrillation (i.e., ventricular fibrillation persisting after three or more external defibrillator shocks) (12, 13). The American Heart Association still recommends a lidocaine bolus followed by a maintenance infusion for several hours, during which any correctable causes are assessed (1, 14); however, this strategy has not been evaluated in placebo-controlled trials. We believe that amiodarone, which is usually characterized by satisfactory hemodynamic tolerance, is probably more effective than lidocaine (15, 16). Beta-blockers have been widely used for acute coronary syndrome and have recently been shown to induce benefits in a swine model of prolonged ventricular fibrillation (17). Nevertheless, beta-blockers have not been studied in the acute and unstable phase following cardiac arrest in humans. Available data do not warrant a recommendation to use beta-blockers, even those with very short half-lives, after cardiac arrest.

Thrombolytic Therapy

Because of the risk of severe bleeding, thrombolysis has been contraindicated during and after CPR. Increasing experience and data from open studies now suggest that thrombolysis during CPR may contribute to achieving hemodynamic stabilization and survival in patients with massive pulmonary embolism or acute myocardial infarction that fails to respond to conventional CPR (18). The risk of bleeding associated with the use of thrombolytic agents may be far smaller than anticipated. Studies are under way to evaluate the use of thrombolytic agents during CPR. After spontaneous circulation is restored, thrombolysis may be beneficial when the 12-lead electrocardiogram shows acute myocardial infarction with ST-segment elevation (14). However, when available, immediate coronary angiography with angioplasty, if necessary, may be the best course of action (10, 14). This treatment may be attempted on a case-by-case basis after successful resuscitation of cardiac arrest due to severe pulmonary embolism. Massive coagulation activation with subsequent fibrin generation leads to microcirculatory reperfusion disorders. Thrombolytic agents (in combination with heparin) have been shown to decrease the "no reflow" phenomenon commonly seen in a cat model of successfully resuscitated cardiac arrest (19). However no controlled studies are available on this treatment strategy.

Percutaneous Transluminal Coronary Angioplasty

Early coronary reperfusion is the cornerstone of management in acute myocardial infarction. When prolonged cardiac arrest occurs in this setting, immediate angioplasty, when readily available, may be the best reperfusion procedure. Immediate angioplasty was clearly superior to thrombolysis in patients with cardiogenic shock related to myocardial infarction. Thrombolysis seems less effective in patients with shock and may be associated with a substantially higher bleeding risk after CPR. The incidence of acute coronary occlusion and the potential benefits of immediate coronary angiography and angioplasty, when indicated, were evaluated in a prospective series of 84 patients who were successfully resuscitated after out-of-hospital cardiac arrest with no detectable noncardiac cause (10). In this highly selected population, 60 patients had significant coronary disease by angiography, including 40 of 84 (48%) with coronary artery occlusion. The in-hospital survival rate (patients without major neurologic sequelae) was 38%. Multivariate logistic-regression analysis revealed that successful angioplasty independently predicted survival (odds ratio [OR], 5.2; 95% confidence interval [CI], 1.1–24.5; $p = .04$) (10). We may expect an additional myocardial salvage over the classic transient, spontaneously reversible myocardial depression (9).

High-Volume Hemofiltration

Various aspects of the homeostasis alterations seen after restoration of spontaneous circulation mimic those observed in severe sepsis. As stated before, the protective role of hypothermia in highly selected patients with a fairly good prognosis (control groups had survival rates close to 35%) suggests that the postresuscitation processes described above may contribute to induce secondary neurologic deterioration and that specific treatments may improve survival rates. High-volume hemofiltration has been found of value in children after extracorporeal circulation for cardiac surgery, another model of whole-body ischemia-reperfusion. We evaluated the potential benefits of high-volume hemofiltration (200 mL/kg/h up to 12.5 L/h of fully balanced ultrafiltration over an 8-hour period) by randomizing 61 patients with out-of-hospital cardiac arrest into three groups: controls, and high-volume hemofiltration with or without hypothermia (20). High-volume hemofiltration improved survival, and adding hypothermia seemed to provide further survival gains. In addition to a potential role in controlling inflammatory processes, this extracorporeal technique readily reduces the body temperature to the desired range (32° to 34°C) within 1 hour in most cases. However, this was a pilot study, and further clinical investigations are needed.

Brain Protection and Hypothermia

A few trials of barbiturates, calcium channel blockers, or corticosteroids failed to show any protective effects against brain damage (14). Induction of moderate hypothermia (28° to 32°C) before cardiac arrest has been used successfully since the 1950s to protect the brain against the global ischemia that occurs during some open-heart surgical procedures. The beneficial effect of hypothermia may be related to the 6% decrease in cerebral oxygen consumption for every 1°C reduction in brain temperature above 28°C, which is ascribable to a reduction in normal electrical activity. Mild hypothermia is also thought to reduce many of the chemical reactions associated with reperfusion injury, such as free radical production, excitatory amino acid release, and calcium shift, which lead to mitochondrial damage and apoptosis.

Therapeutic hypothermia after cardiac arrest in humans was described as helpful in the late 1950s but was subsequently abandoned because the benefits were uncertain and practical implementation was difficult. Subsequently, mild hypothermia (32° to 34°C) was shown to improve functional recovery and to reduce cerebral histologic damage in various animal models of cardiac arrest. More recently, mild hypothermia was found to improve neurologic outcomes in comatose patients after cardiac arrest, compared to normothermia (49% vs. 26%, respectively, in an Australian Study; and 55% vs. 39% in a European study) (4). Both of these studies were conducted in selected populations obtained by excluding up to 92% of patients with out-of-hospital cardiac arrest assessed for eligibility, a fact that explains the good survival in the controls (normothermia groups) (4).

Cooling should probably be initiated as soon as possible and continued for 12 to 24 hours using external cooling methods in combination with a neuromuscular blocker and sedation to avoid shivering. Other cooling techniques based on more invasive procedures may be more efficient in decreasing core temperature but have not been proven superior over external and noninvasive methods. Careful monitoring of body temperature (rectal or bladder temperature probes) is important during therapeutic hypothermia because the incidence of complications such as arrhythmias, infection, and coagulopathy is likely to increase if the core temperature falls considerably below 32°C. Once again, these trials were performed in highly selected patients after ventricular fibrillation. Whether hypothermia is also beneficial in patients with other rhythm disorders, in-hospital cardiac arrest, or longer times to treatment remains to be determined. Therapeutic hypothermia is discussed in greater detail in another chapter.

Neurological Evaluation and Life Support Withdrawal

Most survivors of cardiac arrest are comatose after resuscitation, and meaningful recovery occurs in only a small proportion of cases. Physical examination may contribute useful information for helping physicians and families make decisions about treatment or life support withdrawal. In 1993, a panel of experts stated that the prognosis for adults in permanent vegetative state following cardiac arrest could be predicted with high accuracy after 3 to 7 days. Withdrawal of life support, including artificially administered nutrition and hydration, is ethically permissible when the prognosis is poor (21). In a meta-analysis of 33 studies of anoxic-ischemic coma, Zandbergen et al. (22) identified three factors associated with death or survival in a vegetative state: absence of pupillary light reflexes on the third day, absence of a motor response to pain by the third day, and bilateral absence of early cortical somatosensory evoked potentials within the first week. Because somatosensory evoked potentials show little sensitivity to metabolic changes and drugs, they are extremely useful for outcome prediction. Withdrawal of life support is ethically acceptable when the results of the evaluation after the first week indicate a prognosis of death or survival in a vegetative state.

Conclusion

Detectable causes of cardiac arrest must be treated to prevent recurrences (15). Coronary revascularization has been shown to prevent recurrent ventricular tachycardia/fibrillation but may provide incomplete protection from sudden death in patients with structural heart disease, particularly those with healed myocardial infarction. Cardiac arrest survivors should be carefully evaluated in order to identify the high-risk profile described above, hypertrophic cardiomyopathy, and congenital long QT syndrome. Implantation of a cardioverter defibrillator has been found superior over the best antiarrhythmic drug therapy (predominantly amiodarone) in cardiac arrest survivors (15).

References

1. Eisenberg MS, Mengert TJ. Cardiac resuscitation. N Engl J Med 2001;344:1304–13.
2. Negovsky VA. The second step in resuscitation—the treatment of the "post-resuscitation disease". Resuscitation 1972;1:1–7.
3. Bernard SA, et al. Treatment of comatose survivors of out-of-hospital cardiac arrest with induced hypothermia. N Engl J Med 2002;346:557–63.
4. The Hypothermia after Cardiac Arrest Study Group. Mild therapeutic hypothermia to improve the neurologic outcome after cardiac arrest. N Engl J Med 2002;346:549–56.
5. Adrie C, et al. Successful cardiopulmonary resuscitation after cardiac arrest as a "sepsis-like" syndrome. Circulation 2002;106:562–8.

6. Gorcsan J 3rd, et al. Rapid estimation of left ventricular contractility from end-systolic relations by echocardiographic automated border detection and femoral arterial pressure. Anesthesiology 1994;81:553–62; discussion 27A.
7. Adrie C, et al. Coagulopathy after successful cardiopulmonary resuscitation following cardiac arrest: implication of the protein C anticoagulant pathway. J Am Coll Cardiol 2005;46:21–8.
8. Hekimian G, et al. Cortisol levels and adrenal reserve after successful cardiac arrest resuscitation. Shock 2004;22:116–9.
9. Laurent I, et al. Reversible myocardial dysfunction in survivors of out-of-hospital cardiac arrest. J Am Coll Cardiol 2002;40:2110–6.
10. Spaulding CM, et al. Immediate coronary angiography in survivors of out-of-hospital cardiac arrest. N Engl J Med 1997;336:1629–33.
11. Richard C, et al. Early use of the pulmonary artery catheter and outcomes in patients with shock and acute respiratory distress syndrome: a randomized controlled trial. JAMA 2003;290:2713–20.
12. Dorian P, et al. Amiodarone as compared with lidocaine for shock-resistant ventricular fibrillation. N Engl J Med 2002;346:884–90.
13. Kudenchuk PJ, et al. Amiodarone for resuscitation after out-of-hospital cardiac arrest due to ventricular fibrillation. N Engl J Med 1999;341:871–8.
14. Guidelines 2000 for Cardiopulmonary Resuscitation and Emergency Cardiovascular Care. Part 6: advanced cardiovascular life support: section 8: postresuscitation care. The American Heart Association in collaboration with the International Liaison Committee on Resuscitation. Circulation 2000;102:I166–71.
15. Callans DJ. Management of the patient who has been resuscitated from sudden cardiac death. Circulation 2002;105:2704–7.
16. Levine JH, et al. Intravenous amiodarone for recurrent sustained hypotensive ventricular tachyarrhythmias. Intravenous Amiodarone Multicenter Trial Group. J Am Coll Cardiol 1996;27:67–75.
17. Killingsworth CR, et al. Short-acting beta-adrenergic antagonist esmolol given at reperfusion improves survival after prolonged ventricular fibrillation. Circulation 2004;109:2469–74.
18. Böttiger BW, Martin E. Thrombolytic therapy during cardiopulmonary resuscitation and the role of coagulation activation after cardiac arrest. Curr Opin Crit Care 2001;7:176–83.
19. Fischer M, et al. Thrombolysis using plasminogen activator and heparin reduces cerebral no-reflow after resuscitation from cardiac arrest: an experimental study in the cat. Intensive Care Med 1996;22:1214–23.
20. Laurent I, et al. High-volume hemofiltration after out-of-hospital cardiac arrest: a randomized study. J Am Coll Cardiol 2005;46:432–7.
21. Guidelines for cardiopulmonary resuscitation and emergency cardiac care. Emergency Cardiac Care Committee and Subcommittees, American Heart Association. Part VIII. Ethical considerations in resuscitation. JAMA 1992;268:2282–8.
22. Zandbergen EG, et al. Systematic review of early prediction of poor outcome in anoxic-ischaemic coma. Lancet 1998;352:1808–12.

2.9
Acute Heart Failure Syndrome Management in Heart Failure Clinics

78
Role of the Pharmacist in the Management of Acute Heart Failure Syndrome

Wendy A. Gattis Stough, J. Herbert Patterson, and Jo E. Rodgers

Managing pharmacotherapy is a complex process in patients with acute heart failure syndrome (AHFS). Focus should be placed on ensuring that evidence-based therapies are prescribed, and that heart failure (HF) medications are prescribed appropriately. Many adverse effects and medication errors occur due to a failure to recognize pharmacodynamic and pharmacokinetic alterations that are present in the patient with AHFS. Pharmacists are uniquely trained to focus on the appropriate use of medications in challenging clinical scenarios. These individuals can be extremely helpful in selecting and monitoring medical regimens, as well as providing focused patient education. This chapter reviews the role of the pharmacist in the care of patients with AHFS.

Pharmacists as Care Providers in Heart Failure

The multidisciplinary approach to managing HF has been studied, and it has been proven to reduce rehospitalization.[1] Multidisciplinary care has demonstrated a significant reduction in readmission, improvement in quality of life, and a reduction in health care costs. In fact, several studies have assessed multidisciplinary intervention in HF patients. Data from 29 randomized trials of multidisciplinary management strategies for patients with HF revealed that these programs are associated with a 27% reduction in HF hospitalization rates and a 43% reduction in total number of HF hospitalizations.[2] Multidisciplinary interventions for patients with HF not only reduce hospital admission but also provide an effective method for reducing mortality. A systematic review of the literature assessing such interventions found a 20% reduction in mortality, a 13% reduction in all-cause hospital admission, and a 30% reduction in HF hospital admission.[3] In addition, patients with HF who have the opportunity to participate in a peridischarge program have been shown to benefit from a reduced risk of readmission with a 21% relative risk reduction.[4]

While most of the studies evaluated a nurse-directed multidisciplinary intervention, a few studies have also assessed the value of adding a pharmacist to the HF team. Study results emphasize the need for a multidisciplinary approach for successful treatment of patients to reduce mortality and decrease hospitalization. These studies have been conducted in the outpatient chronic setting, and there are no data available for review in the acute setting. However, one would anticipate the contributions of the pharmacist to be similar in both settings, and perhaps more pronounced in the acute setting. The literature supporting the role of the pharmacist in the outpatient setting will be reviewed in the absence of data in the AHFS patient.

The Pharmacist Assessment Recommendation and Monitoring (PHARM) study was the first randomized trial to evaluate the effect of including a clinical pharmacist on the HF team.[5] The study randomized 192 patients to pharmacist intervention or usual care. Patients randomized to the intervention arm had a pharmacist review their medical regimen and current symptoms,

TABLE 78.1. Clinical events

Event	No. of events		OR (95% CI)	p value
	Intervention group ($n = 90$)	Control group ($n = 91$)		
Nonfatal HF	1	11	0.08 (0.004–0.4)	.005
Total nonfatal cardiovascular	8	23	0.31 (0.13–0.69)	.004
All-cause mortality	3	5	0.59 (0.12–2.49)	.48
All-cause mortality and nonfatal HF	4	16	0.22 (0.06–0.63)	.005
Total	29	36	0.73 (0.39–1.33)	.3

HF, heart failure; OR, odds ratio; CI, confidence interval.

recommend changes in pharmacotherapy to the attending cardiologist, provide patient education, and contact the patient by telephone to identify new symptoms, side effects, and to reinforce education principles. Patients in the usual care group received only standard follow-up. The primary outcome of the study was the combined end point of all-cause mortality and hospitalization or emergency department visit for HF. Secondary end points included an evaluation of angiotensin-converting enzyme (ACE) inhibitor use and dose prescribed.

Patients randomized to the intervention group had a lower rate of death or hospitalizations for HF as compared to the usual care group (odds ratio [OR], 0.22; 95% confidence interval [CI], 0.07–0.65, $p = .005$). This effect was primarily due to a reduction in rehospitalization. Additionally, patients in the intervention group were closer to the target ACE-inhibitor dose as compared to the usual care group ($p < .001$).[5] The results of this study are summarized in Table 78.1.

A similar study was conducted by Rainville.[6] All patients hospitalized for HF from July 1996 to July 1997 in one hospital were evaluated for inclusion in the study. Patients were randomly assigned to a control or intervention group. Patients in the control group received routine care and discharge procedures and a nurse reviewed diet and medications. The intervention group received the same care; however, the pharmacist also reviewed the patients' medication regimen, recommended changes to the physicians, and provided patient education. The primary end point of this study was death or hospital readmission for HF within 1 year after discharge. The study was small, including only 38 patients. However, the investigators observed a readmission rate of 59% in the control group compared to 24% in the intervention group ($p < .05$). Death or readmission was 82% in the control group and 29% in the intervention group ($p < .01$).

Other studies have evaluated the impact of pharmacists on medication appropriateness,[7] diuretic compliance,[8] and patient education.[9] In one of these studies, medication appropriateness was assessed using the medication appropriateness index. Although scores were not statistically higher in the intervention group, directive guidance of patients by pharmacists was found to be beneficial.[7] "Directive guidance" was defined as activities like providing information, giving feedback, and giving advice, with the expectation that this activity would improve adherence to medication and therefore control disease.[7] Overall, these studies consistently found the addition of a pharmacist to the HF team to be effective at improving outcomes, medication use, and patients' knowledge regarding their condition. Patient education is a part of the multidisciplinary care that should include close clinical follow-up, telemanagement or telemonitoring, and home visits where available. Pharmacists can be essential in providing such services to ensure optimal patient education and care.

Optimizing Medication Prescribing by the Physician

Pharmacists are uniquely trained to participate in the care and management of HF patients, especially the patient with AHFS. There are several areas that the pharmacists' expertise can be particularly useful in the management of these patients.

TABLE 78.2. Starting and target doses for heart failure medications

Class	Medication	Starting dose	Target dose
ACE inhibitors	Ramipril	1.25 to 2.5 mg bid	5 mg bid
	Enalapril	2.5 mg bid	10 mg bid
	Lisinopril	2.5 to 5 mg daily	10–20 mg daily
	Fosinopril	5 to 10 mg daily	40 mg daily
	Trandolapril	1 mg daily	4 mg daily
	Perindopril	2 mg daily	8 to 16 mg daily
	Quinapril	5 mg bid	20 mg bid
	Captopril	6.25 mg tid	50 mg tid
Beta-blockers	Bisoprolol	1.25 mg daily	10 mg daily
	Carvedilol	3.125 mg bid	25 mg bid
	Metoprolol succinate XL/CR	12.5 to 25 mg daily	200 mg daily
Aldosterone antagonists	Spironolactone	12.5 to 25 mg daily	25 mg daily
	Eplerenone	25 mg daily	50 mg daily
ARB	Candesartan	4 to 8 mg daily	32 mg daily
	Valsartan	20 to 40 mg daily	160 mg twice daily
Vasodilator/nitrate	Hydralazine/isosorbide dinitrate	37.5/20 mg tid	75/40 mg tid

Drug Selection

Pharmacists can assist in selecting the most optimal medication for a given patient. Pharmacologic properties of medications differ, even among agents from within the same class. Pharmacists can match patients to medications for which there are many examples. For a renally excreted medication, it is important to avoid or to dose adjust such medications in patients with declining renal perfusion and function or to simply select a nonrenally excreted medication. In patients with liver disease, use of medications that require metabolism for activation should be avoided. Within a given drug class, certain medications may have properties that are absolutely or relatively contraindicated. Later in this chapter, we discuss specific examples of each of the above. Overall, a pharmacist's knowledge can aid in proper medication selection, which acts to minimize side effects and improve drug tolerability.

Dose Initiation and Titration

Pharmacists can ensure that drugs are appropriately dosed, accounting for patient specific characteristics, comorbid conditions, concomitant medications, and patient response to therapy. Pharmacists can provide recommendations on optimal starting doses based on patient specific characteristics, which will optimize tolerability and response. Similarly, prescribers should appreciate that target doses of various HF medications should be attained if at all possible. To reach doses that have demonstrated improvement in outcomes, drug therapy needs to be titrated properly so as to avoid possible side effects. For example, ACE inhibitors can be titrated every 3 to 7 days based on tolerability, whereas beta-blockers should not be titrated more frequently than every 2 weeks. Starting and target doses are listed in Table 78.2 for medications with proven benefit for HF patients. Pharmacists not only can assist with initiation and up-titration periods, but also can be helpful in managing tolerability issues that may occur between these crucial periods. Prompt recognition and response to side effects to up-titration can ensure that target doses are achieved in a more optimal and timely manner.

Pharmacokinetic Alterations

The pharmacokinetic properties of medications can be altered in AHFS due to changes in absorption, distribution, metabolism, and excretion. The pharmacist's understanding of these potential changes can aid in selecting appropriate medications and doses for patients.

Absorption

The absorption of medications in patients with AHFS may be altered by several mechanisms. These alterations typically result in a lower systemic bioavailability. As HF progresses, cardiac output is reduced, leading to organ hypoperfusion. Blood flow is redirected to vital organs such as the brain and kidney. Some organ systems, such as the gastrointestinal tract, may remain hypoperfused. Drug absorption may be reduced in this circumstance as a result of this reduced perfusion. Reduced gastrointestinal motility and delayed gastric emptying may also contribute to suboptimal bioavailability. In the setting of fluid overload, gastrointestinal edema may further compromise absorption. Each of these processes may also be responsible for symptoms of gastrointestinal discomfort and cachexia reported by many patients with AHFS

Given the above changes, the efficacy of oral loop diuretics often declines in patients with AHFS. Clinicians often observe worsening HF symptoms despite increasing diuretic doses. The mechanism for diuretic resistance is twofold: pharmacokinetic and pharmacodynamic. While diuretic bioavailability remains normal in HF, the rate of absorption is prolonged and thus peak concentrations are reduced. Given the sigmoid-shaped concentration response curve of loop diuretics, these lower concentrations often result in a reduction in clinical response. Pharmacists can assist with ensuring that diuretic resistance is prevented or overcome through several mechanisms, including increasing diuretic doses, utilizing intravenous administration, or adding a diuretic with a different mechanism of action such as a distally acting thiazide diuretic. In addition, loop diuretic administration may result in distal tubule hypertrophy due to high concentrations of sodium reaching this part of the nephron, further compromising diuretic efficacy. Finally, low cardiac output states may cause reduced renal perfusion, which results in reduced drug delivery to the site of action, the kidney.

Realizing precisely when and how to intervene on a patients' routine diuretic regimen is critical to avoiding the very rapid downward spiral toward fluid overload, and a pharmacist can be instrumental in monitoring this process and responding to it. In addition, patients who struggle with fluid status are optimal candidates for frequent follow-up by telephone to ensure daily weighing and monitoring for fluid overload is ongoing. These steps can help ensure proper diuretic dose titration, which can prevent hospitalization. Intense patient education can assist in identifying appropriate patients who may be optimal candidates for diuretic self-titration. This education can potentially result in patients' learning to titrate their own diuretic; they contact health care professionals only when initial attempts are unsuccessful. Pharmacists can assist with the above educational efforts and monitoring.

Acute heart failure syndrome may also affect the absorption of topically administered medications. Peripheral perfusion may be compromised in patients with low cardiac output. Oral administration may be favored in these patients. For example, oral isosorbide may be preferable to nitroglycerin patches in the advanced HF patient with low cardiac output. Other commonly used topical products to be cautious and aware of in this patient population include clonidine and nicotine.

Data are not widely available evaluating drug absorption in AHFS patients; however, reduced absorption should be considered a potential cause of inadequate response to drug therapy in these patients. One potential mechanism to assess absorption is obtaining a serum digoxin concentration. A subtherapeutic concentration may suggest inadequate absorption based on digoxin pharmacokinetic calculations of expected concentrations and assured compliance. Pharmacists can play a significant role in assisting with such calculations.

Distribution

The volume of distribution (V_d) of drugs can also be altered in patients with AHFS. The V_d may be increased or decreased. Most commonly, V_d is reduced in both central and peripheral compartments. This reduction may be due to reduced cardiac output. Theoretically, the V_d may be increased for hydrophilic drugs in patients with volume overload and preserved cardiac output because these drugs may be widely distributed in the periphery. Conversely, V_d may be reduced for lipophilic drugs given the same scenario. Data evaluating changes in V_d in AHFS patients are not widely available for drugs commonly used to treat these patients.

In addition, protein binding can affect V_d for highly protein-bound drugs. As HF progresses, patients may become cachectic. Subsequently, a reduction in albumin may affect drugs that are highly protein bound, and result in a higher free fraction of active drug. The clinical significance of this has not been well described in the HF literature. Drugs with a narrow therapeutic index that are highly protein bound, such as phenytoin, should be closely monitored in the AHFS patient.

Metabolism

Drugs that are highly protein bound may be affected by the AHFS state. Hepatic metabolism may decrease due to volume overload and hepatic congestion. It may also be reduced in the low cardiac output state due to decreased perfusion. In these scenarios, decreased metabolism, higher concentrations of free drug, and long half-lives may be observed. Patients treated with medications that rely on hepatic metabolism such as warfarin, beta-blockers, and amiodarone should receive close monitoring in the setting of AHFS. For example, patients receiving warfarin for anticoagulation may experience significant elevations in bleeding times during episodes of acute HF. The exact impact of pharmacokinetic alterations is extremely difficult to predict, and close monitoring is warranted.

Excretion

Patients with AHFS may also experience changes in the excretion of medications, particularly those excreted renally. In the low-output state, renal perfusion may be reduced, resulting in a decline in renal function. In addition, aggressive diuretic administration may also worsen renal function. Thus, particular monitoring should be given to serum creatinine, and doses of medications that are renal excreted should be adjusted accordingly. This focused monitoring approach may be particularly important with medications with narrow therapeutic ranges such as digoxin and aminoglycosides as well as other renally eliminated medications that HF patients may be receiving. Milrinone is an example of a medication whose half-life may be prolonged in renal insufficiency. Therefore, caution should be exercised with rapidly up- or down-titrating a milrinone continuous infusion in patients with HF with concomitant renal dysfunction.

Changes in renal function can impact medications by increasing the risk of side effects and toxicity. Side effects can also occur at an increased rate due to changes in renal function. For example, patients taking ACE inhibitors and aldosterone antagonists are at a greater risk for hyperkalemia in the setting of renal dysfunction. Due to worsening renal function, toxicity can occur in drugs with small therapeutic windows, such as digoxin.

Pharmacokinetic Drug Interactions

Due to the number of drugs patients are prescribed, the potential for drug interactions is high in HF patients and especially high in those with AHFS. Interactions may also occur with noncardiac drugs the HF patient is taking, and the pharmacist can recognize these interactions and offer suggestions to avoid or minimize the interaction. Heart failure patients are commonly treated with digoxin, amiodarone, and warfarin, all of which have a high potential for drug interactions. Including a team member with the ability to recognize such interactions can protect against medication errors related to drug interactions.

Amiodarone is a well-characterized inhibitor of many cytochrome P-450 (CYP) enzymes, including 3A4, 1A2, 2C9, and 2D6. There are several important drug interactions that can occur when using amiodarone in HF patients. Patients receiving simvastatin should receive no more than 20 mg daily to prevent the increased risk of myopathy and rhabdomyolysis due to increased simvastatin concentrations through amiodarone-medicated CYP-3A4 inhibition. The same concern exists with use of the other hepatic hydroxymethylglutaryl coenzyme A (HMG CoA) reductase inhibitors that are eliminated through the CYP 3A4 enzyme. Upon initiation of amiodarone, warfarin should be reduced by approximately 25% to 40% depending on the amiodarone dose being administered and bleeding times closely monitored. Also, digoxin dose should be reduced by

50% and patients counseled to monitor for signs and symptoms of digoxin toxicity. For patients taking warfarin, a pharmacist is instrumental in instructing patients on signs and symptoms of bleeding and how to reduce this risk, the importance of regular international normalized ratio (INR) monitoring, and a stable dietary vitamin K intake as well as potential drug interactions, including over-the-counter medications and herbal therapies. Finally, combining digoxin with atorvastatin results in inhibition of p-glycoprotein, an important pathway for the excretion of digoxin, with the net result of a 20% increase in serum digoxin concentrations. These are just a few of the many potential drug interactions that may be present in the typical HF patient.

Pharmacodynamic Interactions

In addition to pharmacokinetic interactions, pharmacodynamic interactions can also occur. Heart failure patients are treated with multiple medications that have similar pharmacodynamic effects. The ACE inhibitors, beta-blockers, and diuretics can all result in hypotension, and low blood pressure is common in patients with AHFS. If patients are having difficulties with dizziness and postural hypotension due to low blood pressure, the doses of medications that lower blood pressure may be spaced in such a way as to minimize this side effect. The pharmacists' knowledge of the onset of action for various ACE inhibitors and beta-blockers may be helpful in most optimally spacing these medications. By activating the release of renin, diuretics may increase a patient's sensitivity to blood pressure–lowering effects of the above-mentioned agents. Ensuring optimal volume status in patients prior to medication initiation or up-titration is essential in assuring tolerability. Finally, pharmacists are uniquely aware of additional properties various agents may possess. For example, in addition to its beta-blocking effects, carvedilol has alpha effects that may be of benefit to a patient with uncontrolled hypertension or a detriment to a patient with borderline low blood pressure. Being aware of differences between the various agents within a medication class can assist with prescribing a given patient the most optimal medication regimen.

The ACE inhibitors, angiotensin receptor blockers, and aldosterone antagonists can each cause hyperkalemia, and the risk of hyperkalemia is likely higher when these agents are used in combination. In addition, patients may be receiving potassium supplementation or no-salt substitutes, which can further increase serum potassium. When initiating aldosterone antagonists, taking into consideration various factors can minimize the risk of hyperkalemia, including avoiding such agents in patients with a creatinine clearance less than 30 mL/min, avoiding concomitant nonsteroidal antiinflammatory drugs (NSAIDs) and cyclooxygenase-2 inhibitors, discontinuing or reducing potassium supplementation, and avoiding dehydration, among others. Being aware of these increased risks for hyperkalemia is essential in ensuring patient safety.

Bradycardia can be caused by beta-blockers, digoxin, and the calcium channel blockers verapamil and diltiazem, especially when used in combination. Pharmacists can assist with developing strategies for the timing of drug administration or provide other recommendations that may minimize the risk for this pharmacodynamic interaction.

Managing Comorbidities

The patient with HF may have multiple comorbidities including pulmonary disease, arthritis, gout, diabetes, and atrial fibrillation, to name just a few. Each of these comorbid conditions increases the difficulty in managing HF in these patients. The pharmacist can be helpful in selecting medications to optimize medication tolerability and the overall outcome. For example, selection of a β_1-selective agent for a patient with bronchospastic pulmonary disease may be critical to ensuring tolerability when initiating this therapy. Despite retaining β_1-selectivity at lower doses, such agents may lose this selectively as up-titration occurs. It is essential that patients be educated to monitor for symptoms of worsening airway control and what actions to take if it occurs. Pharmacists can assist with ensuring that the optimal beta-blocker is selected from the start and educating the patient on monitoring and developing a plan of action.

In the patient with osteoarthritis, the pharmacist can suggest alternatives to NSAIDs, such as acetaminophen, that would be less apt to aggravate fluid control. Gout is a common occurrence in patients receiving aggressive diuretic regimens that are common in the management of AHFS. The NSAIDs are also commonly used to manage acute gout, as are steroids. Safer alternatives can be recommended in these patients. In addition, the chronic medications frequently used to prevent gout, allopurinol and colchicine, should be significantly dose reduced or avoided altogether in patients with worsening renal function. As patients with AHFS have reduced renal perfusion, such medication adjustments may be essential to avoiding important toxicities, such as myelosuppression.

In HF patients with diabetes, many opportunities for pharmacy intervention exists. First, selection of agents that are less prone to worsening glycemic control is important in optimizing cardiovascular risk reduction. In addition, monitoring for fluid retention in the diabetic patient treated with thiazolididones is necessary. Currently, metformin remains contraindicated in HF patients due to the potential risk of lactic acidosis. Pharmacists can assist with selecting safer alternative antidiabetic agents when one or both of the above therapies should be avoided. Pharmacists can also be instrumental in diabetic teaching, including setting blood glucose monitoring guidelines, blood glucose goals, diet and exercise goals, as well as monitoring overall response to antihyperglycemic therapy.

As left ventricle remodeling occurs, many patients develop atrial fibrillation. Antiarrhythmic agents are frequently prescribed in such patients. Amiodarone and dofetilide are safe antiarrhythmic agents to use in HF patients. Unfortunately, both agents have unique limitations. Dofetilide carries a high risk of torsades de pointes. Minimizing the risk of this life-threatening arrhythmia requires dose adjustment for renal dysfunction, dose adjustment for QT prolongation, optimal electrolyte repletion, avoiding drug interactions, and firm compliance. Prescribers can look to pharmacists for assistance with initial dosing and dose adjustments, and patient education regarding compliance and drug interactions. Amiodarone does not carry the same risk of polymorphic ventricular tachycardia; however, it does distribute significantly into tissues of various organs and thus requires close monitoring to avoid disabling and potentially life-threatening toxicities. Regular monitoring for pulmonary, hepatic, thyroid, and ocular toxicity is essential, and a definite area for pharmacy intervention.

Overall, the pharmacist's expertise can assist with developing a care plan to minimize adverse effects of HF medications that may cause difficulties managing comorbid conditions as well as most optimally treat comorbid conditions so as to avoid complicating HF management.

The Elderly

A pharmacist can aid in managing pharmacokinetic alterations that may occur in the aging population. Compared to younger adults, the elderly may have reduced lean body mass, reduced total and percentage body water, and an increase in fat as a percentage of body mass. In addition, older patients frequently experience slower gastric emptying. These changes may be important to consider when prescribing various HF medications. The age-related decline of renal functional capacity is also an important consideration. It is important to note that this decline is often not reflected in an equivalent rise in serum creatinine in this population since the production of creatinine may be reduced as muscle mass declines with age. Therefore, having a pharmacist on the management team can add value with their understanding of the pharmacokinetic changes in the elderly population.

Optimizing Medication Use by the Patient

Medication Reconciliation

An accurate drug history should be obtained as soon as possible after a patient is admitted for AHFS. The history may provide insight into a factor that may have precipitated the hospitalization, and it will ensure that all components of the therapy are addressed during the hospitalization. All drug histories should include over-the-counter products, such as pain relievers, as well as herbal products. Herbal products are important to elucidate, as most have unknown and potentially adverse effects and drug interactions, and none is currently regulated by the Food and Drug Administration.

Upon review of the medication list, the clinical importance of potential pharmacokinetic alterations should be assessed for each medication. In addition, the clinical need for each medication should be evaluated. Patients may be receiving unnecessary medications or medications that can potentially worsen HF.

Obtaining serum concentrations of certain medications may be indicated for those with narrow therapeutic ranges in which a pharmacokinetic alteration is anticipated. For example, obtaining serum digoxin concentrations would be appropriate in a patient with new or worsening renal insufficiency, particularly in elderly patients. Medication doses should be adjusted as indicated to account for significant alterations in absorption, distribution, metabolism, and excretion, as well as the presence of other interacting medications.

Therapies should also be readjusted once the acute HF symptoms such as congestion have been treated. Often, patients are discharged on higher doses of diuretics than needed on a chronic basis because they were receiving higher doses during the admission to overcome gastrointestinal edema as well as other causes of diuretic resistance. Similarly, if doses of other medications were decreased, such as warfarin, because of hepatic congestion or decreased metabolism, they may need to be increased to the preadmission dose. An area for pharmacist intervention exists for therapies such as warfarin, where the INR should be monitored and the dose adjusted as indicated. Pharmacist can also follow-up by telephone to remind patients of the discharge instructions, to assess medication tolerability, and assist with further medication adjustment as necessary.

Patient Education

Patient education is a key component of successful HF management. Patients need to know that their ACE inhibitor or beta-blocker is more than a "heart pill." Education on the purpose of medications, how to take them appropriately, and how to identify medication-related side effects is extremely important to successful patient management. It is also important to stress that although taking medication regularly may not make patients feel better immediately, it will ultimately decrease the risk of death and hospitalization. Comprehensive education and counseling are the foundation for all HF management and preventing AHFS. The goals of education and counseling are to help patients and their families and caregivers acquire the knowledge, skills, strategies, and motivation necessary for adherence to the treatment plan and effective participation in self-care.[10] Heart failure disease-management programs vary in their content, but in general they include intensive patient education, encouragement of patients to be more aggressive participants in their care, close monitoring of patients through telephone follow-up or home nursing, careful review of medications to improve adherence to evidence-based guidelines, and multidisciplinary care.[11] Pharmacists can be instrumental in each of the above activities.

Patient Assistance

The majority of HF patients are over the age of 65, and many do not have prescription coverage. Thus, identifying cost-effective regimens and applying for pharmaceutical company–sponsored patient assistance programs is a valuable contribution the clinical pharmacist can make to the HF patient. In many cases, there are less expensive alternatives with similarly proven efficacy.

Process Implementation

In health care systems, implementing processes and pathways is a successful approach that ensures patients receive evidence-based therapies. Pharmacists can aid in writing drug protocols, standard orders, and participating on quality improvement teams to ensure the best care is provided in managing AHFS patients. A pharmacist can be involved in making sure that a set of standards, called performance measures, are adhered to. These measures can be set up either within an institution or as a means of comparison between institutions to ensure that an adequate level of care is achieved, in order to optimize patient outcomes. These measures can vary, but for each HF patient it can include proper medication use, sharing of educational material, patient follow-up, side-effect monitoring, and proper ejection fraction documentation.[11] Ideally, these outcomes would improve patient outcomes.

End-Stage Patients

Patients with AHFS who are considered to be in the end stage are frequently difficult to manage in the inpatient setting. Diuretic resistance is common in such end-stage patients. Further optimizing diuretic regimens by changing intravenous loop diuretic regimens to continuous infusion, adding oral or intravenous thiazide diuretics, or adding intravenous venodilators may be necessary. Patients with low cardiac output may be refractory to weaning inotropes. Optimizing afterload reduction in the setting of ACE escape may aid in discontinuing these agents. Doing so in patients with low blood pressures in the AHFS setting may prove difficult. Selecting afterload reducing agents with short onset and offset is helpful in assessing efficacy and minimizing adverse effects. Pharmacists can assist with managing these very difficult scenarios in AHFS.

Many patients with AHFS should be considered for heart transplantation. If elevated filling pressures are present, reversal of pulmonary hypertension with nitroprusside or other agents may be required. Pharmacists can assist with nitroprusside titration or assisting with getting access to other agents that may be considered in this setting such as prostacyclin. Smoking cessation is an absolute requirement for all patients undergoing transplant evaluation. Pharmacists can assist with educating patients on various smoking cessation therapies and strategies for success as well as monitoring outcomes. Finally, ensuring medication compliance is critical to the success of any transplant recipient. Pharmacists are uniquely trained in assisting with this assessment.

Conclusion

Pharmacists can play a key role as a member of the HF management team. The unique expertise regarding drug therapy can impact multiple components of HF management. Specific considerations must be given to drug therapy in the advanced HF setting. These considerations have not been well described in the literature, and data are generally unavailable to guide decisions in these situations. Thus, having a care provider knowledgeable in pharmacology can be extremely helpful to successfully managing these patients.

References

1. Rich MW, Beckham V, Wittenberg C, Leven CL, Freedland KE, Carney RM. A multidisciplinary intervention to prevent the readmission of elderly patients with congestive HF. N Engl J Med 1995; 333:1190–5.
2. McAlister FA, Stewart S, Ferrua S, McMurray JJ. Multidisciplinary strategies for the management of HF patients at high risk for admission: a systematic review of randomized trials. J Am Coll Cardiol 2004;44:810–9.
3. Holland R, Battersby J, Harvey I, Lenaghan E, Smith J, Hay L. Systematic review of multidisciplinary interventions in HF. Heart 2005;91:899–906.
4. Gwadry-Sridhar FH, Flintoft V, Lee DS, Lee H, Guyatt GH. A systematic review and meta-analysis of studies comparing readmission rates and mortality rates in patients with HF. Arch Intern Med 2004;164:2315–20.
5. Gattis WA, Hasselblad V, Whellan DJ, O'Connor CM. Reduction in HF events by the addition of a clinical pharmacist to the HF management team: results of the pharmacist in HF assessment recommendation and monitoring (PHARM) study. Arch Intern Med 1999;159:1939–45.
6. Rainville EC. Impact of pharmacist interventions on hospital readmissions for HF. Am J Heath Syst Pharm 1999;56:1339–42.
7. Bucci C, Jackevicius C, McFarlane K, Liu P. Pharmacist's contribution in a heart function clinic: Patient perception and medication appropriateness. Can J Cardiol 2003;19:391–6.
8. Bouvy ML, Heerdink ER, Urquhart J, Grobbee DE, Hoe AW, Leufkens HGM. Effect of a pharmacist-led intervention on diuretic compliance in HF patients: a randomized controlled study. J Cardiac Fail 2003;9:404–11.
9. Fradette M, Bungard TJ, Simpson SH, Tsuyuki RT. Development of educational materials for congestive HF patients. Am J Health Syst Pharm 2004;61: 386–9.
10. Adams KF, Lindenfeld J, Arnold JMO, et al. Executive Summary: HFSA 2006 Comprehensive

HF Practice Guideline. J Cardiac Failure 2006;12:10–38.

11. Hunt SA, Abraham WT, Chin MH, et al. ACC/AHA 2005 guideline update for the diagnosis and management of chronic HF in the adult: a report of the American College of Cardiology/American Heart Association Task Force on Practice Guidelines (Writing Committee to Update the 2001 Guidelines for the Evaluation and Management of HF). J Am Coll Cardiol 2005;46(6):e1–82.

79 Role of Nursing in the Management of Acute Heart Failure Syndromes

Nancy M. Albert

When patients are treated for severe acute heart failure (HF) syndromes in a HF clinic, they are either acutely symptomatic and in need of urgent therapies or recovering from an acute decompensation episode and in need of follow-up monitoring and treatments to prevent hospitalization and worsening clinical status. Many pharmacologic and nonpharmacologic therapies can be delivered by nurses, especially advanced practice nurses with prescribing privileges. This chapter focuses on two topic areas that affect the nursing care of patients with severe acute HF in a clinic setting. First, nurse caregiver expectations should be developed to match a nurse's education level and licensure. Second, nursing roles are based on the type and level of services offered and how well services specifically promote quality care and patient safety. When nurses are active members in a collaborative team and have the autonomy to make treatment decisions based on consensus guideline evidence and best practices, patients' conditions can steadily improve, resulting in decreased mortality and morbidity and a good quality-of-life outcome.

Nursing Roles by Education and Licensure Level

A Two-Step Approach

There is a two-step approach in nursing roles based on education and licensure levels of practitioners. The lower step involves registered nurses with a diploma or associate, bachelor's, or master's degree who have licensure to practice at a basic level. Nurses at this lower level may have achieved basic certification through an approved accreditation group. Basic specialty certification ensures a specific degree of knowledge and decision-making skills in the nurse's specialty area. While nurses at this lower level can carry out many nursing role services, they may have clinical practice limitations due to the rules or regulations beyond the scope of the clinical team, such as policies set by a state or country licensure board, HF clinic (or hospital) standards of practice or policies, and job role or pay grade.

The higher step is an advanced practice nurse. An advanced practice nurse is a registered nurse with a master's degree who is either a clinical nurse specialist or nurse practitioner. A clinical nurse specialist has specialty training in cardiac patient populations and in the roles of researcher, consultant, educator, and expert clinician. A nurse practitioner may have a generalist (internal medicine or family practice) or specialty (geriatrics, pediatrics) focus and receives extensive training in physical examination and in developing an impression and plan of care. In many states, both types of advanced practice nurses may have prescription privileges. Registered nurses at an advanced practice level can complete nursing services at a lower level, but they have advanced knowledge and expertise to practice independently at a higher level.

Patients with severe, acute HF present with varying signs, symptoms, and characteristics (elevated, normal, or low systolic blood pressure; abrupt, rapid, or gradual pulmonary edema;

cardiogenic shock; isolated right heart failure; postcardiac surgery HF; and acute coronary syndromes[1]), each of which may have different treatment plans. The advanced practice nurse is better able to recognize characteristics of the different presentations and coordinate care to the fullest.

There are no nursing standards of practice or consensus guidelines that provide specific expectations of HF care delivered by a nurse in a HF clinic setting. Moreover, there are no recent nursing guidelines available that provide direction in a broader patient population with cardiovascular disease. The American Heart Association (AHA) developed a scientific statement on team management of patients with heart failure[2]. The guideline specifies that services across the continuum from inpatient to outpatient care should have an integrated management approach. Nurses can capably spearhead or be team members in providing the following continuum services: patient assessment and management, education and counseling, compliance with the therapeutic plan of care, discharge planning, community outreach, and HF outpatient management programs.

The team guideline provides further delineation of nursing care in community outreach and HF clinics using two models that are consistent with the two steps of registered nurse licensure. The two models are the nurse coordinated/facilitated model and the nurse managed/directed model of care[2]. In both models, it is assumed that nursing care is delivered by nurses with HF expertise. In a coordinated/facilitated care model, a licensed nurse assists other health care providers, usually a cardiologist, by coordinating or facilitating the plan of care as devised by a higher level of authority. This model is suited to nurses with education and licensure levels that do not allow for full autonomy in care planning and decision making. In a managed/directed care model, a licensed nurse, usually an advanced practice nurse, devises and revises the plan of care and has primary responsibility for patient care and outcomes[2]. Table 79.1 provides an overview of nine nursing roles in an HF clinic that can be delivered through the coordinated/facilitated or managed/directed model.

Maximizing Nursing Services

While nursing education and licensure level is associated with prespecified roles that may limit nurse capabilities, all nurses should work to the highest level of their capabilities to ensure that patients with HF receive optimal care and services. There are a myriad of subjective decisions influencing a nurse's role in clinical practice that may or may not be based on nurse education and licensure level. Some subjective decisions that affect a nurses' scope of practice are physician or office manager preferences, the nurse/patient ratio, and time allotted per patient; availability of treatment and conference room space; availability of resources to supplement patient education; nurses' knowledge and skill in managing severe acute HF; use of assistants or technical personnel to facilitate paperwork, testing, and room coordination; and congruence between nurse and physician beliefs about patient care and service expectations and priorities.

When resources are the influencing factors that limit the scope of a nurses' role, the office administrator should consider modifying office practices to redirect nurses toward roles that use their skills to the fullest. Thus, HF clinic teams can redevelop or redefine their systems and approach to care in ways that support improved patient outcomes.

From Table 79.1, it is apparent that effective implementation of multiple nursing roles requires administrative support (indirect care) time. Patients with severe acute HF have more unmet needs than patients who are stable and require only routine maintenance and assessment. Systems that choose the coordinated/facilitated model, in part or for all the nursing roles, can expect nurses to spend a majority, but not all, of their time on direct patient care. While the direct caregiver role is essential to meeting patient needs, key components associated with systems and processes planning, execution, and maintenance will be lost if time is not allotted for completion of indirect care responsibilities. The need to allot indirect care time to nurses in the managed/directed model becomes even more critical since key components require a review of the literature; time to meet with key stakeholders; time for process improvement, research,

Table 79.1. Nurses role by education and licensure level

Nursing roles	Nurse coordinated/facilitated	Nurse managed/directed (in addition to nurse coordinated/facilitated care)
Patient education	• Provider to patients and families; documents education delivery	• Routinely reviews and revises content of resource materials • Educator to nurses • Uses current research to guide education themes
Initiator and facilitator of ongoing communication to meet patient care needs; including need to die peacefully and the need to receive advanced care by surgical or electrophysiologist (EP) services	• Develops and delivers ongoing services (telephone, in-person, electronic) to patients based on predetermined time intervals or patient-specific situations • Uses algorithms to determine when consults are needed; facilitates consults to hospice, palliative care, surgeon, and EP (or to HF caregiver with prescribing authority) based on algorithms that specify inclusion and exclusion criteria • Develops and uses systems to maintain ongoing communication	• Develops algorithms for content of services that are based on evidence; considers patient wishes as well as technology capabilities and risk to benefit ratio when making decisions about advanced care opportunities • Performs quality monitoring of delivery of services given by new, inexperienced or unlicensed personnel • Is a resource to other nurses in complex cases • Maintains systems, once developed, by providing ongoing assessment, open communication, and team education • Develops consensus among consulting teams regarding limits of care expectations for each
Patient assessment including psychosocial, physical, and emotional health	• May perform physical exam of cardiac, vascular, and respiratory systems • Performs initial assessment of socioeconomic status and emotional health • Obtains medication history, vital signs, weight, recent history of signs and symptoms	• Performs physical exam and assessment of psychosocial and economic health. • Uses knowledge of comorbid conditions, adherence to the plan of care, past medical history and other findings of the patient assessment to develop or revise the plan of care
Pharmacologic care management	• May proactively suggest up-or-down titration of drug dose or addition of new drugs to caregivers with prescriptive privileges based on HF medication algorithms • Delivers medication management per written orders (as needed) • Assesses and documents causes of medication nonadherence	• Makes changes in pharmacologic plan of care using consensus guidelines based on evidence • Initiates orders for serum electrolyte or blood coagulation monitoring based on consensus guideline recommendations • Develops plan of care that takes into account financial and psychosocial constraints
Case management: transition to hospital or transition from hospital to skilled nursing facility	• Consults experts or makes plans for hospital admission, as needed • Makes decisions about transitional care based on algorithm inclusion and exclusion criteria	• Writes admission orders; specifies plan of care and expected length of stay • Develops algorithms used by others to facilitate transitional care
Quality improvement champion and data collector	• Acts as a team member in quality improvement methodology that provides continuous assessment, planning, checking and replanning to ensure performance measure outcome achievement	• Team leader/chair in quality improvement methodology • Develops performance improvement plan • Assures team involvement in processes and decision making
Coordination and triage of incoming patient care calls and incoming data from cardiac monitoring devices	• Uses algorithms and procedures to triage incoming patient requests, issues, concerns and cardiac monitoring device data appropriately	• Develops algorithms • Oversees quality monitoring of nurse responses to callers • Innovator, with team leaders in developing efficient and effective strategies to handle patient care calls
Program and interface maintenance	• Communicates issues that interfere with efficient and effective patient care services to team leaders	• Develops responses and processes/systems to overcome barriers to efficient and effective services • Communicates regularly with interfaces (hospital, emergency care, care consultants—nutrition, cardiac rehabilitation, social work) to ensure optimal care is delivered in all settings
Researcher (nursing and medical)	• Collects data for researchers, as needed • Assesses patients for inclusion in institutional review board–approved studies	• Translates research into practice after reviewing the quality of the findings • Develops research questions that will advance the practice of nursing care of patients with HF; conducts research to answer questions

HF, heart failure.

algorithm development, and review of each; and time to educate colleagues. Ultimately, there is a cost for facilitating optimal quality care and patient safety through evidence-based practices.

This cost of optimizing nursing roles involves more than just provision of indirect care time. When developing or redesigning an office system that allows nurses to participate in the care of patients with severe acute HF, the right mix of nurses working in each model or the right mix of responsibilities that nurses take on when they are hired to work in one model should be considered at the forefront. Before a nurse interviews for a job in this setting, nursing roles should be developed so that they can be explicitly described and discussed at the job interview. Not all nurses are comfortable taking on nursing roles beyond their core or base responsibilities. Some nurses might be uncomfortable in speaking assertively about drug up-titration or about referral to an electrophysiology cardiologist for potential cardiac resynchronization therapy. Nurses might not want to challenge the status quo by making suggestions for more efficient or effective services, especially if they feel the change process is a burden rather than an opportunity. In the nurse managed/directed model, nurses must be leaders in their field before they can successfully carry out the roles listed in Table 79.1. By discussing expectations regarding nursing roles up front, the right team can be developed. Team members will be more cohesive in ensuring that patient care needs are a first priority and that optimization of processes and systems are an important element in high-quality care.

Nursing Services

Before discussing the specific service roles of nurses in an HF clinic, it is important to note that there is no research literature on the hierarchy of nursing roles in relation to patient outcomes. First, nurses generally do not work in isolation; thus, outcomes achievement is due to collaborative efforts of interdisciplinary teams. Second, many patients, especially the elderly, have comorbid conditions that affect the course of a severe acute HF decompensation and HF outcomes. Third, in published studies, the teams that developed and reported the outcomes of an outpatient clinic disease management model each used unique interventions. For example, education, patient self-management, and care coordination could have been conducted through a specialty clinic visit, by telephone by a third party, by office telephone, or through a home care team. Fourth, in these studies there was great heterogeneity in many aspects of individual programs or of the research plan. Caregiver training, level of cardiologist involvement, type and levels of services by nurses (as described in Table 79.1), length of interaction time of the nurse with the patient, financial and social factors, sample inclusion and exclusion, data definitions of interventions and outcomes, and level of support the control group received varied or were not well described in these reports[3–6]. Thus, meta-analyses could be conducted to determine the overall effect of disease management programs on outcomes, but it was impossible to ascertain the specific aspects of the disease management process that demonstrated the greatest benefit. Reports that were included in meta-analyses were generally single-center studies[3–6] or multicenter studies with the same care team[7]. To determine the aspects of nursing care that positively affect patient outcomes, a randomized, multicenter study needs to be conducted.

Patient Education

Patients require education in medication administration, signs and symptoms of worsening condition, daily weight monitoring, activity, and low-sodium diet in order to be adequately prepared to care for themselves at home. Even though the American College of Cardiology/American Heart Association (ACC/AHA) and the Joint Commission on Accreditation of Healthcare Organizations (JCAHO) include patient education as part of their inpatient[8,9] and outpatient[8] performance measures of quality care, patients may not receive the intensity of training that they need to make sense of HF and self-care initiatives. In a qualitative study of 19 patients with HF, researchers found that patients did not connect chronic symptoms with their chronic condition, they did not recognize that these symptoms could worsen over time and lead to acute decompensation, and they did not manage symptoms on a routine basis to prevent or minimize episodes of exacerbation[10]. In a study of 90-day follow-up in a HF disease management program, 32 patients with severe decompensated HF made 37 phone calls to the health care team[11]. All patients were recently discharged after a severe acute HF hospitalization and were given education in medications and symptom monitoring prior to discharge. Patients were treated at regular intervals in the clinic, beginning an average of 10 days after discharge, and received a telephone call from an HF nurse practitioner at regular intervals, beginning at 7 days after discharge[11]. While the number of calls per patient was not provided in the report, the overall number of patients' telephone calls in an environment of close follow-up reflected unmet patient needs.

When HF education and counseling are delivered in a systematic, thorough manner (Table 79.2), whether one-to-one or in a group setting, patients may achieve better clinical outcomes than when they receive written literature alone. In a study of education prior to discharge, patients received either the usual care or a 1-hour, one-to-one nurse–patient education session. At 30 days, self-care practices were significantly improved and beta-blocker therapy was more likely to be maintained in the education group. At 6 months, time to first HF or cardiac hospitalization was significantly reduced in the education group, with relative risk reductions of 51% and 41%, respectively. Additionally, patients were more likely to be maintained on an angiotensin-converting enzyme inhibitor at 6 months in the education group[12]. In a randomized study of two dietary counseling sessions or usual care (dietary modification literature), patients receiving dietary counseling had a significant decrease in sodium intake at 3 months[13].

Nurses must be adequately educated in the HF principles listed in Table 79.2 to effectively teach patients. In two studies that used the same 20-item yes/no survey of nurse knowledge of HF education, the mean survey scores were around 75%, reflecting gaps in knowledge about important subjects patients need to be taught[14,15]. Thus, it should not be assumed that nurses caring for patients with HF have sufficient knowledge.

Table 79.2. Basic principles of patient education program content

Topic	Specifics
What HF is and rationale for pharmacologic therapies	▪ What HF is, its causes and symptoms, timeline (chronic), consequences (poor prognosis; premature death; greater risk for hospitalization) and measures to control it (self-care actions and monitoring) ▪ Why drugs are used in HF; how they improve survival or reduce hospitalization; common side effects and what to do when they occur; how to take medications for greatest effectiveness
Intravascular volume overload and effects of diuretics	▪ Causes of intravascular volume overload; can occur silently (without symptoms) ▪ How diuretics work ▪ Rationale for maintaining a diuretic schedule if on daily/twice daily dosing
Dietary modifications	▪ Role of sodium in diet and need for restriction even when feeling fine ▪ Tips on dining at restaurants or in another person's home ▪ Reading labels; salt used in packaged products ▪ Salt used in cooking ▪ High- and low-salt foods ▪ Sodium alternatives
Daily fluid limitation	▪ Why patients are thirsty ▪ Daily fluid limit to about 64 ounces ▪ How to monitor fluid intake ▪ What foods are considered fluids
Self-care behaviors	▪ Rationale for self-care behaviors: smoking cessation; daily weight monitoring; avoidance of heavy alcohol intake; avoidance of nonsteroidal antiinflammatory drugs and other over-the-counter herbal therapies and drugs, especially decongestants and sodium-based antacids ▪ Monitoring for changes in HF signs and symptoms; what to do if symptoms worsen (first person to call for all issues or when to call which member on the team) ▪ Rationale for activity and exercise; easy warm up/cool down exercises; getting started; when to stop or slow down

HF, heart failure.

Pharmacologic Management, Communication, and Consultation

The management of severe acute HF in an outpatient clinic requires a blending of therapies that target multiple pathophysiologic mechanisms. Patients have myocardial damage and hemodynamic, neurohormonal, and cytokine abnormalities that can worsen renal function and complicate the treatment regime. Every encounter is an opportunity to initiate or optimize core HF drug and device therapies. Registered nurses can proactively make suggestions to advance drug therapies or can prescribe therapies if licensure allows. Likewise, nurses can make suggestions for consultations that could improve patients' quality of life, ameliorate acute symptoms, or decrease the severity of HF.

Consultations, whether to prolong survival or promote palliation, allow specialty teams to recommend or provide services that benefit patients and their families. Use of physician or specialty service consultants may be delayed when the primary provider of HF care is uncertain about the timing of a consultation, reimbursement for consultative care, or drug interaction effects. Nurses can be the mediators of these uncertainties by meeting with consultants to determine the scope and limitations of services, the best time to initiate them, and reimbursement details. When consultants have uncertainties regarding the interaction of their services with HF services, educational opportunities can be planned. For example, a palliative medicine team might not understand the difference between an implantable cardioverter defibrillator and cardiac resynchronization therapy and believe that a dual device must be totally disabled to prevent unwanted shocks when a patient is receiving hospice care.

Patients also have uncertainties about whom to notify when symptoms worsen. Do they contact their primary care team, the electrophysiology team, the HF team, or a specialty physician for a noncardiac problem? Patients do not want to bother a busy physician and may choose to delay contact with any health care provider. Patient confusion about whom to notify when symptoms worsen leads to frustration and also creates a missed opportunity to treat symptoms early and prevent a hospitalization. Most HF symptoms are broad in scope, and patients may have difficulty understanding that what they are experiencing is abnormal. When nurses on the HF team become the first contact person, no matter what the symptoms are, patients gain confidence in their decision to make the call early on. Nurses must have confidence in being able to triage over the telephone and must have the authority to give specific directions to patients other than to go to the local emergency department. Directions can include drug titration algorithms, ordering a consultation service, ordering serum laboratory or other testing, and scheduling an urgent office visit.

Patient Assessment

Nurses, especially advanced practice nurses, are trained in subjective and objective patient assessment and physical examination. At minimum, vital signs, neurologic, cardiovascular, and respiratory examination should be conducted at each visit. Subjective data about recent history, medication plan adherence, diet, fluid management, activity, and barriers to self-care adherence provide a foundation for patient education priorities and the need for consultative services. The combination of physical examination, subjective findings, patients' understanding of HF self-care expectations, and comparison of current treatment-to-treatment plan goals determines the need for alteration of therapies.

Emotional needs are an important aspect of patients' perceptions of health and the meaning of their HF, especially in patients with severe acute HF. Fear of death and feelings of hopelessness[16] and resignation[17] emerged in research. The emotional consequences of HF changed as patients learned to live with their condition. Early emotions of fear, anxiety, and nervousness changed to later emotions of agony, depression, and increased irritation with physical inabilities[18]. When patients believed HF to be a fatal condition with poor prognosis, maladaptive emotional responses occurred. Additionally, fears of death were prompted by the sensations of dyspnea[18]. Thus, nurses must make the time to assess patients' emotional responses to HF and learn if these emotions are prompted by personal beliefs that there is nothing that can be done to improve quality or length of life. Nurses must teach patients that they have control of self-care behaviors. Self-care planning and interventions should be targeted to promote a positive meaning of the illness experience. Since depression in ambulatory patients was associated with diminished physical ability[19,20], worsening HF symptoms, worsening social functioning, and a decline in quality of life[20], nurses need to conduct research that supports valid and simple assessment measures and interventions that improve outcomes.

Case Management-Transition Care

Severe acute HF is a time of risks—risks to viable myocardium, coronary and vascular perfusion, renal function, electrolyte equilibrium, and social, emotional, and financial issues. Transition planning from hospital to home or, once ambulatory, from home alone to home care support provides patients, especially the elderly, and their caregivers with support during a vulnerable period. Nurses are in a position to be part of a multidimensional individualized plan to prolong the time to readmission and lower the total medical costs. When an advanced practice nurse–directed discharge plan was compared to usual care, patients in the intervention group had fewer readmissions at 1 year and a 3-month improvement in quality of life[21]. There are many ways that nurses can promote smooth transitions when HF is in a severe acute stage (Table 79.3). Nurses must conduct research in the intensity of services needed to meet the multiple serious health problems and risk factors faced by patients so that resources are maximized and patients have the best hope of remaining ambulatory with improved functional status, quality of life, survival, and satisfaction with care.

Table 79.3. Multidimensional transitional care nursing roles

- Coordinate care with nutritionist, social worker, cardiac rehabilitation, pharmacist, specialty physicians and others who can target coexisting medical, social, and financial issues
- Facilitate behavioral strategies that ease patient and caregiver burdens related to adherence to the medication, diet, fluid monitoring, and management plans
- Educate on advance directives planning and community services that meet learning needs
- Promote continuity of care between HF clinic and home or palliative care services
  - —Foster collaborative relationships
  - —Coach collaborators to use evidence-based therapies
  - —Ensure open communication
  - —Position patients and caregivers to proactively assess and manage signs and symptoms of worsening condition
- Assess goal progression
- Recognize and target unresolved HF issues

Quality Improvement and Maintenance

Evidence-based clinical performance measures facilitate the delivery of quality care that reflects current practice. Performance measures were developed by the ACC/AHA, JCAHO, Centers for Medicare and Medicaid (CMS), and the Ambulatory Care Quality Alliance for chronic HF teams managing patients in an ambulatory care setting[22–25]. Process and outcome data prompt enhanced quality of care delivery to patients when an improvement plan cycle is implemented. Nurses can champion quality improvement initiatives and promote collaborative, multidisciplinary teamwork that decreases the burden of all HF team members. By comparing individual data to past reports or regional/national data, teams can promote excellence and consistency of care.

When organizations used expert teams to develop performance measures, the measures were aimed at physician care. Many measures are carried out by nurses (volume assessment of signs and symptoms, patient education, smoking cessation counseling, flu shot, Pneumovax shot, taking the patient's weight and vital signs) and can be ordered by advanced practice nurses (drug therapies, assessment of ejection fraction, laboratory monitoring), but nurses are generally not the sole facilitators of quality care and patient safety based on the nationally documented measures. The current measures have been associated with improved outcomes. However, process measures, for example, documentation of delivery of education, do not ensure excellent outcomes. Nurses must work collaboratively with physicians and other team members to develop and test new performance measures that focus on outcomes, including those that reflect unique nursing care.

An ongoing quality improvement program is an essential element of quality assurance; however, the HF clinic must also interface with collaborators and care extenders in order to maintain optimal outreach program capabilities. The HF clinic must work with laboratories and testing centers, home care, hospitals, emergency and urgent care centers, and palliative care providers, to name a few. Maintenance of systems and collaborative programs developed to augment patient care services require constant attention, especially if the collaborating group does not have internal leaders who want the collaborative effort to succeed or internal experts in HF care. Heart failure clinic nurses can become the intermediary with outreach service groups. Nurses who are comfortable in program development, planning and evaluation, and in communication and negotiation will have the greatest success.

Patient Data: Patient Calls and Cardiac Monitoring Devices

Traditionally, patient data was derived from patients' telephone calls to the health care team. Asking patients to notify the health care team when HF signs and symptoms worsened helps patients learn the importance of, and have control of, self-monitoring and ongoing communication.

Cardiac devices with internal monitoring features are growing in use. Devices can monitor hemodynamics, heart rhythm abnormalities, autonomic function, cardiac resynchronization and implantable defibrillator activity, general activity level, and fluid status. In patients with severe acute HF, a monitoring device might serve as an early warning system and minimize or prevent complications and morbidity.

Nurses are generally the recipients of incoming patient data, whether by telephone or cardiac device. They must be trained to understand new hemodynamic and fluid status concepts, such as right ventricular outflow pressure and thoracic impedance. Systems must be developed to handle patients' urgent calls, written reports of data received from the monitoring unit, and outgoing communication to patients. This can be cumbersome, especially when reimbursement for telephone communication is not provided, when hardcopy monitoring reports need to be converted to an electronic health record, or when dedicated time is not created for incoming communication follow-up.

The scope of device monitoring must be considered as well. Since patients may require a device assessment of their hemodynamic or cardiac function status at any time, system planning must include placement of multiple computers and other equipment needed to download device data in around-the-clock environments, such as an emergency department, coronary care unit, or third-party telephone monitoring service.

Ultimately, device monitoring brings additional objective data into the hands of health care providers. Traditional signs and symptoms of HF decompensation are moderately to very specific, but often lack sensitivity. Therefore, they are not always reliable in diagnosing decompensation in patients with acute dyspnea[26]. Since cardiac device monitoring is relatively new, there is much to be learned. Research on sensitivity and specificity of data, frequency of downloading data, aggressiveness in reacting to data findings, and results of other diagnostic tools that support cardiac device findings will help nurse practitioners understand how to use the data to the fullest. Standardized treatment regimes have not been developed for cardiac device alterations. If thoracic impedance levels drop dramatically, reflecting volume overload, the timing and dose of loop or other diuretics is determined after individual care planning. However, research could lead to a standardized drug therapy approach and might include a patient-mediated flexible diuretic (or other agent) regime. Technology is changing rapidly in the HF clinic. Nurses must embrace it, learn from it, and ensure that patient safety and care quality are maintained as data capabilities expand.

Research

Research is essential in strengthening the foundation of both medical and nursing science. Nurses are often study coordinators for medical research; however, there is a great need to advance nursing care and basic science in the practice of HF. Additionally, nurses must become proficient in translating medical and nursing research findings into practice to optimize care quality and patient safety. There are multiple ways nurses can participate in achieving evidence-based practices through research. Journal clubs are useful in discussing new developments and using a team approach to incorporating findings into practice. Nurses who are not skilled in research can collaborate with HF experts in the community to conduct clinical research. It is essential to publish findings to strengthen HF science.

Conclusion

Nurses are capable of carrying out multiple roles in a HF clinic. Collaborative practices with other HF clinic providers and outreach centers can improve patient services, promote smooth transitions between service providers, and increase patient care quality and safety. In addition to direct care, nurses can be leaders in assuring optimal quality and use of evidence based-therapies. Nurses can develop new services and then lead in ensuring service maintenance. Nursing research should be encouraged to assess program outcomes and further nursing science in HF care.

References

1. Gheorghiade M, Zannad F, Sopko G, et al. Acute Heart Failure Syndromes. Current state and framework for future research. Circulation 2005;112: 3958–68.
2. Grady KL, Dracup K, Kennedy G, et al. Team management of patients with heart failure. A statement for healthcare professionals from the Cardiovascular Nursing Council of the American Heart Association. Circulation 2000;102:2443–56.
3. Holland R, Battersby J, Harvey I, et al. Systematic review of multidisciplinary interventions in heart failure. Heart 2005;91:899–906.
4. McAlister FA, Stewart S, Ferrua S, et al. Multidisciplinary strategies for the management of heart failure patients at high risk for admission. A systematic review of randomized trials. J Am Coll Cardiol 2004;44:810–9.
5. Phillips CO, Wright SM, Kern DE, et al. Comprehensive discharge planning with postdischarge support for older patients with congestive heart failure. A meat-analysis. JAMA 2004;291:1358–67.
6. Whellan DJ, Hasselblad V, Peterson E, et al. Meta-analysis and review of heart failure disease management randomized controlled clinical trials. Am Heart J 2005;149:722–9.
7. Atienza F, Anguita M, Martinez-Alzamora N, et al. Multicenter randomized trial of a comprehensive hospital discharge and outpatient heart failure management program. European J Heart Fail 2004; 6:643–52.
8. American College of Cardiology/American Heart Association Task Force on Performance Measures. ACC/AHA clinical performance measures for adults with chronic heart failure. J Am Coll Cardiol 2005; 46:1144–78.
9. Joint Commission on Accreditation of Healthcare Organizations. Overview of the heart failure core measure set. http://jcaho.org/pms/core+measures/hf_overview.htm.
10. Horowitz CR, Rein SB, Leventhal H. A story of maladies, misconceptions and mishaps: effective management of heart failure. Social Sci Med 2004; 58:631–43.
11. Shah MR, Flavell CM, Weintraub JR, et al. Intensity and focus of heart failure disease management after hospital discharge. Am Heart J 2005;149:715–21.
12. Koelling TM, Johnson ML, Cody RJ, et al. Discharge education improves clinical outcomes in patients with chronic heart failure. Circulation 2005;111: 179–85.
13. Arcand JA, Brazel S, Joliffe C, et al. Education by a dietician in patients with heart failure results in improved adherence with a sodium-restricted diet: a randomized trial. Am Heart J 2005;150:716.e1–716.e5.
14. Albert NM, Collier S, Sumodi V, et al. Nurses' knowledge of heart failure education principles. Heart Lung 2002;31:102–12.
15. Washburn SC, Hornberger CA, Klutman A, et al. Nurses' knowledge of heart failure topics as reported in a small Midwestern community hospital. J Cardiovasc Nurs 2005;20:215–20.
16. Evangelista LS, Kagawa-Singer M, Dracup K. Gender differences in health perceptions and meaning in persons living with heart failure. Heart Lung 2001;30:167–76.
17. Mårtensson J, Karlsson J, Fridlund B. Male patients with congestive heart failure and their conception of the life situation. J Adv Nurs 1997;25:579–86.
18. Europe E, Tyni-Lenné R. Qualitative analysis of the male experience of heart failure. Heart Lung 2004;33:227–34.
19. Rumsfeld JS, Havranaek E, Masoudi FA, et al. Depressive symptoms are the strongest predictors of short-term declines in health status in patients with heart failure. J Am Coll Cardiol 2003;42:1811–7.
20. Skotozo CE, Krichten C, Zietowski G, et al. Depression is common and precludes accurate assessment of functional status in elderly patients with congestive heart failure. J Card Failure 2000;6:300–4.

21. Naylor MD, Brooten DA, Campbell RL, et al. Transitional care of older adults hospitalized with heart failure: a randomized, controlled trial. J Am Geriatr Soc 2004;52:675–84.
22. American College of Cardiology/American Heart Association Task Force on Performance Measures. ACC/AHA clinical performance measures for adults with chronic heart failure. J Am Coll Cardiol 2005;46:1144–78.
23. Joint Commission on Accreditation of Healthcare Organizations. Disease specific care. Request for public comment on disease-specific care standardized heart failure measure set. http://jcaho.org/dscc/dsc/performance+measures/heart+failure+measure+set.htm.
24. Toth MM. MedQIC Content and Collaboration Team. Transform: The MedQIC approach to Change. Owings Mills, MD: 2004. [Medicare Quality Improvement Community]. http://www.medqic.org/heartfailure.
25. American College of Physicians. About the Ambulatory Care Quality Alliance. http://www.acponline.org/quality/aboutaqa.htm.
26. Mueller C, Frana B, Rodriguez D, et al. Emergency diagnosis of congestive heart failure: impact of signs and symptoms. Can J Cardiol 2005;21:921–4.

80
Psychological Support in Acute Heart Failure Syndrome

Karen E. Joynt, Wei Jiang, and Christopher M. O'Connor

Clinical Case

Mr. L. is a 62-year-old Native American with a past medical history significant for coronary artery disease status post–myocardial infarction and four-vessel coronary artery bypass grafting 2 years ago, as well as known heart failure with a left ventricular ejection fraction of 30%, type 2 diabetes, and hyperlipidemia. He presents to the emergency room complaining of shortness of breath with exertion, orthopnea, lower extremity edema, and dull chest pain. On initial evaluation he is hypotensive at 86/40 mm Hg, and lung exam reveals rales halfway up the posterior fields. A third heart sound is present. He is admitted to the inpatient cardiology service; the cardiology team notes that this is his third admission for similar symptoms in the past 7 months. What further information might help his clinicians maximize therapy for his chronic heart failure, and prevent future acute exacerbations?

The story of Mr. L. is an increasingly common one. Over 500,000 new cases of heart failure (HF) are diagnosed annually, and experts predict that this number will reach 1.5 million by 2040 as the population continues to age and an increasing number of people survive acute myocardial infarction (MI).[1] More than five million Americans are currently living with HF,[1] and the lifetime risk for the development of HF is now 20%[2]; HF is now the most common discharge diagnosis for Medicare beneficiaries.[1] Many advances in the care of patients with HF, including angiotensin-converting enzyme (ACE) inhibitors, beta-blockers, and aldosterone receptor antagonists, have improved both long- and short-term survival.[3] However, the mortality rate still approaches 20% annually, particularly in patients with New York Heart Association (NYHA) class III or IV symptoms.[4] Morbidity is also high, with hospital readmission rates of 25% to 50% within 6 months after discharge.[5] Managing heart failure is a costly undertaking; in 2006, HF costs are projected to total over $29 billion in direct and indirect costs, and HF is the single largest Medicare expenditure category.[1] Clearly, efforts to identify factors that may affect the prognosis of patients with HF, and in turn to develop ways in which to address these factors, are worthwhile. This chapter discusses the potential contribution of psychological factors—specifically depression, anxiety, and social support—to outcomes in HF, and offers recommendations for intervention, when indicated.

The Impact of Depression on Outcomes in Heart Failure

Depression is perhaps the most frequently studied psychological factor in cardiac disease, and has consistently been found to be highly prevalent in HF. Between 35% and 70% of inpatients with HF, and between 11% and 25% of outpatients,[5–12] have been demonstrated to suffer from depression; in the general population, only 5% to 10% of individuals meet the criteria for depression.[13] Within the HF population, there does not appear to be a difference in the frequency of depression when comparing patients by etiology of HF, that is, ischemic versus nonischemic.[5] Perhaps even more importantly, depression has been shown to be independently associated with poor outcomes in patients with HF. For example, a 2001 study by Jiang et al.[5] demonstrated significant increases in mortality in HF patients with depression over the 12 months following admission for a cardiac event compared to patients without depression. Patients with depression had a 12-month mortality rate of 26.1%, compared with only 13.7% for patients without depression (odds ratio [OR], 2.23; $p = .04$). Similarly, 12-month rehospitalization rates were 80.4% for depressed patients and 52.3% for nondepressed patients (OR, 3.07; $p = .005$).[5] These effects were independent of established risk factors such as age, NYHA class, and left ventricular ejection fraction (LVEF).

Other investigators have noted negative outcomes attributable to depression in HF as well, and these findings have not been limited to the inpatient setting or to patients with ischemic disease. Murberg et al.,[8] in a sample of stable outpatients with HF, found that depression conferred a twofold increased risk of mortality over 2 years of follow-up, and Vaccarino et al.[10] found a strong graded relationship between severity of depression and risk of functional decline or death in elderly HF inpatients. In an exclusively nonischemic population, findings have been similar: Faris et al.[7] reported on outcomes for nearly 400 patients with dilated cardiomyopathy, and showed that depression was associated with a hazard ratio for mortality of 3.0 over 4 years of follow-up, controlling for demographics and usual clinical predictors of outcome; depressed patients in this study also reported more symptoms, demonstrated worse exercise capacity, and had poorer left ventricular (LV) function.[7] In addition to mortality, functional status can be negatively impacted by depression; Clarke et al.,[14] studying a sample of 2992 HF patients, found depression to be associated with an OR of 1.96 for severe functional impairment even after adjusting for baseline demographic and clinical characteristics.

The Impact of Anxiety on Outcomes in Heart Failure

Although anxiety is not nearly as well studied as depression in HF, the research suggests that its prevalence in HF is increased in comparison with the general population. In a sample of 100 stable outpatients with HF, 18.4% were found to suffer from anxiety[15]; in a study enrolling 87 patients with depressed LVEF, the prevalence of anxiety was 31%.[16] In comparison, data from the National Institute of Mental Health suggests that the 1-year prevalence rate of any anxiety disorder in the general population of the United States is roughly 13%.[17]

Anxiety has been suggested to increase the risk of developing ischemic heart disease as well as the risk of sudden death,[18] but the impact of anxiety on outcomes in patients with established ischemic heart disease[19,20] is less clear, and there are very little data available on the impact of anxiety in patients with heart failure.[16,21] Jiang et al.[22] reported on 291 hospitalized HF patients, and noted the prevalence of anxiety to be 29%; measurements of depression and anxiety were highly correlated. At 12-month follow-up, anxiety was not correlated with outcomes in this population, although depression was strongly correlated with both hospital readmission and mortality.

Similarly, Denollet and Brutsaert[16] noted that anxiety was associated with an OR for mortality of 3.7 in a population of post-MI patients with depressed LVEF, but this association disappeared when type D personality (characterized by negative affectivity and social inhibition) was added to the model. Ingle et al.,[23] examining a group of patients with left ventricular systolic dysfunction, found that both self-reported depression and anxiety were negatively correlated with performance on the 6-minute walk test, and both were related to performance in a dose-response relationship. Although anxiety is clearly a discrete emotional experience, it is also worth noting that anxiety frequently co-occurs with depression, particularly in older individuals and medically ill populations; one recent study of elderly patients in the Netherlands demonstrated that 47.5% of those with major depressive disorder also met criteria for anxiety disorders, while 26.1% of those with anxiety disorders also met criteria for major depressive disorder.[24]

Possible Mechanisms Connecting Depression, Anxiety, and Outcomes in Acute Heart Failure Syndrome

Many researchers have postulated that underlying physiologic mechanisms, such as sympathetic nervous system hyperactivity, arrhythmogenicity, inflammation, and platelet reactivity, explain the connection among depression, anxiety, and the development and progression of heart failure.[25,26] Depression and anxiety have been shown to augment the release of catecholamines such as norepinephrine; for example, depressed patients have been shown to have elevated plasma norepinephrine as well as a hypersecretory catecholamine response to orthostatic challenge.[27] Mortality in HF has been correlated with increased levels of circulating catecholamines[28]; this is likely the result of myocardial cell death due to hypercontracture, myocardial remodeling, and increased frequency of arrhythmias, particularly ventricular arrhythmias.[28–30]

Catecholamine release in turn may increase the risk of arrhythmias, promote elaboration of proinflammatory cytokines, and exacerbate platelet activation—processes that are widely believed to influence prognosis in HF. Depressed patients have been found to have lower heart rate variability (HRV) than patients without depression, suggesting a decreased relative parasympathetic influence on the heart and therefore an increased susceptibility to arrhythmias[31,32]; further, some investigators have noted a dose–response effect, that is, patients with more severe depression have lower HRV.[33] Other rhythm disturbances have been reported as well; in patients with recent internal cardioverter defibrillator (ICD) implantation, the presence of a mood disorder was shown to be a significant predictor of arrhythmic events at 3 and 6 months even after controlling for LVEF, arrhythmia history, and medication use,[34] and Carney et al.[35] showed that depression was an independent risk factor for ventricular tachycardia during ambulatory monitoring (relative risk [RR], 8.2; 95% confidence interval [CI], 2.14–31.70).

Patients with depression and/or anxiety also exhibit elevated levels of serum markers of inflammation. Plasma concentrations of interleukin-6 and C-reactive protein have been shown to be more than twice as high in depressed patients as compared with controls,[36–39] and the presence of even mild to moderate depressive symptoms in patients without a diagnosis of major depression has been correlated with elevated inflammatory markers, suggesting that depression may begin to have a significant physiologic impact well before it becomes clinically apparent.[40] Likewise, anxiety has been correlated with elevated levels of C-reactive protein, homocysteine, and interleukin-6.[41] Similar to catecholamines, circulating levels of proinflammatory cytokines are correlated with disease severity as well as with outcomes in HF patients.[42,43]

Studies have shown consistently that patients with depression have increased platelet aggregation, with platelet reactivity up to 40% greater than control subjects as well as elevated β-thromboglobulin, platelet factor 4, and anti-ligand–induced binding-site antibody levels.[44–46] Although the role of platelet reactivity is less well established in HF than in coronary disease, antiplatelet therapy has been shown to be of benefit in patients with HF,[47] suggesting that platelet aggregation may be an important factor in this disease.

The impact of depression on patients' compliance with medical recommendations should also be considered. Particularly in a chronic disease like HF, complicated prescription drug regimens, special diets, exercise, and home monitoring can play a large role in the success of outpatient disease management. Depressed patients have a threefold increased risk of noncompliance with medical recommendations in a range of medical illnesses, including heart disease, renal disease, rheumatoid arthritis, and cancer,[48] and patients who are depressed have been shown to have lower adherence rates to cardiac rehabilitation programs after MI.[49,50] In heart failure in particular, one recent study found that mental health was predictive of both behavioral and pharmacologic compliance,[51] pointing out the importance of assessing compliance particularly carefully in patients with depression. Noncompliance with medical recommendations is high in HF; this may be related to the complexity of and frequent changes in HF medical regimens.[52] Noncompliance with ACE inhibitors in the short-term immediately following a hospitalization for HF is on the order of 20% to 30%,[53,54] and as few as 10% of HF patients may comply with medications consistently throughout any given year.[55] Compliance has been shown to be important for prognosis in HF,[56,57] and may be a factor in as many as 20% to 60% of hospital readmissions.[58–61]

Interventions Addressing Depression and Anxiety in Heart Failure

Pharmacologic Treatment of Depression

Although physiologic intermediaries such as HRV, inflammation, and platelet reactivity are thought to contribute to the relationship between depression and HF, there is little data regarding the impact of treatment of depression on these parameters, and the data that exist are largely in the post-MI population. One small trial showed that depressed post-MI patients treated with sertraline showed progressive improvement, paralleling the improvement seen in nondepressed patients, in their HRV after treatment, while those who received placebo experienced ongoing decline in HRV.[62] Similarly, a small trial of doxepin and fluoxetine demonstrated increased HRV in the subset of patients whose symptoms improved following treatment, as measured by a greater than 50% change in the Hamilton Depression Rating Scale; patients whose symptoms did not improve demonstrated a progressive decline in HRV over the study period.[63] Findings regarding inflammatory markers have been mixed, with some investigators reporting decreased inflammation in patients treated with selective serotonin reuptake inhibitors (SSRIs),[39,64] and others reporting no impact.[36] Platelet reactivity has similarly been shown to normalize after paroxetine[65] or sertraline[66] therapy.

Only one reported trial has examined the impact of treatment of depression in a population with cardiac disease, and again this was in the post-MI population. The Sertraline Anti-Depressant Heart Attack Trial (SADHART) enrolled 369 patients with major depressive disorder and either acute MI or unstable angina in a randomized, double-blind, placebo-controlled trial. Sertraline was demonstrated to be safe; no changes were seen in mean LVEF, prolonged QTc interval, or other cardiac measures.[67] Sertraline was superior to placebo on the Clinical Global Impression Improvement (CGI-I) scale (measured over 24 weeks, 2.57 vs. 2.75, p = .049) but not on the Hamilton Depression (HAM-D) change score (measured over 16 weeks, −8.4 vs. −7.6, p = .14). However, in a predefined subgroup analysis examining patients with recurrent or severe depression, sertraline was shown to be more efficacious than placebo on both CGI-I and HAM-D measurements, and was associated with improvements in quality of life and functional status in this group as well.[67,68] One very interesting outcome from this trial was a numerically lower incidence of severe cardiac events (death, myocardial infarction, congestive heart failure, stroke, and recurrent angina) among patients receiving sertraline than among those receiving placebo (14.5% vs. 22.4%; RR, 0.77; 95% CI, 0.51–1.16), although this result did not reach statistical significance, and the trial was not powered to detect a difference in these parameters.[67] One substudy of this data set demonstrated that sertraline was associated with decreased platelet activation markers, echoing previous findings noted above and suggesting one mechanism by which sertraline might confer a morbidity and mortality advantage.[69] However, this trial was not specifically conducted in patients with HF, and conclusions are therefore risky to draw.

Nonpharmacologic Treatment of Depression

Nonpharmacologic treatment of depression or anxiety, including programs focused on stress management, has shown mixed results in its ability to impact morbidity and mortality for depressed or anxious post-MI patients, and little data exist specific to HF patients. Frasure-Smith and Prince[70] randomized 461 men in the post-MI period to a stress-reduction intervention or usual care and showed that those men receiving the intervention had a 50% decrease in cardiac mortality (4.5% vs. 9%), although no change was found in hospital readmission rates. Blumenthal et al.[71] enrolled stable ischemic heart disease (IHD) patients in a stress management program and demonstrated a relative risk for cardiac events of 0.26 compared to controls; however, the patient population was not assessed for depression.[71] The Montreal Heart Attack Readjustment Trial (M-HART), on the other hand, found that women receiving a home-based nonpharmacologic anxiety-reducing nursing intervention after MI actually had higher mortality than the control group, with the worse outcomes primarily related to an increased risk of sudden death.[72] Jones and West[73] enrolled over 2000 patients in a post-MI rehabilitation program that included stress management training, and found no impact on anxiety, depression, or mortality. However, a 1999 meta-analysis suggested that programs incorporating stress management and health education led to a 34% reduction in cardiac mortality and a 29% reduction in recurrence of MI, and a positive impact on blood pressure, cholesterol, body weight, smoking, physical exercise, and eating habits.[74]

The ENRICHD (ENhancing Recovery In Coronary Heart Disease) trial enrolled 2481 post-MI patients with depression and/or low perceived social support, and randomized subjects to usual care versus an individually tailored cognitive-behavioral therapy (CBT)-based intervention, initiated 2 to 3 weeks after MI and continued over 6 months. Pharmacologic treatment was permitted; patients scoring higher than 24 on the Hamilton Rating Scale for Depression (HRSD) or demonstrating a less than 50% reduction in Beck Depression Inventory (BDI) scores after 5 weeks were eligible to receive an SSRI.[75] The intervention group demonstrated improved psychological outcomes in comparison with the control group, with mean BDI score 9.1 in the intervention group at the 6-month follow-up visit vs. 12.2 in the control group ($p < .001$), but these effects did not persist to the 30-month evaluation. No mortality difference was noted (event-free survival 75.9% vs. 75.8%, p = ns).[75] Interestingly, depression was an independent risk factor for death after MI in this trial (HR [hazard ratio], 2.4; 95% CI, 1.2–4.7),[76] despite the fact that treatment of depression was not associated with a mortality benefit. The concomitant use of antidepressant medication, which reached 20.6% in the control group and 28% in the intervention group by the end of follow-up, may have been a major confounder; antidepressant medication use was associated with a significant decrease in risk of death or nonfatal MI (adjusted HR, 0.57; 95% CI, 0.38–0.85).[75]

Recommendations for the Clinician

Appropriate treatment of depression in patients with cardiac disease is essential, not only because these are serious and debilitating conditions, but also because treatment may reduce associated cardiac morbidity and mortality. A wide range of effective antidepressant agents is available, and many of these agents also have efficacy against anxiety. However, when choosing treatment for patients with ischemic heart disease or heart failure, the clinician needs to consider both their antidepressant efficacy and their safety profiles, in particular any known effects on cardiac conduction, contractility, and heart rhythm.

Tricyclic antidepressants (TCAs) show good clinical efficacy against depression, although they are less frequently used nowadays because of their association with cardiovascular, sedative, anticholinergic, and weight-gain side effects. The cardiovascular effects of TCAs are well characterized, and include orthostatic hypotension, slowed cardiac conduction, type 1A antiarrhythmic activity, and increased heart rate.[77] Orthostatic hypotension is a particular concern in the elderly, and slowing of cardiac conduction contraindicates the use of TCAs in patients with preexisting conduction problems. Moreover, results of the Cardiac Arrhythmia Suppression Trials (CAST) suggest that agents with type 1A antiarrhythmic activity, including TCAs, should not be used in patients with ischemic heart disease.[78] More recently, a comparison of nortriptyline and paroxetine provided clear evidence that therapeutic plasma levels of a TCA can cause a sustained increase in heart rate in patients with ischemic heart disease. Nortriptyline caused a sustained 11% increase in heart rate ($p < .001$), 14% reduction in HRV ($p < .01$), and 12% increase in supine and standing pulse rates ($p < .001$). Standing systolic blood pressure was also significantly reduced at week 2 ($p < .01$).

Overall, 18% of the nortriptyline group discontinued treatment due to adverse cardiovascular events compared with 2% in the paroxetine group.[79]

As discussed above, randomized controlled trials of SSRIs for the treatment of depression in the setting of ischemic heart disease have shown encouraging results. Therefore, when selecting antidepressant therapy in the setting of heart failure, SSRIs should be favored, and TCAs should be second-line therapy at best. The ongoing SADHART-CHF trial, funded by the National Institute of Mental Health, is examining whether sertraline treatment may reduce mortality and rehospitalizations in HF patients with depression. Results forthcoming from this trial should provide important insights into the appropriate management of these patients.

Clinical Case, Revisited

At this point let us return to the case of Mr. L. His astute clinicians asked him a set of simple questions about his mood, compliance with medications, and social support, and identified a number of factors that might have been contributory to his readmission to the hospital. He reluctantly admitted to having difficulty taking his medications as prescribed, and endorsed low mood and anhedonia since the death of his wife a year prior. With the help of the psychiatry consult team and the cardiology social worker, Mr. L. was started on an SSRI for his newly diagnosed depression and set up with community resources to provide social support. His medical regimen was simplified to daily dosing when possible. He received education about his heart failure and about how he could positively impact his prognosis, and was receptive to the information presented to him.

Conclusion

The clinical case presented here is informative because it reminds us of the importance of assessing psychological factors in patients with HF. Depression and anxiety are common in HF, and, as outlined above, have been shown to have a striking negative impact on outcomes in HF. Failing to address these factors may lead to suboptimal outcomes in this particularly vulnerable population. Conversely, providing appropriate interventions when depression or anxiety is noted in patients with HF may improve morbidity and even mortality in this chronic, progressive, and costly disease. Clinicians, therefore, should consider assessment of depression and anxiety to be an essential component in the thorough evaluation of a patient with HF.

References

1. American Heart Association Heart Disease and Stroke Statistics—2006 Update. Dallas: AHA, 2005.
2. Lloyd-Jones DMM: Lifetime risk for developing congestive heart failure: the Framingham Heart Study. Circulation 2002;106:3068–72.
3. Yan AT, Yan RT, Liu PP Narrative review: pharmacotherapy for chronic heart failure: evidence from recent clinical trials. Ann Intern Med 2005;142: 132–45.
4. Packer M, Coats AJ, Fowler MB, et al. Effect of carvedilol on survival in severe chronic heart failure. N Engl J Med 2001;344:1651–8.
5. Jiang W, Alexander J, Christopher E, et al. Relationship of depression to increased risk of mortality and rehospitalization in patients with congestive heart failure. Arch Intern Med 2001;161:1849–56.
6. Koenig HG Depression in hospitalized older patients with congestive heart failure. Gen Hosp Psychiatry 1998;20:29–43.
7. Faris R, Purcell H, Henein MY, Coats AJ Clinical depression is common and significantly associated with reduced survival in patients with non-ischaemic heart failure. Eur J Heart Fail 2002;4: 541–51.
8. Murberg TA, Bru E, Svebak S, Tveteras R, Aarsland T Depressed mood and subjective health symptoms as predictors of mortality in patients with congestive heart failure: a two-years follow-up study. Int J Psychiatry Med 1999;29:311–26.
9. Havranek EP, Ware MG, Lowes BD Prevalence of depression in congestive heart failure. Am J Cardiol 1999;84:348–50, A9.
10. Vaccarino V, Kasl SV, Abramson J, Krumholz HM Depressive symptoms and risk of functional decline and death in patients with heart failure. J Am Coll Cardiol 2001;38:199–205.
11. Freedland KE, Rich MW, Skala JA, Carney RM, Davila-Roman VG, Jaffe AS Prevalence of depression in hospitalized patients with congestive heart failure. Psychosom Med 2003;65:119–28.

12. Turvey CL, Schultz K, Arndt S, Wallace RB, Herzog R Prevalence and correlates of depressive symptoms in a community sample of people suffering from heart failure. J Am Geriatr Soc 2002;50:2003–8.
13. American Psychiatric Association. Let's Talk Facts About Depression. Washington, DC: APA, 1998.
14. Clarke SP, Frasure-Smith N, Lesperance F, Bourassa MG Psychosocial factors as predictors of functional status at 1 year in patients with left ventricular dysfunction. Res Nurs Health 2000;23:290–300.
15. Haworth JE, Moniz-Cook E, Clark AL, Wang M, Waddington R, Cleland JG Prevalence and predictors of anxiety and depression in a sample of chronic heart failure patients with left ventricular systolic dysfunction. Eur J Heart Fail 2005;7: 803–8.
16. Denollet J, Brutsaert DL Personality, disease severity, and the risk of long-term cardiac events in patients with a decreased ejection fraction after myocardial infarction. Circulation 1998;97:167–73.
17. National Institute of Mental Health. Facts About Anxiety Disorders. Publication OM-99 4152. Bethesda, MD: NIMH, 1999.
18. Kawachi I, Colditz GA, Ascherio A, et al. Prospective study of phobic anxiety and risk of coronary heart disease in men. Circulation 1994;89:1992–7.
19. Lane D, Carroll D, Ring C, Beevers DG, Lip GY Mortality and quality of life 12 months after myocardial infarction: effects of depression and anxiety. Psychosom Med 2001;63:221–30.
20. Strik JJ, Denollet J, Lousberg R, Honig A Comparing symptoms of depression and anxiety as predictors of cardiac events and increased health care consumption after myocardial infarction. J Am Coll Cardiol 2003;42:1801–7.
21. Frasure-Smith N, Lesperance F Depression and other psychological risks following myocardial infarction. Arch Gen Psychiatry 2003;60:627–36.
22. Jiang W, Kuchibhatla M, Cuffe MS, et al. Prognostic value of anxiety and depression in patients with chronic heart failure. Circulation 2004;110:3452–6.
23. Ingle L, Rigby AS, Nabb S, Jones PK, Clark AL, Cleland JG: Clinical determinants of poor six-minute walk test performance in patients with left ventricular systolic dysfunction and no major structural heart disease. Eur J Heart Fail 2005;8:321–5.
24. Beekman AT, de Beurs E, van Balkom AJ, Deeg DJ, van Dyck R, van Tilburg W Anxiety and depression in later life: Co-occurrence and communality of risk factors. Am J Psychiatry 2000;157:89–95.
25. Joynt KE, Whellan DJ, O'Connor CM Why is depression bad for the failing heart? A review of the mechanistic relationship between depression and heart failure. Arch Intern Med 1994;154:433–7.
26. Konstam V, Moser DK, De Jong MJ Depression and anxiety in heart failure. J Card Fail 2005;11:455–63.
27. Gold PW, Gabry KE, Yasuda MR, Chrousos GP Divergent endocrine abnormalities in melancholic and atypical depression: clinical and pathophysiologic implications. Endocrinol Metab Clin North Am 2000;31:37–62.
28. Francis GS, Cohn JN, Johnson G, Rector TS, Goldman S, Simon A Plasma norepinephrine, plasma renin activity, and congestive heart failure. Relations to survival and the effects of therapy in V-HeFT II. The V-HeFT VA Cooperative Studies Group. Circulation 1993;87:VI40–8.
29. Pepper GS, Lee RW Sympathetic activation in heart failure and its treatment with beta-blockade. Arch Intern Med 1999;159:225–34.
30. Kjaer A, Hesse B Heart failure and neuroendocrine activation: diagnostic, prognostic and therapeutic perspectives. Clin Physiol 2001;21:661–72.
31. Gorman JM, Sloan RP Heart rate variability in depressive and anxiety disorders. Am Heart J 2000; 140:77–83.
32. Yeragani VK, Rao KA, Smitha MR, Pohl RB, Balon R, Srinivasan K Diminished chaos of heart rate time series in patients with major depression. Biol Psychiatry 2002;51:733–44.
33. Agelink MW, Boz C, Ullrich H, Andrich J Relationship between major depression and heart rate variability. Clinical consequences and implications for antidepressive treatment. Psychiatry Res 2002;113: 139–49.
34. Dunbar SB, Kimble LP, Jenkins LS, et al. Association of mood disturbance and arrhythmia events in patients after cardioverter defibrillator implantation. Depress Anxiety 1999;9:163–8.
35. Carney RM, Freedland KE, Rich MW, Smith LJ, Jaffe AS Ventricular tachycardia and psychiatric depression in patients with coronary artery disease. Am J Med 1993;95:23–8.
36. Maes M, Meltzer HY, Bosmans E, et al. Increased plasma concentrations of interleukin-6, soluble interleukin-6, soluble interleukin-2 and transferrin receptor in major depression. J Affect Disord 1995; 34:301–9.
37. Sluzewska A, Rybakowski J, Bosmans E, et al. Indicators of immune activation in major depression. Psychiatry Res 1996;64:161–7.
38. Seidel A, Arolt V, Hunstiger M, Rink L, Behnisch A, Kirchner H Cytokine production and serum proteins in depression. Scand J Immunol 1995;41: 534–8.

39. Lanquillon S, Krieg JC, Bening-Abu-Shach U, Vedder H Cytokine production and treatment response in major depressive disorder. Neuropsychopharmacology 2000;22:370–9.
40. Suarez EC, Krishnan RR, Lewis JG The relation of severity of depressive symptoms to monocyte-associated proinflammatory cytokines and chemokines in apparently healthy men. Psychosom Med 2003;65:362–8.
41. Pitsavos C, Panagiotakos DB, Papageorgiou C, Tsetsekou E, Soldatos C, Stefanadis C Anxiety in relation to inflammation and coagulation markers, among healthy adults: The ATTICA Study. Atherosclerosis 2006;185:320–6.
42. MacGowan GA, Mann DL, Kormos RL, Feldman AM, Murali S Circulating interleukin-6 in severe heart failure. Am J Cardiol 1997;79:1128–31.
43. Wollert KC, Drexler H The role of interleukin-6 in the failing heart. Heart Fail Rev 2001;6:95–103.
44. Markovitz JH, Matthews KA Platelets and coronary heart disease: potential psychophysiologic mechanisms. Psychosom Med 1991;53:643–68.
45. Nair GV, Gurbel PA, O'Connor CM, Gattis WA, Murugesan SR, Serebruany VL Depression, coronary events, platelet inhibition, and serotonin reuptake inhibitors. Am J Cardiol 1999;84:321–3.
46. Nemeroff CB, Musselman DL Are platelets the link between depression and ischemic heart disease? Am Heart J 2000;140:S57–62.
47. Al Khadra AS, Salem DN, Rand WM, Udelson JE, Smith JJ, Konstam MA Antiplatelet agents and survival: a cohort analysis from the Studies of Left Ventricular Dysfunction (SOLVD) trial. Circulation 1998;31:419–25.
48. DiMatteo MR, Lepper HS, Croghan TW Depression is a risk factor for noncompliance with medical treatment: meta-analysis of the effects of anxiety and depression on patient adherence. Arch Intern Med 2000;160:2101–7.
49. Blumenthal JA, Williams RS, Wallace AG, Williams RB Jr, Needles TL Physiological and psychological variables predict compliance to prescribed exercise therapy in patients recovering from myocardial infarction. Psychosom Med 1982;44:519–27.
50. Glazer KM, Emery CF, Frid DJ, Banyasz RE Psychological predictors of adherence and outcomes among patients in cardiac rehabilitation. J Cardiopulm Rehabil 2002;22:40–6.
51. Evangelista LS, Berg J, Dracup K Relationship between psychosocial variables and compliance in patients with heart failure. Heart Lung 2001;30: 294–301.
52. Cline CM, Bjorck-Linne AK, Israelsson BY, Willenheimer RB, Erhardt LR Non-compliance and knowledge of prescribed medication in elderly patients with heart failure. Eur J Heart Fail 1999;1: 145–9.
53. Bohachick P, Burke LE, Sereika S, Murali S, Dunbar-Jacob J Adherence to angiotensin-converting enzyme inhibitor therapy for heart failure. Prog Cardiovasc Nurs 2002;17:160–6.
54. Roe CM, Motheral BR, Teitelbaum F, Rich MW Compliance with and dosing of angiotensin-converting-enzyme inhibitors before and after hospitalization. Am J Health Syst Pharm 2000;57: 139–45.
55. Monane M, Bohn RL, Gurwitz JH, Glynn RJ, Avorn J. Noncompliance with congestive heart failure therapy in the elderly. Arch Intern Med 1994;28: 154(4):433–7.
56. DiMatteo MR, Giordani PJ, Lepper HS, Croghan TW Patient adherence and medical treatment outcomes: a meta-analysis. Med Care 2002;40:794–811.
57. Miura T, Kojima R, Mizutani M, Shiga Y, Takatsu F, Suzuki Y Effect of digoxin noncompliance on hospitalization and mortality in patients with heart failure in long-term therapy: a prospective cohort study. Eur J Clin Pharmacol 2001;57:77–83.
58. Chin MH, Goldman L Factors contributing to the hospitalization of patients with congestive heart failure. Am J Public Health 1997;87:643–8.
59. Ghali JK, Kadakia S, Cooper R, Ferlinz J Precipitating factors leading to decompensation of heart failure. Traits among urban blacks. Arch Intern Med 1988;148:2013–6.
60. Michalsen A, Konig G, Thimme W Preventable causative factors leading to hospital admission with decompensated heart failure. Heart 1998;80:437–41.
61. Tsuyuki RT, McKelvie RS, Arnold JM, et al. Acute precipitants of congestive heart failure exacerbations. Arch Intern Med 2001;161:2337–42.
62. McFarlane AM Effect of sertraline on the recovery rate of cardiac autonomic function in depressed patients after acute myocardial infarction. Am Heart J 2001;142:617–23.
63. Khaykin Y, Dorian P, Baker B, et al. Autonomic correlates of antidepressant treatment using heart-rate variability analysis. Can J Psychiatry 1998;43: 183–6.
64. Mikova O, Yakimova R, Bosmans E, Kenis G, Maes M Increased serum tumor necrosis factor alpha concentrations in major depression and multiple sclerosis. Eur Neuropsychopharmacol 2001;11:203–8.
65. Musselman DL, Marzec UM, Manatunga A, et al. Platelet reactivity in depressed patients treated with paroxetine: preliminary findings. Arch Gen Psychiatry 2000;57:875–82.

66. Serebruany VL, Glassman AH, Malinin AI, et al. Platelet/endothelial biomarkers in depressed patients treated with the selective serotonin reuptake inhibitor sertraline after acute coronary events: the Sertraline AntiDepressant Heart Attack Randomized Trial (SADHART) Platelet Substudy. Circulation 2003;108:939–44.
67. Glassman AH, O'Connor CM, Califf RM, et al. Sertraline treatment of major depression in patients with acute MI or unstable angina. Sertraline Antidepressant Heart Attack Randomized Trial. JAMA 2002;288:701–9.
68. Swenson JR, O'Connor CM, Barton D, et al. Influence of depression and effect of treatment with sertraline on quality of life after hospitalization for acute coronary syndrome. Am J Cardiol 2003;92: 1271–6.
69. Serebruany VL, Glassman AH, Malinin AI, et al. Platelet/endothelial biomarkers in depressed patients treated with the selective serotonin reuptake inhibitor sertraline after acute coronary events: the Sertraline AntiDepressant Heart Attack Randomized Trial (SADHART) Platelet Substudy. Circulation 2003;108:939–44.
70. Frasure-Smith N, Prince R Long-term follow-up of the Ischemic Heart Disease Life Stress Monitoring Program. Psychosom Med 1989;51:485–513.
71. Blumenthal JA, Jiang W, Babyak MA, et al. Stress management and exercise training in cardiac patients with myocardial ischemia. Effects on prognosis and evaluation of mechanisms. Arch Intern Med 1997;157:2213–23.
72. Frasure-Smith N, Lesperance F, Prince RH, et al. Randomised trial of home-based psychosocial nursing intervention for patients recovering from myocardial infarction. Lancet 1997;350:473–9.
73. Jones DA, West RR Psychological rehabilitation after myocardial infarction: multicentre randomised controlled trial. BMJ 1996;313:1517–21.
74. Dusseldorp E, van Elderen T, Maes S, Meulman J, Kraaij V A meta-analysis of psychoeduational programs for coronary heart disease patients. Health Psychol 1999;18:506–19.
75. Writing Committee for the ENRICHD Investigators. The effects of treating depression and low perceived social support on clinical events after myocardial infarction: The Enhancing Recovery in Coronary Heart Disease Patients (ENRICHD) Randomized Trial. JAMA 2003;289:3106–16.
76. Carney RM, Blumenthal JA, Catellier D, et al. Depression as a risk factor for mortality after acute myocardial infarction. Am J Cardiol 2003;92:1277–81.
77. Roose SP, Spatz E Treatment of depression in patients with heart disease. J Clin Psychiatry 1999; 60(suppl 20):34–7.
78. Preliminary report: effect of encainide and flecainide on mortality in a randomized trial of arrhythmia suppression after myocardial infarction. The Cardiac Arrhythmia Suppression Trial (CAST) Investigators. N Engl J Med 1989;321: 406–12.
79. Roose SP, Laghrissi-Thode F, Kennedy JS, et al. Comparison of paroxetine and nortriptyline in depressed patients with ischemic heart disease. JAMA 1998;279:287–91.

81 Nutrition in Acute Decompensation of Patients with Acute Heart Failure Syndrome

Roberto Aquilani, Cristina Opasich, Simona Viglio, Paolo Iadarola, and Evasio Pasini

Nutrition therapy in patients with acute heart failure syndrome (AHFS) is rarely acknowledged medically or cardiologically as being important for either a patient's quality of life or survival prognosis. We cannot correlate nutrition with AHFS due to several factors: (1) it is unclear whether or not even a short-term (days/week) underfeeding/starvation has a negative impact on cardiac function (1); (2) we underestimate nutrition as a factor that may contribute to the clinical decline of patients; and (3) the difficulty of isolating the role that nutrition status plays a in patient's prognosis, independent of associated disease(s). Given the wide spectrum of clinical features that usually characterize AHFS patients, a great deal of experience is required of physicians to provide patients with individually tailored nutrition therapies. This chapter discusses the pathophysiologic alterations induced by undernutrition, the possible beneficial effects that may result from the prescription of an appropriate nutrition therapy, and the impact of nutrition on AHFS patients with chronic heart failure (CHF) secondary to ischemic, valvular, hypertensive, or idiopathic dilated cardiomyopathies admitted to general medical and cardiac wards. Although the prevalence of CHF is progressively increasing, very little is yet known on the appropriate nutrition therapy that should be supplied to these patients (2). Conversely, there is more certainty in nutrition therapy for AHFS patients in postoperative phases admitted to intensive care units (3, 4).

Why Should Physicians Be Concerned About Nutrition in Treating a Patient with Acute Heart Failure Syndrome?

Inadequate protein-calorie intake in a state of fasting/starvation is a common feature of patients with CHF in acute decompensation phase or in preoperative periods, particularly if patients are elderly (>65 years). In fact, days/weeks of inadequate nutrition may lead to important systemic alterations including cardiac, pulmonary, and immunologic dysfunctions as well as to changes of distribution of water and electrolyte compartment. These undernutrition-caused alterations may add to primary disease(s), thus providing a relevant contribution to both clinical time course and prognosis of patients with AHFS, particularly if they are malnourished (up to 50% of patients with CHF) (3), or are in a postoperative period. As a consequence, short-term nutritional inadequacy keeps the patient in AHFS at high risk of developing life-threatening complications such as cardiac dysfunction, infections, increased imbalance of the Na/K ratio, increased water retention, respiratory failure, and pulmonary edema. In the postoperative state, nutrition alterations are associated with increased incidence of mediastinitis, wound infection, ventricular arrhythmias, pneumonia, mechanical ventilation for respiratory failure, and renal insufficiency (5). The fact that refeeding or nutritional support can generally reverse organ

TABLE 81.1. Negative impact of short-term undernutrition on multiorgan functions in patients with chronic heart failure (CHF)

Effects of undernutrition on myocardium tissue and function (1, 5–9)
• Loss of myocardial mass proportional to the loss of skeletal muscle
• Decreased global ventricular contractility
• Decrease in stroke volume and cardiac output proportional to myocardial mass
• Increased incidence of arrhythmias
Effects of undernutrition on respiratory function (10–19)
• Impaired respiratory muscle efficiency → muscle fatigue
• Alteration of surfactant composition and functions:
—Alveolar collapse
—Impairment of the clearance of inhaled or aspirated organisms
—Loss of antimicrobial effects of surfactant lipids
• Reduced lung defenses:
—Increased bacterial adherence to oral and airway cells (colonization with gram-negative bacilli)
—Alteration in mucociliary function
—Alteration in alveolar macrophage function
—Impaired recruitment of leukocytes
• Increased risk for pulmonary edema by increasing fluid accumulation in the lung interstitial space secondary to increased total body sodium and/ or reduced serum albumin level
Effects of undernutrition on systemic immunity (20)
• Decrease in cell-mediated immunocompetence: reduction in circulating T-lymphocytes, reduction in helper T-cells and suppressor cells, reduction in helper/suppressor T ratio
• Diminution of secretory immunoglobulin A
Effects of under-nutrition on electrolyte and water compartment distribution
• Change in electrolyte distribution:
—Relative increase in the total exchangeable sodium (Na^+_e)
—Decrease in the total exchangeable potassium (K^+_e)
—Consequent increase in Na^+_e/ K^+_e ratio
—Positive sodium balance
• Consequent expansion of the extracellular fluid compartment (ECF)[a]
• Contraction of the intracellular fluid compartment

[a]The expansion of ECF is associated with a progressive fall in levels of serum proteins.

alterations caused by undernutrition is clinically extremely important and should encourage physicians to consider appropriate nutrition intervention for all patients with AHFS.

The short-term organ alterations induced by undernutrition and clinically relevant for the prognosis of a patient with AHFS are listed in Table 81.1.

Nutrition Assessment in Patients with Acute Heart Failure Syndrome

Malnutrition refers to an inadequate intake of energy, proteins, vitamins, or minerals. Therefore, in theory, a nutrition assessment should be performed by measuring quantitative alterations either in body energy-protein content (alterations in body composition) or in cellular vitamin and mineral store. Clinically, however, only indirect measures of alterations in body composition (anthropometric parameters), of visceral protein synthesis (serum albumin, transferrin, prealbumin concentration) and of immunocompetence (blood total lymphocyte count) can be used. In addition, a nutrition assessment in patients with CHF may be more challenging because an excess of extracellular fluid (ECF) may mask weight loss and produces a dilution of serum proteins. In practice: for an objective nutritional assessment of CHF, the clinician may rely on (1) measure of actual dry body weight (BW) as a percentage of usual BW or, when this is not available, of ideal BW; (2) upper arm anthropometric parameters such as triceps skinfold thickness (TST) and arm muscle area (AMA); or (3) blood lymphocyte count.

In an acute decompensation phase, however, only upper arm anthropometric parameters are

Table 81.2. Distribution of altered nutritional parameters in patients with CHF stratified for body weight expressed as percentage of usual/ideal body weight

Altered nutritional parameters	Usual/ideal BW		
	<90% BW	90–110% BW	>110% BW
AMA <5th percentile	100%	59%	3.7%
TST <5th percentile	30%	–	–
Albumin <3.5 g/dL	20%	8.1%	3.8%
Prealbumin <20 mg/dL	60%	22.4%	7.5%

AMA, arm muscle area; BW, body weight; TST, triceps skinfold thickness.

useful for diagnosing malnutrition as they are not influenced by excessive ECF, unless the individual is anasarcous. As an indicator of severe alterations in body compartments, we generally use a value lower than 5th percentile (6). As for the use of serum proteins in acute decompensation, albumin concentration can be adopted to monitor the changes in ECF during diuretic therapy. In addition, since prealbumin responds rapidly to short-term (24- to 36-hour) energy restriction and to refeeding, in the absence of gross fluid retention and/or infection repeated measurements of prealbumin levels over a week may be useful to measure both protein depletion and repletion. The distribution of nutrition alteration indicators found by our group in a population of patients with CHF classified as malnourished (BW <90% ideal BW), normo-nourished (BW = 90% to 110% ideal BW), and overweight (BW >110% ideal BW) is listed in Table 81.2.

Nitrogen balance (NB) is useful as an indirect evaluation of dynamic processes of endogenous protein synthesis (anabolism) and breakdown (catabolism) during acute decompensation. It is expressed as

$$NB\ (g/d) = N_I - N_V + 2\,g$$

where

Table 81.3. Nutritional assessment form adopted by the authors in patients with CHF

Name:		Diagnosis:		Date:	
Height: . . . . cm	Weight: . . . . . . kg	Usual weight (UBW): . . . . kg		Ideal weight (IBW): . . . . . kg	
Parameters of normal status of nutrition	**Observed**	**Applicable in AHFS**	**Significance of observed alterations**	**Altered: Yes**	**Altered: No**
Actual body weight: ≥90% I/U BW	. . . . . . %	Yes, in absence of clinical edema	Reduction in total energy stores	☐	☐
Anthropometrics TST = 5th percentile . . . . mm	. . . . mm	Yes	Severe reduction in fat stores	☐	☐
AMA = 5th percentile . . . . . . cm²	. . . cm²	Yes	Severe reduction in muscle proteins	☐	☐
Immunity Lymphocytes ≥1500/mm³	. . . . . mm³	Yes	Reduction in immunologic defense	☐	☐
Visceral protein concentrations					
Albumin ≥3.5 g/dL	. . . . g/dL	No	It can be used as a marker of hydration	☐	☐
Prealbumin 20–40 mg/dL	. . . . . . mg/dL	Yes (if repeated)	Inadequate current protein intake	☐	☐
Nitrogen balance 0 ± 1 g/day	. . . . g/d	Yes	Information on general protein synthesis/catabolism	☐	☐

AMA, arm muscle area; TST, triceps skinfold thickness.

TABLE 81.4. Anthropometric values corresponding to 5th percentile observed in healthy subjects in authors' metabolic service

	Tricipital skinfold thickness (mm)	
Age (years)	Males	Females
<75	5	11
75	7	11.5
80	6	11
85	5	9
90	4	8
	Arm muscle area (cm^2)	
Age (years)	Males	Females
<75	46	34
75	40	33
80	38	33
85	36	32
90	34	31

N_I is the nitrogen intake/supply (in g/d); it is obtained as protein intake (or amino acid infusion) (g/d): 6.25

N_V is the urinary nitrogen excretion (in g/d) + 20% N_V for nonurea N excretion

2 g is the nitrogen lost in feces and sweat

$$\text{NB in equilibrium} = \pm 1\text{ g/d}$$

$$\text{NB} > +1\text{ g/d} = \text{Prevalence of protein synthesis}$$

$$\text{NB} < -1\text{ g/d} = \text{Prevalence of protein degradation}$$

The layout adopted in our cardiac division to report nutritional assessment and anthropometric values corresponding to 5th percentile (7) are reported in Tables 81.3 and 81.4, respectively.

Furthermore, anamnesis on patient digestive capacity during clinical stability, collected directly by the patient or by their relatives, is a useful tool used to check for possible eating-related symptoms in AHFS (Table 81.5).

TABLE 81.5. Brief outline to check for eating-related possible symptoms in patients with CHF during acute decompensation

	Yes	No
Hiccup	☐	☐
Nausea	☐	☐
Feeling of fullness	☐	☐
Gastroesophageal reflux	☐	☐
Vomiting	☐	☐
Abdominal distention	☐	☐
Diarrhea	☐	☐
Dyspnea	☐	☐
Sweating	☐	☐
Paleness	☐	☐
Dizziness	☐	☐

Practical Approach to Nutrition Therapy in Acute Heart Failure Syndrome

Very often, delivery routes providing adequate nutrition therapy in AHFS are undermined by (1) the need to reduce fluids and substrates; (2) the presence of important digestive difficulties existing in a vast population of CHF patients, yet in clinical stable conditions (Tables 81.6a and 81.6b); and (3) the lack of knowledge of nutrition requirements during acute decompensation. As a consequence, very rarely standard nutritional guidelines/recommendations can be applied in toto to AHFS patients.

Maldigestion, particularly when associated with breathlessness, may preclude the possibility of providing an adequate enteral nutrition by

TABLE 81.6A. Distribution of digestive symptoms usually complained by patients with CHF during the periods of clinical stability

Symptom	%
Fullness after meal	39.7
Fast chewing	34.6
Dry mouth	28.2
Dyspnea after meal	28.2
Tasteless eating in the mouth	24.3
Impression that food stops in the stomach	23
Meal interrupted	23
Reduced appetite	19.2
Dry feces	19.2
Difficulty in deglutition	17.9
Meal interrupted >2 times/week	17.9
Getting tired of chewing	16.7
Feeling of sweetened food in the mouth	16.7
Salty food in the mouth	14.1
Feeling of swallowing hard food	12.8
Foam in feces	11.5
Bitter food in the mouth	10.2
Nausea after a meal	10.2
Gastroesophageal reflux over/after meal	10.2
Dyspnea during meal	10.2
Soft feces	9.0
Fullness during meal	7.2
Normal feces	7.7
Nausea at seeing food	5.0
Vomiting after a meal	4.0

Table 81.6b. Main causes of early interruption of meal in clinically stable patients with CHF (one or more cause/s may be present)

Cause	%
Nausea	64.0
Tachycardia	35.7
Getting tired in chewing	35.7
Asthenia	28.6
Reduced visual capacity	28.5
Sweating	21.4
Feeling of faint	14.3
Pain at right hypochondrium	7.0

nasogastric/duodenum tube, the main and relatively safe route for nutrition therapy. In addition, at least in our experience, many conscious patients refuse feeding tubes. As a consequence, we combine voluntary alimentation with parenteral nutrition whenever possible.

The strategies and program of a nutrition therapy adopted in our cardiac divisions for patients in AHFS secondary to ischemic, valvular, hypertensive, or idiopathic dilated cardiomyopathies are reported below.

Strategy

Based on our clinical experience, it is not possible to stop hypercatabolism in most patients with AHFS. Thus, a nutrition therapy for CHF patients in acute decompensation should be provided over two phases: (1) acute decompensation itself (metabolic therapy) in which, usually, lower than recommended calories (kcal), carbohydrates (CHO), proteins (Prot), vitamins (Vit), and minerals (Min) can be supplied; and (2) postacute decompensation recovery (metabolic rehabilitation) in which we need to restore nutritional reserves.

Aims of Metabolic Therapy

The main aims of metabolic therapy are to sustain the metabolism of stressed vital organs (brain, heart, kidney, liver) and, if otherwise impossible, to decrease body wasting and minimize it as much as possible.

Aim of Metabolic Rehabilitation

The main aim of metabolic rehabilitation is to restore as much as possible the nutritional status that the patient had before acute decompensation. In this way, the patient will be able to face a possible new episode of acute decompensation with better nutritional reserves. Therefore, a patient's nutrition needs to be assessed both at admission and in the postacute recovery period.

Modalities for Nutrition Therapy in Acute Heart Failure Syndrome

First Day from Patient Admission: Evaluation Phase

1. Nutrition assessment (Table 81.1).
2. Enforcement of test meal (Table 81.7) providing about 800 kcal, carbohydrates 73 g, proteins 48 g, lipids 32 g, water 600 ml over a day. From Table 81.7 it is easy to calculate the amount of calories, macronutrients, and water that a patient can ingest. If a patient eats <800 kcal (hence less water), the same amount of water can be added to fluids to calculate the amount of nutritional support.
3. Check for possible digestive difficulties during or after the test meal (as shown in Table 81.5).

Second Day of Admission: Nutrition Therapy

1. Maintain, when possible, a patient's oral intake.

Table 81.7. Test meal (800 kcal/day) adopted for patients with CHF in acute decompensation period

Breakfast	
Biscuits 20 g	kcal 113; CHO 26 g; prot. 1.5 g;
Sugar 10 g	water 50 mL
Tea 50 mL	Time of ingestion: 10 minutes
Lunch	
Vegetable soup (150 mL) with:	kcal ~266; CHO 10.5 g; prot. 22.4 g;
Maize flour 15 g or semolina	water 150 mL
15 g or spelt 25 g	Time of ingestion: 20 minutes
Butter or oil 10 g	
Cooked lean meat 70 g*	
Snack	
See breakfast	
Dinner	
See lunch	

CHO, carbohydrate; prot., protein.
*The weight refers to minced cooked meat, before adding the meat to vegetable soup.

82
Classification of the Level of Evidence in International Guidelines for Acute and Chronic Heart Failure

John G.F. Cleland

Over the centuries, medicine has evolved as a system of care dependent on magic and superstition, fashion, a large placebo effect, self-confident physicians, the fears of patients, and some astute observations. More recently, attempts have begun to put medical care on a more scientific basis by making observations on large numbers of patients to evolve rational constructs for why treatments are effective or fail and ultimately by putting theory and observation to the test in randomized controlled trials. It will be a long time before the science of medicine has eliminated, replaced, or endorsed the current practices and dogma of medical treatment, but a start must be made if future generations of patients are to avoid potentially unnecessary or harmful traditional treatments. Chronic aspirin therapy (1–4), cosmetic angioplasty (5), and intravenous inotropic therapy (6,7) are just three examples of unproven and potentially wasteful or harmful interventions that are widely practiced due to the failure of doctors to understand the evidence presented to them. The lack of clarity of guidelines due to the archaic and redundant system for ranking evidence is partly to blame (8–11). This system is now in urgent need of overhaul.

The purpose of the evidence-based approached to medicine is to create a scientific basis to support the art of applying medical care to the individual patient. The evidence base can rarely create universal rules that always apply. It can provide general guidance that allows an experienced and wise clinician to make the best decision for the patient in light of all the available evidence. Guidelines can speed the learning process by ensuring that less experienced staff focus on what is considered good practice and what is unimportant or harmful. Also, by gathering information on what is known, guidelines can demonstrate gaps in the evidence requiring more research. A good guideline stimulates research and fills in a few blanks with educated guesswork. A bad guideline pontificates on areas of ignorance, perpetuates bad practice, and stifles research. Guideline writers should be careful about what they do.

Critical to the guidelines process is the need for a consistent and systematic way to gauge the evidence. An arbitrary set of rules that was never widely discussed as far as I am aware was created in the early 1980s, possibly by the Agency for Health Care Policy and Research (AHCPR) in the United States. This system of classification has at least four important shortcomings: the importance placed on different forms of evidence, the system used for classifying evidence and recommendations, the failure to specify a hierarchy of outcomes, and the failure to report the estimated size of benefit. The system also fails to deal adequately with topics such as the timing and duration of therapy.

The Importance Placed on Different Forms of Evidence

First, the existing classification puts meta-analysis as the highest level of evidence. This is an important misconception. Meta-analysis of small trials is usually biased in favor of intervention. Investigators often abandon small trials that are failing to show differences. Even if the trial is finished, the author may not feel that a small neutral result is worth reporting. Worse still, even if the investigator does submit a manuscript for publication, there is a good chance that the editor will reject it on the basis that it was not powered to show a difference. This contrasts with the frequent publication of small and inadequately powered studies with a positive outcome. Meta-analysis has several important roles, but as stand-alone evidence of a drug effect, it should be relegated to the minor leagues (12–18). Meta-analysis is useful for confirming whether the mass of available evidence is consistent with that of an adequately powered study. Consistent effects of treatment, preferably in more than one adequately powered study supported by meta-analysis of other relevant trials, should be considered the highest form of evidence, followed by a single adequately powered study alone, followed by meta-analysis of inadequately powered studies, followed by observational data or case-control studies. Meta-analysis is also useful for highlighting differences among trials that require further investigation as to cause, for planning adequately powered studies, and for ascertaining if variability in outcome among patient subgroups in large trials is likely to be due to chance.

System for Classifying Evidence

A major problem with both European and American guidelines is their adherence to outmoded criteria for the assessment and classification of evidence inherited from a system that was never subjected to proper scrutiny or debate (Table 82.1). Given the large number of recommendations being made and the growing body of evidence, a clearer and more robust system that highlights what is well proven and what is mainly expert opinion seems advisable. Description of the classification using plain language would be much clearer than the present alphanumeric system. The use of the roman numeral III to make a recommendation not to do something is particularly perplexing even among guideline experts. For example, the American College of Cardiology/American Heart Association (ACC/AHA) guidelines make a recommendation *not to not recommend* the use of angiotensin-converting enzyme (ACE) inhibitors, angiotensin-receptor blockers (ARBs), and aldosterone antagonists in combination. How should physicians, or indeed a lawyer, interpret such double-negative statements? We all think we know what they mean but the classification system has tied the language in knots! Table 82.2 outlines a method for condens-

Table 82.1. Classification of recommendations and evidence in guidelines

European Society of Cardiology (ESC)		American College of Cardiology/American Heart Association	
Class I	Evidence and/or general agreement that a given diagnostic procedure/treatment is beneficial, useful, and effective	Class I	Conditions for which there is evidence and/or general agreement that a given procedure/therapy is beneficial, useful, and/or effective
Class II	Conflicting evidence and/or a divergence of opinion about the usefulness/efficacy of the treatment	Class II	Conditions for which there is conflicting evidence and/or a divergence of opinion about the usefulness/efficacy of a procedure/therapy
Class IIa	Weight of evidence/opinion is in favor of usefulness/efficacy	IIa	Weight of evidence/opinion is in favor of usefulness/efficacy
Class IIb	Usefulness/efficacy is less well established by evidence/opinion	IIb	Usefulness/efficacy is less well established by evidence/opinion
Class III*	Evidence or general agreement that the treatment is not useful/effective and in some cases may be harmful	Class III	Conditions for which there is evidence and/or general agreement that a procedure/therapy is not useful/effective and in some cases may be harmful
Level of Evidence A	Data derived from multiple randomized clinical trials or meta-analyses	Level of Evidence A	Data are derived from multiple randomized clinical trials or meta-analyses
Level of Evidence B	Data derived from a single randomized clinical trial or large nonrandomized studies	Level of Evidence B	Data are derived from a single randomized trial, or nonrandomized studies
Level of Evidence C	Consensus of opinion of the experts and/or small studies, reprospective studies, registries	Level of Evidence C	Only consensus opinion of experts, case studies, or standard of care

*Use of class III is discouraged by the ESC.

TABLE 82.2. Suggested revised classification system for guidelines

Treatment effect being considered	Primary: symptoms, quality of life, disability or mortality Surrogate: exercise capacity, morbid events (e.g., myocardial infarction, stroke, or hospitalization)
Clinical setting	For example, relevant to acute heart failure: acute pulmonary edema, severe chronic heart failure with progressively worsening peripheral edema, cardiogenic shock
Strength of evidence:	
Robust	At least one adequately powered clinical trial supported by meta-analysis
Adequate	Only one adequately powered clinical trial unsupported by meta-analysis
Inadequate	Meta-analysis unsupported by an adequately powered clinical trial, including single inadequately powered trials
Opinion only	Expert opinion based on other forms of evidence
Recommendation	Recommended or not recommended
Strength of recommendation	Strong, moderate, or weak
Basis for recommendation	Examples: Evidence of benefit, evidence of harm, evidence of safety, lack of evidence of benefit, lack of evidence of harm Lack of evidence of benefit as well as evidence of harm should be taken into account when making recommendations
Estimated size of effect	Give numerical value as proportion of responders for outcomes such as symptoms (state whether placebo subtracted) or rate for outcomes such as death (e.g., lives saved over 1 or 5 years)
Cost per life year gained and cost per quality-adjusted life-year	Describe in low-wage and high-wage economies; for instance, surgery may be more affordable in poor countries than rich countries if health care staff have low wages

ing information in a systematic way to provide clarity on the nature of the recommendation, the strength of recommendation, the size of effect, and cost-effectiveness.

Clinical Outcomes

Clinical trialists have diverse interests and often investigate the underlying mechanisms of disease, such as exercise capacity or ventricular function. While improvement in surrogate markers is encouraging, if this improvement is not evident to the patient in terms of well-being or longevity, then it has little practical value. However, what about morbid events? These are more clinically relevant measures that are frequently used as surrogate measures for disability or mortality, both of which can also be measured. A small troponin increase or a transient neurologic episode clearly does not have the same implications as an extensive Q-wave myocardial infarction or a dense persistent hemiparesis. Trials need to improve their capacity to report disability. Less emphasis should be put on nonfatal morbid events that are often used just to drive up the event rate to try to get a statistical result.

Ultimately, there are three types of primary outcome measures that are of interest. The first type is related to the well-being of the patient. Traditionally, this has focused on symptoms of the disease in question, but as the contribution of treatment side effects and comorbidity to overall patient well-being has become better recognized and measures of quality of life and disability have received more attention. The second type is mortality. Ideally, this should be all-cause mortality. Although cause-specific death, such as cardiovascular death, might be better able to show a treatment effect, from a patient's perspective dead is dead. For example, defibrillators reduce sudden death by about 80% but have a much smaller impact on overall mortality because patients go on to die of other things. The cause-specific outcome shows that the intervention treats the problem it was designed for but does not show the overall outcome for the patient. The third type of primary outcome is controversially the most important and ignored by guidelines so far: cost-effectiveness (cost per life-year gained) and cost-utility (cost per quality adjusted life-year gained). There are good grounds for saying that this latter sort of outcome is the one that best reflects the usefulness of the treatment. Expensive treatments that are highly effective get ranked higher than cheap and ineffective treatments. In other words, defibrillators are probably more cost-effective and a better choice of where to spend money than chronic aspirin therapy beyond 3 months after an acute coronary event. Note that in this system, events such as stroke or heart attack are not given great importance compared to any measure of subsequent disability or death.

TABLE 82.3. Application of new guidelines system to patients with heart failure due to left ventricular systolic dysfunction

Question	Relevant comparisons	Response	Strength	Level of evidence	Absolute effect size*	Basis for recommendation
Should patients intolerant of ACEI receive an ARB to improve symptoms?	ARB vs. placebo in ACEI intolerant patients	Yes	Strong	Robust	Symptoms improve (+) ~ 1 in 3 (–) ~ 1 in 14	Evidence of benefit from one landmark trial plus substantial meta-analysis. No evidence of important risk
Should patients intolerant of ACEI receive an ARB to reduce death or hospitalization for heart failure?	ARB vs. placebo in ACEI intolerant patients	Yes	Strong	Robust	10% over ~3 years	
Should patients intolerant of ACEI receive an ARB to improve mortality?	ARB vs. placebo in ACEI intolerant patients	Yes	Strong	Robust	6% over ~3 years	
Are the effects of ARB, used in adequate doses similar to those of ACEI on symptoms, morbidity, and mortality?	ARB vs. placebo ACEI vs. placebo ARB vs. ACEI	Yes	Moderate	Adequate	Not applicable	RCTs vs. placebo suggest similar benefits Head-to-head comparisons suggest equivalence when adequate doses used
Should ARBs be added to ACEI to improve symptoms?	ARB vs. placebo in patients taking ACEI	Yes	Strong	Robust	Symptoms improve (+) ~ 1 in 2.5 (–) ~ 1 in 16	Evidence of benefit from two landmark trials plus substantial meta-analysis. No evidence of important risk
Should ARBs be added to ACEI to reduce death or HF hosp?	ARB vs. placebo in patients taking ACEI	Yes	Strong	Robust	3.3% over ~3 years	
Should ARBs be added to ACEI to reduce mortality?	ARB vs. placebo in patients taking ACEI	No	Weak	Weak	0.9% over ~3 years	
Should ARAs be added to ACEI to reduce mortality in mild heart failure?	ARA vs. placebo in patients taking ACEI	Yes	Moderate	Adequate	3.3% over 16 months	One key trial (EPHESUS–postinfarction LVSD) in a relevant population supported by another trial in more advanced heart failure; some safety concerns.
Should ARAs be added to ACEI to reduce mortality in moderate to severe HF?		Yes	Strong	Robust	11.4% over 2 years	Two key trials (RALES and EPHESUS) in relevant populations; some safety concerns
Should ARBs and ARAs both be added routinely to ACEI for greater benefit?	Use of all three agents versus only two	No	Weak	Opinion	NA	Subgroup analysis from CHARM study Risk of hyperkalemia and renal dysfunction
Should ARBs and ARAs both be added in selected patients to ACEI for greater benefit?	Use of all three agents versus only two	Yes	Weak	Opinion	NA	Subgroup analysis from CHARM study Risks of combination may be low in younger patients with higher blood pressure without renal dysfunction

ACEI, angiotensin-converting enzyme inhibitor; ARA, ARB, angiotensin-receptor blocker; HF, heart failure; RALES, Randomised ALdactone Evaluation Study; RCT, randomized controlled trial; CHARM, Candesartan in Heart failure-Assessment of Reduction in Mortality and morbidity; EPHESUS, Eplerenone post-acute myocardial infarction heart failure efficacy and survival study.

*The absolute rate on the active agent minus placebo except for symptoms where the comparison with baseline (+) and placebo-subtracted (–) values are shown, reflecting respectively the patient and the scientific perspective of therapy. Overall estimate from large relevant randomized controlled trials.

Size of Benefit

Sometimes we can be certain that a treatment is effective but uncertain whether the treatment is worthwhile. For instance, giving patients with vascular disease an ACE inhibitor clearly reduces mortality, but the effect is so small that in the absence of other reasons to give these agents, such as hypertension, symptoms of heart failure, or left ventricular dysfunction, such treatment may be of little practical value (19). Guidelines should attempt to quantify benefit. An example of such an exercise is shown for ARBs in chronic heart failure (Table 82.3).

Unfortunately, there are no robust data to show the value of agents for acute heart failure in terms of mortality. The size of benefit in terms of symptoms might be quantified by estimating the proportion of patients whose symptoms improve, corrected for the control group, but data are also lacking. Symptom assessment should preferably take place at a time when differences in mortality have not appeared.

Another aspect of assessing the size of benefit is assessing the patient's risk. A 50% reduction in risk of an event in patients who has only a 2% absolute risk of that event will result in an absolute benefit of 1%. In contrast, a 25% reduction in events in a group of patients at 40% risk of an event will reduce the absolute risk by 10%. Guidelines committees should give guidance on identifying risk as well as absolute and relative benefit.

One other important factor that may have an important impact on the size of effect of treatment in a clinical trial is unplanned crossovers. Crossover may occur by patients stopping active treatment (drop-outs) or by stopping placebo and starting active therapy (drop-ins). Although it can be argued that those patients who come off of active therapy (drop-outs) for side effects are a reasonable reflection of clinical reality, it is possible that adherence to medication is better in clinical practice because in the trial the patients are told that the treatment may not work or they may be on a placebo, but in clinical practice they are told the treatment works. Common sense suggests, although evidence is lacking, that patients are more likely to take something once it is proved to be safe and effective. Also, in clinical practice the patient is getting not only the benefits of the medicine but also, in effect, the benefits of the placebo. Indeed, since patients are told in a clinical trial setting that they may be on a placebo or an ineffective or even risky treatment, the placebo effect in clinical practice may be much smaller than in clinical practice. An even greater factor diluting the observed effect of interventions in clinical trials are patients crossing over from the control group to active therapy (drop-ins). If both the control and intervention group end up on similar therapy it would be surprising to find a difference even if the treatment is effective. The extent to which clinical trials underestimate benefit might be quantified by reporting their crossover rates (i.e., rate per day or per year depending on the time-frame for the intervention).

The Clinical Setting

Care should be taken in evaluating the context of clinical trials. For instance, the Levosimendan Infusion versus DObutamine (LIDO) study compared the effects of levosimendan and dobutamine in patients with chronic severe heart failure to assess their hemodynamic effects (20). Levosimendan was associated with a lower mortality. Another study compared levosimendan and placebo in patients with postinfarction pulmonary edema and also showed a reduction in mortality (21). These trials were then extrapolated to acute heart failure with many patients verging on cardiogenic shock. Two much larger trials, one compared to placebo and the other compared to dobutamine, failed to show an effect on mortality. It is now unclear whether levosimendan is effective in reducing mortality, and the initial smaller trials were wrong or whether the change in clinical setting is critical, perhaps related to acute reduction in arterial pressure in unstable hypotensive patients (7). Guideline writers need to take care when making recommendations that they are clear about the clinical setting to which the recommendations apply.

However, cardiovascular disease is part of a continuous spectrum and does not generally constitute discrete, immutable entities. Patients included in clinical trials are highly selected, and if their results were applied strictly to clinical practice, guidelines would apply to very few patients. Trials should be used as a compass providing a general direction of travel. The skill and wisdom of the guidelines committee is in extrapolating data from trials correctly but not too far. Large effects can be extrapolated further or with greater confidence than small effects. Of particular interest to guidelines on heart failure and left ventricular systolic dysfunction (LVSD) are trials, especially long-term trials, after myocardial infarction. In these trials, patients spent only a few weeks in a postinfarction state but months or years with chronic LVSD and heart failure. Provided that the treatment is not considered only to have a short-term effect, which can of course still lead to long-term benefit, these studies should be used to guide clinical practice in patients with chronic disease. Guidelines should actively seek to include information, where reasonable, from trials of associated conditions in order to give the best advice.

Conclusion

It is time to modernize the way we assess evidence for clinical practice. The scheme suggested here might be a good starting point. Clearly, recommendations under either the old or the new scheme are going to be complex, given the mass of data. This may be partly resolved by focusing on those populations and interventions that offer the greatest benefit in terms of symptoms, mortality, cost-effectiveness, or cost-utility.

References

1. Cleland JGF. Chronic aspirin therapy for the prevention of cardiovascular events: a waste of time or worse? Nat Clin Pract Cardiovasc Med 2006;3(5): 234–5.
2. Cleland JGF. No reduction in cardiovascular risk with NSAIDs—including aspirin? Lancet 2002; 359(9301):92–3.
3. Cleland JGF. For debate: preventing atherosclerotic events with aspirin. BMJ 2002;324(7329):103–5.
4. Cleland JGF. Is aspirin "the weakest link" in cardiovascular prophylaxis. The surprising lack of evidence supporting the use of aspirin for cardiovascular disease. Prog Cardiovasc Dis 2002; 44:275–92.
5. Yusuf S. Call for a moratorium on and re-evaluation of the risk/benefit of elective angioplasty. World Congress of Cardiology, 2006.
6. Thackray S, Eastaugh J, Freemantle N, Cleland JGF. The effectiveness and relative effectiveness of intravenous inotropic drugs acting through adrenergic pathways in patients with heart failure—a meta-regression analysis. Eur J Heart Fail 2002;4(4):515–29.
7. Cleland JG, Freemantle N, Coletta AP, Clark AL. Clinical trials update from the American Heart Association: REPAIR-AMI, ASTAMI, JELIS, MEGA, REVIVE-II, SURVIVE, and PROACTIVE. Eur J Heart Failure 2006;8(1):105–10.
8. Hunt SA, Abraham WT, Chin MH, et al. ACC/AHA 2005 guideline update for the diagnosis and management of chronic heart failure in the adult: a report of the American College of Cardiology/American Heart Association Task Force on Practice Guidelines. Circulation 2005;112:154–235.
9. Nieminen MS, et al. Executive summary of the guidelines on the diagnosis and treatment of acute heart failure: the Task Force on Acute Heart Failure of the European Society of Cardiology. Eur Heart J 2005:384–416.
10. Swedberg K, Cleland JGF, Dargie H, et al. Guidelines for the diagnosis and treatment of chronic heart failure. Eur Heart J 2005;26:1115–40.
11. Heart Failure Society of America (HFSA) practice guidelines. HFSA guidelines for management of patients with heart failure caused by left ventricular systolic dysfunction—pharmacological approaches. J Card Failure 1999;5:357–82.
12. McAuley L, Pham B, Tugwell P, Moher D. Does the inclusion of grey literature influence estimates of intervention effectiveness reported in meta-analyses? Lancet 2000;356(9237):1228–31.
13. ioannidis JPA, Cappelleri JC, Lau J. Meta-analyses and large randomised, controlled trials. N Engl J Med 1998;338:59.
14. Bailar JCI. The promise and problems of meta-analysis. N Engl J Med 1997;337:559–61.
15. Editorial. Meta-analysis under scrutiny. Lancet 1997;350:675.
16. Egger M, Smith GD, Schneider M, Minder C. Bias in meta-analysis detected by a simple graphical test. BMJ 1997;315:629–34.
17. LeLorier J, Gregoire G, Benhaddad A, Lapierre J, Derderian F. Discrepancies between meta-analyses and subsequent large randomised, controlled trials. N Engl J Med 1997;337:536–42.
18. Rothwell PM, Robertson G. Meta-analysis of randomised controlled trials. Lancet 1997;350:1181–2.

19. Shelton R, Velavan P, Nikitin NP, et al. Clinical trials update from the American Heart Association meeting: ACORN-CSD, primary care trial of chronic disease management, PEACE, CREATE, SHIELD, A-HeFT, GEMINI, vitamin E meta-analysis, ESCAPE, CARP, and SCD-HeFT cost-effectiveness study. Eur J Heart Fail 2005;7(1):127–35.
20. Follath F, Cleland JGF, Just H, et al. Efficacy and safety of intravenous levosimendan compared with dobutamine in severe low-output heart failure (the LIDO study): a randomised double-blind trial. Lancet 2002;360(9328):196–202.
21. Cleland JGF, Nikitin NP, McGowan J. Levosimendan: first in a new class of inodilator for acute and chronic severe heart failure. Expert Rev Cardiovasc Ther 2004;2(1):9–19.

83
Drug Development for Acute Heart Failure Syndromes: European Regulatory View

Edmond Roland and Eric Abadie

Despite the high prevalence of acute heart failure syndrome (AHFS) associated with its very high rates of morbidity and mortality, little progress has been made in developing new therapies for treatment of this specific clinical condition. Compared with the development of new therapies for other cardiovascular diseases, the lack of progress is striking. Many AHFS trials have displayed negative results and also have raised specific safety concerns in this patient population. To provide regulatory guidance, the European Medicines Agency has recently released Guidance on Clinical Investigations of Medicinal Products for the Treatment of Acute Cardiac Failure (1). To put this guidance into perspective, this chapter discusses issues that are critical for the design of clinical studies in support of regulatory decisions.

Patient Selection

The heterogeneity of the patient population with AHFS is well recognized. In addition, there is a lack of general agreement with respect to the appropriate nomenclature of the clinical problem (2,3).

The clinical manifestations of AHFS relate to pulmonary congestion with or without reduced cardiac output. In general, the clinical manifestations of AHFS are similar irrespective of the underlying cause, but the type of onset of the symptoms may vary. Heart failure is often difficult to diagnose in the emergency department or urgent care setting. The symptoms may be nonspecific, and physical findings are not sensitive enough to be used as a basis for an accurate diagnosis. Furthermore, physical signs have limited reliability for estimating hemodynamics in AHFS (4). These difficulties may often lead to practical problems in the differential diagnosis or may result in overdiagnosis and the inclusion of inadequate patients in clinical trials. Up to one half of heart failure diagnoses made in primary health care may be incorrect (5). In particular, differentiation of patients with dyspnea due to congestive heart failure from those with dyspnea due to other causes is difficult in the acute care setting. Therefore, it is important to provide confirmation of heart disease, pulmonary congestion, or left ventricular dysfunction by appropriate basic investigations (6).

A normal electrocardiogram (ECG) is very uncommon in AHFS. The ECG provides information on the cardiac rhythm and may help determine the etiology of AHFS, particularly in coronary heart disease (6). Chest x-ray should be performed early for all patients with AHFS to assess preexisting chest conditions and cardiac size, and to document pulmonary congestion. Chest x-ray is used both for confirmation of diagnosis and for follow-up of response to treatment. Echocardiography is an essential investigation for the evolution of the functional and structural changes associated with AHFS. It should be performed in all patients as soon as possible. Echocardiography should be used to evaluate left ventricular function and to differentiate systolic dysfunction (left ventricular ejection fraction [LVEF] ≤40%) and preserved systolic function or diastolic dysfunction

(LVEF >40%) (6). Assessment of B-type natriuretic peptide (BNP) currently is most useful for negative predictive value to exclude heart failure (6).

There are two important subgroups of patients to consider: those with new acute onset of cardiac failure and those with acute exacerbation of chronic heart failure (2,3,6). In the first subgroup, there is a sudden onset of signs of heart failure in patients with no history of heart failure. This is typically the case of AHFS associated with acute coronary syndromes or fulminant myocarditis. More frequent is the second subgroup with an established diagnosis of heart failure, and the patients develop worsening of symptoms. Preferably these two categories should be studied separately. If patients from both categories are included in the same trial, a prespecified and adequately sized subgroup analysis will be needed to explore the consistency of effects (1). The exact definitions and categories of the patient subgroups should be determined explicitly in the study protocol in order to avoid post-hoc definitions of data-derived patient categories (1).

Recently, data from over 150,000 consecutive patients hospitalized for heart failure from the Euro Heart Failure Survey and the Acute Decompensated Heart Failure National Registry (ADHERE) in the Unites States have provided useful information on the clinical profile of AHFS (7,8). These two large registries have shown that over 75% of patients hospitalized with AHFS have worsening of previously diagnosed heart failure, 25% receive a heart failure diagnosis during the index admission, and a minority (less than 8%) have low blood pressure, with presumably low output syndrome. Most patients have evidence of pulmonary congestion and have normal or high blood pressure. Fewer than 8% of patients have blood pressure less than 90 mm Hg. An estimated 90% of patients have signs of elevated filling pressures including some degree of dyspnea, with 40% having dyspnea at rest. Evidence of radiographic congestion is present in 75% of patients admitted with AHFS.

Invasive hemodynamics can confirm the diagnosis by findings of increased filling pressures and reduced cardiac output. Baseline assessment of hemodynamics may be useful to monitor the evolution of patient condition and evaluate the effects of pharmacologic intervention (6). However, invasive hemodynamic measurements are not routinely performed in many clinical centers. Furthermore, invasive hemodynamics have not been shown to be useful in the clinical management of decompensated heart failure (9). Thus, in therapeutic confirmatory trials, patients can be included without those invasive measurements. Invasive hemodynamics are mostly useful in exploratory phase II studies, in particular for dose-determination and pharmacokinetic/pharmacodynamic (PK/PD) modeling.

In decompensated heart failure, left ventricular function is an important covariate. Patients with preserved systolic function or diastolic dysfunction should be identified, as they may have different prognoses and may require specific therapeutic strategies. This patient subgroup should preferably be studied separately or at least in a prespecified subgroup analysis (1). The etiology of chronic heart failure has been shown to be a major determinant of survival (6). Patients with ischemic heart failure have a poor prognosis compared to those with nonischemic etiology (3,6). In the setting of decompensated heart failure, myocardial ischemia may play an important role as a trigger for decompensation. Furthermore, inotropic therapy may adversely affect oxygen demand in these patients. Coronary heart disease is the etiology of AHFS in 60% to 70% of patients, particularly in the elderly (6). Patients with decompensated heart failure and coronary heart disease therefore should be clearly identified. Consistency of effect in this important patient subgroup should be shown (1).

Dose Determination for Confirmatory Studies

Information on doses can initially derive from pharmacologic study results. Further data should be generated from phase II invasive hemodynamic studies. Attempt should be made to determine the minimum effective dose, dose escalation, and the maximum duration on the basis of effect on pulmonary capillary wedge pressure PCWP and safety (1). Regarding this latter, systemic blood pressure and renal function are important parameters (1,6). A dose escalation or a parallel dose-response study may be acceptable, but the appropriate design would depend on the pharmacokinetic characteristics, time of onset, and duration of effect. Pk-pd modeling may help in predicting the effects of several dose levels, which are difficult to evaluate in those critically ill patients.

In the end, there is a clear need for adequate justification of dose(s) selected for the large confirmatory studies (1).

Control Groups

Confirmatory studies are expected to be double blind and randomized (1). The absence of double blinding may compromise the interpretation of signs/symptoms-based studies. This may then require harder clinical end points (e.g., all-cause mortality).

Placebo-controlled studies are required only if the new product is intended as add-on therapy to current conventional treatment and belongs to a new therapeutic class or to a therapeutic class that has not previously been considered for the treatment of AHFS. In this case, the efficacy of the new drug is expected to be shown in placebo-controlled trials where the new drug/placebo is added to an optimized background therapy well defined in the study protocol (1). The absence of placebo-controlled studies in these situations will need to be justified.

Investigating the role of a new drug in AHFS on top of available treatments for AHFS may constitute a reasonable way to elucidate whether such strategy may have an added value for this patient population (1,3). It is well known that standardization of the background therapy in this acute setting is difficult, as a number of features, both clinical and hemodynamic, will drive the therapeutic strategy including background treatment and dosing (3,6). However, a significantly different background therapy in both treatment and control arms might result in extremely confusing study results. This may have impact on the judgment about whether the potential differences observed between treatment arms are due to the investigational drug or to a suboptimized background therapy (1). The relevance of this issue is even more significant considering that despite the double-blind nature of the study, investigators' awareness of the study treatment cannot be ruled out due to the often evident hemodynamic effect of the investigational drug (6,10,11). In addition, demonstration of efficacy could be limited if drugs of similar profile or overlapping mechanism of action are administered as background therapy. Therefore, the background therapy strategy should be standardized as much as possible (1).

If the investigational compound belongs to an existing therapeutic class, a double-blind, randomized, active comparator controlled study against another approved product of the same therapeutic class is necessary (1). In this case, when a hypothesis of noninferiority is the selected approach, the quality of the study design, in order to ensure an adequate assay sensitivity, becomes essential (1).

The choice of the comparator depends on the hemodynamic effects of the compound. For vasodilators, nitroglycerine or nitroprusside are the preferred comparators. For diuretics, furosemide is the most widely used and hence the expected control drug for assessment of a new diuretic. Dobutamine, alone or in combination, is the most widely used inotrope in patients with AHFS. These are the preferred comparators, and the choice of other comparators should be justified (1).

Efficacy End Points and Timing for Evaluation

The treatment immediate objectives for AHFS are to relieve symptoms and to improve the hemodynamic condition. These short-term benefits should also be accompanied by favorable effects on longer term outcomes (3,6).

An improvement in the hemodynamic parameters, primarily a reduction in the PCWP and an increase in cardiac output, have traditionally been regarded as beneficial effects in the treatment of AHFS (6). The PCWP as a clinical end point has several advantages. It reflects pulmonary congestion and is a hemodynamic hallmark of left ventricular dysfunction (2,3,6). This is an objective measurement with little placebo effect (<2 mm Hg) (10,11). The PCWP is a suitable variable for pk-pd modeling. Reduction of PCWP below 16 mm Hg has been associated with improved 2-year survival in a study of patients with advanced heart failure who presented with AHFS (12). In contrast, no difference in survival was observed after improvement in the cardiac output in this group (12). In addition, it has been shown that PCWP was a significant predictor of subsequent survival, whereas cardiac output did not predict outcome (3,12). Decreasing abnormal filling pressures is an important step, to both improve symptoms and potentially improve long-term outcomes, provided that this improvement is not at the expense of decreasing systemic pressure or myocardial perfusion (3,6). To date, no study has shown that increasing cardiac output during AHFS improves clinical outcomes (3).

There are, however, major limitations to the use of PCWP measurements. It requires pulmonary artery catheterization (PAC), which is not performed routinely in the clinical management of AHFS and is not useful in the management of advanced heart failure (6,9). Its use is recommended only in hemodynamically very unstable patients, in cardiogenic shock (6). The PCWP is poorly correlated with symptoms of dyspnea (3,4,10,12,13). Mandatory PAC in large confirmatory trials is difficult to implement and may introduce patient selection bias. The PCWP is a most suitable variable for pharmacodynamic exploratory studies and dose-finding trials. An improvement only in hemodynamic parameters may be misleading, and a concomitant improvement in symptoms or outcomes is generally required (1,6). Therefore, PCWP as a sole primary efficacy end point is unlikely to be sufficient for drug approval if no symptomatic or clinical outcome benefit is shown (1).

Dyspnea is the dominant symptom in AHFS. The difficulty of assessing dyspnea at baseline in patients who are acutely ill should not deter physicians from inclusion of this end point for demonstration of symptomatic improvement (13). In practice, the improvement in clinical condition is judged largely by the assessment of dyspnea, by both patients and investigators. This should be seen in conjunction with hemodynamic improvement (6). Various indexes of dyspnea and visual analogue scales have been used in clinical trials (13). However, many of these grading systems relate to chronic dyspnea, and the use of these tools in the acute setting has not been fully validated (13). Whatever method is chosen, it should be well validated, justified, and defined a priori (1). Although dyspnea reflects clinical benefit, it is subjective and subject to a high placebo effect. Improvement of dyspnea has been reported in 62% of placebo patients (10). A global assessment of the patient's clinical status may be useful complementary information to the assessment of dyspnea. Its use as co-primary end point is highly recommended (1,10). Any impact of standard care on potential benefit should be addressed. However, any reduction in need for up-titration of background therapy is not considered an appropriate component of a combined end point related to symptomatic improvement (1). The effect of a drug on symptoms should be seen in conjunction with its hemodynamic effects. Necessary precautions should be taken in order to avoid that the investigator's awareness of the hemodynamic drug effect on each individual patient may influence the evaluation of symptoms (10,13).

Patients with AHFS have a very poor prognosis. In patients hospitalized with decompensated heart failure, a 60-day mortality rate of 9.6% and a combined rate of mortality and rehospitalization of 35% have been reported (6). Likewise, in acute pulmonary edema a 12% in-hospital and 40% one-year mortality have been reported (6). The predictors for mortality are high PCWP ($\geq$16 mm Hg), low serum sodium, increased left ventricular dimensions, and low peak oxygen consumption (2,3,6). Besides the acute symptomatic/hemodynamic improvements, an effective drug in AHFS should also provide longer term benefit (6). The most relevant benefit is improved patient survival. In this context, the preferred primary efficacy end point is all-cause mortality (1). This should include in-hospital mortality during admission for the acute episode and mortality data at 30 days from the randomization/initiation of investigational drug administration (1). The time evaluation of 30 days has been suggested because it is close to the acute therapeutic intervention and therefore less subject to confounding factors relating to the impact of chronic therapies and subsequent acute episodes on longer term survival. In case the reference drug has not demonstrated an improvement in survival in patients with AHFS, a noninferiority approach is not considered appropriate (1).

The need for co-interventions for worsening heart failure symptoms has been proposed as an efficacy end point (3). There are, however, strong limitations to using these criteria. The threshold for changes in background therapy or use of unplanned co-interventions such as continuous positive airway pressure (CPAP), intubation, inotropes, or vasoactive drugs varies among centers and countries (6). In addition, hemodynamically active drugs introduce confounding factors in the threshold for intervention, choice of co-interventions, and blinding (3). Therefore, co-interventions as efficacy end points even as part of a composite score are not currently acceptable to European agencies (1).

Thus, regarding primary efficacy end points, the total mortality is preferred. Improvement in dyspnea with reduction in PCWP, either from the same or different studies, would be acceptable evidence for efficacy, provided that deleterious effects on mortality and morbidity, both immediate and delayed, are ruled out. Hemodynamic findings are useful and needed, but not enough as sole basis for drug approval (1).

Cardiovascular deaths should be identified as a secondary efficacy end point. These should include sudden death, death due to myocardial infarction, arrhythmic deaths, and deaths due to worsening heart failure (1). Duration of hospital stay may be another secondary end point. This includes number of days in intensive care units and total inpatient stay. During long-term follow-up of acute treatment, the number of rehospitalizations (all-cause, cardiovascular, and secondary to new episodes of heart failure) may be considered an additional secondary end point (1). These along with cardiac and noncardiac deaths are considered most important secondary efficacy end points (1). Improvement in quality of life or patient self-assessed global clinical status could be measured as secondary end points. In patients with AHFS due to myocardial ischemia, reduction in recurrent ischemic events may be an important secondary end point. The BNP measurements may be used for monitoring therapy. However, at present BNP is most useful for the negative predictor value for diagnosis of heart failure. It cannot be used as clinical end point to measure efficacy (1).

Safety Data

Early clinical studies in AHFS have reported significant initial responses to vasodilators or agents that stimulate contractility. However, the inability to sustain early improvements with inotropic agents was accompanied by increased mortality (3,6,14,15). Vasodilators or inotropic agents may all have detrimental effects depending on the clinical and hemodynamic profile of AHFS (3,6,14–16). Potential aggravation of myocardial ischemia by inotropic drugs in the setting of myocardial infarction is well recognized (6,14). In addition, critical hypotension itself compromises myocardial perfusion. Markedly elevated left ventricular filling pressures also increase oxygen requirement and further decrease coronary perfusion gradient. The safety issues that could arise from the use of a drug in AHFS include life-threatening arrhythmias, hypotension, myocardial ischemia, and sudden death (3,6). Increased short- or medium-term mortality have been reported with several agents (3,6,15,16). Therefore, even if the claim is made for symptomatic benefit only, mortality data over 6 months are required to exclude the possibility of any deleterious effect (1). The safety data for each group of patients characterized by the indication should be large enough to rule out a detrimental effect on mortality and morbidity (1). For example, if a claim is made for patients with acute decompensation on chronic heart failure, the database in this specific group should be sufficient.

The severity of renal dysfunction in patients with AHFS provides important prognostic information for in-hospital and postdischarge mortality (6,17). Renal dysfunction can prevent adequate diuresis and thereby hamper symptomatic relief. Therefore, there are many reasons to be concerned about the deterioration in renal function in AHFS (17,18). Effects on renal function are critical safety measurements. These data collected prospectively should be provided in addition to the 30-day and the 6-month mortality data (1).

Conclusion

Acute heart failure syndrome is a complex clinical setting. It has a distinct epidemiology and it affects a heterogeneous patient population. The lack of agreement on clinical definitions and the appropriate goals of therapy has delayed advances in the management of these patients. The results of recent clinical trials have been disappointing, with no agent tested to date able to improve survival. The basic regulatory requirements for a drug in AHFS would be to demonstrate predictable favorable hemodynamic effects, with a clear clinical benefit and no safety concern in the short and long term.

Acknowledgment. The views expressed are those of the authors and do not necessarily reflect those of the Agence Française de Sécurité Sanitaire des Produits de Santé (AFSSAPS), Saint-Denis, France.

References

1. Committee for Medicinal Products for Human Use (CHMP), European Medicines Agency (EMEA). Note for guidance on clinical investigation of medicinal products for the treatment of cardiac failure, addendum on acute cardiac failure. Report No. CPMP/EWP/2986/03. www.emea.europa.eu.
2. Felker GM, Adams KF, Konstam MA, et al. The problem of decompensated heart failure: nomenclature, classification and risk stratification. Am Heart J 2003;145:S18–25.
3. Gheorghiade M, Zannad F, Sopko G, et al. Acute heart failure syndromes: current state and framework for future research. Circulation 2005;112: 3958–68.
4. Stevenson LW, Perloff JK. The limited reliability of physical signs for estimating hemodynamics in chronic heart failure. JAMA 1989;261:884–8.
5. Remes J, Miettinen H, Reunanen A, Pyorala K. Validity of clinical diagnosis of heart failure in primary health care. Eur Heart J 1991;12:315–21.
6. Nieminen MS, Böhm M, Cowie MR, et al. The Taskforce on Acute Heart Failure of the European Society of Cardiology. Executive summary of the guidelines on the diagnosis and treatment of acute heart failure. Eur Heart J 2005;26:384–416.
7. Cleland JG, Swedberg K, Follath F, et al. for the study group on diagnosis of the working group on heart failure of the European society of Cardiology. The Euro Heart Failure Survey Programme: a survey on the quality of care among patients with heart failure in Europe, part I: patient characteristics and diagnosis. Eur Heart J 2003;24:442–63.
8. Adams KF, Fonarow GC, Emerman CL, et al. for the ADHERE Scientific Advisory Committee and Investigators. Characteristics and outcomes of patients hospitalized for heart failure in the United States: rationale, design and preliminary observations from the first 100 000 cases in the Acute Decompensated Heart Failure National Registry (ADHERE). Am Heart J 2005;149:209–16.
9. The ESCAPE investigators and ESCAPE study coordinators for the ESCAPE trial. Evaluation Study of Congestive Heart Failure and Pulmonary Artery Catheterization Effectiveness (ESCAPE). JAMA 2005;294:1625–33.
10. Publication Committee for the VMAC Investigators. Intravenous nesiritide vs nitroglycerin for treatment of decompensated congestive heart failure: a randomized controlled trial. JAMA 2002;287:1531–40.
11. Cuffe MS, Califf RM, Adams KF, et al. for the Outcomes of a Prospective Trial of Intravenous Milrinone for Exacerbation of Chronic Heart Failure (OPTIME-CHF) investigators. Effects of short-term, intravenous milrinone on acute exacerbation of chronic heart failure: a randomized controlled trial. JAMA 2002;287:1541–7.
12. Stevenson LW, Tillisch JH, Hamilton M, et al. Importance of hemodynamic response to therapy in predicting survival with ejection fraction ≤20% secondary to ischemic or non ischemic dilated cardiomyopathy. Am J Cardiol 1990;66:1348–54.
13. Teerlink JR. Dyspnoea as an endpoint in clinical trials of therapies for acute decompensated heart failure. Am Heart J 2003;145:S26–33.
14. Stevenson LW. Clinical use of inotropic therapy for heart failure: looking backward or forward? Part I: inotropic infusions during hospitalization. Circulation 2003;108:367–72.
15. Abraham WT, Adams KF, Fonarow GC, et al. for the ADHERE study group. In-hospital mortality in patients with acute decompensated heart failure requiring intravenous vasoactive medication: analysis from the acute decompensated heart failure national registry (ADHERE). J Am Coll Cardio 2005;46:57–64.
16. Sackner-Bernstein JD, Kowalski M, Fox M, Aaronson K. Short-term risk of death after treatment with nesiritide for decompensated heart failure. A pooled analysis of randomized controlled trials. JAMA 2005;293:1900–5.
17. Fonarow GC, Adams KF Jr, Abraham WT, et al. for the ADHERE scientific advisory committee, study group and investigators. Risk stratification for

in-hospital mortality in heart failure using classification and regression (CART) methodology: analysis of 33 046 patients in the ADHERE registry. JAMA 2005;293:572–80.

18. Sackner-Berstein JD, Skopicki HA, Aaronson KD. Risk of worsening renal function with nesiritide in patients with acutely decompensated heart failure. Circulation 2005;111:1487–91.

84 Drug Approval Process for Acute Heart Failure Syndrome in the United States

Ileana L. Piña and Shari L. Targum

The history of drug approval that targets the heart failure (HF) population has been subject to the advancements that have been made in the field of HF. A better understanding of the pathophysiology of the HF syndrome, with its complexity and an ever-growing number of patients, has led to an evolution in thinking at the Food and Drug Administration (FDA) Division of Cardiovascular and Renal Products. Once thought of as a terminal disorder without much hope even of palliation, heart failure therapies have emerged as powerful agents that can impact mortality and morbidity and may alter the course of the disease. The therapeutic choices through the years have targeted the concepts that were "in vogue" in each era. As an example, when inotropic derangement was thought to be the primary cause of HF, several inotropic therapies emerged and were approved based on a small amount of data.[1] As the neurohormonal hypothesis was tested, drugs were targeted to this important axis, and the mortality and morbidity improved. The price to pay for a better survival in populations with HF is that larger patient trials and sicker patients were needed to detect statistically significant changes. Furthermore, as therapies such as angiotensin-converting enzyme (ACE) inhibitors demonstrated remarkable safety and efficacy, subsequent trials needed to add the previously successful drug to further reduce mortality and morbidity.

To complicate the pharmacotherapy arena, the field of heart failure therapies has been fraught with frustrations since drugs targeted at the specific points of abnormalities, for example, endothelin antagonists, have been met with great disappointment.[2] In addition, drugs that appeared to improve parameters of ventricular function or functional capacity were often accompanied by an increase in mortality.[3,4] Some of these agents had inotropic properties as well. Flosequinan, a vasodilator that improved short-term exercise function and symptoms, increased mortality when tested in a prospective randomized control trial, perhaps due to its inotropic effects.[4]

Given these difficulties, it is evident that the field of acute heart failure (AHF) has not been replete with new drugs that alter outcome acutely or in the immediate postacute time period. One potential dilemma is determining a mechanism of drug action that will lead to an effective target of therapy. For example, if one is developing an AHF drug that will lead to a particular clinical benefit, one faces the issue of finding the right drug mechanism that will lead to this benefit. Another issue in drug approval is determining the net clinical benefit for a particular drug. In the case of AHF, reductions in mortality and improvements in symptoms result in the need to perform larger studies of new therapies in order to detect smaller incremental benefits. In this regard, a small clinical benefit in these larger trials may be offset by potential safety concerns.

From the perspective of cardiovascular researchers, difficulties lie in the lack of a uniform definition for the acute heart failure syndrome (AHFS), and the lack of agreement about what to measure, how much excess mortality to accept, if any, and what biomarkers are meaningful.

This chapter broadly reviews the requirements for drug approval by the FDA and applies them to AHFS. This chapter also presents the proceedings of two FDA Cardiorenal Advisory Committee meetings held in 1997 and 1998, which discussed the approval of drugs for heart failure and the intermittent or chronic infusion of inotropes. The small group of drugs commonly used for treatment of AHFS is reviewed, along with the history and date of its approval as well as the multiple generics available. The reader might find this list surprising.

Drug Approval

The cardiorenal section of the FDA reviewed its approval process for acute heart failure drugs in 1997 in an open session chaired by Dr. Milton Packer. The session developed as a general discussion about the evaluation, development, and approval of intravenous drugs for the treatment of heart failure. The following is a synopsis of the discussion that occurred:

There are several scenarios in which an intravenous agent for HF would be used:

1. A given patient is temporarily unable to take a medication by mouth. Therefore, the intravenous formulation would make continued therapy possible by bridging the gap of a small number of missed oral doses.
2. A given patient sustains an acute decompensation of heart failure. The intravenous formulation would be administered for a day or two in the intensive care unit.
3. Myocardial dysfunction develops during cardiopulmonary bypass in a patient with or without heart failure. The intravenous formulation can facilitate the weaning from the bypass pump.
4. The patient is moderately stable. The intravenous formulation would be used intermittently or continuously for maintenance or for prophylaxis against deterioration.

Not all of the above settings were anticipated when many of the drugs that are presently approved for intravenous use were made commercially available. Moreover, up to that time intravenous drugs for the treatment of heart failure had been approved after adequate demonstration of dose dependent and appropriate hemodynamic effects, that is, a decrease in filling pressures or an increase in cardiac output or other effects in patients with acute or chronic heart failure.

In drug approval decisions, several assumptions had been made: First, the drug would be used only occasionally and for a short period of time, always during hospitalization and for the treatment of severe acute heart failure. Second, a useful dosing range could be defined and dose response obtained by observing hemodynamic effects or through another physiologic or clinical variable that predicted dose and response. Third, when a safe and effective chronic oral regimen had been defined, the benefits to acute HF could be extrapolated from the patient with chronic disease. Therefore, there would be concurrence between the intravenous and the oral drug effects. Fourth, when no oral regimen existed, the short-term hemodynamic effects would be suitable surrogates, for short-term symptomatic benefit and for mortality.

The committee then reviewed approved intravenous agents and whether the assumptions made to that date were still relevant and valid. The challenge of approvability based on hemodynamics alone and a dose–response relationship was then brought to the floor.

Up to that time, approval of intravenous drugs for heart failure had been based not on clinical outcomes but on hemodynamics. The committee agreed that some drugs that benefit patients in the short term may not work as well chronically and vice versa. In addition, it was recommended that outcomes beyond hemodynamics should be considered. Some of those outcomes could include length of stay, 30-day readmission rate, days in the intensive care unit, use of other intravenous agents, and dose of diuretics, among others. Therefore, the spirit of the committee was that hemodynamics might be necessary but not sufficient for approval. In addition, the committee recommended that agents that had initially been approved for short-term intravenous use in hospitalized patients have their labels modified to include a statement of lack of data on long-term or intermittent use. Safety also needed to be proven.

Drug Approval (Table 84.1)

Safety and Efficacy

Regardless of the type of drug that is being considered for approval, there must be a demonstration of safety and efficacy. In addition, there must be plausible instructions for drug use to accompany the indications. The burden of proof for safety and efficacy is in the hands of the pharmaceutical industry.

Efficacy

Drugs are approved either because they make the patient live longer, feel better, or both. Contrary to popular opinion, drugs that make patients feel better but live a shorter time could also be approved as long as there is demonstration of a reasonable point estimate for mortality.

The definition of "live longer" may include the following:

1. Prolongation of time to lethal events
2. Prolongation of time to irreversible morbid events
3. Prolongation of time to potentially lethal events

For heart failure, this list could be translated into a decreased rate of mortality, decrease in hospitalization rate, days alive out of hospital, decreased myocardial infarctions, and stroke reduction, among others. For a patient with acute heart failure, these "live longer" end points may relate to survival during the index hospitalization, improved 6-month survival rate for those who are discharged, reduction in rehospitalizations for acute heart failure, and others.

The "feel better" end points specifically for patients with AHFS may mean better functional capacity, improved symptoms of dyspnea and fatigue, shorter hospital stays, or improved quality of life.

Instructions for use include a description of the target population for the indication, and how the drug should be administered, whether by bolus or infusion, titration, initial dose, and dosing range. Dosing instructions should include how long to wait before up-titration. Can add-on treatments be administered? Finally methodology to monitor effects should also be a part of the approval process; see Table 84.2.

Efficacy could also be supported by information about change in surrogate end points that are favorable to the patient and to the disease process. Surrogate end points could include changes in B-type natriuretic peptide (BNP), echocardiographic parameters, lack of troponin rise, and need for inotropic therapy, among others; see Table 84.3).

End-point selection continues to be a challenge. To make the number of patients required more manageable and feasible, composite end points, which usually include mortality and some form of morbidity assessment, have become popular. Important issues include which component (or components) of the composite end point constitutes a "win" and how to interpret components of unequal weight. Although there is no firm consensus on these points, this chapter summarizes a

TABLE 84.1. Drug approvals and drug effect

Drug	Class	Year	Drug Effect
Dobutamine	Cardioselective β-adrenergic agonist	1978	↓PCW, ↓SVR, ↑CO, HR
Amrinone	Phosphodiesterase inhibitor	1984	↓PCW, ↓SVR, ↑CI, ↓dyspnea
Milrinone	Phosphodiesterase inhibitor	1987	↓PCW, ↑CI, ↓SVR
Nitroprusside	Nitrovasodilator	1991	↓PCW, ↓BP
Nesiritide	Human B-type natriuretic peptide	2001	↓PCW, ↓dyspnea

BP, blood pressure; CI, cardiac index; CO, cardiac output; HR, heart rate; PCW, pulmonary capillary wedge; SVR, systemic vascular resistance.
Source: Targum.

Table 84.2. Efficacy and instructions for use applied to acute heart failure syndrome (AHFS)

	General	Specific to AHFS
Efficacy end points for drug approval: "live longer"	1. Prolongation of time to lethal events 2. Prolongation of time to irreversible morbid events 3. Prolongation of time to potentially lethal events	1. Reduction in inpatient mortality 2. Reduction in mortality postdischarge 3. Increase in days alive out of hospital 4. Decrease in total hospitalizations 5. Decrease in 30-, 60-, or 90-day hospitalization rate 6. Reduced time in intensive care
Efficacy end points for drug approval: "feel better"	1. Performance enhancement 2. Symptomatic improvement 3. Less duration of hospitalization	1. Improved functional capacity 2. Decreased dyspnea 3. Less fatigue 4. Shorter hospitalizations 5. Preservation of renal function 6. Improved hemodynamics
Instructions for use	1. How should it be used? 2. Who should use it? 3. Bolus? 4. Titrate? 5. Initial dose and dose range 6. How long to wait before dose change? 7. Add-on treatments? 8. How to monitor?	1. Population indication 2. Intravenous or oral 3. Loading dose vs. constant infusion 4. Titration instruction 5. Initial dose and dosing range 6. Type of hemodynamic effect 7. Time to hemodynamic effect 8. Timing prior to up-titration 9. Add-on treatment recommendation and drug–drug interaction 10. Monitoring of effectiveness guideline 11. Need for hemodynamic monitoring

document from a meeting of heart failure professionals and the Center for Drug Evaluation and Research (CDER)[5] branch of the FDA held in 1997 to discuss these very issues.

Safety

The safety profile of any drug must be well characterized. Examples include onset or offset of blood pressure changes, mortality estimates, renal function effects, and stimulation of the renin-angiotensin axis. Safety also includes interactions with commonly used drugs that the population being tested is likely to be taking, for example, lipid-lowering agents. Figure 84.1 depicts a few safety end points that can be applied to drugs for AHFS. It is important to remember that although the length of stay for a hospitalized patient with AHFS may be short, the higher mortality that occurs subsequently necessitates safety assessment beyond the discharge and at least for 90 days.[6]

To recap, the approval process includes understanding the effects of the drug, such as the hemodynamics. However, the hemodynamics are not sufficient for approval, and demonstration of clinical benefit is required along with point estimates of mortality. As in any approval process, the balance of benefit vs. risk, at the end, can win the day.

Table 84.3. Surrogate end points

General	Specific to AHFS
1. Improved biomarkers 2. Stabilization of myocardial changes 3. Less myocardial oxygen demands	1. Decrease in BNP 2. No troponin leak 3. Less ventricular dilatation or stabilization of remodeling (LVEDV, LVES, EF) 4. Need for inotropes

BNP, B-type natriuretic peptide; EF, ejection fraction; LVEDV, left ventricular end-diastolic volume; LVES, left ventricular end systolic volume.

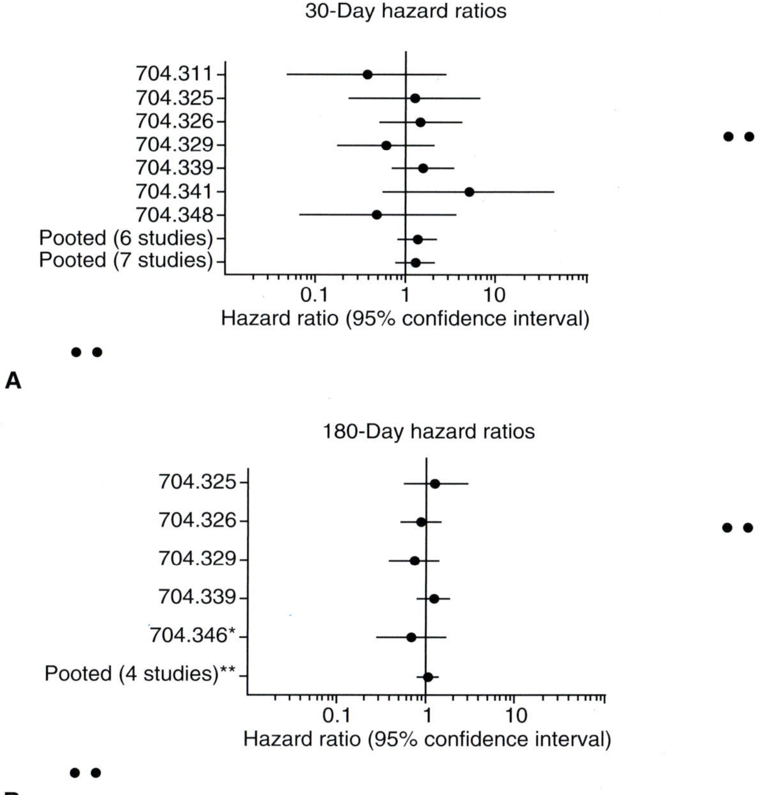

Figure 84.1. Safety end points that can be applied to drugs for acute heart failure syndrome (AHFS). (A) The figure (on logarithmic scale) contains a plot for the six studies involving hospitalized or emergency department patients combined ($n = 1507$), and for all 7 studies combined ($n = 1717$). The percentage is the Kaplan-Meier estimate. (B) The figure represents 180-day mortality hazard ratios for randomized and treated patients from all four individual studies where 180-day data were collected, 16-week hazard ratios for study 348 (180-day data were not collected), and the four studies with 180-day data pooled ($n = 1167$). There were few deaths in these studies, so the confidence limits around the hazard ratios for mortality are wide. The studies are also small, so some potentially important baseline imbalances exist among the treatment groups, the effects of which cannot be ascertained.

Specific Agents by Class

Table 84.4 is a list of drugs by types which are currently used in the treatment of AHFS, although their approval might not include AHFS in the label. The pharmacologic profile and the hemodynamic effects of these agents are beyond the scope of this chapter. The information on drug approval and indication was taken from the FDA Web site and from the *Physicians' Desk Reference*.

Table 84.4. Usual intravenous (IV) treatment for acute heart failure

Inotropes
Dobutamine
Dopamine
Milrinone
Vasodilators
Nitroglycerine
Nitroprusside
Nesiritide
Diuretics
Furosemide
Bumetanide
Torsemide
Ethacrynic acid

Inotropic Agents

In the 1990s, a series of outpatient clinics had developed in the United States to administer intermittent inotropic therapy. On January 27, 1998, the Cardiorenal Committee of the FDA met in a public meeting to evaluate long-term treatment with cyclic adenosine monophosphate (cAMP)-dependent positive inotropic agents.[5] The purpose of the meeting was to summarize the data available from clinical trials on the efficacy and safety of long-term positive inotropic therapy for heart failure. Several trials had suggested that the continuous or intermittent treatment with positive inotropic agents could produce symptomatic improvement. The question was whether those agents were safe and effective when administered for longer periods. The agents that were discussed included dobutamine, ibopamine, milrinone, xamoterol, flosequinan, enoximone, pimobendan, and vesnarinone. Trials were reviewed that fit the criteria of randomization and controls.[7–18] Regarding efficacy, the panel concluded that it was "difficult to draw conclusions from the existing database about the effect of long-term treatment with positive inotropic agents on symptoms and clinical status of patients with heart failure." It further concluded,

> If only trials of class III–IV heart failure are considered, there is no evidence of a favorable effect of treatment on symptoms or clinical status. . . . Treatment failed to have any favorable effect on the 3 measures of efficacy most commonly evaluated in class III–IV patients. . . . Treatment was associated with either no effect or a significant increase in the frequency of hosp italization. . . . It would be difficult to determine how much symptom improvement would be needed to offset the increase in the risk of death.

Regarding safety, the panel concluded,

> An increase in mortality risk was not readily apparent early in the development of each drug. Early trials reported very few deaths and did not have the power to discern an adverse effect on survival. . . . All subgroups of patients appeared to have an increased risk of death, but patients with class IV . . . appeared to be at particularly enhanced risk as a result of treatment with a positive inotropic drug. This finding is of interest, since physicians are most likely to utilize intermittent intravenous positive inotropic therapy in class IV patients.

Some of the agents discussed at the specially convened meeting of the FDA are not available on the market today. It should also be noted that the panel was evaluating the constant or intermittent infusion therapy and not the use of inotropes as short-term agents. The prospective randomized milrinone survival evaluation (PROMISE) trial of milrinone vs. placebo, however, in hospitalized patients with AHFS failed to show a reduction in length of stay or in readmission rates. However, inotropes continue to be used either as palliative agents for patients who are at end of life or for bridging to transplantation.

The following subsections discuss the inotropic agents that are available and still commonly used for AHFS.

Dobutamine

Dobutamine was approved on July 18, 1978, as Dobutrex (Eli Lilly & Co.). There are currently at least eight generic forms. Dobutamine is only available in injectable form.

The indications for dobutamine, as listed on the Lilly product information, are as follows:

> The treatment of adults with cardiac decompensation due to depressed contractility resulting from organic heart disease or following cardiac surgical procedures in which parenteral therapy is necessary for inotropic support. . . . Most clinical experience with dobutamine is short-term—up to several hours in duration. In a limited number of patients who were studied for 24, 48, and 72 hours, a persistent increase in cardiac output occurred in some, whereas the output of others returned toward baseline values.

Dopamine

Dopamine was approved on February 25, 1974, as Intropin (Mayne Pharma USA). There are currently at least five generic forms of dopamine. Dopamine is only available in injectable form. The indications for dopamine, as listed on the Mayne Pharma product information, are as follows:

> For the correction of hemodynamic imbalances present in the shock syndrome due to myocardial infarction, trauma, endotoxic septicemia, open heart surgery, renal failure, and chronic cardiac decompensation as in congestive failure. Where appropriate, restoration of blood volume with a suitable plasma expander or whole blood should be instituted or completed prior to dopamine administration.

Milrinone

Dopamine was approved on December 31, 1987, as Primacor (Sanofi Aventis, USA). There are at least six generic forms of milrinone. Milrinone is only available in injectable form. The indications for milrinone, as listed on the Sanofi Aventis product information, are as follows:

For the short term intravenous treatment of patients with acute decompensated heart failure. Patients receiving milrinone should be observed closely with appropriate electrocardiographic equipment. The facility for immediate treatment of potential cardiac events, which may include life threatening ventricular, arrhythmias must be available. The majority of experience with intravenous milrinone has been in patients receiving digoxin and diuretics. There is no experience in controlled trials with infusions or milrinone for periods exceeding 48 hours.

Vasodilators

Vasodilators continue to be popular agents for the treatment of AHFS. Vasodilators are seen to be "safe" particularly given the mortality increase reported with inotropes. However, the recent reports concerning nesiritide have also raised caution about these agents. There are no large randomized trials of either nitroprusside or nitroglycerin in patients with AHFS. Nonetheless, these agents are commonly used to decrease afterload and preload in patients acutely ill. The rapidity of effect on hemodynamics makes them attractive agents as long as there is adequate blood pressure.

Nitroprusside

Nitroprusside was approved prior to January 1, 1982, as Nipride (Roche). The indications for nitroprusside, as listed on the Roche product information, are as follows:

Treatment of acute hypertension refractory to standard therapeutic measures.... Nitroprusside is also indicated for producing controlled hypotension during anesthesia in order to reduce bleeding in surgical procedures where surgeon and anesthesiologist deem it appropriate. In each case, the benefit-risk ratio should be carefully considered on an individual basis.

Nitroglycerin

Nitroglycerin exists in many forms. The intravenous form (Baxter) was approved on December 29, 1989. There are at least 10 generic forms. It should be noted that a randomized controlled trial of nitroglycerine vs. placebo in heart failure has not been reported. Nonetheless, the drug is used often to lower left ventricular (LV) filling pressures acutely. The indications for nitroglycerine intravenous use, as listed on the Baxter product information, are as follows:

Nitroglycerin in 5% dextrose injection is indicated for treatment of peri-operative hypertension; for control of congestive heart failure in the setting of acute myocardial infarction; for treatment of angina pectoris in patients who have not responded to sublingual nitroglycerin and β-blockers; and for induction of intraoperative hypotension.

Nesiritide

This human recombinant natriuretic peptide, named Natrecor (Scios) came before the Cardiorenal Advisory Committee for approval in 1999. The drug failed to meet regulatory approval at that time based on the lack of definitive symptomatic benefit, lack of information on up-titration and on use with concomitant medications for decompensated heart failure, and the need for more information on the risk of hypotension. In 2001, based on the Vasodilatation in the Management of Acute CHF (VMAC) trial, the drug was approved based on a reduction in pulmonary capillary wedge pressure ($p < .05$), improvement in dyspnea ($p = .03$), and acceptable hypotension profile when compared with nitroglycerine. The drug, therefore, met the "feel better" criterion.[19] The original indications for use, as listed on the Scios product information, were as follows:

For the intravenous treatment of patients with acutely decompensated congestive heart failure who have dyspnea at rest or with minimal activity. In this population, the use of Natrecor reduced pulmonary capillary wedge pressure and improved dyspnea.

Other statements that accompanied the approval included the following:

[The co-administration of] Natrecor with enalapril did not have significant effects on the PK [pharmacokinetic] of Natrecor. The PK effect of co-administration of Natrecor with other IV vasodilators such as nitroglycerin, nitroprusside, milrinone, or IV ACE inhibitors has not been evaluated. During clinical studies, Natrecor was administered concomitantly with other medications, including: diuretics, digoxin, oral ACE inhibitors, anticoagulants, oral nitrates, statins, class III antiarrhythmic agents, beta-blockers, dobutamine, calcium channel blockers, angiotensin II receptor antagonists, and dopamine. Although no PK interactions were specifically assessed, there did not appear to be evidence suggesting any clinically significant PK interaction.

More recently nesiritide came into the spotlight after a publication pointed to worsening renal function and a higher mortality in patients treated with nesiritide.[20,21]

Scios convened a panel of experts to review all the data. Subsequently, the recommendations of the panel were as follows:

> The use of nesiritide should be strictly limited to patients presenting to the hospital with acutely decompensated congestive heart failure who have dyspnea at rest, as were the patients in the largest trial that led to approval of the drug (VMAC). Physicians considering the use of nesiritide should consider its efficacy in reducing dyspnea, the possible risks of the drug summarized above, and the availability of alternate therapies to relieve the symptoms of congestive heart failure.

The panel furthermore concluded, "Ongoing trials should continue," and "A large mortality end point trial should be initiated without delay," In addition, the data available "does not support intermittent outpatient infusion" or "scheduled repetitive use" or its use "to 'improve' renal function" or to "'enhance' diuresis."

Subsequently, the FDA gave a label modification as follows:

> Data from all seven studies in which 30-day data were collected are presented in the chart below. The data depict hazard ratios and confidence intervals of mortality data for randomized and treated patients with Natrecor relative to active controls through day 30 for each of the 7 individual studies. The figure [Fig. 84.1] (on logarithmic scale) also contains a plot for the six studies involving hospitalized or emergency department patients combined ($n = 1507$), and for all 7 studies combined ($n = 1717$). The percentage is the Kaplan-Meier estimate.

See Fig. 84.1 for Kaplan Meier estimates and hazard ratios.

A large trial is currently planned to address the issue of mortality with nesiritide in a prospective randomized controlled fashion. This trial will complement the ongoing Follow-Up Serial Infusions of Nesiritide (FUSION) II study of outpatient nesiritide administration.

Loop Diuretics

Intravenous diuretics are the most commonly used drugs for the treatment of AHFS in spite of lack of randomized controlled trials and new information about the potential harmful effects of large doses of loop diuretics.

Furosemide

Furosemide was approved as Lasix (Sanofi Aventis, USA) on March 20, 1968. There are at least 15 generic forms. Not all are currently on the market. The indications for furosemide, as listed on the Sanofi Aventis product information, are as follows:

> For the treatment of edema associated with congestive heart failure, cirrhosis of the liver, and renal disease, including the nephrotic syndrome. Also for the treatment of hypertension alone or in combination with other antihypertensive agents.

Bumetanide

Bumetanide was approved as Bumex on February 28, 1983 (Roche). There are at least five generic forms. The indications for bumetanide, as listed on the Roche product information, are as follows:

> Bumex is indicated for the treatment of edema associated with congestive heart failure, hepatic and renal disease, including the nephritic syndrome. Almost equal diuretic response occurs after oral and parenteral administration of bumetanide. Therefore, if impaired gastrointestinal absorption is suspected or oral administration is not practical, bumetanide should be given by the intramuscular or intravenous route. Successful treatment with Bumex following instances of allergic reactions to furosemide suggests a lack of cross-sensitivity.

Torsemide

Torsemide was approved as Demadex on August 23, 1993 (Roche). There are four generic forms of torsemide approved. The indications for torsemide use, as listed on the Roche product information, are as follows:

For the treatment of edema associated with congestive heart failure, renal disease or hepatic disease. Use of torsemide has been found to be effective for the treatment of edema associated with chronic renal failure. Chronic use of any diuretic in hepatic disease has not been studied in adequate and well-controlled trials. Demadex intravenous injection is indicated when a rapid onset of diuresis is desired or when oral administration is impractical. Demadex is indicated for the treatment of hypertension alone or in combination with other antihypertensive agents.

Ethacrynic Acid

Ethacrynic acid was approved as Edecrin (Aton) on January 10, 1967. The indications for ethacrynic acid use, as listed on the Aton product information, are as follows:

Indicated for treatment of edema when an agent with greater diuretic potential than those commonly employed is required. 1. Treatment of the edema associated with congestive heart failure, cirrhosis of the liver, and renal disease, including the nephrotic syndrome. 2. Short-term management of ascites due to malignancy, idiopathic edema, and lymphedema. 3. Short-term management of hospitalized pediatric patients, other than infants, with congenital heart disease or the nephrotic syndrome. 4. Intravenous Edecrin is indicated when a rapid onset of diuresis is desired, e.g., in acute pulmonary edema, or when gastrointestinal absorption is impaired or oral medication is not practicable.

References

1. Cohn, JN. Inotropic therapy for heart failure: paradise postponed. N. Engl. J. Med. 1989;320(11): 729–31.
2. O'Connor, CM, et al. Tezosentan in patients with acute heart failure and acute coronary syndromes: results of the Randomized Intravenous TeZosentan Study (RITZ-4). J. Am. Coll. Cardiol. 2003;41(9): 1452–57.
3. Massie, BM, et al. Can further benefit be achieved by adding flosequinan to patients with congestive heart failure who remain symptomatic on diuretic, digoxin, and an angiotensin converting enzyme inhibitor? Results of the flosequinan-ACE inhibitor trial (FACET). Circulation 1993;88(2):492–501.
4. Packer, M. PROFILE abstract. Circulation 88(suppl I), I-301 (1993).
5. Center for Drug Evaluation and Research Advisory Committee: Cardiovascular and Renal Drugs Advisory Committee. Evaluation of Long-term Treatment with Cyclic AMP Dependent Positive Inotropic Agents. Food and Drug Administration. January 27, 1998.
6. Gheorghiade, M, et al. Acute heart failure syndromes: current state and framework for future research. Circulation 2005;112(25):3958–68.
7. Hampton, JR, et al. Randomised study of effect of ibopamine on survival in patients with advanced severe heart failure. Second Prospective Randomised Study of Ibopamine on Mortality and Efficacy (PRIME II) Investigators. Lancet 1997; 349(9057):971–77.
8. Szabo, BM, et al. Clinical and autonomic effects of ibopamine as adjunct to angiotensin-converting enzyme inhibitors in chronic heart failure. J. Card. Fail. 1996;2(3):185–92.
9. van Veldhuisen, DJ, et al. Double-blind placebo-controlled study of ibopamine and digoxin in patients with mild to moderate heart failure: results of the Dutch Ibopamine Multicenter Trial (DIMT). J. Am. Coll. Cardiol. 1993;22(6):1564–73.
10. Double-blind placebo-controlled comparison of digoxin and xamoterol in chronic heart failure. The German and Austrian Xamoterol Study Group. Lancet 1988;1(8584):489–93.
11. Xamoterol in severe heart failure. The Xamoterol in Severe Heart Failure Study Group. Lancet 1990;336(8706):1–6.
12. Waller, DG, et al. Clinical efficacy of xamoterol, a beta 1-adrenoceptor partial agonist, in mild to moderate heart failure. U.K. Xamoterol Study Group. Eur. Heart J. 1989;10(11):1003–10.
13. DiBianco, R, et al. A comparison of oral milrinone, digoxin, and their combination in the treatment of patients with chronic heart failure. N. Engl. J. Med. 1989;320(11):677–83.
14. Packer, M, et al. Effect of oral milrinone on mortality in severe chronic heart failure. The PROMISE Study Research Group. N. Engl. J. Med. 1991;325(21): 1468–75.
15. Uretsky, BF, et al. Multicenter trial of oral enoximone in patients with moderate to moderately severe congestive heart failure. Lack of benefit compared with placebo. Enoximone Multicenter Trial Group. Circulation 1990;82(3):774–80.
16. Gottlieb, SS, et al. Sustained hemodynamic response to flosequinan in patients with heart failure receiving angiotensin-converting enzyme inhibitors. J. Am. Coll. Cardiol. 1993;22(4):963–7.
17. Massie, BM, et al. Can further benefit be achieved by adding flosequinan to patients with

congestive heart failure who remain symptomatic on diuretic, digoxin, and an angiotensin converting enzyme inhibitor? Results of the flosequinan-ACE inhibitor trial (FACET). Circulation 1993;88(2): 492–501.

18. Packer, M, et al. Double-blind, placebo-controlled study of the efficacy of flosequinan in patients with chronic heart failure. Principal Investigators of the REFLECT Study. J. Am. Coll. Cardiol. 1993;22(1): 65–72.
19. Intravenous nesiritide vs nitroglycerin for treatment of decompensated congestive heart failure: a randomized controlled trial. JAMA 2002;287(12): 1531–40.
20. Sackner-Bernstein, JD, et al. Short-term risk of death after treatment with nesiritide for decompensated heart failure: a pooled analysis of randomized controlled trials. JAMA 2005;293(15):1900–5.
21. Sackner-Bernstein, JD, Skopicki HA, Aaronson, KD. Risk of worsening renal function with nesiritide in patients with acutely decompensated heart failure. Circulation 2005;111(12):1487–91.

Further Reading

Burger, AJ, et al. Effect of nesiritide (B-type natriuretic peptide) and dobutamine on ventricular arrhythmias in the treatment of patients with acutely decompensated congestive heart failure: the PRECEDENT study. Am. Heart J. 2002;144(6):1102–8.

Butler, J, et al. The efficacy and safety of B-type natriuretic peptide (nesiritide) in patients with renal insufficiency and acutely decompensated congestive heart failure. Nephrol. Dial. Transplant. 2004;19(2): 391–9.

Peacock, WF, et al. Observation unit treatment of heart failure with nesiritide: results from the proaction trial. J. Emerg. Med. 2005;29(3):243–52.

Yancy, CW, Singh A. Potential applications of outpatient nesiritide infusions in patients with advanced heart failure and concomitant renal insufficiency (from the Follow-Up Serial Infusions of Nesiritide [FUSION I] trial). Am. J. Cardiol. 2006;98(2):226–9.

Index